Register Now for Online Access to Your Book

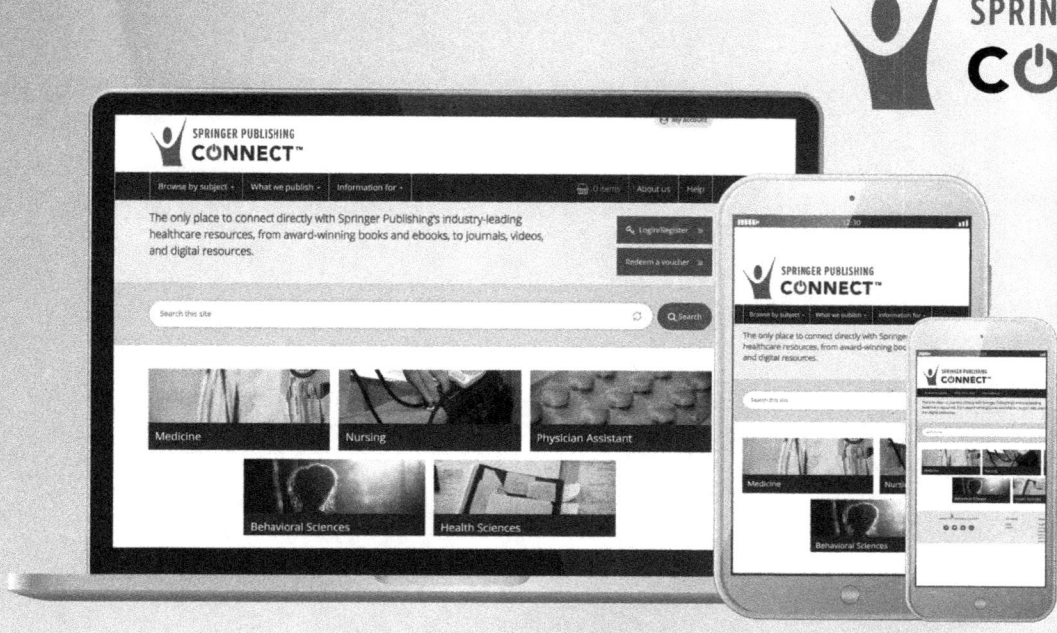

SPRINGER PUBLISHING CONNECT™

Your print purchase of *Psychiatric-Mental Health Guidelines for Advanced Practice Nurses* **includes online access to the contents of your book**—increasing accessibility, portability, and searchability!

Access today at:
http://connect.springerpub.com/content/reference-book/978-0-8261-6229-8
or scan the QR code at the right with your smartphone. Log in or register, then click "Redeem a voucher" and use the code below.

N84J71GA

Scan here for quick access.

Having trouble redeeming a voucher code?
Go to https://connect.springerpub.com/redeeming-voucher-code

If you are experiencing problems accessing the digital component of this product, please contact our customer service department at cs@springerpub.com

The online access with your print purchase is available at the publisher's discretion and may be removed at any time without notice.

Publisher's Note: New and used products purchased from third-party sellers are not guaranteed for quality, authenticity, or access to any included digital components.

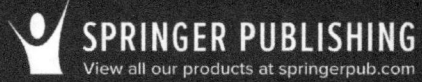

# PSYCHIATRIC-MENTAL HEALTH GUIDELINES FOR ADVANCED PRACTICE NURSES

Brenda Marshall, EdD, PMHNP-BC, APN, ANEF, FAANP, is a full professor in the School of Nursing at Montclair State University. She is a Fulbright Scholar Specialist in mental health with a hospital affiliation at Holy Name Medical Center in Teaneck, New Jersey, and a private practice (Learn 2 Choose Inc.) in Wayne, New Jersey. She has been recognized by multiple organizations for innovative teaching methods in research and was awarded the National Excellence in Research Award (2018) by the American Psychiatric Nurses Association.

Julie Bliss, EdD, RN, is a graduate of Teachers College, Columbia University. She is Professor Emerita at William Paterson University of New Jersey, where she served as the chairperson of the Department of Nursing for many years. Under her leadership, the department fostered a key partnership with St. Joseph's Regional Medical Center and initiated the Doctor of Nursing Practice (DNP) degree, the first doctoral program at the University. Further, she ushered the transition of the department to a School of Nursing in 2023. She is the author of numerous research and journal articles and has been featured in state and national discussions on nursing education, including an Associated Press article "Nursing Educators in Critical Demand," where she highlighted the profession's educational gap compared to other healthcare fields. Dr. Bliss continues to advocate for advancing nursing education, emphasizing the importance of graduate degrees to support critical thinking and competent decision-making in the profession.

Suzanne Drake, PhD, PMHCNS-BC, APN, is a psychiatric-mental health advanced practice nurse with a career spanning more than 40 years as owner/principal of her private practice, The Wellness Group of NJ, LLC. In addition to her clinical work, she has held leadership positions on various advisory, trustee, and executive boards. Currently, she leads as the executive director and cofounder of Advanced Practice Nurses of New Jersey (APN-NJ), a large statewide grassroots organization promoting active campaigns to eliminate legislative barriers to APN practice and monitoring regulatory changes to empower APNs to improve healthcare accessibility. Among honors, Dr. Drake has received the Society of Psychiatric Advanced Practice Nurses's 2013 Leadership Award, the 2019 Lifetime Achievement Award, the American Association of Nurse Practitioners (AANP) 2014 State Award For Excellence, and a 2022 Institute for Nursing Diva Award for Outstanding Achievement in Nursing.

PSYCHIATRIC-MENTAL HEALTH GUIDELINES FOR ADVANCED PRACTICE NURSES

Brenda Marshall, EdD, PMHNP-BC, APN, ANEF, FAANP
Julie Bliss, EdD, RN
Suzanne Drake, PhD, PMHCNS-BC, APN

Editors

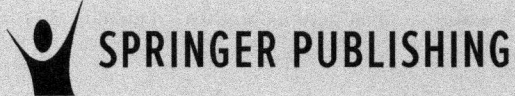

Copyright © 2025 Springer Publishing Company, LLC
All rights reserved.

No part of this publication may be reproduced, stored in a retrieval system, or transmitted in any form or by any means, electronic, mechanical, photocopying, recording, or otherwise, without the prior permission of Springer Publishing Company, LLC, or authorization through payment of the appropriate fees to the Copyright Clearance Center, Inc., 222 Rosewood Drive, Danvers, MA 01923, 978-750-8400, fax 978-646-8600, info@copyright.com or at www.copyright.com.

Springer Publishing Company, LLC
902 Carnegie Center, Princeton, NJ 08540
www.springerpub.com
connect.springerpub.com

Senior Acquisitions Editor: John Zaphyr
Senior Director, Content Development: Taylor Ball
Compositor: Exeter Premedia Services Pvt Ltd.
Production Editor: Rachel Haines

ISBN: 978-0-8261-8051-3
ebook ISBN: 978-0-8261-8052-0
DOI: 10.1891/9780826180520

24 25 26 27 / 5 4 3 2 1

Medicine is an ever-changing science. Research and clinical experience are continually expanding our knowledge, in particular our understanding of proper treatment and drug therapy. The authors, editors, and publisher have made every effort to ensure that all information in this book is in accordance with the state of knowledge at the time of production of the book. Nevertheless, the authors, editors, and publisher are not responsible for any errors or omissions or for any consequence from application of the information in this book and make no warranty, expressed or implied, with respect to the content of this publication. Every reader should examine carefully the package inserts accompanying each drug and should carefully check whether the dosage schedules therein or the contraindications stated by the manufacturer differ from the statements made in this book. Such examination is particularly important with drugs that are either rarely used or have been newly released on the market. The publisher has no responsibility for the persistence or accuracy of URLs for external or third-party internet websites referred to in this publication and does not guarantee that any content on such websites is, or will remain, accurate or appropriate.

Library of Congress Cataloging-in-Publication Data

Names: Marshall, Brenda, editor. | Bliss, Julie, editor. | Drake, Suzanne, editor.
Title: Psychiatric-mental health guidelines for advanced practice nurses / edited by Brenda Marshall, Julie Bliss, Suzanne Drake.
Description: Princeton, NJ : Springer Publishing Company, [2025] | Includes bibliographical references and index. |
Identifiers: LCCN 2024028359 (print) | LCCN 2024028360 (ebook) | ISBN 9780826180513 (paperback) | ISBN 9780826180520 (ebook)
Subjects: MESH: Psychiatric Nursing--methods | Advanced Practice Nursing--methods | Mental Disorders--nursing
Classification: LCC RC440 (print) | LCC RC440 (ebook) | NLM WY 160 | DDC 616.89/0231--dc23/eng/20240909
LC record available at https://lccn.loc.gov/2024028359
LC ebook record available at https://lccn.loc.gov/2024028360

Contact sales@springerpub.com to receive discount rates on bulk purchases.

Publisher's Note: **New and used products purchased from third-party sellers are not guaranteed for quality, authenticity, or access to any included digital components.**

Printed in the United States of America.

*To Lewis, Olivia, Megan, Nhat, Brett, and Theodore
"Teddy" Shell (July 11, 1972–April 13, 2022)*
—Brenda Marshall

*I dedicate this work to the many individuals who have recognized
and implemented change in the thinking about mental health.
We must be aware of not only the role it plays in others' lives
but unequivocally in our own. The need for competent advanced
practice psychiatric-mental health nurse practitioners is urgent.*
—Julie Bliss

*To Richard, Amy, Chris, Ed, Passa, Megan, Brian, Samantha, Kevin,
and all my precious grandchildren. And to Carolyn and
my incredible colleagues whose inspiration, support, and collaboration
have been invaluable throughout my nursing journey.*
—Suzanne Drake

CONTENTS

Contributors ix
Foreword xiii
Preface and Acknowledgments xv

PART I: PSYCHIATRIC NURSING GUIDELINES

1. Psychiatric-Mental Health Nursing: An Overview 3
   Lucille A. Joel

2. Therapeutic Communication 9
   Faith Atte

3. Trauma-Informed Care 18
   Brayden N. Kameg

4. Conducting the Adult Psychiatric Assessment 33
   Kim K. Johnson

5. Conducting the Pediatric Psychiatric Assessment 47
   Michelle A. Peralta Westland, Carole Gionet, Julia Farquharson, John Westland, Maria Manalo, Hillary J. Chan, and ValLori R. Abad

6. Conducting the Geriatric Psychiatric Assessment 75
   Kenneth Berc and Brenda Marshall

7. Psychiatric Assessment Scales 85
   Brenda Marshall, Rosita Rodriguez, Veronica Betts, and Elizabeth Fitzgerald

8. Psychotherapy 93
   Sara Jones and Sattaria "Tari" Dilks

PART II: DIAGNOSIS-SPECIFIC PROCEDURES AND PATIENT TREATMENT PLANNING

9. Anxiety Disorders 113
   Brenda Marshall and Nhat Nguyen

10. Feeding and Eating Disorders 137
    Kim K. Johnson

11. Mood Disorders, Depression Disorders, and Bipolar Disorders 157
    Shaquita Starks

12. Perinatal Mental Health 175
    Barbara Caldwell and Mamilda Robinson

13. Personality Disorders 196
    Alex Cheng

14. Sleep–Wake Disorders 215
    Rosa Landinez

15. Somatic Symptom and Related Disorders 239
    Nataliya Pilipenko and Kimberly A. Muellers

16. Substance Use Disorders 261
    Rabia Hanif, Jack Spencer, and Brenda Marshall

17. Thought and Psychotic Disorders 282
    Rosa Landinez and Yovan Gonzalez

PART III: SPECIAL POPULATIONS AND CARE SETTINGS

18. Cultural Considerations 305
    Marie Smith-East

19. Special Considerations for the LGBTQ+ Population 308
    Dallas Ducar, Hyun-Hee Kim, and Kai Camara

20. Special Considerations for Childhood and Adolescent Populations 326
    Michelle A. Peralta Westland, Hillary J. Chan, John Westland, Julia Farquharson, Carole Gionet, Maria Manalo, and ValLori R. Abad

21. Aging and Older Adult Populations 342
    Suzanne Drake and Helen Jones

22. Physical and Mental Disabilities in the Pediatric Population 350
    Steven E. Curtis

23. Mental and Physical Disabilities in Adults 359
    Colin Hemmings

24. Homeless and Indigent Populations 369
    Rosa Landinez and Sandra Ojurongbe

25. Veterans and Survivors of War 392
    Pamela Herbig Wall, Connie Braybrook, and Katie St. Pierre

26. Provision of Psychiatric Care in Acute Settings 403
    Se Min Um

27. Provision of Care in the Community 417
    Christy Perry and Shirley Griffey

PART IV: CONCEPTION TO LAUNCH AND ESTABLISHING A PRACTICE

28. Establishing a Psychiatric APRN Practice 429
    Suzanne Drake

29. Electronic Health Records and Telehealth 445
    Suzanne Drake

30. **Advocacy, the Law, and Mental Illness** 464
    Denise Snow

PART V: SPECIAL CONSIDERATIONS

31. **Intersection of Health Comorbidities and Mental Health** 471
    Brenda Marshall, Kathleen T. McCoy, Melanie R. Baker, and Kirsten E. Pancione

32. **Symptom Sharing Between Medical and Psychiatric Disorders** 477
    Lewis Marshall and Brenda Marshall

33. **Movement, Nutrition, and Mental Health** 487
    Katherine J. Roberts

34. **Ethical Considerations for the Advanced Practice Registered Nurse** 495
    Shaquita Starks, Nia Josiah, and Freida Outlaw

35. **Caregiver and End-of-Life Issues** 500
    Denise Snow

Appendix: Coding Reference for Psychiatric Conditions 503
Index 507

CONTRIBUTORS

VaLori R. Abad, DNP, MSN-Ed, RN
Regional Nurse Administrator
François-Xavier Bagnoud Center—Child Health Program
Rutgers University School of Nursing
Newark, New Jersey

Faith Atte, PhD, RN
Assistant Professor
Department of Nursing
College of Science and Health
William Paterson University
Wayne, New Jersey

Melanie R. Baker, DNP, PMHNP-BC
Department of Community and Mental Health
College of Nursing
University of South Alabama
Mobile, Alabama

Kenneth Berc, MD
Emeritus Faculty
Columbia Medical School
Mt. Sinai Medical School
Hunter Brookdale Graduate School of Social Work
New York, New York

Veronica Betts, DNP, RN, CMGT-BC
Assistant Professor
Montclair State University School of Nursing
Montclair, New Jersey

Connie Braybrook, DNP, PMHNP-BC
CAPT, NC, USN
Program Director
Graduate School of Nursing, PMH
Uniformed Services University of the Health Sciences
Bethesda, Maryland

Barbara Caldwell, PhD, APN-BC
Rutgers, The State University of New Jersey
Newark, New Jersey

Kai Camara, DNP, APRN, PMHNP-BC
Transhealth, Inc.
Northampton, Massachusetts

Hillary J. Chan, RN, MN, BScN
Clinical Nurse Specialist
Psychiatric Emergency Services
Sinai Health
Toronto, Ontario, Canada

Alex Cheng, MD
Department of Psychiatry
Holy Name Medical Center
Teaneck, New Jersey

Steven E. Curtis, PhD, NCSP, MSCP
PsyD Clinical Psychology Program
Antioch University
Seattle, Washington

Sattaria "Tari" Dilks, DNP, APRN, PMHNP-BC, FAANP
Professor and Department Head of Graduate Nursing
College of Nursing and Health Professions
McNeese State University
Lake Charles, Louisiana

Suzanne Drake, PhD, PMHCNS-BC, APN
The Wellness Group of New Jersey, LLC
Advanced Practice Nurses of New Jersey (APN-NJ)
Edison, New Jersey

Dallas Ducar, MSN, RN, APRN, PMHNP-BC, CNL, FAAN
Instructor in Clinical Nursing
Columbia University School of Nursing
New York, New York;
Clinical Instructor of Nursing
University of Virginia School of Nursing
Charlottesville, Virginia;
Faculty
Mass General Brigham Institute of Health Professions School of Nursing
Boston, Massachusetts

Julia Farquharson, PHC-NP, MN, BScN, BSc
Nurse Practitioner
Department of Psychiatry
The Hospital for Sick Children
Toronto, Ontario, Canada

Elizabeth Fitzgerald, PhD, MSN, RN
Assistant Professor
Montclair State University School of Nursing
Montclair, New Jersey
Regional Educational Specialist
Prime Healthcare
Lake Hopatcong, New Jersey

Carole Gionet, BSc, BScN, NP Cert, MN
Nurse Practitioner
Department of Psychiatry
The Hospital for Sick Children
Lawrence S. Bloomberg Faculty of Nursing
University of Toronto
Toronto, Ontario, Canada

Yovan Gonzalez, DNP, PMHNP-BC, FNP-BC, CARN-AP
Psychiatric Nurse Practitioner
Behavioral Health Department
NYC Health + Hospitals/Gotham Health, Gouverneur
New York, New York

Shirley Griffey, DNP
College of Nursing
Southeastern Louisiana University
Baton Rouge, Louisiana

Rabia Hanif, PhD
Post-Doctoral NIDA-INVEST Fellow
International Certified Addiction Professional (ICAP-II)
Associate Professor, PhD Psychology, MPhil Clinical Psychology
Fulbright/Humphrey Alumni (Substance Use Disorders Education, Prevention, Treatment, and Rehabilitation)
Department of Applied Psychology
Riphah International University
Islamabad, Pakistan;
Institute for Women's Health
Virginia Commonwealth University School of Medicine
Richmond, Virginia

Colin Hemmings, BSc, MBBS, MSc, MA, MD(Res), MRCPsych
Consultant Psychiatrist and Clinical Lead
Mental Health of Learning Disability Service
Kent and Medway Partnership NHS Trust
Associate Teacher
Kent and Medway Medical School
Kent, United Kingdom

Lucille A. Joel, EdD, RN, APN, FAAN
Distinguished Professor
School of Nursing
Rutgers, The State University of New Jersey
Newark, New Jersey

Kim K. Johnson, DNP, PMHNP-BC, FNP-C, RN
Associate Professor
Department of Nursing
Middle Georgia State University
Macon, Georgia

Sara Jones, PhD, APRN, PMHNP-BC, FAAN, FAANP
Associate Professor
College of Nursing and Health Professions
McNeese State University
Lake Charles, Louisiana

Helen Jones, PhD, APN-C
Professor Emeritus
Health Science Education
Raritan Valley Community College
North Branch, New Jersey

Nia Josiah, DNP, PMHNP
Assistant Professor
School of Nursing
Columbia University
New York, New York

Brayden N. Kameg, PhD, DNP, PMHNP-BC, CARN-AP, CNE, FIAAN
Assistant Professor of Nursing
Department of Health and Community Systems
University of Pittsburgh School of Nursing;
Coordinator, Psychiatric-Mental Health Nurse Practitioner Area of Concentration
Director, Mental Health Nurse Practitioner Residency Program
Veterans Administration Pittsburgh Healthcare System
Pittsburgh, Pennsylvania

Hyun-Hee Kim, MD
Massachusetts General Hospital
Boston, Massachusetts

Rosa Landinez, DNP, APMHNP-BC, MS, MA
Adjunct Faculty
The College of Nursing and Public Health
Adelphi University
Garden City, New York

Maria Manalo, NP-PHC, MN, BScN
Nurse Practitioner
Eating Disorders Program
Division of Adolescent Medicine
The Hospital for Sick Children
Toronto, Ontario, Canada

Brenda Marshall, EdD, PMHNP-BC, APN, ANEF, FAANP
Professor
Montclair State University School of Nursing
Montclair, New Jersey
Psychiatric Nurse Practitioner
Holy Name Medical Center
Teaneck, New Jersey

Lewis Marshall, MD, JD, FACHE
Chief Medical Officer
Lincoln Medical Center
Bronx, New York

Kathleen T. McCoy, DNSc, PMHNP-BC, PMHCNS-BC, FNP-BC, FAANP
Department of Community and Mental Health
College of Nursing
University of South Alabama
Mobile, Alabama

Kimberly A. Muellers, MPH, MS
Doctoral Student
Department of Psychology
Pace University
Psychology Extern
Farrell Center for Family Medicine
New York Presbyterian Hospital
New York, New York

Nhat Nguyen, MSN, APN-C, DO
Medicine Resident
Riverside, California

Sandra Ojurongbe, PhD, APRN, PMHNP-BC
Associate Professor
School of Nursing
Palm Beach Atlantic University
West Palm Beach, Florida

Freida Outlaw, PhD, RN, APRN, PMH, FAAN
Professor
Department of Family and Community Medicine
Meharry Medical College
Nashville, Tennessee

Kirsten E. Pancione, DNP, PMHNP-BC, FNP-C, MCST
Department of Community and Mental Health
College of Nursing
University of South Alabama
Mobile, Alabama

Michelle A. Peralta Westland, NP-PHC, RP, Post-MN NP Dip, MN, BScN, BHSc Hon.
Primary Care Lead
Youth Wellness Hubs Ontario
Toronto, Ontario, Canada
Nurse Practitioner-Primary Care
Registered Psychotherapist
Centre for Addiction and Mental Health;
Adjunct Lecturer
Lawrence S. Bloomberg Faculty of Nursing
University of Toronto;
Practice-Based Researcher
Li Ka Shing Knowledge Institute of St. Michael's Hospital at Unity Health Toronto
Toronto, Ontario, Canada

Christy Perry, DNP, PMHNP, ANP
College of Nursing
Southeastern Louisiana University
Baton Rouge, Louisiana

Nataliya Pilipenko, PhD, ABPP
Director of Behavioral Medicine for Family Medicine Residency
Assistant Professor of Behavioral Medicine (in Medicine, in Psychiatry)
Center for Family and Community Medicine
College of Physicians and Surgeons
Columbia University
New York, New York

Katherine J. Roberts, EdD, MPH, MCHES, CPH
Department of Health and Behavior Studies
Teachers College
Columbia University
New York, New York

Mamilda Robinson, DNP, APN, PMHNP-BC
Specialty Director and Clinical Assistant Professor
Division of Advanced Nursing Practice
Rutgers, The State University of New Jersey
Newark, New Jersey

Rosita Rodriguez, DNP, PMHNP-BC, AGPCNP-BC, FNP-BC, WHNP-BC, CDCES, CNE, RYT
Associate Professor
Montclair State University School of Nursing
Montclair, New Jersey;
Psychiatric-Mental Health Nurse Practitioner
Family Psychiatry and Therapy
Paramus, New Jersey

Marie Smith-East, PhD, DNP, PMHNP-BC
Director of the Psychiatric-Mental Health Nurse Practitioner Program
Assistant Professor
Brooks College of Health, School of Nursing
University of North Florida
Jacksonville, Florida

Denise Snow, JD, RN
Clinical Associate Professor
School of Nursing
Stony Brook University
Stony Brook, New York

Jack Spencer, MSN, PMHMP-BC
New York, New York

Shaquita Starks, PhD, APRN, FNP-BC, PMHNP-BC
Assistant Professor
Nell Hodgson Woodruff School of Nursing
Emory University
Atlanta, Georgia

Katie St. Pierre, DNP, PMHNP-BC, FNP-BC
Owls Head, Maine

Se Min Um, DNP, RN-BC
Nurse Manager
Holy Name Pavilion
Teaneck, New Jersey

Pamela Herbig Wall, PhD, PMHNP, FAANP
Clinical Associate Professor
Department of Nursing
University of New Hampshire
Jackson Springs, North Carolina

John Westland, MSW, RSW
Social Worker
Substance Use Program
Division of Adolescent Medicine
The Hospital for Sick Children
Toronto, Ontario, Canada

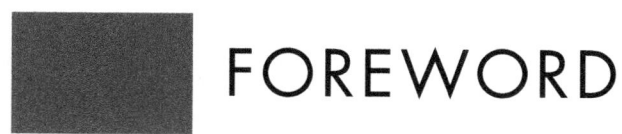
FOREWORD

It is no simple thing to offer a foreword to *Psychiatric-Mental Health Guidelines for Advanced Practice Nurses*. It provides the psychiatric assessment tools and diagnostic conclusions that advanced practice registered nurses (APRNs) will commonly deal with in their day-to-day encounters with patients. This has not always been the case, and many of the conditions highlighted here have often been ignored, untreated, and relegated to the status of the expected side effects of illness. This does not have to be the case, and if the APRN is competent and the care is relevant to the times, there are endless options. Such examples are evidenced in eating and feeding disorders, thought disorders, the integration of mental and physical symptoms, indigent and homeless populations, and trauma-informed care for the survivors of war and violence. All of these and more are populations that require nursing care for maintenance and recovery. And the growing complexity of life is predictive of even more special populations and settings for care.

Cultural competence holds real meaning for the nurse, whether entry level or advanced practice. There are many resources in the literature, and it is our responsibility to be current, well-versed, and oriented to the populations most frequently served. These populations include diversities in race, religion, and gender identity, as well as older adults, individuals experiencing homelessness, and the LGBTQ+ constituency.

Within these pages, you will find a thorough orientation to mental health conditions across the life span. The life span is changing. For further proof, just include the local obituaries in your daily reading. It is not unusual to live well into the 90s today. This brings special care issues for both the primary patient and their caregivers.

Among the most daunting challenges is the growing use of electronic devices and systems in the delivery of care: The electronic health record, telehealth, and artificial intelligence are examples. And with these systems in common use come advocacy and ethical dilemmas. To rely on incorrect electronic information or to overlook a patient's need for advocacy or right to autonomy could result in disciplinary action against the nurse's professional license. This varies from state to state but is rapidly appearing as a major cause of disciplinary action for professionals.

The complexity that has been identified here creates an environment well-suited to independent practice for APRNs, those specializing in psychiatric-mental health being one among many specialties. The most serious impediment to independent practice is the absence/presence of prescriptive authority. Prescriptive authority holds both federal and state implications. Many states require a joint protocol with a physician to prescribe either drugs or medical devices. More than half of states have done away with the joint protocol for APRNs to practice, but this requirement will only be completely abolished over time and with significant political action by APRNs.

This text offers a comprehensive look at the complex psychiatric-mental health environment. It provides new insights yet supports the traditional therapeutic use of self and environmental manipulation as the primary vehicles for healing.

Lucille A. Joel, EdD, RN, APN, FAAN
Distinguished Professor
School of Nursing
Rutgers, The State University of New Jersey
New Brunswick, Newark, Blackwood, New Jersey

PREFACE AND ACKNOWLEDGMENTS

This guidelines book was created to support the ongoing needs and practice change requirements that allow advanced practice registered nurses (APRNs) and psychiatric-mental health advanced practice registered nurses (PMH-APRNs) to provide the best, evidence-based care to patients with lived experiences. There are a few vocabulary choices that have been made purposefully by the editors, for example, using *patient* instead of *client*, and referring to patients diagnosed with psychiatric illnesses as "persons with lived experiences." We have chosen to use only patient-centered/patient-first language. Finally, we use the term *APRN* rather than *nurse practitioner* (*NP*) or *clinical nurse specialist* (*CNS*) to be more inclusive.

CONTENT

This guidelines book is divided into five parts:

- **Part I, "Psychiatric Nursing Guidelines,"** contains guidelines, general assessments, scales, and skills for therapeutic communication.
- **Part II, "Diagnosis-Specific Procedures and Patient Treatment Planning,"** covers psychiatric conditions, including mood and anxiety disorders, feeding disorders, and thought disorders, and the skills needed for diagnosis and treatment planning.
- **Part III, "Special Populations and Care Settings,"** features chapters related to cultural considerations for nonmajority populations requiring mental healthcare, such as LGBTQ+, veterans, and persons without homes.
- **Part IV, "Conception to Launch and Establishing a Practice,"** takes the reader through the necessary support for establishing an APRN practice. We explore subjects like telepsychiatry, electronic health records, and other technological advancements changing how healthcare is provided.
- **Part V, "Special Considerations,"** covers important topics such as the role of nutrition, comorbidities, pain, and end-of-life issues in persons with lived experiences.

USING THE GUIDELINES

Psychiatric nursing is a challenging and rewarding field that necessitates not only scientific skills backed by theory and knowledge, but also empathy and resilience. To tackle the difficulties and challenges encountered in this field, we hope to provide a comprehensive examination of evidence-based psychiatric care methods, ethical concerns, patient assessment, and management strategies. It is our hope that these guidelines will be used by APRNs and other healthcare providers as an accessible reference tool designed to support those clinicians working in various settings when concerns regarding a patient's mental health arise. Mental illness is seen in all aspects of healthcare; however, it is often overlooked, misdiagnosed, or identified as the sole problem. These guidelines bring together solid empirical methods, professional knowledge, and useful recommendations to assist and enhance the clinician's psychiatric skills, ensuring the provision of the highest level of professional care.

PERSONAL NOTE FROM THE EDITORS

This book is the result of years of hard work from authors reflecting expertise from numerous subspecialties and international collaborations. Clinicians from diverse practice fields, along with nursing experts, have carefully crafted every chapter of this book, combining current evidence-based practice and advanced research with practical, humanistic approaches.

It is truly an endeavor of love for the specialty and those of us who care every day for persons with lived experiences.

Finally, we hope that everyone who utilizes this book will see it as a helpful partner supporting their effort to provide expert-informed care. This is more than just a "guidelines" to us; we see it as a journey through the specialty of mental health nursing. We enthusiastically stand alongside you, confident that the knowledge shared will inspire, complement, and fortify your skills. We encourage readers to actively engage with colleagues, mentors, and the community to foster learning and self-reflection, ultimately improving patient outcomes.

Within these pages you will discover many thought-provoking ideas, shared by the various authors, and we would love to hear from you regarding how you have applied information from this guidebook in your practice.

ACKNOWLEDGMENTS

Thanks to our families, colleagues, Springer Publishing Company—especially Taylor Ball and John Zaphyr—and those to whom we have had the honor of providing care. We have learned so much from all of you.

Brenda Marshall
Julie Bliss
Suzanne Drake

PSYCHIATRIC-MENTAL HEALTH GUIDELINES FOR ADVANCED PRACTICE NURSES

I PSYCHIATRIC NURSING GUIDELINES

1 PSYCHIATRIC-MENTAL HEALTH NURSING: AN OVERVIEW

Lucille A. Joel

INTRODUCTION

In order to understand psychiatric-mental health nursing, it is necessary to appreciate the history of this specialty, the documents that continue to confer credibility, the treatment options through which we serve the public, and the debates that continue to promote controversy.

DEFINING TERMS

The first step in our journey to understand psychiatric-mental health nursing is to distinguish it from psychosocial nursing. Every patient and every presenting problem carry psychosocial implications that must be addressed, whether these can be put in perspective and managed by the patient themselves, or if—like the proportion dominating the nurse–patient relationship—they require psychiatric-mental health specialty care.

Stress and anxiety become the companion of anyone facing hospitalization, surgery, childbirth, or a medical condition, prompting them to seek professional help. Knowing this—and being holistic in their approach to practice—nurses anticipate such reactions and know not to wait until the medical issues have resolved in order to address them.

Building upon a thorough assessment of the presenting problem, evidence-based practice becomes the standard for intervention in any clinical situation. Evidence-based practice leads the healthcare provider to best practice through research, evidence-based theory, expert opinion, one's own clinical experience as well as that of others, and patient preference (Melnyk & Fineout-Overholt, 2023). This is not only applicable to psychiatric-mental health nursing, but to all specialties in practice.

To hold vigorously to this standard demands skill in research. It is a developed talent to sift and sort through primary sources and data determining best practice or recognizing when there is not enough evidence to decide. At best, this requires an environment that is open to clinical inquiry and thus attracts colleagues who value intellectual curiosity.

THE DEVELOPMENT OF PSYCHIATRIC-MENTAL HEALTH NURSING

The first educational program for psychiatric nursing—setting aside mental health for the moment—occurred in the late 19th century. It was based in a mental hospital and catered to male students. The first psychiatric nursing text was published in 1920, but accredited schools of nursing were not required to offer psychiatric nursing experiences until much later. This did not happen until after World War II and was most likely the result of the experiences of war, including the mental health problems that surfaced among soldiers during the conflict and the treatment/care provided to combatants. For many, the care provided while in the military surpassed what they had encountered as civilians, and they wanted these services in peacetime.

The definitive breakthrough for advanced practice into the nursing profession came with the 1952 publication of Hildegard Peplau's book, *Interpersonal Relations in Nursing*, and the subsequent establishment of the first graduate program in a nursing specialty (psychiatric-mental health) at Rutgers University in 1954 with Peplau as Director. This was shortly followed by the publication of Standards of Practice by the American Nurses Association (ANA) and certification of generalists in the specialty by the American Nurses Credentialing Center (ANCC) in 1967, and the addition of specialist certification in 1979 (Boyd & Luebbert, 2022). The ANCC is an arm of the ANA that credentials practitioners, accredits healthcare providers of continuing education, and awards Magnet® status to hospital nursing services. The ANCC's certification was predated (1966) by certification awarded for psychiatric nursing advanced practice through the New Jersey State Nurses Association, and subsequently recognized by the New Jersey Board of Nursing as the credential for advanced practice in this specialty. See Box 1.1 for more details on the historical development of psychiatric-mental health nursing.

BOX 1.1 HISTORY OF PSYCHIATRIC-MENTAL HEALTH NURSING

- **Late 19th century:** Reform movements for mental asylums lead to the beginning of the psychiatric-mental health nurse role.
- **1882:** The first training school for nurses in the psychiatric setting is established by Edward Cowles at McLean Asylum in Massachusetts.
- **1913:** Psychiatric nursing educational program is organized by nurses at Johns Hopkins University.
- **Post-World War I:** The National League for Nursing Education adds nursing in nervous and mental diseases to curriculum guides.
- **1920:** The first psychiatric nursing textbook, *Nursing Mental Disease*, is written by Harriet Bailey and published.
- **1944:** The American Psychiatric Association commissions Laura Fitzsimmons to evaluate psychiatric nursing educational programs.
- **1946:** The National Mental Health Act names psychiatric nursing as one of the four core mental health disciplines and includes funding to develop advanced educational programs for mental health nursing.
- **1950s:** Process of deinstitutionalization of psychiatric care begins.
- **1952:** Hildegard Peplau publishes *Interpersonal Relations in Nursing*.
- **1954:** Hildegard Peplau establishes the first psychiatric nursing graduate program at Rutgers University in New Jersey.
- **1963:** The Community Mental Health Centers Act helps expand the psychiatric-mental health clinical nurse specialist (PMHCNS) practice into community and ambulatory care settings.
- **1963:** The first psychiatric-mental health nursing research journals are published.
- **1965:** The psychiatric-mental health registered nurse (PMHRN) practice expands over the next two decades due to the establishment of Medicare and Medicaid.

(continued)

BOX 1.1 HISTORY OF PSYCHIATRIC-MENTAL HEALTH NURSING (CONTINUED)

- **1973:** The American Nurses Association publishes the first issue of the *Standards of Psychiatric Nursing Practice* and begins to certify PMHRNs.
- **1974:** The first American Nurses Credentialing Center (ANCC) Psychiatric-Mental Health Clinical Nurse Specialist Exam is offered.
- **1986:** The American Psychiatric Nurses Association is founded.
- **1990s:** Decade of the brain, recovery-oriented systems begin to gain traction.
- **2000:** The first ANCC Psychiatric-Mental Health Nurse Practitioner Exam is offered.
- **2003:** The National Organization of Nurse Practitioner Faculties releases the Psychiatric-Mental Health Nurse Practitioner Competencies.
- **2007:** ANCC logical job analysis of PMHCNS and psychiatric-mental health nurse practitioner (PMHNP) roles is conducted.
- **2008:** The Consensus Model for APRN Regulation: Licensure, Accreditation, Certification, and Education is developed.
- **2010:** The Institute of Medicine releases the *Future of Nursing: Leading Change to Advance Health Report*.
- **2014:** The second edition of *Psychiatric-Mental Health Nursing: Scope and Standards of Practice* is published.
- **2017:** The ANCC administers the final PMHCNS certification exam. Previously certified PMHCNS continue to practice.
- **2022:** The third edition of *Psychiatric-Mental Health Nursing: Scope and Standards of Practice* is published.

Source: Adapted from American Psychiatric Nurses Association. (n.d.). *History of psychiatric-mental health nursing.* Accessed August 23, 2024. https://www.apna.org/history/

PSYCHIATRIC-MENTAL HEALTH NURSING CERTIFICATION

The ANCC Psychiatric-Mental Health Nursing Certification exam evaluates the foundational clinical knowledge and abilities of registered nurses (RNs) specializing in psychiatric-mental health, following their initial RN licensure. After meeting the eligibility criteria and passing the exam, nurses receive the designation *Psychiatric-Mental Health Nurse-Board Certified* (PMH-BC™), which remains valid for 5 years. The Accreditation Board for Specialty Nursing Certification provides accreditation for this particular ANCC certification, a standard practice for similar "entry-level" specialty certifications.

PSYCHIATRIC-MENTAL HEALTH NURSING CERTIFICATION FOR ADVANCED PRACTICE

Advanced practice nursing certification in psychiatric-mental health nursing has a more convoluted history. The ANCC originally awarded certification as either a nurse practitioner (PMHNP) or a clinical nurse specialist (PMHCNS). Currently, the PMHCNS certification and credential are available for renewal only. This certification can be renewed every 5 years and healthcare providers can continue to use the credential by maintaining their license to practice and fulfilling the certification renewal requirements that were in effect at the time they submitted their application.

The growing demand for mental health services necessitates access to highly trained professionals. Advanced certifications in psychiatric-mental health nursing, which include roles such as clinical nurse specialist (CNS) and nurse practitioner (NP), carry the recommended credential of psychiatric-mental health advanced practice registered nurse (PMH-APRN). These professionals are educated at the graduate level, focusing on research, system management, and direct patient care. They are equipped to conduct psychiatric evaluations and treatments; offer individual, family, and group therapies; manage psychopharmacologic treatments; and implement preventive measures at primary, secondary, and tertiary levels throughout the patient's life. Both CNS and NP roles are crucial in addressing the mental health needs of the community. The credential is modified by the term *suggested* since the stated credential is left to the discretion of the state under states' rights. One such example is New Jersey, where all newly credentialed advanced practice nurses carry the modifier NP (PMHNP), the exclusion being those APRNs who were awarded another modifier (PMH-APRN or PMHCNS) that predated the regulation and have consistently maintained this credential by conforming to the recertification requirements as they existed for them originally. Had they allowed the original certification to lapse, they would be bound to use the new credential.

Before the PMHNP certification in the early 2000, there was certification for psychiatric-mental health certified nurse specialist (1974). Having two such certifications was confusing with regard to defining the scope of practice between the CNS and the NP.

The distinction between a PMHNP and a PMHCNS has historically created some confusion, particularly before the establishment of the PMHNP certification in the early 2000s. This confusion was compounded by variations in state licensure and professional titles.

The American Psychiatric Nurses Association (APNA), along with other professional organizations such as the ANA and the International Society of Psychiatric-Mental Health Nurses (ISPN), has taken a stance on this issue. Their position, as of 2022, emphasizes that both PMHCNS and PMHNPs share core competencies in clinical and professional practice (APNA, 2022a).

According to this stance, PMHCNS and PMHNPs are both equipped to fulfill essential roles in various clinical settings, including providing psychotherapy, administering psychopharmacologic interventions, and offering clinical supervision. Additionally, they are expected to be accountable for their own practice and be capable of providing services independently across a range of delivery settings.

In essence, while there may be differences in educational preparation and professional titles, both PMHCNS and PMHNPs are recognized as APRNs with the expertise of providing high-quality psychiatric-mental healthcare (ANA et al., 2022).

The following data further reinforce this position:

A. In 2005, the ANCC and the APNA conducted a logical job analysis of PMHCNS and PMHNP roles. This analysis revealed that 99% of identified competencies were shared between NPs and CNS (Rice et al., 2007).

B. PMHCNS gained title rights, prescriptive authority, and direct care billing of Current Procedural Terminology (CPT) codes starting in 1978 in the Pacific Northwest. As of 2020, CNS can practice independently in 28 states and prescribe independently in 19 states (NACNS, 2020). CNS can bill for services in states where they are licensed to practice as APRNs (CMS, 2022).

C. Reimbursement from Medicare to ANCC-certified PMHCNS for CPT codes related to psychotherapeutic evaluation and treatment continues. Notably, certified PMHNPs were also recognized and added for reimbursement in 2007 (APNA, 2022a, 2022b).

D. ANCC data reveal a concerning trend: Pass rates for CNS exams have been declining for the past decade by a rate of 41% per year. If this continues, the new number of CNS certificates awarded will drop to zero.

The APNA Workforce Survey (2022b) has revealed approximately 27% of PMH-APRNs will be retiring over the next 6 years, with 7% of them retiring within the next 2 years (APNA, 2022b, p. 25). These figures are consistent with the fact that 40% of PMH-APRN respondents are over 60 years old. Retirement plans vary by certification, with a higher percentage of PMHCNS indicating intentions to retire in the next 6 years, including 55% of adult PMHCNS and 51% of child and adolescent PMHCNS. Given the higher mean age of the CNS group, this retirement rate is not unexpected.

One solution, already discussed here, is to permit currently licensed and certified PMH-APRNs who demonstrate their competency by continuing recertification to either practice under their current license and certification, or to use the PMH-APRN credential.

PSYCHIATRIC-MENTAL HEALTH NURSING SCOPE AND STANDARDS

The Scope and Standards Revision Joint Task Force, comprising members from the APNA and the ISPN, has undertaken a comprehensive revision and update of all sections of the Scope and Standards document. This includes significant revisions such as the following:

A. Refinement of the definition of psychiatric-mental health nursing to reflect contemporary practices and perspectives
B. Reorganization and expansion of the scope of practice section to align with evolving roles and responsibilities within the field of psychiatric-mental health nursing
C. Introduction of a new standard on cultural humility, emphasizing the importance of cultural competence and sensitivity in the delivery of psychiatric-mental healthcare

These revisions aim to ensure that the Scope and Standards document remains current, relevant, and reflective of the complexities and nuances of psychiatric-mental health nursing practice in today's healthcare landscape.

The following lists some of the main changes/additions made in the third edition:

A. Emphasis on population health and social determinants: The document now places a greater emphasis on population health and the social determinants of health/mental health. This entails an expanded focus on assessing and addressing these factors within psychiatric-mental health nursing practice.
B. Inclusion of disparities and inequities: There is an expanded review of disparities and inequities in psychiatric-mental healthcare. This underscores the importance of addressing and mitigating disparities to ensure equitable access to quality care for all individuals.
C. Recognition of substance use disorders: Substance use disorders are now recognized as psychiatric disorders within the Scope and Standards. Consequently, there is an increased emphasis on the importance of all psychiatric-mental health nurses being competent in providing comprehensive care for substance use disorders.
D. Identification of new/expanded roles: The document identifies new and expanded roles for psychiatric-mental health RNs/APRNs. These roles include integrated care, transdisciplinary collaboration, case management, telehealth practice, and more. This reflects the evolving landscape of psychiatric-mental health nursing and acknowledges the diverse settings and modalities in which psychiatric-mental health nurses practice (ANA et al., 2022).

None of these revisions/additions are surprising and are in keeping with what has been proposed for nursing in general: Movement toward population health and the social determinants of health, and new models of practice.

EDUCATION FOR PRACTICE

The APNA 2022 Psychiatric-Mental Health Nursing Workforce Study highlights two notable trends in PMH-APRN educational preparation. First, there is a significant increase in the percentage of content delivered online within PMH-APRN programs. More than a quarter of participants in their 20s reported that 100% of their didactic coursework was online, while for those in their 30s a quarter reported that 85% of their coursework was online (APNA, 2022b). However, it is essential to note that while the shift to online education is evident, there remains a lack of direct study on the effectiveness of this delivery method.

Second, there is a continued interest in the development of clinical competencies among PMH-APRNs. This includes a growing movement toward adapting the competency-based education model advocated by the American Association of Colleges of Nursing (AACN). This model emphasizes the acquisition of specific, measurable competencies that align with the skills and knowledge required for effective psychiatric-mental health nursing practice.

These trends underscore the evolving landscape of PMH-APRN education, with a shift toward online delivery methods and a continued emphasis on the development of clinical competencies to ensure high-quality patient care (National Task Force on Quality Nurse Practitioner Education, 2012).

The second trend highlighted in the APNA 2022 Psychiatric-Mental Health Nursing Workforce Study is the increasing number of recent PMH-APRN graduates with Doctor of Nursing Practice (DNP) preparation. This trend reflects the broader national movement toward adopting the DNP as the entry-level degree for advanced practice nursing. Specifically, the PMHNP population focus has emerged as a top priority in the transition from Master of Science in Nursing (MSN) to DNP programs (APNA, 2022b).

Research by Baldyga and DePaepe (2021) underscores the substantial growth (74% change) in PMHNP programs linked to Bachelor of Science in Nursing (BSN) to DNP programs since 2010. DNP preparation equips graduates with advanced skills in outcome evaluation and quality improvement, offering a significant opportunity to enhance the evidence base and scholarly output of psychiatric-mental health nursing.

This shift in educational preparation not only prepares PMH-APRNs to address complex service issues but also provides a platform to leverage DNP project research to advance our understanding of nursing approaches in mental healthcare. By utilizing DNP projects to contribute to the knowledge and evidence base, psychiatric-mental health nurses can play a pivotal role in driving improvements in patient outcomes and the quality of mental health services (Redman et al., 2015).

Indeed, the slow growth in the number of PMH-APRNs with PhD preparation is a concern echoed by research, such as that by Vance et al. (2020). Our own data further underscore this issue, revealing that only 6% of respondents hold a PhD degree, with a decreasing percentage of PMH-APRNs holding a PhD among those graduating since 2010.

Nursing research plays a crucial role in improving mental health services and informing policy development. Therefore, it is imperative for the profession to prioritize the cultivation of a sufficient number of PhD-prepared psychiatric-mental health nurses. These individuals contribute not only to advancing the scientific understanding of mental health but also to shaping evidence-based practices and policies that promote optimal outcomes for individuals and communities affected by mental illness.

Maintaining focus on increasing the number of PMH-APRNs with PhD preparation ensures a robust research workforce capable of addressing the multifaceted challenges within mental healthcare. By investing in the education and development of PhD-prepared psychiatric-mental health nurses, we can bolster the profession's capacity to drive innovation, promote equity, and enhance the overall quality of mental healthcare delivery.

TOOLS OF PSYCHIATRIC-MENTAL HEALTH NURSING PRACTICE

Norman Keltner, in *Keltner's Psychiatric Nursing,* eloquently proposes that the real-world approach to psychiatric-mental health nursing practice lies in "me, meds, and milieu" (Steele, 2022).

Simply put, the use of words from which the nurse–patient relationship springs; psychotropic medications that the nurse administers and that have worked miracles in modifying behavior and symptoms since their introduction around 1955; and the ever-present environment that is our oldest and most unpredictable tool.

PSYCHOTHERAPY/THERAPEUTIC USE OF SELF (ME)

The nurse–patient relationship is the backbone of psychiatric-mental health nursing practice, regardless of whether the nurse is at the entry phase or an advanced practitioner. For the RN, this takes the form of creating a therapeutic milieu for the patient and being a therapeutic presence in their lives. For the APRN, it is psychotherapy, a more active and directed therapeutic use of self.

The use of psychotherapy is an essential part of the practice of the PMH-APRN role. It is a standard of practice for PMH-APRNs in the Psychiatric-Mental Health Standards published by the ANA, the APNA, and the ISPN, and is included in the psychiatric-mental health competencies developed by the National Organization of Nurse Practitioner Faculties (NONPF). Both PMHCNS and PMHNPs are educationally prepared to provide psychotherapy, and the approaches to psychotherapy are transferable to relationships with families and groups. Groups may be constituted based on some common characteristics or concerns. It may be because people are living together in an institutional unit or in a home or other arrangement of convenience, or obtaining outpatient services at a common time and place. It is fair to say that patients may often resist coming together in a group, and the nurse must reexamine the reason group is a chosen modality and discuss this with their patient.

The first requisite for the nurse-psychotherapist is to know themselves. Well-developed self-awareness can only come with the often-painful process of self-examination and introspection. This involves understanding your own beliefs, thoughts, motivation, biases, and limitations, and recognizing the effect they have on others. The introspection must go further. The nurse brings their unique biopsychosocial self to each encounter and must be aware of how physical characteristics and qualities affect the patient. Body language is a large element in the equation, and closely aligned with culture. "Know thyself" is the basic tenet of psychiatric-mental health nursing (Boyd, 2018, p. 106). It is absolutely essential for advanced practice.

In these days of financial stress and noninstitutional treatment, it becomes necessary that the healthcare provider relinquish a great deal of autonomy to the patient and educate patients on how to use that autonomy therapeutically, according to their own priorities and goals. This is not only a value endorsed by the profession, but also guaranteed by law. Patients must understand their treatment and its expected outcome.

Psychotherapy, or more commonly the nurse–patient relationship, is divided into three phases: orientation, working, and resolution/termination. Each is characterized by therapeutic communication, active listening, and continuing assessment to move toward the patient's goals. These topics are covered in other sections of this book.

PSYCHOPHARMACOLOGY (MEDS)

Psychopharmacology revolutionized the treatment for those with psychiatric and mental health problems. Psychotropic drugs, with advent around 1955, calmed patients and reduced some of their socially unacceptable symptoms. This opened the door for legislation to support deinstitutionalization and the creation of a community mental health system. There have been very few studies on the outcomes of community treatment. What we do know is that the concept was never developed adequately and funded sufficiently to test its credibility. We do know that from a peak in the pretranquilizer era, state mental hospital population today has declined more than 85% (Steele, 2022). This should not be construed as a victory but is the shifting of care to social programs concerned with homelessness, poverty, and occupational development. We are in the midst of a period of transinstitutionalization, where individuals with mental illness are commonly housed in nursing homes, prisons, board-and-care homes, or with family. This transinstitutionalization creates other practice areas for PMH-APRNs, as well as presenting unique, new practice challenges.

The use of psychotropic drugs in the care of individuals with mental illness is not always desirable nor appropriate. What we can say is that it places individuals as being more open to other therapies, most especially those that require one-to-one receptiveness, such as psychotherapy. Patients usually respond more rapidly than they would without drugs. Psychotropic drugs have enabled millions of people to lead increasingly independent lives. This creates an invaluable role for RNs/APRNs, not limited to psychiatric-mental health practice. The nurse is responsible for educating the patient, and with their permission other responsible people in their lives, about their medication regimen, including side effects, interactions, desired effects, and dietary requirements.

ENVIRONMENTAL MANAGEMENT (MILIEU)

The word *milieu,* which is often used in psychiatric nursing, is a French word that means *environment.* The environment has been a primary concern of nurses since Florence Nightingale. It forges therapeutic benefits from the patient's surroundings wherever they may be. For Nightingale, the first concern was *safety,* and it is still today. Safety may be interpreted as harm in the broadest sense: infection, accident, or whatever threatens or is seen by patients as holding danger. Safety outweighs all other environmental concerns.

The *structure* of the physical environment may be a formidable challenge. Are rules, regulations, and schedules acceptable to the patient? Are there *norms* of conduct and behavioral expectations that create problems? These are present in any treatment setting and may be expressed or implied. Is violence or "speaking out" tolerated? What are the expectations for privacy and acceptance of unusual behavior of any type? Who imposes *limits* on behavior and how is it done? And closely related, how is *balance* achieved? Where is the line between dependence and independence? Who and how are *environmental modifications* carried out, no matter how seemingly insignificant? The preceding concerns characterize the milieux wherever the nurse and the patient may find themselves. It also makes sense that different issues may be involved where we are confronted with an outpatient as compared with an inpatient situation.

INTERDISCIPLINARY/TRANSDISCIPLINARY CARE

Transdisciplinary practice is the newest addition to our psychotherapeutic repertoire, and is here to stay, although growing slowly. The future of nursing and healthcare depends on partnerships. The nursing approach to practice is holistic, but no one professional can address every dimension of need. This point is well taken as we look at current healthcare legislation and the models that have been instituted in some of our most revered hospitals, private practices, and rehabilitation centers.

There are many emergent models of shared professional practice; one of the most noteworthy is facilitated by the Patient Protection and Affordable Care Act (PPACA) of 2010. Accountable care organizations (ACOs), created in that legislation, are collaboratives between primary care and specialist clinicians, hospitals, and other health professionals accepting joint responsibility for both quality and cost of care provided to a patient. Although the ACO targets Medicare, there is the potential for private plans to pick up the idea, and they have through state-based legislation (Joel, 2022). The ACO is highly dependent on team leadership and case management, and APRNs would seem uniquely suited to function in such holistic roles.

Another related concept is the patient-centered medical home (PCMH), which is a move away from the primary care model and looks to provide coordinated care through an interprofessional team of healthcare providers, which is likely to include APRNs, RNs, physicians, social workers, occupational therapists, and more. Again, the holistic view and educational skills of APRNs place them in a unique position to lead "team" development in this instance.

The most recent model for health system redesign puts patients at the center of treatment decisions. Labeled as *shared decision-making* (SDM), the model places the APRN/RN at the center of the model as educator, advocate, and facilitator during the exchange of information with the larger team to find a plan of care and treatment mutually acceptable to the patient and their healthcare providers. This model was first pioneered at Harlem Hospital in New York but has grown to other locations, becoming known as the Patient Navigator Program. The navigator role is again very suited to an APRN but need not even be someone in the medical field. Some patients have reported a preference for laypersons with good interpersonal skills, and some experience in service-oriented fields (Joel, 2022). All these partnership models are particularly suited to managed care arrangements, which have grown in both the public and private domains through insurance.

BARRIERS TO PRACTICE

The most significant barrier to APRN practice is continued physician supervision over aspects of the ability to prescribe. In some states, this means the maintenance of a joint protocol for the prescription of some or all drugs and treatments. Regardless of how extreme or lenient the restrictions are, which reduce or eliminate the PMH-APRN's right to prescribe, they are an undue obstacle to the public.

The legislative language for a National Licensure Compact for APRNs (NLC-APRN) has been authorized and published by the National Council of State Boards of Nursing (NCSBN). It will be functional once seven states have ratified their intent to go ahead and have language that would eliminate such obstacles. Delaware and North Dakota are the only two states whose legislators have formally endorsed the NLC-APRN. Both Maryland and Utah are somewhere in the process. Proponents of the NLC-APRN claim that changing practice patterns, including telehealth and travel across state borders to work, requires this accommodation (NCSBN, 2022). Strong resistance comes from the medical community, which claims jeopardy of safety. However, by withholding a multistate license and full scope of practice, we are reducing the health services available to the public, primarily in underserved medical areas. In the face of these objections arises the issue of states' rights and the organizational and political affiliations that come with our current government structure.

Of 4,780 PMH-APRN respondents involved in the APNA 2022 Psychiatric-Mental Health Nursing Workforce Report, 86% showed they provide telehealth services in their employment settings. On average, they supply these services in two states, to an average of 25 patients per week (APNA, 2022b). Since the survey was conducted at the start of the COVID-19 pandemic, these numbers may only be a fraction of telehealth services provided in the last 2 years.

Of these 4,780 respondents, 88% reported having prescriptive authority. Those holding PMHNP certifications had much higher rates of prescriptive authority (98%), while those with PMHCNS certifications had significantly lower rates; however, a substantial number of PMHCNS do prescribe (66%). Prescriptive authority decreases with years since graduation and increases with those graduating since 2010; 97% of these more recent graduates have prescriptive authority. This is because most PMH-APRN graduates during this period completed PMHNP programs.

SUMMARY

This abbreviated view of psychiatric-mental health nursing practice serves as the background for the extensive knowledge presented in the chapters that follow. References to PMHRN are included, but only to set the context. The historical development of the specialty is detailed, as is discussion on credentialing, the scope and standards of the PMH-APRN, and education for practice. The therapeutic tools used in practice are presented, as well as the emergence of new models of care and the barriers that prevent the PMH-APRN from functioning in full scope of practice.

REFERENCES AND BIBLIOGRAPHY

American Nurses Association, American Psychiatric Nurses Association, & International Society of Psychiatric-Mental Health Nurses. (2022). *Psychiatric-mental health nursing: Scope and standards of practice* (3rd ed.). American Nurses Association.

American Psychiatric Nurses Association. (2022a, June). *APNA position: Psychiatric-mental health advanced practice nurses.* https://www.apna.org/pmh-aprns-position-statement

American Psychiatric Nurses Association. (2022b). *Psychiatric-mental health nursing workforce report.* https://omsapaprod.wpenginepowered.com/wp-content/uploads/2022/08/APNA-Workforce-Survey-Data-Report-8.15.22.pdf

Baldyga, J., & DePaepe, C. (2021). *Doctor of nursing practice: Trends in program growth, enrollment and graduation across population foci.* AANP Research Brief. https://www.aanp.org/practice/practice-related-research/research-reports/doctor-of-nursing-practice-research-brief

Boyd, M. A. (2018). *Psychiatric nursing: Contemporary practice* (6th ed.). Wolters Kluwer.

Boyd, M. A., & Luebbert, R. (2022). *Psychiatric nursing: Contemporary practice* (7th ed.). Wolters Kluwer.

Centers for Medicaid & Medicare Services. (2022). *Advanced practice registered nurses, anesthesiologist assistants, & physicians assistants.* MLN Booklet. https://www.hhs.gov/guidance/sites/default/files/hhs-guidance-documents/Advanced_Practice_Registered_Nurses__Anesthesiologist_Assistants_Physician_Assistants_MLN901623.pdf

Joel, L. A. (2022). *Advanced practice nursing: Essentials for role development* (5th ed.). F. A. Davis Company.

Melnyk, B. M., & Fineout-Overholt, E. (2023). *Evidence-based practice in nursing & healthcare: A guide to best practice* (5th ed.). Wolters Kluwer.

National Association of Clinical Nurse Specialists. (2020, July 31). *CNS scope of practice and prescriptive authority as of 7.31.2020.* https://nacns.org/wp-content/uploads/2020/08/PractPrescAuthority7.31.2020.pdf

National Council of State Boards of Nursing. (2022, July). *Multistate licensure for telephonic practice (telehealth) - July 2022.* https://www.ncsbn.org/recorded-webinar/multistate-licensure-for-telephonic-practice-telehealth

National Task Force on Quality Nurse Practitioner Education. (2012). *Criteria for evaluation of nurse practitioner programs 2012: A report of the National Task Force on Quality Nurse Practitioner Education* (4th ed.). American Association of Colleges of Nursing & National Organization of Nurse Practitioner Faculties. https://www.aacnnursing.org/Portals/0/PDFs/Teaching-Resources/Criteria-Evaluation-NP-2012.pdf

Redman, R. W., Pressler, S. J., Furspan, P., & Potempa, K. (2015). Nurses in the United States with a practice doctorate: Implications for leading in the current context of health care. *Nursing Outlook, 63*(2), 124–129. https://doi.org/10.1016/j.outlook.2014.08.003

Rice, M. J., Moller, M. D., DePascale, C., & Skinner, L. (2007). APNA and ANCC collaboration: Achieving consensus on future credentialing for advanced practice psychiatric and mental health nursing. *Journal of the American Psychiatric Nurses Association, 13*(3), 153–159. https://doi.org/10.1177/1078390307305171

Steele, D. (2022). *Keltner's psychiatric nursing* (9th ed.). Mosby.

Vance, D. E., Heaton, K., Antia, L., Frank, J., Moneyham, L., Harper, D., & Meneses, K. (2020). Alignment of a PhD program in nursing with the AACN report on the research-focused doctorate in nursing: A descriptive analysis. *Journal of Professional Nursing, 36*(6), 604–610. https://doi.org/10.1016/j.profnurs.2020.08.011

2 THERAPEUTIC COMMUNICATION

Faith Atte

INTRODUCTION

Therapeutic communication is the major tool of the APRN. Skillful use of strategies and expertise facilitates the treatment and outcomes of the patients they encounter. Practicing effective communication allows for individuals to connect with empathy and understanding, leading to a therapeutic relationship. Many things can interfere with this process. Factors such as the patient's disease process, cultural beliefs, and language differences can hinder establishing a genuine rapport with the patient. Implicit bias and stereotyping can create barriers to effective care and must be continually part of the healthcare provider's self-reflection. How statements or questions are phrased is paramount to establishing and maintaining the patient relationship.

THERAPEUTIC COMMUNICATION

The root of the word *communication* is derived from the Latin word *communicare*, which means to share, or to make common, to convey, or to transmit (Weekley, 1967). In nursing, communication embodies different variables, including the message (what we say), the delivery (how it is said), and the recipient (to whom it is said). Establishing a therapeutic relationship with our patients, especially with a patient who has a psychiatric diagnosis, is our primary goal, as such the goal of the interaction between a patient facing mental health challenges and a healthcare provider is therapeutic communication. Communication is a nonlinear, dynamic process.

Thich Nhat Hanh, a Vietnamese Buddhist monk, states that both parties should be open to change in an authentic dialogue or communication. He further affirms the importance of appreciating that truth can be received from within and without. When a healthcare provider communicates with a patient, understanding becomes a fundamental and crucial part of the conversation. By engaging in a dialogue with a patient, the clinician creates a shift in thinking. If the patient misinterprets or fails to understand what is being conveyed, effective communication has not occurred. Therapeutic communication is planned, deliberate, purposeful, helpful, patient-centered, and goal-directed. It is a learned skill that improves with practice focusing on patient needs.

Social interaction is often a chance occurrence without the constraints of time and outcomes. It can be flamboyant, nondirectional, and without a specific goal. This social communication may include sharing information, feelings, and ideas, but is not directed toward actively clinically helping another person.

Communication exists between healthcare providers when discussing therapies and patient planning. Evidence suggests that ineffective communication among healthcare providers is one of the leading causes of medical errors and patient harm. According to The Joint Commission, it is estimated that communication failures were responsible at least in part for 30% of medical malpractice claims, 1,744 deaths, and $1.7 billion in malpractice costs for 5 years (Budryk, 2016). Data from the National Institutes of Health (NIH) show that $12 billion is lost from ineffective communication in hospitals (Agarwal et al., 2010).

In summary, the outcomes of effective therapeutic communication may include:

A. Improved relationships between the healthcare provider and the patient
B. Increased patient satisfaction
C. Better patient understanding of the disease process through psychoeducation
D. Reduction of healthcare costs and burden of diseases within an economy

ELEMENTS OF THE COMMUNICATION PROCESS

A. Communication is an engaging process of sending and receiving messages involving two or more individuals intending to create an understanding.
B. The initial stages of communication often involve conceptualizing ideas and thoughts and the need to communicate with other individuals for different purposes, such as sharing information and offering comfort or advice.
C. The communication process is divided into seven major elements:
  1. Sender
  2. Encoding
  3. Message
  4. Channel
  5. Receiver
  6. Decoding
  7. Feedback

D. Sender: The sender is the person initiating the conversation. The great philosopher Aristotle said that, for in-depth communication to occur, the three critical elements of ethos, pathos, and logos are required.
  1. Ethos involves the sender's credibility and authenticity. Why should people believe in you and what you are saying? What is your expertise?
  2. Pathos establishes an emotional connection with the audience. Why should the audience believe in your content? This skill involves being present with the audience and providing undivided attention.
  3. Logos is the process of appealing to logic and reason. The sender must employ strategic thinking and problem-solving skills when expressing ideas that will influence the conversation's outcome.

E. Encoding: Encoding is converting thoughts, ideas, and information into an understandable message. The sender's knowledge of the subject (e.g., background and body gestures) dramatically impacts how the message is received.

F. Message: After the encoding process, the sender then relays the intended message. *Message* can be defined as the information sent or expressed to another. This information can be communicated orally, written, or nonverbal visually to elicit the receiver's response. The most straightforward messages are well-organized and communicated in a manner familiar to the receiver (Table 2.1).

G. Channel: The sender decides what channel would be appropriate for the message to be well-received. The channel must be carefully selected in order for the message to be effectively interpreted. The message can be relayed through various channels depending on the interpersonal relationship between the sender and the receiver and the message's urgency.

H. Receiver: The receiver is the person for whom the message is intended. The degree of comprehensibility depends on the receiver's relationship with the sender, knowledge of the subject, and the degree to which they are willing and able to engage in the communication process.

I. Decoding: Decoding is the process of interpreting the sender's message as it was intended. Effective communication occurs only when the sender and the receiver understand the message.

J. Feedback: Feedback validates the sender's message and increases the effectiveness of the communication process. It allows the sender to establish the efficacy of the message. Feedback can be established through clarification of the message.

FACTORS AFFECTING THERAPEUTIC COMMUNICATION

Several factors may impact therapeutic communication. Multiple factors may impede therapeutic communication, including patient-centered factors, healthcare provider factors, and environmental factors. A genuine therapeutic relationship will develop when the patient perceives they are being heard and understood with empathy, respect, and dignity.

PATIENT-CENTERED FACTORS

Culture

A. Betancourt (2004) defined *culture* as a pattern of learned beliefs, values, and behavior shared within a group. These include language, modes of communication, practices, customs, and views on roles and relationships.

B. Not identifying, understanding, or accepting cultural differences and norms can negatively impact the communication process. For example, a person's culture may have specific gender roles in caring for the ill. Other cultures do not believe in the existence of mental illness and challenges, such that a person having clinical depression may be termed as being *lazy*, and a person having symptoms of schizophrenia may be said to have *evil spirits*. Therefore, as healthcare providers, we must have the cultural competence to care for patients effectively. Deardorff defined *competence* as "the ability to communicate effectively and appropriately in intercultural situations based on one's intercultural knowledge, skills, and attitudes" (Deardorff, 2006, pp. 247–248).

C. Cultural competence and understanding cultural consistency ensure that healthcare providers respect, interact, and communicate effectively and without judgment with patients across cultures.

Disease Process

A. A patient's disease process can interfere with the communication process. If a patient is agitated and shows signs of aggression, it will be challenging to establish an alliance through therapeutic communication. Safety of the patient, the clinician, and the environment is the first and most important intervention.

B. Another symptom that may present as a challenging communication factor is psychosis, with hallmark symptoms of hallucinations and delusions.

C. Developing a shared understanding between the patient and the healthcare provider in a psychotic experience can become particularly challenging from the patient's perspective ▶

TABLE 2.1 NONVERBAL BEHAVIOR VISUAL CUES

Nonverbal Behavior	Visual Cues	Common Behaviors
Body movement	*Body movement* is the broadest term used to elaborate nonverbal communication. It includes posture, body language, and gait.	Crossed arms, body turned away from the speaker, slouching, pacing
Hand gestures	The movement of the hands can impact how information is decoded. Of the nonverbal behaviors, hand gestures may have the most cultural capriciousness.	Throwing hands in the air (defeat or dismissing the message), peace sign
Eye contact or eye expression	Eye contact can show the degree to which the receiver is paying attention. Attention can be expressed by intense gaze and lowering of brows.	Darting of eyes, intense and intimidating eye stare
Touch	With consent and cultural appropriateness, touch can be therapeutic; for example, open to touch.	Hugs, pat on the hand, a firm squeeze on the shoulder
Space	Personal space—accessible to close friends and family. It can be culturally driven; for example, standing far away or too close to the speaker.	Needs increased space during a conversation
Voice	The voice of the speaker can be a source of emotional connection and healing; for example, tone, pauses, silences, and fluency.	Using a loud voice during communication, whispering, sing-song voice
Personal appearance and physical characteristics	Presentation of oneself may influence how we are addressed; for example, casual dressing, routine grooming, and hygiene. Physical attributes include physical physique, height, and weight.	Dressed in a dirty outfit, malodorous, grossly obese, short or tall

on communicating their concerns and how the healthcare provider decodes them.

D. The healthcare provider must provide reality to the patient throughout the communication. However, a conflict can occur from the health provider's standpoint on whether to challenge the psychotic experiences or agree with the patient.

E. To develop a shared understanding with a patient experiencing psychosis, the clinician's capacity to assess the situation and the patient's experience increases the likelihood of improved communication.

Developmental Level

A. A patient's developmental level can significantly impact the overall outcome of the conversation. The developmental level can include patients with autism (e.g., delayed speech and intellectual disability) and other psychiatric diagnosis. Assessment and evaluation of the developmental level is critical to establishing communication.

B. Establishing therapeutic communication with patients who have complex communication needs may be challenging. Several researchers (Ganz, 2015) have recommended using communication therapy, referred to as *augmentative and alternate communication* (*AAC*), to assist in the communication process.

   1. AAC involves using various modalities that can replace a person's speech.
   2. Some modalities include graphic symbols displayed in books, music/sounds, smell, and touching.
   3. other modalities include communication boards or devices such as speech-generating devices or manual signs.

HEALTHCARE PROVIDER FACTORS

Knowledge Level

A. A clinician's level of experience and knowledge in the diagnostics of psychiatric illnesses, conducting a thorough patient assessment, and awareness of personal bias can affect the clinician–patient communication process. As clinicians gain more experience in formulating therapeutic communication, they tend to individualize care and center more on the subjective presentation of the disease. Novice clinicians focus on the patient's diagnosis, relying primarily on the disease process when communicating with patients.

B. There is often a progression and refinement of knowledge and experience as clinicians develop expertise within their specialized practice.

C. Experienced clinicians rely more on interactive and conditional reasoning to determine the patient's treatment plan.

Credibility

A. *Credibility* refers to the quality, capability, or power to elicit belief from others and plays a vital role in influencing the audience's thoughts and beliefs. It is the extent to which the patient believes their healthcare provider. *Why should I agree or comply with what you are telling me?*

B. According to Engleberg and Daly (2004), credibility can be categorized into three: (a) *character*: Is the individual sincere, honest, friendly, and ethical?; (b) *competence*: What qualification and experience does the person have?; (c) *caring*: Is there empathy, compassion, and sensitivity from the speaker? The healthcare providers' credibility, or lack thereof, is essential in effective patient communication. These are consistent with the elements of ethos, pathos, and logos referenced in the discussion about the sender in the "Elements of the Communication Process" section.

ENVIRONMENT (ATMOSPHERIC) FACTORS

A. Environmental (atmospheric) factors that hinder or enhance therapeutic communication include physical space, noise, climate, and safety.

   1. The physical distance between the patient and the healthcare provider may affect messages sent and received.
   2. When the physical distance is too close, the patient may feel threatened and afraid.
   3. A lack of trust and credibility may occur when the distance is too far apart.

B. External noise is one of the most recognized environmental factors that can create barriers to communication. When two individuals are engaged in a conversation and there is noise, the communication process will be impossible as it will be challenging to hear each other. Noise is particularly a barrier if the patient has psychotic features of hallucinations and delusions. The patient might struggle with differentiating between internal and external voices.

C. It is vital for the healthcare provider to consciously and intentionally provide an environment conducive to communication, avoiding distractions and promoting progression toward treatment goals.

D. By creating a therapeutic environment, patients will be more at ease and more likely to talk about the disease process and how it impacts their lives because of a subconscious sense of safety.

MEDIUMS AND CHANNELS OF COMMUNICATION

A. A medium of communication refers to the physical methods whereby the message can be delivered from the messenger to the receiver. The mediums are interpersonal, print, and broadcast. There are four channels of communication. These are verbal, nonverbal, visual, and written.

   1. Interpersonal: This is described as two-way communication between the sender and the receiver(s) and can be done on a 1:1 basis or a group setting. It can also be done in-person or online. This is an immediate response channel.
   2. Print: This includes flyers, pamphlets, texts, emails, and letters. This is a delayed response channel.
   3. Broadcast: This medium of communication is less personalized and utilizes mass media to deliver the message. It is described as one-way communication without requiring a response.

B. Communication between the clinician and the patient is crucial in determining the correct diagnosis, planning, and executing the treatment plan. According to Barry and Fulmer (2004), the key to effective communication is to match the communication channel with the goal of the message.

C. The choice of channel and the concept are particularly vital when caring for patients with psychiatric challenges.

   1. Verbal: This includes face-to-face conversations, telephone conversations, voicemail, in-person conferences, and video conferences. It consists of spoken words that often transmit emotions. When we use our voices to convey a message, we communicate our beliefs, perceptions, expectations, feelings, understanding, conflicts, and interests.
   2. Nonverbal: This includes physical appearance, physical barriers such as distance, tone of voice, eye contact, hand gestures, and reaction to sadness and happiness. What we say is an integral part of any communication. What is not said can also impact the outcome of the message transmission. Purposeful and implicit nonverbal cues can send essential messages.

3. **Visual:** This includes the use of images to deliver added meaning to a message. This is used commonly in mass media and personal communications, including an emoticon used in text communication. They may have a different meaning to the recipient than to the sender, so care must be taken to ensure the message is received as intended.
4. **Written:** This includes email, text, slide presentations, and/or flyers and mass media (e.g., billboards). Organization of the message is important, putting the substance of the message in the beginning sentence and keeping the message succinct. Care must be taken to avoid miscommunication or undesired tone.

The Interaction Between Verbal and Nonverbal Cues

A. To become an effective communicator, a clinician must employ verbal and nonverbal cues.
   1. Congruence between the clinician's verbal and nonverbal communication is essential. This is especially true during a patient's stressful period when it can be challenging for them to interpret the clinician's subtle nonverbal communication changes.
   2. Patients with mental health challenges often have incongruence between verbal and nonverbal communication, much of which can also serve as a diagnostic tool if examined, identified, and clarified by the clinician.
   3. Patients as well as healthcare providers may have unique nonverbal characteristics and cues that are influenced by their culture, behavior, or disease process, which can interfere with clear messaging. The most common and traditional interpersonal communication channel in psychiatric care is face-to-face. This form of communication between the clinician and the patient, as well as clinician to clinician, puts into practice the interaction between verbal and nonverbal cues. Interpersonal, face-to-face communication is also the most effective.
   4. Gaining popularity since the COVID-19 pandemic is web-based and online communication. This channel allows for "face-to-face" without the communicators having to be in the same place at the same time.
   5. Significant differences between virtual and face-to-face modes of communication include the following:
      a. Some critical facets of face-to-face conversation (e.g., body-to-body interactions) in online communication with patients with mental challenges can be lost.
      b. Healthcare providers need to engage in consciously compensating for such losses.
      c. Another significant challenge of online communication is the possible loss of a felt therapeutic presence.
         i. *Therapeutic presence* can be defined as bringing one's whole self to the engagement with the patient and being fully in the moment with and for the patient.
         ii. It is the state of having oneself in full interaction with the patient by successfully transforming an intention into action (Lemma, 2017).
   6. When the healthcare provider is fully present (e.g., physically, emotionally, cognitively, and spiritually) with the patient, it sends a message to the patient that they are being heard, understood, and most importantly a safe platform has been provided for them, thus strengthening the therapeutic presence and relationship.
   7. Despite the challenges, it is possible to create an online therapeutic presence. Healthcare providers can reinforce their online presence by using self-disclosure to increase credibility and responsibility. Using the self as a therapeutic tool for understanding the patient, the healthcare provider can provide sufficient support for patients to feel safe in expressing their emotional vulnerabilities.

THERAPEUTIC COMMUNICATION TECHNIQUES

To make a clinical decision regarding patient concerns, a healthcare provider must employ a variety of communication techniques. The treatment plan for an individual with mental illness can be fraught with uncertainties as each patient presents differently. The healthcare provider needs to have the skills and knowledge that will assist the patient in communicating their thoughts and feelings. Having strong communication skills will enhance the patient interaction process. These skills are called *therapeutic communication techniques*, including verbal and nonverbal cues, which help achieve the established goal (Table 2.2).

ACTIVE LISTENING

A. Active listening is an art. This sophisticated communication technique can be learned and understood with considerable practice. The process of active listening or improving one's listening skills can be tedious, challenging, and demanding; however, it can be rewarding. Listening accomplishes the following:
   1. Demonstrates acceptance
   2. Promotes problem-solving abilities
   3. Increases a speaker's receptiveness to the ideas and thoughts of others
   4. Helps prevent head-on emotional collisions

B. Giving undivided attention to the patient provides a safe platform for them to express their feelings. It is essential to remember that in a conversation every person involved is trying to find a solution to a problem. The clinician seeks to understand the patient's challenges, while the patient wants to be understood, to seek clarity of thoughts, link ideas, and together come up with a feasible treatment plan that actively involves the patient's input.

SILENCE

A. Silence is one of the most potent forms of communication. It is described as the absence of words but an effective communication tool. When we pause in a conversation, we allow ourselves, as healthcare providers, time to focus and reflect on what the patient is trying to communicate before responding. When used at specific points in the conversation, silence can relay confidence and strength and allow the patient space to formulate new ideas and gain a new perspective. Ultimately, healthcare providers can assess patient needs effectively.

B. Silence may be uncomfortable at the beginning of a conversation, and both patients and healthcare providers may try to fill the void with questions or chatter. It is important to note that some patients may present with profound depression, paranoia, or shyness, and may be acutely aware of the silence. In such a situation, the healthcare provider should recognize and acknowledge the patient's discomfort and focus on building a therapeutic foundation to further the conversation.

C. Despite its numerous benefits, using silence as a communication technique can have some unintended, nontherapeutic consequences. Silence can cause miscommunication. Some cultures regard silence as a form of disrespect or expression of anger. If this type of situation occurs, the healthcare provider should incorporate other therapeutic techniques to allow the patient to feel safe enough to express themselves.

TABLE 2.2 THERAPEUTIC COMMUNICATION TECHNIQUES

Therapeutic Techniques	Definition	Rationale
Acceptance	This technique acknowledges the patient's emotions or message and affirms they have been heard.	Patients who feel their nurses are listening to them and taking them seriously are more likely to be receptive to care.
Clarification	This technique asks the patient for further information. It demonstrates the healthcare provider actively listening.	Clarification helps nurses ensure they understand what is actually being said and can help patients process their ideas more thoroughly.
Focusing	This technique directs attention to a specific remark made by the patient.	Patients do not always have an objective perspective on their situation or past experiences, but as impartial observers nurses can pick out important topics on which to focus.
Exploring	This technique gathers more information about what the patient is communicating.	Exploring helps the patient examine a statement or idea by providing added information.
Giving recognition	This technique acknowledges and validates the patient's positive health behaviors.	Recognition acknowledges the patient's behavior and highlights it without giving an overt compliment.
Open-ended questions/ offering general leads	Using open questions or offering general leads provides keywords to "open" the discussion while also seeking more information.	Giving patients a broad opening such as "What would you like to talk about?" encourages them to discuss what is on their mind.
Paraphrasing	This technique rephrases the patient's words and key ideas.	Paraphrasing is a clarifying technique to encourage additional communication.
Presenting reality	This technique establishes current reality.	This technique restructures the patient's distorted thoughts with valid information.
Restating	This technique uses different word choices for the same.	Restating is a strategy to encourage patient elaboration.
Reflecting	This technique encourages the patient to verbalize a resolution to their quandary.	Reflecting encourages the patient to be accountable for their own actions. It helps patients come up with solutions.
Providing silence	This technique provides patients time for self-reflection.	This technique provides time for patient reflection.
Making observations	Observations about the appearance, demeanor, or behavior of patients can help draw attention to areas that might pose a problem for them.	This technique acknowledges external indicators of possible problems.
Offering self/providing presence	This means being present and offering healthcare providers' physical time.	This technique promotes a caring connection and patient value.
Encouraging descriptions of perceptions	Asking about perceptions in an encouraging, nonjudgmental way is important for patients experiencing sensory issues or hallucinations. It gives patients a prompt to explain what they are perceiving without casting their perceptions in a negative light.	This technique establishes safety by ensuring the hallucinations are not encouraging the patient to harm themselves or others.
Encouraging comparisons	Encourage comparisons of previous situations in which they have coped effectively.	This technique helps patients discover solutions to their problems.
Offering hope	Offering hope encourages the patient to persevere and be resilient.	This technique encourages positive thinking, not a promise of an outcome.
Offering humor	Humor can lighten the mood and contribute to feelings of togetherness, closeness, and friendliness. Care must be taken to tailor to the patient's sense of humor.	This technique can lighten the mood and contribute to friendliness, and may facilitate a therapeutic relationship.
Confronting	Confrontation, when used correctly, can help patients break destructive routines or understand the state of their current situation.	This technique challenges the patient's assumptions. Nurses should only apply this technique during the working phase after they have established trust.
Summarizing	This technique allows the healthcare provider to verify information.	Summarizing provides the patient with explicit permission to make corrections, if necessary.

THERAPEUTIC CLARIFYING TECHNIQUES

Clarification can be most effective by seeking feedback from the listeners. The clinician should ask the patient if what was communicated is what was meant. When the patient begins to withdraw from communication, it is crucial to find out what is happening and validate their feelings. Several strategies can be employed in seeking clarification:

A. Paraphrasing: Paraphrasing is the process of rewording the patient's message to seek further clarification. To build a therapeutic relationship, the patient needs to know that they are not only being listened to but are also understood and valued as a human being. The healthcare provider can use simple, concise, and culturally appropriate phrases to clarify the patient's message. Paraphrasing allows the healthcare provider to exercise *empathy*—the art of putting oneself in another person's shoes. Empathy is the capacity to accurately understand another person's internal perspective, along with the emotions and meanings attached to it, while still maintaining the awareness that you are not that person.

B. Reflection: Reflection involves assisting the patient in understanding their thoughts and feelings. Reflection should consider the emotional tone of what the patient is expressing, including verbal and nonverbal cues. It shows the patient that you, the healthcare provider, have *heard, seen, felt, and listened* to what has been shared. When you use reflection, you allow the patient to listen to themselves by being aware of their inner feelings. Reflection is comparable to holding a mirror to the patient, repeating what they have said to gain more clarity. You can repeat the whole sentence or parts of the sentence.

C. Restating: This form of active listening technique helps the healthcare provider understand what the patient is saying. Restating involves repeating and phrasing what the patient has said in a question format. Restating allows the patient to further expound on what they have said to offer clarity to the healthcare provider. While this technique is valuable, it should be used cautiously and sparingly. If used repeatedly, restating may be interpreted as inattention or lack of interest.

D. Exploration: This technique allows the healthcare provider to develop and examine a specific area of concern and essential ideal experiences brought forth by the patient. Some examples of conversation openers to explore a concern include the following: (a) Tell me more about how you feel when you are about to do an exam. (b) Can you recall when you felt confident prior to doing an exam? These statements will enable the patient to reflect on when the anxiety was not as pronounced. In addition, asking for a specific example can clarify a general statement made by the patient.

E. Open-ended questioning: This type of questioning helps the healthcare provider see things from the patient's point of view. These questions also allow you, the healthcare provider, to practice active listening and validating the patient's answers. These are questions that cannot be answered with a "yes" or "no." Most of the open-ended questions begin with "what and how." Open-ended questions are ideal for establishing a trusting rapport with the patient. This technique is especially important at the beginning of an interview as they are not intrusive and can put the patient at ease to talk about themselves.

F. Closed-ended questioning: This questioning elicits a short answer. Healthcare providers are often encouraged to ask open-ended questions to explore a question further. However, the use of closed-ended questions can provide crucial and specific information. For example, if a patient presents with signs and symptoms of depression, it is imperative to use a closed-ended question to ascertain if there are thoughts of harming or killing oneself.

G. Projective questioning: This questioning is intended to uncover a deeper understanding of emotional needs, feelings, desires, barriers, and motivators. These questions often begin with a *"What if…"* scenario *and* can provide insight into inner thoughts that are not forthcoming from direct questioning.

H. The miracle question: This solution-focused communication technique guides patients in envisioning their lives if the problem no longer exists. This type of question allows the patient to discover the fundamental goal in their lives. It also helps the healthcare provider know what the patient wants and how to assist them effectively.

    1. The miracle question is most beneficial when the patient has a goal they want to pursue or a problem to be solved. It helps the patient to be conscious of what life would be like sans the problem.

SUMMARIZING

Summarization is putting together vital points of the healthcare provider and the patient to enhance communication. It allows and ensures that the highlights of communication are captured and further clarifications are made. A good summary can ascertain that the healthcare provider and the patient have a similar understanding of the conversation.

NONTHERAPEUTIC COMMUNICATION TECHNIQUES

During social interactions with other people (e.g., friends, coworkers, and family), it is not uncommon to use nontherapeutic communication. However, using such techniques during a patient–healthcare provider interaction might lead to an unintended conversation that will impede achieving the treatment goal (Table 2.3).

TABLE 2.3 NONTHERAPEUTIC COMMUNICATION TECHNIQUES

Technique	Rationale
Giving advice	This technique gives the patient the impression that they are incapable of self-direction. It can be considered intrusive by the patient.
Giving approval or disapproval	This implies the healthcare provider judges the patient's actions and behavior. It is heavily rooted in healthcare providers' biases and stereotypical views about a group of people.
Excessive questioning in succession	This can be perceived as demanding and accusatory. The patient may feel that the healthcare provider is unwilling to engage in a discussion but is seeking answers.
Using clichés	These statements hold little meaning and have lost their originality. A feeling of being "put in a box" may be experienced using cliché words.
Changing the subject	This technique causes the healthcare provider to be the deciding factor in how the conversation progresses. This can be perceived as dismissive.
Asking "why"	Asking "why" demands an explanation and may lead to the patient defending their stance.
Agreeing and disagreeing	This implies that the healthcare provider decides the rightfulness and wrongness of the patient's ideas, resulting in a halt in conversation.
Belittling	This causes the patient to feel insignificant.

GIVING ADVICE

A. Giving and receiving advice is a common phenomenon in regular human interaction. However, when a healthcare provider advises a patient, the healthcare provider may inevitably interfere with the patient's autonomy to make personal decisions.

B. Giving advice fosters dependency in that the patient feels inadequate to make decisions on their own. Instead of giving advice, the healthcare provider can offer information that assists the patient in making informed decisions.

GIVING APPROVAL OR DISAPPROVAL

A. In regular conversations, we often approve or disapprove of various things (e.g., how people dress, cook, and take compliments). It is a way of making others feel good about themselves or sometimes belittle them. Such compliments, when given to a vulnerable patient, can evoke feelings of wanting to please, and in turn patients may become desperate for recognition, attention, and approval.

B. Recognizing the patient's behavior and further exploring how the patient feels suggest to the patient that they have control over how they feel and how to react when they feel scared or uncomfortable in any given situation.

C. Making a statement that implies that the healthcare provider does not condone some behavior indicates disapproval, and the patient may feel hurt and unsure of themselves.

EXCESSIVE QUESTIONING

A. Although questioning can be therapeutic, *excessive* questioning in succession could become nontherapeutic. The patient may feel attacked as the healthcare provider is seen as an interrogator demanding answers, thus impeding communication. Excessive questioning can also sound accusatory to the patient in that the patient may feel at fault for being sick. A more therapeutic approach is the use of open-ended questions.

CHANGING THE SUBJECT

A. In social conversations, changing the subject can occur due to the difficulty of the content being shared or choosing not to participate in a particular conversation. However, when a clinician changes the subject during a conversation, the patient may feel alienated and isolated, leaving the patient feeling alienated. Changing the subject demonstrates a lack of empathy and can impede further communication.

USING CLICHÉS

A. A *cliché* is a sentence or phrase that expresses a popular or common thought that has lost its originality. It takes vigilance and practice to avoid using cliché words and phrases during patient–healthcare provider interaction.

ASKING "WHY" QUESTIONS

A. "Why" questions put a person on the defensive as it demands a justification for actions and implies that something has not been correctly done. When interacting with patients, especially those with depression or anxiety, such questions are intrusive and may further exacerbate the illness as the patient may feel judged by the healthcare provider.

CULTURAL CONSIDERATIONS

A. Culture defines how healthcare information is provided and received, how rights and protections are exercised, what is considered a health problem, how symptoms and concerns about the problem are expressed, who should provide treatment for the problem, and what type of treatment should be given.

B. Healthcare providers must be culturally competent and sensitive to provide appropriate care to patients from all walks of life without prejudice and assumptions.

C. While it is important to understand culture from the perspective of those who belong to it, healthcare professionals must also be familiar with the cultural meaning of popular verbal and nonverbal cues that may have different interpretations in other cultures.

D. Differences in cultural interpretation may result in unintended bias, disrespect, ineffective communication, and ultimately poor provision of care.

E. Healthcare providers also need to be aware of their own cultural background in terms of attitudes and beliefs that may influence how they interact with the patients as this can have a tremendous effect on the provision of care.

F. Given the diversity among and within cultural groups, communication may be daunting for healthcare providers. It is unfathomable to create and have a list of facts for each culture; however, healthcare providers can treat the patient with respect and dignity, focus on effective communication, and offer individualized care.

G. In mental healthcare, particularly verbal and nonverbal communication styles are critical about culture and should be considered when assessing patients. These include eye contact and the use of touch as a therapeutic agent.

EYE CONTACT

A. In Western culture, eye contact is an expectation as it is considered the hallmark of truthfulness. It is a fundamental ingredient in social conversation as it shows a person's willingness to be engaged and interested in what is being said.

B. Non-Western cultures may associate eye contact or lack of eye contact with forms of disrespect. In some cultures, when conversing with someone of a higher authority, it is proper and respectful to avoid eye contact. Therefore, it would be crude for healthcare providers to use eye contact to assess attentiveness and draw a conclusion on patient engagement during an assessment. Establishing rapport and building trust should be the initial goal when caring for a patient from a different cultural background.

TOUCH

A. Physical touch is a powerful force that can be healing or destructive. The therapeutic use of touch is a fundamental component of a healthcare provider–patient relationship that is generally considered a show of concern, warmth, and support.

B. In a psychiatric setting, touch should be used cautiously as it can elicit a different interpretation from the patient and result in unfavorable outcomes. If a patient is experiencing delusions or hallucinations, touch may further exacerbate their symptoms, leading to aggression or false interpretation of touch.

IMPLICIT BIAS

A. *Implicit bias* is defined as the association, attitude, belief, and/or stereotypes toward any social group that is held in a less than conscious manner and influences an individual's actions and decisions. Bias, whether explicit or implicit, is a complex concept that influences how we see the world and interact with one another as human beings. It is important to remember that there is bias in each of us, but implicit bias operates on an unconscious level. Implicit bias often occurs as a collection of our thought processes that manifest when making decisions or judgments. Explicit bias is conscious, intentional, and controllable.

B. Bias is part of human life as much as is diversity, and not only does it affect how we judge other people but also how we judge ourselves. When implicit bias is viewed in this way, it is closely related to the concept of *stereotype threat*, in that when an individual is reminded of their social identity and the stereotypes associated with it (e.g., gender, race, and nationality), it leads to feelings of anxiety, isolation, and underperformance.

C. Healthcare providers need to think carefully about the definition of bias and its impact on the delivery of care and evaluation of care by patients. Healthcare provider implicit bias is often associated with ineffective communication between the patient and the healthcare provider, leading to poor medical care outcomes.

D. The implicit biases of concern among healthcare providers affect individuals who are already vulnerable. The vulnerable population includes underrepresented ethnic groups (e.g., people of color), immigrants, children, women, older adults, sexual minority groups, and mentally challenged individuals. Unfortunately, the vulnerable population is typically a group already disadvantaged on other levels, a concept referred to as *corrosive disadvantage*.

    1. *Corrosive disadvantage* is a term coined by philosophers Wolff and de-Shalit and refers to a disadvantage that begets more disadvantages. Research indicates that high levels of negative stereotypes and bias, through subtle and often subconscious processes, can influence expectations and interactions with mentally challenged patients in ways that reduce the quality of service provided by clinicians.

THE HEALTHCARE PROVIDER AS A THERAPEUTIC AGENT

A. A therapeutic agent is a person or thing that takes on an active role or produces a specified effect capable of yielding a curative effect in a disease state.

B. A healthcare provider in a psychiatric setting takes on the role of a therapeutic agent during the patient–healthcare provider interaction. It is the use of *self* as a therapeutic agent that further establishes a genuine therapeutic relationship with patients.

    1. A strong sense of *self* allows us to develop resilience in dealing with the difficulties and complexities of human communication and experiences.

    2. The use of *self* is built upon self-awareness and an understanding that you, the healthcare provider, are in a therapeutic relationship with the patient, authentically involved while maintaining boundaries. This approach involves being conscious and aware of one's inner thoughts and feelings and becoming more intentional in our interaction with patients.

C. The healthcare provider must exercise and cultivate empathy to effectively use *self* as a therapeutic agent.

    1. Empathy is the connecting fiber of being human, the fundamental component of human connection. It is a broad concept that refers to an individual's cognitive and emotional reactions as observed and experienced by others.

D. Evidence suggests that empathy potently predicts positive outcomes among patients and society. In addition, empathy is considered a crucial ingredient in alleviating implicit bias.

    1. Empathy in itself is not always an automatic gesture from healthcare providers. Some empathic researchers reckon that developing empathy that helps patients requires intentional strategy as it can be a draining skill if not practiced correctly, a phenomenon referred to as *empathy fatigue*.

    2. To avoid empathy fatigue, healthcare providers may take on the *other-oriented empathy* perspective, where the healthcare provider imagines the patient's perspective by understanding and reflecting upon the patient's feelings and emotions. It is important to remember that the goal of using *self* as a therapeutic agent while employing empathy is not to be the sufferer but to remain the healthcare provider.

CONCLUSION

Mental health providers must be aware of personal biases that can influence and impact implicit bias. We all have conscious and unconscious biases; however, if we make it a personal discipline to self-reflect to uncover ingrained beliefs about a group of people, we can become more intentional about our responsibility, accountability, and our service to others in need. Evidence suggests that biases and ignorance can be better understood through reflection. According to philosopher John Dewey, *reflection* is the "active, persistent, and careful consideration of any belief or supposed form of knowledge in the light of the grounds that support it, and the further conclusions to which it tends" (Dewey, 1910/2011, p. 6). Reflection starts with a state of doubt or reluctance. As we engage in an internal dialogue with ourselves, we search to find evidence that will address our implicit bias toward others.

REFERENCES AND BIBLIOGRAPHY

Abramson, A. (2021, November 1). *Cultivating empathy*. Monitor on Psychology. https://www.apa.org/monitor/2021/11/feature-cultivating-empathy

Agarwal, R., Sands D. Z., & Schneider, J. D. (2010). Quantifying the economic impact of communication inefficiencies in U.S. hospitals. *Journal of Healthcare Management, 55*(4), 265–281; discussion 281–282. PMID: 20812527.

Al Shamsi, H., Almutairi, A. G., Al Mashrafi, S., & Al Kalbani, T. (2020). Implications of language barriers for healthcare: A systematic review. *Oman Medical Journal, 35*(2), e122. https://doi.org/10.5001/omj.2020.40

Allen, L. A. (1958). *Management and organization*. McGraw-Hill.

Asendorpf, J. B., & Baudonnière, P. M. (1993). Self-awareness and other-awareness: Mirror self-recognition and synchronic imitation among unfamiliar peers. *Developmental Psychology, 29*(1), 88–95. https://doi.org/10.1037/0012-1649.29.1.88

Betancourt, J. R. (2004). Cultural competence—marginal or mainstream movement? *The New England Journal of Medicine, 351*(10), 953–955. https://doi.org/10.1056/NEJMp048033

Budryk, Z. (2016, February 1). *Healthcare miscommunication cost $1.7B--and nearly 2,000 lives*. FierceHealthcare. https://www.fiercehealthcare.com/healthcare/healthcare-miscommunication-cost-1-7b-and-nearly-2-000-lives

Craig, P. E. (1986). Sanctuary and presence: An existential view of the therapist's contribution. *The Humanistic Psychologist, 14*(1), 22–28. https://doi.org/10.1080/08873267.1986.9976749

Deardorff, D. K. (2009). Synthesizing conceptualizations of intercultural competence: A summary and emerging themes. In D. K. Deardorff (Ed.), *The SAGE handbook of intercultural competence* (pp. 264–270). Sage.

Dewey, J. (2011, September 14). *How we think*. Project Gutenberg, EBook #37423. https://www.gutenberg.org/files/37423/37423-h/37423-h.htm (Original work published 1910 by D. C. Heath & Co)

Engleberg, I. N., & Daly, J. A. (2004). *Presentations in everyday life: Strategies for effective speaking* (2nd ed.). Pearson.

FitzGerald, C., & Hurst, S. (2017). Implicit bias in healthcare professionals: A systematic review. *BMC Medical Ethics, 18*(1), 19. https://doi.org/10.1186/s12910-017-0179-8

Ganz, J. B. (2015). AAC interventions for individuals with autism spectrum disorders: State of the science and future research directions. *Augmentative and Alternative Communication, 31*(3), 203–214. https://doi.org/10.3109/07434618.2015.1047532

Geller, S. (2021). Cultivating online therapeutic presence: Strengthening therapeutic relationships in teletherapy sessions. *Counselling Psychology Quarterly, 34*(3–4), 687–703. https://doi.org/10.1080/09515070.2020.1787348

Hall, W. J., Chapman, M. V., Lee, K. M., Merino, Y. M., Thomas, T. W., Payne, B. K., Eng, E., Day, S. H., & Coyne-Beasley, T. (2015). Implicit racial/ethnic bias among health care professionals and its influence on health care outcomes: A systematic review. *American Journal of Public Health, 105*(12), e60–e76. https://doi.org/10.2105/AJPH.2015.302903

Halter, M., (2022). *Varcarolis' foundations of psychiatric mental health nursing* (9th ed.). Saunders.

Hanh, T. N. (2010). *Reconciliation: Healing the inner child*. Parallax Press.

Herdtner, S. (2000). Using therapeutic touch in nursing practice. *Orthopedic Nursing, 19*(5), 77–82. https://doi.org/10.1097/00006416-200019050-00013

Iacono, T., Trembath, D., & Erickson, S. (2016). The role of augmentative and alternative communication for children with autism: Current status and future trends. *Neuropsychiatric Disease and Treatment, 12*, 2349–2361. https://doi.org/10.2147/NDT.S95967

Joint Commission on Accreditation of Healthcare Organizations. (2012). Joint Commission Center for Transforming Healthcare releases targeted solutions tool for hand-off communications. *Joint Commission Perspectives, 32*(8), 1–3. PMID: 22928243.

Jost, J. T., Rudman, L., Blair, I. V., Carney, D. R., Dasgupta, N., Glaser, J., & Hardin, C. (2009). The existence of implicit bias is beyond reasonable doubt: A refutation of ideological and methodological objections and executive summary of ten studies that no manager should ignore. *Research in Organizational Behavior, 29*, 39–69. https://doi.org/10.1016/j.riob.2009.10.001

Koloroutis, M. (2014). The therapeutic use of self: Developing three capacities for a more mindful practice. *Creative Nursing, 20*(2), 77–85. https://doi.org/10.1891/1078-4535.20.2.77

Kourkouta, L., & Papathanasiou, I. V. (2014). Communication in nursing practice. *Materia Socio-Medica, 26*(1), 65–67. https://doi.org/10.5455/msm.2014.26.65-67

Lemma, A. (2017). *The digital age on the couch: Psychoanalytic practice and new media*. Routledge.

Martin, A. K., Tavaglione, N., & Hurst, S. (2014). Resolving the conflict: Clarifying 'vulnerability' in health care ethics. *Kennedy Institute of Ethics Journal, 24*(1), 51–72. https://doi.org/10.1353/ken.2014.0005

McCabe, R., & Healey, P. G. T. (2018). Miscommunication in doctor–patient communication. *Topics in Cognitive Science, 10*(2), 409–424. https://doi.org/10.1111/tops.12337

Pearson, J., & Nelson, P. (2000). *An introduction to human communication: Understanding and sharing* (8th ed.). McGraw-Hill.

Sharma, N., & Gupta, V. (2023, August 2). Therapeutic communication. In *StatPearls*. StatPearls Publishing. https://www.ncbi.nlm.nih.gov/books/NBK567775

Unsworth, C. A. (2001). The clinical reasoning of novice and expert occupational therapists. *Scandinavian Journal of Occupational Therapy, 8*(4), 163–173. https://doi.org/10.1080/110381201317166522

Weekley, E. (1967). *An etymological dictionary of modern English*. Dover Publications.

Weinberg, H. (2021). Obstacles, challenges, and benefits of online group psychotherapy. *American Journal of Psychotherapy, 74*(2), 83–88. https://doi.org/10.1176/appi.psychotherapy.20200034

Wolff, J., & de-Shalit, A. (2007). *Disadvantage*. Oxford University Press.

3 TRAUMA-INFORMED CARE

Brayden N. Kameg

INTRODUCTION

Trauma, or exposure to adverse or traumatic events and/or experiences, remains a pervasive public health problem. Given the sheer prevalence of exposure to trauma, APRNs will undoubtedly interact with and provide care for individuals who have experienced or who are currently experiencing trauma. Unique care and consideration must be taken to ensure that trauma survivors feel safe and supported within healthcare environments. Thus, APRNs must not only be familiar with the concept of *trauma-informed care* but must also be capable of and confident in their delivery of high-quality trauma-informed care. This chapter provides an overview of neurobiological theories related to trauma, epidemiologic and etiologic information related to trauma, key concepts and principles related to trauma-informed care, and best practices and practical considerations when implementing a trauma-informed approach.

BACKGROUND

Trauma remains exceedingly common across the United States and globally. Thus, to assure the delivery of high-quality care, it is important that APRNs understand key concepts and definitions related to trauma. The American Psychological Association (2008) defines a *traumatic event* as "one that threatens injury, death, or the physical integrity of self or others and also causes horror, terror, or helplessness at the time it occurs" (p. 2). Traumatic events can include, but are certainly not limited to, physical abuse, sexual abuse, emotional abuse, neglect, intimate partner or other interpersonal violence, community or school-based violence, medical trauma, physical injury, acts of terrorism, war experiences, natural or human-caused disasters, and deaths by suicide. Regardless of the type of traumatic event, the Substance Abuse and Mental Health Services Administration (SAMHSA) conceptualizes trauma and its associated sequelae as resulting "from an event, series of events, or set of circumstances that is experienced by an individual as physically or emotionally harmful or life-threatening and that has lasting adverse effects on the individual's functioning and mental, physical, social, emotional, or spiritual wellbeing" (2014a, p. 7).

THE THREE "ES" OF TRAUMA: EVENT, EXPERIENCE, AND EFFECT

A. The SAMHSA describes three concepts related to trauma exposure, known as "The Three Es," which include a traumatic event, how one experiences the event, and the effects of the event.

B. Traumatic events are described as follows:
   1. Traumatic events can include physical abuse, sexual abuse, emotional abuse, neglect, intimate partner or other interpersonal violence, community or school-based violence, medical trauma, physical injury, acts of terrorism, war experiences, natural or human-caused disasters, and deaths by suicide.
   2. trauma may be isolated or might occur repeatedly over time, which can lead to potential *complex trauma* (see later).
   3. Criterion A for posttraumatic stress disorder (PTSD) in the *Diagnostic and Statistical Manual of Mental Disorders, Fifth Edition, Text Revision* (*DSM-5-TR*; American Psychiatric Association, 2022) references the following within the PTSD diagnostic criteria: exposure to actual or threatened death, injury, or sexual violence as a direct experience; witnessing its occurrence to others; learning that a traumatic event occurred to a close contact; and experiencing repeated exposure to details of the traumatic event. There have long been calls to expand the restrictive definition of "event" in criterion A within the *Diagnostic and Statistical Manual of Mental Disorders* (*DSM*), although a significant revision of criterion A has yet to take place.
      a. PTSD is discussed in detail in Chapter 9, "Anxiety Disorders."

C. Experiences of trauma are described as follows:
   1. Trauma is an inherently subjective phenomenon. What might be deemed traumatic for one person might not be for another person. How someone labels, assigns meaning to, and is physically, psychologically, and emotionally impacted by a potentially traumatic event likely contributes to whether they identify an event as trauma.
   2. Other specific experiences or emotions related to trauma include survivor's guilt, shame or self-blame, humiliation, or betrayal.
   3. Cultural considerations, access to social support, or developmental age are factors that might contribute to how one experiences or perceives a potentially traumatic event.

D. Effects of trauma include the following:
   1. The effects of trauma include both physical and mental health adverse effects.
      a. Effects can occur immediately after the trauma, such as with acute stress disorder, defined as trauma symptoms that occur between 3 and 30 days following traumatic exposure.
      b. Some trauma survivors might experience the effects chronically, and some might experience the effects of trauma throughout the remainder of their life.
      c. Trauma symptoms can occur at any point, even years or decades, following a traumatic event, and might not occur immediately after the event.
   2. Regardless of the timing or onset of symptoms, the effects of trauma are serious and can lead to early morbidity and mortality.
   3. Much progress has been made to advance the understanding of trauma's impacts on mental health outcomes and symptomatology in the past four decades.

a. It was not until 1980 and the release of the *Diagnostic and Statistical Manual of Mental Disorders*, Third Edition (*DSM-III*; American Psychiatric Association, 1980), that PTSD was recognized as a mental health condition, although now known PTSD symptoms have been well-documented in the medical and scientific literature with terms like *soldier's heart*, *traumatic war neurosis*, *shell shock*, and *battle fatigue* (Pomerantz, 2017).

b. Later, the effects of early childhood trauma on myriad physical and mental health problems were described in Felitti and colleagues' landmark study, "The Adverse Childhood Experiences Study" (1998).

ADVERSE CHILDHOOD EXPERIENCES AND HEALTH OUTCOMES

A. Felitti et al. (1998) surveyed 45,000 adults seeking treatment at a managed care organization on their history of certain adverse childhood experiences (ACEs), health behaviors, and health outcomes. More than 50% of the respondents reported exposure to at least one ACE and about 25% reported exposure to two or more ACEs.

   1. A graded, dose–response relationship was highlighted in which a greater number of ACEs, rather than exposure to any one ACE alone, was associated with increased odds of a variety of adverse health behaviors and outcomes.

      a. Individuals who had experienced four or more ACEs, compared with those who had experienced none, had fourfold and twelve-fold increased risks of depression and suicidality, respectively, and a sevenfold and twofold increase for at-risk alcohol use and tobacco use, respectively (Felitti et al., 1998). Similar findings have been replicated consistently thereafter.

B. Recently, Merrick et al. (2019) utilized the Centers for Disease Control and Prevention (CDC) Behavioral Risk Factor Surveillance System (BRFSS) data to compare ACEs and self-reported health outcomes, including coronary artery disease, stroke, asthma, chronic obstructive pulmonary disease, cancer, kidney disease, diabetes, major depressive disorder, current tobacco use, and at-risk alcohol use among respondents from 25 states.

   1. Approximately 15% of adults reported exposure to four or more ACEs, and those with a history of four or more ACEs were at approximately twofold to threefold greater risk for coronary artery disease, stroke, asthma, and chronic obstructive pulmonary disease.

   2. The work of Merrick et al. (2019) was supported by a systematic review and meta-analysis authored by Petruccelli et al. (2019). Based on a systematic analysis of 96 primary research articles related to ACEs and health outcomes, Petruccelli et al. (2019) reported an approximately twofold increase in risk of cardiac diseases, respiratory diseases, and stroke among those with a history of four or more ACEs.

   3. Like the original findings published by Felitti et al. (1998), Petruccelli et al. (2019) also highlighted increased risk, as high as fourfold, for mental health problems, including depression, substance use, and suicidality.

C. These findings clearly support the association between ACEs and adverse health outcomes in adulthood, support how trauma exposure can lead to neurobiological changes, and increase the risk for at-risk health behaviors and associated morbidity and mortality.

D. See Figure 3.1.

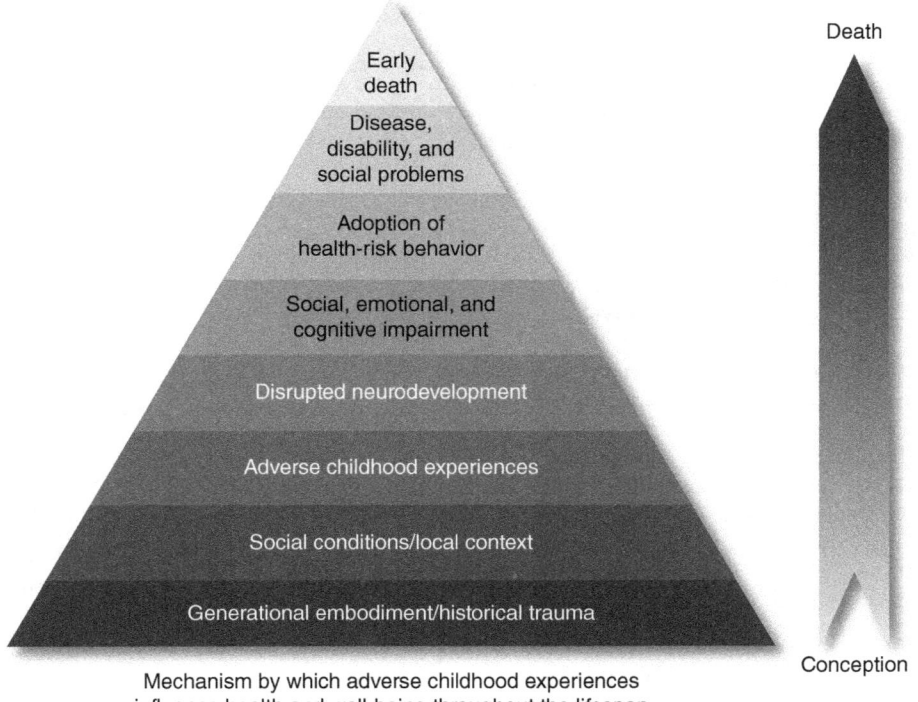

FIGURE 3.1 The adverse childhood experience pyramid.

Source: Centers for Disease Control and Prevention. (n.d.). *About the CDC-Kaiser ACE study*. Reviewed April 6, 2021. https://www.cdc.gov/violenceprevention/aces/about.html.

NEUROBIOLOGICAL THEORIES RELATED TO TRAUMA AND HEALTH RISK BEHAVIORS

Exposure to traumatic events, particularly at vulnerable developmental periods such as during youth, can result in neurobiological changes, including structural and neuroendocrine changes. It is important that APRNs are equipped with a basic understanding of neurobiological changes that can occur secondary to trauma exposure.

STRUCTURAL CHANGES

A. Reduction in hippocampal volume has been noted in multiple structural neuroimaging studies that have compared individuals exposed to ACEs and those not exposed.

  1. Given that the hippocampus plays a significant role in memory processing and emotional regulation, structural changes to the hippocampus in trauma survivors can impact symptomatology.
  2. Other findings have demonstrated structural amygdala alterations in trauma survivors, although the evidence is mixed; some reports indicate an increase in amygdala volume in trauma survivors, while others indicate a decrease.
      a. Results from functional neuroimaging studies in trauma survivors have demonstrated amygdala hyperactivity, in addition to reduced connectivity between structures in the limbic system, including both the hippocampus and the amygdala.
      b. Other evidence has suggested a dysregulation in dorsolateral prefrontal cortex (DLPFC) activity in trauma survivors. Given that the prefrontal cortex is involved in executive functioning, impulse control, and decision-making, alterations in the DLPFC might contribute to some of the adverse health behaviors that trauma survivors are at-risk for, to be discussed in a section henceforth.

NEUROENDOCRINE CHANGES

A. In trauma survivors, particularly those who were exposed to multiple or cumulative traumas, hypothalamic–pituitary–adrenocortical (HPA) axis dysregulation is a well-documented phenomenon.

B. Prolonged activation of the HPA axis, secondary to trauma exposure, can precipitate glucocorticoid dysregulation and blunted cortisol reactivity.

  1. This can lead to chronic inflammation, thereby increasing the risk for a variety of mental and physical health problems.
  2. Chronic inflammation can reduce concentration and availability of brain-derived neurotrophic factor (BDNF), resulting in deficiencies in essential neurotransmitters, including dopamine and serotonin.

C. This pathway, in which trauma precipitates neuroendocrine changes, forms the basis of the toxic stress theory and the cumulative risk model, the latter of which posits that an accumulation of traumatic events confers increased risk for negative health outcomes, rather than any event in isolation.

HEALTH RISK BEHAVIORS

A. Structural and neuroendocrine changes can lead to adverse mental health symptoms, including depression, anxiety, impulsivity, and executive dysfunction. These symptoms can increase the risk of engagement in high-risk behaviors directly (e.g., impulsivity can increase the risk of high-risk sexual behavior and substance use) or indirectly (e.g., mood or anxiety-related symptoms can lead to ineffective coping through the use of substances).

B. Disrupted neurodevelopment, secondary to structural or neuroendocrine changes, can lead to mental health symptoms including social, emotional, and/or cognitive impairment, which in turn can lead to either direct or indirect adoption of health risk behavior (see Figure 3.1).

  1. Engagement in such health risk behavior, such as substance use, self-injurious behavior, or physical inactivity, can thereby lead to premature morbidity and mortality.
  2. Box 3.1 provides a clinical vignette reinforcing the potential trajectory through which trauma exposure can lead to premature morbidity and mortality.

EPIDEMIOLOGY AND ETIOLOGY OF TRAUMA

It is important for APRNs to have a general understanding of the epidemiology and etiology of trauma, with an understanding that trauma can take the shape of many forms, spanning from ACEs to intimate partner or other interpersonal violence, to military or combat-related trauma, among others. Epidemiology and etiology related to common types of trauma exposure for which data are readily available will be briefly reviewed henceforth, including prevalence rates and risk factors. For additional information related to trauma and PTSD, please see Chapter 9, "Anxiety Disorders."

BOX 3.1 TK'S STORY: PART I

TK (she/her/hers) is a 33-year-old woman seeking mental health treatment in the context of depression, anxiety, and substance use-related concerns. She has been struggling with these mental health symptoms for many years and has intermittently been engaged with treatment but historically has been lost to follow-up after initial treatment. Today, TK presents to the mental health clinic after being discharged from the hospital. The advanced practice registered nurse notices that she is polite but seems reticent about engaging in the interview.

TK experienced multiple adverse childhood experiences. TK's mother struggled with mental health and substance-related issues and was ultimately incarcerated for substance use. During her mother's incarceration when TK was about 4 years old, TK was placed in foster care where she experienced physical and sexual abuse at the hands of a caregiver. TK was ultimately reunited with her mother following her mother's release a few years later, although they had a strained relationship thereafter.

TK experienced multiple adverse childhood experiences over a long duration of time. Given the critical developmental age at which point TK experienced these adverse childhood experiences, there were likely neurodevelopmental changes that occurred secondary to toxic stress. These neurodevelopmental changes were evidenced by TK struggling with social, emotional, and cognitive impairment. TK struggled to connect with her mother, as evidenced by their strained relationship, and struggled to connect with peers. Throughout middle and high school, TK struggled with feeling lonely and ostracized, ultimately leading to depressive and anxiety-related symptoms. Later, TK began experimentation with substances, including alcohol and cannabis, in high school. She reports that she historically had used substances to "numb the pain," which she experienced secondary to the trauma that she endured as a child. As TK became older, her substance use evolved from alcohol and cannabis to opioid use, ultimately culminating in intravenous heroin use, for which she was ultimately hospitalized following an opioid overdose. This engagement in health risk behavior (substance use) led to the development of a substance use disorder, but also hepatitis C (i.e., disease/disability).

Additional discussion about *TK's Story* is included in Box 3.2, as it relates to trauma-informed care principles.

ADVERSE CHILDHOOD EXPERIENCES
A. Epidemiology and etiology
1. Adults: At least 60% of adults in the United States report having been exposed to at least one ACE, with approximately 25% of adults reporting exposure to three or more ACEs.
2. Children and adolescents: A recent systematic review highlighted similar rates of ACEs globally, with about two-thirds of children worldwide reporting exposure to at least one ACE.
    a. Research over the last two decades has supported a graded, dose–response relationship between ACEs and adverse health outcomes, with more ACEs accumulating to greater odds of health risk behavior, morbidity, and mortality.
    b. Evidence also suggests that the *types* of ACEs, rather than the number, contribute to subsequent symptomatology.
        i. Evidence suggests that childhood sexual abuse, particularly when coupled with other ACEs, is a strong predictor of the development of future health risk behaviors, morbidity, and mortality.
        ii. Exposure to ACEs can lead to a variety of negative physical and mental health outcomes.
        iii. ACEs are associated with an increased risk for mood disorders, substance use disorders, and anxiety- and trauma-related disorders.
3. In adults, people of color, those who are unemployed/unable to work, those with an income level at or near the poverty line, and those with less than a high school education are at elevated risk for ACEs.
4. Those with diverse sexual orientations or gender identities are more likely to report having experienced ACEs.
5. Children with complex healthcare needs, children of color, those living rurally, and those living in poverty are at higher risk for ACEs.
6. Emotional abuse, parental separation, and household substance use are the most common types of ACEs reported by adults.
7. In children, economic hardship and parental separation are the most cited ACEs.

INTIMATE PARTNER OR OTHER INTERPERSONAL VIOLENCE
A. Epidemiology and etiology
1. There are over 40 million adults in the United States who have experienced intimate partner violence (IPV). Lifetime IPV, including physical violence, sexual violence, and stalking, is experienced by approximately one-third of individuals, with rates higher for females than males.
2. IPV exposure can lead to early morbidity and mortality. Alarmingly, homicide is one of the leading causes of death in women under the age of 45 years, and 55% of all homicide deaths among women were related to IPV, with about 1 in 10 women who died by homicide experiencing violence in the month preceding their deaths.
3. While often conceptualized as an adult health issue, there is emerging evidence to suggest that teenagers, particularly adolescent females assigned at birth, are at elevated risk for experiencing intimate partner or teen dating violence and are at risk of firearm violence related to intimate partner or teen dating violence.
4. IPV impacts individuals across the life span, spanning from adolescents to older adults.
    a. Older adults might be more vulnerable to the physical impacts of IPV, including injuries such as fractures, bruising, or head trauma.
5. Survivors of IPV are at elevated risk for a variety of adverse physical and mental health outcomes, including substance use issues and mood disorders.
6. Those who have experienced IPV are more likely to report their health status as "poor."
7. the estimated cost of IPV exceeds $100,000 per female victim and is about $25,000 per male victim. The total economic burden of IPV in the United States exceeds $3.5 trillion.
8. Exposure to intimate partner or other types of violence as a child is a strong risk factor for experiencing IPV in adulthood.
    a. Those with diverse sexual orientations or gender identities are at elevated risk for experiencing intimate partner and other interpersonal violence.
    b. People of color, those living near or below the poverty line, unmarried individuals, younger people, those who experienced an unplanned pregnancy, and those who did not graduate from high school are also at higher risk of experiencing intimate partner and other interpersonal violence.
    c. Those living in regions with higher rates of gender-based disparities, such as elevated maternal mortality rates, elevated teen birth rates, lower rates of educational attainment or labor force participation among women, and lack of diverse gender representation in government are also at increased risk of experiencing IPV.
9. Social support, help-seeking behavior, and availability of community-based health or social services can reduce morbidity and mortality associated with IPV.

MILITARY-RELATED OR COMBAT TRAUMA
A. Epidemiology and etiology
1. Approximately 7% of all U.S. adults are military veterans, although this number is down from about 18% in 1980 following the inactivation of the draft system in 1973. Among recent-era veterans (Operation Enduring Freedom [OEF], Operation Iraqi Freedom [OIF], and Operation New Dawn [OND]) or post-9/11 veterans, approximately 60% have been deployed to a combat zone.
    a. Among post-9/11 veterans, approximately one-third have experienced posttraumatic stress symptoms. Post-9/11 veterans are more likely to have been deployed and to have served in a combat zone compared with those who served before them.
    b. Older veterans, those with higher combat exposure, enlisted-rank veterans, veterans with a history of depression, and those with a history of physical assault are at higher risk for trauma-related symptoms following military service.
2. Among veterans who have PTSD, there are high rates of comorbid mental health issues.
    a. The prevalence of PTSD, major depressive disorder, and comorbid PTSD with major depressive disorder among a nationally representative sample of veterans was estimated at approximately 2%, 5%, and 3.5%, respectively, indicating that more veterans have comorbid PTSD with major depressive disorder than PTSD alone.

b. Comorbid PTSD with major depressive disorder is predictive of worse mental health outcomes, including higher rates of current suicidal ideation and lifetime suicide attempts.

c. Veterans with comorbid PTSD with major depressive disorder are more than twice as likely to have attempted suicide compared with those with PTSD alone.

d. Older veterans, those who experienced combat, those with anxiety, veterans who have experienced physical assault, those with a disability or bodily pain, and veterans who lack social support are at increased risk for chronicity associated with PTSD and associated mental health comorbidities.

e. Veterans with PTSD are at elevated risk for the development of substance use disorders.

3. In addition to combat-related trauma, veterans may also have experienced military sexual trauma. Defined as sexual assault, sexual harassment, or any unwanted or nonconsensual sexual activity that occurred during military service, military sexual trauma includes being pressured or coerced into sexual activities, with threats of negative treatment or promises of better treatment; nonconsensual sexual contact or rape; being touched in ways that made an individual feel uncomfortable, including during "hazing" or initiation experiences; and comments about an individual's appearance and unwanted sexual advances.

a. Military sexual trauma is exceedingly common, with about 16% of military personnel and veterans reporting having experienced military sexual trauma and with disparate rates by sex and gender.

b. Approximately 40% of female veterans report having experienced military sexual trauma, compared with about 4% of male veterans.

c. LGBTQ+ veterans are at elevated risk for military sexual trauma compared with their heterosexual and cisgender peers.

d. Military sexual trauma increases the risk of adverse mental health outcomes, including mood disorders, suicidality, and substance use issues. For additional information related to trauma as it relates to veterans, please see Chapter 25, "Veterans and Survivors of War."

TRAUMA RELATED TO NATURAL OR HUMAN-CAUSED DISASTERS

A. Epidemiology and etiology

1. Natural disasters are expected to become more frequent and more intense due to ongoing climate change. Natural disasters, including tornadoes, hurricanes, severe storms, floods, wildfires, earthquakes, and droughts, impact thousands of individuals annually in the United States alone, although the exact numbers and rates of those impacted by natural disasters are difficult to discern.

2. Individuals who have been impacted by natural disasters are at higher risk for psychological distress, including depression and posttraumatic stress symptoms (Beaglehole et al., 2018).

a. As many as 30% will develop acute stress symptoms following the event.

b. About one in three individuals will develop PTSD after experiencing certain natural disasters.

c. Evidence suggests that individuals who have experienced a natural disaster are at elevated risk for suicidality, including ideation, attempts, and death by suicide, particularly among those with underlying mental health disorders, with low social support and economic status, and who lost family or loved ones following the natural disaster.

3. Protective factors for those struggling following the trauma of a natural disaster include social or familial support, in addition to economic resources such as access to housing or treatment services.

4. Human-caused disasters, or "man-made" disasters, include industrial accidents, shootings, acts of terrorism, and incidents of mass violence. Exposure to such events is inherently traumatic and can lead to adverse mental health outcomes.

a. Risk factors for the development of trauma-related symptoms following exposure to a human-caused disaster include preexisting conditions, the severity of disaster exposure, gender, and socioeconomic status. In fact, there is evidence that low socioeconomic status is not only associated with the development of future mental health symptoms, but also with chronic inflammation (i.e., elevated levels of interleukin 6) following exposure to a human-caused disaster, and this chronic inflammation might mediate future mental health symptoms.

b. Mass shootings and other firearm-related violence have garnered significant public health attention within the United States in recent years.

i. Firearm-related deaths in the United States increased between 2017 and 2020 across all ages, with death rates rising from 4.47 per 100,000 in 2017 to 5.88 per 100,000 in 2020.

ii. Rates of school shootings, specifically, have increased and have more than tripled between 2017 and 2021.

iii. Survivors of mass shootings and other firearm-related violence are at risk for trauma-related and other mental health symptoms. Recent evidence suggests that as many as 50% of mass shooting survivors report mental health concerns approximately 1 year postincident and as many as one-third have symptoms consistent with PTSD.

iv. Trauma-related symptoms can persist, and do evolve, following exposure to a mass shooting event. In a sample of survivors of the 2007 Virginia Tech shooting, survivors reported initial psychological reactivity following reminders of the event at approximately 8 weeks postevent, whereas at 1 year following the event they noted more anhedonia and physiologic reactivity.

c. Firearm-related violence disproportionately impacts boys, particularly boys of color, as evidenced by a mortality rate of 3.44 per 100,000 among Black youth compared with 1.24 per 100,000 among all races and ethnicities, and 0.86 and 0.83 per 100,000 among Hispanic/Latinx youth and Caucasian youth, respectively. Thus, a chapter on trauma-informed care would be incomplete without outlining trauma in the context of racial injustice and inequities in the United States.

i. Evidence suggests that people of color experience mental health symptoms following events driven by racial injustice and inequities, including police homicides of people of color, some of which have garnered national media attention.

ii. Following the murder of George Floyd in Minnesota, Black individuals reported larger increases in depression and anxiety symptoms compared with their White peers, with evidence suggesting that nearly one million additional Black individuals would have screened positive for depression following Floyd's death.

iii. Following the murder of Michael Brown in Missouri, Black individuals reported higher rates of posttraumatic stress symptoms as compared with their White counterparts. Furthermore, Black individuals were more likely to engage in protest following Brown's death, and protest engagement was an independent risk factor for worsening posttraumatic stress symptoms.

iv. The proliferation of "smartphones" equipped with cameras, coupled with increased social media utilization, has allowed for viral videos of police killings of unarmed citizens. Exposure to such media can also be traumatic. A recent study with adolescents of color indicated that exposure to traumatic events online, including videos of police killings of unarmed citizens, was associated with increases in both posttraumatic stress and depressive symptoms.

v. Racially driven microaggressions are also associated with posttraumatic stress symptoms. It is important for APRNs to understand concepts related to how racial injustice and inequities can contribute to mental health symptoms, including concepts such as *historical trauma* and *collective trauma* (Table 3.1).

vi. It is essential that APRNs incorporate antiracist principles into their own clinical practice and advocacy work.

WAR OR FORCED MIGRATION

A. Epidemiology and etiology

1. Individuals exposed to war or forced migration are at risk of developing adverse mental health outcomes. Globally, approximately one in four individuals reside in a conflict-affected area, and an estimated 84 million individuals were forcibly displaced due to conflict, violence, and/or human rights violations. Further, nearly 275 million individuals globally require humanitarian assistance due to exposure to conflict.

2. APRNs working in the United States will undoubtedly work with immigrants, some of whom are impacted by forced migration. Common countries from which forced migrants originate include Syria, Afghanistan, South Sudan, Myanmar, Somalia, and Venezuela, among others.

3. In conflict-affected areas, evidence suggests that more than one in five individuals struggle with a mental health diagnosis. Following forced migration, rates of PTSD near 10%, while rates of depression and anxiety are estimated at 28% and 23% postmigration, with others suggesting even higher rates.

4. Children may be more vulnerable to the mental health consequences of war and/or forced migration, particularly unaccompanied refugee minors, or refugees who are traveling without a parent or adult caregiver.

5. Forced migrants are at elevated risk for human trafficking, a crime involving the exploitation of a person for labor, services, or commercial sex.

KEY CONCEPTS AND PRINCIPLES RELATED TO TRAUMA-INFORMED CARE

Trauma-informed care is a care delivery model that seeks to acknowledge the need to understand a patient's life experiences, including potentially adverse or traumatic life experiences, to deliver effective, high-quality care that can improve patient engagement, treatment adherence, health outcomes, and healthcare provider and staff wellness. Understanding that not all patients will disclose trauma, it is imperative that trauma-informed care is implemented as a universal intervention, regardless of one's known trauma history. Thus, trauma-informed care is an intervention and organizational approach that focuses on how trauma may affect an individual's life and their response to health services from prevention

TABLE 3.1 HISTORICAL, COLLECTIVE, AND GENERATIONAL TRAUMA

Terminology	Definition	Clinical Examples
Historical trauma*	"A complex and collective trauma experienced over time and across generations by a group of people who share an identity, affiliation, or circumstance" (Mohatt et al., 2014, p. 128)	• The experience of children and/or grandchildren of Holocaust survivors (of note, the concept of historical trauma was originally developed with this population) • The experience of descendants of colonized, Indigenous groups (e.g., Native Americans, among others globally)
Collective trauma	"Psychological reactions to a traumatic event that affect an entire society" (Hirschberger, 2018, p. 1)	• The impact that disasters (e.g., mass shootings, natural disasters) have on members of communities affected • The impact of current wars/conflicts on not only the individuals affected but also unaffected individuals of that origin (e.g., Ukrainian Americans impacted by learning of current conflict in Ukraine) • The impact of the COVID-19 pandemic among nurses and other healthcare workers
Generational trauma*	"A specific experience of trauma across familial generations, but one that does not necessarily imply a shared group trauma" (Mohatt et al., 2014, p. 128)	• An adult woman learns that their mother was sexually abused as a child • A child learns of experiences that their father endured during their time as a combat veteran • A woman who is experiencing intimate partner violence witnessed intimate partner violence between their parents as a child

*See Wolynn, M. (2017). *It didn't start with you: How inherited family trauma shapes who we are and how to end the cycle.* Penguin Books.

through treatment. It is important to note that trauma-informed care is a broader approach, and thus one does not have to be a "trauma therapist" to implement trauma-informed practices.

An effective trauma-informed model requires participation from more than healthcare providers, and a trauma-informed culture must be integrated within organizational operations so that all staff members are engaged. It is essential that APRNs are trauma aware and should anticipate the possibility of trauma when working with patients, including during initial contact and subsequent interactions, with intake processes, and during screening and assessment procedures. According to the SAMHSA's "Treatment Improvement Protocol 57 (TIP 57) Trauma-Informed Care in Behavioral Health Services" (2014b), a trauma-informed approach integrates three key elements: "(1) realizing the prevalence of trauma; (2) recognizing how trauma affects all individuals involved with the program, organization, or system, including its own workforce; and (3) responding by putting this knowledge into practice" (p. 11). Others have suggested the inclusion of respect and resilience as key trauma-informed elements. Each concept is discussed in further detail (Table 3.2).

ELEMENTS OF TRAUMA-INFORMED CARE: REALIZING, RECOGNIZING, RESPONDING

A. *Realizing* the prevalence of trauma
  1. There are various types of traumatic experiences, and thus trauma exposure is exceedingly common among individuals across the life span. For APRNs working in psychiatric settings, it is also important to note that those with mental health or substance use problems are at an even higher risk of trauma when compared with the general population.
     a. APRNs should be familiar with any risk factors for trauma that are specific to the population with whom they work (e.g., those working with military veterans should be cognizant of potential combat or military sexual trauma; those working with youth in foster care settings should be cognizant of ACEs).
     b. Trauma-informed realization includes an understanding that trauma not only influences individuals, but also their environment, social networks, and treatment engagement.
  2. APRNs should also have a general understanding of complex trauma. While not recognized by the *DSM-5-TR* (American Psychiatric Association, 2022), complex trauma, or complex posttraumatic stress disorder (CPTSD), is recognized by the *International Classification of Diseases*, 11th Edition (*ICD-11*; World Health Organization, 2019). For those with complex trauma, the trauma is often repetitive and prolonged, rather than an isolated traumatic incident, although notably not all individuals with repetitive, chronic trauma exposure will go on to develop either PTSD *or* CPTSD.
     a. The *ICD-11* CPTSD diagnostic criteria requires that the PTSD criteria are met. It is *additionally* characterized by severe and persistent (a) problems in affect regulation; (b) beliefs about oneself as diminished, defeated, or worthless, accompanied by feelings of shame, guilt, or failure related to the traumatic event; and (c) difficulties in sustaining relationships and in feeling close to others (World Health Organization, 2022).
     b. There is significant symptom overlap between PTSD, CPTSD, and borderline personality disorder (Maercker, 2021). See Table 3.3 for differentiating PTSD from CPTSD and borderline personality disorder.
     c. PTSD is discussed in greater detail in Chapter 9, "Anxiety Disorders," and borderline personality disorder is discussed in greater detail in Chapter 13, "Personality Disorders."
B. *Recognizing* how trauma affects all individuals involved with the program, organization, or system
  1. APRNs must recognize how trauma might impact the individuals they care for, including how trauma-related symptoms and behaviors originate from adapting to traumatic experiences.
     a. When working with patients, APRNs should utilize a framework of "What happened to you… What did ▶

TABLE 3.2 KEY TRAUMA-INFORMED ELEMENTS

Key Elements	Trauma-Informed Care	Trauma-Informed Primary Care
Recognition	Recognition of trauma history	Screening and trauma recognition: In a calm and empathic manner, ask about exposure to trauma. Acknowledge that disclosure is difficult and that the patient may disclose when comfortable.
Realization	Trauma influences individuals, their environment, social network, and treatment	Understanding the health effects of trauma: Empower the patient by education about the effects of trauma on health and health-related behaviors.
Response	Patient-centered and controlled care	Patient-centered communication and care: Patients are in control of their care and decisions about their health.
Respect	Respect for emotional safety; avoiding retraumatization	Emphasize emotional safety and avoid triggers: Identify examinations and procedures that may result in anxiety, flashbacks, or other retraumatization and create care that is acceptable to the patient.
Resilience	Base care approach on individual strengths	Knowledge of helpful treatment for trauma patients: Recognize individual strengths in managing health. Encourage resilience by focusing on positive aspects of patients' lives (what is going well) to reduce physical and psychological symptoms and improve disease management.

Source: Adapted with permission from Roberts, S. J., Chandler, G. E., & Kalmakis, K. (2019). A model for trauma-informed primary care. *Journal of the American Association of Nurse Practitioners, 31*(2), 139–144.

TABLE 3.3 DIFFERENTIATING POSTTRAUMATIC STRESS DISORDER, COMPLEX POSTTRAUMATIC STRESS DISORDER, AND BORDERLINE PERSONALITY DISORDER

Posttraumatic Stress Disorder	Complex Posttraumatic Stress Disorder	Borderline Personality Disorder
Exposure to actual or threatened death, serious injury, or sexual violence		While not part of the diagnostic criteria, a history of trauma or adverse childhood experiences common in those with borderline personality disorder A pervasive pattern of instability of interpersonal relationships, self-image, and affect, and marked impulsivity

• Reexperiencing/intrusive symptoms
  • Intrusive memories of the event
  • Nightmares
  • Flashbacks
  • Psychological or physiologic reactions to reminders of the event
		Transient, stress-related paranoid ideation or dissociative symptoms

• Avoidance symptoms
  • Avoidance of memories, thoughts, or feelings about the event
  • Avoidance of external reminders of the event		

• Negative alterations in cognitions and mood associated with the event
  • Inability to remember an important aspect of the traumatic event
  • Persistent and exaggerated negative beliefs or expectations about oneself, others, or the world
  • Persistent, distorted cognitions about the cause or consequences of the traumatic event that lead to self-blame
  • Persistent negative emotional state (e.g., fear, horror, anger, guilt, or shame)
  • Markedly diminished interest or participation in significant activities
  • Feelings of detachment or estrangement from others
  • Persistent inability to experience positive emotions
	• Severe and pervasive problems in affect regulation
	• Persistent beliefs about oneself as diminished, defeated, or worthless, accompanied by deep and pervasive feelings of shame, guilt, or failure related to the stressor
	• Persistent difficulties in sustaining relationships and in feeling close to others
		• Frantic efforts to avoid real or imagined abandonment
		• A pattern of unstable and intense interpersonal relationships
		• Identity disturbance
		• Recurrent suicidal behavior
		• Affective instability
		• Chronic feelings of emptiness

• Alterations in arousal and reactivity associated with the traumatic event
  • Irritability
  • Recklessness or self-destructive behavior
  • Hypervigilance
  • Exaggerated startle response
  • Problems with concentration
  • Sleep disturbances
		• Inappropriate, intense anger
		• Impulsivity

Clinically significant impairment		

you overcome?" rather than "What's *wrong* with you?" This allows for a shifted paradigm from a "pathology" mind-set to one that focuses on and emphasizes resilience.

b. Trauma survivors might engage in a variety of health risk behaviors as a means of coping with the emotional and psychological burden resulting from trauma. Such health risk behaviors can include substance use, at-risk sexual behavior, and nonsuicidal self-injurious behavior, among others.

c. A trauma-informed framework emphasizes the importance of utilizing a nonstigmatizing approach when working with patients who might engage in health risk behaviors, and recognizes that at one point such behaviors might have been adaptive or protective while one was actively experiencing trauma.

2. Recognition of trauma history when working with patients is important. There are a variety of screening tools that can be utilized to assess for trauma (Table 3.4).

a. When screening for trauma, APRNs should recognize that disclosure of trauma might be difficult and should encourage patients to share as much or as little as they feel comfortable with.

b. The APRN should clarify expectations related to the screening process, approach the patient in a supportive manner, elicit only necessary information related to the trauma, provide the patient with as much control and autonomy as possible, offer feedback about the results of the screen, and avoid phrases or language that implies judgment about the trauma.

c. Evidence suggests that self-administered questionnaires, including both paper and electronic questionnaires, might be more tolerable for trauma survivors as compared with face-to-face interview questions.

d. When screening for trauma history, APRNs should be cognizant of their own emotional and affective response to trauma disclosure and should try to remain calm and supportive of the patient.

TABLE 3.4 SCREENING TOOLS FOR TRAUMA

Screening Tool	Characteristics of the Tool	Population
Did the patient experience a traumatic event?		
Life Stressor Checklist-Revised (Wolfe & Kimerling, 1997)	• Self-report measure that assesses traumatic or stressful life events • Includes 30 life events following a yes-or-no response format o For each item endorsed, respondents are asked to what extent the event has impacted their life within the past year.	• Adults of all genders
Trauma History Questionnaire (Hooper et al., 2011)	• Self-report measure that examines experiences with potentially traumatic events • Includes 24 items following a yes-or-no format o For each event endorsed, respondents are asked to provide the frequency of the event and their age at the time of the event.	• Adults of all genders • Available in multiple languages
Adverse Childhood Experience Questionnaire (Felitti et al., 1998)	• Self-report measure that examines various types of adverse childhood experiences • Includes 10 items following a yes/no format	• Adults of all genders • Evidence that it can be used in children/adolescents
Does the patient have posttraumatic stress disorder?		
Posttraumatic Stress Disorder Checklist for *DSM-5* (Weathers et al., 2013)	• Self-report measure that assesses for 20 *DSM-5* symptoms of posttraumatic stress disorder • Includes 20 items following a Likert-style format	• Adults of all genders
Primary Care Posttraumatic Stress Disorder Screen for *DSM-5* (Prins et al., 2015)	• Self-report measure that briefly assesses for select *DSM-5* symptoms of posttraumatic stress disorder • Includes five items following a yes-or-no format	• Adults of all genders
Child Trauma Screen (Lang et al., 2021)	• Self-report measure that assesses for trauma exposure and posttraumatic stress disorder symptoms • Includes 10 items	• Children ages 6–17 years • Available in multiple languages

DSM-5, *Diagnostic and Statistical Manual of Mental Disorders*, Fifth Edition.

    e. APRNs should be aware of clinical practice guidelines as it relates to screening for trauma:
       i. In 2018, the U.S. Preventive Services Task Force (USPSTF) updated its recommendations related to screening for IPV:
          (a) "The USPSTF recommends that clinicians screen for intimate partner violence (IPV) in women of reproductive age and provide or refer women who screen positive to ongoing support services" (B recommendation; U.S. Preventative Services Task Force, 2018, p. 1678).
          (b) "The USPSTF concludes that the current evidence is insufficient to assess the balance of benefits and harms of screening for abuse and neglect in all older or vulnerable adults" (I statement; U.S. Preventative Services Task Force, 2018, p. 1678).
       ii. The American Academy of Child and Adolescent Psychiatry recommends that psychiatric assessment should routinely include questions about traumatic experiences and PTSD symptoms.
          (a) The American Academy of Child and Adolescent Psychiatry recommends that for "children with a history of foster care, adoption, or institutional rearing, clinicians should inquire routinely about a) whether the child demonstrates attachment behaviors and b) whether the child is reticent with strangers" (Zeanah et al., 2016, p. 996).

C. *Responding* by putting trauma-related knowledge into practice

    1. In utilizing a trauma-informed approach, APRNs should seek to develop collaborative and patient-centered relationships with those they care for.
       a. They should utilize patient-centered communication and should empower patients to remain in control of their care and decisions about their health.
          i. A trauma-informed response is different from the traditional authoritarian model of medical care, and leverages patients' strengths and encourages a partnership between patients and healthcare providers, through which the patient has equal or greater control in healthcare decisions.
       b. They should be aware of evidence-based treatment strategies to treat trauma-related symptoms and should be able to implement or make referrals for such treatments, when desired by the patient (Table 3.5).
       c. They should follow clinical practice guidelines related to the treatment of trauma-related disorders.
          i. The American Academy of Child and Adolescent Psychiatry has active clinical practice guidelines related to (a) assessment and treatment of children and adolescents with PTSD and (b) assessment and treatment of children and adolescents with reactive attachment disorder and disinhibited social engagement disorder.
          ii. The U.S. Department of Veterans Affairs has active clinical practice guidelines related to the management of posttraumatic stress (2023) that propose three levels of PTSD.

TABLE 3.5 EVIDENCE-BASED TRAUMA TREATMENT MODALITIES

Pharmacologic Treatment	
Medication	**FDA indication**
Sertraline	Posttraumatic stress disorder in adults
Paroxetine	Posttraumatic stress disorder in adults
Fluoxetine	Can be used off-label; evidence that it is effective, although not FDA-approved for posttraumatic stress disorder in children, adolescents, or adults
Venlafaxine	Can be used off-label; evidence that it is effective, although not FDA-approved for posttraumatic stress disorder in children, adolescents, or adults
Mirtazapine	Can be used off-label; evidence that it is effective, although not FDA-approved for posttraumatic stress disorder in children, adolescents, or adults
Prazosin	Can be used off-label for nightmares; evidence that it is effective, although not FDA-approved for posttraumatic stress disorder-related nightmares in children, adolescents, or adults
Psychotherapies	

- Cognitive processing therapy
- Cognitive behavioral therapy
- Prolonged exposure for posttraumatic stress disorder
- Eye movement desensitization and reprocessing
- Written or narrative exposure therapy

FDA, U.S. Food and Drug Administration.

PRINCIPLES OF TRAUMA-INFORMED CARE

In addition to the aforementioned *elements* of trauma-informed care (i.e., realization, recognition, and response), there are six *principles* of trauma-informed care. These are (a) safety; (b) trustworthiness and transparency; (c) peer support; (d) collaboration and mutuality; (e) empowerment, voice, and choice; and (f) cultural, historical, and gender issues (Centers for Disease Control and Prevention, 2018).

A. Safety
    1. APRNs must promote and ensure physical, psychological, social, and moral safety within a trauma-informed approach.
    2. aprns must seek to understand what safety *means* to the individual patients that they serve. This requires them to challenge their assumptions and ask patients directly: "Do you feel safe?" and/or "What can we do to assure that you feel safe here?" Assessing for feelings of safety is dynamic and thus should be a fluid, ongoing assessment. Individuals may have varying definitions and experiences of safety based on their trauma history.
        a. Example: A person with a history of sexual abuse might feel unsafe during invasive procedures, such as during mammography or pelvic exams, while other individuals might feel more comfortable during these types of procedures. Recognizing that some seemingly routine medical procedures and interventions might be retraumatizing for those with a history of trauma, APRNs, including those who work in mental health, should explore the source of any anxiety or discomfort and should offer interventions to help individuals overcome these concerns. Examples include offering an as-needed anxiolytic prior to medical interventions or can include accommodations such as allowing a trusted support person to accompany them to medical interventions, should the patient wish to do so.
    3. An individualized care plan must be implemented to effectively promote patient safety. In promoting a feeling of safety for patients within medical settings, APRNs are seeking to actively avoid retraumatization.

B. Trustworthiness and transparency
    1. APRNs need to gain the trust of the patients they serve, and this is especially critical when working with patients who have a history of trauma exposure.
    2. Negative beliefs about oneself and/or other people are a potential characteristic of PTSD, and thus trauma survivors may be mistrustful of others, particularly those who are in a position of authority.
    3. Given the historical authoritarian medical model, trauma survivors might be particularly uncomfortable around or mistrustful of medical providers.
    4. Gaining the trust of these individuals is paramount in developing a collaborative and effective therapeutic relationship. When working with patients, consistency and transparency are key.
    5. While a trauma-informed approach seeks to develop a collaborative relationship with patients, there are times that an APRN may be required to make difficult decisions surrounding a patient's care. When these situations arise, APRNs should be transparent with the patients that they serve and provide an explanation and rationale for the decision made (Box 3.2).

C. Peer support
    1. Peer support or mutual self-help organizations can be essential in establishing safety and hope, building trust, and enhancing collaboration. "Peer" refers to not only individuals with lived experiences of trauma but also their caregivers.

BOX 3.2 TK'S STORY: PART II

TK has been working with an APRN for the last 6 months to address depressive, anxiety-related, and substance use symptoms. She is stable on the following medication regimen: buprenorphine/naloxone 8 mg/2 mg twice daily for opioid use disorder, duloxetine 60 mg twice daily for major depressive disorder, and buspirone 10 mg three times daily for anxiety-related symptoms. Her treatment plan includes routine medication management appointments, in addition to trauma-focused psychotherapy. She has developed a trusting, therapeutic relationship with the APRN, and together they have utilized a collaborative, shared decision-making model as it relates to treatment planning.

TK's mental health symptoms have been well-controlled for the last 3 months, including anxiety-related symptoms. Nonetheless, TK asks the APRN if she could be prescribed alprazolam for anxiety, as a friend had used it in the past and found it to be effective. The APRN is aware that alprazolam should be avoided with buprenorphine due to risk of respiratory depression. Further, TK's anxiety has been manageable, and TK denies recent panic attacks.

In a shared decision-making model, patients have equal or great power as it relates to treatment planning. That said, APRNs will certainly encounter difficult clinic issues that occur when a patient requests a particular type of treatment that might be unsafe. **The key is to proceed with transparency and to negotiate an alternative.**

The APRN explains to TK the risks of combining benzodiazepines with an opioid medication. While TK is initially disappointed, she has a trusting relationship with the APRN, and ultimately appreciates the APRN's transparency and concern for TK's safety. They agree to an alternative of utilizing hydroxyzine as needed for anxiety, which is generally safer when combined with medications like buprenorphine.

a. Multiple models of peer support include coaching, group therapy or other group approaches, and internet-based approaches, among others.
   b. this allows individuals from diverse backgrounds, who share similar common experiences, to come together to (a) build relationships, (b) share their strengths, and (c) support healing and growth.
   c. Peer support utilizes a strengths-based approach and thus is not focused on diagnoses, symptoms, or deficits.
   d. Peer support allows participants to learn from one another, build connections, and grow and foster resilience.
   2. There are elements essential to assuring the success of a peer support model.
      a. Foremost, peer support is *voluntary*. The voluntary nature of peer support encourages individuals to connect and share their ideas and experiences freely.
         i. It is essential that peer support participants be free of coercion to participate.
         ii. For individuals who might be engaged with the legal or criminal justice system, engagement in peer support programming should not be required or mandated as a treatment.
      b. Further, peer support services foster a nonjudgmental, empathetic, and respectful approach to promote safety and avoid retraumatization.
         i. Peer support services require honesty, mutual responsibility, and are reciprocal in their approach in that all participants share ideas and learn from one another.
   3. APRNs should familiarize themselves with resources in their community that offer peer support services.
   4. Additionally, the SAMHSA houses the *Peer Recovery Center of Excellence* (www.samhsa.gov/peer-recovery-center-of-excellence), which is a useful resource for APRNs.
D. Collaboration and mutuality
   1. A trauma-informed approach seeks to develop collaborative, patient-centered relationships with patients that are based on a foundation of mutual respect.
   2. One important way to foster collaborative relationships is through the utilization of motivational interviewing techniques (Table 3.6).
E. Empowerment, voice, and choice
   1. Trauma-informed practices should utilize "strengths-based approaches that are empowering and support individuals to take control of their lives and service use. Such approaches are vital because many trauma survivors will have experienced an absolute lack of power and control" (Sweeney et al., 2018, p. 324).
   2. APRNs should empower patients by focusing on adaption to trauma and associated resiliency, rather than pathologizing trauma symptoms.
      a. The strengths and experiences of trauma survivors should not only be recognized but should be leveraged to improve health outcomes.
      b. Trauma survivors should be encouraged to practice self-advocacy skills, both within the healthcare setting and in other facets of their own lives.
F. Cultural, historical, and gender issues
   1. APRNs must be cognizant of potential implicit biases when working with diverse groups.
      a. Seek to challenge cultural stereotypes and biases.
      b. Offer gender-responsive services.
      c. Leverage the healing value of traditional cultural practices.
      d. Respond to the racial, ethnic, and cultural needs of the individuals that they serve.
      e. Be cognizant of historical or collective trauma, as outlined in Table 3.1.

BEST PRACTICES AND PRACTICAL CONSIDERATIONS WHEN IMPLEMENTING A TRAUMA-INFORMED APPROACH

There are a variety of considerations when implementing trauma-informed practices in healthcare settings. Trauma-informed care should comprise a cultural change within an organization, and thus all healthcare providers, policies, and procedures should be trauma-informed, rather than an individual healthcare provider alone.

A. Practical recommendations when implementing a trauma-informed approach include the following:
   1. Organizational policies and procedures should be grounded in a trauma-informed approach. Trauma-informed care should be "hard-wired" into organizational culture.

TABLE 3.6 ESSENTIAL ELEMENTS OF MOTIVATIONAL INTERVIEWING

Skill	Examples
Open-ended questions allow a patient to freely share their experiences, perspectives, and ideas. Information is then often offered within a structure of open-ended questions (elicit-provide-elicit) that (a) explore what the patient already knows, (b) seek permission to offer what the advanced practice registered nurse knows, and (c) explore the patient's response.	• "What brings you in to the clinic today?" • "How are you feeling about treatment?" • "What is your level of comfort in what we discussed today?"
Affirmation of strengths, efforts, and past successes helps build the patient's hope and confidence in their ability to change.	• "I appreciate that you were willing to talk with me today." • "It sounds like you handled what was a really stressful situation."
Reflections are based on careful listening and trying to understand what the patient is saying by repeating or rephrasing.	• "It sounds like you are telling me that, when you're feeling more anxious, you tend to use cannabis more regularly."
Summarizing ensures shared understanding and reinforces key points made by the patient.	• "Based on what we talked about today, it sounds like you have been on the fence about trying medication but are now willing to begin."

a. Organizations should offer ongoing continuing education and training events related to best practices in trauma-informed care. Additionally, APRNs should seek out additional training and continuing education opportunities as it relates to trauma-informed care.

b. Example: McLean Hospital has recently launched its *Institute for Trauma-Informed Systems Change*, which offers regular workshops and continuing education opportunities for healthcare providers, including APRNs (https://home.mcleanhospital.org/ce-itisc).

2. APRNs should utilize a strengths-based, rather than a deficit- or symptom-based, approach when working with patients across the life span. This includes:

a. Gathering information about positive, healthy coping skills

b. Eliciting information about social support systems

c. Acknowledging specific strengths and seeking to foster resiliency

d. Applauding individuals for positive progress made

3. APRNs should foster an attitude and promote a healthcare environment that is inclusive of all patients. This includes the following:

a. Antiracist practices and culturally sensitive care should be utilized for people of color and all diverse racial/ethnic groups.

b. An approach that celebrates those with diverse sexual orientations or gender identities should be utilized. This means assuring that all policies, procedures, and paperwork are inclusive and challenge heteronormative, binary models of care (see Chapter 19, "Special Considerations for the LGBTQ+ Population," for additional details).

c. A healthcare environment that is accessible for those with physical and mental health disabilities should be assured. Thus, intake paperwork, reading material, and so forth should be tailored to the literacy and health literacy of individuals, and for those with hearing impairments, visual impairments, or for whom English is not their primary language accommodations should be made to assure adequate communication.

4. APRNs should ask permission before discussing potentially sensitive topics, including trauma history. While screening for trauma should occur universally, APRNs should inquire first as to whether the patient feels comfortable answering questions about trauma history. If the patient declines, the APRN can visit the discussion later after additional trust and rapport have been built and developed.

5. For APRNs conducting physical examinations or other medical procedures, consent should not only be obtained prior to the examination or procedure but also throughout. APRNs should take time to explain each part of the examination or procedure and should assure that the patient is comfortable along the way. Should the patient request to discontinue the examination or procedure, the APRN should make efforts to immediately grant this request.

6. For patients presenting with trauma-related symptoms or trauma-related disorders, the APRN should utilize evidence-based treatment interventions, including pharmacologic and nonpharmacologic interventions, as appropriate and as tolerated by the patient. If referrals are needed to access trauma treatment, a warm handoff approach should be utilized.

7. For APRNs working on inpatient psychiatric or medical-surgical units, consideration should be made as it relates to retraumatization via the use of restraints and/or seclusion. Restraints and seclusion are inherently dehumanizing and restrictive interventions. Individuals with a history of trauma exposure might be particularly susceptible to retraumatization or psychological distress secondary to the use of restraints and/or seclusion. Thus, APRNs should make all efforts to avoid the use of restraints and/or seclusion and should use less restrictive measures, if possible.

CONCLUSION

It is imperative that APRNs have a thorough understanding of the elements and principles of trauma-informed care. Trauma-informed care is a well-established, evidence-based intervention that can improve health outcomes and quality of life among trauma survivors. In utilizing a trauma-informed approach, APRNs can seek to foster effective therapeutic relationships with the patients that they serve.

REFERENCES AND BIBLIOGRAPHY

Abu Suhaiban, H., Grasser, L. R., & Javanbakht, A. (2019). Mental health of refugees and torture survivors: A critical review of prevalence, predictors, and integrated care. *International Journal of Environmental Research and Public Health*, 16(13), 2309. https://doi.org/10.3390/ijerph16132309

American Psychiatric Association. (1980). *Diagnostic and statistical manual of mental disorders* (3rd ed.). Author.

American Psychiatric Association. (2022). *Diagnostic and statistical manual of mental disorders* (5th ed., text rev.). https://doi.org/10.1176/appi.books.9780890425787

American Psychological Association Presidential Task Force on Posttraumatic Stress Disorder and Trauma in Children and Adolescents. (2008). *Children and trauma: Update for mental health professionals*. American Psychological Association.

Armenta, R. F., Rush, T., LeardMann, C. A., Millegan, J., Cooper, A., & Hoge, C. W. (2018). Factors associated with persistent posttraumatic stress disorder among US military service members and veterans. *BMC Psychiatry*, 18, Article 48. https://doi.org/10.1186/s12888-018-1590-5

Bacchus, L. J., Ranganathan, M., Watts, C., & Devries, K. (2018). Recent intimate partner violence against women and health: A systematic review and meta-analysis of cohort studies. *BMJ Open*, 8(7), e019995. https://doi.org/10.1136/bmjopen-2017-019995

Beaglehole, B., Mulder, R. T., Frampton, C. M., Boden, J. M., Newton-Howes, G., & Bell, C. J. (2018). Psychological distress and psychiatric disorder after natural disasters: Systematic review and meta-analysis. *The British Journal of Psychiatry*, 213(6), 716–722. https://doi.org/10.1192/bjp.2018.210

Beckman, K., Shipherd, J., Simpson, T., & Lehavot, K. (2018). Military sexual assault in transgender veterans: Results from a nationwide survey. *Journal of Traumatic Stress*, 31(2), 181–190. https://doi.org/10.1002/jts.22280

Bender, A. K., Koegler, E., Johnson, S. D., Murugan, V., & Wamser-Nanney, R. (2021). Guns and intimate partner violence among adolescents: A scoping review. *Journal of Family Violence*, 36(5), 605–617. https://doi.org/10.1007/s10896-020-00193-x

Benevolenza, M. A., & DeRigne, L. (2019). The impact of climate change and natural disasters on vulnerable populations: A systematic review of literature. *Journal of Human Behavior in the Social Environment*, 29(2), 266–281. https://doi.org/10.1080/10911359.2018.1527739

Blanch, A., Filson, B., & Penney, D. (2012, April). *Engaging women in trauma-informed peer support: A guidebook*. Center for Mental Health Services, National Center for Trauma-Informed Care. https://www.nasmhpd.org/sites/default/files/PeerEngagementGuide_Color_REVISED_10_2012.pdf

Briggs, E. C., Amaya-Jackson, L., Putnam, K. T., & Putnam, F. W. (2021). All adverse childhood experiences are not equal: The contribution of synergy to adverse childhood experience scores. *American Psychologist*, 76(2), 243–252. https://doi.org/10.1037/amp0000768

Bush, A. M. (2020). A multi-state examination of the victims of fatal adolescent intimate partner violence, 2011–2015. *Journal of Injury and Violence Research*, 12(1), 73–83. https://jivresearch.org/jivr/index.php/jivr/article/view/1197/854

Carlson, J. S., Yohannan, J., Darr, C. L., Turley, M. R., Larez, N. A., & Perfect, M. M. (2020). Prevalence of adverse childhood experiences in school-aged youth: A systematic review (1990–2015). *International Journal of School & Educational Psychology*, 8(Suppl. 1), 2–23. https://doi.org/10.1080/21683603.2018.1548397

Charlson, F., van Ommeren, M., Flaxman, A., Cornett, J., Whiteford, H., & Saxena, S. (2019). New WHO prevalence estimates of mental disorders in conflict settings: A systematic review and meta-analysis. *The Lancet*, 394(10194), 240–248. https://doi.org/10.1016/S0140-6736(19)30934-1

Chen, J., Walters, M. L., Gilbert, L. K., & Patel, N. (2020). Sexual violence, stalking, and partner violence by sexual orientation, United States. *Psychology of Violence*, 10(1), 110–119. PMID: 32064141.

Centers for Disease Control and Prevention. (2018, June 28). *Six guiding principles to a trauma-informed approach*. https://stacks.cdc.gov/view/cdc/56843

Cohen, J. A., Bukstein, O., Walter, H., Benson, S. R., Chrisman, A., Farchione, T. R., Hamilton, J., Keable, H., Kinlan, J., Schoettle, U., Siegel, M., Stock, S., Medicus, J., & American Academy of Child and Adolescent Psychiatry Work Group On Quality Issues. (2010). Practice parameter for the assessment and treatment of children and adolescents with posttraumatic stress disorder. *Journal of the American Academy of Child & Adolescent Psychiatry*, 49(4), 414–430. PMID: 20410735.

Cohen, G. H., Tamrakar, S., Lowe, S., Sampson, L., Ettman, C., Kilpatrick, D., Linas, B. P., Ruggiero, K., & Galea, S. (2019). Improved social services and the burden of post-traumatic stress disorder among economically vulnerable people after a natural disaster: A modelling study. *The Lancet Planetary Health*, 3(2), e93–e101. https://doi.org/10.1016/S2542-5196(19)30012-9

Crouch, E., Probst, J. C., Radcliff, E., Bennett, K. J., & McKinney, S. H. (2019). Prevalence of Adverse Childhood Experiences (ACEs) among US children. *Child Abuse & Neglect*, 92, 209–218. https://doi.org/10.1016/j.chiabu.2019.04.010

Eichstaedt, J. C., Sherman, G. T., Giorgi, S., Roberts, S. O., Reynolds, M. E., Ungar, L. H., & Guntuku, S. C. (2021). The emotional and mental health impact of the murder of George Floyd on the US population. *Proceedings of the National Academy of Sciences*, 118(39), e2109139118. https://doi.org/10.1073/pnas.2109139118

Engel, R. J., Lee, D. H., & Rosen, D. (2020). Psychiatric sequelae among community social service agency staff 1 year after a mass shooting. *JAMA Network Open*, 3(8), e2014050. https://doi.org/10.1001/jamanetworkopen.2020.14050

Felitti, V. J., Anda, R. F., Nordenberg, D., Williamson, D. F., Spitz, A. M., Edwards, V., & Marks, J. S. (1998). Relationship of childhood abuse and household dysfunction to many of the leading causes of death in adults: The Adverse Childhood Experiences (ACE) Study. *American Journal of Preventive Medicine*, 14(4), 245–258. https://doi.org/10.1016/s0749-3797(98)00017-8

Felix, E., Rubens, S., & Hambrick, E. (2020). The relationship between physical and mental health outcomes in children exposed to disasters. *Current Psychiatry Reports*, 22, Article 33. https://doi.org/10.1007/s11920-020-01157-0

First, J. M., Danforth, L., Frisby, C. M., Warner, B. R., Ferguson Jr, M. W., & Houston, J. B. (2020). Posttraumatic stress related to the killing of Michael Brown and resulting civil unrest in Ferguson, Missouri: Roles of protest engagement, media use, race, and resilience. *Journal of the Society for Social Work and Research*, 11(3), 369–391. https://doi.org/10.1086/711162

Geoffrion, S., Goncalves, J., Robichaud, I., Sader, J., Giguère, C. E., Fortin, M., Lamothe, J., Bernard, P., & Guay, S. (2022). Systematic review and meta-analysis on acute stress disorder: Rates following different types of traumatic events. *Trauma, Violence, & Abuse*, 23(1), 213–223. https://doi.org/10.1177/1524838020933844

Gerino, E., Caldarera, A. M., Curti, L., Brustia, P., & Rollè, L. (2018). Intimate partner violence in the golden age: Systematic review of risk and protective factors. *Frontiers in Psychology*, 9, Article 1595. https://doi.org/10.3389/fpsyg.2018.01595

Giano, Z., Wheeler, D. L., & Hubach, R. D. (2020). The frequencies and disparities of adverse childhood experiences in the US. *BMC Public Health*, 20(1), Article 1327. https://doi.org/10.1186/s12889-020-09411-z

Goldberg, S. B., Livingston, W. S., Blais, R. K., Brignone, E., Suo, Y., Lehavot, K., Simpson, T. L., Fargo, J., & Gundlapalli, A. V. (2019). A positive screen for military sexual trauma is associated with greater risk for substance use disorders in women veterans. *Psychology of Addictive Behaviors*, 33(5), 477–483. https://doi.org/10.1037/adb0000486

Golitaleb, M., Mazaheri, E., Bonyadi, M., & Sahebi, A. (2022). Prevalence of post-traumatic stress disorder after flood: A systematic review and meta-analysis. *Frontiers in Psychiatry*, 13, 890671. https://doi.org/10.3389/fpsyt.2022.890671

Hakamata, Y., Suzuki, Y., Kobashikawa, H., & Hori, H. (2022). Neurobiology of early life adversity: A systematic review of meta-analyses towards an integrative account of its neurobiological trajectories to mental disorders. *Frontiers in Neuroendocrinology*, 65, Article 100994. https://doi.org/10.1016/j.yfrne.2022.100994

Herzog, J. I., & Schmahl, C. (2018). Adverse childhood experiences and the consequences on neurobiological, psychosocial, and somatic conditions across the lifespan. *Frontiers in Psychiatry*, 9, Article 420. https://doi.org/10.3389/fpsyt.2018.00420

Hirschberger, G. (2018). Collective trauma and the social construction of meaning. *Frontiers in Psychology*, 9, Article 1441. https://doi.org/10.3389/fpsyg.2018.01441

Hooper, L., Stockton, P., Krupnick, J., & Green, B., (2011). Development, use, and psychometric properties of the Trauma History Questionnaire. *Journal of Loss and Trauma*, 16(3), 258–283. https://doi.org/10.1080/15325024.2011.572035

Hou, W. K., Liu, H., Liang, L., Ho, J., Kim, H., Seong, E., Bonanno, G. A., Hobfoll, S. E., & Hall, B. J. (2020). Everyday life experiences and mental health among conflict-affected forced migrants: A meta-analysis. *Journal of Affective Disorders*, 264, 50–68. https://doi.org/10.1016/j.jad.2019.11.165

Jafari, H., Heidari, M., Heidari, S., & Sayfouri, N. (2020). Risk factors for suicidal behaviours after natural disasters: A systematic review. *The Malaysian Journal of Medical Sciences*, 27(3), 20–33. https://doi.org/10.21315/mjms2020.27.3.3

Jiang, Y., Zilioli, S., Rodriguez-Stanley, J., Peek, K. M., & Cutchin, M. P. (2020). Socioeconomic status and differential psychological and immune responses to a human-caused disaster. *Brain, Behavior, and Immunity*, 88, 935–939. https://doi.org/10.1016/j.bbi.2020.05.046

Katsiyannis, A., Rapa, L. J., Whitford, D. K., & Scott, S. N. (2022). An examination of US school mass shootings, 2017–2022: Findings and implications. *Advances in Neurodevelopmental Disorders*, 7(1), 66–76. https://doi.org/10.1007/s41252-022-00277-3

Lang, J. M., Connell, C. M., & Macary, S. (2021). Validating the child trauma screen among a cross-sectional sample of youth and caregivers in pediatric primary care. *Clinical Pediatrics*, 60(4–5), 252–258. https://doi.org/10.1177/00099228211005302

LaNoue, M. D., George, B. J., Helitzer, D. L., & Keith, S. W. (2020). Contrasting cumulative risk and multiple individual risk models of the relationship between Adverse Childhood Experiences (ACEs) and adult health outcomes. *BMC Medical Research Methodology*, 20, Article 239. https://doi.org/10.1186/s12874-020-01120-w

Maercker, A. (2021). Development of the new CPTSD diagnosis for ICD-11. *Borderline Personality Disorder and Emotion Dysregulation*, 8, Article 7. https://doi.org/10.1186/s40479-021-00148-8

Mancini, A. D., Littleton, H. L., Grills, A. E., & Jones, P. J. (2019). Posttraumatic stress disorder near and far: Symptom networks from 2 to 12 months after the Virginia Tech campus shootings. *Clinical Psychological Science*, 7(6), 1340–1354. https://doi.org/10.1177/2167702619859333

McGuire, A. P., Gauthier, J. M., Anderson, L. M., Hollingsworth, D. W., Tracy, M., Galea, S., & Coffey, S. F. (2018). Social support moderates effects of natural disaster exposure on depression and posttraumatic stress disorder symptoms: Effects for displaced and nondisplaced residents. *Journal of Traumatic Stress*, 31(2), 223–233. https://doi.org/10.1002/jts.22270

Menschner, C., & Maul, A. (2016, April). *Key Ingredients for successful trauma-informed care implementation* (Issue Brief). Center for Health Care Strategies. Robert Wood Johnson Foundation. https://www.samhsa.gov/sites/default/files/programs_campaigns/childrens_mental_health/atc-whitepaper-040616.pdf

Merrick, M. T., Ford, D. C., Ports, K. A., & Guinn, A. S. (2018). Prevalence of adverse childhood experiences from the 2011–2014 behavioral risk factor surveillance system in 23 states. *JAMA Pediatrics*, 172(11), 1038–1044. https://doi.org/10.1001/jamapediatrics.2018.2537

Merrick, M. T., Ford, D. C., Ports, K. A., Guinn, A. S., Chen, J., Klevens, J., Metzler, M., Jones, C. M., Simon, T. R., Daniel, V. M., Ottley, P., & Mercy, J. A. (2019). Vital signs: Estimated proportion of adult health problems attributable to adverse childhood experiences and implications for prevention—25 States, 2015–2017. *Morbidity and Mortality Weekly Report, 68*(44), 999–1005. https://doi.org/10.15585/mmwr.mm6844e1

Miller, K. K., Brown, C. R., Shramko, M., & Svetaz, M. V. (2019). Applying trauma-informed practices to the care of refugee and immigrant youth: 10 clinical pearls. *Children, 6*(8), 94. https://doi.org/10.3390/children6080094

Mohatt, N. V., Thompson, A. B., Thai, N. D., & Tebes, J. K. (2014). Historical trauma as public narrative: A conceptual review of how history impacts present-day health. *Social Science & Medicine, 106*, 128–136. https://doi.org/10.1016/j.socscimed.2014.01.043

Monteith, L. L., Holliday, R., Schneider, A. L., Forster, J. E., & Bahraini, N. H. (2019). Identifying factors associated with suicidal ideation and suicide attempts following military sexual trauma. *Journal of Affective Disorders, 252*, 300–309. https://doi.org/10.1016/j.jad.2019.04.038

Morina, N., Akhtar, A., Barth, J., & Schnyder, U. (2018). Psychiatric disorders in refugees and internally displaced persons after forced displacement: A systematic review. *Frontiers in Psychiatry, 9*, Article 433. https://doi.org/10.3389/fpsyt.2018.00433

Mothersill, O., & Donohoe, G. (2016). Neural effects of social environmental stress—an activation likelihood estimation meta-analysis. *Psychological Medicine, 46*(10), 2015–2023. https://doi.org/10.1017/S0033291716000477

Nadal, K. L., Erazo, T., & King, R. (2019). Challenging definitions of psychological trauma: Connecting racial microaggressions and traumatic stress. *Journal for Social Action in Counseling & Psychology, 11*(2), 2–16. https://doi.org/10.33043/JSACP.11.2.2-16

Nichter, B., Norman, S., Haller, M., & Pietrzak, R. H. (2019). Psychological burden of PTSD, depression, and their comorbidity in the US veteran population: Suicidality, functioning, and service utilization. *Journal of Affective Disorders, 256*, 633–640. https://doi.org/10.1016/j.jad.2019.06.072

Parker, K., Igielnik, R., Barroso, A., & Cilluffo, A. (2019, September 10). *The American veteran experience and the post-9/11 generation*. Pew Research Center. https://www.pewresearch.org/social-trends/2019/09/10/the-american-veteran-experience-and-the-post-9-11-generation

Peitzmeier, S. M., Malik, M., Kattari, S. K., Marrow, E., Stephenson, R., Agénor, M., & Reisner, S. L. (2020). Intimate partner violence in transgender populations: Systematic review and meta-analysis of prevalence and correlates. *American Journal of Public Health, 110*(9), e1–e14. https://doi.org/10.2105/AJPH.2020.305774

Peterson, C., Kearns, M. C., McIntosh, W. L., Estefan, L. F., Nicolaidis, C., McCollister, K. E., Gordon, A., & Florence, C. (2018). Lifetime economic burden of intimate partner violence among US adults. *American Journal of Preventive Medicine, 55*(4), 433–444. https://doi.org/10.1016/j.amepre.2018.04.049

Petrosky, E., Blair, J. M., Betz, C. J., Fowler, K. A., Jack, S. P., & Lyons, B. H. (2017). Racial and ethnic differences in homicides of adult women and the role of intimate partner violence—United States, 2003–2014. *Morbidity and Mortality Weekly Report, 66*(28), 741–746. https://doi.org/10.15585/mmwr.mm6628a1

Petruccelli, K., Davis, J., & Berman, T. (2019). Adverse childhood experiences and associated health outcomes: A systematic review and meta-analysis. *Child Abuse & Neglect, 97*, 104127. https://doi.org/10.1016/j.chiabu.2019.104127

Pomerantz, A. S. (2017). Treating PTSD in primary care: One small step is one giant leap. *Families, Systems, and Health, 35*(4), 505–507. https://doi.org/10.1037/fsh0000318

Prins, A., Bovin, M. J., Kimerling, R., Kaloupek, D. G., Marx, B. P., Pless Kaiser, A., & Schnurr, P. P. (2015). *The Primary Care PTSD Screen for DSM-5 (PC-PTSD-5)*. U.S. Department of Veterans Affairs: National Center for PTSD. https://www.ptsd.va.gov/professional/assessment/documents/pc-ptsd5-screen.pdf

Rhee, T. G., Barry, L. C., Kuchel, G. A., Steffens, D. C., & Wilkinson, S. T. (2019). Associations of adverse childhood experiences with past-year DSM-5 psychiatric and substance use disorders in older adults. *Journal of the American Geriatrics Society, 67*(10), 2085–2093. https://doi.org/10.1111/jgs.16032

Roberts, S. J., Chandler, G. E., & Kalmakis, K. (2019). A model for trauma-informed primary care. *Journal of the American Association of Nurse Practitioners, 31*(2), 139–144. https://doi.org/10.1097/JXX.0000000000000116

Sanz-Barbero, B., Barón, N., & Vives-Cases, C. (2019). Prevalence, associated factors and health impact of intimate partner violence against women in different life stages. *PLoS One, 14*(10), e0221049. https://doi.org/10.1371/journal.pone.0221049

Schaeffer, K. (2023, November 8). *The changing face of America's veteran population*. Pew Research Center. https://www.pewresearch.org/fact-tank/2021/04/05/the-changing-face-of-americas-veteran-population

Selous, C., Kelly-Irving, M., Maughan, B., Eyre, O., Rice, F., & Collishaw, S. (2020). Adverse childhood experiences and adult mood problems: Evidence from a five-decade prospective birth cohort. *Psychological Medicine, 50*(14), 2444–2451. https://doi.org/10.1017/S003329171900271X

Shonkoff, J. P., Garner, A. S., Committee on Psychosocial Aspects of Child and Family Health, Committee on Early Childhood, Adoption, and Dependent Care, and Section on Developmental and Behavioral Pediatrics, Siegel, B. S., Dobbins, M. I., Earls, M. F., & Wood, D. L. (2012). The lifelong effects of early childhood adversity and toxic stress. *Pediatrics, 129*(1), e232–e246. https://doi.org/10.1542/peds.2011-2663

Spencer, C. M., Stith, S. M., & Cafferky, B. (2019). Risk markers for physical intimate partner violence victimization: A meta-analysis. *Aggression and Violent Behavior, 44*, 8–17. https://doi.org/10.1016/j.avb.2018.10.009

Strathearn, L., Mertens, C. E., Mayes, L., Rutherford, H., Rajhans, P., Xu, G., Potenza, M. N., & Kim, S. (2019). Pathways relating the neurobiology of attachment to drug addiction. *Frontiers in Psychiatry, 10*, 737. https://doi.org/10.3389/fpsyt.2019.00737

Straus, E., Norman, S. B., Haller, M., Southwick, S. M., Hamblen, J. L., & Pietrzak, R. H. (2019). Differences in protective factors among US veterans with posttraumatic stress disorder, alcohol use disorder, and their comorbidity: Results from the National Health and Resilience in Veterans Study. *Drug and Alcohol Dependence, 194*, 6–12. https://doi.org/10.1016/j.drugalcdep.2018.09.011

Substance Abuse and Mental Health Services Administration. (2014a, October). *SAMHSA's concept of trauma and guidance for a trauma-informed approach* (Publication No. SMA14-4884). Department of Health and Human Services. https://store.samhsa.gov/product/samhsas-concept-trauma-and-guidance-trauma-informed-approach/sma14-4884

Substance Abuse and Mental Health Services Administration. (2014b, March). *TIP 57: Trauma-informed care in behavioral health services* (Publication No. SMA13-4801). Department of Health and Human Services. https://store.samhsa.gov/product/tip-57-trauma-informed-care-behavioral-health-services/sma14-4816

Substance Abuse and Mental Health Services Administration. (2022). *Types of disasters*. https://www.samhsa.gov/find-help/disaster-distress-helpline/disaster-types

Sweeney, A., Filson, B., Kennedy, A., Collinson, L., & Gillard, S. (2018). A paradigm shift: Relationship in trauma-informed mental health services. *British Journal of Psychiatry Advances, 24*(5), 319–333. https://doi.org/10.1192/bja.2018.29

Tynes, B. M., Willis, H. A., Stewart, A. M., & Hamilton, M. W. (2019). Race-related traumatic events online and mental health among adolescents of color. *Journal of Adolescent Health, 65*(3), 371–377. https://doi.org/10.1016/j.jadohealth.2019.03.006

United Nations. (2022, March 30). *"War's greatest cost is its human toll," secretary-general reminds peacebuilding commission, warning of "perilous impunity" taking hold* [Press release]. https://press.un.org/en/2022/sgsm21216.doc.htm

United Nations Refugee Agency. (2019). *Global trends: Forced displacement in 2018*. https://www.unhcr.org/5d08d7ee7.pdf

U.S. Department of Veteran Affairs. (2022). *Mental health: Military sexual trauma*. https://www.mentalhealth.va.gov/msthome/index.asp

U.S. Department of Veterans Affairs. (2023). *VA/DoD clinical practice guideline: Management of posttraumatic stress and acute stress disorder 2023*. https://www.healthquality.va.gov/guidelines/mh/ptsd

U.S. Preventative Services Task Force. (2018, October 23/30). Screening for intimate partner violence, elder abuse, and abuse of vulnerable adults: US Preventive Services Task Force final recommendation statement. *Journal of the American Medical Association, 320*(16), 1678–1687. https://doi.org/10.1001/jama.2018.14741

Van der Kolk, B. A. (2014). *The body keeps the score: Brain, mind, and body in the healing of trauma*. Penguin Books.

von Werthern, M., Grigorakis, G., & Vizard, E. (2019). The mental health and wellbeing of Unaccompanied Refugee Minors (URMs). *Child Abuse & Neglect, 98*, 104146. https://doi.org/10.1016/j.chiabu.2019.104146

Vujanovic, A. A., Farris, S. G., Bartlett, B. A., Lyons, R. C., Haller, M., Colvonen, P. J., & Norman, S. B. (2018). Anxiety sensitivity in the association between posttraumatic stress and substance use disorders: A systematic review. *Clinical Psychology Review, 62*, 37–55. https://doi.org/10.1016/j.cpr.2018.05.003

Weathers, F. W., & Keane, T. M. (2007). The Criterion A problem revisited: Controversies and challenges in defining and measuring psychological trauma. *Journal of Traumatic Stress, 20*(2), 107–121. https://doi.org/10.1002/jts.20210

Weathers, F. W., Litz, B. T., Keane, T. M., Palmieri, P. A., Marx, B. P., & Schnurr, P. P. (2013). *The PTSD Checklist for DSM-5 (PCL-5)*. U.S. Department of Veterans Affairs, National Center for PTSD. https://www.ptsd.va.gov/professional/assessment/adult-sr/ptsd-checklist.asp

Weems, C. F., Russell, J. D., Herringa, R. J., & Carrion, V. G. (2021). Translating the neuroscience of adverse childhood experiences to inform policy and foster population-level resilience. *American Psychologist, 76*(2), 188–202. https://doi.org/10.1037/amp0000780

Willie, T. C., & Kershaw, T. S. (2019). An ecological analysis of gender inequality and intimate partner violence in the United States. *Preventive Medicine, 118*, 257–263. https://doi.org/10.1016/j.ypmed.2018.10.019

Wilson, L. C. (2018). The prevalence of military sexual trauma: A meta-analysis. *Trauma, Violence, & Abuse, 19*(5), 584–597. https://doi.org/10.1177/1524838016683459

Wolfe, J., & Kimerling, R. (1997). Gender issues in the assessment of posttraumatic stress disorder. In J. Wilson & T. M. Keane (Eds.), *Assessing psychological trauma and PTSD* (pp. 192–238). Guilford Press.

Wolynn, M. (2017). *It didn't start with you: How inherited family trauma shapes who we are and how to end the cycle*. Penguin Books.

World Health Organization. (2019). *International statistical classification of diseases* (11th rev.). https://icd.who.int

World Health Organization. (2022). ICD-11 *for mortality and morbidity statistics*. https://icd.who.int/browse11/l-m/en#/http://id.who.int/icd/entity/585833559

Yakubovich, A. R., Stöckl, H., Murray, J., Melendez-Torres, G. J., Steinert, J. I., Glavin, C. E., & Humphreys, D. K. (2018). Risk and protective factors for intimate partner violence against women: Systematic review and meta-analyses of prospective–longitudinal studies. *American Journal of Public Health, 108*(7), e1–e11. https://doi.org/10.2105/AJPH.2018.304428

Zeanah, C. H., Chesher, T., Boris, N. W., & American Academy of Child and Adolescent Psychiatry Committee on Quality Issues. (2016). Practice parameter for the assessment and treatment of children and adolescents with reactive attachment disorder and disinhibited social engagement disorder. *Journal of the American Academy of Child & Adolescent Psychiatry, 55*(11), 990–1003. https://doi.org/10.1016/j.jaac.2016.08.004

4 CONDUCTING THE ADULT PSYCHIATRIC ASSESSMENT

Kim K. Johnson

INTRODUCTION

The terms *psychiatric assessment* and *psychiatric evaluation* are commonly used interchangeably when discussing mental healthcare. Both describe the thorough procedure carried out by an APRN, psychiatrist, or other mental health professional to diagnose and formulate a plan for an individual's mental health condition. This procedure includes obtaining specific data about the individual's past and present symptoms, evaluation of current mental condition, diagnostic screening tools and instruments with the aim of gaining insight into the individual's mental processes, and determining the best course of treatment. For this chapter, we use the term *psychiatric assessment*.

The psychiatric assessment is the most important diagnostic tool an APRN employs to make an accurate diagnosis, case formulation, and treatment plan. The psychiatric assessment is primarily subjective, but also uses objective observation, which begins when the patient enters the office. The nurse practitioner (NP) must consider the patient's appearance and actions at the outset and in an ongoing manner, including gait, personal grooming, demeanor, and any unusual behaviors. The NP should observe whether the patient is dressed appropriately for the season. For example, the NP should note whether the patient presents to the clinic in the winter wearing summer clothes or whether the patient is wearing too many layers for comfort in the summer. Observable behaviors include the patient's hygiene, restlessness, body and facial demeanor or disposition, talking to themselves in the waiting area, pacing outside the office door, or having slowed body movements as with psychomotor impairment. These small indicators noted by an astute clinician will offer insight into the patient's illness, help guide questions for the interview, and provide indications for treatment.

A perceptive, sympathetic, and sensitively constructed psychiatric assessment can be a powerful therapeutic tool. Therapeutic assessment and communication aptitude will build over time. Obtaining a comprehensive history from the patient and, if necessary, from informed sources (e.g., family, past healthcare providers) is essential to making an accurate diagnosis to develop a specific, culturally sensitive case formulation and treatment plan (Sadock et al., 2017). Components of the psychiatric assessment include the reason for evaluation; history of present illness (HPI); past psychiatric history; history of substance use; general medical history; developmental, psychosocial, and sociocultural history; occupational and military history; family history; review of systems; mental status exam; values and belief systems; differential diagnosis; and case formulation. The NP may include a genogram in later sessions to provide the patient insight into familial patterns. The goals for the psychiatric assessment are to build a therapeutic alliance, gather data, demonstrate an understanding of the patient as a person with unique needs, and arrive at the most accurate understanding of how the NP can help the patient. When the patient and NP are fully engaged during the assessment process, comprehensive information leads to an accurate diagnosis and treatment plan. Decisions regarding treatment planning must be made by the NP in light of clinical data presented by the patient and the availability of diagnostic and treatment options available.

THE PSYCHIATRIC ASSESSMENT

PURPOSE
A. The psychiatric assessment is the start of a dialogue with patients upon which future assessments evolve.
B. With the increased prevalence of chronic medical conditions, the emphasis on healthcare delivery must shift to the ongoing management of chronic conditions.
C. Modifications applied by the NP to the psychiatric assessment offered in this guideline should be consistent with the purpose of the assessment, the practice setting, the patient's presenting problem, and the progressing information regarding the patient's symptomology (American Psychiatric Association, 2016).

OBJECTIVES
A. Establish the presence of a mental condition that requires management by an NP.
B. Collect sufficient data to support differential diagnoses and a comprehensive diagnosis.
C. Collaborate with the patient to develop an initial treatment plan that will encourage treatment compliance.
D. Consider any immediate interventions that may be needed to address the safety of the patient and others.
E. Identify longer term issues (e.g., personality disorder traits) that need to be considered in follow-up care.
F. Certain areas of the evaluation may need to be prioritized in consideration of the patient's reason for seeking evaluation and the patient's presenting problem.

GOALS
A. Identify psychiatric signs and symptoms, psychiatric disorders (including substance use disorders), and medical conditions (that could affect the treatment of a psychiatric diagnosis).
B. Identify patients who are at increased risk for suicide, self-harm, and violent or aggressive behaviors.
C. Identify factors that influence the therapeutic alliance, enrich clinical decision-making, provide for safe and appropriate treatment planning, and strengthen treatment outcomes.
D. Improve collaborative decision-making between patients and the clinician regarding treatment-related decisions, as well as increase coordination of psychiatric treatment with other clinicians who may be involved in the patient's care.

INPATIENT SETTINGS

A. Inpatient settings provide a structured and controlled setting in which patient safety can be monitored.
B. It allows continuous or frequent observation of symptoms while the patient is treated for psychiatric and general medical conditions through the collaboration of the multidisciplinary treatment team.
C. The level of observation in the inpatient environment is enhanced, which may aid the assessment of co-occurring medical and psychiatric conditions or evaluation for procedures such as electroconvulsive therapy. This is particularly relevant to individuals with complex psychiatric presentations.
D. It aids in resolving diagnostic dilemmas and may help determine the patient's ability to function safely and independently in a less restrictive setting.
E. If the patient has an unclear sensorium, such as delirium, hallucinations, or cognitive impairments, it is critical to interview people in the patient's familial network to understand if these are new or reoccurring symptoms, and to note previous treatment methods and outcomes. It is very useful to discuss their beliefs about the patient's illness and treatment, the patient's record of adherence to medication treatment, and concerns about discharge planning.
F. If family members do not perceive themselves as allies in treatment, the patient's treatment is likely to be compromised once they leave the inpatient setting.
G. Documentation of psychiatric evaluations in general medical charts should be sensitive to the standards of confidentiality of the nonpsychiatric medical sector and the possibility that charts may be read by persons who are not well-informed about psychiatric confidentiality, evaluation, and treatment.
   1. Information written in general medical charts should be limited to only information necessary for the medical team and should be conveyed with a level of detail that will be most helpful to the overall management of the patient.
   2. Documentation should offer sufficient detail to establish a diagnosis and treatment plan (American Psychiatric Association, 2016).

OUTPATIENT SETTINGS

A. Outpatient settings may include office-based practices, assertive community treatment from mental health centers, intensive outpatient, and partial hospital programs.
B. Evaluation in the outpatient setting usually differs in intensity from inpatient evaluation due to less frequent interviews, less immediate availability of laboratory or diagnostic services, and reduced availability of prompt consultation from other medical specialties.
C. The NP in the outpatient setting has fewer opportunities to systematically observe the patient's behavior and to quickly implement protective interventions.
   1. During frequent periods of evaluation, the clinician must reassess whether the patient requires hospitalization or more intensive outpatient care (e.g., greater visit frequency, intensive outpatient or partial hospital programs, or programs of assertive community treatment).
   2. Unresolved questions about the patient's medical status may require a rapid assessment in a structured setting (e.g., EDs or urgent care centers).
   3. If the patient's presentation is atypical (e.g., with respect to symptoms, symptom severity, or age at onset), a thorough medical workup may be required or coordinated with the patient's primary care provider (PCP). Patients who do not have a PCP will need assistance in obtaining an appropriate referral.
D. A change to the care setting should be considered, dependent on observation of the patient's current mental status and behavior, the patient's history of psychiatric symptoms and treatment, and the status of co-occurring medical conditions or substance use. Advantages of the outpatient setting include greater patient autonomy and the potential for a prolonged evaluation of the patient's symptoms.
   1. Evaluation of the patient in the context of psychoeducational or group therapy can augment one-to-one interviews.
   2. With the patient's permission, the clinician should note whether family and significant others are supportive of the patient's psychiatric treatment.
      a. If the patient states that family issues are problematic, an evaluation session with the family can provide valuable information, clarify treatment issues, and promote education regarding the use of therapy and biopsychological treatment.
E. When substance use is suspected, screening for substances and obtaining information and support from other involved persons (e.g., family, close friends), or regular testing for substances may be needed to improve treatment planning.

CONSULTATION IN THE AMBULATORY CARE SETTING

A. Consulting psychiatric assessments are conducted in the ED, urgent care, inpatient units, and other nonpsychiatric settings.
B. The level of behavioral observation and potential intervention in outpatient or ambulatory care settings must be continuously measured and assessed in consideration of a change in treatment setting.
C. Interruptions and lack of privacy can compromise evaluations performed in ambulatory care settings.
   1. Use a space in which the patient and the NP can meet privately. Developing an ongoing rapport with staff in ambulatory care settings will increase the likelihood of obtaining accurate behavioral data and ensuring that staff implements clinician recommendations.
D. Consider engaging staff for education to improve interactions in cases of noticeable hostility or anxiety with the patient.

BEGINNING THE ADULT PSYCHIATRIC ASSESSMENT

A. Patients' initial care experience and involvement in their care planning will impact behaviors (e.g., compliance with medicines as prescribed, returning for subsequent visits, remaining in care). The first few minutes of the meeting with a new healthcare provider are critical to establishing the patient–clinician relationship. Building rapport contributes to a better care experience and alleviates anxiety and distress, enriching the patients' ability to be involved in their care decisions.
B. The first moments of an initial assessment are vital to accomplishing alliance-building tasks:
   1. Provide appropriate greeting.
   2. Indicate preferred seating.
   3. Offer a brief introduction to the assessment process.
   4. Provide an open-ended invitation for the patient to explain how the NP can be of best service (Wheeler, 2020).
C. A prepared, well-organized, sequential approach to the interview will make the best use of the time, promote trust, and allow the patient to feel unrushed.

OBSERVATION

A. Mirroring the patient's body language can assist in establishing rapport. Allowing the patient to determine where they would like to sit and then sitting in an opposite manner mirrors their sitting posture. There are a variety of verbal and nonverbal techniques to maximize the assessment interview. Some of these include attentive listening, making eye contact, establishing equal body level (e.g., sitting or standing as the patient does, and leaning slightly toward the patient expressing interest in the comments).

ESTABLISHING RAPPORT

A. Create a safe space. Set a comfortable temperature, provide white noise for privacy, and offer water to ease apprehension.
B. Provide comfort objects like tissues, pillows, and a fidget toy, with soothing decor.
C. Place a wall clock behind the patient so as to monitor time.
D. Make a clear introduction—speak sincerely and warmly when stating name, role, and interview purpose.
E. Speak directly to the patient, noting their eye contact. Maintain appropriate eye contact throughout the interview, leaning toward the patient from a comfortable distance.
F. Maintain an open and inviting posture at a comfortable distance, establishing equal body level (e.g., sitting or standing as the patient does).
G. Concentrate on the patient's words, respond appropriately, and consistently show understanding and concern by nodding and gesturing.
H. Adopt a calm approach if the patient speaks quietly, reflecting reserved confidence—similar personalities between patients and healthcare providers can improve symptom reduction.

ACTIVE LISTENING

A. Ask understandable, open-ended questions to encourage comprehensive sharing. Give the patient time to respond.
B. Demonstrate genuine warmth, comfort, and caring in the interview process.
C. Validate the patient's thoughts and ideas.
D. Tools for active listening include the following:
   1. Summarizing and repeating what the patient says
   2. Adjusting communication to the patient's language
   3. Asking clarifying questions

IDENTIFY THE PATIENT

A. Note the patient's identity, including legal name and preferred name, preferred gender and pronoun as appropriate, birth date and age, marital status, race, ethnicity, and language.

INFORMED CONSENT

A. A psychiatric assessment conducted and documented against the patient's will is considered assault with battery.
B. Secure the patient's permission to assess and enter the psychiatric information.
C. If the assessment is performed in an emergency and consent cannot be acquired, document why it cannot be acquired and why the assessment is being done without the patient's approval.
D. Introductory statements and questions that meet this criterion can begin with: "Hello, John. It is nice to meet you in person. Please, sit down where you would like. I am a nurse practitioner, and I would like to understand your difficulties in today's session. With your permission, I will ask questions about important areas of your life and take notes as I do not want to miss anything."

THE ADULT PSYCHIATRIC ASSESSMENT

CHIEF COMPLAINT

A. The initial focus should center on the chief complaint or main issue prompting the examination. The chief complaint should be documented in quotations using the patient's own words. After the introduction, allow the patient to sit and observe the patient's behavior.
   1. The clinician may begin the process by asking "Can you tell me what brings you in today?"
   2. The patient's response should be documented as the chief complaint. An example of a written chief complaint would be "I'm here for my anxiety."
   3. Look for a chronological account of what led up to the chief complaint, when it started, and how long it has lasted. Note the severity, timing, context, what makes it better or worse, and the associated signs or symptoms.

HISTORY OF PRESENT ILLNESS

A. The HPI should include sufficient detail on the reason for the patient visit, the chronological history of current symptoms, recent exacerbations, and remissions. Note onset, duration, severity, timing, context, associated symptoms, and what makes it better or worse.
   1. Elicit descriptions of worries, changes in mood, changes in patterns of pleasure (anhedonia), libido, helplessness/hopelessness/regret, preoccupations, delusions, or hallucinatory experiences, as well as recent changes in energy level, fatigue, motivation, sleep, appetite, concentration, memory, or behavior, including suicidal or aggressive behaviors. Individuals experiencing anxiety may progressively find diminished pleasure in activities that provoke anxiety, subsequently catalyzing the emergence of depressive symptoms.
   2. Document symptoms that are positive (present) and negative (not present).
   3. Explore recent onset and exacerbation of the severity of symptoms and possible causes for the new onset (e.g., onset after use of licit or illicit substances, variation in symptoms with the menstrual cycle, postpartum onset).
   4. Note new environmental influences believed to precipitate, aggravate, or modify the current presenting symptoms (e.g., taking a challenging course or new responsibilities at work or home).
   5. Obtain details of previous treatments and the patient's response to those treatments to steer the course of future treatment.
   6. Note duration of symptoms; if long-standing, the reason for seeking treatment at this specific time is relevant. If a hospitalization precipitates the evaluation, the reason for the hospitalization is needed.
   7. Note the reason for the requested assessment if the patient did not initiate the evaluation.
   8. Seek input from other sources as needed (e.g., with patients experiencing psychosis or those who are less communicative).
   9. Consider that many psychiatric patients present in crisis from undiagnosed and untreated psychiatric symptoms. They may minimize their symptoms until you build a trusting relationship.
   10. Document descriptions of the patient's significant symptoms. The interview may determine the following:
      a. Symptoms the patient is experiencing (e.g., worries, preoccupations, changes in mood, delusions or

hallucinatory experiences, recent changes in sleep, appetite, libido, concentration, memory, appetite, or behavior, including suicidal or aggressive behaviors)
b. Severity of the patient's symptoms (Have the symptoms gotten worse or fluctuated?)
c. Associated features of specific psychiatric syndromes (i.e., pertinent positive or negative factors) present or absent during the present illness
d. Factors that the patient believes precipitate, aggravate, modify the illness, or are related to the current symptoms
e. Prior treatment for this episode or a similar illness
f. Existing relationships with clinicians who care for the patient (Note an information release form must be signed if the patient consents to collaboration.)
g. Chronological order or timeline of symptoms, when they worsened, and any precipitating events
h. Patient's baseline functioning (An example would be "I used to be so energetic.")
i. Repeating above components if there is more than one possible diagnosable disorder
j. Last period of and length of stability, perceived reason the patient was able to maintain stability at that time
k. Reasons given by other involved parties (e.g., family, friends) for seeking help
   i. When the patient responds to questioning with disagreement that there is a problem or by withholding information, the NP may reword their initial question.
      (a) For example: "Why does your family feel you need to be seen?" The patient may respond, "My family says I stay in bed all day, and they think I'm depressed." The clinician should ask the patient what the patient believes about this concern. For example: "Are you staying in bed all day?" or "What do you think about their concern?"
      (b) Allowing the patient to share their feelings regarding why they presented builds trust and helps them understand that the clinician is their advocate.
l. Obtain information regarding the patient's goal for seeking treatment. Discuss and educate how the clinician can help the patient achieve their goals while detailing limitations to care. Assisting patients to set frequent, realistic targets increases their chances of success by maximizing time and resources toward their primary objective. Accomplishing frequent goals (even small) helps keep the patient motivated to participate in care.
   i. "What is your goal for seeking help?" or "How would you like me to help you?"
   ii. Patients with depression have more difficulty setting goals and are less likely to believe they can achieve them. The NP can encourage and make evident how their needs can be met. The NP can provide resources for care needed outside their scope of practice.

HISTORY OF PSYCHIATRIC ILLNESS
A. The past psychiatric history includes a chronological summary of all past episodes of mental illness, including substance use disorders and treatment.

1. It includes prior hospitalizations, suicide attempts, self-harm, or other self-destructive behavior.
2. The interview should assess any psychiatric illness not formally diagnosed at the time, previously established diagnoses, treatments offered, and responses to and satisfaction with treatment.
3. Concerning psychotherapy, it is essential to ascertain the type (e.g., psychodynamic, cognitive, behavioral, supportive), format (e.g., individual, group, couple), frequency, duration, patient's perception of the alliance, and compliance.
4. Obtain a complete list of medications the patient has been prescribed in the past and present. The dose, efficacy, side effects, treatment duration, and adherence are essential to ascertain while understanding that compliance mistakes are more likely when treatment involves more than one medication.
5. When medical records are available and readily accessible, they must be consulted for supplementary information. The chronological timeline should describe the most recent periods of stability and episodes when the patient was functionally impaired or distressed by behavioral symptoms, even if no formal treatment occurred. Such episodes can be identified by asking the patient about the past use of psychotropic medications prescribed by other clinicians, including unexplained episodes of social, school, or occupational dysfunction.
6. Knowledge of prior psychiatric diagnoses helps the clinician update current diagnoses because there may be a continuation of a previous disorder or may now have a different condition that is commonly comorbid with the first. Information on treatment-related side effects is essential to predict tolerance and safety of future treatment (e.g., agranulocytosis with clozapine, neuroleptic malignant syndrome, serotonergic syndromes, tardive dyskinesia, severe dystonic reactions) and/or discontinuation concerns,
7. If adherence to medication treatment has been troublesome, inquire about past reactions, length of taking medication, and side effects. These will suggest the tolerability or feasibility of future medication treatment. For example, the patient states, "I've tried every medication, and nothing works." The clinician should prod the patient to discuss how the medication was prescribed (e.g., started on too high of a dose), the length of time they took each medication (e.g., took medication a few weeks and saw no results, so discontinued), and whether the patient had side effects (after starting at too high of a dose, the patient had intolerable nausea, or the medication made them too tired during the day, so they discontinued). Education by the clinician regarding starting medication at lower doses, scheduling drugs at more appropriate times, or the time frame the clinician expects the side effects to subside should increase compliance. Some medication treatment is less likely to benefit the patient or could be harmful depending on the prior psychiatric diagnoses or comorbidities (e.g., antidepressants in depressive episodes that occur in the context of bipolar disorder, use of bupropion in patients with an eating disorder).
8. Note previous procedures and therapies such as electroconvulsive therapy; information on the number of treatment sessions, treatment course duration, technical parameters, efficacy, and side effects is similarly helpful to obtain.

9. Document descriptions of the following:
   a. Past psychiatric treatment and precipitating factors for past treatment
      i. Treatment setting (e.g., inpatient, intensive outpatient, partial hospitalization, outpatient)
      ii. Number of treatments and duration of treatment
      iii. History of violence, self-harm, and trauma
      iv. Compliance with past and current pharmacologic and nonpharmacologic psychiatric treatments
         (a) What treatment worked, what treatment did not work, allergic or adverse reactions to medication treatment, type, duration, and, where applicable, doses
   b. History of therapy
      i. Therapeutic provider
      ii. Duration of therapy
      iii. Outcome of therapy, noting any unpleasant reaction to therapy and reconsidering the initial diagnosis if the patient has not responded well to past treatments
      iv. Previous coping skills developed in or out of therapy (e.g., What has helped you cope with past adversity?)
         (a) Obtain an example (helps build a list of strengths).
         (b) What has sustained the patient during this stressful time?

HISTORY OF SUBSTANCE ABUSE

A. The history of substance use includes past and present legal and illicit psychoactive substances, including but not limited to alcohol, caffeine, nicotine, marijuana, synthetic cannabinoids, opiates (e.g., heroin, opioid medications), sedative-hypnotic agents, stimulants (e.g., methamphetamine, cocaine), solvents, methylenedioxymethamphetamine (MDMA), androgenic steroids, and hallucinogens (e.g., lysergic acid diethylamide [LSD], peyote), as well as psychoactive herbs such as *Salvia divinorum*, kratom, kava, and morning glory seeds.
B. Assess the patient's use or misuse of prescribed or over-the-counter medications or supplements. Ensuring that initial psychiatric evaluations include an assessment of substance use may clarify differential diagnoses that present as other disorders (e.g., the use of ginseng or kava may exacerbate or cause anxiety).
C. Relevant information includes the quantity and frequency of use; route of administration; the pattern of use (e.g., intermittent vs. continual, private vs. social); functional, interpersonal, or legal consequences of use; tolerance during use and withdrawal after discontinuation; and any self-perceived benefits of use.
D. Inquire about prior treatment decision-making for substance use disorders and periods of abstinence, including the current and past duration and factors contributing to relapse or supporting sobriety. Obtaining a substance use history often involves a gradual, nonjudgmental approach by asking several questions that seek the same information differently. If necessary, use slang terminology to determine the types of substances used, gather patterns of use, and establish drug effects for accuracy. Patients are particularly likely to underestimate their level of substance use and misjudge related functional impairments; thus, corroboration by other sources may be necessary.
E. Inquire about patterns of substance use by family members or those who live in the home with the patient. Naming potential substances can remind the patient of substances not previously considered when answering the question.
F. Assessing the patient's substance use history requires a documented description of the following:
   1. History of substances used, and the start and end of use
      a. Note substances used, including quantity, frequency, and pattern of use. Determining route of administration can herald present or future physical conditions (e.g., intravenous drug use can progress to infectious disease).
      b. Determine functional, social, occupational, or legal consequences or self-perceived benefits of use.
      c. Explore whether tolerance or withdrawal symptoms have been noted.
      d. Note whether substance use has been associated with psychiatric symptoms.
   2. Family members available to provide corroborating information about the patient's use and its consequences (e.g., car accidents, falls, family problems)
   3. Daily caffeine, nicotine, vaping
   4. Use of any natural substances in protein powders for working out
   5. Use of aggression, problems with the law, injuries, or depression when using

GENERAL MEDICAL HISTORY

A. Clinical training and education equips the clinician in understanding the complex relationship between psychiatric and other medical illnesses. The clinician must evaluate medical and psychological data, make diagnoses, and work with patients to develop treatment plans.
B. Medical history should include available information on known medical illnesses (e.g., hospitalizations, procedures, treatments, and medications), drug sensitivities, and health problems that have caused the patient distress or functional impairment.
   1. Any episodes of physical injury, trauma, sexual and reproductive history, endocrine disorders, infectious disease (including but not limited to HIV, tuberculosis, and hepatitis C), neurologic disorders, sleep disorders (including sleep apnea), and conditions causing emotional distress
      a. Any specific history regarding physical symptoms that may impact the patient's mental health is particularly important.
      b. Examples of pertinent psychiatric medical health information include an infectious disease caused by intravenous drugs, a pulmonary disorder with a patient who smokes marijuana, or an untreated chronic medical illness due to psychosis.
C. Medical information should include all current and recent medications, including hormonal replacement, birth control pills, side effects, over-the-counter medicines, vitamins, complementary medical treatments, and trialed or failed psychiatric drugs.
D. With all aspects of the medical history, obtaining corroborating information (e.g., medical records, treating clinicians, and family) can be helpful since details or difficulties in recall can lead to omission.
E. The initial psychiatric evaluation should initially include an assessment of the patient's constitutional evidence (e.g., fever, weight loss, energy level), height, weight, body mass index (BMI), vital signs, skin (including any signs of trauma, self-injury, or drug use), sexually transmitted disease, history

of vitamin deficiency, and locally endemic infectious diseases (e.g., Lyme disease). If the patient cannot recall medical illnesses, ask what conditions they take medication for, how often, and who prescribed their current medication. This will remind the patient of medically treated disease (e.g., "Yes, I do have diabetes").

F. Medical history inquiries should include the following areas:
1. Constitutional symptoms, particularly energy levels, hygiene, and eye contact
2. BMI
   a. Monitor for food restriction, eating disorder, or weight gain that could contribute to metabolic syndrome.
   b. Proper psychiatric medication therapy must include weight gain or loss considerations.
3. Vital signs
   a. Blood pressure and heart rate as blood pressure changes or tachycardia may indicate caution is needed when considering psychiatric medication therapy.
4. Pulmonary and cardiovascular disorders
   a. Elevated blood pressure, tachycardia, or arrhythmias may limit stimulants.
   b. Cigarette smoking is the most potent risk factor for chronic obstructive pulmonary disease (COPD), development of structural lung disease, airflow obstruction, and functional outcomes. Indicate the number of years the patient has smoked and packs per day.
5. Endocrine disease
   a. Glycated hemoglobin (A1c) test and thyroid levels should be taken before psychiatric medication therapy to rule out a medical reason for unexpected rapid and unpredictable mood changes.
   b. Common mood problems related to endocrine disorders may include overactivity, nervousness, and heart rate elevation with anxiety or underactivity that precipitates low mood, loss of appetite, poor energy, or disturbed sleep.
6. Sexual and reproductive history
   a. Determine the patient's developmental sexual orientation and gender identity to best organize a plan of care for the patient.
   b. The stability of relationships, risky sexual behavior, and sexually transmitted infection (STI) must be noted. An STI can mimic psychiatric disorders, including irritability, confusion, psychosis, and dementia (e.g., neurosyphilis).
   c. Determine the number of pregnancies, current children, and history of postpartum depression and postpartum psychosis in the patient or family.
7. Head, eyes, ears, nose, throat (HEENT)
   a. Determine hearing or sight deficits that impair the quality of therapeutic interventions.
8. Neurologic history
   a. Determine history of head injury, concussion, repetitive damage from sports, loss of consciousness, episodes of short- or long-term memory loss, headaches, and neuroimaging, including the outcome of the imaging.
9. Dermatologic issues
   a. The overall reduced physical condition of many mentally ill patients is associated with a reduced immune defense and increased susceptibility to skin infections. Examples of skin conditions that should be observed include the following:
      i. Scars or cigarette burns from self-injury, abuse
      ii. Obliteration of peripheral veins, hyperpigmentation of the overlying skin, punched-out scars, persistent edema following thrombophlebitis, and any excoriations due to intravenous drug use or heroin, pruritus
      iii. Multiple sores and scabs from an excoriation disorder
      iv. Severe acne or skin disfiguring skin resulting in decreased self-esteem, depression, or social phobias
      v. Parasitic infectious skin diseases as they are commonly comorbid with mood disorders
      vi. Psoriasis, atopic dermatitis, eczema, leg ulcers, or wounds that fail to heal, which can be associated with depression and anxiety
      vii. Darkened or stained fingertips or nails from smoking illicit drugs or cigarettes or drugs
10. Further exploration of history of hospitalizations, trauma, and surgeries and other conditions
    a. Obstructive sleep apnea (OSA): Repeated cessations in breathing and ongoing sleep deprivation can lead to behavior changes, stress disorders, memory loss, anxiety and depression, headaches, and low energy. Proper treatment of OSA, including the use of continuous positive airway pressure (CPAP) when indicated, can help maintain adequate oxygen levels during sleep. Compliance is often an issue due to discomfort, inconvenience, or other factors.
    b. Hospitalizations, ED visits, frequent doctor's visits, or surgery from accidents, abuse, injury, rape, or somatic complaints
11. Medication history
    a. History of side effects of medications, drug sensitivities, hormonal replacement, birth control pills, androgens, use of natural substances
    b. Trialed or failed psychiatric medications, side effects, duration of use, dosages, discontinuation syndrome, serotonin syndrome
    c. Over-the-counter medications, vitamins, natural substances, and complementary or alternative medical treatments
12. Pain, ambulation, accessibility of care, or difficulty getting to appointments
    a. Does chronic medical or psychiatric illness prevent daily functioning?
    b. Does pain exacerbate the psychiatric illness or prevent the patient from seeking treatment?
    c. Does chronic medical or psychiatric illness prevent care of recurring disease (e.g., the patient has schizophrenia, untreated diabetes, and elevated blood pressure and cannot afford to seek treatment for all three comorbidities)
13. Allergies and sensitivity to medication

DEVELOPMENTAL HISTORY

A. Suboptimal life functioning is highly correlated with chronic mental illness. Thus, an assessment of trauma should be included in the initial fact-finding interview.

B. Diagnostic accuracy requires gathering information about the development and duration of prodromal signs and symptoms, which may indicate the early onset of mood disorders, schizophrenia, neurodevelopmental disorders, personality disorders, and attention deficit disorder.

C. Adverse childhood events include early-age trauma, including parental neglect, food insecurity, living in a home ▶

where alcohol or drugs were used, loss of a parent, and witnessing domestic violence.

D. The peak age of incidence for many psychiatric disorders, including depression, coincides with life transitions (e.g., hormonal changes associated with puberty are likely to have the most significant impact in adolescence, a period when depression rises).

E. A developmental perspective is essential to investigate risk exposures, protective factors, and resilience to trauma. This information helps the NP establish interventions specific to the patient (e.g., "When you had severe anxiety in your teens, you removed yourself from anxiety-provoking situations and listened to music. How can you use that past action in this scenario?").

F. Developmental history inquiries should include the following areas:
  1. Assess developmental milestones and academic and social development.
  2. Seek patient perception of adverse childhood experiences (ACEs) as evidence supporting adult physical and mental health sequela is documented. Some of these include parental or sibling serious illness or death, sudden accidental or violent death of a loved one, and hospitalization; parental divorce, separation, remarriage, and relocation; physical, emotional, and sexual abuse; severe human suffering; life-threatening illness or injury to self or close others; serious accidents; physical and/or sexual assaults; captivity; combat or exposure to a war zone; and natural disasters.
  3. Does the patient have any of the following risk factors for ACEs (e.g., multiracial and native peoples, less than a high school education, low income, unemployed or underemployed, and LGBTQ+ community)?
  4. What has been the patient's capacity to maintain interpersonal relationships, and what is the patient's history of and satisfaction with marital and other significant relationships?
  5. What is the patient's sexual history, including sexual orientation, beliefs, and practices?
  6. What past or current psychosocial stressors have affected the patient (including the primary support group, social environment, education, occupation, housing, economic status, and access to healthcare)?
  7. What strategies for coping have the patient used successfully during times of stress?
  8. What is the patient's capacity for self-care? What are the patient's sociocultural supports (e.g., family, friends, work, religious, and other community groups)?
  9. What are the patient's preferences and values regarding their health?

PSYCHOSOCIAL HISTORY

A. The clinician must assess family, peer networks, and other support systems as an essential part of the psychiatric assessment due to the potential positive or negative role of these support systems in the patient's mental health. This is particularly true when assessing individuals with multilayered biopsychosocial or cultural challenges, chronic mental illness, and medical conditions (e.g., an Asian patient with depression who is far from their family and has a language barrier).

B. Ask about the patient's social network, such as size, proximity, and engagement of spouse, children, parents, aunts and uncles, and siblings, as well as current living situations, divorce, death, and births.

C. Culturally competent care must be integrated into the treatment plan to support system beliefs about treatment and medication therapy as this may influence compliance (e.g., "My husband doesn't believe I need psychiatric medicine").

D. While the NP generates a treatment plan for the patient's diagnosis and individual healthcare needs, the evaluation may suggest the need for education for family support systems and coordination with psychiatric professionals (e.g., therapists), medical providers, or governmental agencies (e.g., community mental health centers or family service agencies).

E. The patient's capacity to maintain stable and gratifying interpersonal relationships should be noted, including the patient's capacities for attachment, trust, and intimacy.

F. A sexual history is obtained and includes consideration of sexual orientation and practices, past sexual experiences (including unwanted experiences), and cultural beliefs about sex.

G. Psychosocial history also ascertains the patient's past and present levels of interpersonal functioning in family and social roles such as marriage and parenting. For patients with children (including biological, foster, adopted, or stepchildren), the psychosocial history should include information about these individuals, their relationship to the patient, and relational stressors.

H. As part of psychosocial history, past or current stressors are assessed, including social environment (e.g., discrimination and acculturation), education, occupation, housing, economic status, and access to healthcare.

I. Specific information obtained during evaluating psychosocial stressors should include details about the patient's living arrangements, access to transportation, sources of income, insurance or prescription coverage, and use of social agencies.

J. The NP should assess the patient's self-care to consider money management skills and gambling behavior.

K. Psychosocial history inquiries should include the following areas:
  1. Presence of legal issues (Is the patient in trouble legally? On parole? Probation? Pending or incarcerated?)
  2. Financial (What is the patient's financial status?)
     a. The challenges that adults with mental illness face are made more difficult if they are living in poverty. Limited financial resources may need services from social services to access behavioral healthcare.
  3. Housing, cultural, school/occupational, or interpersonal/relationship problems
  4. The presence or lack of support from family or other support systems
  5. Psychosocial stressors that affect the patient's mental health
  6. How social support influence patients' compliance with medication and treatment

SOCIOCULTURAL HISTORY

A. The sociocultural history establishes the patient's past and current sociocultural influences and stressors and other significant cultural and religious effects on the patient's life.

B. Balancing factors: What gives meaning to the patient's life? Does the patient have hobbies or interests? How do they recreate? What are they good at? Do they participate in sports? Healthy lifestyle factors: diet, exercise, meditation? Who does the patient love and feel loved by? Friendships? Emphasis is given to familial and nonfamilial relationships and to religion and spirituality, which may have meaning and purpose in the patient's life.

C. Depending on the focus and extent of the initial psychiatric assessment, a complete sociocultural evaluation based on the findings of the initial interview may not be possible. However, when sociocultural issues emerge, they may be explored further during subsequent meetings with the patient. This analysis begins with a review of the individual's ethnicity, acculturation/biculturality, language, age, gender, socioeconomic status, sexual orientation, religious and spiritual beliefs, disabilities, political orientation, and health literacy, among other factors.

D. This analysis looks at how the patient's culture affects how they express (display) and understand their symptoms and problems. It also takes into account how the patient describes their own feelings of distress and compares these descriptions with what is considered normal in their culture.

E. Treatment experiences and preferences must be identified, including complementary and alternative medicine and indigenous approaches. Each patient presents for a psychiatric assessment with their preferences and value systems for treatment, which may involve cultural explanatory models of illness that affect attitudes, expectations, and priorities for professional and popular therapies (e.g., "I prefer Christian counseling provided by my church").

F. Sociocultural history inquiries should include the following areas:
  1. Patient's cultural, religious, and spiritual beliefs, and how these developed or changed over time
  2. The effect of sociocultural, cultural, religious, or spiritual beliefs on treatment decisions
  3. The sources the patient prefers for decision-making (e.g., spiritual leader, patriarchal, or matriarchal figures)
  4. Should include influential partners in treatment education and decision-making sessions
  5. Should incorporate all social values into care

OCCUPATIONAL, EDUCATIONAL, AND MILITARY HISTORY

A. Educational history: What is the patient's highest level of education? This information informs the clinician on how to interact with the patient. Were there any disciplinary issues at school? Academic? Social? Bullying?

B. Occupational history describes the patient's previous jobs in the past 5 years, if the patient was ever fired or let go, and current or most recent employment, including quality and fulfillment of work and work relationships, and whether present or recent jobs have involved shift work, a toxic or perilous environment, exposure to hazardous materials, unusual physical or psychological stress, or injury or exposure to trauma while in the dangerous occupations (e.g., nursing, fire and rescue, law enforcement). Work skills, strengths, and the patient's relationships with coworkers and work supervisors are noted.
  1. Past or current experience with the workers' compensation and patterns of recovery or disability following episodes of illness should be determined.
  2. A history of preparation for and adjustment to retirement is included when appropriate.
  3. Relevant data about military experience include volunteer, recruited, or draftee status; combat exposure; disciplinary actions; and discharge status. Occupational and military history inquiries should include the following areas:
     a. Identify the patient's current and past occupations, jobs the patient held, and any history of job loss.
     b. Identify the patient's work skills and strengths.
     c. How important is the patient's work to their identity?
     d. What is the quality of the patient's work relationships?
     e. Is the patient unable to work due to a disability?
  4. Regarding military service, what was the patient's status (volunteer, recruit, or draftee)? Did the patient experience combat or war zone? Did the patient suffer injury or trauma?
  5. Is the patient preparing for or adjusting to retirement?

FAMILY HISTORY

A. The family history includes available information about the patient's family constellation, family dynamics, the strength of relationships, and familial and genetic medical and psychiatric history. Information obtained about close family members, including parents, siblings, spouse, and children, will include general information (e.g., current age or age at time of death, the position of siblings, and occupation), quality of relationship to the patient, and health status.

B. General medical and psychiatric illness in close relatives is noted, including disorders that may be familial or strongly affect the family environment. Family history information will include any history of psychiatric hospitalizations, illness, or significant symptoms, including suicide and attempted suicide in first- and second-degree relatives.

C. A history of adoption or foster care or disruptions in the family environment due to divorce, remarriage, prolonged absences of family members (e.g., occupational absences, hospitalization, incarceration), or deaths may be helpful to elicit.

D. Depending on the patient's clinical presentation, more specific questions are essential, given the heritability of psychosis; mood disorders; anxiety disorders; cognitive disorders; learning disabilities; developmental disabilities, including autism, hyperactivity, or attention deficit disorder; substance use disorders; and personality disorders.

E. For family members who have experienced psychiatric symptoms, it is helpful to ascertain the treatment received and their response to treatment. It is also essential to determine first- and second-degree relatives' history of medical disorders relevant to psychiatric illness and treatment, such as cardiac, neurologic, and endocrine disorders.

F. If family health problems are current, this may contribute to psychological or financial stress for the patient. The construction of a formal genogram is often helpful in delineating family relationships and identifying a family history of illness.

G. Family history inquiries should include the following areas:
  1. Family composition, the strength of relationships, and sibling order
  2. Past family history of diagnosed or undiagnosed mental illness, treatment successes, and failures (Does the family support the person with mental illness? How do they support that person?)
  3. Familial psychiatric symptomology (e.g., hallucinations, bizarre behavior, cognitive problems, memory loss), treatment, and collective belief regarding psychiatric illness
  4. Familial psychiatric genetic history (e.g., schizophrenia, bipolar disorder, mood disorders, developmental delays, and neuropsychiatric disorders)
  5. Current or past family members' use of substances, treatment, familial attitudes toward substances (e.g., Does the family use substances together?)
  6. Current family members with psychiatric treatment, including medications used and efficacy of medication treatment
  7. Common side effects observed with prescribed or over-the-counter medications and other treatments, including complementary or alternative therapies

MENTAL STATUS EXAMINATION

A. The clinician will assess the patient's mental status by describing the patient's clinical presentation and cognitive functioning. The mental status exam assists with accurate diagnosis and establishes baseline functioning information in the initial interview.

B. The skilled clinician will have evaluated mental status throughout history taking and then focus upon specific areas of concern at the end of the interview. The mental status exam will be performed again in each session to determine and document improvement or worsening of symptoms.

C. Sensorium and level of cognitive function
  1. Orientation, attention, concentration, short- and long-term memory, level of intelligence, and executive functioning
  2. Patient's level of insight, judgment, and capacity for abstract reasoning
  3. Patient's motivation to change their health risk behaviors

D. Appearance and behavior
  1. Approximate age, dress, grooming, hygiene, and distinguishing features (e.g., scars, tattoos)
  2. Level of distress, degree of eye contact, and attitude toward the interviewer

E. Psychomotor activity
  1. Presence of any gait abnormalities, purposeless, repetitive, or unusual postures or movements (e.g., tremors, dyskinesias, akathisia, mannerisms, tics, catatonic posturing, echopraxia, responses to hallucinations)

F. Speech
  1. Rate, rhythm, volume, slurred, accent, inflection, fluency, articulation, and pressure

G. Mood and affect
  1. Expressions of mood in reference to the patient's internal, subjective, and more sustained emotional state
  2. Affect relating to the patient's externally observable and changeable emotions; affect range, intensity, stability, appropriateness, and congruence with the topic discussed in the interview

H. Thought processes
  1. Includes speech and flow of ideas, self-contradiction, incoherence, circumstantiality, tangentiality, perseveration, neologisms, loose associations, and flight of ideas

I. Thought content
  1. Spontaneously expressed worries, concerns, thoughts, and impulses
  2. Delusions (e.g., delusions of persecution, grandeur, poverty, somatic illness, guilt)
  3. Thought insertion, thought broadcasting, ideas of reference, ruminations, obsessions, compulsions, and phobias
  4. Safety assessment of suicidal, homicidal, aggressive, or self-injurious thoughts, feelings, or impulses essential in determining the patient's risk to self or others; if such thoughts are present, must elicit intensity and specificity, when they occur, and what prevents the patient from acting on the thoughts

J. Perceptual disturbances
  1. Hallucinations and type: visual, auditory, olfactory, tactile, and gustatory
  2. Illusions: presence of a flawed perception (e.g., hearing the wind and mistaking it for someone crying)
     a. Depersonalization
     b. Derealization

K. Sensorium and cognition: level of consciousness and stability
  1. Orientation (e.g., person, place, time, situation)
  2. Attention and concentration
  3. Memory (e.g., short-term, long-term)
  4. Language function with naming, comprehension, repetition, and reading
  5. Abstract reasoning (e.g., explaining similarities or interpreting proverbs)
  6. Executive function (e.g., list-making, inhibiting impulsive answers, resisting distraction, recognizing contradictions)

L. Insight
  1. Awareness of problems and their implications (e.g., recognize psychosis, that behavior affects their relationships, potential benefits of treatment)
  2. Motivation to change their health risk behaviors
     a. Motivation often fluctuates over time from denial and resistance to ambivalence to commitment

M. Judgment
  1. The quality of the patient's judgment may be assessed by asking for the patient's response to a hypothetical situation (e.g., smelling smoke in a theater).
  2. Assess the patient's responses and decision-making in terms of self-care, interactions, and other aspects of recent or current situations and behavior.
  3. If the patient reports having aggressive ideas, assess the patient's impulsivity, including anger management issues.
  4. Determine the patient's access to firearms; identify specific persons toward whom homicidal or aggressive ideas or behaviors have been directed.
  5. Ask about history of violent behaviors in the patient's biological relatives. There is no evidence that the risk of aggression is increased by asking about past experiences, symptoms such as impulsivity, or current aggressive and homicidal ideas or plans.

N. The intended course of action if symptoms worsen

O. Patient's access to suicide methods, including firearms

P. Possible motivations for suicide (e.g., attention or reaction from others, revenge, shame, humiliation, delusional guilt, command hallucinations) and reasons for living or protective factors against suicide (e.g., sense of responsibility to children or others, religious beliefs)
  1. The American Psychiatric Association recommends that clinicians evaluate the patient's current suicidal ideas, plans, and intent, including active or passive thoughts of suicide or death, such as:
     a. Prior suicidal ideas, plans, and attempts, including attempts that were aborted or interrupted
     b. Prior intentional self-injury in which there was no suicide intent
     c. Current hopelessness and impulsivity
     d. Current or recent substance use disorder or change in use of alcohol or other substances
     e. Aggressive or unbalanced ideas, including thoughts of physical or sexual aggression or homicide
     f. The intended course of action if symptoms worsen (e.g., patient's access to suicide methods, including firearms); possible motivations for suicide (e.g., attention or reaction from others, revenge, shame, humiliation, delusional guilt, command hallucinations) and reasons for living (e.g., sense of responsibility to children or others, religious beliefs)
     g. Details of each attempt (e.g., context, method, damage, potential lethality, intent), if the patient has attempted suicide in the past

h. Patient's possible motivations for suicide (e.g., attention or reaction from others, revenge, shame, humiliation, delusional guilt, command hallucinations)
i. Reasons for living (e.g., sense of responsibility to children or others, religious beliefs)

SELF-REPORT QUESTIONNAIRES AND RATING SCALES

A. Forms and surveys (e.g., Beck Depression Inventory, General Anxiety Disorder-7, Vanderbilt Rating Scale, Alcohol Use Disorders Identification Test) may be used to screen and monitor improvement or worsening of baseline symptomology.
B. Rating scales may be used to detect prodromal symptoms or symptoms that are not yet severe enough for diagnosis. To be most useful, rating scales need to be valid and reliable and demonstrate practical utility in inpatient, outpatient, and ambulatory psychiatric clinical settings.
C. The patient or concerned parties may complete the forms (e.g., teachers, advisors) or with the clinician.
D. Questionnaires or rating scales may be computerized or documented with written responses. The need for these surveys decreases over time, but they remain valuable reference points during subsequent visits (e.g., the patient does not notice they are improving; however, their self-report responses demonstrate otherwise). Self-report of improvement in subsequent interviews discloses which areas the patient no longer has trouble (e.g., psychopathologic sleep issues, appetite, hopelessness) and clarifies areas that are reticent and need attention.

RISK ASSESSMENT

A. Risk assessment formulation involves assessing the patient's risk of harm to self or others, which is the primary concern. It is vital to analyze the patient's risk to self or others. Predictions can be difficult; however, clinical judgment is necessary when considering the patient's stated danger, present mental status, risk factors, and protective factors (e.g., the individual whose thought content is not reality-based).
B. The risk formulation should consider suicide or homicide risk, as well as other forms of self-injury (e.g., cutting behaviors, accidents), aggressive behaviors, neglect of self-care, or neglect of the care of dependents.
C. The risk assessment should identify specific factors that may increase or decrease the patient's degree of risk, the clinician's ability to plan specific interventions that may modify particular risk factors, and the clinician's ability to address the safety of the patient or others.
D. Specific risk factors may include demographic considerations (e.g., age, gender), past behavior (e.g., suicide attempts, self-injury, aggression), psychiatric diagnoses, presentation (e.g., anger, despair, hopelessness), co-occurring chronic medical conditions (e.g., pain, inability to care for selves), sociocultural factors, psychosocial stressors, and individual vulnerabilities.
E. Standardized rating scales for suicidal or aggressive behaviors may suggest helpful lines of clinical inquiry.
F. For individuals with dependent children, the risk assessment also includes an evaluation of the patient's ability to meet the needs of dependent children during psychiatric crises. Consideration of the number and ages of any children in terms of vulnerability, and overall health, including mental health, is relevant. Care must be given to how the patient's psychiatric condition may affect children genetically or psychosocially and whether the patient can recognize and attend to the needs of their child.

DIAGNOSIS FORMULATION

A. The main goal of psychiatric assessment is to diagnose and plan treatment accurately. To diagnose accurately, the clinician must gather a clear description of the patient's symptoms. The information is collected and integrated into a comprehensive evaluation of symptoms, behaviors, and psychosocial factors to formulate a diagnosis considering a framework that recognizes the complexities of psychiatric-mental health disorders. The diagnostic analysis is derived from the observed and reported patient's clinical symptoms, considering the presentation timeline.
B. To make an appropriate diagnosis, the clinician must be versed in the constellation of symptoms connected with each clinical diagnosis or be familiar with patterns of symptoms that fall in a particular category (e.g., nervousness, inability to control worry, restlessness, irritability, and sense of impending doom that prevents functioning would be associated with generalized anxiety disorder). The clinician must be able to discern symptoms, ask appropriate questions during the assessment, and recognize deviance, distress, and dysfunction in the patient's presentation.
C. The clinician might use the following steps to diagnose:
1. Identify complaints, symptoms, and observations.
2. Identify cluster-related symptoms and observations.
3. Identify a potential diagnosis.
4. Locate the potential diagnosis and the criteria needed in the *Diagnostic and Statistical Manual of Mental Disorders*, Fifth Edition, Text Revision (*DSM-5-TR*; American Psychiatric Association, 2022) or the *International Classification of Diseases*, 11th Revision (*ICD-11*; World Health Organization [WHO], 2019).
5. Affirm or invalidate the diagnosis based on the cluster of symptoms observed in the *DSM-5-TR* (American Psychiatric Association, 2022) or *ICD-11* (WHO, 2019) assessment.
6. Confirm and clarify diagnostic symptoms with the patient if necessary.
7. Using the *ICD-11*, write the diagnostic code in your patient's chart (e.g., 6A71 is the *ICD-11* diagnostic code for depressive disorder, recurrent, which includes a history of at least two depressive episodes, which may include a current episode, separated by several months without significant mood disturbance).
8. There is no history of manic, mixed, or hypomanic episodes, which would indicate the presence of bipolar disorder.
9. Electronic health records and the availability of computerized decision support tools may enhance the development of differential diagnoses and diagnostic formulations. These need to be compared with face-to-face clinical observations and evaluations.

D. To make an appropriate diagnosis, the clinician must be versed in the constellation of symptoms connected with each clinical diagnosis or be familiar with symptoms that fall under a particular category (e.g., nervousness, inability to control worry, restlessness, easily annoyed, irritability, and sense of impending doom that prevents functioning would be associated with generalized anxiety disorder).

CASE FORMULATION

A. The case formulation comprises the clinician's clinical judgment about the cause, precipitants, and influences of the patient's psychological behavior problems, considering the patient's environment, strengths, challenges, and coping skills. ▶

B. The formulation includes synthesized information specific to the patient, including neurobiological, sociocultural, and genetic issues; family history of mental illness; medical conditions; quality of interpersonal relationships; coping strategies; patterns of behavior; current struggles; conflicts; and defense mechanisms involved in diagnosis and management.
C. The clinician presents diagnostic and therapeutic implications of the assessment findings and the plan for future treatment, including medication management, therapy, lifestyle changes, and safety considerations.
D. Elements of the treatment plan will depend on individual needs and preferences and will generally include treatment that addresses the patient's primary and co-occurring diagnoses. Often co-occurring psychiatric symptoms may not respond to the treatment for the primary disorder (e.g., psychotic symptoms in mood disorders, cognitive impairment in schizophrenia). Prior diagnoses of a co-occurring personality disorder may signal a need for a different approach to psychotherapy than for an individual without such comorbidity. For individuals with past trauma, their ability to establish a trusting relationship may need to be considered in terms of building a therapeutic alliance.
E. The impression and plan should include the following:
  1. Documentation of the estimated risk of suicide, violence, or aggressive behavior (including homicide), including factors influencing risk
  2. Documentation of the rationale for treatment selection, including discussion of the specific factors that influenced the treatment choice
  3. Explanation to the patient of the differential diagnosis, risks of untreated illness, treatment options, and benefits and risks of treatment
  4. Collaboration between the clinician and the patient about decisions pertinent to treatment
  5. Measurements of symptoms, level of functioning, and quality of life using surveys, standardized measures, and rating scales
  6. Documentation of the rationale for clinical tests (e.g., vitamin D level to rule out deficiency)

PRIVACY AND CONFIDENTIALITY

A. Considerations of privacy, dignity, and confidentiality are vital components of the psychiatric encounter. The clinician must maintain confidentiality unless the patient consents to a specific intervention or communication.
B. Safety of the patient and others, the ability to communicate necessary information about the patient to medical personnel, and emergencies may preclude confidentiality and must be carefully weighed.
C. The clinician may listen to information provided by family members and other important people in the patient's life as long as the clinician does not reciprocate with confidential information. The Health Insurance Portability and Accountability Act (HIPAA) contains guidelines for releasing the results of psychiatric evaluations.
D. State laws may be more restrictive, and if so state laws take precedence over HIPAA. According to HIPAA, information can be released without a specific consent form for "treatment, payment, and health care operations" (HIPAA, 2013). Otherwise, patients must sign an authorization form indicating what information is to be disclosed, the purposes for the disclosure, the recipient, and the expiration date.
E. HIPAA gives special protection to psychotherapy notes, and they must be kept in a separate part of the medical chart. The interpretation of HIPAA and other federal and state laws about confidentiality is continually evaluated. Legal or risk management consultation should be sought if there are questions about releasing information and protecting psychiatric records.
F. According to HIPAA, necessary information may be disclosed to medical personnel when treating a condition that poses an immediate threat to the health of any individual. Under such circumstances, documentation in the medical record needs to include the name of the medical personnel to whom the disclosure was made, their affiliation with any healthcare facility, the name of the individual making the disclosure, the date and time of the disclosure, and why the emergency called for the disclosure.
G. Medical records may also be viewed by the clinician writing the note or other members of an interdisciplinary treatment team. These include third-party payers, quality assurance and peer review evaluators, and the patient. Medical records with confidential information may be part of future or current legal or administrative hearings, including disability litigation, divorce and custody adjudication, competency determinations, and actions of medical licensing boards. The potential for other parties who may access a patient's medical records in the future must be considered when documenting the assessment, case formulation, impression, diagnosis, and treatment plan.

USE OF TECHNOLOGY AND TELEHEALTH

A. Research has focused on the impact of technology on information gathering and the clinician–patient encounter.
  1. Some studies have examined differences in the information elicited by face-to-face interviews compared with computer-aided assessments or telephone interviews.
  2. Other studies have assessed computerized documentation by physicians at the time of evaluation and its effect on patient perceptions.

B. Patients and family members are increasingly learning about possible diagnoses and treatments through consumer advertising and internet-based educational resources and bring these perceptions to the initial assessment.
C. The clinician must be aware of the influence of virtual information sources on the assessment and treatment planning processes. Template-based electronic health records, as compared with narrative-based health records, influence the assessment process, impression, and plan. With the increasing use of technology in medicine, including computer-based interviews and telepsychiatry, the influence of such technologies is worthy of additional study in the full range of psychiatric settings.

RESOURCES

CLINICAL INTERVIEW WITH PSYCHIATRIC EVALUATION

Although useful, no diagnostic screening test or rating scale can replace a thorough clinical interview, a carefully considered differential diagnosis, a comprehensive case conceptualization, and an individualized treatment plan. The clinical interview by an experienced practitioner is the most effective tool in advanced practice psychiatric nursing.

A. Structured Clinical Interview for *DSM-5* Disorders—Clinician Version (SCID-5-CV): The SCID-5-CV provides helpful guidance for a well-organized diagnostic interview and covers common diagnoses most often seen in clinical settings.

B. Structured Clinical Interview for *DSM-5* Personality Disorders (SCID-5-PD) and Structured Clinical Interview for *DSM-5* Alternative Model for Personality Disorders (SCID-5-AMPD): These scales assess personality disorders using either the 10 *DSM-5* (American Psychiatric Association, 2013) personality disorders or the *DSM-5* Alternative Model for Personality Disorders.

C. *The Psychiatric Interview*, Fifth Edition, by Daniel Carlat: *The Psychiatric Interview* offers a concise approach to the psychiatric interview and brings you up-to-date with the *DSM-5-TR* (American Psychiatric Association, 2022) and current research.

D. Level 1 and Level 2 Cross-Cutting Symptom Checklists: Supplemented with clinical history, the *DSM-5* (American Psychiatric Association, 2013) Level 1 and Level 2 Cross-Cutting Symptom Checklists have good specificity, although with less sensitivity. Note: The American Psychiatric Association's "emerging measures" can be used for clinical assessment, designed for initial interviews, and tracking treatment progress. These tools aim to support clinical decisions but should not be the sole diagnostic basis. They come with instructions, scoring, and interpretation guides, with more details in *DSM-5* (American Psychiatric Association, 2013). The American Psychiatric Association encourages feedback on these instruments' effectiveness in assessing and enhancing patient care.

E. Mental Status Exam (MSE) Checklist: The MSE is used for a wide range of psychiatric and neurologic evaluations to understand comprehensively a patient's mental state. The Mini-Mental State Examination (MMSE) is specifically designed to screen for cognitive impairment and monitor its progression, particularly in the context of dementia. One of the many free MSE downloadable templates can be found on the internet. Here is an example: www.soapnote.org/category/mental-health.

INITIAL SCREENING TESTS AND RATING SCALES

These scales and instruments should always be interpreted in the context of the patient's clinical presentation obtained during the clinical interview and should not be used as a solitary criterion for making decisions. Navigating the complexities of copyrights and infringement patents in mental health assessments can be daunting as it takes time to sift through countless options. The following is a list of the most commonly used validated, free-to-use mental health assessments. Most are available in both digital and paper forms. To check a tool's copyright status, (a) check the publisher's website, (b) contact the authors, (c) use online copyright databases, or (d) search the internet for usage information. Remember, copyrighted tools require the holder's permission for use.

A. Risk assessment tools
  1. Violence Risk Assessment Tools: There is no gold standard for measuring workplace violence risk; however, the Centers for Disease Control and Prevention (CDC) Violence Risk Assessment Tools provide a standard against which to evaluate individuals for potential violence, enabling all healthcare providers to share a common frame of reference and understanding, minimizing the possibility that communications regarding a person's potential for violence will be misinterpreted.
  2. DATools (Danger Assessment Tools): This 20-item instrument uses a weighted system to score risk factors associated with intimate partner homicide: www.dangerassessment.org/DATools.

B. Suicidality
  1. Columbia-Suicide Severity Rating Scale (C-SSRS): The C-SSRS offers various versions and assesses suicidal behaviors, intensity of thoughts, and severity of ideation. Studies have validated its effectiveness as a predictive indicator of suicide risk in both children and adults.

C. Anxiety disorders screening tools
  1. General Anxiety Disorder-7 (GAD-7): GAD-7 is a reliable tool used to assess severity of generalized anxiety disorder. It is commonly used in clinical and research settings, but is not suitable for posttraumatic stress disorder (PTSD) or phobias.
  2. Hamilton Anxiety Rating Scale (HAM-A): The HAM-A scale was developed in 1959 and is used to measure anxiety severity. It is widely used internationally despite some criticism. The scale is helpful in tracking treatment progress rather than diagnosing.
  3. Penn State Worry Questionnaire (PSWQ): The PSWQ is a self-administered 16-item questionnaire with high reliability. It is useful in distinguishing GAD from other anxiety disorders.
  4. Zung Self-Rating Anxiety Scale: The Zung Self-Rating Anxiety Scale is a 20-item self-report scale that measures anxiety levels across cognitive, autonomic, motor, and central nervous system (CNS) symptoms. It is scored on a Likert-type scale.

D. Adjustment disorders
  1. International Adjustment Disorder Questionnaire (IADQ): The IADQ identifies symptoms of adjustment disorder in adults.

E. Substance use disorders and screening tools
  1. CAGE Questionnaire: The CAGE Questionnaire is a brief, four-question screening tool for adult alcohol dependency, focusing on behavior rather than consumption amounts. Its questions, symbolized by "**C**ut down, **A**nnoyed, **G**uilty, **E**ye-opener," lack specificity in differentiating active from former users.
  2. Alcohol Use Disorders Identification Test (AUDIT): AUDIT screens for recent heavy drinking and alcohol dependence. It is more sensitive than the CAGE Questionnaire in screening for heavy drinking and/or active alcohol abuse or dependence.
  3. Michigan Alcohol Screening Test (MAST): The MAST is a detailed 25-item questionnaire used to identify lifetime alcohol-related issues, with scores indicating nondependence to probable alcoholism. It covers a wide range of alcohol's negative impacts, but does not distinguish between past and current drinking.
  4. CRAFFT 2.1 Interview: The CRAFFT (**C**ar, **R**elax, **A**lone, **F**orget, **F**riends, **T**rouble) 2.1 Interview is designed for adolescents (12–21 years) to detect substance use and associated risks, supporting early intervention in high-demand settings.
  5. Brief Addiction Monitor (BAM): The BAM is a 17-item tool used for monitoring substance use disorder treatment progress, assessing risk and protective factors and substance use in the past 30 days, individualizing care plans.
  6. Drug Abuse Screening Test (DAST-10)
  7. Fagerstrom Test for Nicotine Dependence (FTND)

F. Mood disorders screening tools
  1. Beck Depression Inventory (BDI): The BDI is a widely used, validated, self-reported questionnaire used to assess the severity of depressive symptoms and monitor changes over time.

2. Hamilton Rating Scale for Depression (HAM-D): The HAM-D is a clinician-administered depression assessment tool, also known as the Hamilton Depression Rating Scale, developed in the 1950s. It takes 15 to 20 minutes to complete.
   3. Patient Health Questionnaire-9 (PHQ-9): The PHQ-9 is a self-administered depression screening tool used for diagnostic help and progress monitoring, including tracking patient outcomes.
   4. Mood Disorder Questionnaire (MDQ): The MDQ is a widely used screening instrument for bipolar disorder, consisting of 13 yes-or-no questions and two additional questions. It takes about 5 minutes to complete and is available in 19 languages.
   5. Zung Self-Rating Depression Scale (SDS): The SDS is a 20-item self-report questionnaire to measure depression severity and is widely used in clinical and research settings.
   6. Geriatric Depression Scale (GDS): The GDS is a self-report screening tool for depression in older adults, focusing on psychiatric symptoms rather than somatic symptoms. It is commonly used in various settings, including comprehensive geriatric assessment.
   7. Young Mania Rating Scale (YMRS): The YMRS is a clinician-administered scale for evaluating manic symptoms and is used throughout the treatment course. It takes 15 to 30 minutes to complete depending on complexity.
G. Eating disorders
   1. Eating Disorder Diagnostic Scale (EDDS): The EDDS is a 22-question assessment tool for eating disorders, validated against *DSM-IV* criteria (American Psychiatric Association, 1994), ensuring accurate diagnosis.
H. Trauma
   1. Posttraumatic Stress Disorder Checklist (PCL-5): The PCL-5 is a self-administered questionnaire consisting of 20 items, aligning with the *DSM-5* (American Psychiatric Association, 2013) criteria for PTSD symptoms, and is crucial for accurately assessing the prevalence of PTSD.
   2. International Trauma Questionnaire (ITQ): The ITQ is a self-report measure evaluating traumatic experiences and PTSD symptoms, and is useful in screening, monitoring, and assessing treatment effectiveness.
I. Behavioral and emotional disorders
   1. Adult ADHD Self-Report Scale: This is an 18-item self-report questionnaire developed by WHO to assess ADHD symptoms in adults. It is available in multiple languages and is used for screening, diagnosis, and treatment monitoring.
   2. Adverse Childhood Experiences Questionnaire: This is a self-report measure consisting of 10 items to assess the frequency of ACEs. It is helpful in identifying individuals at risk of poor health outcomes and in evaluating intervention effectiveness.
J. Personality disorders
   1. Borderline Personality Screener (BPS): The BPS screens for symptoms of borderline personality disorder in adults.
   2. Personality Inventory for *DSM-5* (PID-5): PID-5 is a useful tool to enhance clinical decision-making, but is not the sole basis for making a clinical diagnosis.
K. Cognitive disorders
   1. Six-Item Cognitive Impairment Test (6CIT): The 6CIT screens for cognitive impairment in adults.
L. Movement disorders
   1. Abnormal Involuntary Movement Scale (AIMS): The AIMS monitors movement disorders in individuals taking antipsychotic medication, detecting tardive dyskinesia early.

FUNCTIONAL ASSESSMENTS

A. GAIN Short Screener (GSS): The GSS is a brief, self-administered tool published by the Substance Abuse and Mental Health Services Administration (SAMHSA) in 2001, as part of GAIN assessment. It identifies individuals needing substance abuse or mental health services.
B. Katz Index of Independence in Activities of Daily Living (Katz ADL Index): The Katz ADL Index is a six-item scale used to evaluate functional independence in older adults. It is commonly used in geriatric research and clinical practice.
C. Quality of Life Scale (QOLS): The QOLS measures overall well-being across life domains, scored from 16 to 112 and widely used in research and clinical settings.
D. Satisfaction With Life Scale (SWLS): The SWLS is a five-item measure used to assess overall life satisfaction. It is useful in identifying individuals at risk for mental health disorders.

FAMILY ASSESSMENTS

A. Marital Status Inventory (MSI): The MSI assesses marital relationship quality and is used in research and clinical settings to improve relationship satisfaction.
B. Parental Stress Index (PSI): The PSI measures stress levels in parents of children with developmental or behavioral disorders, aiding intervention evaluation.

DEVELOPMENT DISORDERS

A. Ritvo Autism Asperger Diagnostic Scale (RAADS): The RAADS diagnoses autism spectrum disorder symptoms in adults and consists of 84 items across four scales.

REFERENCES AND BIBLIOGRAPHY

American Psychiatric Association. (1994). *Diagnostic and statistical manual of mental disorders* (4th ed.). Author.

American Psychiatric Association. (2013). *Diagnostic and statistical manual of mental disorders* (5th ed.). https://doi.org/10.1176/appi.books.9780890425596

American Psychiatric Association. (2022). *Diagnostic and statistical manual of mental disorders* (5th ed., text rev.). https://doi.org/10.1176/appi.books.9780890425787

American Psychological Association. (2016). *Practice guidelines for the psychiatric evaluation of adults* (3rd ed.). https://psychiatryonline.org/doi/full/10.1176/appi.books.9780890426760.pe02

Bovendeerd, B. (2021, June 21). *Presentation society for psychotherapy research congress 2021 in Heidelberg. Paper presented at SPR 52nd International Annual Meeting, Heidelberg, Germany*. University of Groningen. https://research.rug.nl/en/publications/presentation-society-for-psychotherapy-research-congress-2021-in-

Carlat, D. J. (2023). *The psychiatric interview: A practical guide* (5th ed.). Wolters Kluwer.

First, M. B., Williams, J. B. W., Benjamin, L. S., & Spitzer, R. L. (2016). *Structured clinical interview for DSM-5 Screening Personality Questionnaire (SCID-5-SPQ)*. American Psychiatric Association.

Harvey, P. D., Depp, C. A., Rizzo, A. A., Strauss, G. P., Spelber, D., Carpenter, L. L., Kalin, N. H., Krystal, J. H., McDonald, W. M., Nemeroff, C. B., Rodriguez, C. I., Widge, A. S., & Torous, J. (2022). Technology and mental health: State of the art for assessment and treatment. *American Journal of Psychiatry Online*. https://ajp.psychiatryonline.org/doi/10.1176/appi.ajp.21121254

Health Insurance Portability and Accountability Act, 45 C.F.R. § 164.520 (2013). https://www.ecfr.gov/current/title-45/subtitle-A/subchapter-C/part-164/subpart-E/section-164.520

Heitzman, A., Perfitt, L. L., & Ziegler, A. (2023). Nonverbal communication. In M. S. Courey, S. K. Rapoport, L. Goldberg, & S. K. Brown (Eds.), *Voice and communication in transgender and gender diverse individuals* (pp. 103–111). Springer. https://doi.org/10.1007/978-3-031-24632-6_9

Sadock, B. J., Sadock, V. A., Ruiz, P., & Kaplan, H. I. (2017). *Kaplan and Sadock's comprehensive textbook of psychiatry* (10th ed.). Wolters Kluwer.

Substance Abuse and Mental Health Services Administration. (2016, November 15). *Serious mental illness among adults below the poverty line.* https://www.samhsa.gov/data/sites/default/files/report_2720/Spotlight-2720.pdf

Tusaie, K. R., & Fitzpatrick, J. J. (Eds.). (2022). *Advanced practice psychiatric nursing: Integrating psychotherapy, psychopharmacology, and complementary and alternative approaches across the life span* (3rd ed.). Springer Publishing Company.

Weathers, F. W., Blake, D. D., Schmurr, P. P., Kaloupek, D. G., Marx, B. P., & Keane, T. M. (2013). *The life events checklist for DSM-5 (LEC-5).* U.S. Department of Veterans Affairs, National Center for PTSD. https://www.ptsd.va.gov/professional/assessment/te-measures/life_events_checklist.asp

Wheeler, K. (2020). *Psychotherapy for the advanced practice psychiatric nurse: A how-to guide for evidence-based practice* (3rd ed.). Springer Publishing Company.

World Health Organization. (2019). *International statistical classification of diseases* (11th rev.). https://icd.who.int/

5 CONDUCTING THE PEDIATRIC PSYCHIATRIC ASSESSMENT

Michelle A. Peralta Westland, Carole Gionet, Julia Farquharson, John Westland, Maria Manalo, Hillary J. Chan, and VaLori R. Abad

INTRODUCTION

An age-appropriate and developmentally appropriate psychiatric interview is imperative for assessing youth (children and adolescents) with mental health challenges. Sharing difficult, intimate details about one's life with a healthcare provider can be very tough and emotional at any age. Interviewing children and adolescents can simultaneously be stimulating, thought-provoking, interesting, surprising, and inspiring, as well as puzzling and sometimes heart-wrenching. APRNs should conduct developmentally appropriate interviews. Understanding the developmental stage of patients allows the APRN to tailor the interview to the patient's needs and abilities, communication capacity, and learning styles. Knowledge and familiarity with developmental milestones are the key to evaluating the pertinence of behaviors and patient responses. The use of developmentally appropriate language and engagement style is central to the pediatric psychiatric assessment. Developmentally appropriate engagement is critical. For example, using cartoons, drawing, and play is a great way to work with younger children but will likely not appeal to adolescent patients. Depending on the assessment, it may also be beneficial to interview the entire family to provide the APRN with an opportunity to observe relationships and interactions. Healthcare providers working with youth must adapt the interview to ensure patient understanding and participation. This focus on the youth's comprehension of questions can prevent patient frustration during the assessment, which might result in challenging behaviors that interfere with proper diagnosis. The more individualized the APRN's approach, the easier it will be to obtain the information needed to discern a diagnosis. One of the goals of the initial interview is to work on building an alliance with the patient and the family, facilitating an understanding of the patient's symptoms, examining the information through a biopsychosocial lens, and collaborating with the team on the development of a multidisciplinary, comprehensive treatment plan.

Although each APRN develops a personal application of the psychiatric interview, there remains the framework of beginning (building therapeutic rapport), middle (collecting the necessary information to achieve diagnosis and develop a treatment plan), and end (summarizing to the patient and the family the outcomes of the assessment and recommendations for next steps). Structuring the interview is important, and as the APRN moves from novice to expert the interview style becomes more organic. Meeting the needs and evaluating the capacity of each patient provide opportunities throughout the interview to build rapport and trust and establish a therapeutic alliance. Conducting the psychiatric youth (child and adolescent) assessment using a template helps ensure the collection of all necessary, required data for establishing the diagnosis and crafting the treatment planning. This chapter provides the APRN with a road map for the pediatric psychiatric interview.

THE ASSESSMENT PROCESS

A. There are seven phases of the interview process: preparation, building therapeutic rapport, information collecting, psychiatric review of systems, mental status exam, physical health assessment, and summary. Table 5.1 summarizes each phase of the psychiatric assessment.

B. When starting an interview with a youth and their family, it is good practice to start off the interview together. However, it may be advantageous to meet with the child/adolescent on their own to gather more information, as well as in cases when the APRN observes nonverbal cues indicating interpersonal conflict within the family in the waiting room.

C. Use the initial time together to build therapeutic rapport, then the next few minutes to ascertain a sense of the patient's and legal guardian's understanding of why they have been referred for a mental health/psychiatric assessment and what they hope to get out of the assessment.

    1. Use this time for introduction, icebreaker, seeking permission for use of name/nicknames, and establishing pronouns.
    2. "Why do you think you are here to see me?"
    3. "What do you hope to get out of this interview?"

D. Once the patient's legal guardian's needs and wants are understood, the interviewer uses the next bit of time to describe how the interview process will unfold and how long the interview may take.

    1. The interviewer provides information on confidentiality and the limits to confidentiality.
    2. The interviewer asks if those in the room understand and answers any questions before continuing.

E. Paying attention to topics of interest provided by the patient allows them to reveal more about themselves to the healthcare provider.

    1. This information makes the approach more relevant to the desires of the patient.
    2. Reflection on this information demonstrates that the APRN is listening to the needs of the patient.
    3. The APRN can use this information as the bridge to the information-collecting phase of the interview.

F. After meeting together with the youth and the family, the APRN will meet with the youth alone and then with the legal guardian(s) alone.

    1. In certain situations, the APRN may want to have another clinician present during the interview with the youth.
    2. When another adult is not available, the APRN might ask for permission to record the interview. This provides security for both the APRN and the patient.

G. Finally, during the formulation and synthesis phase, the APRN will bring everyone back together, meeting simultaneously with the patient and the family/legal guardians. Legal ▶

TABLE 5.1 THE ASSESSMENT PROCESS

Phases of Assessment	Clinical Activity
Phase 1: preparation	After receiving the patient referral, request any documentation pertaining to the reason for referral from referring sources. This can include: 1. Primary care provider's notes 2. School reports 3. Assessment or follow-up notes from any other mental health provider the youth has seen in the past (e.g., psychological reports, assessment notes from a specialist) Having the opportunity to review these documents ahead of the initial interview assists in better understanding the patient's history and presentation. If obtaining historical information about the patient is not possible prior to the interview, consent can be obtained during the interview, and this information can be requested following the interview. When reviewing collateral information following the interview, ensure historical information is included in the formulation and diagnosis. Schedule a follow-up appointment with the patient and legal guardians to present the formulation and diagnosis, using the appointment to collaborate on a treatment plan. Assess the patient's ability to cope during interview. If there are concerns for aggression or agitation in an in-person interview, consider the need for additional security or pivoting to a virtual interview for the safety and well-being of everyone. If it is necessary to bring the patient into the interview in person and these concerns persist, create a plan with the legal guardians and the healthcare team ahead of the interview to ensure safety and success for the patient and healthcare team.
Phase 2: the interview: building therapeutic rapport	At the beginning of the interview, time for the APRN and the patient to get to know each other is imperative. Individuals feel more engaged, safe, and interested in building an alliance with the interviewer if given the time to connect.
Phase 3: the interview: information gathering	Begin the interview by including the youth and legal guardians. Introduce appropriate topics that will yield information from everyone in the room. Prepare separate topics to ask the youth during the individual interview time. Topics to cover during the assessment include: History of presenting illness Developmental history Social history Past medical/surgical history Past and current medications Family psychiatric history
Phase 4: the interview: psychiatric review of systems	During the psychiatric review of systems phase of the interview, the APRN will use the information collected from questions regarding the history of presenting illness to guide decisions around what psychiatric conditions may need more focus and attention as the APRN interviews diagnostically for these conditions. Consider including screening and assessment questions to discern if the patient is presenting with any one of the following psychiatric problems: Anxiety Adjustment disorders Feeding and eating disorders: anorexia nervosa, bulimia, avoidant restrictive food intake disorder Gender dysphoria Mood disorders: major depressive disorder, bipolar disorder, dysthymia disorder, mood disorders due to medical conditions or substance use Neurodevelopmental/behavioral conditions: attention deficit hyperactivity disorder, autism spectrum disorder Oppositional defiance disorder/conduct disorder Psychotic disorders (organic vs. nonorganic presentations) Somatic symptoms and related disorders Substance use disorders Trauma
Phase 5: the mental status exam	During this phase, consider observations of the patient during the interview and describe the patient's behavior and cognition using a structured approach.
Phase 6: physical health assessment	In this phase of the interview, focus attention on the physical assessment. The physical assessment plus the symptoms that the patient is presenting with should guide decision-making about further investigations (e.g., laboratory, imaging).
Phase 7: summary	• Formulation • Diagnosis • Treatment planning

APRN, advanced practice registered nurse.

guardians and youth must be asked the same psychiatric review of system interview questions, providing the APRN more insight into the problem to aid in the formulation and diagnosis.

H. Bidirectional integration of systems: The mind and body are integrated and can affect one another; this must be factored into the interview. Consider all possible contributing factors, including medical problems that might affect the youth's psychiatric presentation. Additionally, the APRN's understanding of the potential for youth substance use is imperative for establishing a comprehensive evaluation of the patient's symptomology.

GENERAL PRINCIPLES OF PEDIATRIC HISTORY TAKING

A. Use developmentally appropriate language and questions (e.g., Do you have a lack of interest vs. Are you bored?).
B. Use open-ended questions where possible.
C. Where possible, allow patient experience and expression to guide assessment (e.g., order of questions from clinician assessment).
D. Be empathic and understanding.
E. Ask clear and specific questions about patient experience to inform the APRN's understanding of possible psychopathology (do not be afraid to ask tough questions!). Restate questions until the youth understands what is being asked.
  1. Clarify the youth's understanding of the question.
  2. Restate what the youth says and ask for assurance that what was heard was what the youth meant to say.
  3. If English is not the youth's first language, be certain to have translation support available.

F. History taking should be collaborative (e.g., patient, parental figures, family, friends, legal guardians, school), respecting the Health Insurance Portability and Accountability Act of 1996 (HIPAA), or the Personal Information Protection and Electronic Documents Act (PIPEDA), or whatever legislation is appropriate in your jurisdiction, when possible and appropriate.

THE BIOPSYCHOSOCIAL MODEL TO ASSIST IN FORMULATION

A. The biopsychosocial model considers the "4 Ps"—predisposing factors, precipitating factors, perpetuating factors, and protective factors—for each of the biological, psychological, and social factors.
  1. This information is collected throughout the interview and then organized under these headings when formulating the problem and summarizing findings and treatment plan to the family.
  2. Listen for information from the patient and family/legal guardians that describes each one of the 4 Ps. This model is the framework that will be used to formulate treatment planning. The next few sections further discuss the 4 Ps (Table 5.2).

CHARACTERISTICS PROMOTING OR HINDERING DEVELOPMENTAL COMPETENCIES

A. Mental health in youth can be promoted or hindered by specific contextual variables that the youth is exposed to.
B. Identification of these variables can either improve or negatively impact the youth's physical and emotional development.
C. Two types of variables that have been identified are protective factors, which can increase developmental well-being; and risk factors, which increase the likelihood of negative developmental outcomes.
D. Understanding of the impact of risk and protective factors can reduce and sometimes prevent the occurrence of mental, emotional, and behavioral disorders in youth.

PROTECTIVE FACTORS FOR MENTAL HEALTH CONDITIONS IN CHILDREN AND ADOLESCENTS

A. Protective factors are conditions and/or attributes that foster and protect the well-being of the youth and their families. They can be individual, within the family system, or from the community.
B. Protective factors can positively protect a person from the likelihood of developing mental illness.
C. Assess for protective factors during the interview (Box 5.1).

TABLE 5.2 THE 4 PS OF THE BIOPSYCHOSOCIAL MODEL

Predisposing factors	Areas of vulnerability that increase the risk of the presenting problem (e.g., family history, prenatal exposure to tobacco/alcohol)
Precipitating factors	Stressors or other events (they could be positive or negative) that may be precipitants of the symptoms (e.g., death in the family, transitions)
Perpetuating factors	Conditions in the patient, family, community, or larger systems that exacerbate rather than solve the problem (e.g., unaddressed relationship conflicts, lack of education, financial stresses, occupational stress or lack of employment)
Protective factors	Patient's own areas of competency, skill, talents, interest, and other supportive elements; counteract the predisposing, precipitating, and perpetuating factors

Source: Adapted from Winters, N.C., Hanson, G., & Stoyanova, V. (2007). The case formulation in child and adolescent psychiatry. *Child and Adolescent Psychiatric Clinic of North America, 16*(2007), 111–132. https://doi.org/10.1016/j.chc.2006.07.010.

RISK FACTORS FOR MENTAL HEALTH CONDITIONS IN CHILDREN AND ADOLESCENTS

A. Many factors can place a person at risk of mental illness. Early recognition of risk factors will provide the clinician with better opportunities for early prevention or intervention to prevent or mitigate further risk for mental health issues.
B. Examples of risk factors that should be screened for in child and adolescent patients are shown in Box 5.2.

WHAT TO INCLUDE IN A CHILD/ADOLESCENT PSYCHIATRIC ASSESSMENT

A. Youth psychiatric assessments are challenging for healthcare providers and mental health clinicians.

BOX 5.1 PROTECTIVE FACTORS IN DEVELOPMENT

Genetic predisposition
Being future-/goal-oriented
Being resilient
Having active coping skills (e.g., journaling, art, music)
Having healthy and stable relationships
Having motivating factors
Having opportunities for engagement and participation in group activities
Having opportunities to explore religious and spiritual practices
Having school or work in one's life
Having social connections
Living in clean and well-kept housing
Having parents or legal guardians with knowledge of parenting, who have resilience, and who know how to access support
Parents or caregivers who have knowledge of child and youth development
Relationships that are nurturing and promote positive attachment
Safe, supportive space (e.g., affirming, free of violence, supportive family/friend relationships)

BOX 5.2 RISK FACTORS IN DEVELOPMENT

Affective response: affective involvement, behavioral control, general function
Family problems: problem-solving, communication
Gender discrimination
Heritability
Housing and food insecurity
Human rights conditions
Medical conditions
Persistent economic pressures
Physical illness
Problems between parents or legal guardians and the patient
Parents with existing mental health condition
Problems with peer groups or school friends
Race (e.g., BIPOC—Black, Indigenous, people of color)
Rapid social change
Refugee status
Role
Stressful environmental conditions
Sexuality
Social determinants of health (e.g., family stress—abuse, neglect, domestic violence, income/stability, education access and quality, healthcare access and quality; supports—social, community)
Social exclusion
Substance use
Trauma
Unhealthy lifestyles
Untreated symptoms of anxiety and depression
Victim of bullying
Violence (recipient or witness)

   1. Youth may not be able to report the nature of their mental health symptoms.
   2. Depending on the diagnosis and on age, gender, education, and culture, the youth might not be able to provide accurate information related to the presenting problems.
B. Children and adolescents may be reluctant to participate because they often present for care that they did not seek on their own.
   1. They may feel embarrassed to disclose their problems for fear they will be judged negatively.
   2. Where possible, the APRN can use multiple sources to obtain information (e.g., legal guardians, teachers) and settings (home, school).

PHASE 1: PREPARATION

A. Identify the reason(s) for the referral, including any primary care provider notes, school reports, or other assessments.
B. Collateral information is taken into consideration when formulating a plan and arriving at a diagnosis.
C. Include information related to any concern of aggression or agitation observed to ensure the safety and well-being of everyone.

PHASE 2: BUILDING THERAPEUTIC RAPPORT

A. Building a good therapeutic rapport with the patient will aid in the interview process. The relationship between the clinician and the youth can affect intervention outcomes.
B. It is important to establish rapport with the youth and not assume that all the information can be gathered from the legal guardian(s). Patients are always the expert of their own life and experiences. A paternalistic view will lead to misdiagnosis.
C. Being empathic, having awareness, and being oneself are key elements in rapport building. Being aware of oneself, one's patient, and the family/legal guardians will aid in the process of relationship building.
D. APRNs should be aware of personal implicit and explicit biases or judgments that can interfere with proper rapport building and challenge themselves to grow beyond these.
E. Create an environment of comfort and trust.
   1. This will help promote the patient's and the family's engagement in the interview process.
   2. A good rapport with the youth provides a safe, confidential, nonjudgmental place where they can disclose their problems and begin to work with the APRN to resolve their problems.
F. Take note of the youth's learning style.
   1. Assess sensory needs (visual, auditory, or kinetic approaches) and communication techniques. These observations will inform how the rest of the interview is approached.
   2. The APRN should describe their observations and conclusions during the interview simply, using plain language whenever possible for both the patient and the legal guardians.
G. Tips to build strong, positive therapeutic rapport include the following:
   1. Be yourself.
   2. Respect the patient's autonomy.
      a. Interview the patient alone.
      b. Offer choices to the patient when possible.
   3. Offer opportunities for shared decision-making.
   4. Be empathic and nonjudgmental.
   5. Be an active listener—paraphrase throughout the interview to ensure understanding of what is being said.
   6. Use reflective statements (e.g., "You sound angry when you talk about your friend.")

PHASE 3: INFORMATION-GATHERING PHASE

HISTORY OF PRESENTING ILLNESS

A. Obtaining the chief complaint
   1. This is a record of the reason the patient is pursuing psychiatric assessment, evaluation, and treatment.
   2. Ideally, it is a verbatim record from both the patient and the legal guardian and can provide understanding into the capacity of the patient, as well as the level of insight the patient and the legal guardian have about the current issue.
B. History of presenting illness
   1. This is a chronological description of the chief complaint, including all symptoms and when and how they emerged.
   2. It is vital to the psychiatric assessment to obtain the history of presenting illness from both the patient and the legal guardian.
   3. It may also be necessary to obtain collateral history from the patient's school or current mental health clinicians.
C. Social environment information
   1. It is important to gather information about home, school, and social life from the patient and legal guardians to obtain a full picture and a richer understanding of the range of factors that can be affecting the patient's mental health.
   2. These conversations also give APRNs the opportunity to engage with the patient and establish a connection and a therapeutic relationship.
   3. This is especially important given the developmental age of some patients as well as the complex subject matter of many assessments.

4. Ask about current symptoms (onset, provocation, duration, course).
   a. What is your understanding of why you are here today? (Clarify for the patient if needed.)
   b. When did this (symptoms) start for you? How long has this been happening?
   c. What makes it worse? What makes it better?
   d. Have you noticed any change recently?
   e. What else can you tell me about how you have been feeling lately?
   f. What do you think causes this (symptoms) for you?
5. Ask about functional status (past and present).
   a. Any past history of similar symptoms?
   b. Do you feel you were able to manage to do what you needed/wanted to do in the past?
   c. Were you able to care for yourself the way you wanted (e.g., shower, eat)?
   d. Were you able to play the sports you wanted?
   e. Were you able to focus the way you wanted without distraction? Were you able to eat and sleep the way you wanted?
   f. Do you think your ability to do the things you want to do has changed? In what way?
6. Identify associated symptoms (pertinent positive and negative symptoms).
   a. Have you noticed any other symptoms/changes? Has anyone mentioned noticing a difference in your behavior?
   b. What do you think has changed in your life recently?

DEVELOPMENTAL HISTORY

A. Legal guardians are usually the best sources of information for the youth's developmental history.
   1. This part of the interview is often conducted together with the patient.
   2. Depending on the age of the patient and their developmental stage, the patient can sometimes be an additional source of information here.
   3. With the information that the legal guardians provide, the goal is to identify if the patient has experienced any developmental delay or regression in their history.

B. The following questions are helpful to ask the patient's mother during a developmental assessment:
   1. Please tell me more about your pregnancy.
      a. Did you deliver your baby vaginally or by cesarean section?
      b. How many weeks did you carry the baby before delivery?
      c. Were there any delivery complications?
   2. How was your health during your pregnancy?
   3. Did you take any medications during pregnancy? If so, which ones?
   4. Did you use any substances during your pregnancy (e.g., alcohol, nicotine, marijuana)? If so, did you use this throughout the pregnancy, or did you stop and if so in what trimester?
   5. What was the birth weight of your child?
   6. Can you recall the nurse telling you a number that they called an Apgar score? If so, do you recall the number?
   7. I would like to ask you questions about nutrition: Were you able to breastfeed? If so, for how long? Follow up: What age was the child when you stopped breastfeeding?
   8. Were there any complications during the first year of life? If so, what were they? How were they resolved? (Here one may learn about medical or surgical interventions required. Remember to ask who made any diagnosis, any special procedures the patient had to have and where, and the date[s] of any interventions/treatments.)
   9. Ask about language milestones.
      a. When did your child start to babble?
      b. What was the age of the first single words?
      c. What was the age your child first strung two words together?
      d. What was the age when your child started to make phrased speech?
      e. When did your child start to make social use of speech?
   10. Ask about motor milestones.
      a. When did your child first sit on their own?
      b. When did your child start to walk?
      c. When was your child toilet-trained (bowel, bladder)?
   11. Ask the legal guardians if they, the day care, or the school have had any concerns about the child's development or if they have had to involve any resources in the past to help with aspects of development (e.g., involvement of speech-language pathology, occupational therapy, or a developmental pediatrician).
   12. Ask the legal guardians if they currently require, or have required in the past, any extra support at school, such as an individual education plan. Is it helpful? (For more information about this, please see Chapter 20, "Special Considerations for Childhood and Adolescent Populations.")
   13. Ask the legal guardian(s) if they have had any concerns about their child's growth, a slowing down of growth, or a rapid catchup in growth.
      a. As your child has grown, is your child able to take care of their own personal care/hygiene? If not, what help does your child require?
      b. As your child has grown, is your child able to take care of their own health and healthcare?

SOCIAL HISTORY

A. A social history provides a context for the patient's life: where they live, who they spend time with and how they get along with these individuals, and how they are doing with school and, for some, part-time work.

B. It can be helpful to start the interview off with social history. This can be completed when meeting with the youth alone. Following is a list of topics, with suggested questions for each topic, that are important to gather information about during the interview.
   1. Home
      a. What is the patient's place of birth?
      b. Where does the patient live?
      c. Who do they live with? Any pets at home?
      d. Have there been any changes to living situation recently?
      e. Do they feel safe at home?
      f. How is their relationship with various family members at home?
      g. Do they have responsibilities at home (e.g., chores)? What are they? Are they able to complete them?
      h. What types of chores or activities in daily life does the patient find difficult?
      i. What chores or activities do they like to have help with?

2. Family relationships
   a. Ask about the patient's relationship with legal guardians.
   b. Ask about the patient's relationship with sibling(s).
   c. Ask about any conflict in the family. How does the patient get along with each member of the family (e.g., mother, father, brother, sister)?
   d. Ask what the patient likes to do with their family.
3. School
   a. Where do they go to school and how long have they been attending school there?
   b. What grade are they in?
   c. Do they enjoy school? Do they have any issues at school (e.g., difficulties adjusting to school)?
   d. Do they get any extra help in school? From whom? Is it helpful?
   e. What is their favorite subject in school?
   f. What is their least favorite subject in school?
   g. What are their grades like in school (e.g., do they get As, Bs, Cs, Ds)?
   h. Have they missed days at school? If so, what interfered with them getting to school?
   i. Have they had any trouble at school (e.g., failing classes, detention, expulsion, encounter with law enforcement)?
   j. Do they find it difficult to go to school?
   k. Do they have difficulties getting up on time to go to school?
   l. Do they find it difficult to keep up with schoolwork?
   m. Are they able to complete their schoolwork on time?
   n. Does the youth have accommodations or an individual education plan? If asking the youth directly: "Do you get any extra help at school?" (Information about the individual education plan can be found in Chapter 20, "Special Considerations for Childhood and Adolescent Populations.")
4. Vocational
   a. Do they volunteer or have a part-time job?
   b. Do they like their job?
5. Peer relationships
   a. Do they have close friends they trust at school?
   b. Would they say that they have a tough time figuring out how to socialize/get along with others at school/work/home?
   c. Do they experience challenges interacting with people at school/work/home?
   d. Have they experienced any bullying at school?
6. Social time/relaxation
   a. What do they like to do for fun or when they have free time?
   b. What do they like to do to relax?
   c. Who are their friends?
   d. What do they like to do with their friends at school, after school, on weekends?
7. Religious beliefs
   a. Do they have any religious affiliation?

PSYCHIATRIC HISTORY

A. Assess for any prior psychiatric, psychological, or educational evaluations or interventions that may have been sought for the chief concern.
B. Assess the outcome of any such interventions, as well as the patient's and legal guardians' attitude toward such earlier attempts to obtain help.
C. The following questions are helpful to ask when assessing psychiatric history:
   1. When did you first notice the symptoms?
   2. Did you seek treatment for the symptoms?
   3. Did you fully recover?
   4. Have you ever been hospitalized? How many times? What were the reasons for the hospitalizations and how long were you hospitalized?
   5. Do you receive outpatient mental health services?

PAST/CURRENT MEDICATIONS

A. Assess current and past medications. Pay particular attention to current and past psychiatric medications.
B. The following questions are helpful to ask:
   1. Do you take medications for a mental illness?
   2. Which medications have helped the most?
   3. Did you have any negative side effects from any medications?
   4. What was the reason for stopping prior medications?
   5. How long were you taking each medication and how often did you take it?
   6. Do you know the name, strength, and number of doses per day of medicines and supplements you are currently taking?

FAMILY PSYCHIATRIC HISTORY

A. Inquire about family members' past and current history of medical and psychiatric disorders that have potential environmental or genetic consequences for the patient.
B. The following questions are helpful to ask:
   1. Have any of your relatives ever have mental or behavioral health problems such as attention deficit hyperactivity disorder (ADHD), anxiety, depression, bipolar disorder (BD), psychosis, problems with drinking or other drugs, suicide attempts, or psychiatric hospitalizations?
   2. Does anyone in your family have any long-standing medical problems?
   3. Does the patient know about/has the patient witnessed any of the illnesses? How did they respond to it?

REFERENCES AND BIBLIOGRAPHY

American Psychiatric Association. (2013). *Diagnostic and statistical manual of mental disorders* (5th ed.). https://doi.org/10.1176/appi.books.9780890425596

American Psychiatric Association. (2022). *Diagnostic and statistical manual of mental disorders* (5th ed., text rev.). https://doi.org/10.1176/appi.books.9780890425787

Boland, R. J., Verduin, M. L., & Ruiz, P. (2022). *Kaplan & Sadock's synopsis of psychiatry* (12th ed.). Wolters Kluwer.

Carlat, D. J. (2005). *Practical guides in psychiatry: The psychiatric interview* (2nd ed.). Lippincott Williams & Wilkins.

Cepeda, C., & Gotanco, L. (2017). *Psychiatric interview of children and adolescents*. American Psychiatric Association Publishing.

Gardner, H., & Randall, D. (2012). The effects of the presence or absence of parents on interviews with children. *Nurse Researcher*, 19(2), 6–10. https://doi.org/10.7748/nr2012.01.19.2.6.c8902

Hilt, R., & Nussbaum, A. (2016). DSM-5 *pocket guide for child and adolescent mental health*. American Psychiatric Association Publishing.

Katzenellenbogen, R. (2005, March). HEADSS: The "review of systems" for adolescents. *Virtual Mentor: Ethics Journal of the American Medical Association*, 7(3), 231–233. https://doi.org/10.1001/virtualmentor.2005.7.3.cprl1-0503

Pashak, T. J., & Heron, M. R. (2022). Build rapport and collect data: A teaching resource on the clinical interviewing intake. *Discover Psychology*, 2, Article 20. https://doi.org/10.1007/s44202-022-00019-5

Zimmerman, M. (1994). *Interview guide for evaluating DSM-IV psychiatric disorders and the mental status examination*. Psych Product Press.

PHASE 4: PSYCHIATRIC REVIEW OF SYSTEMS

ASSESSING FOR MOOD DISORDERS

Major Depressive Disorder

A. Screen all children and adolescents for major depressive disorder (MDD) to ensure timely access to mental health services.
  1. The U.S. Preventive Services Task Force (USPSTF) recommends screening in adolescents 12 to 18 years of age.
  2. Although the USPSTF does not recommend screening in youth 11 years of age and younger, early identification can facilitate early intervention.

B. During mood assessment, the APRN will identify symptoms; frequency of symptoms; severity; onset and duration; degree of associated distress and functional impairment; developmental deviations; and physical signs/factors predisposing, precipitating, or protecting the patient from the symptom presentation.

C. Symptoms consistent with a diagnosis of MDD include the following:
  1. Discrete episode of at least 2 weeks in duration with clear changes in mood (sadness/irritability, feelings of emptiness or boredom)
  2. Lack of interest/pleasure
  3. Changes in cognition and neurovegetative functions
  4. Suicidality: may or may not be present

D. Except for suicidality, symptoms of depression must be present for most of the day, nearly every day, and must result in clinically significant distress or functional impairment.

E. The Patient Health Questionnaire-9 (PHQ-9) is the preferred screening tool for office visits to address suicidality. The Patient Health Questionnaire-2 (PHQ-2) can be used virtually, but if it is positive an in-person visit is needed. For younger children, clinicians can use the Short Mood and Feelings Questionnaire (SMFQ) virtually and the Mood and Feelings Questionnaire (MFQ) in person.

F. Screening questions for MDD include the following:
  1. Have you been feeling sad, blue, depressed, down, or irritable? If yes, does feeling this way make it hard for you to concentrate or sleep? Are you angry most of the time?
  2. If yes to above, ask: Did those times ever last at least 2 weeks? Did these periods ever cause you significant troubles with your friends or family, at school, or in another setting?
  3. If yes to above, screen for MDD: During this period when you have been feeling depressed or when you have been experiencing an inability to experience pleasure (anhedonia):
     a. Significant weight loss or gain: Did you notice a change in appetite? Did you notice a change in your weight?
     b. Insomnia or hypersomnia: Did you have any difficulty with sleep? Any problems falling or staying asleep?
     c. Psychomotor agitation/retardation: Has anyone told you that you seem to be moving more slowly or faster than usual?
     d. Fatigue or loss of energy: What has your energy been like? Has anyone told you that you look less energetic than usual?
     e. Feelings of worthlessness or excessive guilt: Do you feel tremendous regret or guilt about current or past events or relationships?
     f. Diminished concentration: Were you able to make decisions like you normally do?
     g. Recurrent thoughts of death and suicide: Did you think about death more than usually do? Have you thought about hurting yourself or taking your life?

Bipolar Disorder

A. There continues to be controversy in terms of what symptoms constitute BD in children and adolescents.
  1. Some believe that youth with severe irritability, mood swings, emotional instability, and severe temper outbursts have BD, while others feel this narrow definition of BD is better explained by other diagnoses, such as ADHD, oppositional defiant disorder (ODD), MDD, or generalized anxiety disorder (GAD).
  2. A history of emotional trauma such as physical or sexual abuse can lead to symptoms like those found in BD.

B. When assessing BD in children and adolescents, the APRN may need to consider observing and obtaining collateral information from legal guardians over an extended period. This evaluation for BD must be done by an APRN with extensive experience in mental health. Novice APRNs must consider referral to a psychiatrist or trained mental health specialist if they suspect their patient has symptoms consistent with BD.

C. Screening questions for mania/hypomania include the following:
  1. Has there been a time when, for many days straight, your mood was super happy, you were more self-confident, and you had more energy than usual?
  2. If yes to the above question, then ask:
     a. During those times, did you feel this way all day or most of the day?
     b. Did something happen that started these feelings?
     c. Did these times ever last a week or result in you being hospitalized?
     d. Did these times ever cause significant trouble with your friends or family, at school, or another setting?

Psychiatric Rating Scales for Mood Disorders

A. PHQ-9 Modified for Adolescents (PHQ-A)
B. Mood Disorder Questionnaire (MDQ)

REFERENCES AND BIBLIOGRAPHY

American Academy of Child and Adolescent Psychiatry. (2007). Practice parameters for the assessment and treatment of children and adolescents with bipolar disorder. *Journal of the American Academy of Child & Adolescent Psychiatry, 36*(10), 157S–176S. https://doi.org/10.1097/00004583-199710001-00010

Walter, H. J., Abright, A. R., Bukstein, O. G., Diamond, J., Keable, H., Ripperger-Suhler, J., & Rockhill, C. (2022). Clinical practice guideline for the assessment and treatment of children and adolescents with major and persistent depressive disorder. *Journal of the American Academy of Child & Adolescent Psychiatry, 62*(5), 479–502. https://doi.org/10.1016/j.jaac.2022.10.001

Youngstrom, E. Y., Freeman, A., & McKeown Jenkins, M. (2009). The assessment of bipolar disorder in children and adolescents. *Child and Adolescent Psychiatric Clinics of North America, 18*(2), 353–390. https://doi.org/10.1016/j.chc.2008.12.002

ASSESSING FOR ANXIETY DISORDERS

A. Anxiety disorders (ADs) are among the most common psychiatric diagnoses in youth.

B. While fear and anxiety behaviors can be a normative part of development during infancy and childhood (e.g., fear of strangers, fear of the dark), ADs can be defined by extreme perceptions of threat or fear that are significantly out of proportion to risk.

C. ADs cause recurrent physiologic and emotional arousal that can occur beyond the existence of a perceived threat and can impair the day-to-day functioning of the individual.
D. When assessing for AD, the APRN must distinguish everyday worries and fear, which are common, from anxiety symptoms that are causing significant distress and functional impairment.
  1. Identify symptoms, symptom frequency, severity, onset, and duration.
  2. Determine the degree of associated distress and functional impairment, developmental deviations, physical signs, and factors predisposing, precipitation, or protecting from the symptom presentation.
E. The most common ADs in children and adolescents are GAD, separation anxiety, panic disorder, social anxiety disorder (SAD), and selective mutism.
F. General screening questions for all ADs include the following (Hilt & Nussbaum, 2016, p. 106, pp. 109–110):
  1. Would you say you worry more than other kids your age?
  2. Do people say you worry too much or you are too shy?
  3. Do you feel afraid when you are alone or away from your family?
  4. Do you get scared about going to school?
  5. Is it hard for you to control or stop your worrying?
  6. Are there specific places or situations that make you feel very anxious or scared?
  7. Have you ever felt suddenly frightened, nervous, or anxious for no reason at all? If yes, can you tell me about that?
  8. If yes to any of the above, ask: Do these experiences ever cause you trouble with your friends or family, at school, or in another setting?

Generalized Anxiety Disorder

A. Symptoms consistent with GAD include the following:
  1. Excessive worry and anxiety, occurring more days than not for at least 6 months in several different situations (e.g., work, school)
  2. Difficulty controlling the worry
  3. Worry and anxiety associated with at least three or more (one for children) of the following:
      a. Restlessness or feeling "keyed up" or "on edge"
      b. Being easily fatigued
      c. Difficulties with concentration
      d. Irritability
      e. Muscle tension
      f. Sleep disturbance (e.g., issues with sleep initiation and/or maintenance)
B. Screening questions for GAD include the following:
  1. When you think about activities or situations that make you anxious or worried, do you feel restless or on edge?
  2. Do you often tire easily?
  3. When you are anxious or worried, do you often find it hard to concentrate, or do you find that your mind goes blank?
  4. When you are anxious or worried, do you often feel irritable or easily annoyed?
  5. When you are anxious or worried, do you often experience muscle tightness or tension?
  6. Do you find it difficult to fall asleep or stay asleep, or do you experience restless sleep?

Separation Anxiety

A. Separation anxiety is developmentally normal for infants from about 6 months of age to 2 years and reflects a child's understanding of separation from their primary caregiver.
B. Throughout childhood, there may be normative brief separation anxiety in transition periods, such as when starting school or being away from caregivers for the first time. The main symptom of separation anxiety disorder is an excessive fear or anxiety when separated from the primary caregiver that is not developmentally appropriate. The child or adolescent will also avoid situations in which they are separated from their primary caregiver. The fear and anxiety must be persistent and lasting at least 4 weeks in children and 6 months or more in adolescents. For diagnosis of separation anxiety, a child or adolescent must also experience three of the following:
  1. Recurrent extreme distress when anticipating or experiencing separation from home or from major attachment figures
  2. Persistent or excessive worry about losing major attachment figures or about possible harm to them (e.g., illness, injury, disasters, death)
  3. Persistent or excessive worry about experiencing a negative event (e.g., getting lost, being kidnapped, being in an accident, becoming ill) that causes separation from a major attachment figure
  4. Persistent reluctance or refusal to go out, away from home, to school, to work, or elsewhere due to fear of separation
  5. Persistent and excessive fear of or reluctance about being alone or without major attachment figures at home or in other settings
  6. Persistent reluctance or refusal to sleep away from home or to go to sleep without being near a major attachment figure
  7. Repeated nightmares involving the theme of separation
  8. Repeated complaints of physical symptoms (e.g., headaches, stomachaches, nausea, vomiting) when separation from major attachment figures occurs or is anticipated
C. Screening questions for separation anxiety include the following:
  1. Extreme fear of separation from legal guardian(s):
      a. Do you worry a lot when you know you will be away from your parents/caregiver?
      b. Do you worry that something bad will happen to your parents/caregiver (e.g., illness, injury, death)?
      c. Do you worry that something bad will happen to you when you are away from your parent/caregiver (e.g., getting lost, kidnapping, injury, illness)?
      d. Do you have bad dreams about being away from your parent/caregiver? How often?
      e. Do you worry so much about being away from your parent/caregiver that you do not want to leave their side? Do you insist on sleeping in the same bed?
      f. Do you refuse to go to school or other places outside the home?
      g. When you are worried about being away from your parent/caregiver, how does your body feel? Does your stomach hurt, or do you get headaches?
  2. Impairment in daily functioning:
      a. How do you feel at school when you are away from your parent/caregiver?
      b. How are your grades? Are you able to concentrate/complete your work at school?

c. How do you feel about being away from your parents/caregivers when you are doing something fun with your friends?

Social Anxiety Disorder

A. Social anxiety disorder (SAD) usually starts in late childhood. It is characterized by extreme shyness or avoidance of many social interactions for fear the person will be scrutinized or judged by others.

B. Symptoms consistent with SAD include the following:
   1. Excessive fear or anxiety about one or more social situations in which the individual is exposed to possible scrutiny by others (e.g., class presentations, meeting new people, being observed while eating). For youth, the anxiety must also occur in peer settings.
   2. The individual fears that their behavior will be negatively evaluated (i.e., that they will be humiliated or rejected by others).
   3. Social situations almost always provoke fear or anxiety (e.g., children may cry, have tantrums, or fail to speak in social situations).
   4. Social situations are avoided or endured with intense fear or anxiety.
   5. The fear or anxiety is out of proportion to the actual threat posed by the social situation and to the sociocultural context.
   6. Fear, anxiety, or avoidance is persistent, typically lasting 6 months or more.

C. Screening questions for SAD (reference, or original) include the following:
   1. Extreme fear in social settings:
      a. How do you feel about being in a big crowd?
      b. When you go to the mall, or to a busy store, do you feel scared or anxious being around a lot of people?
      c. How do you feel about meeting and speaking with strangers?
      d. Do you tend to avoid parties and/or family gatherings or places where there are a lot of people?
      e. How do you feel about speaking in front of a crowd of people?
      f. Do these social situations always cause you to feel scared/anxious?
      g. Legal guardians: Have you noticed increased or excessive crying, tantrums, or clinginess of the youth in social situations? Have you noticed that the youth tends to freeze up or shy away from social situations? Is this a change from before?
   2. Fear of negative judgment from others:
      a. Do you worry about how people will judge you for what you say or do in social situations?
      b. Do you worry about doing something that will make you feel embarrassed or bad about yourself when you are with other people?
   3. Anxiety in social situations causing functional impairment:
      a. What do you feel in your body when you are worried in these situations?
      b. Do you feel your heart beating fast? Do you feel like there is a weight, like an elephant on your chest? Do you feel hot or sweaty?
      c. Does your fear of these situations cause you to miss school or miss out on socializing with friends/family/peers?
      d. Have your grades suffered because of your fears?
      e. Has any other part of your life been affected by your fear of being in these social situations?

Panic Disorder

A. Panic disorder is a common anxiety disorder in children and adolescents. It is characterized by abrupt, unexpected, and repeated periods of intense fear or discomfort with at least four or more of the following symptoms:
   1. Racing or pounding heartbeat
   2. Sweating
   3. Dizziness or lightheadedness
   4. Feelings of choking
   5. Chest pain or discomfort
   6. Chills or heat sensations
   7. Nausea or abdominal distress
   8. Shortness of breath or feeling of being smothered
   9. Trembling or shaking
   10. Sense of things being unreal (derealization) and/or the person feeling unreal (depersonalization)
   11. Fear of dying
   12. Fear of losing control

B. At least one of the panic attacks must be followed by 1 month (or more) of one of the following:
   1. Persistent concern or worry about additional panic attacks or their consequences (e.g., losing control, having a heart attack)
   2. A significant maladaptive change in behavior related to the attacks

C. Screening questions for panic disorder include the following:
   1. How often do you have these times of extreme worry/fear/anxiety?
   2. When did these symptoms start?
   3. When do these symptoms come on?
   4. Between panic attacks, do you worry you will have another attack?
   5. When you have these symptoms, do you feel afraid you cannot escape a situation or place?
   6. Do these feelings cause you to want to stay home more often or avoid doing new things?
   7. How do you feel in your body when these symptoms start?
   8. Do you feel like it is hard to breathe and you are breathing faster?
   9. Do you feel like you are choking?
   10. Do you feel your heart beating harder or faster?
   11. Do you feel pain anywhere?
   12. Do you feel like you want to throw up, or does your stomach hurt?
   13. Do you feel hot or cold? Sweaty?
   14. Do you feel dizzy, shaky, or numb?
   15. Do you ever have feelings of tingling, like pins and needles, or numbness?
   16. Have you ever felt so worried or scared that you felt like you could not move or think for a period of time? Or that you were not in your own body?
   17. Do you have feelings of future disaster/trouble? Fear of dying? Fear of "going crazy"?

Selective Mutism

A. Selective mutism refers to the persistent failure to speak in social situations, where speech is expected, even though the youth is speaking in other situations (e.g., at home). The APRN should consider a diagnosis of selective mutism if the failure to speak persists longer than 1 month (excluding the first month of school), it cannot be better explained by a language barrier, and it interferes with educational and social functioning. Age of onset is typically 3 to 6 years, but it is usually noticed when a child starts school.

B. Screening questions for selective mutism include the following:
   1. Does your child have trouble speaking with adults or at school?
   2. Have you noticed your child will not speak in certain situations?
   3. Does your child converse well when they have no fear or anxiety? In what environments do they speak well/fluently/easily?
   4. Has your child's school spoken to you about issues with speaking in public?
   5. Has your child's not speaking interfered with their learning?
   6. Has your child's not speaking interfered with them making friends or doing activities they like?
   7. Any issues with learning language? Any developmental delay/disorders?
   8. Any medical issues or diagnosis that affected language development?
   9. Any history of psychological disorders/diagnoses?
   10. Is English a second language? Is it possible your child does not feel comfortable speaking in English?

Specific Phobias

A. Specific phobias are characterized by intense, excessive fear of certain things or situations (e.g., flying, heights, elevators, animals, receiving an injection, seeing blood) that has lasted for at least 6 months. In children, the fear or anxiety may be expressed by crying, tantrums, freezing, or clinging. Exposure to the object or situation almost always provokes immediate fear or anxiety.

B. Questions for screening specific phobia include the following:
   1. Is there anything that you really feel scared of (e.g., an animal, the dark, needles)?
   2. Have legal guardians noticed extremely fearful behaviors? Around what objects or situations?
   3. What happens in your body when you feel afraid?
   4. What do you do when you feel afraid?
   5. Do you try to not go near the object/situation you are afraid of?
   6. What do you think will happen to you when you are near the object/situation?
   7. Ask legal guardians if they identify their child's fear as being out of proportion or more extreme than it usually would be for a youth?
   8. Do you always feel this scared of the object/situation, or is it sometimes okay?
   9. Do you find this fear of the object/situation is causing problems in your life every day? Do you feel like you are not able to do the things you like to do because of this fear?
   10. Is this fear affecting your school or time spent doing activities you like?
   11. Does it affect how you spend time with your friends or family?

C. Psychiatric rating scales for anxiety include the following:
   1. Panic Disorder Severity Scale (PDSS)
   2. Screen for Child Anxiety Related Disorders (SCARED)
   3. Spence Children's Anxiety Scale (SCAS)
   4. Preschool Anxiety Scale
   5. Generalized Anxiety Disorder-7 (GAD-7; for teens/adults)

REFERENCES AND BIBLIOGRAPHY

Binesh-Marvasti, T. B., & McQueen, S. (2018). *Essential Med Notes 2018: Comprehensive medical reference and review for USMLE II and MCCQE* (34th ed.). Thieme.

Hilt, R. & Nussbaum, A. (2016). *DSM-5 pocket guide for child and adolescent mental health*. American Psychiatric Association Publishing.

Vecchio, J. L., & Kearney, C. A. (2005). Selective mutism in children: Comparison to youths with and without anxiety disorders. *Journal of Psychopathology and Behavioral Assessment, 27*(1), 31–37. https://doi.org/10.1007/s10862-005-3263-1

Walter, H. J., Abright, A. R., Bukstein, O. G., Diamond, J., Keable, H., Ripperger-Suhler, J., & Rockhill, C. (2022). Clinical practice guideline for the assessment and treatment of children and adolescents with anxiety disorders. *Journal of the American Academy of Child & Adolescent Psychiatry, 59*(10), 1107–1124. https://doi.org/10.1016/j.jaac.2020.05.005

ASSESSING FOR OBSESSIVE-COMPULSIVE DISORDER

A. Obsessive-compulsive disorder (OCD) in children and adolescents is a disabling condition characterized by unwanted, repetitive, intrusive thoughts, and/or distressing, time-consuming rituals (compulsions).

B. Children or adolescents suffering from OCD may have intrusive thoughts they are unable to stop and develop obsessions to mitigate these thoughts.

C. Some of the most common obsessions in children and youths include fear of harm to themselves or family members/loved ones, fear of uncleanness or contamination, obsessions with symmetry, sexual obsessions, hoarding obsessions, and obsessions with religious or moral matters.

D. Onset of OCD symptoms in the pediatric population may be subtle, and the youth may hide their symptoms as long as is reasonably possible. OCD is frequently associated with diagnoses of tic disorders, anxiety disorders, and ADHD.

E. Screening questions for OCD include the following:
   1. Do you sometimes have thoughts that come into your head even though you do not want them to? What are these thoughts?
   2. Do you have images that you see in your head that you do not want to see?
   3. Do you have the urge to do something you do not want to do? What types of things do you have urges to do?
   4. To stop unwanted thoughts or urges, some people might do things repeatedly to make themselves feel better, for example, counting, praying, or repeating words or phrases. Do you feel the need to do anything like this repeatedly?
      a. Do you feel the need to clean a lot or repeatedly?
      b. Do you feel the need to organize or arrange things often just the way you like it?
      c. Does it upset you if anyone moves your things or changes the order of something you have arranged?
      d. Do you avoid doing certain things because you know it will cause unwanted thoughts or feelings?
   5. How long every day would you say you spend with your mind stuck on something or on these repeated activities?
   6. Are you unable to complete tasks or slow down because you feel the need to repeat any of the behaviors previously described?

7. Legal guardian: Ask all above questions, specifically around severity of obsessions and compulsive rituals. Ask about the effect on youth's ability to function daily and how they are doing in school and social situations.

Psychiatric Rating Scale for Obsessive-Compulsive Disorder
A. Yale-Brown Obsessive Compulsive Scale (Y-BOCS)

ASSESSING PSYCHOSIS IN CHILDREN AND ADOLESCENTS
A. Determining the presence of a psychotic disorder in children and adolescents is a complex and challenging task. APRNs must pause and review clinical cases with a developmental lens to fully appreciate the presenting signs or symptoms before making any determinations or treatment recommendations.
B. Misdiagnosis can often occur due to the delicate interplay between normal developmental attributes and other emotional, behavioral, developmental, or medical conditions that may distort the findings of a psychotic condition.
C. A patient presents with symptoms of psychosis that have been present for a brief period. A *brief period* can be defined as less than 1 month or if the onset is sudden with no history of previous symptoms, and requires a complete, thorough medical assessment, including investigations to rule out any organic causes of this presentation of psychosis (e.g., due to a medical condition like encephalopathy). In some medical conditions, the patient can experience some psychiatric prodromal symptoms before presenting with medical symptoms.
D. Children and adolescents may exhibit various clinical conditions requiring a differential diagnosis, such as psychotic mood disorders, schizophrenia, schizoaffective disorder, and organic psychoses that are caused by other medical conditions or psychoactive substances.
  1. APRNs who are unfamiliar with normal developmental processes may find themselves misinterpreting typical emotional, mental, or behavioral responses as psychotic presentations.
  2. For example, young children have overactive imaginations and magical thinking. The presence of fantasy is a normal part of development. A child who imagines themselves going into space and flying to the moon while playing on the playground is typical. However, an adult exhibiting a similar ideation, believing they are an astronaut who has gone to the moon, may be experiencing a delusional disorder.
  3. Although the diagnostic criteria for psychosis do not change between children and adults, the context in which symptoms are reviewed dramatically changes the outcome of the findings.
  4. Studies have shown that the onset of childhood schizophrenia (12 years or younger) is possible, but it is also exceedingly rare, with a prevalence of 0.2 to 0.4 per 10,000.
  5. Delusional disorders are also less frequently observed in children.
  6. Most children younger than 12 years who report psychotic-like symptoms suggestive of hallucinations or delusions likely do not truly have a psychotic illness.
E. Atypical behaviors for a youth's developmental stage are always a cause for concern and should be assessed carefully. The APRN's assessment of symptoms should be done with social and environmental contexts in mind as they may change or impact how the youth behaves or reacts to stimuli.
F. Asking legal guardians questions about when the behaviors occur, how long they last, and who is present when they appear can be extremely helpful in determining the likelihood of psychosis.
G. Careful review of patients with trauma histories may also support understanding atypical behaviors.
  1. For example, a 13-year-old who speaks with an imaginary friend may not necessarily be experiencing a hallucination or a delusion rooted in psychosis but exhibiting behavioral regression as a comfort/protective measure related to trauma.
H. Often, consistency in behavioral presentations, including hallucinations or delusions, regardless of changes in social or environmental contexts and in conjunction with disorganized thoughts and behaviors, will be more indicative of a psychotic condition in youth.
I. Screening questions for psychosis/delusions include the following:
  1. Have you ever had an unusual experience that you could not explain?
  2. Do you see things that others cannot see?
  3. Do you hear things that others cannot hear (e.g., voices of people talking or whispering, noises that cannot be explained by something naturally occurring in the space)?
  4. Have you ever felt something on your skin/body (e.g., bugs crawling on your skin)?
  5. Have your ever experienced seeing a shadow in the room and feeling like someone else was there? Do you feel like someone is bothering you? Does this experience make you feel afraid?
  6. Have you ever felt that characters on television are talking to you and that their messages are only intended for you?
  7. Have you ever seen a sign or billboard and felt that the message on it was directed to you only?

REFERENCES AND BIBLIOGRAPHY
Courvoisie, H., Labellarte, M. J., & Riddle, M. A. (2001). Psychosis in children: Diagnosis and treatment. *Dialogues in Clinical Neuroscience, 3*(2), 79–92. https://doi.org/10.31887/DCNS.2001.3.2/hcourvoisie

Dulcan, M. K. (Ed.). (2010). *Dulcan's textbook of child and adolescent psychiatry.* American Psychiatric Publishing, Inc.

Griswold, K. S., Del Regno, P. A., & Berger, R. C. (2015). Recognition and differential diagnosis of psychosis in primary care. *American Family Physician, 91*(12), 856–863. PMID: 26131945.

Reimherr, J. P., & McClellan, J. M. (2004). Diagnostic challenges in children and adolescents with psychotic disorders. *The Journal of Clinical Psychiatry, 65*(Suppl. 6), 5–11. PMID: 15104521.

ASSESSING FOR ADJUSTMENT DISORDER
A. When people are exposed to extreme amounts of stress, they can develop an adjustment disorder in response to the stress. This is a transient condition, limited to a duration of 2 years maximum, but usually improving within 6 months after eliminating the stressor.
B. Individuals who have adjustment disorders have maladaptive behaviors and emotions that develop from this exposure to a nontraumatic psychosocial stress, which can contribute to the development of a stress response.
C. Adjustment disorder is more commonly seen in children and adolescents who have medical conditions, but it should not be excluded from the differential list in patients without a comorbid medical illness. Other differentials to consider when thinking about adjustment disorder are posttraumatic stress disorder (PTSD) and prolonged grief disorder.

D. Screening tools for adjustment include the following:
1. The APRN can use the Adjustment Disorder-New Module 20 as a screening instrument if there is suspicion of an adjustment disorder. This instrument can help identify low, moderate, or high symptomatology.
   a. This tool is based on the *International Classification of Diseases*, 11th Revision (*ICD-11*; World Health Organization [WHO], 2019), criteria for diagnosis. This tool is best used with adolescents and adults and may not translate well for use with children.
2. Assessing for adjustment disorder should be done in the context of a larger mental health/psychiatric assessment. It is essential to ensure that the symptoms of adjustment are not better explained by another psychiatric diagnosis.

E. Criteria for diagnosis of adjustment disorder include the following:
1. Ask questions based on the information sought related to the following criteria:
   a. The patient presents with clinically significant emotional or behavioral symptoms that are a reaction to a stressor that the patient can identify.
   b. Symptoms develop within the first 3 months of the stressor's start.
   c. The patient may become preoccupied or hyperfocused on the stressor and fail to adapt to the stressor.
   d. The patient experiences significant distress that is disproportionate to the severity of the stressor, and these emotional or behavioral symptoms cause the patient significant functional impairments (e.g., socially, at school, at work).
   e. It is important to consider that the stress that the patient is experiencing is not related to the following:
      i. Another mental health condition
      ii. A worsening of a preexisting psychiatric problem
      iii. Normal grief from loss

F. Once the patient experiences relief from the stressor, the emotional or behavioral symptoms improve. These symptoms should not persist longer than 6 months following the stressor's termination.

G. Screening questions for adjustment disorder include the following:
1. Have you experienced any recent stressful events? What has been happening in your life over the last month? (Ask the patient to describe the stressor.)
2. Have you felt more emotional or acted in a way that is different from you usually act since you have been experiencing the stressor?
3. When did these symptoms start?
4. Has your distress impacted you at school, home, or with your friends? If so, can you share with me how it has affected you in these areas?

REFERENCES AND BIBLIOGRAPHY

Lorenz, L., Bachem, R. C., & Maercker, A. (2016). The adjustment disorder—new module 20 as a screening instrument: Cluster analysis and cut-off values. *The International Journal of Occupational and Environmental Medicine*, 7(4), 215–220. https://doi.org/10.15171/ijoem.2016.775

Maercker, A., & Lorenz, L. (2018). Adjustment disorder diagnosis: Improving clinical utility. *The World Journal of Biological Psychiatry*, 19(sup1), S3–S13. https://doi.org/10.1080/15622975.2018.1449967

O'Donnell, M. L., Agathos, J. A., Metcalf, O., Gibson, K., & Lau, W. (2019). Adjustment disorder: Current developments and future directions. *International Journal of Environmental Research and Public Health*, 16(14), 2537. PMID: 27651082.

World Health Organization. (2019). *International classification of diseases* (11th rev.). https://icd.who.int

Zelviene, P., & Kazlauskas, E. (2018). Adjustment disorder: Current perspectives. *Neuropsychiatric Disease and Treatment*, 14, 375–381. https://doi.org/10.2147/NDT.S121072

ASSESSING FOR SOMATIC SYMPTOM DISORDER AND RELATED DISORDERS

A. Somatic symptoms refer to physical symptoms that can be caused by psychological stress, pain, or anxiety.

B. Everyone experiences somatization in their lives. Some examples are feeling muscle tension or headaches after a difficult or stressful day, blushing when feeling embarrassed, or having "butterflies" in the stomach if feeling anxious, such as when giving a presentation.

C. Most people can manage these somatic symptoms effectively and move on with their lives; however, these symptoms become disordered when there is significant impairment or disruption in a person's daily life.

D. In the pediatric population, somatic symptoms may develop from existing medical illnesses or traumatic events, as a response to stress and strong emotions, and many times the trigger for symptoms is not clear.
1. A diagnosis of somatic symptom disorder and related disorders is no longer considered one of the symptoms that are medically unexplained, as this is not useful or reliable.
2. The individual's distress is genuine regardless of medical explanation.
3. Mental health clinicians frequently treat patients with recognized medical diagnoses who have significant preoccupation with symptoms and distressing physical symptoms.

E. Diagnosis of somatic symptom disorder is centered around assessment for positive signs and symptoms such as intense or abnormal thoughts and behaviors related to physical symptoms.

F. An assessment using the biopsychosocial approach is helpful in exploring the factors contributing to a youth's mental state and how this may be causing physical symptoms.

G. Significant medical and psychiatric comorbidity can occur among individuals with somatic disorders. Consequently, any individual who is being assessed for somatization should also be assessed for other mental health concerns such as anxiety or depression.

H. Typically, pediatric patients with somatic symptoms present in medical or primary care settings before they present in a psychiatric setting. It is also common for multiple health professionals to be involved in both assessment and diagnosis, depending on the individual's symptoms. Interdisciplinary communication and teamwork are thus especially important for somatizing individuals.

I. Among the related disorders in this category are factitious disorder and illness anxiety disorder.
1. *Factitious disorder* is a disorder in which the individual purposefully fabricates or misrepresents medical or psychiatric symptoms and seeks treatment for such (refer to the *Diagnostic and Statistical Manual of Mental Disorders, Fifth Edition* [*DSM-5*; American Psychiatric Association, 2013] for diagnostic criteria).
2. *Illness anxiety disorder*, previously classified as hypochondriasis, occurs when an individual does not have somatic symptoms or other psychological or medical symptoms but has a preoccupation with and high anxiety about developing or having a medical condition (refer to

the *DSM-5* [American Psychiatric Association, 2013] for diagnostic criteria).
3. The assessment for these diagnoses will be similar to other somatic symptom disorders but is not discussed in this chapter because incidents in the pediatric population are quite low for both illness anxiety disorder and factitious disorder.

Somatic Symptom Disorder
A. Individuals with somatic symptom disorder typically have persistent thoughts, feelings, and behaviors that are associated with their physical symptoms.
B. These symptoms cause excessive and unexpected distress and impairment of daily life.
C. These individuals tend to have elevated levels of anxiety about their health and may be concerned that a medical diagnosis has been missed.

Conversion Disorder (Functional Neurologic Symptom Disorder)
A. Individuals with conversion disorder present with some kind of loss of function—motor or sensory (e.g., limb weakness, vision loss, speech symptoms, nonepileptic seizures).
B. Clinical findings are not clarified by physical exam, are conflicting, and are unexplained by currently known neurologic or medical etiology.
C. As with somatic symptom disorder, the symptoms of conversion disorder can cause significant impairment and loss of function and independence in an individual's life.
D. Often, physiologic distress from conflict may precede symptoms of conversion disorder, but this is not necessary for diagnosis.
E. Patients may seem unconcerned with loss of function or functional change (called *la belle indifference*). Although this is not a diagnostic criterion, la belle indifference has been most associated with conversion disorders and should be assessed.

Psychological Factors Affecting Medical Conditions
A. Individuals with this diagnosis must have a medical condition present that is negatively impacted or exacerbated by psychological factors.
B. An example is asthma attacks or exacerbation in the context of anxiety or stress.
C. A diagnosis of psychological factors affecting medical conditions can range from mild to extreme.

Screening Questions for Somatic Symptom Disorder and Related Disorders
A. Biological factors
  1. Have you had any recent injuries or medical diagnoses? What is your understanding of these diagnoses?
  2. What are your physical symptoms?
  3. Do these symptoms worry you? How has it been for you?
  4. What is your understanding of the reason you are in clinic/hospital being assessed?
  5. Are there any other physical conditions you have that you feel are affecting you currently?
  6. Do you feel your symptoms are affecting your ability to do day-to-day things (e.g., getting dressed, going to school/work, playing sports, eating meals, sleeping, participating in normal activities)?
  7. How long have you had these symptoms?

B. Psychological factors
  1. How do you feel about your medical diagnoses?
  2. How do you feel your illness has affected your life?
  3. Is there any stress in your life currently?
  4. Was there any stressful event that happened right before you got sick?
  5. How do you usually manage your stress?
  6. Are there any emotions you have that you feel uncomfortable with?
  7. What does a healthy life look like to you?

C. Social factors
  1. How are things at your home? How would you describe your relationship with your parents/siblings/family?
  2. Do you feel safe at home? Is there anything that bothers you at home?
  3. How is school? Do you like school? Are there any parts of school you do not like?
  4. Is there anything about school that you find worrisome or stressful?
  5. Do you have many friends? Do you feel you can trust your friends?
  6. Is there anything about your friendships/relationships that you find stressful or hurtful?
  7. Are there other parts of your life that you wish could change? What are those things?
  8. Are there other parts of your life you find stressful or worrisome? What are they?

Psychiatric Rating Scale
A. Currently, there are no valid psychometric pediatric scales for somatic disorders.
B. The Somatic Symptom Scale (SSS-8) has been used in the *DSM-5* (American Psychiatric Association, 2013) as a reference measure to aid diagnosis.

REFERENCES AND BIBLIOGRAPHY

American Academy of Child and Adolescent Psychiatry. (2023). *Physical symptoms of emotional distress: Somatic symptoms and related disorders.* https://www.aacap.org/AACAP/Families_and_Youth/Facts_for_Families/FFF-Guide/Physical_Symptoms_of_Emotional_Distress-Somatic_Symptoms_and_Related_Disorders-124.aspx

American Psychiatric Association. (2013). *Diagnostic and statistical manual of mental disorders* (5th ed.). https://doi.org/10.1176/appi.books.9780890425596

Barkley, R. A. (2022). *Treating ADHD in children and adolescents: What every clinician needs to know.* Guilford Press.

Erskine, H. E., Ferrari, A. J., Nelson, P., Polanczyk, G. V., Flaxman, A. D., Vos, T., Whiteford, H. A., & Scott, J. G. (2013). Epidemiological modelling of attention-deficit/hyperactivity disorder and conduct disorder for the Global Burden of Disease Study 2010. *Journal of Child Psychology and Psychiatry, 54*(12), 1263–1274. https://doi.org/10.1111/jcpp.12144

Gierk, B., Kohlmann, S., Kroenke, K., Spangenberg, L., Zenger, M., Brähler, E., & Löwe, B. (2014). The Somatic Symptom Scale-8 (SSS-8): A brief measure of somatic symptom burden. *JAMA Internal Medicine, 174*(3), 399–407. https://doi.org/10.1001/jamainternmed.2013.12179

Gorkarakonda, S. B., & Kumar N. (2024, May 7). *La belle indifference.* StatPearls Publishing. https://www.ncbi.nlm.nih.gov/books/NBK560842

Kelty Mental Health Resource Centre. (n.d.). *Somatization and the mind-body connection.* BC Children's Hospital. https://keltymental health.ca/somatization

Kelty Mental Health Resource Centre. (2014, November 5). *Body talk: Stories of somatization* [Video]. BC Children's Hospital. YouTube. https://www.youtube.com/watch?v=3wycDLD0Bxo

Nair, S. S., Kwan, S. C., Ng, C. W. M., & Teo D. C. L. (2021). Approach to the patient with multiple somatic symptoms. *Singapore Medical Journal, 62*(5), 252–258. https://doi.org/10.11622/smedj.2021059

Owens, E. B., & Hinshaw, S. P. (2020). Adolescent mediators of unplanned pregnancy among women with and without childhood ADHD. *Journal of Clinical Child and Adolescent Psychology, 49*(2), 229–238. https://doi.org/10.1080/15374416.2018.1547970

Pliszka, S., & American Academy of Child and Adolescent Psychiatry. (2007). Practice parameter for the assessment and treatment of children and adolescents with attention-deficit/hyperactivity disorder. *Journal of the American Academy of Child & Adolescent Psychiatry, 46*(7), 894–921. https://doi.org/10.1097/chi.0b013e318054e724

ASSESSING FOR ATTENTION DEFICIT HYPERACTIVITY DISORDER

A. Attention deficit hyperactivity disorder (ADHD) is one of the most common childhood psychiatric conditions, as well as the best researched disorder in medicine. It is a neurobiological condition that can cause significant impairment in children and adolescents.

B. There is abundant evidence to conclude that ADHD comprises serious deficits in the development and use of executive function, which lead to significant problems with time management, self-restraint, working memory and self-organization, planning and problem-solving toward a goal, and self-regulation of emotion.

C. Untreated ADHD in children and adolescents can result in profound consequences, such as early mortality due to accidental injury, substance use disorder, difficulty with relationships, and poor performance at work and school.

D. ADHD is a pattern of behavior, with onset before 12 years of age, that is present in multiple settings and gives rise to social, educational, and work performance difficulties. The symptoms must be persistently present for at least 6 months to a degree inconsistent with developmental level.

Screening Questions for Attention Deficit Hyperactivity Disorder

A. For inattentive type, the patient must have at least six of the following symptoms:
  1. Overlook details: Over the last 6 months, have other people told you that you have often overlooked or missed details or that you made careless mistakes in your work?
  2. Task inattention: Do you often have difficulty staying focused on a task or activity, such as reading a book or listening to a lecture or conversation?
  3. Appears not to listen: Do other people tell you when they speak to you that your mind seems to be elsewhere or that it seems like you are not listening?
  4. Fails to finish tasks: Do you often struggle to finish schoolwork, chores, or work assignments because you lose focus or are easily distracted?
  5. Difficulty organizing tasks: Do you often find it difficult to organize tasks or activities? Do you struggle with time management or fail to meet deadlines?
  6. Avoid tasks requiring sustained mental activity: Do you often avoid tasks that require sustained focus?
  7. Often loses things necessary for tasks: Do you often lose things that are essential for tasks or activities, such as school materials, books, tools, wallets, keys, paperwork, eyeglasses, or phone?
  8. Easily distracted: Do you find that you are often distracted by things or thoughts unrelated to the activity or task you are supposed to be doing?
  9. Often forgetful: Do you find, or do other people find, that you are often forgetful in your daily activities?

B. For hyperactive/impulsive type, the patient must have at least six of the following symptoms:
  1. Fidgets: Over the past 6 months, have you often found yourself fidgeting with your hands or feet? Do you find it hard to sit without squirming?
  2. Leaves seat: When you are in a situation where you are expected to sit, do you often leave your seat?
  3. Runs or climbs: Do you often find yourself running around or climbing in a situation where doing so is inappropriate?
  4. Unable to maintain quiet: Do you often find yourself unable to work or play quietly?
  5. Hyperactivity: Do you often feel as if you are or do other people describe you as always being or acting as if you were "driven by a motor"? Is it hard to sit still for an extended period?
  6. Talks excessively: Do you often talk excessively?
  7. Blurts answers: Do you often struggle to wait your turn in a conversation? Do you often complete other people's sentences or blurt out an answer before a question has been completed?
  8. Struggles to take turns: Do you often have difficulty waiting your turn or waiting in line?
  9. Interrupts or intrudes: Do you often "butt into" other people's activities, conversations, or games? Do you often use other people's things without permission?

Psychiatric Rating Scale

A. Child Behavior Checklist-Attention Problem Scale
B. Conners' Parent Rating Scale-Revised Short Form
C. Conners' Teacher Rating Scale-Revised Short Form
D. Conners' Abbreviated Symptoms Questionnaire
E. Vanderbilt ADHD Diagnostic Parent Rating Scale

REFERENCES AND BIBLIOGRAPHY

Barkley, R. A. (2022). *Treating ADHD in children and adolescents: What every clinician needs to know.* Guilford Press.

Erskine, H. E., Ferrari, A. J., Nelson, P., Polanczyk, G. V., Flaxman, A. D., Vos, T., Whiteford, H. A., & Scott, J. G. (2013). Epidemiological modelling of attention-deficit/hyperactivity disorder and conduct disorder for the Global Burden of Disease Study 2010. *Journal of Child Psychology and Psychiatry, 54*(12), 1263–1274. https://doi.org/10.1111/jcpp.12144

Owens, E. B., & Hinshaw, S. P. (2020). Adolescent mediators of unplanned pregnancy among women with and without childhood ADHD. *Journal of Clinical Child and Adolescent Psychology, 49*(2), 229–238. https://doi.org/10.1080/15374416.2018.1547970

Pliszka, S., & American Academy of Child and Adolescent Psychiatry. (2007). Practice parameter for the assessment and treatment of children and adolescents with attention-deficit/hyperactivity disorder. *Journal of the American Academy of Child & Adolescent Psychiatry, 46*(7), 894–921. https://doi.org/10.1097/chi.0b013e318054e724

ASSESSING FOR AUTISM SPECTRUM DISORDER

A. Autism spectrum disorder (ASD) is a developmental disability that is characterized by patterns of delay in the development of social, communicative, and cognitive skills. It also includes limited and repetitive patterns of behavior.

B. Some children will display symptoms of autism in early infancy, but others will show signs later in life. Signs are usually seen by 2 years of age.

C. People with autism have some degree of difficulty with social interaction and communication. Other characteristics are atypical patterns of activities and behaviors, such as difficulty with transition from one activity to another, a focus on details, and unusual reactions to sensations.

D. It is important to be aware that individuals with autism often have co-occurring conditions, including epilepsy, depression, anxiety, and ADHD, as well as challenging behaviors such as difficulty sleeping and self-injury. The level of intellectual functioning among people with autism varies widely, extending from profound impairment to superior levels of functioning.

E. The diagnosis requires persistent deficits in social communication and social interaction, across multiple contexts, that are present in early childhood (before 5 years of age), but may not be apparent until social demands exceed limited capacities, causing clinically significant impairment in functioning.

F. An ASD diagnosis is made from clinical interview and use of the Autism Diagnostic Observation Schedule and the Autism Diagnostic Interview-Revised.

G. For APRNs who are not qualified to use the assessment tools or have limited experience assessing individuals for ASD, referral to a specialist (e.g., developmental pediatrician, child psychiatrist, psychologist, clinician expert) to make this diagnosis is recommended.

Screening Questions for Autism Spectrum Disorder

A. The patient must meet all of the following criteria:
  1. Deficits in social-emotional reciprocity
     a. How do you introduce yourself to other people?
     b. Do you find it hard to greet another person?
     c. Do you find it hard to share your interests, thoughts, and feelings with other people?
     d. Do you dislike hearing what other people are interested in or how they feel?
  2. Deficits in nonverbal communicative behaviors used for social interaction
     a. These are observed by the APRN.
     b. Observations can range from poorly integrated verbal and nonverbal communication to abnormalities in eye contact and body language, to deficits in understanding and use of nonverbal communication, to total lack of facial expression or gestures.
  3. Deficits in developing and maintaining friendships
     a. Are you disinterested in other people?
     b. Are you unable to engage in imaginative play with other people?
     c. Do you find it difficult to make new friends?
     d. When a situation changes, do you find it hard to adjust what you do in response?

B. In addition to meeting the criteria mentioned previously, the patient must also have at least two of the following signs of restricted, repetitive patterns of behaviors, interests, or activities:
  1. Stereotyped or repetitive speech, motor movements, or use of objects, such as simple motor stereotypies, echolalia, repetitive use of objects, or idiosyncratic phrases
  2. Insistence on sameness and excessive adherence to routines or avoidance of change
     a. Do you have any special routines or patterns of behavior?
     b. What happens when you cannot follow these routines or engage in these behaviors?
     c. Do you struggle to change?
  3. Restricted interests of abnormal intensity or focus
     a. Do you intensely focus on, or find yourself extremely interested in, just a few things?
  4. Hyper- or hypoactivity to sensory input
     a. Do you have intense responses to something that is painful? Something hot? Something cold?
     b. Are there particular sounds, textures, or smells to which you respond strongly?
     c. Do you find yourself fascinated with lights or spinning objects?

Psychiatric Rating Scale

A. Autism Diagnostic Observation Schedule
B. Autism Diagnostic Interview-Revised
C. Modified Checklist for Autism in Toddlers
D. Childhood Autism Spectrum Test
E. Autism Spectrum Quotient

REFERENCES AND BIBLIOGRAPHY

Kamp-Becker, I., Tauscher, J., Wolff, N., Küpper, C., Poustka, L., Roepke, S., Roessner, V., Heider, D., & Stroth, S. (2021). Is the combination of ADOS and ADI-R necessary to classify ASD? Rethinking the "Gold Standard" in diagnosing ASD. *Frontiers in Psychiatry, 12*, 727308–727308. https://doi.org/10.3389/fpsyt.2021.727308

Volkmar, F., Siegel, M., Woodbury-Smith, M., King, B., McCracken, J., State, M., & American Academy of Child and Adolescent Psychiatry Committee on Quality Issues. (2014). Practice parameter for the assessment and treatment of children and adolescents with autism spectrum disorder. *Journal of the American Academy of Child & Adolescent Psychiatry, 53*(2), 237–257. https://doi.org/10.1016/j.jaac.2013.10.013

World Health Organization. (2023, November 15). *Autism*. https://www.who.int/news-room/fact-sheets/detail/autism-spectrum-disorders

ASSESSING FOR OPPOSITIONAL DEFIANCE DISORDER AND CONDUCT DISORDER

Oppositional Defiant Disorder

A. Oppositional behavior in children and adolescents is a normal aspect of development and is often required so young people can gain perspective on their social and environmental constructs and understand their limits.

B. There are times when oppositional behaviors become more disruptive than helpful in normal development and are seen as a symptom of something potentially more problematic.

C. Youth experiencing increased frequency or patterns of anger, irritability, arguing, and general defiance toward legal guardians or other authority figures (e.g., teachers) could be displaying early signs of oppositional defiant disorder (ODD). Other behavioral presentations such as being spiteful or revenge seeking may also be warning signs of ODD.

D. In many situations, if not addressed, these behavioral challenges can often lead to severe impacts on a patient's social, academic, or occupational functioning.

E. Symptoms of ODD can include, but are not limited to, the following:
  1. Frequently exhibits temper tantrums
  2. Engages in excessive arguing with adults
  3. Often challenges or repeatedly questions rules
  4. Actively defies and refuses to comply with adult requests and rules
  5. Engages in deliberate attempts to annoy or upset others
  6. Blames others for their own mistakes or misbehavior
  7. Easily annoyed by others
  8. Frequently experiences anger and resentment toward others
  9. Uses mean and hateful language when angry
  10. Exhibits a spiteful attitude and seeks revenge (vindictive)

TABLE 5.3 SCREENING QUESTIONS FOR OPPOSITIONAL DEFIANCE DISORDER

Frequently exhibits temper tantrums	• What happens when you get angry or mad? • Do you get angry or mad often? • Would you say that you have a temper? Tell me about it. • Does your temper get so big you feel like you can't stop it? • Have you ever had a temper tantrum? • What causes them and how often does it happen?
Engages in excessive arguing with adults	• Do you frequently argue with your parents/caregiver or teachers? • Do you always find something to argue about?
Actively defies and refuses to comply with adult requests and rules	• Is it hard for you to follow rules? • Do you think most rules are stupid? Tell me about it. • Do you like to break rules on purpose? • Is your first instinct to say "no" when your parents or teachers ask you to do something? • How does this impact your home life?
Engages in deliberate attempts to annoy or upset others	• Do you like to do things that annoy or bother others? • How often do you do things like that? • Has it caused you to lose friends?
Blames others for their own mistakes or misbehavior	• Is it hard for you to admit you are wrong? • Have you ever blamed someone else for your mistake? • Do you sometimes blame others if you have done something wrong or misbehaved to avoid getting into trouble?
Frequently experiences anger and resentment toward others	• Do you get angry often? • Does it bother you if people boss you around or tell you what to do? • Do you think you get treated unfairly by others?
Exhibits a spiteful attitude and seeks revenge (vindictive)	• When you feel like you are being treated unfairly, how do you respond to the other person?

Source: Adapted from Zimmerman, M. (1994). *Interview guide for evaluating DSM-IV psychiatric disorders and the mental status examination.* Psych Product Press, pp. 80–81.

F. ODD is one of the most common behavioral disorders among children and is associated with significant parent/caregiver strain.
G. Children and adolescents with ODD are also more likely to exhibit symptoms at home with family members; however, the degree to which behaviors are observed outside of the home is often an indicator of the disorder's severity. It is therefore important to assess the youth from a multitude of social perspectives. If left unaddressed, ODD is also associated with an increased risk of suicidal behaviors.
H. Screening questions for ODD are summarized in Table 5.3.
I. Risk factors include the following:
  1. Home environment that lacks stability
  2. Disruptions in childcare by several different caregivers in the home
  3. Parent or caregivers with harsh or inconsistent parenting/disciplinary methods
  4. History of neglect or abuse
  5. History of ADHD

Conduct Disorder

A. The diagnostic term *conduct disorder* (CD) refers to a series or cluster of persistent maladaptive or antisocial behaviors observed in young children that can also endure into late adolescence (Table 5.4).
B. Youth who present with CD often experience emotional problems and dysregulation that severely impact their ability to function in socially acceptable ways. They often have difficulty appreciating rules or demonstrating empathy toward others, making it difficult for them to build or sustain healthy social relationships and/or follow the law (AACAP, 2018). These youth are often described as difficult, delinquent, or purposefully defiant.
C. The presence of a CD often stems from deeper root causes, both physiologic (e.g., traumatic brain injury) and environmental (e.g., neglect, abuse).
D. Children and adolescents with CD often exhibit other concurrent or comorbid presentations, such as mood and anxiety disorders, PTSD, substance use, attention deficit disorders, and learning difficulties.
E. Risk factors include the following:
  1. Being assigned male at birth
  2. Residing in an urban area
  3. Having a low socioeconomic status (e.g., living in poverty)
  4. Having a family history of mental illness, especially CD
  5. Having comorbid psychiatric conditions
  6. Having parents who misuse drugs or alcohol
  7. Challenges within the home environment during the child's upbringing (e.g., dysfunctional home environment)
  8. Past history of trauma, abuse, or neglect
F. Screening questions for CD include the following:
  1. Assessing for a CD can be a challenging task as the youth may reveal difficult or sensitive information. Table 5.5 provides example questions for evaluation of this psychiatric disorder.

TABLE 5.4 MALADAPTIVE AND ANTISOCIAL BEHAVIORS IN CHILDREN AND ADOLESCENTS WITH A CONDUCT DISORDER

Aggression toward people and/or animals	- Engages in bullying, threats, or intimidating of others - Initiates physical altercations or fights - Has wielded a weapon that poses a serious physical threat to others, such as a knife, gun, bat, or broken bottle - Inflicts physical harm on individuals or animals - Commits theft while causing harm or pain to the victim - Coerces people into engaging in sexual activity - Takes enjoyment in being unkind and/or malicious toward others - Displays no authentic remorse following an aggressive outburst
Destruction of property	- Engages in intentional fire-setting with the purpose of causing damage - Purposely damages the property of others
Deceitful behaviors, lying, or theft	- Illegally enters another person's building, house, or car - Deceives others to obtain goods, services, or favors, or to evade responsibilities - Steals items without confronting the victim, such as shoplifting or theft without breaking and entering
Serious violation of regulations, laws, or rules	- Frequently stays out at night, disregarding parent's/caregiver's objections (before 13 years of age) - Runs away from home - Regularly stays away from home for extended periods of time

Source: Adapted from American Academy of Child and Adolescent Psychiatry. (2018). *What is conduct disorder?* https://www.aacap.org/AACAP/Families_and_Youth/Facts_for_Families/FFF-Guide/Conduct-Disorder-033.aspx.

Screening Tools for Conduct Disorder
A. Child Behavior Checklist (CBCL)
B. Strengths and Difficulties Questionnaire (SDQ)
C. Eyberg Child Behavior Inventory
D. Behavior Assessment System for Children (BASC)

REFERENCES AND BIBLIOGRAPHY

American Academy of Child and Adolescent Psychiatry. (2013). *Oppositional defiant disorder.* https://www.aacap.org/App_Themes/AACAP/docs/resource_centers/odd/odd_resource_center_odd_guide.pdf

American Academy of Child and Adolescent Psychiatry. (2018, June). *Conduct disorder.* https://www.aacap.org/AACAP/Families_and_Youth/Facts_for_Families/FFF-Guide/Conduct-Disorder-033.aspx

Cohan, S. L. (2022, January 6). Conduct disorder. *Healthline.* https://www.healthline.com/health/conduct-disorder

Loeber, R., Burke, J. D., & Pardini, D. A. (2009). Perspectives on oppositional defiant disorder, conduct disorder, and psychopathic features. *Journal of Child Psychology and Psychiatry, 50*(1–2), 133–142. https://doi.org/10.1111/j.1469-7610.2008.02011.x

Mayo Clinic Staff. (2021). *Oppositional Defiant Disorder (ODD).* Mayo Clinic. https://www.mayoclinic.org/diseases-conditions/oppositional-defiant-disorder/symptoms-causes/syc-20375831

TABLE 5.5 EXAMPLES OF ASSESSMENT QUESTIONS FOR CONDUCT DISORDERS

Aggression toward people and/or animals	- Do you pick on kids younger or smaller than you? Can you describe? - Are you a bully? - Do you ever threaten other kids so they will get you things or do things for you? How often? - Do you get into fights at home or school? - How often do you start the fight? - Have you ever used a weapon in a fight? For what reason? What type of weapon? - Have you ever physically hurt someone? - Have you ever hurt or killed an animal on purpose? - Have you ever stolen anything? - Have you ever forced someone to do something with you or for you? Have those acts ever been sexual in nature?
Destruction of property	- Have you ever set anything on fire? Why? - Have you ever damaged property, like spraying graffiti or tagging walls, breaking windows, or breaking someone's possession?
Deceitful behaviors, lying, or theft	- Have you ever broken into someone's house, business, or car? Why? Were you alone? - Sometimes kids do not tell the truth and make up stories because they might get in trouble. Have you ever done that before? - Do you often lie to get things you want? - Do you often lie to avoid chores or other responsibilities? - Have you ever stolen from your parents/caregiver/loved one?
Serious violation of regulations, laws, or rules	- Do you ever argue with your parents/caregiver about how late you can stay out? - Do you often stay out later than they said you could? - Have you ever stayed out all night? How old were you when this first started? - Have you ever run away from home? How long did you stay away? - Have you ever skipped school? How often do you do it? How old were you when this first started?

Source: Adapted from Zimmerman, M. (1994). *Interview guide for evaluating DSM-IV psychiatric disorders and the mental status examination.* Psych Product Press, pp. 76–78.

ASSESSING FOR GENDER DYSPHORIA

A. Gender dysphoria (GD) refers to the psychological distress that results when one experiences a mismatch between their gender identity and their assigned gender at birth.
B. *ICD-11* defines *gender dysphoria* as "gender incongruence of adolescence and adulthood" and "gender incongruence of childhood" (WHO, 2019, "Gender incongruence").
C. Adolescents or children experiencing GD may derive comfort from presenting and being perceived as their identified gender. The diagnosis of GD in children is controversial, and the degree to which the *DSM-5* (American Psychiatric Association, 2013) criteria reflect an illness or social bias against gender nonconformity has been debated.
D. According to the *Diagnostic and Statistical Manual of Mental Disorders*, Fifth Edition, Text Revision (*DSM-5-TR*; American Psychiatric Association, 2022), there must be clinically significant distress or impairment in activities of daily living directly related to the incongruence between the assigned sex and the gender affiliation. GD is not experienced by all persons who are gender-diverse or transgender.
E. The following are key points to remember:
  1. Advocate for and help the patient navigate the healthcare system as it relates to all care, including transgender care.
  2. Monitor for risk of self-harm and substance use because patients younger than 18 years are at particularly high risk for distress, leading to self-harm and substance use, especially in the months following coming out to family and friends.
F. Practice points: It may take a few visits to gain rapport and trust.
  1. Assess mental health and other diagnoses.
  2. Ensure optimal psychosocial readiness (check for safety and social supports, whether living in desired gender role).
  3. Assess whether the patient fulfills the diagnostic criteria for GD; rule out psychotic or dissociative disorders.
G. Screening questions for GD include the following:
  1. Are you uncomfortable with your assigned gender? If yes: Has this discomfort lasted at least 6 months, to the point where your assigned gender does not match with your gender identity?
  2. Do the people who live with you know that you are 2SLGBTQ? If yes: Who?
  3. How did they find out, and how did they react?
  4. Do you feel you can be yourself at home/school and with friends?
  5. Do people at school know that you are 2SLGBTQ? If yes: Who?
  6. How did they find out, and how did they react?
  7. Are you able to express your gender and orientation safely at school?
  8. Do teachers and classmates use your preferred name and pronouns?
  9. Do you have access to a bathroom that fits with your gender identity?
  10. Have you ever been harassed or attacked at school/work?
  11. Do you ever worry about your academic/work future as a 2SLGBTQ person?
  12. Do you attend any groups/drop-ins for 2SLGBTQ youth?
  13. Has anyone ever threatened to out you as 2SLGBTQ?
  14. Do you worry about this happening?
  15. Have you ever been threatened or attacked because you are 2SLGBTQ, or for other reasons? Do you worry about this happening?
  16. How safe do you feel in your neighborhood or the places where you hang out?
  17. Has anyone offered you money, clothes, alcohol, or drugs in exchange for sex? Has anyone tried to get you involved in the sex trade?

REFERENCES AND BIBLIOGRAPHY

Adelson, S. L., & American Academy of Child and Adolescent Psychiatry. (2012). Practice Parameter on gay, lesbian, or bisexual sexual orientation, gender nonconformity, and gender discordance in children and adolescents. *Journal of the American Academy of Child & Adolescent Psychiatry*, 51(9), 960–973. https://doi.org/10.1016/j.jaac.2012.07.004

American Psychiatric Association. (2013). *Diagnostic and statistical manual of mental disorders* (5th ed.). https://doi.org/10.1176/appi.books.9780890425596

American Psychiatric Association. (2022). *Diagnostic and statistical manual of mental disorders* (5th ed., text rev.). https://doi.org/10.1176/appi.books.9780890425787

Toban, J. (2022, August). *What is gender dysphoria?* American Psychiatric Association. https://www.psychiatry.org/patients-families/gender-dysphoria/what-is-gender-dysphoria

World Health Organization. (2019). *International classification of diseases* (11th rev.). https://icd.who.int

ASSESSING FOR SUICIDE AND NONSUICIDE SELF-INJURY

A. Nonsuicidal self-harm and suicidal behaviors are on a spectrum classified as self-injurious behavior. Some may suggest that eating disorder (ED) and substance use behaviors can be on this continuum of self-harm.
B. There is a strong relationship between suicidal behavior and a number of different psychiatric conditions. (These are listed in the "Risk Factors for Suicidal Behavior" section of this chapter.) *Suicidal behavior* is defined as an intentional act to hurt one's body with the intent to end life.
C. People experience suicidal ideation before attempting suicide. Suicidal ideation is a range of thoughts involving death and suicide (e.g., wishes, preoccupations). These thoughts can wax and wane depending on how the person is doing from a mental health perspective.
D. Suicidal ideation can be described as being on a continuum from passive to active. Passive suicidal ideation is the act of wishing for and thinking about death without actual plans to end their life. On the other hand, active suicidal ideation is the act of wishing for and thinking about death and making specific plans to end their life.
E. *Nonsuicidal self-injury* is defined as "the deliberate, self-inflicted destruction of body tissue without suicidal intent and for purposes not socially sanctioned" (Zetterqvist, 2015, p. 1). Nonsuicidal self-injury is often associated with individuals who have cluster B personality traits, as well as individuals with cognitive disorders, such as autism. What sustains self-harm behavior is the positive and negative reinforcement attained from the act of harming oneself. Nonsuicidal self-injurious behavior is discussed in more detail in the next section.
F. The APRN has a significant opportunity to detect risk of nonsuicidal self-harm and suicide in pediatric patients. Patients are often screened for depression and anxiety but not for suicide risk. APRNs may find it challenging to assess this type of risk. Barriers to assessment can include discomfort when reviewing suicide risk with patients, inadequate training on the subject, lack of time to complete lengthy assessments, ambiguity around resources for patients who may be

at risk, and lack of access to these resources. All of these can impact the APRN's integration of suicide risk screening into routine primary care.

Nonsuicidal Self-Injurious Behaviors

A. Nonsuicidal self-injurious behaviors (NSSIs) are intentional self-inflicted actions to cause harm to one's body without the intent to die. Cutting, burning, biting, hitting, and scratching are some of the typical manifestations of NSSI and are performed without lethal intent often used as a means of coping with intense emotional pain or distress.
B. In recent years, children as young as 10 years have been observed engaging in this type of behavior. It is the youth's experience of pain associated with the behaviors that acts as a catalyst to achieving a sense of relief or control over emotional distress. The sensation of regaining calm and control can be very powerful and supports why these behaviors may continue if the root cause of emotional pain is not uncovered or treated.
C. The most concerning risk with NSSI is that, although there is no intention to die, studies have argued that the persistence of the behavior(s) over time may lead to habituation of the experience of pain/relief, causing further escalation in behaviors and resulting in eventual, accidental, lethal self-injury.
D. Similar to a substance use paradigm, once tolerance develops and the intended purpose of the behavior begins to lose effect, the youth may then engage in more painful, harmful, or lethal behaviors to find comfort.
E. When assessing NSSI, it is important to determine the history of exhibiting NSSI behaviors, the number of methods used to engage in NSSI, and the youth's experience with pain tolerance.
F. NSSI can also be a symptom of various other mental health conditions, such as depression, anxiety, PTSD, substance use disorders, and borderline personality disorder; therefore, careful screening and monitoring of these behaviors is important.

Screening Tools for Self-Harm
A. Self-Injurious Thoughts and Behaviors Interview-Revised (SITBI-R)
B. Inventory of Statements About Self-Injury (ISAS)

Suicidal Behavior

Risk Factors for Suicidal Behavior
A. Psychiatric conditions that can be associated with suicidal behavior
   1. Depression (e.g., MDD)
   2. EDs
   3. BD
   4. Schizophrenia and schizoaffective disorder
   5. Anxiety (e.g., panic disorder)
   6. PTSD
   7. Substance use disorders
   8. Borderline personality disorders
   9. Adjustment disorders
   10. Antisocial personality disorder
B. Current ideation, intent, plan, access to means
C. Previous suicide attempt or attempts
D. Impulsivity and poor self-control
E. Hopelessness: presence, duration, severity
F. Recent losses: physical, financial, personal
G. PTSD flashbacks
H. Increased risk of reattempt in patients diagnosed with a mood disorder within the first 3 months postdischarge
I. Family history of suicide
J. History of abuse (physical, sexual, or emotional; bullying)
K. Comorbid chronic/acute medical problems, especially a newly diagnosed problem or worsening symptoms
L. Age, gender, ethnicity
   1. Increased risk among individuals 10 to 40 years of age
   2. Increased risk among non-Hispanic American Indian, Alaska Native, and White individuals
   3. Increased risk among males
M. Sexual orientation (e.g., LGBTQ+), with increased risk for self-injurious behavior among youth

Warning Signs of Suicidal Behavior
A. Expressing suicidal ideation (e.g., in a note, by text, verbally)
B. Searching for means to kill oneself (e.g., looking online, buying pills, buying a gun)
C. Changes in behavior (e.g., behaving recklessly, being agitated, increasing anxiety behavior)
D. Changes in sleep pattern (sleeping too much or too little)
E. Hopelessness
F. Sadness
G. Changes in mood (e.g., extreme mood swings, sudden cheerfulness)
H. Withdrawing/isolating self/anhedonia
I. Giving away belongings
J. Increased use of substances (e.g., drugs, alcohol)
K. Recent changes in behaviors (e.g., making a will)

Screening for Suicide in Primary Care
A. Horowitz et al. (2022) suggest that universal screening for suicide risk in pediatric patients is valuable and can be feasibly implemented in primary care settings.
B. When considering the implementation of a mental health screening tool, it is critical to form connections with mental health providers in the community and create referral pathways so that appropriate referrals can be made as needed, dictated by the APRN's clinical assessment and treatment planning. The Ask Suicide-Screening Questions (ASQ) is a reliable suicide risk screening tool in primary care settings for youth and adults. If the patient screens positive on the ASQ, it is important to move on to a more comprehensive assessment or refer the patient for a further assessment by a mental health professional. The following section guides assessment and further decision-making.
C. The risk assessment is intended to guide the decision-making process around level of risk for further self-harm behavior at and following the suicidal behavior (Figures 5.1 and 5.2).

Screening Tools
A. The ASQ (Figure 5.3) can be found online at www.nimh.nih.gov/research/research-conducted-at-nimh/asq-toolkit-materials.

Risk Assessment Interview
A. During a risk assessment, it is essential to explore the patient's beliefs around the intent of the behavior or action. The risk assessment should be completed in the context of a fuller psychiatric-mental health assessment.
B. During this conversation about risk, the APRN should investigate the following:

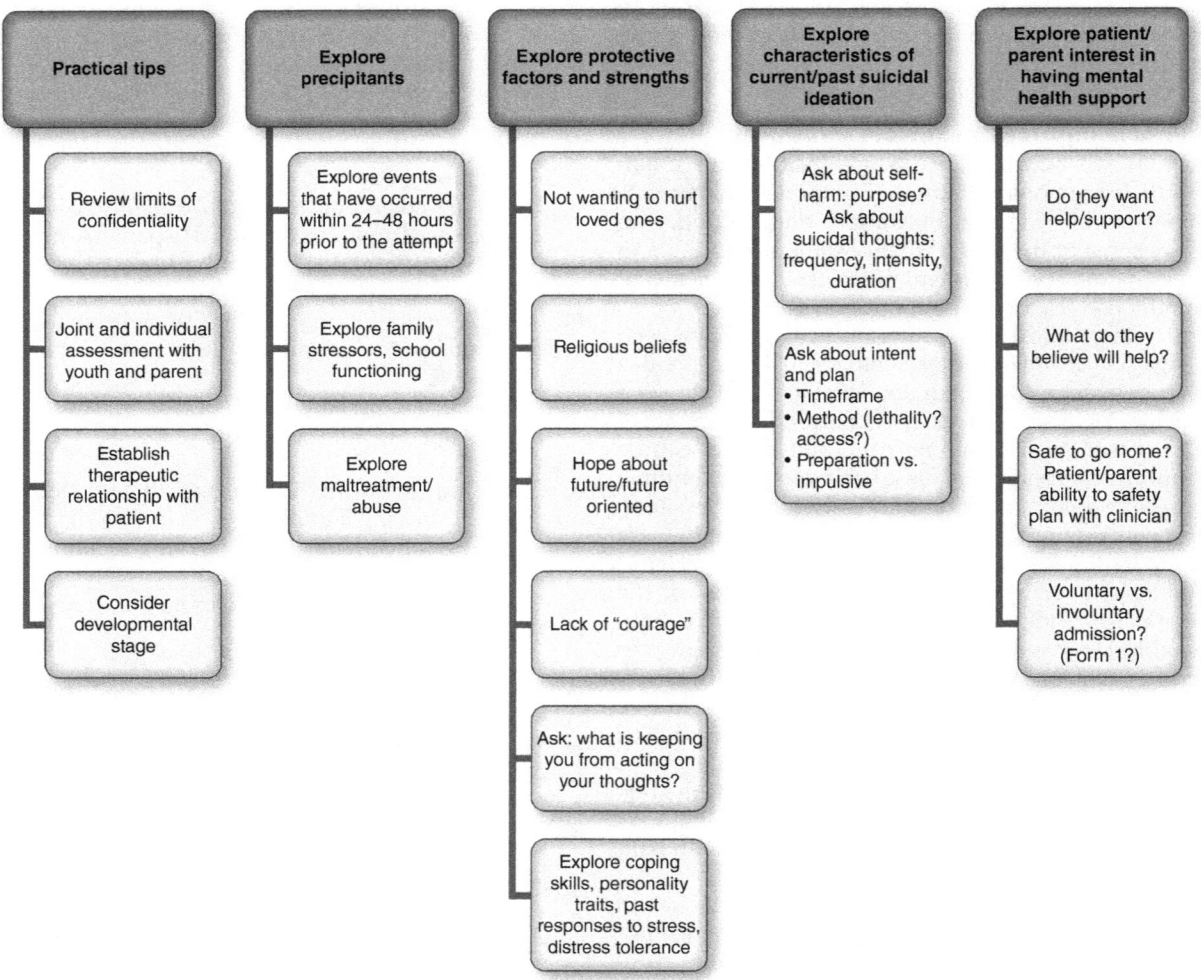

FIGURE 5.1 Suicide risk screening process map.

1. Ask if the patient is having active or passive suicidal thoughts.
   a. For passive ideation: The patient may say "I hope I don't wake up tomorrow."
   b. For active ideation: The patient may say "I want to just die, I'm going to wrap a cord around my neck and just do it."
2. Has the patient experienced prior suicidal ideation, and if so how long (ask for dates or time frames)?
   a. In the past few weeks, have you thought about killing yourself? How often?
   b. What is the frequency of the suicidal thoughts?
   c. Do things ever get so bad for you that you think about dying?
   d. Do you ever think about ending your life?
   e. How often do thoughts like that happen?
   f. How long do the thoughts last?
   g. When you have a thought like that, how difficult is it for you to distract yourself?
3. Explore suicidal intent.
   a. Have you ever thought of acting on your thoughts?
   b. Do you want to end your life?
   c. Have you thought that you might try and end your life?
   d. What has stopped you from trying to end your life/attempting to end your life?
4. Consider if this suicidal ideation or attempt was planned or impulsive.
   a. Do you have a plan?
   b. What is your plan?
5. If the patient has disclosed that they have attempted suicide, the APRN will ask the above questions and also the following:
   a. When did you decide to attempt suicide?
6. Explore the plan further.
   a. What method would you consider using to end your life?
   b. How close have you come to attempting to end your life?
   c. What means do you have access to (e.g., pills, a gun, rope)?
   d. What was the intended plan?
   e. How close have you come to ending your life?
   f. Have you done anything to reduce the chances of being discovered by someone?
7. Explore the context in which the behavior has occurred.
   a. What has been happening in the last few days, weeks, or months that has led to these feelings?

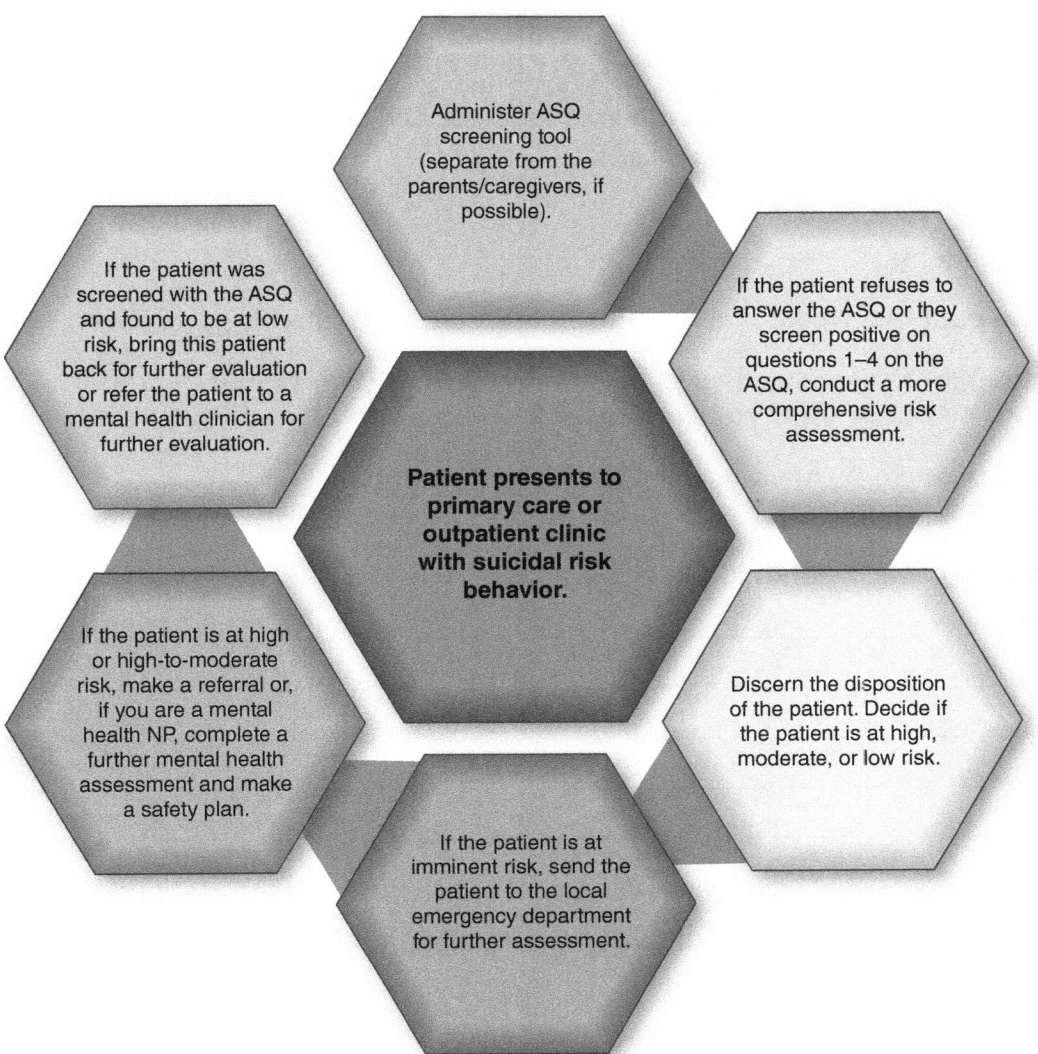

FIGURE 5.2 Clinical algorithm for suicidal risk.

ASQ, Ask Suicide-Screening Questions; NP, nurse practitioner.

Source: Adapted from Horowitz, L. M., Bridge, J. A., Tipton, M. V., Abernathy, T., Mournet, A. M., Snyder, D. J., Lanzillo, E. C., Powell, D., Schoenbaum, M., Brahmbhatt, K., & Pao, M. (2022). Implementing suicide risk screening in a pediatric primary care setting: From research to practice. *Academic Pediatrics*, 22(2), 217–226. https://doi.org/10.1016/j.acap.2021.10.012.

8. If the patient has told you that they have attempted suicide, explore the patient's feelings about being alive, reasons to live, and feelings around regret of the suicide attempt.
   a. Are you hopeful that things will get better for you?
   b. What are reasons to live for?
   c. Do you regret attempting suicide?
9. Consider what type of coping strategies the patient has to deal with suicidal thoughts and how effective the patient perceives these to be.
   a. What coping strategies do you use to help you deal with your suicidal thoughts?

Suicide Risk Assessment Disposition Planning

Disposition planning should occur following the risk assessment or following a fuller psychiatric interview. This should be incorporated in the biopsychosocial formulation of the patient. Following are descriptions of the level of risk that may be associated with the patient and the next steps associated with the level of risk, to be used as a guide in the summary phase of the mental health assessment.

A. Levels of risk

1. Imminent risk: Is the person at imminent risk to harm themselves? If the patient is at imminent risk, the APRN would initiate safety precautions and recommend the family take the patient immediately to the local emergency department. If the family cannot safely transport the patient, the APRN can consider the following: (a) call 911 to transport the patient safely to the emergency department at the local hospital; and/or (b) consider involuntary status (information found in the country's Mental Health Act) based on the APRN's scope in the jurisdiction where they practice, and then call local emergency service to assist in the safe transport of the patient to the hospital for an emergency psychiatric evaluation.

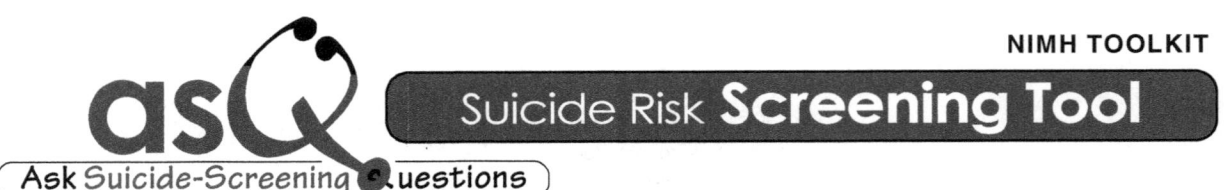

NIMH TOOLKIT

Suicide Risk Screening Tool

Ask the patient:

1. In the past few weeks, have you wished you were dead? ◯ Yes ◯ No
2. In the past few weeks, have you felt that you or your family would be better off if you were dead? ◯ Yes ◯ No
3. In the past week, have you been having thoughts about killing yourself? ◯ Yes ◯ No
4. Have you ever tried to kill yourself? ◯ Yes ◯ No
   If yes, how? _____
   _____
   When? _____
   _____

If the patient answers Yes to any of the above, ask the following acuity question:

5. Are you having thoughts of killing yourself right now? ◯ Yes ◯ No
   If yes, please describe: _____

Next steps:

- If patient answers "No" to all questions 1 through 4, screening is complete (not necessary to ask question #5). No intervention is necessary *(Note: Clinical judgment can always override a negative screen).*
- **If patient answers** "Yes" **to any of questions 1 through 4, or refuses to answer, they are considered a** positive screen. **Ask question #5 to assess acuity:**
   ☐ "Yes" to question #5 = acute positive screen (imminent risk identified)
      - **Patient requires a** STAT **safety/full mental health evaluation.** Patient cannot leave until evaluated for safety.
      - Keep patient in sight. Remove all dangerous objects from room. Alert physician or clinician responsible for patient's care.
   ☐ "No" to question #5 = nonacute positive screen (potential risk identified)
      - **Patient requires a brief suicide safety assessment to determine if a full mental health evaluation is needed. If a patient (or parent/guardian) refuses the brief assessment, this should be treated as an "against medical advice" (AMA) discharge.**
      - Alert physician or clinician responsible for patient's care.

Provide resources to all patients

- 24/7 National Suicide Prevention Lifeline: 988
- 24/7 Crisis Text Line: Text "HOME" to 741741

asQ Suicide Risk Screening Toolkit   NATIONAL INSTITUTE OF MENTAL HEALTH (NIMH)   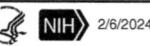   2/6/2024

FIGURE 5.3 The Ask Suicide-Screening Questions (ASQ).

Source: From National Institute for Mental Health (2023). *Ask Suicide-Screening Questions (ASQ) toolkit.* https://www.nimh.nih.gov/research/research-conducted-at-nimh/asq-toolkit-materials.

2. High to moderate risk: If the patient is deemed at high risk from the initial screening, further evaluation is necessary to determine the next steps for this patient. Further evaluation should take the form of a full psychiatric evaluation that can be done by an expert mental health APRN or psychiatrist. A referral for an urgent (within 72 hours) assessment by one of these experts may be required if the APRN is not able to complete this fuller evaluation. If the patient cannot get an appointment within 3 days, they should be seen again by the APRN every 2 to 3 days to reassess the level of risk until they can get an appointment with a mental health clinician. Before sending the patient home, the APRN will need to complete a safety plan and ensure that caregivers are included in the planning of the youth's safety.

3. Low risk: This patient may be screened with the ASQ questionnaire and, when assessed further, been found to have mental health concerns and may have a positive risk of suicidal behavior. This may not have been what brought the patient to the clinic initially. The APRN should book this patient for a further evaluation or refer the patient to a mental health clinician for further evaluation.

REFERENCES AND BIBLIOGRAPHY

Aguinaldo, L. D., Sullivant, S., Lanzillo, E. C., Ross, A., He, J. P., Bradley-Ewing, A., Bridge, J. A., Horowitz, L. M., & Wharff, E. A. (2021). Validation of the Ask Suicide-Screening Questions (ASQ) with youth in outpatient specialty and primary care clinics. *General Hospital Psychiatry, 68*, 52–58. https://doi.org/10.1016/j.genhosppsych.2020.11.006

Brahmbhatt, K. (2017). *Pediatric suicide risk screening and management: Outcomes from implementation of a national clinical pathway.* Morressier.

Brahmbhatt, K., Kurtz, B. P., Afzal, K. I., Giles, L. L., Kowal, E. D., Johnson, K. P., Lanzillo, E., Pao, M., Plioplys, S., & Horowitz, L. M. (2019). Suicide risk screening in pediatric hospitals: Clinical pathways to address a global health crisis. *Psychosomatics, 60*(1), 1–9. https://doi.org/10.1016/j.psym.2018.09.003

Cash, J. C., Glass, C. A., Fraser, D., Corcoran, L., & Edwards, M. (2020). *Canadian family practice guidelines.* Springer Publishing Company.

Curtin, S. C., & Hedegaard, H. (2019). Suicide rates for females and males by race and ethnicity: United States, 1999 and 2017. *NCHS Health E-Stat.* https://www.cdc.gov/nchs/data/hestat/suicide/rates_1999_2017.htm

Felthous, A. R., Kulkarni, N., & Belean, C. (2023). DSM-5-TR diagnosis as a guide to suicide risk assessment. *Behavioral Sciences & the Law, 41*(5), 373–396. https://doi.org/10.1002/bsl.2617

Harmer, B., Lee, S., Duong, T. V. H., & Saadabadi, A. (2024, April 20). *Suicidal Ideation.* StatPearls Publishing. https://www.ncbi.nlm.nih.gov/books/NBK565877/

Horowitz, L. M. (2019, June 4). *Suicide risk screening training: How to manage patients at risk for suicide* [Video]. National Institute for Mental Health. YouTube. https://youtu.be/P4_-SF9lQuc

Horowitz, L. M., Bridge, J. A., Tipton, M. V., Abernathy, T., Mournet, A. M., Snyder, D. J., Lanzillo, E. C., Powell, D., Schoenbaum, M., Brahmbhatt, K., & Pao, M. (2022). Implementing suicide risk screening in a pediatric primary care setting: From research to practice. *Academic Pediatrics, 22*(2), 217–226. https://doi.org/10.1016/j.acap.2021.10.012

Hughes, D., & Kleespies, P. (2011). Suicide in the medically ill. *Suicide & Life-Threatening Behavior, 31*(s1), 48–59. https://doi.org/10.1521/suli.31.1.5.48.24226

Hatchel, T., Polanin, J. R., & Espelage, D. L. (2021). Suicidal thoughts and behaviors among LGBTQ youth: Meta-analyses and a systematic review. *Archives of Suicide Research, 25*(1), 1–37. https://doi.org/10.1080/13811118.2019.1663329

Korczak, D., Charach, A., & Andrews, D. (2024, January 11). *Practice point: Suicidal ideation and behaviour.* Canadian Paediatric Society. https://cps.ca/en/documents/position/suicidal-ideation-and-behaviour

National Institute of Mental Health. (2023). *Ask Suicide-Screening Questions (ASQ) toolkit.* https://www.nimh.nih.gov/research/research-conducted-at-nimh/asq-toolkit-materials

Nock, M. K., Joiner Jr, T. E., Gordon, K. H., Lloyd-Richardson, E., & Prinstein, M. J. (2006). Non-suicidal self-injury among adolescents: Diagnostic correlates and relation to suicide attempts. *Psychiatry Research, 144*(1), 65–72. https://doi.org/10.1016/j.psychres.2006.05.010

Oldham, J. M. (2015). The spectrum of self-injurious behavior. *Journal of Psychiatric Practice, 21*(3), 179. https://doi.org/10.1097/PRA.0000000000000069

Ruengorn, C., Sanichwankul, K., Niwatananun, W., Mahatnirunkul, S., Pumpaisalchai, W., & Patumanond, J. (2011). Incidence and risk factors of suicide reattempts within 1 year after hospital discharge in mood disorder patients. *Clinical epidemiology, 3*(1), 305–313. https://doi.org/10.2147/CLEP.S25444

Whitlock, J., & Knox, K. L. (2007). The relationship between self-injurious behavior and suicide in a young adult population. *Archives of Pediatrics & Adolescent Medicine, 161*(7), 634–640. https://doi.org/10.1001/archpedi.161.7.634

Zetterqvist, M. (2015). The DSM-5 diagnosis of nonsuicidal self-injury disorder: A review of the empirical literature. *Child and Adolescent Psychiatry and Mental Health, 9*(1), Article 31. https://doi.org/10.1186/s13034-015-0062-7

ASSESSING FOR SUBSTANCE USE DISORDERS

A. Signs and symptoms of substance use in children and adolescents include the following:

1. Signs and symptoms can be suggestive of acute use, such as reddened eyes or dilated pupils, or indicative of chronic use (e.g., having track marks and changes in behaviors).

2. The signs and symptoms seen with substance use can also be suggestive of a mental health condition.

3. When assessing for substance use, it is essential to assess for other mental health issues, such as trauma, anxiety, and depression.

a. Often, substance use can be seen concurrently with other psychiatric conditions, such as GAD or MDD.

b. It can be difficult for adolescents to share details of their substance use. They will be concerned about confidentiality.

B. The substance use portion of the interview may be better when conducted near the end of the assessment, after the APRN has had the opportunity to build rapport with the patient.

1. Conduct the assessment of substance use when the adolescent is alone (in the absences of parents/legal guardians or caregivers).

2. Providing a safe, confidential environment allows the youth to be more candid in responses.

Criteria for Substance Use Disorder

A. To be described as having a substance use disorder, the patient needs to have the following characteristics:

1. Impaired control over their use of substances

a. The person is using substances to excess.

2. Use of substances impairing the person's ability to fulfill obligation at school, home, or work

3. Continued use of the substance even though it is contributing to significant social impacts and impairments with interpersonal relationships

4. Use of substances placing the individual at risk

a. Risk of harm by placing self in physically unsafe environments

b. Continued use of substances even though the person is aware that the substance is harmful

i. The person reduces or stops their involvement in recreational, social, or school activities due to substance use.

ii. The person develops a tolerance for the substance or experiences withdrawal symptoms from the substance.

Signs and Symptoms of Substance Use
A. Awkward physical movements, tremors
B. Change in peer group, withdrawal from friends or family and activities
C. Decrease in academic performance
D. Frequent minor illnesses (colds, flu)
E. Gastrointestinal upset (diarrhea or pain)
F. History of bizarre behavior
G. Needle track marks
H. Wounds on the skin due to intravenous drug use
I. Reddened eyes, dilated or pinpoint pupils
J. Restlessness or drowsiness, hallucinations, disorientation
K. Runny or stuffy nose (constant)
L. Slurred speech
M. Unusual sleep patterns
N. Weight loss or gain, change in eating pattern

Substance Use Screening
A. The CRAFFT (**C**ar, **R**elax, **A**lone, **F**orget, **F**riends, **T**rouble) is a validated screening tool that can be used to screen adolescents for substance-related problems and disorders (https://crafft.org/about-the-crafft).
   1. It is recommended that the APRN review local, state/provincial, and national guidelines on substance use screening in adolescents.
   2. A positive response to two or more of the CRAFFT questions requires further investigation. Often, APRNs will opt to investigate further even if only one positive item is identified on the CRAFFT.
B. APRNs without experience with mental health screening should consider involving a mental health professional for a fuller mental health screening.

The CRAFFT Screening Tool (https://crafft.org/get-the-crafft/#repro)
A. C: Have you ever ridden in a car driven by someone (including yourself) who was "high" or had been using drugs or alcohol?
B. R: Do you ever use alcohol or drugs to relax, feel better about yourself, or fit in?
C. A: Do you ever use alcohol or drugs while you are by yourself, alone?
D. F: Do you ever forget things you did while using drugs or alcohol?
E. F: Do your family or friends ever tell you that you should cut down on your drinking or drug use?
F. T: Have you ever gotten into trouble while using drugs or alcohol?

Substance Use Assessment Questions
A. Do you use tobacco? How do you use tobacco (e.g., smoke cigarettes, chew)? How often do you use tobacco daily, weekly, monthly? When did you start to use tobacco?
B. Have you ever tried marijuana? If so, how often do you use marijuana? When did you first start to use marijuana? How much do you use daily, weekly, monthly?
C. Have you ever tried or continue to use vape? What substances are in your vape (e.g., nicotine, marijuana)? How often do you use your vaping device?
D. Have you ever used alcohol? If so, when was the first time? How often do you use alcohol (how many drinks daily, weekly, monthly)?
E. Have you used prescription drugs for other reasons than for what is prescribed or not prescribed to you (such as pain medication, Xanax, or Adderall)? If so, what did you use them for? How often have you tried prescription drugs?
F. In the past year, have you tried other types of substances (e.g., cocaine, crystal meth, ecstasy)?
G. Have you ever tried inhalants? If so, how often have you used inhalants in the past year?
H. Have you ever used herbs or synthetic drugs (such as salvia, "K2," or bath salts)? If so, when? What happened when you tried these substances?
I. Have you ever tried substances that you have to inject into your body with a needle?
J. Do any of the people you hang out with use substances? If so, how much? How often?
K. Has anything bad happened to you because you were using these substances?
L. Is your family or are your friends aware that you have tried or are continuing to use any of these substances?
M. Does anyone in your family have a problem with substances? (You may need to simplify this question and ask about specific substances.)

Resources
A. https://crafft.org/resources
B. https://crafft.org/resources/#clin-res

REFERENCES AND BIBLIOGRAPHY
American Psychiatric Association. (2013). Substance-related and addictive disorders. In *Diagnostic and statistical manual of mental disorders* (5th ed., pp. 483–484). American Psychiatric Association. https://dsm.psychiatryonline.org/doi/book/10.1176/appi.books.9780890425596

Knight, J. R., Sherritt, L., Shrier, L. A., Harris, S. K., & Chang, G. (2002). Validity of the CRAFFT substance abuse screening test among adolescent clinic patients. *Archives of Pediatrics & Adolescent Medicine, 156*(6), 607–614. https://doi.org/10.1001/archpedi.156.6.607

Levy, S. J. L., Kokotailo, P. K., & Committee on Substance Abuse. (2011). Substance use screening, brief intervention, and referral to treatment for pediatricians. *Pediatrics, 128*(5), e1330–e1340. https://doi.org/10.1542/peds.2011-1754

Substance Abuse and Mental Health Services Administration. (2023). *Risk and protective factors.* https://www.samhsa.gov/sites/default/files/20190718-samhsa-risk-protective-factors.pdf

ASSESSING FOR EATING/FEEDING DISORDERS AND EATING/FEEDING DISORDER BEHAVIORS
A. Eating/feeding disorders are serious, with life-threatening physical and psychological complications.
   1. It is vital that APRNs have the knowledge and skill to screen for these disorders.
   2. Untreated, eating/feeding disorders can lead to life-threatening consequences.
B. Diagnosis of an eating disorder (ED) is based on clinical assessment using a combination of self-report, legal guardian report, and clinical observation.
   1. A comprehensive assessment of a youth with a suspected eating disorder includes a thorough medical, nutritional, and psychiatric history, followed by a detailed physical examination.
   2. A collateral history from a legal guardian may reveal additional relevant information about abnormal eating-related behaviors, developmental history, and weight loss/exercise pattern that were denied or minimized by the patient.

a. APRNs are in a unique position to detect EDs early and interrupt their progression.
b. Routine visits are an excellent opportunity to screen for eating/feeding disorders.
3. Review history for reports of dieting, body image dissatisfaction, experiences with weight-based stigma, or changes in eating and/or exercise patterns and positive responses on standard review of symptoms (e.g., amenorrhea). This section includes screening questions for anorexia nervosa (AN), binge eating disorder (BED), and avoidant restrictive food intake disorder (ARFID). It does not address feeding problems in infancy, such as failure to thrive; other feeding disturbances, such as pica, rumination disorder, or purging disorder; or evaluation of obesity.

Assessing for an Eating/Feeding Disorder

A. Assessing for the presence of an ED can be a challenging task. Consider evaluating a youth for an eating/feeding disorder who presents with any of the following:
1. Significant weight loss or gain (precipitous fluctuations)
2. Sudden changes in eating behaviors (new vegetarianism, gluten-free, lactose-free, uncontrolled binge eating, elimination of certain food or food groups)
3. Sudden changes in exercise patterns
4. Body image disturbance
5. Electrolyte abnormalities without an identified medical cause

B. Pay close attention to specific populations such as the following:
1. Preteens
2. Males
3. Adolescents with larger body habitus
4. Adolescents with chronic health conditions requiring dietary control
5. Patients with orthorexia
6. Elite athletes
7. Gender-diverse youth

Screening Questions for Eating Disorders

A. What do you think about your appearance? Do you ever restrict or avoid certain foods so much that it negatively affects your health or weight? If yes, ask:
1. Do you consider your body shape or weight the most important aspect of yourself? If yes, proceed to AN. If no, proceed to ARFID.

Screening Questions for Anorexia Nervosa-Restricting Type

A. Diagnosis of an requires the presence of all three of the following:
1. Eating restriction leading to significantly low body weight:
    a. Have you limited the food you eat in order to lose weight?
    b. What was the least you ever weighed?
    c. What do you weigh now?
2. Fear of weight gain or behavior interfering in weight gain:
    a. Do you have an intense fear of gaining weight or becoming fat?
    b. Has there ever been a time when you were already at a low weight and still did things to interfere with gaining weight?
3. Disturbance in self-perceived weight or shape:
    a. What do you think about your current weight and shape of your body?
    b. How do you think a significantly low body weight will affect your physical health?

Screening Questions for Anorexia Nervosa-Binge Eating/Purging Type

A. Binge eating
1. Do you ever feel out of control when you eat? If so, with what foods?
2. How much? How often? Any triggers?

B. Purging
1. Do you vomit (includes self-induced and involuntary)?
2. What do you use to vomit (e.g., finger, toothbrush)?
3. How often? How soon after eating?
4. Do you use other methods to lose weight, such as laxatives, diuretics, diet pills, or caffeine? If so, what types, when was the last use, how many, and how often?

Avoidant/Restrictive Food Intake Disorder

A. The youth must experience significant disturbance in eating or feeding characterized by persistent failure to meet appropriate nutritional and/or energy needs associated with at least one of the following:
1. Faltering growth or significant weight loss:
    a. Do you avoid certain foods or restrict what you eat to the extent that you have not grown at the expected rate or have experienced significant weight loss?
2. Significant nutritional deficiency:
    a. Do you avoid or restrict food to the extent that it has negatively affected your health, as in experiencing a significant nutritional deficiency?
3. Dependence on enteral feeding or oral supplements:
    a. Have you avoided or restricted food to the extent that you depend on tube feedings or oral supplements to maintain nutrition?
4. Marked interference with psychosocial functioning:
    a. Can you eat with other people or take part in social activities when food is present? b. Has avoiding or restricting food affected your ability to participate in your usual activities or made it difficult to form or maintain relationships?

Eating Disorder Measures

A. The following are self-report instruments that have been used to assess disordered eating in children and adolescents:
1. Eating Disorder Examination Questionnaire (EDE-Q 6.0)
2. SCOFF (**S**ick, **C**ontrol, **O**ne, **F**at, **F**ood) Questionnaire

REFERENCES AND BIBLIOGRAPHY

Academy of Eating Disorders. (2016). *Eating disorders: A guide to medical care* (3rd ed.). AED Report 2016. https://www.massgeneral.org/assets/mgh/pdf/psychiatry/eating-disorders-medical-guide-aed-report.pdf

Katzman, D. K., & Findlay, S. M. (2011). Medical issues unique to children and adolescents. In D. Le Grange & J. Lock (Eds.), *Eating disorders in children and adolescents: A clinical handbook* (pp. 137–147). Guilford Press.

Mairs, R., & Nicholls, D. (2016). Assessment and treatment of eating disorders in children and adolescents. *Archives of Disease in Childhood, 101*(12), 1168–1175. https://doi.org/10.1136/archdischild-2015-309481

Rosen, D. S., & American Academy of Pediatrics Committee on Adolescents. (2010). Identification and management of eating disorders in children and adolescents. *Pediatrics, 126*(6), 1240–1253. https://doi.org/10.1542/peds.2010-2821

PHASE 5: THE MENTAL STATUS EXAM

A. The mental status exam (MSE) is an essential tool in making psychiatric diagnoses. It includes a historical report from the patient and observational data gathered by the APRN throughout the patient encounter. It includes the elements in Table 5.6.

REFERENCES AND BIBLIOGRAPHY
Mental Status Exam. (2017). *The Calgary guide to understanding disease.* https://calgaryguide.ucalgary.ca/mental-status-exam-mse/

Snyderman, D., & Rovner, B. (2008). Mental status examination in primary care: A review. *American Family Physician, 80*(8), 809–814. PMID: 19835342.

PHASE 6: PHYSICAL HEALTH ASSESSMENT

PAST MEDICAL AND SURGICAL HISTORY
A. Since child and adolescent psychiatry straddles pediatric medicine and neurology, the APRN needs to take a detailed medical history and conduct a physical examination and the appropriate laboratory investigations in order to support or rule out the provisional diagnosis from a biopsychosocial perspective.

B. Ask patients and their families the following questions:
  1. Any chronic medical problems?
  2. Any illnesses that affected you emotionally?
  3. Any surgeries? Any seizures?
  4. Any concussions with loss of consciousness?

PHYSICAL EXAMINATION
A. It is essential to complete a focused physical examination on patients who are newly presenting with psychiatric symptoms. Please remember to follow the general principles of pediatric physical examinations. For children and adolescents, also consider including the following:
  1. Assess for orthostatic vital signs.
  2. Assess for marked weight loss or gain in a child or adolescent who is still growing and developing (obtain growth history whenever possible).
  3. Assess for deviation from growth trajectory based on weight and height measurements plotted on appropriate growth charts.
     a. Assess for delayed or interrupted pubertal development.
  4. Assess for angular stomatitis, palatal scratches, and dental enamel erosions.
  5. Assess for salivary gland enlargement (parotid and submandibular).
  6. Assess for amenorrhea or oligomenorrhea (absent or irregular menses) as appropriate.
  7. Consider assessing bone mineral density (consider for patients with amenorrhea for more than 6–12 months).
  8. Inspect for pallor, dry skin, and carotenemia (yellowish discoloration of skin, particularly palms and soles), which may be signs of an ED.
  9. Inspect for dry, brittle hair and nails; thin scalp hair; lanugo (fine hair growth on the body and face); and alopecia, which may be signs of an ED.
  10. Assess for evidence of Russell's sign (abrasion or callous on knuckles from self-induced emesis), which may be a sign of an ED.
  11. When performing inspection, look for marks on the skin that could be indicative of self-harm (scarring, burns, cuts). Look for lesions at various stages of healing. Make sure to look at the arms, legs, thighs, shoulders, under breasts, and abdomen.
  12. Inspect for cachexia and facial and muscle wasting.
  13. Inspect for edema (hypoalbuminemia-related).
  14. Inspect the spine for scoliosis and kyphosis.
  15. Assess for bruising or abrasions over the spine (related to excessive sit-ups or other exercise).

INVESTIGATIONS
A. Performing specific investigations will be largely contingent on a comprehensive history taking, certain risk factors (e.g., family history, drug use), as well as physical and psychological assessment findings. Targeting investigations through history and examination will avoid unnecessary tests, false positives, and anxiety for the patient that may come with investigations. When performing a psychiatric evaluation, routine laboratory tests can be considered if they have not already been completed by the patient's healthcare team.

B. Clinical investigations are very useful when exploring or ruling out organic causes. Many illnesses of medical etiology may present with psychiatric symptoms. Illnesses, such as infections, cancers, and metabolic disorders, and polypharmacy can frequently have psychiatry symptoms and sequelae. There may even be some misdiagnosis and premature referral to psychiatry when clinical data are missing or incomplete. Some common examples of medical illness with psychiatric symptoms are infection or drug use associated with delirium, anemia and thyroid disorders associated with anxiety, and systemic lupus erythematosus associated with depression.

Routine Laboratory Investigations to Consider
A. Complete blood count (CBC)
B. Extended electrolytes, urea, creatinine, liver function tests (LFTs), blood urea nitrogen (BUN)
C. Beta-human chorionic gonadotropin (βhCG), prolactin
D. Thyroid-stimulating hormone (TSH), vitamin B_{12}, vitamin D, folate, amylase, fasting lipids, glucose, hemoglobin A1c (HbA1c)
E. Autoimmune serology, antinuclear antibodies (ANA), erythrocyte sedimentation rate (ESR), C-reactive protein (CRP), anti-double stranded DNA (anti-dsDNA)
F. Sexually transmitted infection screening: HIV, hepatitis B, hepatitis C, syphilis
G. Heavy metals: lead, mercury, copper
H. Urinalysis
I. Blood cultures

Psychiatric Medication Screening and Monitoring
A. Lithium: monitoring of drug levels and thyroid function, CBC
B. Antipsychotics: baseline EKG, continuous monitoring of EKG for QTc prolongation
C. Benzodiazepines: monitoring of LFTs
D. Stimulants: monitoring of blood pressure, pulse, weight

Laboratory Monitoring of Drug and Alcohol
A. Toxicology screening
B. Urine drug screen
C. Blood alcohol level
D. Blood toxicology screen (including screening for synthetic substances)

TABLE 5.6 ELEMENTS OF THE MENTAL STATUS EXAM

Appearance and general behavior	Grooming, dress, and appearance • Abnormalities: disheveled appearance suggestive of schizophrenia; provocative dress may be suggestive of bipolar disorder; unkempt appearance may be suggestive of depression, psychosis Eye contact: note good, fleeting, sporadic, avoidant, none • Abnormalities: poor/avoidant; may occur with psychotic disorders (responding to internal voices)
Behavior and motor activity	Observing how the patient responds to you, family, and the environment Body posture and movement, facial expressions • Abnormalities: akathisia (restlessness), psychomotor agitation (can occur in anxiety or mania): excessive motor activity (e.g., pacing, wringing hands, inability to sit still), bradykinesia, psychomotor retardation: generalized slowing of physical and emotional reactions (can occur in depression, negative symptoms in schizophrenia) • Changes in motor activity: may be related to treatment response secondary to antipsychotic medications
Speech	Quantity: talkative, expansive, paucity, poverty of speech (alogia) Rate: fast, pressured, slow, normal Volume and tone: loud, soft, monotone, weak, strong, mumbled Fluency and rhythm: slurred, clear, hesitant, aphasic, stutter Coherent/incoherent • Abnormalities: can be caused and seen in schizophrenia, substance use disorders, severe depressive disorder, bipolar disorder, stroke, multiple sclerosis, amyotrophic lateral sclerosis
Mood and affect	Mood: the subjective report of the patient's emotional state Affect: the APRN's objective impression of the patient's expressed emotional state (e.g., labile, restricted range, appropriate); should assess emotional range (broad or restrictive), intensity (blunted or flat), and stability; affect may or may not be congruent to mood Can indicate depression, bipolar, anxiety, and schizophrenia (inappropriate affect)
Thought process	Patient's form of thinking, how are their thoughts expressed Rate of thoughts (e.g., flight of ideas, as seen in bipolar disorder) Are they goal-directed? Need to describe their thoughts as logical, tangential, circumstantial, and closely or loosely associated
Thought content	What the patient is thinking; need to include presence or absence of delusional or obsessional thinking Delusions: fixed; false beliefs differ from obsessions because persons recognize these intrusive thoughts as not normal Includes suicidal ideation and homicidal ideation
Perceptual disturbances	Hallucinations that occur in the absence of a sensory stimulus; includes auditory, visual, olfactory, gustatory, tactile, and visceral (symptoms of a schizophrenic disorder, bipolar disorder, severe unipolar depression, acute intoxication) Is the patient responding to internal stimuli?
Sensorium and cognition	Assessment of the patient's level and stability of consciousness (e.g., alert, clouded, somnolent, lethargic, comatose); disturbance or fluctuation of consciousness a probable indication of delirium Cognition: includes attention, concentration, and memory; overall intelligence based on vocabulary, grammar, executive functioning, and inferred level of education Can use the Montreal Cognitive Assessment or Mini-Mental State Examination to formally assess the patient
Insight	Patient's awareness and understanding of their illness and need for treatment (fair, good, partial, poor) Highly determined by the age of the youth

Judgment	Patient's ability to identify the consequences of actions (e.g., ability to act in ways that are safe and in the interest of self and others)
	Child/adolescent's capacity to consent to treatment needs APRN assessment; *capacity to consent to treatment* is a legal term that describes the ability to understand relevant information and appreciate the consequences of accepting or refusing the treatment in question
	Assessing capacity to consent:
	• Explain to the patient, in detail, the condition for which you are proposing treatment and how it will affect them.
	• Explain to the patient the proposed treatment and its risks and benefits.
	• Ask the patient the following questions to assess their capacity:
	  o Do you know why we are proposing treatment for you?
	  o Do you understand the treatment we are proposing? Please tell me what you know about it.
	  o What is your understanding of the expected benefits of the treatment?
	  o Are you aware of any risks of the treatment?
	  o Are you aware of any other types of treatment?
	  o Are you having problems right now for which you might benefit from treatment?
	  o How do you think the proposed treatment will affect you?
	  o What will happen if you don't take the treatment?

APRN, advanced practice registered nurse.

Source: Data from Geist, R., & Oplet, S. E. (2010). A guide for health care practitioners in the assessment of young people's capacity to consent for treatment. *Clinical Pediatrics, 49*(9), 834–839. https://doi.org/10.1177/0009922810363610.

Imaging, Neurologic, and Other Investigations

A. Head imaging: CT scan/MRI/ultrasound: patients with new or worsening psychological symptoms as well as history of recent trauma, weakness, headache, delirium, seizures
B. EEG: seizures
C. Lumbar puncture: check for fever, headaches, delirium, meningitis
D. Chest x-ray: cough, fever, low oxygen
E. EKG: arrhythmias, low oxygen, syncope, dizziness, chest pain, drug monitoring
F. Psychoeducational assessment: measure of intellect and functional abilities

REFERENCES AND BIBLIOGRAPHY

McAllister-Williams, R. H., Cousins, D., & Lunn, B. (2016). Clinical assessment and investigation in psychiatry. *Medicine, 44*(11), 630–637. https://doi.org/10.1016/j.mpmed.2016.08.004

McKee, J., & Brahm, N. (2016). Medical mimics: Differential diagnostic considerations for psychiatric symptoms. *Mental Health Clinician, 6*(6):289–296. https://doi.org/10.9740/mhc.2016.11.289

Srinath, S., Jacob, P., Sharma, E., & Gautam, A. (2019). Clinical practice guidelines for assessment of children and adolescents. *Indian Journal of Psychiatry, 61*(Suppl. 2), 158–175. https://doi.org/10.4103/psychiatry.IndianJPsychiatry_580_18

PHASE 7: SUMMARY

PROCESS OF FORMULATION

A. Formulating a plan for a patient with mental health issues is complex and requires more than providing the patient with a diagnosis. The process of formulation involves the deliberate conceptual organization of the information collected at all phases of the interview process. This integrative process aids in the synthesis of the information to understand the problem with the aim of identifying the diagnosis that fits the patient's symptoms and guides the clinical treatment plan. The formulation helps to explain the different perspectives of the patient, including the youth as a biological system, as a developing individual, as a person, as a member of a family, as a school member, and as a member of larger social systems.

B. During the formulation phase of the interview process, the APRN is creating a road map for the patient and legal guardians that includes the synthesis of information collected, the diagnosis, and the treatment plan. The APRN can use the biopsychosocial model, which combines biological, psychological, and social factors, to understand the patient in order to guide the development of a treatment plan. The APRN must explore all factors (e.g., biological, psychological, social) that may be contributing to the patient's clinical presentation. It is the contribution of these interacting factors that can trigger mental illness. When approaching the treatment plan, both individual patient and family strengths and abilities should be considered as they can help with the development of a fuller care plan.

How to Assemble a Formulation and the Treatment Plan

A. Step 1: Summarize the demographic information, history of presenting illness, chief complaint, and presenting problem from both the patient and the legal guardian perspective.
B. Step 2: Describe the precipitating stressor(s).
C. Step 3: Describe the biological, psychological, and social factors that can be affecting the patient's presentation.
D. Step 4: Consider the patient's risk factors and protective factors.
E. Step 5: Consider the patient's level of functioning and how it weaves into the construction of the formulation and diagnosis.
F. Step 6: Identify the patient's and the legal guardians' strengthens and abilities.
G. Step 7: Identify a list of differential diagnoses and create a rule-in or rule-out chart with the information collected to help narrow down the list to the best possible diagnosis or diagnoses.
H. Step 8: Outline the findings and final diagnosis to the patient and legal guardians.
I. Step 9: Collaborate with the patient and the legal guardians to determine a treatment plan.
J. Step 10: Create a plan for follow-up.
K. Taking a structured approach to the formulation, diagnosis, and treatment planning for the patient and the family will always ensure that all the necessary information has been integrated into the decision-making. It is essential to remember that as more is learned about the patient in subsequent follow-up visits, the APRN may adapt the formulation, diagnosis, and treatment plan.

REFERENCES AND BIBLIOGRAPHY

Cepeda, C., & Gotanco, L. (2017). *Psychiatric interview of children and adolescents*. American Psychiatric Association Publishing.

DeMaso, D., Martini, D. R., Sulik, L. R., Hilt, R., Marx, L., Pierce, K., Sarvet, B., Becker, E., Kendrick, J., Kerlek, A. J., Biel, M., & Ptakowski, K. K. (2010, June). *A guide to building collaborative mental health care partnerships in pediatric primary care*. American Academy of Child and Adolescent Psychiatry. https://www.aacap.org/App_Themes/AACAP/docs/clinical_practice_center/guide_to_building_collaborative_mental_health_care_partnerships.pdf

Sharifi, A., Shahrivar, Z., Zarafshan, H., Beiky Ashezary, S., Stuart, E., Mojtabai, R., & Wissow, L. (2019). Collaborative care for child and youth mental health problems in a middle income country: Study protocol for a randomized controlled trial training general practitioners. *Trials, 20*(1), Article 405. https://trialsjournal.biomedcentral.com/articles/10.1186/s13063-019-3467-4

Winters, N. C., Hanson, G., & Stoyanova, V. (2007). The case formulation in child and adolescent psychiatry. *Child and Adolescent Psychiatric Clinics of North America, 16*(1), 111–132. https://doi.org/10.1016/j.chc.2006.07.010

World Health Organization. (2003). *Caring for children and adolescents with mental disorders: Setting WHO directions*. https://apps.who.int/iris/bitstream/handle/10665/42679/9241590637.pdf

GENERAL RESOURCES

A. American Academy of Child and Adolescent Psychiatry: www.aacap.org
B. American Psychiatric Association: www.psychiatry.org/patients-families/somatic-symptom-disorder
C. Anxiety Canada: www.anxietycanada.com
D. Anxiety & Depression Association of America: www.adaa.org
E. Kelty Mental Health Resource Centre: https://keltymentalhealth.ca/somatization

6 CONDUCTING THE GERIATRIC PSYCHIATRIC ASSESSMENT

Kenneth Berc and Brenda Marshall

INTRODUCTION

Geriatric psychiatry, also known as psychogeriatrics, is a subspecialty of medicine that focuses on the cognitive, neurodegenerative, and mental disorders of old age. This field covers people over the age of 55 years. There are three major subdivisions: 55 to 65 years, 65 to 75 years, and very old age, more than 75 years. As medical progress and human awareness and avoidance of life-shortening toxins have evolved over the past 150 years, the percentages of people in these groups have changed considerably. Many can no longer believe that middle age ends at 55 years of age.

The high geriatric death toll from the COVID-19 pandemic, along with the isolation secondary to government lockdown measures, has resulted in increased levels of anxiety and depression in older adults and should be investigated in all new geriatric patients.

Because this field views all mental illness under the compound influence of overall medical, social, socioeconomic, and chronicity, initial evaluation may be much more complex and time-consuming than similar evaluations of younger people.

GERIATRIC PSYCHIATRIC ASSESSMENT

A. As with all exemplary medical diagnostic interviews, the first 10 or more minutes should be general surveys and an attempt to do the following:
  1. Bridge empathic communication with the patient.
  2. Engage in verbal and nonverbal communication as well as information gathering.
      a. Utilize open-ended questions.
      b. Be flexible and diverse.
      c. Assess orientation between the lines in an informal way.
      d. Why did this person come for the evaluations?
          i. At their own volition?
          ii. At someone else's insistence/recommendation?
          iii. Do they have a "hoped for" outcome?
  3. Connect with caregivers, relatives, and referral sources, including doctors who are present in person or available for consult.
      a. Who is on the patient's "team"?
      b. Assess the relationships.
      c. Do not assume they are unbiased or without mental illness.
  4. Assess any psychiatric impairment, which may preclude breaking the interview into multiple shorter sessions.
  5. Utilize a structured interview approach.
      a. Interview: Collect a complete psychiatric-mental health history.
      b. Assess diagnostic criteria utilizing the *Diagnostic and Statistical Manual of Mental Disorders*, Fifth Edition (*DSM-5*; American Psychiatric Association, 2013).
      c. Assess patient knowledge of illness, treatment, and prognosis.
B. Use external time-limited computer algorithms.
  1. Conserve initial assessment time, assisting the healthcare provider in preventing missed topics
  2. May serve as much to distort what must be learned
  3. Do not replace the clinician's breadth of knowledge and interviewing skills
      a. Are adjunctive to the interview technique
      b. Must be used with great care and finesse lest they lead the examiner into a seemingly satisfying but medically vapid corner
C. Conduct assessment of healthy aging.
  1. One should assess overall aging success or failure.
  2. Questions should be simple, friendly, and generally inquisitive.
      a. "Did you come alone?"
      b. "Do you have friends or family who are waiting or who would like to join us?"
  3. Assess patient response to current event or change in mental status.
      a. "Before this event, how was your overall health and ability to have a life as good as you'd hoped for?"
      b. "How long has this new problem persisted?"
      c. "In what ways are these problems interfering with your life, specifically with regard to hours/day, days/week, task-specific behaviors and interactions, etc.?"
  4. If others have come to the exam (after obtaining the patient's consent with/without visitors) it is best that the patient get the first 5 to 10 minutes without added comments or corrections by others present.
      a. Ask the helpers to hold comments and promise to add their comments and edits soon.
      b. One should never assume the other commentators are more reliable or less biased or distorted, perhaps negatively, than the patient themselves.

EXPLORATION OF DIFFERENTIAL EVALUATION

The differential evaluation should briefly explore the indirect psychiatric avenues for disease and disruption, such as recent or chronic trauma, infection, endocrine disorders, metabolic disorders, and severe persistent disorders such as cancer, which may commandeer pressure over the entire cluster of findings. Carefully list all medications taken by the patient, including vitamins and folk remedies, as these can often have an effect on the disease process. Prescribed medications are thought by some to be the most common cause of delirium and new mental symptoms.

A. Diagnosis-directed questions
  1. As a diagnosis forms from the interview questions, the clinician should ask specific symptom questions to narrow down the criteria to arrive at an evidence-based diagnosis.

2. Utilize the *DSM-5* (American Psychiatric Association, 2013) criteria in formulating and asking specific symptom related questions.
    a. "Do you find yourself not needing to sleep?" (*DSM-5* [American Psychiatric Association, 2013] bipolar disease)
    b. "Are you sad or depressed most of the day and most days?" (*DSM-5* [American Psychiatric Association, 2013] depression).
3. Craft questions to funnel from general to more specific criteria.

B. The structured interview
  1. Some of the structured interview guides are specifically adapted for use in the geriatric population.
      a. In 2000, there were multiple scales available to assess depression specifically in the geriatric population.
      b. Patient healthcare experiences may impact the geriatric patient's willingness to comply with treatment plans. Assessing past experiences related to psychiatric hospitalization is important.
  2. As the clinician examines the patient, utilization of symptom measures can guide the structured interview.
      a. The *DSM-5* (American Psychiatric Association, 2013) Cross-Cutting Symptom Measures evaluate mental illness across the life span. They are standardized, valid, and reliable questionnaires that are available online for free.
      b. The National Institutes of Health (NIH) Screening and Assessment Tools Chart used to assess drug, tobacco, and alcohol use across the life span can be found on the NIH website.
  3. The combination of the diagnostic questions and the results from valid, reliable measures will assist the clinician in determining the best-fit diagnosis related to the patient's experience of symptoms.
      a. Other examples of structured interview guides include the following:
          i. Composite International Diagnostic Interview (CIDI)
          ii. Mini International Neuropsychiatric Interview (MINI-Plus)

C. Utilizing the *International Classification of Diseases*, 10th Revision (*ICD-10*; World Health Organization [WHO], 1990) billing coding:
  1. The 2023 *ICD-10* code for encounter for general psychiatric examination is Z04.6, with the code type "diagnosis."

COMMON CONDITIONS IN THE GERIATRIC POPULATION

Treatment planning for the geriatric patient often involves the caretakers, and the modes of treatment—especially pharmacotherapy—must often take into account other medical and social complexities.

The following common diagnoses in the geriatric population are arranged by highest prevalence. It is hoped that by searching for the most common causes first, the most efficient route to diagnosis will be found. However, due to cultural differences, economic differences, and other shifting modifiers, even prevalence can be a changing measure. For general assessment of each of these diagnoses, please refer to the "Geriatric Psychiatric Assessment" section at the start of this chapter. Any additional, specific questions or interventions that need to be considered specific to the diagnosis are listed under that diagnosis.

LATE LIFE PSYCHOSIS

DEFINITION
Late life psychosis often results as a complication for patients who have been diagnosed with bipolar disorder (BD) and depression earlier in life. Psychosis does not have a formal definition in the *ICD* classification (WHO, 1990) or the *DSM-5* (American Psychiatric Association, 2013). Rather, the features associated with psychosis, including delusions, hallucinations, and positive and negative symptoms, are included under schizophrenia spectrum and other psychotic disorders. Late onset (LOS) is considered between 40 and 60 years of age, while very late-onset schizophrenia-like psychosis (VLOS) is after 60.

ETIOLOGY
A. There are varied etiologies for the older adult.
B. Development can be due to biological, social, psychological, and environmental interactions, which might be very complex.

PREVALENCE AND INCIDENCE
A. The prevalence of late-onset psychosis/schizophrenia is between 0.1% and 0.5%, and the incidence of psychosis/schizophrenia after 65 years of age is 7.5 per 100,000.
B. The prevalence of schizoaffective disorder in adults more than 60 years of age is 0.14%.
C. The prevalence of psychotic features in older adults with neurocognitive disorders is as high as 40%. Those with Alzheimer disease (AD) are identified at 41% and those with vascular dementia are reported at 15%.
D. Lewy bodies disorder has a prevalence of 78% visual and auditory hallucinations and 25% delusions.
E. The overall incidence of affective psychosis (secondary to depression and BD) is 30.9 per 100,000.

HISTORY AND PHYSICAL
A. Conduct a full geriatric psychiatric assessment (see earlier in this chapter).

DESIRED OUTCOMES
A. There are significant levels of morbidity and mortality when psychosis affects an older adult. Comprehensive workups are required to diagnose.
B. Recognition of the desired outcome for the patient, in addition to the etiology of symptoms, needs to be considered.
C. Utilization of multimodal approach with sensitivity to polypharmacy is required.
  1. Nonpharmacologic management strategies
  2. Psychotropic medication
      a. Cautious use of antipsychotic medications
      b. Regular monitoring of all aspects of additional psychotropic medications for efficacy as well as adverse effects

SPECIFIC CONCERNS
A. Assess for suicide: Older adults with schizoaffective disorders, depression-related psychosis, and schizophrenia are more isolated, have increased treatment resistance, and are at increased risk for death by suicide.
B. Psychotic features of depression in older adults are not uncommon and can begin around 51 years of age. Delusions

have been identified in 45% of these older adults when admitted to the hospital.
C. Patients with AD and/or vascular neurocognitive disorders commonly have persecutory delusions and visual hallucinations.

TREATMENT
A. Currently, there is no cure for AD. The medications that are listed here are specifically for temporary reduction of the symptoms of AD and may slow the progression. Six drugs have U.S. Food and Drug Administration (FDA) approval; however, tacrine was removed in 2013 due to serious side effects that outweighed the benefits.
B. Pharmacologic treatments for cognitive changes include the following:
    1. Acetylcholinesterase (AChE) inhibitors: for early to midstage and can be continued into late stage
        a. Donepezil
        b. Galantamine
        c. Rivastigmine
    2. Memantine: N-methyl-D-aspartate (NMDA) receptor antagonist that blocks glutamate effects; can be taken with AChE inhibitors for moderate to severe dementia
        a. Side effects usually transitory:
            i. Headaches
            ii. Dizziness
            iii. Constipation
            iv. Gastrointestinal (GI) upset
    3. Aducanumab: amyloid-targeting monoclonal antibody
        a. Used in early AD; requires strict monitoring and multiple adverse effects
        b. Requires the clinician to review the diagnostic evaluation to determine if the patient's profile is appropriate for this drug
C. Pharmacologic treatments are available for behavioral and psychological symptoms in dementia (BPSD).
    1. BPSD can include the following:
        a. Anxiety, wandering, and depression
        b. Increased agitation, delusions, and hallucinations
    2. Medications to treat BPSD include the following:
        a. Antipsychotics
            i. Risperidone
            ii. Haloperidol
            iii. Antidepressants: L-deprenyl: selegiline, selective monoamine oxidase B (MAO-B) inhibitor
        b. Other medications
            i. Vitamin E
            ii. Estrogen replacement therapy
            iii. Ergoloid mesylates: Hydergine
            iv. Anticonvulsants (carbamazepine has a few studies)
D. Nonpharmacologic treatments include the following:
    1. Cognitive stimulation therapy (e.g., group activities)
    2. Cognitive rehabilitation (e.g., occupational therapy, relearning or learning to do everyday tasks like using the phone, or using apps on a mobile device)
    3. Life story work/reminiscence therapy: reviewing photos, memorabilia, music, and stories to improve mood
    4. Somatic treatments
        a. Electroconvulsive therapy (ECT; no substantial literature supports ECT)
        b. Light therapy

DELIRIUM IN OLDER ADULTS

DEFINITION
Delirium is a common, often fatal, acute transient condition that impacts consciousness or state of mind. It is marked by an alteration in baseline cognition and attention.

ETIOLOGY
A. The exact etiology is not well-understood. It is believed that delirium results from disturbed neurotransmitter (acetylcholine, dopamine, glutamate, noradrenaline), and gamma-aminobutyric acid (GABA) interaction.
B. The etiology of delirium in the older adult is considered multifactorial.
    1. Susceptibility (advanced age, dementia) as well as precipitating factors (polypharmacy, chronic medical conditions) interact for a cumulative effect.
    2. The more severe the precipitating factors, the higher the risk of delirium.
    3. The more vulnerable the patient, even stimulus considered mild in other adults can result in delirium or extend the length of time the adult experiences it.
C. In the older adult, consider predisposing factors of advanced age, neurocognitive disorders, visual and/or hearing impairment, malignancy, coronary artery disease, chronic obstructive pulmonary disease (COPD), anemia, and any past psychiatric disorders.

PREVALENCE AND INCIDENCE
A. Prevalence: Between 11% and 42% of hospitalized older Americans experience delirium compared with 1% to 2% in the nonhospitalized general older community.
B. Incidence: 20% to 29% of older Americans (more than 65 years), more than 1.6 million adults, experience delirium.
C. Delirium is seen in 15% to 53% of postop older adults, and 70% to 87% of older adults in the ICU.
D. 60% of older adults living in nursing homes and postacute care experience delirium, which increases to up to 83% at end of life.

HISTORY AND PHYSICAL
A. Conduct a full geriatric psychiatric assessment (see earlier in this chapter).
B. Screening instruments include the following:
    1. 4 AT (4 A's test)
        a. Brief and easy to administer
        b. Provides score that suggests cognitive impairment
    2. Confusion Assessment Method (CAM)
        a. 3D-CAM (3-minute assessment time): a brief assessment
        b. CAM-S (10- to 15-minute assessment time): quantifies the intensity of delirium but not diagnosis
C. Look for etiology in a medical condition or effects of medications. Examine for history of falls, alcohol and drug use/misuse, and long-term use of medications (including prescribed, over-the-counter [OTC], and nonprescribed).
D. Utilize the National Institute for Health and Care Excellence (NICE) guidelines to evaluate for prevention and management of delirium in patients older than 65 years.
E. Clinical presentation in the older adult include the following:
    1. Clouding of consciousness with behavioral and cognitive changes

2. Limited in its course and resulting from an external stimulus
3. Diurnal fluctuation in confusion resulting in changes in awareness, psychomotor behaviors, emotions, and sleep–wake cycle
4. May last for hours or days when treated
5. May last for weeks or months if left untreated

DESIRED OUTCOMES
A. Early diagnosis and treatment reduces the long-term impact on health and well-being.
B. Engage in prevention protocols and patient screening.
1. Hospital Elder Life Program (HELP): https://geriatricscareonline.org/ProductAbstract/Hospital-Elder-Life-Program/M0011#
2. Maintenance of physical and cognitive function of the older patient

C. Utilize the NICE guidelines implemented by an interdisciplinary team.

SPECIFIC CONCERNS
A. Advanced age as well as presence of dementia are risk factors. The older adult is the fastest growing demographic group globally.
B. The older hospitalized adult is the most vulnerable group for delirium, which may often be prevented.
C. Hospitalization may be when delirium presents in the older patient, or the patient might be brought to the ED due to change in consciousness.
D. Delirium is often underrecognized and not adequately managed in the older adult.
E. Delirium is rarely confirmed by a psychiatric specialist provider.
F. Use of antipsychotic drugs has the following risks:
1. May prolong the delirium
2. May accelerate functional as well as cognitive decline in older adults with AD
3. Should only be used after nonpharmacologic interventions have been deemed unsuccessful
4. Should only be used in persons who are a danger to themselves or others

G. Delirium may have a long-term sequelae in the older adult, increasing the following risks threefold.
1. Risk of functional decline
2. Cognitive dysfunction
3. Increased likelihood of long-term care needs
4. Increased risk of death

TREATMENT
A. Early diagnosis with confirmation by a specialized psychiatric provider is important.
B. There are no groups of medications that have been approved for treatment of delirium, nor has any evidence been provided demonstrating that any drug regimen benefits the patient in relieving its symptoms. Treatment of the cause of the patient's delirium is the first line of treatment.
C. Consider short-term use of medication to reduce some symptoms (less than 1 week).
1. Consider low-dose antipsychotics for patients who are considered a risk to themselves and after other nonpharmacologic efforts have failed in de-escalation.
2. Haloperidol has been seen to correct some acute behavioral changes, but second-generation antipsychotics have not been demonstrated to reduce the severity or duration of delirium.

D. Identify and treat the causative factors (e.g., polypharmacy, medical conditions, infections). Consider nonpharmacologic interventions first.
1. Ensure nutrition and adequate fluid intake.
2. Closely monitor responses to medication, as well as physical and psychological changes.
3. Reduce stimuli.
4. Reduce the need to move the patient frequently.
5. Provide reorientation when needed, as well as clear instructions.
6. Arrange care to reduce interruptions with sleep.
7. Avoid catheterization when possible.
8. Ensure availability of aids.
   a. Dentures that fit
   b. Glasses
   c. Hearing aids
9. Encourage mild exercise (walking, range of motion).

SLEEP DISORDERS

DEFINITION
Any disruption in normal sleep pattern is considered a sleep disorder and can include all aspects of the sleep regimen, from falling asleep to staying in undisturbed sleep, or sleeping too much. Abnormal behaviors during and surrounding the sleep regimen are also considered part of the sleep disorder cluster. Some changes in sleeping patterns are part of the normal aging process; they become a disorder when they are related to pathologic processes and when they impact the individual's activities of daily living. Insomnia is the most common sleep disorder.

ETIOLOGY
A. Causes of sleep disorders in older adults are varied; however, obstructive sleep apnea (OSA) and periodic limb movements (PLMS) have been identified as the primary precipitators, with rapid eye movement (REM) sleep behavior disorder and circadian rhythm sleep–wake disorders as other primary sleep disorders.
B. Other causes of sleep disorders and insomnia include acute and chronic medical illnesses, behavioral and psychological physical stressors, medications, and environmental causes.
C. Pathophysiology: In the aging adult, there is an increase in stage 1 non-REM sleep (light sleep) and a decrease in stages 3 and 4 (deep sleep).
D. Sex differences: Older females have been assessed to have normal and sometimes increased stage 3 sleep, while males either have normal or reduced stage 3. In adults more than 90 years, there might be no stages 3 and 4 at all.

PREVALENCE AND INCIDENCE
A. The prevalence of insomnia symptoms in adults more than 65 years is 50%.
B. The incidence rates are estimated at 3% to 5% and remission has been achieved as high as 50%.

HISTORY AND PHYSICAL
A. Conduct a full geriatric psychiatric assessment (see earlier in this chapter).
B. Evaluate by referral to a sleep disorder center for evidence-based diagnosis.

DIFFERENTIAL DIAGNOSIS
A. Psychiatric: anxiety disorders, BD, depression, delirium, posttraumatic stress disorder (PTSD), schizophrenia
B. Pulmonary: COPD
C. GI: gastroesophageal reflux disease (GERD)
D. Other: Parkinson plus syndromes, periodic limb movement disorders (PLMBs), restless legs syndrome

DESIRED OUTCOMES
A. Assisting the patient in achieving a restorative pattern of sleep
B. Increased daytime performance
C. Increased cognitive function
D. Decreased risk of falls and memory impairments

SPECIFIC CONCERNS
A. Insomnia in the older patient is often associated with other medical and/or psychiatric conditions beyond OSA and PLMS, including depression, chronic pain, stroke, congestive heart failure, and anxiety.
B. Sleep disorders, especially in older adults, have been correlated with higher mortality rates.
  1. Presence of sleep disorders that cause increased intermittent hypoxia increases daytime hypersomnolence, hypertension, cor pulmonale, arrythmias including atrial fibrillation, complex ventricular ectopy (CVE), sleep disordered breathing, cognitive decline, and even sudden death.
  2. Use of benzodiazepines has been associated with increased dementia in patients more than 65 years.

TREATMENT
A. Balance of risk and benefits to increase daytime performance
B. Nonpharmacologic treatment
  1. Patient education
  2. Sleep hygiene
  3. Cognitive behavioral therapy (CBT)
  4. Bright light therapy
  5. Pharmacologic treatments when nonpharmacologic treatments do not work adequately 1. Assess for comorbid depression, anxiety, or other psychiatric diagnosis prior to considering medications (Table 6.1).
  6. Use any hypnotic at the lowest effective dose and only in the short term.
  7. For sleep onset issues, use ultra-short-acting or short-acting medications, such as nonbenzodiazepine hypnotics (i.e., zolpidem).

MILD COGNITIVE DISORDERS/MILD COGNITIVE IMPAIRMENTS

DEFINITION
Mild cognitive impairment (MCI) is considered a preclinical decline in memory, assessed as greater than the patient's

TABLE 6.1 PHARMACOLOGIC TREATMENT FOR INSOMNIA

Class	Type	Generic Name	Dose (mg)	Half-Life (hours)
Benzodiazepine	Ultra-short-acting	Triazolam	0.125–0.25	2–4
	Short-acting	Etizolam	0.5–1	6
		Brotizolam	0.25	7
		Rilmazafone	1–2	10
		Lormetazepam	1–2	10
	Intermediate-acting	Flunitrazepam	0.5–2	24
		Estazolam	1–4	24
		Nitrazepam	5–10	28
	Long-acting	Quazepam	15–30	36
		Flurazepam	10–30	65
Nonbenzodiazepine	Ultra-short-acting	Zolpidem	5–10	2
		Zopiclone	7.5–10	4
		Eszopiclone	1–3 (older adult 1–2)	Adults: 5 Older adults: 7
Melatonin receptor agonist		Ramelteon	8	1–2
Dual orexin receptor antagonist		Suvorexant	20 (older adult 15)	12

Source: Data from Suzuki, K., Miyamoto, M., & Hirata, K. (2017). Sleep disorders in the elderly: Diagnosis and management. *Journal of General and Family Medicine, 18*(2), 61–71. https://doi.org/10.1002/jgf2.27.

peers, and is usually seen as a transitional stage between age-appropriate cognitive decline and the onset of dementia. It impacts memory, language, and/or judgment, but is not as debilitating as AD or other neurocognitive disorders. Often, those with MCI are capable of conducting their activities of daily living.

A. There are two types of MCI:
1. Amnestic: related predominantly with memory issues
2. Nonamnestic: focused on other issues of cognition, such as language, executive function, and visual/spatial abilities
3. Four subtypes have been identified:
   a. Amnestic MCI single domain
   b. Amnestic MCI multiple domains
   c. Nonamnestic MCI single domain
   d. Nonamnestic MCI multiple domains

ETIOLOGY
A. No single cause has been identified in MCI, but genetics is an important factor influencing its development.
B. Medication side effects can cause MCI, as can dysfunction in metabolic and/or endocrine systems.
C. MCI can be part of the sequalae from delirium that have been produced due to an illness, like urinary tract infection (UTI) or COVID-19.

PREVALENCE AND INCIDENCE
A. Prevalence: 12% to 18% of adults more than 60 years have MCI.
1. The prevalence increases with age, with those less than 70 years having between 7% and 9% MCI and those more than 70 years between 10% and 25.2%.

B. Incidence: The overall incidence of MCI is 22.6%.
1. Annually, 10% to 15% of persons with MCI will develop dementia.
2. 30% to 50% of persons with MCI due to AD will progress to Alzheimer's dementia over a period of 5 to 10 years.

HISTORY AND PHYSICAL
A. Conduct a full geriatric psychiatric assessment (see earlier in this chapter).
B. There are no cognitive assessments or screening tools or tests for MCI.
C. Rule out other systemic and neurocognitive disorders:
1. Parkinson disease
2. Lewy bodies dementia
3. MCI due to AD: should look for biomarker tests (e.g., beta-amyloid deposits, pathologic tau in imaging, or cerebrospinal fluid [CSF]).

DIFFERENTIAL DIAGNOSIS
A. Psychiatric: depression, pseudodementia
B. Medication side effects: analgesics, sedative-hypnotics, anticholinergics, psychotropics, alcohol overuse/misuse
C. Sleep disturbances: sleep apnea, restless leg syndrome, nocturnal hypoxemia
D. Deficiencies: hypothyroidism, vitamin B_{12} deficiency
E. Neurologic: Parkinson disease, multiple sclerosis (MS), epilepsy, cerebrovascular accident (CVA), brain tumor

DESIRED OUTCOMES
A. Prevention of cognitive decline through patient education
1. Reduce alcohol consumption.
2. Reduce risk of head injury.
3. Management of diabetes, obesity, hypertension, and psychiatric comorbidities
4. Engaging in good sleep hygiene practices

B. Early diagnosis and treatment to slow or halt the progression to dementia
1. Lifestyle changes
2. Medications

SPECIFIC CONCERNS
A. Limited expertise in MCI by nonpsychiatric care providers can lead to misdiagnosis and delay in treatment.
B. Chronic conditions in minority and underserved populations, language barriers, and culturally insensitive cognitive assessments for aging populations impact diagnosis and treatment.

TREATMENT
A. No specific treatments identified currently for MCI
B. Follow-up appointments every 6 to 12 months to monitor any changes in memory or cognitions
C. Patient and family education on decreasing influences that can accelerate cognitive decline (e.g., alcohol and substance use, falls/traumatic brain injury [TBI], isolation)
D. Medications
1. AChE inhibitors: Donepezil may be necessary for symptomatic relief from memory problems but has not been demonstrated to have any significant impact on MCI.

MOOD DISORDERS IN OLDER ADULTS

DEFINITION
Mood disorders, persistent emotional disturbances, like unipolar depression and bipolar subtypes, although less frequent in the older adult, are an important public health dilemma as these disorders are correlated with comorbid medical conditions and cognitive decline. The most common mood disorders are major depressive disorder, dysthymic disorder, BD, mood disorder due to a medical condition, and mood disorder due to substance use/misuse.

ETIOLOGY
A. Neurobiological correlates have been identified with depression in older adults, including neuroendocrine dysfunction on the hypothalamic–pituitary–adrenal (HPA) axis, structural and functional changes in the frontal cortical–subcortical pathways, and reduced hippocampal volume.
B. Vascular depression hypothesis identifies white matter lesions that impact the delivery of blood to the orbital and dorsolateral prefrontal regions, depressing executive functioning, which results in lack of interest, slowed processing speed, less motivation, depressive ideation, and limited insight.
C. Structural and functional neuroimaging has not indicated neurobiological bases for BD; however, in patients with more than 10 episodes of hospitalization related to depression and/or mania in BD, hippocampal atrophy was present. HPA dysfunction, secondary to increased proinflammatory cytokines underlying serotonin and dopamine neurotransmitters in specific areas of the brain including the hippocampus, amygdala, and nucleus accumbens, is present in advanced age BD.

PREVALENCE AND INCIDENCE
A. Unipolar depression: prevalence of 10% to 38%, with 35.5% of older adult depression as mild, 51.9% as moderate, and 12.7% as severe

B. BD: prevalence of 0.1% to 0.5% and represents 4% to 8% of admissions to geropsychiatric units
C. Incidence: 5% more than 65 years reporting depression, with 10% having had depression during their lifetime
D. Suicide: highest rate of suicide in the United States in persons more than 80 years of age

HISTORY AND PHYSICAL
A. Conduct a full geriatric psychiatric assessment (see earlier in this chapter).
B. Assess suicidality.
C. Examine for more sleep disturbances, presence of psychomotor retardation, and a sense of hopelessness in the future.
D. For those with bipolar disease, in those older patients experiencing an early onset, the presentation has more mixed episodes. Those with late onset have greater psychosocial functional deficits and cognitive impairment, but less acute psychopathology.

DIFFERENTIAL DIAGNOSIS
A. Dementia
B. Pseudobulbar
C. OSA
D. Medication-induced depression and/or mania
E. Hypothyroid

DESIRED OUTCOMES
A. To support euthymia by increasing patient understanding of early signs and symptoms and engagement in treatment
B. To reduce high-risk behaviors associated with hypomania and mania and to decrease suicidal ideation

SPECIFIC CONCERNS
A. Older adults may have multiple age-related conditions, all of which increase with further aging. Diagnostic tools as well as treatments need to take into consideration age-appropriate cognitive functioning, physical abilities, and daily level of functioning.
B. The clinician maintains a respectful therapeutic relationship, assessing how chronic and acute illnesses impact functionality and can disrupt mood.
C. Consideration must be paid to the coexisting comorbidities and their impact on function, medication efficacy and risk, and alternate modalities of treatment.

TREATMENT
A. Similar to treatment guidelines for depression and BD in middle-aged adults
B. Psychotherapy
  1. CBT
  2. Dialectical behavioral therapy (DBT)
C. Medications
  1. Consider the following for unipolar depression:
     a. Selective serotonin reuptake inhibitors (SSRIs): Sertraline, citalopram, escitalopram, and desvenlafaxine, which are drugs less likely to cause a drug–drug reaction and are not associated with any sedative effects or anticholinergic effects, are better for the older patient.
     b. Electroconvulsive therapy (ECT): ECT demonstrates improvement in greater than 80% of patients. Take into consideration loss of memory, cardiac events/complications, and the possibility of delirium. Although the cognitive impact is usually transient, there are some patients for whom it is permanent.
  2. There are better medications to be utilized for older adults, especially for those who are older and have polypharmacy and multiple comorbidities.
D. Transcranial magnetic stimulation for depression
E. Increased physical exercise, which has been effective in treating depression in older patients
F. Bipolar—special consideration
  1. Be alert for extrapyramidal symptoms in older adults.
     a. BD depression: Lamotrigine trials have demonstrated some improvement (Sajatovic & Chen, 2011).
     b. BD mania, hypomania, and mixed episodes: Lithium and quetiapine have demonstrated efficacy.

ANXIETY DISORDERS

DEFINITION
Anxiety disorders appear in all stages of life; however, special consideration should be given to the impact of anxiety disorders on older adults. Anxiety disorders, especially general anxiety disorder (GAD), are common in older adults; however, the identification of the disorder might be complicated by other medical comorbidities and therefore be untreated. The general definition for anxiety disorders can be found in Chapter 9, "Anxiety Disorders." Within the geriatric community, the threshold for arriving at this diagnosis relies upon the clinician's clinical judgment. In the older population, anxiety has been identified as more prevalent than depression in the community and in the clinical milieu. The presence of anxiety also impacts other areas of daily living, such as recovery from other illnesses, increased disability levels, and decreased quality of life. The symptoms of anxiety in the geriatric population are often misunderstood by the patient due to poor insight and blaming the worry on medical conditions or medications. Most often, the clinician looks for excessive, consistent state of worrying that lasts for over 6 months, including motor tension, scanning, and vigilance. There is a high comorbidity with depression.

ETIOLOGY
Anxiety in the older adult has been identified as different, qualitatively, from that of the younger adult. There is decreased autonomic nervous system activation, which hinders detection of anxiety and panic. The existence of other medical conditions, such as lung diseases, cardiovascular diseases, thyroid diseases, and diabetes, increases the older adult's risk for anxiety. Sleep disturbances, use/misuse of alcohol and drugs, and increasing physical limitations in activities of daily living are also considered risk factors for anxiety. The National Council on Aging also identifies that for some adults, experiencing extreme stress and anxiety can bring about a chemical imbalance in the brain resulting in an anxiety disorder. In addition, the older adult is more concerned about the attached stigma of reporting psychiatric symptoms to their healthcare providers.

PREVALENCE AND INCIDENCE
A. The prevalence of anxiety disorders in persons over 65 years of age who are not institutionalized is 30%.
  1. The prevalence rate for anxiety is 14% and for phobias 11%.
B. 14.5% of adults over 85 years of age experience anxiety.
  1. the prevalence is higher in females than in males.
  2. Recent death of friends or family in the past 18 months doubles the risk of experiencing anxiety.

HISTORY AND PHYSICAL

A. Conduct a full geriatric psychiatric assessment (see earlier in this chapter).
B. Increase awareness of symptom sharing with other neurologic, cardiovascular, GI, metabolic/endocrine disorders, and vitamin deficiencies.
  1. Neurologic: stroke, epilepsy, MS, tumors, parkinsonism
  2. Cardiovascular: angina, cardiac arrythmia, acute asthma, mitral valve prolapse
  3. GI: irritable bowel syndrome (IBS), Crohn's disease, acute diverticulitis
  4. Metabolic/endocrine: diabetes, hypoglycemia, hyperthyroidism, hepatic failure, hypercalcemia
  5. Vitamin deficiencies: B vitamins (B_1, B_6, B_{12}, folic acid)
C. Older patients are part of a vulnerable population—examine also for elder abuse.
D. Investigate for medications that can bring on anxiety; the more common are listed in the following:
  1. Levodopa
  2. Amantadine
  3. Bromocriptine
  4. Monoamine oxidase (MAO) inhibitors
  5. Tricyclic antidepressants (TCAs)
  6. Theophylline
  7. Interferon
  8. Thyroid hormones
  9. Caffeine, amphetamines
E. Examine for distinct clinical features in the older population.
  1. Lower cognitive and somatic distress, even during panic attack
  2. Higher religiosity, religious obsessions, and contamination obsessions
  3. Increased physical rather than psychological symptoms (e.g., fatigability, sleep disturbances, muscle tension)
  4. Increased use of avoidance as a coping mechanism
F. Environmental and psychological risk factors associated with anxiety disorder in the older adult include the following:
  1. Low socioeconomic status
  2. Female
  3. Low educational level
  4. Chronic medical illnesses
  5. Single, widowed, childless
  6. Functional impairment
  7. History of adverse childhood experiences (ACEs)
  8. Neuroticism
  9. Poor coping skills
  10. Low self-efficacy
  11. Small or impaired social networking
  12. Cognitive impairment or other psychiatric diagnosis
  13. Living with a partner with a major illness
G. Examine the three categories of anxiety disorders before diagnosing.
  1. Worry/distress disorders
     a. GAD (7.3%)
     b. PTSD
     c. Acute stress disorder
  2. Fear disorders
     a. Panic disorder
     b. Phobia (3.1%)
  3. Obsessive-compulsive disorder (OCD; 0.6%)

SPECIFIC RATING SCALES FOR ANXIETY IN THE OLDER ADULT

A. Geriatric Anxiety Scale (gold standard)
B. Hamilton Anxiety Rating Scale
C. Beck Anxiety Inventory
D. Anxiety Status Inventory

DIFFERENTIAL DIAGNOSIS

A. Medication use, misuse, abuse
B. Substance use, misuse, abuse
C. Anxiety resulting from medical comorbidities
D. Anxiety resulting from other psychiatric disorders inclusive of neurogenerative and cognitive disorders

DESIRED OUTCOMES

A. To support the patient to a comfortable, higher functioning level in activities of daily living, without the debilitation of anxiety symptoms
B. Duration of treatment for older adults usually 12 months to 2 years, with ongoing examination for new cognitive symptoms, remission, or exacerbation of anxiety-related symptoms

SPECIFIC CONCERNS

A. Caregiver reflections as well as the concerns of the patient are important. Significant others and the patient might underreport or attempt to normalize the symptoms for fear of stigma of a psychiatric diagnosis or dementia.
B. Underreporting of the severity of symptoms can increase the likelihood of decreased functioning.

TREATMENT

A. Lifestyle modifications
  1. Sleep hygiene, nutrition exercise
  2. Socialization with a focus on reducing anxiety-provoking situations
  3. Slow introduction/reintroduction to structured daily activities and moderate exercise
B. Therapy
  1. Relaxation therapies, breathing exercises, guided imagery, yoga, art therapy, dance therapy, music therapy, complementary and alternative therapies (e.g., reflexology, massage, reiki)
  2. Desensitization
  3. Exposure and response prevention (especially good for OCD)
  4. Eye movement desensitization and reprocessing (EMDR) for PTSD and stress response
  5. Mindfulness therapy
  6. CBT: demonstrated to have lower efficacy in older adults
C. Three common medications for GAD in the older adult
  1. Antidepressants
     a. Citalopram and venlafaxine have good efficacy in this population even in the absence of major depression.
     b. Escitalopram, paroxetine, and trazodone have also been demonstrated to be effective for later in life GAD.
  2. Benzodiazepines
     a. Benzodiazepines have limited role and can cause neurocognitive effects and paradoxical agitation.
     b. If utilized, either lorazepam or oxazepam has more favorable pharmacokinetic considerations.
     c. There is increased risk for abuse or dependence. If abuse is suspected, engage the patient in detoxification or a taper method.
  3. Buspirone
     a. Buspirone has limited role.

SOMATIZATION DISORDER IN THE OLDER PATIENT

DEFINITION
The *DSM-5* (American Psychiatric Association, 2013) definition of somatic symptoms disorder includes the patient's focus on a physical symptom, which impairs the person's ability to think about other things, leading to excessive feelings, behaviors, and thoughts that are related to that physical symptom. These complaints of the physical symptoms are to an extent that disrupts the patient's activities of daily living. The symptoms may or may not be explained by a medical condition. The patient demonstrates more concern related to the symptom rather than to the potential medical condition.

ETIOLOGY
A. There is no clear etiology for somatization disorder; however, risk factors have been identified. There is an association with increased awareness of physical, body sensations.
B. Genetic and biological factors include increased sensitivity to pain and family influence (may be environmental, genetic, or both).
C. Risk factors include the following:
  1. ACEs
  2. Sexual abuse
  3. Chronic alcohol and substance use, misuse, and abuse
  4. Chaotic lifestyle
  5. Comorbid anxiety and depression

PREVALENCE AND INCIDENCE
A. The NIH reflects that few studies assess the presence of somatoform disorders in the older population.
B. Prevalence rates in older adults vary from 1.5% to 13% (Yates & Xiong, 2019).
C. An international study including six countries and 3,142 persons aged 65 to 84 years identified a prevalence rate at 3.8% (Dehoust et al. 2017).

HISTORY AND PHYSICAL
A. Conduct a full geriatric psychiatric assessment (see earlier in this chapter).
B. The Somatic Symptom Index is a scale used to assess somatic symptoms disorder.
  1. Four unexplained complaints of a somatic nature in men and six unexplained complaints in women

DESIRED OUTCOMES
A. Reduction in somatic symptoms, pain, depression, and anxiety
B. Increase in quality of life

SPECIFIC CONCERNS
A. Studies have demonstrated a strong association between physical illness and abridged somatization (combination of psychopathology and physical disability). A person with abridged somatization is 50 times more likely to have experienced a comorbid physical medical diagnosis. This indicates the need for the practitioner to carefully consider overlapping diagnosis in the older patient.
B. Musculoskeletal and inflammatory diseases cause joint, muscle, and bone pain, as can the polypharmacy that is used to treat other comorbidities in older adults. Co-occurring medical conditions in the older population can also be an underlying cause of pain.

TREATMENT
A. CBT
  1. Reattribution CBT: Encourage the patient to associate the symptoms to a physiologic or psychological cause.
     a. Increase patient understanding and insight.
     b. Develop mutual agenda between the healthcare provider and the patient.
     c. Link the psychosocial problems with the physical symptoms.
B. Behavior therapy
  1. Biofeedback: Look at the heart rate, respirations, or muscle response/tension, in relation to the physical symptoms. Increase strategies to control responses.
C. Mindful-based therapy
  1. Has potential to improve severity of pain symptoms and quality of life; does not appear to relieve depressive or anxiety symptoms
  2. Mindful-based stress relief (MBSR): limited evidence to demonstrate effectiveness
D. Psychoeducation
  1. Educate patients that physical symptoms may be increased by emotional problems.
  2. Older adults did not have significant improvement with psychoeducation; however, the approach was evaluated as positive by older adults.

REFERENCES AND BIBLIOGRAPHY

American Psychiatric Association. (2013). *Diagnostic and statistical manual of mental disorders* (5th ed.). https://doi.org/10.1176/appi.books.9780890425596

Bryant, C., Mohlman, J., Gum, A., Stanley, M., Beekman, A. T., Wetherell, J. L., Thorp, S. R., Flint, A. J., & Lenze, E. J. (2013). Anxiety disorders in older adults: Looking to *DSM-5* and beyond. *The American Journal of Geriatric Psychiatry, 21*(9), 872–876. https://doi.org/10.1016/j.jagp.2013.01.011

Busse, A., Hensel, A., Gühne, U., Angermeyer, M. C., & Riedel-Heller, S. G. (2006). Mild cognitive impairment: Long-term course of four clinical subtypes. *Neurology, 67*(12), 2176–2185. https://doi.org/10.1212/01.wnl.0000249117.23318.e1

Cummings, J., Aisen, P., Apostolova, L. G., Atri, A., Salloway, S., & Weiner, M. (2021). Aducanumab: Appropriate use recommendations. *The Journal of Prevention of Alzheimer's Disease, 8*(4), 398–410. https://doi.org/10.14283/jpad.2021.41

Dehoust, M. C., Schulz, H., Härter, M., Volkert, J., Sehner, S., Drabik, A., Wegscheider, K., Canuto, A., Weber, K., Crawford, M., Quirk, A., Grassi, L., DaRonch, C., Munoz, M., Ausin, B., Santos-Olmo, A., Shalev, A., Rotenstein, O., … Andreas, S. (2017). Prevalence and correlates of somatoform disorders in the elderly: Results of a European study. *International Journal of Methods in Psychiatric Research, 26*(1), e1550. https://doi.org/10.1002/mpr.1550

Flint, A. J. (2005). Generalized anxiety disorder in elderly patients. *Drugs & Aging, 22*, 101–114. https://doi.org/10.2165/00002512-200522020-00002

Kukreja, D., Günther, U., & Popp, J. (2015). Delirium in the elderly: Current problems with increasing geriatric age. *Indian Journal of Medical Research, 142*(6), 655–662. https://doi.org/10.4103/0971-5916

Lakhan, S. E., & Schofield, K. L. (2013). Mindfulness-based therapies in the treatment of somatization disorders: A systematic review and meta-analysis. *PLoS One, 8*(8), e71834. https://doi.org/10.1371/journal.pone.0071834

Los Angeles Department of Mental Health. (n.d.). *Dementia: Specific therapies*. Adapted from "The American Psychiatric Association's Practice Guideline for the Treatment of Patients With Alzheimer's Disease and Other Dementias of Late Life," American Psychiatric Association, 2000. https://dmh.lacounty.gov/for-providers/clinical-tools/web-based-training-meeting-solution/dementia-therapies

Oh, E. S., Fong, T. G., Hshieh, T. T., & Inouye, S. K. (2017). Delirium in older persons: Advances in diagnosis and treatment. *JAMA, 318*(12), 1161–1174. https://doi.org/10.1001/jama.2017.12067

Sachdev, P. S., Mohan, A., Taylor, L., & Jeste, D. V. (2015). *DSM-5* and mental disorders in older individuals: An overview. *Harvard Review of Psychiatry, 23*(5), 320–328. https://doi.org/10.1097/HRP.0000000000000090

Sajatovic, M., & Chen, P. (2011). Geriatric bipolar disorder. *Psychiatric Clinics of North America, 34*(2), 319–333. https://doi.org/10.1016/j.psc.2011.02.007

Stafford, J., Howard, R., & Kirkbride, J. B. (2018). The incidence of very late-onset psychotic disorders: A systematic review and meta-analysis, 1960–2016. *Psychological Medicine, 48*(11), 1775–1786. https://doi.org/10.1017/S0033291717003452

Subramanyam, A. A., Kedare, J., Singh, O. P., & Pinto, C. (2018). Clinical practice guidelines for Geriatric Anxiety Disorders. *Indian Journal of Psychiatry, 60*(Suppl. 3), S371–S382. https://doi.org/10.4103/0019-5545.224476

Suzuki, K., Miyamoto, M., & Hirata, K. (2017). Sleep disorders in the elderly: Diagnosis and management. *Journal of General and Family Medicine, 18*(2), 61–71. https://doi.org/10.1002/jgf2.27

Tampi, R. R., Young, J., Hoq, R., Resnick, K., & Tampi, D. J. (2019). Psychotic disorders in late life: A narrative review. *Therapeutic Advances in Psychopharmacology, 9*. https://doi.org/10.1177/2045125319882798

Targum, S. D. (2001). Treating psychotic symptoms in elderly patients. *Primary Care Companion to the Journal of Clinical Psychiatry, 3*(4), 156–163. https://doi.org/10.4088/pcc.v03n0402

Valiengo, L. d. C. L., Stella, F., & Forlenza, O. V. (2016). Mood disorders in the elderly: Prevalence, functional impact, and management challenges. *Neuropsychiatric Disease and Treatment, 12*, 2105–2114. https://doi.org/10.2147/NDT.S94643

Wahl, A.-S., Benson, G., Hausner, L., Schmitt, S., Knoll, A., Ferretti-Bondy, A., Hefter, D., & Froelich L. (2021). Rapid support for older adults during the initial stages of the COVID-19 pandemic: Results from a geriatric psychiatry helpline. *Geriatrics (Basel), 6*(1), 30. https://doi.org/10.3390/geriatrics6010030

Welzel, F. D., Stein, J., Röhr, S., Fuchs, A., Pentzek, M., Mösch, E., Bickel, H., Weyerer, S., Werle, J., Wiese, B., Oey, A., Hajek, A., König, H. H., Heser, K., Keineidam, L., van den Bussche, H., van der Leeden, C., Maier, W., Scherer, M., ... Riedel-Heller, S. G. (2019). Prevalence of anxiety symptoms and their association with loss experience in a large cohort sample of the oldest-old. Results of the geCoDe/AgeQualiDe study. *Frontiers in Psychiatry, 10*, 285. https://doi.org/10.3389/fpsyt.2019.00285

World Health Organization. (1990). *International statistical classification of diseases* (10th rev.). https://icd.who.int/browse10/2019/en

Yates, W. R., & Xiong, G. L. (Ed.). (2019, April 23). *Somatic symptom disorders*. Medscape. https://emedicine.medscape.com/article/294908-overview

7 PSYCHIATRIC ASSESSMENT SCALES

Brenda Marshall, Rosita Rodriguez, Veronica Betts, and Elizabeth Fitzgerald

INTRODUCTION

This chapter is divided into two categories: initial assessment and specific diagnostic scales. Within each category, the scales are divided into free scales and those that must be purchased. Scales are constantly being developed, revised, and tested for reliability and validity. The scales that are presented here are the most up-to-date at the time of publication.

A. Primary initial assessment scales and secondary initial diagnosis-specific scales: Each scale that is presented will be assessed on the following criteria:
   1. For whom is the scale intended?
   2. What specific purpose does the scale have?
   3. Has the scale been validated with the intended population?
   4. Can the scale be conducted prior to the first interview or is it part of the initial interview?

B. Diagnosis-specific scales (adult and pediatric):
   1. Anxiety disorders
   2. Assessment for adults with cognitive and neurodegenerative disorders
   3. Assessments for patients with substance use disorders
   4. Mood disorders
   5. Attention deficit hyperactivity disorder (ADHD)

INITIAL SYMPTOM ASSESSMENT SCALES

Screening tools are important in the evaluation of symptoms and the clinician's determination of diagnosis and evidence-based treatments, especially in light of the current prevalence of anxiety, depression, and substance use. Incorporation of valid and reliable screening scales to assist the clinician during the clinical interview and to assess patient progress during treatment is invaluable. Utilization of scales like the Cross-Cutting Symptom Measures or the Brief Psychiatric Rating Scale can aid the clinician and serve as adjuncts during the initial assessment period. During treatment, incorporation of valid, reliable scales that are specific to the patient's identified challenges and diagnoses can help monitor progress and support clinical decision-making, thereby adding another dimension to treatment assessment. Use of scales, however, is adjunctive and not to replace the in-depth psychiatric interview and assessment that is critical to proper diagnosis and treatment.

FREE INITIAL ASSESSMENT SCALES

Brief Psychiatric Rating Scale

A. The Brief Psychiatric Rating Scale (BPRS) assists the clinician who suspects that the patient is presenting with a psychotic disorder.
B. The scale includes 18 symptom constructs (including, but not limited to, suspiciousness, hallucinations, grandiosity, and hostility) and can be used at the initial assessment or throughout treatment to gauge treatment impact.
C. The clinician or rater, if completed by a family member or significant other, assesses each symptom on a Likert scale of 1 to 7, where 1 means the symptom is not present and 7 indicates extreme severity. It can usually be completed in less than 30 minutes.
D. The scale can be accessed online at www.physio-pedia.com/images/5/5d/Brief-Psychiatric-Rating-Scale_BPRS.pdf.

Brief Psychiatric Rating Scale (Version 4)

A. The revised, expanded version of the BPRS is a 24-item scale, with responses ranging from 1 to 7, with 2 indicating very mild and 7 indicating extreme severity.
B. The expanded version has also been tested for sensitivity in patients with unipolar depression (Zanello et al., 2013). It has improved the coverage of symptoms and has demonstrated increased interrater reliability.
C. The scale can be accessed online at https://cdn.sanity.io/files/0vv8moc6/psychtimes/5468a2f9b6b34b9ae55de3621ce55d57d20bc59b.pdf/bprsinstructions.pdf.

Diagnostic and Statistical Manual of Mental Disorders, Fifth Edition, Self-Rated Level 1 Cross-Cutting Symptom Measure

A. The *Diagnostic and Statistical Manual of Mental Disorders, Fifth Edition* (*DSM-5*; American Psychiatric Association, 2013), Level 1 Cross-Cutting Symptom Measure is a product of the American Psychiatric Association and assesses thresholds for further inquiry related to symptoms.
B. This one-page brief assessment evaluates for symptoms of depression, anger, mania, anxiety, somatic symptoms, suicidal ideation, psychosis, sleep problems, memory, repetitive thoughts and behaviors, dissociation, personality functioning, and substance use.
C. This measure includes a scoring and interpretation explanation and can be used at regular points during patient treatment to examine changes in symptoms over time.
D. As long as the patient can fill out the survey, it is suggested that they do so. If the person lacks capacity to fill out the form, another adult who is knowledgeable about the patient's symptoms can do so.
E. The score has 23 items and takes about 10 to 15 minutes to complete. The assessment asks the patient how frequently the symptoms were present within the past 2 weeks and the patient responds on a Likert scale, ranging from none at all (0); slight—rare, less than a day or 2 (1); mild—several days (2); moderate—more than half the days (3); and severe—nearly every day (4). The clinician adds the scores up for each of the 13 transdiagnostic mental health domains, revealing insight as to the severity of the patient's symptoms. Any domain with a score of 2 or greater identifies a possible problem area.
F. Currently, this is the only transdiagnostic screening instrument.

G. The Cross-Cutting Symptom Measure has three versions: adult self-report, child self-report (for children 11–17 years of age), and a parent/guardian report, which can be used for children between the ages of 6 and 17 years.
H. This measure can be accessed online at www.psychiatry.org/File%20Library/Psychiatrists/Practice/DSM/APA_DSM5_Level-1-Measure-Adult.pdf.

Child Self-Report Version
A. The child version has 25 questions that cover 12 transdiagnostic mental health domains. These domains include depression, anger, irritability, mania, anxiety, somatic symptoms, inattention, suicidal ideation/attempt, psychosis, sleep disturbance, repetitive thoughts and behaviors, and substance use.
B. The American Psychiatric Association makes this scale available online for any researcher or clinician to use with their patients as one of the many tools utilized to formulate a diagnosis.
C. Like the adult version, it uses a 5-point Likert scale assessing how much or how often a specific symptom bothered the youth during the past 2-week period. Some questions, like suicidal ideation, are a binary choice (i.e., yes/no).
D. The *Diagnostic and Statistical Manual of Mental Disorders*, Fifth Edition, Text Revision (*DSM-5-TR*; American Psychiatric Association, 2022) Self-Rated Level 1 Cross-Cutting Symptoms Measure for children ages 11 to 17 can be accessed online at www.psychiatry.org/File%20Library/Psychiatrists/Practice/DSM/APA_DSM5_Level-1-Measure-Child-Age-11-to-17.pdf.
E. *DSM-5-TR* Parent/Guardian-Rated Level 1 Cross-Cutting Measure for children ages 6 to 17 can be accessed online at www.psychiatry.org/getmedia/1e799501-f718-4d06-817e-ce98e35c6bdd/APA-DSM5TR-Level1MeasureParentOrGuardianOfChildAge6To17.pdf.

Diagnostic and Statistical Manual of Mental Disorders, Fifth Edition, Level 2 Cross-Cutting Symptom Measure
A. This measure can be used during the initial interview after the level 1 indicator or can be used during treatment to assess patient progress.

Level 2 Cross-Cutting Symptom Measures for Adults
A. The eight level 2 cross-cutting symptom measures for adults can be used to follow up on severity of symptoms for those areas that tested positive on level 1. This adult level 2 scale is free to access and includes:
  1. Depression (8 items)
  2. Anger (5 items)
  3. Mania (5 items)
  4. Anxiety (7 items)
  5. Somatic symptoms (15 items)
  6. Sleep disturbances (8 items)
  7. Repetitive thoughts and behaviors (5 items)
  8. Substance use (10 items)
B. This measure can be accessed online at www.psychiatry.org/psychiatrists/practice/dsm/educational-resources/assessment-measures#section_1.

Level 2 Cross-Cutting Symptom Measures for Parents of Children Ages 6 to 17
A. Assessments can be provided to parents to help the clinician focus on the specific domain that has been identified in the level 1 scale.
B. Level 2 measures include somatic symptoms, sleep disturbances, inattention, depression, anger, irritability, mania, anxiety, and substance use.
C. The measure can be accessed online at www.psychiatry.org/psychiatrists/practice/dsm/educational-resources/assessment-measures#section_1.

Level 2 Cross-Cutting Symptom Measures for Children Ages 11 to 17
A. Cross-cutting measures provide a deeper assessment of the domains that have been identified in the level 1 cross-cutting questionnaire.
B. Each of the scales provides an explanation of how to measure the responses and interpret the results.
C. Utilization of level 2 scales provides a dimensional approach to not only diagnosing the presentation of symptoms, but also continuing to assess the symptoms as the patient undergoes treatment.
D. These assessments also allow the clinician to assess comorbid symptoms in addition to those presented by the primary diagnosis. It can be accessed online at www.psychiatry.org/psychiatrists/practice/dsm/educational-resources/assessment-measures#section_1.

OTHER FREE MEASURES

Early Development and Home Background—Parent/Guardian
A. For parents/guardians whose children are between 6 and 17 years old; to be completed by the parent or guardian
B. Assists the clinician in clinical decision-making and can be administered at the time of initial evaluation as well as throughout treatment to track progress
C. Consists of 19 items with responses of yes, no, can't remember, or don't know; can be completed prior to the first intake
D. Can be accessed online at www.psychiatry.org/getmedia/ef4ce2bb-ae0e-4270-a8de-dfbb20e5d2f6/APA-DSM5TR-EarlyDevelopmentAndHomeBackgroundFormParentOfChildAge6To17-pdf.pdf

Early Development and Home Background—Clinician-Rated
A. The early development and home background-clinician rated measure is used by clinicians in addition to the EDHB parent/guardian form.
B. The eight clinician-rated items should be completed after a thorough review of the parent/guardian-rated EDHB form. Clarification through follow-up questions to the parent/guardian can fill in any missing information.
C. It can be accessed online at www.psychiatry.org/getmedia/b06aa42b-5b39-40f0-8ac1-d24815d44343/APA-DSM5TR-ClinicianRatedEarlyDevelopmentAndHomeBackground.pdf.

Cultural Formulation Interviews Supporting and Enhancing Cultural Competence
Cultural Formulation Interview-With Patient
A. The Cultural Formulation Interview-With Patient is an interview guide to assist the clinician in clarifying key aspects of the problem presented by the patient, from the point of view of the patient and their social network. A written opening statement is provided in the interview explaining how the

clinician wants to see the problem from the patient's point of view.
B. It includes the cultural definition of the problem, the cultural perception of the cause, context and support (e.g., social networks), stressors, role of cultural identity, cultural factors affecting self-coping and past help-seeking behavior, and cultural factors affecting current help-seeking behavior.
C. Clinician prompts are provided in each category to support the acquisition of information from the patient.
D. It can be accessed online at www.psychiatry.org/getmedia/5cc5329d-3bd4-4c6a-bae1-dfd0d6496f44/APA-DSM5TR-CulturalFormulationInterview.pdf.

Cultural Formulation Interview-Informant Version

A. The Cultural Formulation Interview-Informant version is an interview guide intended for the family member/significant other who is providing information on the patient; it assists the clinician in obtaining information from the point of view of the informant.
B. It covers the topics of the relationship with the patient, cultural definition of the problem, cultural perceptions of cause, context and support, cultural factors affecting self-coping and past help-seeking behavior, and cultural factors affecting current help-seeking behavior.
C. Clinician prompts are provided in each category to support the acquisition of information from the informant; it includes indication when more probing may be necessary.
D. It can be accessed online at www.psychiatry.org/getmedia/4b37a60b-dcbd-402c-9ee2-3af7f5c9dc70/APA-DSM5TR-CulturalFormulationInterviewInformant.pdf.

Supplementary Modules to the Core Cultural Formulation Interview

A. These serve as a guide to support a more comprehensive assessment of the patient's culture. There are two ways to use these interview guides:
   1. As adjuncts to the Cultural Formulation Interview (CFI) information
   2. As deeper examination tools for the core CFI

B. Each module has an explanation for the clinician as well as prompts to be used when interviewing the patient.
   1. Eight supplementary models devoted to a deeper exploration of the domains of the CFI
   2. Three modules on special populations like children and adolescents, older adults, and immigrants and refugees
   3. One module that examines the caregiver experience

C. These modules can be accessed online at www.psychiatry.org/getmedia/aca8f5a2-9b1b-456c-a3b7-f7f852edcf7c/APA-DSM5TR-CulturalFormulationInterviewSupplementaryModules.pdf.

FEE-BASED INITIAL SCALES AND MEASURES

Structured Clinical Interview for DSM-5

A. The Structured Clinical Interview for *DSM-5* (SCID-5) is for trained clinicians to implement. The structured clinical interviews—SCID-5-CV (Clinician Version) and SCID-5-RV (Research Version)—are not free and can be purchased for use.
B. Osorio et al. (2019) assessed the clinical validity and intrarater and test–retest reliability of the SCID-CV and determined that the reliability and specificity of the measure were excellent. Its clinical validity was also confirmed.
C. It can be purchased online at www.appi.org/Products/Interviewing/Structured-Clinical-Interview-for-DSM-5-Disorders.

DIAGNOSIS-SPECIFIC SCALES

ANXIETY DISORDERS ASSESSMENT SCALES FOR ADULTS

Patient-Reported Outcomes Measurement Information System Emotional Distress—Anxiety—Short Form

A. The *DSM-5-TR* Level 2—Anxiety—Adult measure is a seven-item Patient-Reported Outcomes Measurement Information System (PROMIS)—Anxiety—Short Form that assesses the pure domain of anxiety in individuals 18 years of age and older.
B. The form is completed by the individual prior to a visit with the clinician. If the individual receiving care is of impaired capacity and unable to complete the form (e.g., an individual with dementia), a knowledgeable informant may complete the measure as done in the *DSM-5* Field Trials. However, the PROMIS—Anxiety—Short—Form has not been validated as an informant report scale by the PROMIS group. Each item asks the individual receiving care (or informant) to rate the severity of the individual's anxiety during the past 7 days. It can be reprinted without permission by clinicians for use with their patients.
C. The form can be accessed online at www.psychiatry.org/getmedia/f284f967-ed9e-4754-99fc-b32765b1c4a0/APA-DSM5TR-Level2AnxietyAdult.pdf.

General Anxiety Disorder-7

A. The General Anxiety Disorder-7 (GAD-7) is a self-administered, seven-item instrument that incorporates some of the *DSM-5* (American Psychiatric Association, 2013) criteria for GAD to identify possible cases of GAD along with measuring anxiety symptom severity.
B. It can also be used as a screening measure for panic, social anxiety, and posttraumatic stress disorder (PTSD).
C. It can be used quickly and effectively within a primary care setting. The scale takes less than 5 minutes to complete and is best to be self-administered by the patient, but can be completed by an interviewer in person or over the phone.
D. It can be accessed at https://adaa.org/sites/default/files/GAD-7_Anxiety-updated_0.pdf.

Liebowitz Social Anxiety Scale

A. The Liebowitz Social Anxiety Scale (LSAS) is a 24-item, self-report scale used to determine the role social anxiety plays in a patient's life across a variety of situations. The LSAS has been shown to be an efficient and effective scale to identify patients with problems with social anxiety.
B. The scale is free to use and is readily available. The results need to be interpreted by a trained licensed professional to determine the extent of social anxiety. The scale takes about 8 to 10 minutes to complete and is meant for patients 18 years of age and older.
C. It can be accessed online at https://nationalsocialanxietycenter.com/liebowitz-sa-scale.

Penn State Worry Questionnaire

A. The Penn State Worry Questionnaire (PSWQ) is a 16-item, self-report scale that is designed to measure the level of worry in adults.
B. Worry is generally recognized as a dominant feature of GAD.
C. The PSWQ has been found to distinguish patients with GAD from other anxiety disorders.
D. The scale takes about 3 to 5 minutes to complete and is meant for patients 18 years of age and older.

E. It can be accessed online at https://novopsych.com.au/assessments/diagnosis/penn-state-worry-questionnaire-pswq.

Hamilton Anxiety Rating Scale
A. The Hamilton Anxiety Rating Scale (HAM-A) consists of 14 items, each defined by a series of symptoms, and measures both psychic anxiety (mental agitation and psychological distress) and somatic anxiety (physical complaints related to anxiety).
B. The scale has been criticized as it does not discriminate between anxiolytic and antidepressant effects, and somatic anxiety versus somatic side effects. Despite this, the scale is still widely used and has an acceptable level of interrater reliability.
C. The scale takes about 5 to 8 minutes to complete and is meant for patients 18 years of age and older.
D. It can be accessed online at https://dcf.psychiatry.ufl.edu/files/2011/05/HAMILTON-ANXIETY.pdf.

Short Health Anxiety Inventory
A. *Health anxiety* (now referred to as Illness Anxiety Disorder in the *DSM-5-TR* and previously known as hypochondriasis; American Psychiatric Association, 2022) refers to inappropriate or excessive fears about one's health. It is characterized by excessive fears or beliefs that one has a serious illness, and this is often based on the misinterpretation of bodily sensations or symptoms.
B. The Short Health Anxiety Inventory (SHAI) consists of 18 items that assess health anxiety independent of health status. It can be used in both healthy and sick individuals, including those who are acutely ill and those who have been diagnosed with a chronic illness.
C. The scale takes about 3 to 5 minutes to complete and is meant for patients 18 years of age or older.
D. It can be accessed online at https://novopsych.com.au/assessments/health/short-health-anxiety-inventory-shai.

ANXIETY ASSESSMENT SCALES FOR CHILDREN

Screen for Child Anxiety Related Emotional Disorders
A. The Screen for Child Anxiety Related Emotional Disorders (SCARED) is a measure widely used to assess childhood anxiety based on parent and child report.
B. While the SCARED is a reliable, valid, and sensitive measure to screen for pediatric anxiety disorders, informant discrepancy can pose clinical and research challenges.
C. The SCARED comes in the form of a 41-item questionnaire. The items cover the nuances of anxiety, such as separation anxiety, fear of attending school, social anxiety, and more. There is a standard answer pool for the whole questionnaire, so those answering it just need to tick which of the three options best applies to each item.
D. It can be accessed online at www.ohsu.edu/sites/default/files/2019-06/SCARED-form-Parent-and-Child-version.pdf.

Revised Child Anxiety and Depression Scale (and Subscales)
A. The Revised Child Anxiety and Depression Scale (RCADS) is a 47-item, youth self-report questionnaire with subscales including separation anxiety disorder, social phobia, generalized anxiety disorder, panic disorder, obsessive-compulsive disorder, and low mood. It also yields a total anxiety scale (sum of the five anxiety subscales) and a total internalizing scale.
B. The questionnaire takes between 5 and 10 minutes to administer. Both parent and child questionnaires can be given to the appropriate respondent to complete themselves.
C. The scale can be accessed online at www.corc.uk.net/outcome-experience-measures/revised-childrens-anxiety-and-depression-scale-rcads.

Spence Children's Anxiety Scale
A. The Spence Children's Anxiety Scale assesses six domains of anxiety including generalized anxiety, panic, social phobia, separation anxiety, obsessive-compulsive disorder, and physical injury fears.
B. The scale consists of 44 items, 38 of which reflect specific symptoms of anxiety and 6 of which are positive filler items that are intended to reduce negative response bias. Children are asked to rate on a 4-point scale the frequency with which they experience each symptom. The scale takes about 10 minutes to complete.
C. The scale can be accessed online at www.scaswebsite.com.

ASSESSMENT FOR ADULTS WITH COGNITIVE AND NEURODEGENERATIVE DISORDERS

Mental Status Examination
A. Mental status examination is a useful tool to assist physicians in differentiating between a variety of systemic conditions, as well as neurologic and psychiatric disorders ranging from delirium and dementia to bipolar disorder and schizophrenia.
B. The examination itself may comprise a few brief observations made during a general patient encounter or a more thorough evaluation by the physician. It may also include administration of relatively brief standardized tools such as the Mini-Mental State Examination (MMSE) and Mini-Cog.

Montreal Cognitive Assessment
A. The Montreal Cognitive Assessment (MoCA) is a test used to detect mild cognitive decline and early signs of dementia. It can help identify people at risk of Alzheimer disease and screen for conditions like Parkinson disease, brain tumors, substance abuse, and head trauma.
B. The MoCA test is based on scores, with a maximum score of 30. It takes 10 to 12 minutes to complete.
C. The MoCA test examines seven domains (aspects) of cognitive function with a total of 11 different exercises and tasks. Explicit instructions are found when accessing the MoCA test.
   1. Executive and visuospatial function
   2. Naming
   3. Attention
   4. Language
   5. Abstraction
   6. Delayed recall
   7. Orientation
D. The test can be accessed online at www.verywellhealth.com/alzheimers-and-montreal-cognitive-assessment-moca-98617.

ASSESSMENTS FOR ADULTS WITH SUBSTANCE USE DISORDERS

Tobacco, Alcohol, Prescription Medications, and Other Substances Tool
A. The Tobacco, Alcohol, Prescription Medications, and Other Substances (TAPS) Tool consists of a four-item screening for ▶

tobacco use, alcohol use, prescription medication misuse, and illicit substance use in the past year.
B. The instrument is used to assess primary care patients for tobacco, alcohol, prescription drug, and illicit substance use, and problems related to their use, and is available for self-administration and intervieweradministration to detect substance use, subthreshold substance use disorder (i.e., at-risk, harmful, or hazardous use), and substance use disorders.
C. The instrument is available for use in the public domain, and research for the development of the instrument was supported by the National Institute on Drug Abuse.
D. The instrument can be accessed online at https://cde.nida.nih.gov/instrument/29b23e2e-e266-f095-e050-bb89ad43472f.

Opioid Risk Tool-Opioid Use Disorder
A. The Opioid Risk Tool-Opioid Use Disorder (ORT-OUD) should be used to screen patients upon initial visit prior to beginning or continuing opioid therapy for pain management. The score will determine the risk for future opioid risk disorder.
B. The instrument can be given in either a self-report or interview format. The instrument takes about 3 to 5 minutes to complete and consists of 10 items.
C. The instrument can be accessed online at https://nida.nih.gov/nidamed-medical-health-professionals/screening-tools-resources/opioid-risk-tool-oud-ort-oud.

Drug Abuse Screening Test
A. The Drug Abuse Screening Test (DAST-10) provides a brief, self-report instrument for population screening, clinical case finding, and treatment evaluation research. It can be used with adults and older youth.
B. The instrument takes approximately 5 minutes to administer and may be given in either a self-report or interview format.
C. The instrument can be accessed online at https://cde.nida.nih.gov/instrument/e9053390-ee9c-9140-e040-bb89ad433d69.

ASSESSMENTS FOR ADOLESCENTS WITH POSSIBLE ALCOHOL, TOBACCO, AND OTHER SUBSTANCE MISUSE

Brief Screener for Alcohol, Tobacco, and Other Drugs
A. The Brief Screener for Alcohol, Tobacco, and Other Drugs (BSTAD) consists of questions on frequency of use to identify risky substance use by adolescent patients. The screening tool is meant to be used under clinician supervision and is not intended to guide self-assessment. The tool may be administered by either the patient or the clinician.
B. The tool can be accessed online at https://nida.nih.gov/bstad.

Screening to Brief Intervention
A. The Screening to Brief Intervention (S2BI) consists of questions on frequency of use to categorize substance use by adolescent patients into different risk categories. The screening tool is meant to be used under clinician supervision and is not intended to guide self-assessment.
B. The tool can be accessed online at https://nida.nih.gov/s2bi.

CRAFFT (Car, Relax, Alone, Forget, Friends, Trouble)
A. CRAFFT (Car, Relax, Alone, Forget, Friends, Trouble) is a short clinical assessment scale that screens adolescents for substance-related risks and problems.
B. CRAFFT has an internal consistency (Cronbach's alpha) of 0.85 and Spearman correlation coefficient test–retest reliability of 0.979 ($p < .001$; Ola & Atilola, 2017).

C. The scale may be administered by either the patient or the clinician. Variations include CRAFFT, CRAFFT 2.1, and CRAFFT 2.1+N (which includes the "Hooked on Nicotine Checklist–10 items").
D. These questionnaires can be used as a self-report survey or as part of the clinical interview.
E. CRAFFT 2.1 can be accessed online at https://njaap.org/wp-content/uploads/2018/03/COMBINED-CRAFFT-2.1-Self-Admin_Clinician-Interview_Risk-Assess-Guide.pdf.
F. CRAFFT 2.1+N can be accessed online at https://crafft.org/wp-content/uploads/2021/07/CRAFFT_2.1N-HONC_Clinician_2021-07-03.pdf.

ASSESSMENT FOR MOOD DISORDERS
A. There are several validated mood disorder scales available to the APRN to assess various mood-related conditions, including depression and mania. Screening tools allow for timely problem identification, intervention, treatment, and referral to a mental health specialist. These screening tests may also have the added benefits of preventing suicide associated with an untreated mental health disorder.
B. No special training is required for the APRN to complete these assessments. These scales target specific populations such as adults, children, pregnant patients, and older adults. These tools serve as valuable resources for clinicians and researchers in evaluating and monitoring mood disorders.
C. These scales, validated through rigorous research, aid in screening, diagnosing, monitoring, and tailoring treatments for individuals across different age groups dealing with mood disorders. This section provides a compilation of commonly utilized tools for diagnosing mood disorders.
D. Some questionnaires are freely available, while others the clinician or institution may purchase. Additionally, specific screening assessments can be completed by the patient, the informant, or guided by the clinician.

Depression Assessments for Adults
A. Patient Health Questionnaire-2 (free)
  1. The Patient Health Questionnaire-2 (PHQ-2) functions as a concise screening tool for depression and is applicable for self-administration or clinician-led assessment.
  2. It comprises merely two questions, and exhibits a sensitivity of 83% and a specificity of 92% for major depression when scores surpass 3.
  3. Test specifically inquires about two pivotal aspects of depressive disorders: a persistent sad mood and anhedonia experienced within the past 2 weeks, aligning with the diagnostic criteria for depression. However, a positive outcome on this test necessitates further evaluation using the Patient Health Questionnaire-9.
B. Patient Health Questionnaire-9 (free)
  1. The PHQ-9 is a versatile tool utilized for self-administration or guided by clinicians. It serves multiple purposes, encompassing screening, evaluation of disease severity, and monitoring therapeutic responses.
  2. Validation studies indicate that a PHQ-9 score ≥10 demonstrates a sensitivity of 88% and a specificity of 88% for major depression. This questionnaire includes the two screening questions found in PHQ-2, along with other *DSM-5-TR* (American Psychiatric Association, 2022) criteria necessary for diagnosing Major Depressive Disorder (MDD). Additionally, it assesses the potential for suicidal ideation.

3. The Severity Measure for Depression—Adult questionnaire modifies the PHQ-9 by focusing on symptoms experienced by the patient within the last 7 days, contrasting with the PHQ-9 and PHQ-2, which assess symptoms over the past 2 weeks.

C. Hamilton Depression Rating Scale (free)
1. The Hamilton Depression Rating Scale (HAMD) can be conducted during the first visit and periodically to monitor the effectiveness of treatment. It can be completed either through self-reporting or via an interview format. The assessment typically takes about 3 to 5 minutes to complete and comprises 17 categories.
2. The categories include symptoms mood, anxiety, insomnia, motor activity, weight loss, and more.
3. An in-depth analysis of 70 studies revealed that while the HAMD performs acceptably in generating a global score, it shows limitations when it comes to individual items.
4. The scale can be accessed online at www.mdcalc.com/calc/10043/hamilton-depression-rating-scale-ham-d.

D. Geriatric Depression Scale (free)
1. The Geriatric Depression Scale (GDS) is a research-supported measurement tool used to assess and monitor depressive symptoms in older adults, including those who are mildly cognitively impaired.
2. It consists of 15 yes-or-no questions that are worth 1 point each related to symptoms consistent of a depressive disorder. A score greater than 5 may suggest depression and should be followed up with a more comprehensive assessment, whereas a score greater than 10 indicates a diagnosis consistent with depression.
3. Validation studies indicate that the GDS demonstrates a sensitivity of 92% and a specificity of 89% for a diagnosis of depression.
4. The scale can be accessed online at https://hign.org/consultgeri/try-this-series/geriatric-depression-scale-gds.

E. Edinburgh Postnatal Depression (free)
1. The Edinburgh Postnatal Depression (EPDS) stands as a validated screening tool. Validation studies reveal that it exhibits a sensitivity of 81% and a specificity of 87% in diagnosing depression during pregnancy or in the postpartum phase.
2. Comprising 10 questions, a score exceeding 10 necessitates additional exploration for depression. It can be self-administered by individuals aged 18 or older. Alternatively, clinicians can guide its use in an interview format.
3. The tool can be accessed online at https://perinatology.com/calculators/Edinburgh%20Depression%20Scale.htm.

F. Beck Depression Inventory 2 (available for purchase)
1. The Beck Depression Inventory 2 (BDI-2) serves as a depression assessment tool designed to gauge the severity of depression, ranging from minimal to severe. It facilitates symptom tracking over time.
2. Comprising 21 questions, it assesses two subscales: the affective/cognitive, encompassing suicidal ideations, and the physiologic domains of depressive symptoms. Suitable for individuals 13 to 80 years of age, the screening tool is also available in Spanish. Patients can self-administer the questionnaire, or clinicians can guide its use during assessment.
3. It is a validated tool with a robust internal consistency, demonstrating a coefficient alpha of 92% for 500 outpatients and 93% for 500 college students.
4. The tool can be accessed online at www.pearsonassessments.com/store/usassessments/en/Store/Professional-Assessments/Personality-&-Biopsychosocial/Beck-Depression-Inventory/p/100000159.html?tab=overview.

G. Level 2—Depression—Adult (PROMIS Emotional Distress—Depression—Short Form; free)
1. This measurement tool is a 5-point Likert scale questionnaire comprising eight questions that assess a patient's depressive symptoms over the past 7 days. It functions both as an assessment tool for evaluating the severity of depression and for ongoing symptom monitoring. However, it has not been validated when completed by an informant.
2. The scale can be accessed online at www.psychiatry.org/psychiatrists/practice/dsm/educational-resources/assessment-measures.

Mania Assessments for Adults

A. Level 2—Mania—Adult (Altman Self-Rating Mania Scale)
1. The Altman Self-Rating Mania Scale (ASRM) is a five-question self-reporting tool for initial screening and ongoing monitoring of mania within the last 7 days.
2. The ASRM score spans from 5 to 25, where higher scores denote increased severity of manic symptoms.
3. The questionnaire can be completed by the patient, an informant, or facilitated by the clinician.
4. The questionnaire can be accessed online at www.psychiatry.org/psychiatrists/practice/dsm/educational-resources/assessment-measures.

B. Rapid Mood Screener (free)
1. The Rapid Mood Screener (RMS) questionnaire is a rapid assessment tool designed to differentiate between MDD and bipolar I disorder. It consists of six yes-or-no self-reporting items.
2. If four or more items of the RMS are affirmed ("yes"), it results in an 88% sensitivity and an 80% specificity; meanwhile, the positive and negative predictive values stood at 80% and 88%, respectively.
3. The questionnaire can be accessed online at www.nppsychnavigator.com/Clinical-Tools/Psychiatric-Scales/RMS-(Rapid-Mood-Screener)-Tool

Depression Assessments for Children

A. For Parents of Children Ages 6 to 17
1. Level 2—Depression—Parent/Guardian of Child Age 6 to 17 (PROMIS Emotional Distress—Depression—Parent Item Bank; free)
   a. This is an 11-question form designed to assess the level of depression in pediatric patients between 6 and 17 years of age.
   b. It focuses on symptoms experienced in the last 7 days. Parents or guardians are responsible for completing the form, rating their child's depression level over the past week based on each question.
   c. The form can be accessed online at www.psychiatry.org/psychiatrists/practice/dsm/educational-resources/assessment-measures.

B. For Children Ages 11 to 17
1. Level 2—Depression—Child Ages 11 to 17 (PROMIS Emotional Distress—Depression—Pediatric Item Bank; free)
   a. The assessment involves self-reporting by the child before meeting with the healthcare provider.

b. This is a 14-item assessment of depressive symptoms within the last week. The tool may be useful for initial determination of depression and for assessment of the degree of depression. The tool can be administered throughout treatment to monitor for therapeutic effectiveness.

c. The tool can be accessed online at www.psychiatry.org/psychiatrists/practice/dsm/educational-resources/assessment-measures.

2. Severity Measure for Depression—Child Ages 11 to 17 (adapted from PHQ-9, modified for Adolescents [PHQ-A]; free)

a. This adapted version of the validated PHQ-9 is tailored for use in adolescents. The questions focus on activities and social roles relevant to children impacted by depression. Similar to the PHQ-9, this questionnaire comprises nine questions aimed at evaluating the presence or severity of symptoms experienced within the past 7 days.

b. The questionnaire can be accessed online at www.psychiatry.org/psychiatrists/practice/dsm/educational-resources/assessment-measures.

Mania Assessments For Children

A. For Parents of Children Ages 6 to 17

1. Level 2—Mania—Parent/Guardian of Child Ages 6 to 17 (adapted from the ASRM; free)

a. The tool assists in identifying mania by utilizing a five-item scale that parents or guardians can use to assess the presence and intensity of manic symptoms in their child.

b. The five specific items evaluated encompass mood, speech, sleep, activity, and confidence, all of which are dysregulated in mania. A score surpassing 6 may suggest hypomania or mania, necessitating treatment or further investigation.

c. This questionnaire evaluates symptoms experienced by the child within the previous 7 days. The parents can complete the form before meeting with the healthcare provider.

d. The questionnaire can be accessed online at www.psychiatry.org/psychiatrists/practice/dsm/educational-resources/assessment-measures.

B. For Children Ages 11 to 17

1. Level 2—Mania—Child Ages 11 to 17 (ASRM; free)

a. This is a self-reporting assessment that targets mania symptoms in children 11 to 17 years of age. The five-item questionnaire assessing manic symptoms can be completed before the clinician appointment.

b. It serves as a valuable tool to identify or gauge the extent of mania experienced within the past 7 days.

c. The tool can be accessed online at www.psychiatry.org/psychiatrists/practice/dsm/educational-resources/assessment-measures.

ASSESSMENT FOR ATTENTION DEFICIT HYPERACTIVITY DISORDER

A. Several validated scales are accessible to APRNs to assess ADHD. These screening tools not only identify ADHD symptoms but also have the potential to improve social, occupational, and academic performance.

B. Tailored to children, parents, adults, and teachers, these tools have undergone rigorous validation through research, aiding in screening, diagnosis, and ongoing monitoring.

C. This compilation includes commonly utilized ADHD diagnostic tools, with some questionnaires available for free and others requiring purchase.

D. Patients, informants (e.g., parents or teachers), or clinicians can complete specific screening assessments. For simplicity, this section is divided into tools used for children and adults.

Pediatric Assessments

A. Vanderbilt ADHD Rating Scales (free)

1. The Vanderbilt ADHD Rating Scales (VADPRS) is a 45-question screening tool completed by the parent on behalf of the child to provide insight into their child's social functioning and school performance.

2. The Vanderbilt ADHD Diagnostic Teacher Rating Scale (VADTRS) is a 43-question tool focused on school performance and ADHD symptoms.

3. Both scales utilize 4- and 5-point rating systems, where higher scores typically indicate more severe symptoms, except for the performance section, where elevated scores denote better classroom behavior and academic achievement. The scales are available in English and Spanish.

4. The scales can be accessed online at https://chadd.org/for-professionals/clinical-practice-tools-quick-links.

B. Measure: Level 2—Inattention—Parent/Guardian of Child Ages 6 to 17 (free)

1. The Level 2—Inattention—Parent/Guardian of Child Ages 6 to 17 measure (or the Swanson, Nolan, and Pelham Teacher and Parent Rating Scale, Version IV [SNAP-IV]) helps understand if a child has trouble paying attention. A parent or guardian fills it out before visiting the clinician. They rate how much the child seems distracted or unfocused during the past week using numbers from 0 to 3 (0 means "not at all" and 3 means "very much"). When all the ratings are added up, the total can be from 0 to 24. A higher total suggests more difficulties with paying attention.

2. The measure is also helpful in keeping track of how these symptoms change over time.

3. The measure can be accessed online at www.psychiatry.org/psychiatrists/practice/dsm/educational-resources/assessment-measures.

Adults Assessments

A. Adult ADHD Self-Report Scale Symptom Checklist (free)

1. The Adult ADHD Self-Report Scale (ASRS-v1.1) is a short questionnaire used to screen for adult ADHD symptoms. Scoring 4 or higher out of 6 indicates possible ADHD consistency. The screener demonstrates decent sensitivity (68.7%), outstanding specificity (99.5%), and a solid κ value (0.76) at the threshold of four or more out of six positive criteria.

2. The scale can be accessed online at https://chadd.org/for-professionals/clinical-practice-tools.

B. Conners' Adult ADHD Rating Scales (available for purchase)

1. The Conners' Adult ADHD Rating Scales (CAARS™) is used to find out if adults aged 18 and older have ADHD and how severe it might be. These scales come in different versions—long, short, and screening—that help measure the presence and seriousness of ADHD symptoms. They are self-reporting questionnaires.

2. The scales can be accessed online at https://storefront.mhs.com/collections/caars

C. Brown Attention-Deficit Disorder Scales for Children and Adults (available for purchase)

  1. The Brown Attention-Deficit Disorder Scales (BADDS) are used to assess attention deficit disorder across different ages. The scales are clinically validated and comes in versions for preschoolers, school-age children, teenagers, and adults.

  2. The scale can be accessed online at www.pearsonassessments.com/store/usassessments/en/Store/Professional-Assessments/Behavior/Attention-ADHD/Brown-Attention-Deficit-Disorder-Scales/p/100000456.html.

REFERENCES AND BIBLIOGRAPHY

American Academy of Pediatrics. (n.d.). *ADHD: Caring for children with ADHD—A practical resource toolkit for clinicians* (3rd ed.). https://www.aap.org/ADHD-Caring-for-Children-With-ADHD-A-Practical-Resource-Toolkit-for-Clinicians-3rd-Edition

American Psychiatric Association. (2013). *Diagnostic and statistical manual of mental disorders* (5th ed.). https://doi.org/10.1176/appi.books.9780890425596

American Psychiatric Association. (2022). *Diagnostic and statistical manual of mental disorders* (5th ed., text rev.). https://doi.org/10.1176/appi.books.9780890425787

American Psychiatric Association. (2023). *DSM-5-TR online assessment measures.* https://www.psychiatry.org/psychiatrists/practice/dsm/educational-resources/assessment-measures

Chand, S. P., Arif, H., & Kutlenios, R. M. (2023, July 17). *Depression (Nursing)*. StatPearls Publishing. https://www.ncbi.nlm.nih.gov/books/NBK568733

Kroenke, K., Spitzer, R. L., & Williams, J. B. (2001). The PHQ-9: Validity of a brief depression severity measure. *Journal of General Internal Medicine, 16*(9), 606–613. https://doi.org/10.1046/j.1525-1497.2001.016009606.x

Kroenke, K., Spitzer, R. L., & Williams, J. B. (2003). The Patient Health Questionnaire-2: Validity of a two-item depression screener. *Medical Care, 41*(11), 1284–1292. https://doi.org/10.1097/01.MLR.0000093487.78664.3C

McIntyre, R. S., Patel, M. D., Masand, P. S., Harrington, A., Gillard, P., McElroy, S. L., Sullivan, K., Montano, C. B., Brown, T. M., Nelson, L., & Jain, R. (2021). The Rapid Mood Screener (RMS): A novel and pragmatic screener for bipolar I disorder. *Current Medical Research and Opinion, 37*(1), 135–144. https://doi.org/10.1080/03007995.2020.1860358

MDCalc. (n.d.). *Hamilton Depression Rating Scale (HAM-D)*. https://www.mdcalc.com/calc/10043/hamilton-depression-rating-scale-ham-d

National HIV Curriculum. (2023). *Patient Health Questionnaire-2 (PHQ-2)*. https://www.hiv.uw.edu/page/mental-health-screening/phq-2#:~:text=Interpretation%3A,major%20depressive%20disorder%20is%20likely

Norris, D., Clark, M. S., & Shipley, S. (2016). The mental status examination. *American Family Physician, 94*(8), 635–641. PMID: 27929229.

Ola, B., & Atilola, A. (2017). Validation of CRAFFT for use in youth correctional institutions in *Lagos*, Nigeria. *Journal of the American Academy of Psychiatry and the Law Online, 45*(4), 439–446. PMID: 29282234.

Osorio, F. L., Loureiro, S. R., Hallak, J. E. C., Machado-de-Sousa, J. P., Ushirohira, J. M., Baes, C. V. W., Apolinario, T. D., Donadon, M. F., Bolsoni, L. M., Guimarães, T., Fracon, V. S., Silva-Rodrigues, A. P. C., Pizeta, F. A., Souza, R. M., Sanches, R. F., dos Santos, R. G., Martin-Santos, R., & Crippa, J. A. S. (2019). Clinical validity and intrarater and test-retest reliability of the structured Clinical Interview for *DSM-5*—Clinician Version (SCID-5-CV). *Psychiatry and Clinical Neurosciences, 73*(12), 754–760. https://doi.org/10.1111/pcn.12931

Park, S. H., & Kim, J. I. (2023). Predictive validity of the Edinburgh postnatal depression scale and other tools for screening depression in pregnant and postpartum women: A systematic review and meta-analysis. *Archives of Gynecology and Obstetrics, 307*(5), 1331–1345. https://doi.org/10.1007/s00404-022-06525-0

Sharp, R. (2015). The Hamilton rating scale for depression. *Occupational Medicine, 65*(4), 340. https://doi.org/10.1093/occmed/kqv043

Zanello, A., Berthoud, L., Ventura, J., & Merlo, M. C. (2013). The Brief Psychiatric Rating Scale (version 4.0) factorial structure and its sensitivity in the treatment of outpatients with unipolar depression. *Psychiatry Research, 210*(2), 626–633. https://doi.org/10.1016/j.psychres.2013.07.001

8 PSYCHOTHERAPY

Sara Jones and Sattaria "Tari" Dilks

THE NURSE PSYCHOTHERAPIST: HISTORY

The American Psychiatric Association (APA) defines *psychotherapy* as a collaborative treatment between the healthcare provider and the patient that helps with a wide array of psychiatric illnesses and emotional difficulties with the aim of eliminating or controlling troubling symptoms, ultimately supporting the patient to function better in life. Psychotherapy increases emotional well-being and can allow for healing to occur. Problems that may be addressed by psychotherapy include coping with daily life; the psychological impact of trauma; or other life stressors including troubling thoughts, behaviors, and emotions. Psychotherapy is provided by a trained therapist and often includes medication management.

Psychotherapy is intimate work. Psychotherapy can produce positive results when provided safely, but can also cause the patient harm when not properly implemented. The trained psychotherapist is an expert who works collaboratively with the patient. It is the responsibility of the APRN who provides psychotherapy to acquire the proper supervised training in order to achieve and maintain clinical expertise throughout their professional life. Most psychotherapists agree that it takes at least 10 years to become a skilled practitioner. Modern nursing, as established by Florence Nightingale, ensures that patients have the care and compassion needed to achieve health with a focus that includes environmental conditions. Hildegard Peplau (1952) wrote the seminal book on interpersonal relations in nursing, providing a conceptual frame of reference on psychodynamic nursing. Her theory emphasized relational conditions as they apply to patient care. She heavily relied on the work of Harry Stack Sullivan, an American Neo-Freudian psychiatrist known for his interpersonal theory of mental illness. Peplau, the mother of modern psychiatric nursing, espoused the transformative power of relationships in nursing care.

Peplau established a program at Rutgers University in 1954, offering the first master's degree for clinical nurse specialists. This program concentrated on advanced practice psychiatric nursing, leading to the development of the first nurse psychotherapists. Rutgers' master's program emphasized the development of expert theoretical and practical knowledge, leading to improvement in patient outcomes. Graduates of this program focused on psychotherapy and milieu management, which combined the environmental focus of Nightingale and the relational connections of Peplau. Peplau additionally placed emphasis on the nurse knowing themselves as well as they did the patient.

Various disciplines are licensed to provide psychotherapy services, including psychiatrists, social workers, psychologists, licensed professional counselors, marriage and family counselors, and APRNs. What makes psychiatric APRNs different in their approach to psychotherapy? They integrate nursing theories with those of other disciplines like counseling, psychology, social work, or educational counseling. Nursing is, at its core, an interpersonal process that embraces the focus on disease and treatment while simultaneously integrating the experiences of the individual and families around the illnesses. Nursing is a collaborative, mutual, and interpersonal process. With the provision of psychotherapy, nursing values and expertise are combined to bring complex treatment for patients to a different level. APRNs bring a person-centered approach and understanding of the underlying factors (e.g., medical, psychological, cultural) that influence the patient's presentation.

REFERENCES AND BIBLIOGRAPHY

American Psychiatric Association. (2023, April). *What is psychotherapy?* https://www.psychiatry.org/patients-families/psychotherapy

D'Antonio, P., Beeber, L., Sills, G., & Naegle, M. (2014). The future in the past: Hildegard Peplau and interpersonal relations in nursing. *Nursing Inquiry, 21*(4), 311–317. https://doi.org/10.1111/nin.12056

Hurley, J., Lakeman, R., Cashin, A., & Ryan, T. (2020). The remarkable (Disappearing Act of the) mental health nurse psychotherapist. *International Journal of Mental Health Nursing, 29*(4), 652–660. https://doi.org/10.1111/inm.12698

Karimi, H., & Masoudi Alavi, N. (2015). Florence nightingale: The mother of nursing. *Nursing and Midwifery Studies, 4*(2), e29475. PMID: 26339672.

Peplau, H. E. (1952). *Interpersonal relations in nursing: A conceptual frame of reference for psychodynamic nursing.* G. P. Putnam's Sons.

Schimmels, J. Bajjani-Gebara, J., Owen, R., Lewis, T., & Wallace, E. (2015). The service theories and healing leadership of Florence Nightingale and Hildegard Peplau: Their central importance for military psychiatric nurse practitioner education. *Journal of Health and Human Experience, 7*(1), 40–58. https://jhhe.sempervifoundation.org/pdfs/v7n1/03_Schimmels.pdf

Wheeler, K. (2022). Supportive and psychodynamic psychotherapy. In K. Wheeler (Ed.), *Psychotherapy for the advanced practice psychiatric nurse: A how-to-guide for evidence-based practice* (3rd ed., pp. 249–288). Springer Publishing Company.

NURSES AS PSYCHOTHERAPISTS: EDUCATION AND TRAINING

A. The education and training for psychiatric-mental health nurse practitioners (PMHNPs) requires a minimum of two modalities of psychotherapy.
   1. Advanced practice builds on the education and experiences of baccalaureate-prepared registered nurses (RNs) to advanced knowledge of psychiatric neurobiology, neurochemistry, disease processes, and psychopharmacology.
   2. The typical PMHNP academic curriculum provides an introduction to psychotherapy; however, due to academic requirements and time constraints, proficiency in any one psychotherapeutic approach (which includes supervision) is usually not included in training.
   3. Competency through experiential and didactic exposure must be demonstrated in at least two areas.

B. PMHNPs are strongly encouraged to pursue postgraduate training and supervision in specific modalities of psychotherapy to deepen their knowledge base.

C. Supervision is critical for all nurse psychotherapists, especially while developing proficiency in the desired approach.
   1. This helps them develop and maintain clear boundaries while being empathetic but not taking on the patient's issues themselves.

2. Therapy certifications are available for PMHNPs and most require some form of supervision.

D. There is no "one-size-fits-all" approach to psychotherapy, and PMHNPs are encouraged to seek education to understand skills in various modalities.

REFERENCES AND BIBLIOGRAPHY

American Nurses Credentialing Center. (2023). *Psychiatric-mental health nurse practitioner (across the lifespan) certification (PMHNP-BC™)*. https://www.nursingworld.org/our-certifications/psychiatric-mental-health-nurse-practitioner/

Wheeler, K. (2022). Supportive and psychodynamic psychotherapy. In K. Wheeler (Ed.), *Psychotherapy for the advanced practice psychiatric nurse: A how-to guide for evidence-based practice* (3rd. ed., pp. 249–288). Springer Publishing Company.

SCOPE AND STANDARDS OF PRACTICE

A. The Scope and Standards of Practice for psychiatric-mental health nursing are outlined by the American Nurses Association (ANA), the American Psychiatric Nurses Association (APNA), and the International Society of Psychiatric-Mental Health Nurses (ISPN) to "describe the competent level of nursing practice demonstrated by the critical thinking model known as the nursing process… [which] forms the foundation of the nurses' decision-making" and "should be reviewed in conjunction with the state board of nursing regulations" (ANA et al., 2022).

1. Psychotherapeutic interventions are addressed in Standard 5: Implementation and are addressed in Standard 5H: Counseling and Psychotherapy.

B. The Scope and Standards of Practice describes the importance of establishing and maintaining the therapeutic relationship to guide all aspects of nursing care.

1. This includes using patient- and family-centered, culturally competent care to engage patients and families in the context of the nurse–patient relationship.
2. While this is emphasized by the nursing model for all specialties, the care provided by psychiatric-mental health nurses is founded on the principles of psychotherapy to help improve patients' mental health and recovery.

a. Psychiatric-mental health registered nurses (PMHRNs) are tasked with using counseling to assist patients toward recovery. It is through the development of the therapeutic alliance that PMHRNs can build trust, rapport, and actively engage and empower patients in their recovery. Interventions conducted by the PMHRN include suggesting and reinforcing healthy strategies to achieve recovery. They promote awareness of personal reactions to internal and external factors, particularly how they guide unhealthy behaviors. RNs will use the therapeutic relationship to intervene in times of crisis and assist in managing stress, build interpersonal skills, resolve conflict, and develop relaxation skills. Throughout, the PMHRN must be aware of their own emotional and behavioral responses that may impact the therapeutic relationship.

b. PMHNPs utilize their comprehensive knowledge of biopsychosocial development and well-being to select and guide the use of psychotherapy based on patients' needs. Through their graduate education, PMHNPs gain a foundational knowledge of various psychotherapeutic modalities. With this advanced theoretical understanding, they can select, implement, and prescribe therapy most appropriate for patients, their experiences, symptomologies, and needs based on research and evidence-based practice guidelines. They use evidence and clinical judgment to guide referrals to psychotherapists based on their own capabilities to conduct appropriate therapy modalities to best serve the patient. With additional training and certification, PMHNPs can also conduct psychotherapy for various diagnoses and trauma.

REFERENCE AND BIBLIOGRAPHY

American Nurses Association, American Psychiatric Nurses Association, & International Society of Psychiatric-Mental Health Nurses. (2022). *Psychiatric-mental health nursing: Scope and standards of practice*. (3rd ed.). American Nurses Association.

TYPES OF PSYCHOTHERAPY

COGNITIVE BEHAVIORAL THERAPY

A. The founder of cognitive behavioral therapy (CBT) was Aaron Beck, MD, who was originally trained in Freudian psychoanalysis. During the 1960s to 1970s, Beck developed CBT on the premise that all individuals' emotional, behavioral, and psychological reactions are influenced by their personal interpretations of their experiences.

B. In the early years, Dr. Beck's practices demonstrated that patients with depression often presented with the same cognitive distortions. These distortions included misrepresented and inaccurate conclusion of their experiences and created dysfunctional patterns of thoughts, feelings, and behaviors.

C. Beck identified that, by modifying patients' interpretations of their experiences, even slightly, he could improve emotional responses. This aided in the development of a systematic approach to conceptualize how cognitions impact emotional responses.

D. Into the 1970s, Beck incorporated principles of behavioral theories, which integrated the relationship between cognitions and behaviors. Ultimately, this led to what we now know as CBT, which emphasizes how experiences guide cognitions, which ultimately guide emotional and behavioral responses.

E. The following are the constructs of CBT:

1. CBT posits that an individual's previous experiences guide how they interpret every situation, whether that interpretation is accurate or distorted. All individuals maintain memories of situations that serve as the foundation of their core beliefs and automatic thoughts.
2. CBT is used to help patients understand themselves in the context of their experiences, starting with how they view themselves and the world, followed by how they interpret their experiences based on these views.
3. CBT is a time-limited process that relies on a strong therapeutic alliance to facilitate collaboration and problem-solving.

F. A brief overview of this process consists of the following:

1. The psychotherapist assists patients in identifying cognitive distortions and cognitive processes that have resulted from past experiences. Focus is on the interplay between those cognitions and the associated emotions.
2. Therapy then targets correcting these distortions to sustainably change affective responses, followed by behavioral responses, with the goal of modifying symptomologies that are negatively impacting their lives.
3. When able to identify and rectify distorted thinking, patients can better understand their feelings and modify their behaviors to be more adaptive and assist with coping.

IMPORTANT TERMS AND ASSUMPTIONS

A. Essential components of CBT include core beliefs, also known as *schemas*, automatic thoughts, and cognitive distortions. CBT incorporates guided discovery, cognitive restructuring, psychoeducation, and homework.

1. Core beliefs, or *schemas*: These are deeply held beliefs, typically learned in early childhood, about oneself, others, and the world. When there are negative views of self, the world, and the future, this composition is referred to as *the cognitive triad of negative core beliefs*.
2. Automatic thoughts: These are involuntary perceptions of reality that occur habitually and are typically negative and can be difficult to recognize. The thought may be transient but can cause a lasting emotion.
3. Cognitive distortions: These are also referred to as *dysfunctional assumptions*; these are irrational thought patterns that are exaggerated by negative thinking and feelings.
4. Guided discovery, or *Socratic dialogue*: This is a type of collaboration in which the therapist works with the patient by leading them through a process of inquiry and dialogue. This method aims to uncover and explore the patient's spontaneous thoughts and beliefs, scrutinizing their validity and the reasoning and evidence supporting them. This process aims to guide patients in finding their own conclusions after exploring their own automatic thoughts and patterns of behavior.
5. Cognitive restructuring: Cognitive restructuring involves identifying negative schemas and automatic thoughts and then altering them so they are adaptive and reasonable.
6. Psychoeducation: Psychoeducation includes providing patients and families with knowledge about mental health, mental illness, and treatment so that they can work together for improved outcomes, integrated throughout the therapeutic process.
7. Homework: Patients are given assignments to practice and/or complete outside of the therapeutic session to further explore and address what was done during therapy. This may include journaling, deep-breathing exercises, role-play applicable to certain social situations, or abstention from certain activities.

APPLICATION AND EVIDENCE

A. Throughout the years, evidence has supported the use of CBT techniques to address various disease states, even to the point of being identified as the first-line treatment for multiple diagnoses.
B. The American Psychological Association evidence-based practice guidelines recommends CBT as one of the first-line treatments for major depressive disorders across the life span.
C. Evidence also supports its use in treating anxiety disorders, posttraumatic stress disorder (PTSD), and obsessive-compulsive disorders.
D. There is significant evidence for its effectiveness in treating substance use disorders, eating disorders, and somatoform disorders.
E. CBT has shown to significantly decrease suicidality and nonsuicidal self-injurious behaviors.
F. Research has supported the adaptation of CBT for different diagnoses.

1. Trauma-focused CBT (TF-CBT): TF-CBT was developed and tested to show the effectiveness of treating PTSD and other trauma-related disorders.
2. CBT-insomnia (CBT-I): CBT-I is shown to be an effective therapy for assisting patients with sleep disorders.

G. Various medical disorders have been effectively treated with CBT:

1. Tinnitus
2. Sexual dysfunction
3. Chronic fatigue syndrome
4. Some studies even support use for treatment of cardiovascular diseases, such as myocardial infarction

TRAINING AND CERTIFICATION

A. There are multiple certification courses in CBT that range in length of time for didactic and experiential case supervision.
B. The Beck Institute for Cognitive Behavior Therapy has a few levels of certification: certified clinician, certified master clinician, and certified supervisor (https://beckinstitute.org/certification).

REFERENCES AND BIBLIOGRAPHY

Agras, W. S. (2019). Cognitive behavior therapy for the eating disorders. *Psychiatric Clinics of North America, 42*(2), 169–179. https://doi.org/10.1016/j.psc.2019.01.001

An, H., He, R. H., Zheng, Y. R., & Tao, R. (2017). Cognitive-behavioral therapy. In X. Zhang, J. Shi, & R. Tao (Eds.), *Substance and non-substance addiction* (pp. 321–329). Advances in Experimental Medicine and Biology, Vol. 1010. Springer, Singapore. https://doi.org/10.1007/978-981-10-5562-1_16

American Psychological Association. (2019, February). Clinical practice guidelines for the treatment of depression across three age cohorts. https://www.apa.org/depression-guideline

Beck, J. S., & Fleming, S. (2021). A brief history of Aaaron T. Beck, MD, and cognitive behavior therapy. *Clinical Psychology in Europe, 3*(2), e6701. https://doi.org10.32872/cpe.6701

Clevenger, S. M. F. (2022). Cognitive behavior therapy. In K. Wheeler (Ed.), *Psychotherapy for the advanced practice registered nurse: A how-to guide for evidence-based practice* (3rd ed., pp. 359–400). Springer Publishing Company.

Cohen, J. A., & Mannarino, A. P. (2015). Trauma-focused cognitive behavior therapy for traumatized children and families. *Child and Adolescent Psychiatric Clinics of North America, 24*(3), 557–570. https://doi.org/10.1016/j.chc.2015.02.005

D'Anci, K. E., Uhl, S., Giradi, G., & Martin, C. (2019). Treatments for the prevention and management of suicide: A systematic review. *Annals of Internal Medicine, 171*(5), 334–342. https://doi.org/10.7326/m19-0869

Erfanifar, E., Behroozi, N., Latifi, S. M., & Abbaspoor, Z. (2022). The effectiveness of cognitive-behavioural consultation on sexual function and sexual self-efficacy of women after childbirth. *European Journal of Obstetrics & Gynecology and Reproductive Biology: X, 15*, 100157. https://doi.org/10.1016/j.eurox.2022.100157

Fernie, B. A., Murphy, G., Wells, A., Nikčević, A. V., & Spada, M. M. (2016). Treatment outcome and metacognitive change in CBT and GET for chronic fatigue syndrome. *Behavioural and Cognitive Psychotherapy, 44*(4), 397–409. https://doi.org/10.1017/s135246581500017x

Fuller, T., Cima, R., Langguth, B., Mazurek, B., Vlaeyen, J. W., & Hoare, D. J. (2020). Cognitive behavioural therapy for tinnitus. *Cochrane Database of Systematic Reviews, 1*. Article CD012614. https://doi.org/10.1002/14651858.CD012614.pub2

Hofmann, S. G., Asnaani, A., Vonk, I. J., Sawyer, A. T., & Fang, A. (2012). The efficacy of cognitive behavioral therapy: A review of meta-analyses. *Cognitive Therapy and Research, 36*(5), 427–440. https://doi.org/10.1007/s10608-012-9476-1

Katzman, M. A., Bleau, P., Blier, P., Chokka, P., Kjernisted, K., Van Ameringen, M., & Canadian Anxiety Guidelines Initiative Group on behalf of the Anxiety Disorders Association of Canada/Association Canadienne des troubles anxieux and McGill University. (2014). Canadian clinical practice guidelines for the management of anxiety, posttraumatic stress and obsessive-compulsive disorders. *BMC Psychiatry, 14* (Suppl. 1), S1. https://doi.org/10.1186/1471-244x-14-s1-s1

Leahy, R. L. (2008). The therapeutic relationship in cognitive-behavioral therapy. *Behavioural and Cognitive Psychotherapy, 36*(6), 769–777. https://doi.org/10.1017/S1352465808004852

Magán, I., Jurado-Barba, R., Casado, L., Barnum, H., Jeon, A., Hernandez, A. V., & Bueno, H. (2022). Efficacy of psychological interventions on clinical outcomes of coronary artery disease: Systematic review and meta-analysis. *Journal of Psychosomatic Research*, 153, 110710. https://doi.org/10.1016/j.jpsychores.2021.110710

Redeker, N. S., Yaggi, H. K., Jacoby, D., Hollenbeak, C. S., Breazeale, S., Conley, S., Hwang, Y., Iennaco, J., Linsky, S., Nwanaji-Enwerem, U., O'Connell, M., & Jeon, S. (2022). Cognitive behavioral therapy for insomnia has sustained effects on insomnia, fatigue, and function among people with chronic heart failure and insomnia: The HeartSleep Study, zsab252. *Sleep*, 45(1). https://doi.org/10.1093/sleep/zsab252

Thoma, N., Pilecki, B., & McKay, D. (2015). Contemporary cognitive behavior therapy: A review of theory, history, and evidence. *Psychodynamic Psychiatry*, 43(3), 423–461. https://doi.org/10.1521/pdps.2015.43.3.423

Trauer, J. M., Qian, M. Y., Doyle, J. S., Rajaratnam, S. M., & Cunnington, D. (2015). Cognitive behavioral therapy for chronic insomnia: A systematic review and meta-analysis. *Annals of Internal Medicine*, 163(3), 191–204. https://doi.org/10.7326/m14-2841

DIALECTICAL BEHAVIOR THERAPY

A. Dialectical behavioral therapy (DBT) originated when American psychologist Marsha Linehan identified the need for a cognitive behavioral approach to treat individuals who experienced intense emotions and chronic suicidal thoughts. With these more complex presentations, Dr. Linehan identified the importance of acceptance, both conveyed by the psychotherapist and felt by the patients themselves. Still, even with acceptance, there is clear need for change. Hence, she incorporated dialectical philosophy into behavioral therapy, which posits that polarity can coexist.
  1. It becomes the role of the psychotherapist to continually convey acceptance, all while promoting and facilitating strategies to change, even if change is feared.
  2. DBT guides patients in viewing their situations by applying terms and techniques like those in CBT. They are encouraged to analyze their thoughts, feelings, and behaviors, all without judgment. Through this self-assessment and awareness, the therapist assists them in building on their own capabilities to develop skills to improve quality of life.

B. DBT treatment consists of four essential components. Evidence supports the effectiveness of DBT when adhering to the following protocol. Although clinical resources may not always be available, adapting the treatment planning should align with theoretical underpinnings and evidence-based practice.
  1. Weekly individual therapy: Sessions (typically 1 hour) are intended to motivate and assist patients in applying strategies to address specific challenges in their lives. While the patient tries to apply these strategies, the therapist only intervenes when necessary.
  2. Weekly group skills training: Sessions (typically 2.5 hours) focus on developing four skills: mindfulness, distress tolerance, interpersonal effectiveness, and emotion regulation. Homework is often assigned to further assist with skill development outside of the group.
  3. Skills coaching outside of sessions: Unique to DBT, this is typically by phone or electronic messaging. Patients are encouraged to contact their therapists in between sessions when they are in difficult situations. This allows the therapist to coach them to use their learned skills in real-life scenarios.
  4. Team consultations for therapists: Because DBT can be taxing for therapists, this time is used for support and to monitor adherence to treatment planning, increase therapeutic skills, and sustain their motivation to work with this population.

IMPORTANT TERMS AND ASSUMPTIONS

A. The four primary skills taught in DBT, primarily in groups sessions, are defined in the following:
  1. Mindfulness: Patients are taught techniques to practice being fully present and aware in the moment, including breathing exercises, observing self, and ridding of judgment.
  2. Distress tolerance: Based on the concept of acceptance, patients develop strategies to tolerate pain in difficult situations instead of changing it.
  3. Interpersonal effectiveness: Patients learn how to listen to others, ask for what they want, and say *no* when needed, all with self-respect and to maintain healthy relationships.
  4. Emotion regulation: Since emotions can feel intense for patients in DBT, they are taught how to correctly identify their feelings, combat vulnerabilities, and problem-solve.

B. DBT also has critical assumptions. Therapists explain and reiterate these assumptions throughout the therapy process, while also monitoring their own acceptance and application of these concepts.
  1. Patients' lives are unbearable as they are currently living. The therapist must validate this and emphasize that the only solution is to make changes.
  2. Patients are doing the best they can and want to improve. Still, they need to try hard and be motivated to change.
  3. Patients must solve their problems, even if they did not cause them.
  4. Within all contexts, patients need to learn new behaviors.
  5. Patients cannot fail therapy, nor can the therapist. Even if therapy has stalled or stopped, the therapist explores the patient's commitment to treatment and revises the treatment plan to improve engagement.

APPLICATION AND EVIDENCE

A. When initially developing DBT, Dr. Linehan was treating women diagnosed with borderline personality disorder (BPD) and experiencing reoccurring suicidal thoughts. She found that traditional CBT left many of these patients feeling criticized and invalidated, resulting in them dropping out of treatment. While applying constructs that seemed to be dichotomous—full acceptance and the need for change—her research showed better engagement in therapy and improved outcomes.

B. Many consider DBT as the gold standard therapy for individuals diagnosed with BPD.

C. Randomized controlled trials also show its effectiveness in treating parasuicidality, which includes suicide attempts and nonsuicidal self-injury.

D. Compared with treatment as usual, studies find that DBT significantly reduces the number of suicide attempts, self-injury, hospitalizations, and aggressive behaviors.

E. Significant evidence supports the effectiveness of DBT in treating symptoms of depressive disorders, other mood spectrum symptoms (including self-injury), substance use disorders and dependence, and binge eating disorder.

F. For individuals who have experienced significant trauma, such as sexual assault survivors, there is strong evidence on the use of DBT treatment alone or concurrently with trauma-focused therapies, such as eye movement desensitization and reprocessing therapy (EMDR).

G. New protocols have even been developed to treat individuals who have experienced childhood sexual assault and diagnosed with PTSD, called *DBT-PTSD*.

TRAINING AND CERTIFICATION

A. Certification in DBT takes about 6 months to complete. There are four modules: mindfulness, distress tolerance, emotion regulation, and interpersonal effectiveness.
B. There are multiple certification courses and counseling programs that offer classes in DBT certification.
C. The DBT-Linehan Board of Certification identifies healthcare providers and programs as well as certification courses (https://dbt-lbc.org).

REFERENCES AND BIBLIOGRAPHY

Cavicchioli, M., Movalli, M., Vassena, G., Ramella, P., Prudenziati, F., & Maffei, C. (2019). The therapeutic role of emotion regulation and coping strategies during a stand-alone DBT Skills training program for alcohol use disorder and concurrent substance use disorders. *Addictive Behaviors, 98*, 106035. https://doi.org/10.1016/j.addbeh.2019.106035

Chapman, A. L. (2006). Dialectical behavior therapy: Current indications and unique elements. *Psychiatry (Edgmont), 3*(9), 62–68. PMID: 20975829.

Comtois, K. A. (2002). A review of interventions to reduce the prevalence of parasuicide. *Psychiatric Services, 53*(9), 1138–1144. https://doi.org/10.1176/appi.ps.53.9.1138

Görg, N., Priebe, K., Böhnke, J. R., Steil, R., Dyer, A. S., & Kleindienst, N. (2017). Trauma-related emotions and radical acceptance in dialectical behavior therapy for posttraumatic stress disorder after childhood sexual abuse. *Borderline Personality Disorder and Emotion Dysregulation, 4*, Article 15. https://doi.org/10.1186/s40479-017-0065-5

Limandri, B. (2022). Dialectical behavior therapy for complex trauma. In K. Wheeler (Ed.), *Psychotherapy for the advanced practice psychiatric nurse: A how-to guide for evidence-based practice* (3rd ed., pp. 689–709). Springer Publishing Company.

Linehan, M. M., & Wilks, C. R. (2015). The course and evolution of dialectical behavior therapy. *The American Journal of Psychotherapy, 69*(2), 97–110. https://doi.org/10.1176/appi.psychotherapy.2015.69.2.97

May, J. M., Richardi, T. M., & Barth, K. S. (2016). Dialectical behavior therapy as treatment for borderline personality disorder. *Mental Health Clinician, 6*(2), 62–67. https://doi.org/10.9740/mhc.2016.03.62

O'Connell, B., & Dowling, M. (2014). Dialectical Behaviour Therapy (DBT) in the treatment of borderline personality disorder. *Journal of Psychiatric and Mental Health Nursing, 21*(6), 518–525. https://doi.org/10.1111/jpm.12116

Snoek, A., Beekman, A. T. F., Dekker, J., Aarts, I., van Grootheest, G., Blankers, M., Vriend, C., van den Heuvel, O., & Thomaes, K. (2020). A randomized controlled trial comparing the clinical efficacy and cost-effectiveness of Eye Movement Desensitization and Reprocessing (EMDR) and integrated EMDR-Dialectical Behavioural Therapy (DBT) in the treatment of patients with post-traumatic stress disorder and comorbid (Sub)clinical borderline personality disorder: Study design. *BMC Psychiatry, 20*, Article 396. https://doi.org/10.1186/s12888-020-02713-x

INTERPERSONAL THERAPY

A. In the late 20th century, Dr. Myrna Weissman and Dr. Gerald Klerman were testing ways to treat depressive disorders with pharmacotherapy versus pharmacotherapy plus a psychotherapeutic intervention. They developed this intervention based on the works of three theorists prominent in the world of psychopathology and called it *interpersonal therapy* (IPT). Applying the assumptions of Adolf Meyer, John Bowlby, and Harry Stack Sullivan, the primary premise of IPT was that most mental health problems occur within a social context.
   1. Adolf Meyer is recognized as the founder of the biopsychosocial model, which posits the role of social context on physical and mental health.
   2. John Bowlby is known as the founder of attachment theory, in which the most organic interpersonal relationship—that of the mother and the child—has the most evolutionary impact on future relationships.
   3. Harry Stack Sullivan viewed relationships as an integral part of our personal views. As such, psychopathology is a result of anxiety interrupting communication and interactions within interpersonal relationships. His work aligned well with nursing theorist Hildegard Peplau, who is considered the mother of psychiatric nursing.
   4. The works of Meyer, Bowlby, Stack, and Peplau leads to an understanding that all psychiatric problems occur within the context of interpersonal, social contexts. This basic principle guides all of IPT, which is meant to be concentrated on the current distressing situations and symptoms, not open-ended, and not focused on past experiences or relationships.
B. Focus is on interpersonal constructs instead of intrapsychic (i.e., the unconscious), cognitive, or behavioral. The IPT process is brief and structured, typically occurring in 12 to 16 weeks, and within three phases.
C. IPT has three phases:
   1. Phase 1: During this phase, the therapist assesses symptoms and the effects of symptoms on interpersonal relationships. They provide education about the patient's symptoms, "sick role," and their expectations to move toward wellness. Together, the primary focus and goals for treatment are established.
   2. Phase 2: This is considered the *active treatment* phase, in which the therapist offers strategies to maximize opportunities, strengths, and relationships to progress toward wellness. At each appointment, the patient discusses experiences related to the specific problems that have been identified and the therapist leads them toward new strategies to improve problem.
   3. Phase 3: In the termination phase, initial problems and goals are reviewed. Together, the therapist and the patient develop a relapse prevention plan, which entails strategies to manage reoccurrence of problems.

IMPORTANT TERMS AND ASSUMPTIONS

A. A significant factor in the effectiveness of IPT is the therapeutic alliance, or nurse–patient relationship. Important concepts of IPT align with Peplau's interpersonal nursing theory and Sullivan's interpersonal theory and include the following:
   1. The patient, who is in a constant state of imbalance and development and aiming to reduce pathologies caused by personal and environmental needs. This person and their needs are always viewed in a cultural (social) context.
   2. Environment includes all existing forces that are extrinsic to the patient.
   3. Health symbolizes the forward progress of the patient as they process toward equilibrium, which includes interpersonal relationships.
   4. Nursing is the act of facilitating understanding by the patient as it relates to experiences, environment, and health. Within the patient–nurse relationship, therapeutic interpersonal processing progresses toward health.
B. Another important component of IPT is the therapeutic alliance and the role of the psychotherapist. While implementing IPT, therapists should be an ally and advocate in the process of recovery, while providing unconditional positive regard and acceptance. They are encouraged to share personal experiences that may demonstrate important points of discussion and guide patients in developing their own strategies for change.
C. Goals of treatment are met when the patient is able to implement these strategies and report desired changes in their lives. Compared with other therapy modalities, IPT does not typically include homework and, since this is a time-limited intervention, transference is typically not of concern.

APPLICATION AND EVIDENCE

A. IPT was originally developed to treat depressive disorders, and the initial protocols of care reflected this intention. Throughout the years, protocols have been modified to target varying symptoms presentations. IPT continues to effectively reduce major depressive symptoms, as well as symptoms that appear in postpartum depression and eating disorders.

B. In adolescent populations, a systematic review of 42 randomized controlled trials over 16 years showed IPT as an efficacious intervention for treatment of depressive disorders, similar to the effectiveness rates of CBT.

C. IPT also shows significant reduction in suicidal ideations, and alongside social rhythm therapy IPT can effectively increase maintenance time between mood episodes and improve overall functioning.

D. IPT protocols have also been adapted to be utilized by nonmental healthcare providers in medical settings to provide brief counseling to address general life stressors, including work, family, and friendships. This training, along with other IPT protocols, can be obtained through various professional organizations, including medical, nursing, and social work, although there are no standard guidelines for certification.

TRAINING AND CERTIFICATION

A. Multiple programs provide training in IPT and can be located online.

B. The Interpersonal Therapy Institute (IPT Institute) provides international training programs on multiple levels (clinical levels A–D, advanced, and supervisory, as well as IPT for adults, adolescents, and perinatal). The website provides access to training materials. Completion of the IPT Institute-accredited level A IPT course requires 14 to 16 hours of instruction (https://iptinstitute.com/ipt-certification).

REFERENCES AND BIBLIOGRAPHY

Karam, A. M., Fitzsimmons-Craft, E. E., Tanofsky-Kraff, M., & Wilfley, D. E. (2019). Interpersonal psychotherapy and the treatment of eating disorders. *Psychiatric Clinics of North America*, 42(2), 205–218. https://doi.org/10.1016/j.psc.2019.01.003

Lavigne, B., Audebert-Mérilhou, E., Buisson, G., Kochman, F., Clément, J. P., & Olliac, B. (2016). Thérapie interpersonnelle (TIP) en psychiatrie de l'enfant et de l'adolescent [Interpersonal therapy (IPT) in child psychiatry and adolescent]. *L'Encéphale*, 42(6), 535–539. https://doi.org/10.1016/j.encep.2015.06.009

Markowitz, J. C., Svartberg, M., & Swartz, H. A. (1998). Is IPT time-limited psychodynamic psychotherapy? *The Journal of Psychotherapy Practice and Research*, 7(3), 185–195. PMID: 9631340.

O'Hara, M. W., Pearlstein, T., Stuart, S., Long, J. D., Mills, J. A., & Zlotnick, C. (2019). A placebo controlled treatment trial of sertraline and interpersonal psychotherapy for postpartum depression. *Journal of Affective Disorders*, 245, 524–532. https://doi.org/10.1016/j.jad.2018.10.361

Peplau, H. E. (1997). Peplau's theory of interpersonal relations. *Nursing Science Quarterly*, 10(4), 162–167. https://doi.org/10.1177/089431849701000407

Swartz, H. A., Levenson, J. C., & Frank, E. (2012). Psychotherapy for bipolar II disorder: The role of interpersonal and social rhythm therapy. *Professional Psychology: Research and Practice*, 43(2), 145–153. https://doi.org/10.1037/a0027671

van Bentum, J. S., van Bronswijk, S. C., Sijbrandij, M., Lemmens, L., Peeters, F., Drukker, M., & Huibers, M. J. H. (2021). Cognitive therapy and interpersonal psychotherapy reduce suicidal ideation independent from their effect on depression. *Depression and Anxiety*, 38(9), 940–949. https://doi.org/10.1002/da.23151

Weersing, V. R., Jeffreys, M., Do, M. C. T., Schwartz, K. T., & Bolano, C. (2017). Evidence base update of psychosocial treatments for child and adolescent depression. *Journal of Clinical Child & Adolescent Psychology*, 46(1), 11–43. https://doi.org/10.1080/15374416.2016.1220310

Weissman, M. M., Markowitz, J. C., & Klerman, G. L. (2000). *Comprehensive guide to interpersonal psychotherapy*. Basic Books.

Weissman, M. M. (2020). Interpersonal psychotherapy: History and future. *The American Journal of Psychotherapy*, 73(1), 3–7. https://doi.org/10.1176/appi.psychotherapy.20190032

Wheeler, K., & Crowe, M. (2022). Interpersonal psychotherapy. In K. Wheeler (Ed.), *Psychotherapy for the advanced practice psychiatric nurse: A how-to guide for evidence-based practice* (3rd ed., pp. 419–440). Springer Publishing Company.

MOTIVATIONAL INTERVIEWING

A. Motivational interviewing (MI), an evidence-based approach, was developed by Miller and Rollnick in the 1980s. It was originally focused on working with patients diagnosed with substance use disorders. It focuses on the impact of interpersonal processes involved in changing behaviors.

B. While not technically a psychotherapy, MI provides a foundational framework to include the patient in decision-making. MI was originally developed in the field of addiction to motivate individuals to commit to a lifestyle change without the use of alcohol or drugs.

C. The goal of MI is to engage the patient in "change talk" and help them identify motivation to change through use of the therapeutic alliance and specific communication strategies directing the discussion. MI evolved from Carl Rogers's person-centered approach as a way of helping people commit to the difficult process of change. It was introduced by William Miller in 1983, with further refinements working with another psychologist, Stephen Rollnick. In the words of Dr. Rollnick, "The more you try to insert information and advice into others, the more they tend to back off and resist. This was the original insight that generated our search for a more satisfying and effective approach. Put simply, this involves coming alongside the person and helping them to say why and how they might change for themselves" (Rollnick, 2023, para. 1).

D. MI identifies four processes to help practitioners make better progress. The processes are not linear but rather four activities that occur during MI and use the skills of asking, listening, affirming, and summarizing. The following are the four processes:

  1. Engaging: The practitioner listens to the patient's story and develops connections.
  2. Focusing: What changes would the patient be willing to discuss?
  3. Evoking: What changes would the patient be willing to do?
  4. Planning: How will they get there?

IMPORTANT TERMS AND ASSUMPTIONS

A. In MI, it is not the therapist's job to make the changes for the patient, nor do therapists force or manipulate change. Instead, it is the patient who identifies personal motivation for making behavioral changes and ways to progress in that direction to improve their health. It involves four elements, known as PACE:

  1. Partnership: One cannot fix other people's behaviors as it requires side-by-side collaboration.
  2. Acceptance: This is an empathic, nonjudgmental attitude that accepts people where they are and their right to choose their own paths.
  3. Compassion: This is based on the Hippocratic oath to alleviate suffering, do no harm, and promote the patients' health and well-being.
  4. Empowerment: Empowerment is helping patients identify their values, ideas, and motivation to change. It combines the best advice of the healthcare professional and the wisdom of the patient to empower them to decide on ▶

working on behavioral changes. This honors the patient's autonomy and their ability to make changes.

B. OARS is an anacronym to remember the communication skills inherent in MI:
   1. Asking Open questions: Open questions are phrased in such a way that they cannot be answered with yes/no or short answers.
   2. Affirming: Affirmations acknowledge the patient's strengths and their efforts related to the changes they are willing to make.
   3. Reflecting: Reflecting is related to statements that mirror the content and feelings that are either stated by or implied by the patient and may highlight discrepancies in what was said.
   4. Summarizing: Summarization links together what has been said, agreed to by the patient, or to transition to another topic.

APPLICATION AND EVIDENCE
A. MI is a method of communication between the practitioner and the patient acknowledging the patient's power to change. It is an evidence-based approach that helps patients achieve lifestyle changes to improve health and motivate individuals to engage in other forms of psychotherapy.
B. MI is an important and needed skill for all healthcare professionals, not just the PMHNP.
C. Research has shown that MI is effective in the treatment of substance use disorders, including smoking cessation, and chronic disease management, including diabetes.
D. It has also been shown effective in improving medication adherence and physical activity.

TRAINING AND CERTIFICATION
A. While there is no definitive certification for MI, there are online simulations and live programs that can be utilized to practice the techniques of the interventions. One online training resource that has several modules to train clinicians is www.motivationalinterview.org.
B. When seeking training in this approach to engaging with patients, it is wise to look for programs that combine didactic content with experiential and practice sessions.
C. There are a number of programs available online and in-person for MI certification.
D. The Motivational Interviewing Network of Trainers (MINT) is an international organization that provides access to trainers and to certification courses. Certification courses usually run about 4 weeks of didactic full time, and 6 to 12 weeks part time (https://motivationalinterviewing.org/motivational-interviewing-training).

REFERENCES AND BIBLIOGRAPHY
Adams, S., & Hamera, E. (2022). Motivational interviewing. In K. Wheeler (Ed.), *Psychotherapy for the advanced practice psychiatric nurse: A how-to guide for evidence-based practice* (3rd ed., pp. 401–418). Springer Publishing Company.

Ekong, G., & Kavookjian, J. (2016). Motivational interviewing and outcomes in adults with type 2 diabetes: A systematic review. *Patient Education and Counseling, 99*(6), 944–952. https://doi.org/10.1016/j.pec.2015.11.022

Frost, H., Campbell, P., Maxwell, M., O'Carroll, R. E., Dombrowski, S. U., Williams, B., Cheyne, H., Coles, E., & Pollock, A. (2018). Effectiveness of motivational interviewing on adult behaviour change in health and social care settings: A systematic review of reviews. *PLoS One, 13*(10), e0204890. https://doi.org/10.1371/journal.pone.0204890

Lindson-Hawley, N., Thompson, T. P., & Begh, R. (2015). Motivational interviewing for smoking cessation. *Cochrane Database of Systematic Reviews, 3*, Article CD006936. https://doi.org/10.1002/14651858.CD006936.pub3

O'Halloran, P. D., Blackstock, F., Shields, N., Holland, A., Iles, R., Kingsley, M., Bernhardt, J., Lannin, N., Morris, M. E., & Taylor, N. F. (2014). Motivational interviewing to increase physical activity in people with chronic health conditions: A systematic review and meta-analysis. *Clinical Rehabilitation, 28*(12), 1159–1171. https://doi.org/10.1177/0269215514536210

Miller, W. R., & Rollnick, S. (2009). Ten things that motivational interviewing is not. *Behavioural and Cognitive Psychotherapy, 37*(2), 129–140. https://doi.org/10.1017/s1352465809005128

Palacio, A., Garay, D., Langer, B., Taylor, J., Wood, B. A., & Tamariz, L. (2016). Motivational interviewing improves medication adherence: A systematic review and meta-analysis. *Journal of General Internal Medicine, 31*(8), 929–940. https://doi.org/10.1007/s11606-016-3685-3

Rollnick, S. M. (2023). *About motivational interviewing.* https://www.stephenrollnick.com/about-motivational-interviewing

Rollnick, S. M., Miller, W. R., & Butler, C. C. (2022). *Motivational interviewing in health care: Helping patients change behavior* (2nd ed.). Guilford Press.

PSYCHOANALYSIS

A. Sigmund Freud, trained as a neurologist, is considered the pioneer of psychotherapy. He focused his private practice on psychological disorders and is credited with the development of psychoanalysis.
   1. Psychoanalytic theory examines psychopathology, which is rooted in the individual's past and focuses on the consequences of early interactions with others.
   2. Freud developed free association as a method to encourage patient expression from the unconscious mind. This technique led him to uncover the belief in "blockages" or resistance that kept conflicts hidden to the patient.
   3. Freud concluded that resistance usually reflected sexual material, where the patient repressed the sexual nature of some thoughts. This was the etiology, according to Freud, of neurotic symptoms, or the emotional struggle between the wish and the defense.
B. Psychoanalysis is a therapeutic approach that counts the length of treatment in terms of years rather than number of sessions and defines itself by freedom from constraint and preconception.
   1. Training in psychoanalytic psychotherapy usually requires 4 years of didactic training, with an additional 3 to 4 years of case supervision.
   2. This time factor presents profound research limitations that have led academic disciplines to distance themselves from psychoanalytic study.
   3. Freudian psychoanalysis, however, remains as a form of therapy taking years to master and requiring that the therapist themselves be in psychoanalytic therapy.
C. The following are the components of human personality:
   1. Id: primitive source of basic urgers and is unconscious; governed by pleasure seeking and sexual and aggressive urges
   2. Ego: deals with reality and helps satisfy the demands of the id in socially acceptable, realistic, and safe ways
   3. Superego: holds internalized morals and standards
D. The American Psychoanalytic Association (APsA; https://apsa.org/education-research/adult-psychoanalytic-training) lists training programs across the country complete with personal analysis, didactic curriculum, and intensive supervised psychoanalytic clinical work.
E. Other approved training institutes for psychoanalysis include, but are not limited to, the following:
   1. American Institute for Psychoanalysis (New York)
   2. Boston Psychoanalytic Society and Institute, Inc.
   3. Center for Psychoanalytic Studies (Houston)

4. Chicago Psychoanalytic Institute
5. Cincinnati Psychoanalytic Society and Institute
6. Cleveland Psychoanalytic Center

REFERENCES AND BIBLIOGRAPHY

American Psychoanalytic Association. (2023). *About psychoanalysis.* https://apsa.org/content/about-psychoanalysis

Jay, M. (2023). *Sigmund Freud: Austrian psychoanalyst.* Britannica. https://www.britannica.com/biography/Sigmund-Freud

Taubner, S. (2013). Working with unconscious and explicit memories in psychodynamic psychotherapy in patients with chronic depression. In M. R. Linden & K. Rutkowski (Eds.), *Hurting memories and beneficial forgetting: Posttraumatic stress disorders, biographical developments, and social conflicts* (pp. 153–163). Elsevier.

PSYCHODYNAMIC THERAPY

A. In the late 19th century, as Sigmund Freud developed psychoanalytic psychotherapy, psychodynamic therapy also emerged. While the latter originated with Freud, the trajectory of his work alongside colleagues is what eventually differentiated psychoanalytic and psychodynamic therapies. Others recognized in its development include Ernst Wilhelm von Brücke, a German physician who first published papers that drew assumptions from thermodynamics and applied them to psychology; Alfred Adler, Otto Rank, Adolf Meyer, and Carl Jung, Freud's colleagues in the Vienna Psychoanalytic Society; and Melanie Klein, who recognized how early childhood experiences impact our emotions, even into adulthood.

B. Both psychoanalytic and psychodynamic psychotherapies emphasize the importance of the human psyche as a *dynamic* construct. The psychodynamic theory further emphasizes the influence that development (adaptive and maladaptive) has on psychological health. In the simplest terms, what happens in our past affects what we do today.

C. Psychodynamic therapy, like psychoanalytic therapy, is a form of talk therapy. It helps the patient remember the past and gain insight into how those experiences impact their present situation and mind-set.

D. The therapeutic process focuses on exploring parts of self, particularly the parts that are unknown, which are known as the *unconscious*.

1. The process seeks to explore how the unconscious manifests in daily life and how it may be causing maladaptive functioning in various contexts, including emotionally, socially, and occupationally.
2. It is the responsibility of the psychotherapist to facilitate this exploration and expand on how embedded negativity—conflict, fear, and inhibitions—influences emotional reactions.
3. The treatment process can be time-limited, is continuous, and can occur as much as multiple times weekly.
4. The central roles of the psychotherapist include the following:
    a. Establishing a therapeutic alliance with the patient that is a mutual partnership
    b. Understanding the potential for transference, in which the patient experiences feelings, thoughts, or behaviors derived from previous relationships (e.g., caretakers, significant others) and projects those onto the therapist
    c. Identifying when transference occurs and helping the patient accurately interpret the origin, importance, and projection of these feelings
    d. Encouraging reflection so that the patient can understand self and relationship patterns and apply insight to improve personal and relational outcomes

IMPORTANT TERMS AND ASSUMPTIONS

A. When considering transference, the therapist must (a) understand the type of transference that is occurring and (b) be prepared for the possibility of countertransference. The following are the types of transference:

1. Positive transference: The patient projects good aspects onto the therapist, which allows them to see the therapist as helpful, caring, and empathetic. This can be beneficial to the therapeutic process.
2. Negative transference: When the patient projects negative emotions onto the therapist, how the therapist reacts can influence the direction of therapy. If the negativity can be addressed, growth can occur. However, if the therapist is unable to recognize it, it can be detrimental. Even further, if countertransference occurs, the process can be further stifled.
3. Countertransference: This is how the therapist reacts to a patient's projections. If the emotions and relationship associated with those emotions become reciprocal, emotional entanglement can occur and inhibit the therapeutic alliance.

B. Other important concepts associated with psychodynamic therapy include free association, dream analysis, resistance, and defense mechanisms.

1. Free association: This is a technique used in psychodynamic therapy in which the therapist gives a word or idea to the patient. The patient is then encouraged to say anything and everything that comes to mind, understanding there will be no judgment or negative consequences. Freud posited this technique in hopes that repressed memories and emotions will emerge and give insight into the unconscious mind.
2. Dream analysis: This is a technique that gives insight into the unconscious mind. Freud believed that the mind transforms emotions and experiences into dreams so that they are more acceptable and understandable.
3. Resistance: This occurs when a patient withholds information, intentionally or unintentionally, that would otherwise be helpful in the therapeutic process.
4. Defense mechanisms: These are intrinsic traits derived from implicit memories that help mitigate anxiety that occurs due to not meeting developmental (i.e., psychosexual, psychosocial) milestones. These defenses can be used deliberately or unintentionally and can be adaptive or maladaptive.

APPLICATION AND EVIDENCE

A. Since its inception, research has continued to empirically support the efficacy and effectiveness of psychodynamic psychotherapy to treat a myriad of mental health problems.

B. Systematic reviews and meta-analyses have shown that both long-term psychodynamic therapy, defined as at least 50 sessions over 1 year, and short-term therapy, occurring up to 25 to 30 times over 6 to 8 weeks, are effective in the treatment of depressive, anxiety, and somatic disorders, even those with severe pathologies.

C. Evidence also supports its use to treat more complex presentations, such as chronic mental illnesses, co-occurring disorders, and personality disorders.

D. The APA publishes clinical practice guidelines that recommend psychodynamic therapy for treatment of obsessive-compulsive disorder, panic, borderline personality, and PTSD.
E. The APA and the American Psychological Association, along with the Department of Veterans Affairs, recommend psychodynamic therapy to treat depressive disorders.
F. Although it may not be considered first-line therapy, there is evidence that it can reduce suicidal and self-harm behaviors, as well as effectively treat a wide range of problems in pediatric populations.

TRAINING AND CERTIFICATION

A. There are multiple certificate programs available for certification in psychodynamic psychotherapy. The training program is usually 2 years of combined didactic and clinical supervision.
   1. The National Psychological Association for Psychoanalysis (NPAP) provides a practice-based psychodynamic learning center (PPLC), which has a certificate program (https://npap.org/psychodynamic-psychotherapy-program-description).
   2. The program is open to any licensed mental health practitioner.

REFERENCES AND BIBLIOGRAPHY

Baée, J., & Jeyasingam, N. (2019). Short-term psychodynamic psychotherapy: A brief history. *Australasian Psychiatry, 27*(6), 581–583. https://doi.org/10.1177/1039856219859291

Bond, M., & Perry, J. C. (2004). Long-term changes in defense styles with psychodynamic psychotherapy for depressive, anxiety, and personality disorders. *The American Journal of Psychiatry, 161*(9), 1665–1671. https://doi.org/10.1176/appi.ajp.161.9.1665

Briggs, S., Netuveli, G., Gould, N., Gkaravella, A., Gluckman, N. S., Kangogyere, P., Farr, R., Goldblatt, M. J., & Lindner, R. (2019). The effectiveness of psychoanalytic/psychodynamic psychotherapy for reducing suicide attempts and self-harm: Systematic review and meta-analysis. *British Journal of Psychiatry, 214*(6), 320–328. https://doi.org/10.1192/bjp.2019.33

de Maat, S., de Jonghe, F., Schoevers, R., & Dekker, J. (2009). The effectiveness of long-term psychoanalytic therapy: A systematic review of empirical studies. *Harvard Review of Psychiatry, 17*(1), 1–23. https://doi.org/10.1080/10673220902742476

Kernberg, P. F., Ritvo, R., Keable, H., & American Academy of Child and Adolescent Psychiatry Committee on Quality Issues. (2012). Practice parameter for psychodynamic psychotherapy with children. *Journal of the American Academy of Child and Adolescent Psychiatry, 51*(5), 541–557. https://doi.org/10.1016/j.jaac.2012.02.015

Leichsenring, F., & Rabung, S. (2008). Effectiveness of long-term psychodynamic psychotherapy: A meta-analysis. *JAMA, 300*(13), 1551–1565. https://doi.org/10.1001/jama.300.13.1551

Luborsky, L., Barber, J. P., & Crits-Christoph, P. (1990). Theory-based research for understanding the process of dynamic psychotherapy. *Journal of Consulting and Clinical Psychology, 58*(3), 281–287. https://doi.org/10.1037//0022-006x.58.3.281

McLeod, S. (2024, January 25). Psychodynamic approach. *Simply Psychology*. www.simplypsychology.org/psychodynamic.html

Parth, K., Datz, F., Seidman, C., & Löffler-Stastka, H. (2017). Transference and countertransference: A review. *Bulletin of the Menninger Clinic, 81*(2), 167–211. https://doi.org/10.1521/bumc.2017.81.2.167

Shedler, J. (2010). The efficacy of psychodynamic psychotherapy. *American Psychologist, 65*(2), 98–109. https://doi.org/10.1037/a0018378

Wheeler, K. (2022). The nurse psychotherapist and a framework for practice. In K. Wheeler (Ed.), *Psychotherapy for the advanced practice psychiatric nurse: A how-to guide for evidence-based practice* (3rd ed., pp. 3–56). Springer Pusblishing Company.

TRAUMA-INFORMED THERAPIES

A. Trauma-informed therapies emphasize the need to acknowledge and understand that patients' experiences of trauma have multifaceted impacts on health. Trauma can include various experiences, including, but not limited to, child maltreatment, neglect, physical and sexual assault, and emotional abuse. Patient safety during therapy is the priority.
B. There are nine types of therapies most commonly used as trauma therapy: eye movement desensitization and reprocessing therapy (EMDR), comprehensive resource model (CRM), internal family systems therapy (IFS), CBT, cognitive processing therapy (CPT), prolonged exposure therapy (PE), TF-CBT, brief eclectic therapy (BET), and narrative exposure therapy (NET).
C. Additional types of therapies that are somatic (body-based) and cognitive–somatic (body-based and including thought processes) are also employed for treatment of trauma. As with other therapies, certification with didactic and supervision should be attained prior to implementing these therapies. Some of them include mindfulness meditation, mind–body stress reduction (MBSR), mindfulness and self-compassion (MSC), and sensorimotor psychotherapy (SP).
D. In the 1990s, Dr. Vincent Felitti's work with adverse childhood experiences (ACEs) clearly provided the evidence for this impact and revolutionized healthcare. Dr. Felitti's work resulted in the development of the ACEs Scale and includes physical, sexual, and verbal abuse; experiences of parental separation, abandonment, divorce, or death; living with someone with mental illness, substance use disorders, and suicidal behaviors, or who was incarcerated; and feelings of being unloved. His research showed that the higher the score on the ACEs Scale, the higher the likelihood of not only mental health and substance use problems, but also medical problems such as obesity, cancer, and cardiac, liver, and pulmonary diseases.
E. Individuals who score a 4 or more on the ACEs Scale have a 12-fold increased risk of alcohol and drug abuse and suicide attempts. They can also have potential for lifelong consequences and can influence the likelihood of future victimization, as well as higher numbers of sexual partners and sexually transmitted infections.
F. With Dr. Felitti's work, all areas of healthcare are encouraged to utilize trauma-informed strategies when caring for all patients. All healthcare providers should explore and take into account patients' histories of trauma, while remembering that trauma is subjective. That is, there is no universal definition of trauma, and without judgment patients should be asked about experiences that have made a long-term, negative impact on their lives.
G. Evidence shows that healthcare providers must also consider social determinants of health and systemic racism as possible traumas. APRNs should do the following:
   1. Know the research and evidence that has laid the foundation for trauma-informed care.
   2. Ask patients about their experiences and associated long-term effects. Use the ACEs Scale to assess for childhood trauma, but do not forget to ask about adult experiences.
   3. Even if the patient does not relate their symptoms with their trauma, the healthcare provider needs to consider it an underlying factor.
   4. Realize that trauma is subjective. Think of *trauma* as the new pain scale: *It is what the patient says it is.*

H. The board-certified PMHRN may want their one-on-one and group interactions to incorporate trauma-informed strategies. The PMHNP may want to conduct trauma-informed therapy with patients and refer properly. Referral requires a depth of knowledge about the approaches so that the referring clinician can appropriately educate and prepare patients for the therapies they need. This may include trauma-informed CBT (TI-CBT) and two other prominent modalities: EMDR and Somatic Experiencing® therapy.

I. While these therapies may have evidence-based indications to treat trauma disorders—particularly PTSD, even if patients do not meet full criteria for PTSD—these therapies can be effective in processing and resolving trauma.

REFERENCES AND BIBLIOGRAPHY

Bernard, D. L., Calhoun, C. D., Banks, D. E., Halliday, C. A., Hughes-Halbert, C., & Danielson, C. K. (2021). Making the "C-ACE" for a culturally-informed adverse childhood experiences framework to understand the pervasive mental health impact of racism on black youth. *Journal of Child & Adolescent Trauma, 14*(2), 233–247. https://doi.org/10.1007/s40653-020-00319-9

Dube, S. R., Anda, R. F., Felitti, V. J., Chapman, D. P., Williamson, D. F., & Giles, W. H. (2001). Childhood abuse, household dysfunction, and the risk of attempted suicide throughout the life span: Findings from the Adverse Childhood Experiences Study. *JAMA, 286*(24), 3089–3096. https://doi.org/10.1001/jama.286.24.3089

Felitti, V. J., Anda, R. F., Nordenberg, D., Williamson, D. F., Spitz, A. M., Edwards, V., Koss, M. P., & Marks, J. S. (1998). Relationship of childhood abuse and household dysfunction to many of the leading causes of death in adults. The Adverse Childhood Experiences (ACE) study. *American Journal of Preventive Medicine, 14*(4), 245–258. https://doi.org/10.1016/s0749-3797(98)00017-8

Menschner, C., & Maul, A. (2016). *Key ingredients for successful trauma-informed care implementation*. Center for Health Care Strategies. https://www.chcs.org/resource/key-ingredients-for-successful-trauma-informed-care-implementation/

Muller, R. (2013, September 27). *Sensorimoter psychotherapy: A somatic path to treat trauma*. Psychology Today. https://www.psychologytoday.com/us/blog/talking-about-trauma/201309/sensorimotor-psychotherapy-somatic-path-treat-trauma

Salamon, M. (2023). *What is somatic therapy?* Harvard Health Publishing, Harvard Medical School. https://www.health.harvard.edu/blog/what-is-somatic-therapy-202307072951

EYE MOVEMENT DESENSITIZATION AND REPROCESSING THERAPY

A. EMDR was developed by Dr. Francine Shapiro as a behavioral technique to address and process trauma, as well as explicitly integrate neural networks. Over the past two decades, research has consistently shown its effectiveness in treating trauma-related disorders and symptoms, either by itself or as an adjunct therapy alongside other modalities, many of which are discussed in this chapter.

B. Research hypothesizes that the mechanism of action is due to activation of both temporal lobes in the brain, allowing for improved neural connectivity and integration of memories. Multiple evidence-based practice guidelines recommend EMDR as a frontline therapy to treat PTSD and other trauma-related disorders, including the APA, the Department of Veterans Affairs and the Department of Defense, the National Institute for Health and Care Excellence, and the World Health Organization.

C. EMDR has been shown to be effective in treating a myriad of mental health problems (e.g., eating disorders, psychosis, phobias, grief) and shows to be a promising treatment for medical problems such as cancer and phantom limb pain.

D. The protocol for EMDR treatment includes eight phases that have changed very little since its development. Each phase, along with a brief description, is provided in the following:

1. Phase 1: history taking and treatment planning: This phase includes a comprehensive assessment that explores thoroughly the patient's history, as well as their current problems/symptoms and readiness for treatment.

2. Phase 2: preparation: This phase includes the development of the therapeutic alliance and expectations of treatment. The therapist helps patients identify their role in therapy, how to indicate when they want/need to stop during a session, and how to remove self out of the processing when complete. Planning for safety and stability in between sessions also occurs.

3. Phase 3: assessment: During this session, the therapist helps the patient identify which memory should be the *target* for the session. The patient is then encouraged to recognize the most prominent images related to the memory, as well as the thoughts and feelings that are elicited with those images. The patient is asked to rate their level of distress during these memories using both subjective report and an objective assessment.

4. Phase 4: desensitization: The patient is advised to continue thinking about the memory and an associated negative thought/feeling. The therapist initiates bilateral stimulation with the patient, which can include eye movement, sound, and/or tapping. The patient is instructed to focus on the action until they report a decreased level of distress.

5. Phase 5: installation: The bilateral stimulation is continued, and the patient is advised to think of a positive thought/feeling in place of the negative one.

6. Phase 6: body scan: The therapist instructs the patient to cognitively scan their body and pay attention to any physical reactions to the process. If the body is still experiencing distress, such as muscle tension or stomach upset, the sensation becomes the new focus of processing.

7. Phase 7: closure: The therapist brings the patient out of processing using techniques that were previously identified in phase 2. The therapist advises the patient to journal their cognitive and somatic experiences in between sessions and explains what to expect.

8. Phase 8: reevaluation: At the beginning of the next session, the therapist and the patient review the previous session and what target memories were processed, and plan the target(s) for the current session.

TRAINING AND CERTIFICATION

A. There are a number of programs available online and in-person for EMDR certification.

B. The EMDR International Association provides basic training, which is about 12 weeks long (https://www.emdria.org/emdr-training).

REFERENCES AND BIBLIOGRAPHY

Menon, S. B., & Jayan, C. (2010). Eye movement desensitization and reprocessing: A conceptual framework. *Indian Journal of Psychological Medicine, 32*(2), 136–140. https://doi.org/10.4103/0253-7176.78512

Nash, W. P., & Watson, P. J. (2012). Review of VA/DOD Clinical Practice Guideline on management of acute stress and interventions to prevent posttraumatic stress disorder. *Journal of Rehabilitation Research & Development, 49*(5), 637–648. https://doi.org/10.1682/jrrd.2011.10.0194

Portigliatti Pomeri, A., La Salvia, A., Carletto, S., Oliva, F., & Ostacoli, L. (2020). EMDR in cancer patients: A systematic review. *Frontiers in Psychology, 11*, 590204. https://doi.org/10.3389/fpsyg.2020.590204

Rostaminejad, A., Behnammoghadam, M., Rostaminejad, M., Behnammoghadam, Z., & Bashti, S. (2017). Efficacy of eye movement desensitization and reprocessing on the phantom limb pain of patients with amputations within a 24-month follow-up. *International Journal of Rehabilitation Research, 40*(3), 209–214. https://doi.org/10.1097/mrr.0000000000000227

Ursano, R. J., Bell, C., Eth, S., Friedman, M., Norwood, A., Pfefferbaum, B., Pynoos, J. D. R. S., Zatzick, D. F., Benedek, D. M., McIntyre, J. S., Charles, S. C., Altshuler, K., Cook, I., Cross, C. D., Mellman, L., Moench, L. A., Norquist, G., Twemlow, S W., Woods., & Yager, J. (2004). Practice guideline for the treatment of patients with acute stress disorder and posttraumatic stress disorder. *American Journal of Psychiatry*, 161(Suppl. 11), 3–31. PMID: 15617511.

Wheeler, K. (2022). Eye movement desensitization and reprocessing therapy. In K. Wheeler (Ed.), *Psychotherapy for the advanced practice registered nurse: A how-to guide for evidence-based practice* (3rd ed., pp. 329–357). Springer Publishing Company.

SOMATIC EXPERIENCING THERAPY

A. Somatic Experiencing® (SE) therapy is one of the newest trauma-informed therapies. It was developed by Dr. Peter Levine, a pioneer in trauma-informed therapy. SE is a body-oriented model that posits that humans often override natural means of regulating their nervous systems with negative feelings, such as shame, judgment, and fear. Many individuals stay *stuck* in the memory of a traumatic experience and have problems resolving it, which can lead to mental and physical problems. SE helps patients move out of the fight-or-flight (or freeze-or-feign) state that the trauma traps them in. Instead of staying stuck, SE helps patients incrementally process through the trauma by employing their body's natural abilities to regulate and achieve balance.

B. There is no standardized protocol for SE sessions. The progression of the therapy is determined by the patient and how comfortable they are moving forward.

   1. The first step, as is common in all therapies, is to develop a trusting, comfortable space for the patient. It is important that all senses—touch, smell, and sound—feel safe to the patient.

   2. Next, the processing begins by asking the patient to focus on small aspects of their experience, but not the whole experience. Once identified, the therapist guides the patient through assessing their somatic sensations, which may not even be apparent to the therapist. Does the patient feel their breathing or posture change? Are there new tensions, pain, or tightness in their muscles? Do they feel heavy or dizzy? This body scan is done slowly and carefully, as not to retrigger being stuck in the memory. As somatic experiences are identified, the patient is encouraged to use self-regulating strategies.

   3. As the patient slowly moves toward safety and comfort with one aspect of the trauma, they move to another aspect and repeat the process until they, again, feel regulated. By gaining awareness into their body–mind connection, patients improve their abilities to identify and regulate emotions as they occur.

C. As a newer therapy modality, empirical evidence is not as abundant as that for other therapies. One study used a randomized controlled trial to evaluate the effectiveness of SE in treating symptoms of PTSD. The results showed significant effects on PTSD symptom severity and depressive symptoms. In a systematic review conducted in 2021 ($N = 16$), SE was shown to significantly improve affective and somatic symptoms among individuals with histories of trauma, although the quality of the studies was noted to be mixed.

   1. Both SE and SP address issues of stress and trauma by examining the body reaction; SP integrates the somatic with cognitive and emotional processing. There are three levels in SP that must be completed and supervised in order to gain certification.

TRAINING AND CERTIFICATION

A. There are a number of programs available online and in-person for SE therapy certification.

B. The Somatic Experiencing® International provides training in a number of modalities (https://traumahealing.org/training).

C. The following provide additional training for trauma therapies:

   1. Comprehensive resource model (CRM): https://comprehensiveresourcemodel.com/training-modules
   2. Internal family systems therapy (IFS): https://ifs-institute.com/trainings
   3. Prolonged exposure therapy (PE): www.nicabm.com/trauma-courses
   4. Brief eclectic therapy (BET): www.apa.org/ptsd-guideline/treatments/brief-eclectic-psychotherapy
   5. Narrative exposure therapy (NET): www.net-institute.org
   6. Sensorimotor psychotherapy (SP): https://sensorimotorpsychotherapy.org

REFERENCES AND BIBLIOGRAPHY

Brom, D., Stokar, Y., Lawi, C., Nuriel-Porat, V., Ziv, Y., Lerner, K., & Ross, G. (2017). Somatic Experiencing for posttraumatic stress disorder: A randomized controlled outcome study. *Journal of Traumatic Stress*, 30(3), 304–312. https://doi.org/10.1002/jts.22189

Kuhfuß, M., Maldei, T., Hetmanek, A., & Baumann, N. (2021). Somatic Experiencing—effectiveness and key factors of a body-oriented trauma therapy: A scoping literature review. *European Journal of Psychotraumatology*, 12(1), Article 1929023. https://doi.org/10.1080/20008198.2021.1929023

Somatic Experiencing International. (2023). *Somatic Experiencing International*. https://traumahealing.org

TRAUMA-INFORMED COGNITIVE BEHAVIORAL THERAPY

A. TI-CBT was originally developed as a family-focused therapy, aimed at treating children who have experienced trauma. Both the child and the caregivers (although not an offending caregiver) are equally involved in therapy in parallel session, as well as in family sessions. The protocol for TI-CBT is fairly regimented and introduced in phases and components. The exposure to previous trauma should be gradual, as should be the inclusion of parents/caregivers. The first few sessions should include assessment and orientation and education about the method. The three phases TI-CBT are as follows:

   1. Stabilization: This phase occurs in 4 to 12 sessions and primarily includes *psychoeducation* about trauma and responses. The therapist explores reminders, or triggers, of traumas, which may include people, places, smells, or other sensory memories. It also includes parenting skills, which provides the parents the what, why, and when of implanting these skills. Patients are also taught *relaxation* (e.g., grounding techniques, mindfulness), affect *modulation* (i.e., problems-solving, distraction, seeking social support), and *cognitive processing skills*, which help the child connect internal reactions to external responses.

   2. Trauma narration and processing: This phase occurs in two to six sessions and consists of an interactive process in which the child discusses aspects of their trauma, including their thoughts and feelings. They are encouraged to speak about all details so that they master the experience instead of avoiding it. Through this process, the therapist helps the patient feel safe and help them reframe negative cognitive distortions.

3. Integration and consolidation: This phase occurs in two to eight sessions and includes *in vivo mastery*, conjoint child–parent sessions, and enhancing safety. During *in vivo mastery*, the therapist assists in trauma processing through imaginal exposure to situations that are still haunting. The child is encouraged to face the most fearful aspects of the experience (e.g., a specific location), while learning that the anticipated outcome (e.g., abuse happening again) does not occur. Joining the sessions, caregivers are taught communication, modeling, and safety reinforcement skills. Throughout this process, the child may report feelings of abandonment, betrayal of trust, and loss of safety. Together, the therapist helps the parents develop a safety plan that helps the child feel safe.

TRAINING AND CERTIFICATION
A. Beck Institute (http://beckinstitute.org)

REFERENCE AND BIBLIOGRAPHY
Cohen, J. A., & Mannarino, A. P. (2015). Trauma-focused cognitive behavior therapy for traumatized children and families. *Child and Adolescent Psychiatric Clinics of North America*, 24(3), 557–570. https://doi.org/10.1016/j.chc.2015.02.005

OTHER TYPES OF THERAPY

APPLIED BEHAVIORAL ANALYSIS

A. Behaviorism is an early form of therapy based on learning theories developed by Pavlov and Skinner. The following are some terms to know from these theories:
1. Classical conditioning: An association is made between a previously neutral stimulus and a stimulus that evokes a response. This is not an active form of learning. Classical conditioning has several components.
    a. Unconditioned stimulus (US): US is something that naturally provokes a response that does not need any learning (e.g., the smell of food makes a person hungry—the US is the food).
    b. Conditioned stimulus (CS): A stimulus that has been neutral is associated with the US and eventually elicits a conditioned response (e.g., a dinner bell being rung that makes one feel hungry regardless of where the person is or is not hungry—the CS is the bell).
    c. Conditioned response (CR): CR is the learned response to a previously neutral stimulus (the bell).
    d. Other terms associated with classical conditioning include extinction, spontaneous recovery, stimulus generalization, discrimination, and contiguity.
2. Operant conditioning: Operant conditioning is a type of learning in which behavior is influenced by antecedents (things occurring before the behavior) and consequences (things that follow the behavior). This applies reinforcement (reward) or punishment after a behavior that either strengthens the behavior or weakens it. The learner is an active participant.
    a. Negative reinforcement: The removal of an adverse stimulus is what is rewarding and strengthens the behavior.
    b. Punishment: This is different from negative reinforcement and is used to stop behaviors or weaken them.
3. Applied behavioral analysis (ABA): ABA uses operant conditioning to shape and modify behavior and comprises multiple intervention procedures based on the basic principles of motivation and learning. These principles include things such as positive reinforcement, extinction, stimulus control, and generalization.
    a. ABA applies the principles of learning and motivation to allow the solution of socially significant problems, such as those seen with autism. *Autistic spectrum disorder (ASD)* is a term used for all diagnoses falling in the categories of pervasive developmental disorders. ABA treatment programs for individuals with autism have a significant amount of scientific evidence supporting its efficacy. Based on theoretical principles of learning, ABA is based on the theory that the consequences of actions shape behavior, initially introduced by studies done by B.F. Skinner.
4. Early intensive behavioral intervention applies ABA principles and procedures to habilitate young children with ASD. This treatment is administered as early as possible in the child's life, is intensive, and can be applied up to 40 hours per week. This intensive treatment is an attempt to address all impaired areas of functioning.

BASIC PRINCIPLES
A. The procedures utilized in ABA therapy are founded on the behavioral principles of learning and motivation, consisting of reinforcement, stimulus control, and extinction, among others. An assumption in behavioral psychology is that all behaviors, including linguistic, social, adaptive, or maladaptive, can be addressed through the application of ABA.
1. Reinforcement techniques include positive reinforcement, which is something that occurs after a behavior and increases the probability of a behavior occurring again in the future. Positive reinforcement requires the addition of a stimulus following a specified behavior and will increase the behavior to occur in the future. Negative reinforcement is the removal of stimulus following a behavior to increase the probability of that behavior occurring again in the future. Differential reinforcement combines both positive and negative reinforcements to more rapidly change the behavior. This is done by reinforcing only the behaviors that are targeted to increase and applying extinction to all other responses.
2. Extinction occurs when reinforcement for the problem behavior is terminated and the future probability of a particular behavior is reduced.
3. Stimulus control is when a behavior is reinforced in the presence of a particular stimulus and not in its absence. This causes the behavior to occur only in the presence of the stimulus.
4. Generalization is the spreading of the effects of learning from one set of circumstances to another.

PROCEDURES AND STRATEGIES
A. There are four teaching procedures that utilize the previously mentioned principles:
1. Prompting: Prompting presents cues in order to make a behavior occur that otherwise would not. This is a temporary measure and is only used to illicit a particular behavior that can then be reinforced. For example, a child asks for their favorite stuffed bear and is prompted to say "bear" before giving the child the stuffed animal.
2. Fading: Fading is the systematic removal of the prompt so that the behavior continues to occur in the absence of the prompt.

3. Shaping: Shaping is a technique of reinforcing successive approximations of the desired behavior. If a child is learning a particular word, for example, the syllables can be divided and reinforced, until the entire word is learned.
4. Chaining: Chaining involves a long sequence of behaviors that have been broken down into smaller behaviors that are reinforced. Eventually the more complex behavior can be learned as a whole.

EVIDENCE

A. Elena et al. (2018) reviewed meta-analytic studies that showed a substantial improvement in IQ scores and socially adapted behaviors using early intervention ABA therapy. Early intensive behavioral interventions have impacted and reshaped the field of ASD. Most of the reviews focused on ABA interventions. The basis of all forms of ABA is that for learning to occur there are three components that are necessary. First, a stimulus must be present that cues a response; second, the patient should respond with a behavioral demonstration; and third, there should be a consequence that reinforces the frequency of a specific behavior or decrease that behavior through punishment.

B. ABA therapy is now considered first-line in the treatment of ASD.

REFERENCES AND BIBLIOGRAPHY

Granpeesheh, D., Tarbox, J., & Dixon, D. R. (2009). Applied behavior analytic interventions for children with autism: A description and review of treatment research. *Annals of Clinical Psychiatry*, 21(3), 162–173. PMID: 19758537.

Grigorenko, E., Torres, S., Lebedeva, E., & Bondar, Y. (2018). Evidence-based interventions for ASD: A focus on Applied Behavior Analysis (ABA) interventions. *Psychology. Journal of Higher School of Economics*, 15(4), 711–727. https://doi.org/10.17323/1813-8918-2018-4-711-727

Kodak, T., & Bergmann, S. (2020). Autism spectrum disorder: Characteristics, associated behaviors, and early intervention. *Pediatric Clinics of North America*, 67(3), 525–535. https://doi.org/10.1016/j.pcl.2020.02.007

FAMILY THERAPY APPROACHES

A. Family therapy provides the groundwork for an understanding of the family system and its effect on the individual members. It is a complex therapeutic intervention that requires a great deal of training beyond the basics taught in a PMHNP program. There are several different approaches that can be utilized in the provision of family therapy and a select few are presented here.

B. The practical aspects of family therapeutic interventions include assessment strategies, family genograms, and determining the diverse approach that might work with the identified family unit. Families (and couples) experience stressors that may include issues related to infertility, blended families, infidelity, trauma, incarceration, social media effects, and LGBTQ+ identity, among others.

C. The roots of family therapy began with psychoanalysts including Sigmund Freud, Alfred Adler, and Nathan Ackerman. Karl Ludwig von Bertalanffy introduced the general system theory, which viewed problems as the expression of dysfunction within the family. As newer family therapies developed, the foci became systemic, structural, strategic, and emotionally focused types of family therapy. Pitta and Datchi describe integration of different theories that combine the strengths of the approaches into a broader, more effective approach to treatment based on the idea that no one approach works for all patients.

D. The following are a few leaders in the field of family therapy, along with the basic concepts:

1. *Murray Bowen* developed *the family systems theory*: Human behavior defines the family unit. The unit is a social system that is complex with interconnected family members. It is for this reason Bowen's theory sees the family as a whole rather than the members as individuals. This model includes eight concepts (thebowencenter.org).

    a. Triangles: This refers to a three-person relationship system that creates tension that shifts between members.
    b. Differentiation of self: Poor differentiation of self results in a person who relies heavily on the acceptance and approval of others. A person with well-differentiated sense of self can recognize realistic dependence on others but is able to make independent decisions with or without acceptance or approval of others.
    c. Nuclear family emotional process: There are four basic relationship patterns that govern where problems develop: marital conflict, dysfunction in a spouse, impairment of one or more children, and emotional distance.
    d. Family projection processes: This refers to the transmission of emotional problems from a parent to a child.
    e. Multigenerational transmission process: Small differences in differentiation between the parent and the child lead to generational differences in differentiation among members of the extended family.
    f. Emotional cutoff: Emotional contact between family members is cut off due to unresolved emotional issues with other family members.
    g. Sibling position: Sibling position is a concept where people who grow up in a specific sibling position can predictably have important characteristics in common.
    h. Societal emotional process: Societal emotional process is a concept where the emotional system governs behavior in societies as a whole.

2. *Salvador Minuchin* proposed a structural family therapy approach where symptoms and family issues are believed to be part of a dysfunctional family organization. It provides a framework that focuses on the structure, substructure, and imperceptible rules. Key concepts include the following:

    a. Family system: This includes roles and rules, hierarchy and power structures, communication patterns, and decision-making functions that organize the family relationships in recurrent patterns.
    b. Subsystems: These are smaller groups that carry out the function of the family system. Examples are spousal, parental, sibling, and extended family subsystems, among others.
    c. Boundaries: These are emotional barriers that may be physical or invisible and that protect the integrity of the individuals, subsystems, and families.
    d. Enmeshed family: Boundaries in this type of family are diffuse and permeable, causing a loss of personal autonomy and a denial of differences.
    e. Disengage family: Boundaries are rigid and impermeable, causing the family members to be disconnected with one another and unaware of their impact on each other.
    f. Coalition: Coalition is characterized by a dysfunctional alliance of two members against a third member.

g. Parentification: Parentification is a type of role reversal where the child is given the role of a parent, along with the power and authority that belong to the parent.
h. Therapeutic interventions include enactments, structural mapping, and modifying problematic interactions.

3. Strategic family therapy came to the forefront in the 1980s with work by *Jay Haley* and *Cloe Madanes*. Key concepts include the following:
   a. Cybernetics: This is the control process in a system that evaluates the flow of information through feedback loops.
   b. Homeostasis: This refers to a dynamic state of equilibrium within a system.
   c. Feedback loops: A feedback loop is a circular process in which the system's output is continuously reintroduced as input.
   d. Circular causality: This refers to a network of interacting loops in which any cause is seen as the effect of a prior cause.
   e. First-order changes: These are superficial behavioral changes that do not change the system structure.
   f. Second-order changes: These changes require a fundamental revision of the system structure and function.
   g. The goal of therapy is to alter problematic patterns of behavior that maintain the family's dysfunction.
   h. Therapeutic interventions include placing the problem under the family's control, paradoxical techniques, pretend techniques, ordeals, rituals, and invariant prescriptions.

4. Emotionally focused family therapy (EFT), developed by *Leslie Greenburg* and *Sue Johnson*, was based on the realization that families were caught in negative cycles that caused them to be stuck in patterns of behavior. They believed these cycles were impacted by attachment issues and interrupted emotions. It is a short-term, experiential, and evidence-based approach rooted in the humanistic–existential school. Key concepts include the following:
   a. Emotions: Primary emotions are fundamental and initial emotional reactions to a situation. Secondary emotions are reactions to a person's thoughts or feelings rather than to a situation.
   b. Attachment styles: These refer to the emotional bonds in relationships and are classified into four styles: secure attachment, insecure attachment, anxious attachment, and vacillating attachment.
   c. Key interventions are empathic attunement, reflective statements, evocative questions, creative images, and utilization of metaphors.

E. Other types of family therapies include supportive family therapy, CBT, narrative therapy, transgenerational, brief family therapy, and psychodynamic.

EVIDENCE

A. Larson discussed the difficulty in providing evidence-based research for family therapies. While there is much outcome research showing the efficacy of family therapy, it remains on the fringes of mental health practice. The therapies that satisfy the gold standard of evidence require manualized and controlled replication by independent investigators. Many family therapies are patient-directed and focused on the relational process rather than step-by-step techniques.

B. Research based on qualitative studies clearly demonstrates that family therapy works for a variety of problems but is often ignored because it is nonexperimental and the therapy itself is oftentimes multimodal.

REFERENCES AND BIBLIOGRAPHY

Knight, C. (2022). Family therapy. In K. Wheeler (Ed.), *Psychotherapy for the advanced practice psychiatric nurse: A how-to guide for evidence-based practice* (3rd ed., pp. 495–537). Springer Publishing Company.

Pitta, P. J., & Datchi, C. C. (Eds.). (2019). *Integrative couple and family therapies: Treatment models for complex clinical issues*. American Psychological Association.

GROUP THERAPY: PRINCIPLES AND APPROACHES

A. Group therapy allows for the treatment of multiple individuals at the same time, which may decrease wait times and increase the accessibility of psychotherapy. It is a well-validated treatment that can be utilized for treatment of a variety of symptoms, including PTSD, depression, and anxiety. Yalom developed a list of therapeutic factors and goals that many use to guide the application of this type of therapy.

B. The therapeutic factors outlined by Yalom include the following:

1. Universality: Patients feel connected by the realization that others share similar thoughts, feelings, and issues.
2. Altruism: Helping the other patients in the group can improve self-esteem.
3. Instillation of hope: Witnessing the success of others can assist patients in seeing themselves as being able to follow a similar path in their lives.
4. Imparting information: Knowledge and information can be gained from both other group members as well as the healthcare provider.
5. Corrective recapitulation of primary family experience: The opportunity for patients to re-create family dynamics in a controlled environment can be beneficial.
6. Development of socialization techniques: Group therapy allows patients to learn effective and appropriate ways to interact with the others in the group.
7. Imitate behavior: Observing other group members can allow the patient to gain insight and understanding of their own behaviors.
8. Cohesiveness: Therapy can allow patients to experience feelings of belongingness, support, and trust in one another.
9. Existential factors: Group therapy assists patients in realizing that they alone are responsible for their life decisions.
10. Catharsis: The sharing of personal experiences from both the past and the present can aid patients in releasing emotions.
11. Interpersonal learning: Patients learn from one another by obtaining feedback from other members on their impact on others.
12. Self-understanding: Patients can safely uncover covert factors that impact their behavior and emotions.

C. The goals of group therapy assist in facilitating the patient's growth in comfort and function within the group. The outcome of the patient's involvement in group therapy includes being able to apply what they learned regarding the needed behavioral corrections, interpersonal and relationship skills, education, ability to utilize preventive measures and coping skills, and eventually returning to normal functioning within their society. Ideally, group therapy members include those with similar conditions and members at different stages of treatment to help facilitate recovery.

D. The stages of group development include the following:
1. Forming stage: There often are feelings of anxiety, distrust, and uncertainty in the initial group meetings and a heavy reliance on the healthcare provider.
2. Storming stage: Internal conflict is often present in this stage as the patient becomes more comfortable with sharing intimate details. The healthcare provider may have to intervene to decrease disruptive conflict within the group and reinforce the goals and purposes of the group.
3. Norming stage: The patient's commitment to the group process and goals grows stronger and the cohesiveness of the group will increase. The healthcare provider has a less active role and tends to guide the discussion with insight.
4. Performing stage: Healthcare provider intervention is low and the group often functions on its own, with members being aware of each other's strengths and weaknesses. This allows the members to help individual members grow.
5. Adjourning stage: This is the stage where group therapy comes to an end. There may be feelings of anxiety and sadness as the group says goodbye to each other.

E. The following are other types of groups that can be therapeutic:
1. Psychoeducational groups: The healthcare provider acts in the role of an educator in this type of group by providing information on things such as diagnoses, medications, skill development, and others.
2. Skills development groups: This type of group focuses on the development of life skills, coping methods, emotional control, and socialization skills. Development of other skills can be done depending on the specifics of the group's needs.
3. Cognitive behavioral groups: CBT can be helpful in a group format, in addition to the individual therapy discussed earlier. The focus in this type of group is on the individual's beliefs, perceptions, cognitive distortions, coping skills, and behaviors based on the needs of the patients.
4. Person-centered: The provision of unconditional positive regard and empathy by the healthcare providers creates a trusting environment, with honest feedback provided to and among group members.
5. Psychodynamic group therapy: This type of group therapy focuses on assisting the group members in increasing awareness of their unconscious motivations.
6. Support groups: The healthcare provider is less directive and only facilitates the group process. The patients develop connections with one another and emphasize similarities between the group members.
7. Self-help groups: These groups are often made up of people with similar issues and do not include a healthcare provider. Alcoholics Anonymous and other 12-Step programs are good examples of this type of group. As an example, the participants of these groups have substance use disorders and the focus is on maintenance of sobriety.

EVIDENCE

A. Research on group therapy has articulated how it is useful in creating positive changes in patients facing a variety of mental health and physical health issues.
B. Evidence-based research on group therapy has shown it to be effective in patients with diverse conditions such as eating disorders, schizophrenia, personality disorders, obsessive-compulsive disorder, and cancers.
C. It has been linked to reducing the core symptoms of PTSD and reducing experiences of complicated bereavement. A meta-analysis of group therapy indicated that it has been shown to be equally as effective as individual therapy in outpatient populations. This indicates that if group therapy and individual therapies are equally efficacious, group therapy may be much more cost-effective in a variety of situations.

REFERENCES AND BIBLIOGRAPHY

Beck, J. G., Clapp, J. D., Unger, W., Wattenberg, M., & Sloan, D. M. (2021). Moderators of PTSD symptom change in group cognitive behavioral therapy and group present centered therapy. *Journal of Anxiety Disorders, 80*, 102386. https://doi.org/10.1016/j.janxdis.2021.102386

Burlingame, G. M., Svien, H., Hoppe, L., Hunt, I., & Rosendahl, J. (2020). Group therapy for schizophrenia: A meta-analysis. *Psychotherapy, 57*(2), 219–236. https://doi.org/10.1037/pst0000293

Grenon, R., Schwartze, D., Hammond, N., Ivanova, I., McQuaid, N., Proulx, G., & Tasca, G. A. (2017). Group psychotherapy for eating disorders: A meta-analysis. *International Journal of Eating Disorders, 50*(9), 997–1013. https://doi.org/10.1002/eat.22744

Jónsson, H., & Hougaard, E. (2009). Group cognitive behavioural therapy for obsessive-compulsive disorder: A systematic review and meta-analysis. *Acta Psychiatrica Scandinavica, 119*(2), 98–106. https://doi.org/10.1111/j.1600-0447.2008.01270.x

Koppers, D., Van, H. L., Peen, J., & Dekker, J. J. M. (2023). Exploring the effect of group schema therapy and comorbidity on the treatment course of personality disorders. *Current Opinion in Psychiatry, 36*(1), 80–85. https://doi.org/10.1097/yco.0000000000000828

Lai, J., Song, H., Ren, Y., Li, S., & Xiao, F. (2021). Effectiveness of supportive-expressive group therapy in women with breast cancer: A systematic review and meta-analysis. *Oncology Research and Treatment, 44*(5), 252–260. https://doi.org/10.1159/000515756

Malhotra, A., & Baker, J. (2022). *Group therapy*. StatsPearls Publishing. https://www.ncbi.nlm.nih.gov/books/NBK549812/

McLean, C. P., Levy, H. C., Miller, M. L., & Tolin, D. F. (2022). Exposure therapy for PTSD: A meta-analysis. *Clinical Psychology Review, 91*, 102115. https://doi.org/10.1016/j.cpr.2021.102115

Okumura, Y., & Ichikura, K. (2014). Efficacy and acceptability of group cognitive behavioral therapy for depression: A systematic review and meta-analysis. *Journal of Affective Disorders, 164*, 155–164. https://doi.org/10.1016/j.jad.2014.04.023

Piper, W. E., Ogrodniczuk, J. S., Joyce, A. S., Weideman, R., & Rosie, J. S. (2007). Group composition and group therapy for complicated grief. *Journal of Consulting and Clinical Psychology, 75*(1), 116–125. https://doi.org/10.1037/0022-006x.75.1.116

Pessagno, R. (2022). Group therapy. In K. Wheeler (Ed.), *Psychotherapy for the advanced practice registered nurse: A how-to guide for evidence-based practice* (3rd ed., pp. 469–493). Springer Publishing Company.

Shnaider, P., Boyd, J. E., Cameron, D. H., & McCabe, R. E. (2022). The relationship between emotion regulation difficulties and PTSD outcomes during group cognitive processing therapy for PTSD. *Psychological Services, 19*(4), 751–759. https://doi.org/10.1037/ser0000546

Wolgensinger, L. (2015). Cognitive behavioral group therapy for anxiety: Recent developments. *Dialogues in Clinical Neuroscience, 17*(3), 347–351. https://doi.org/10.31887/DCNS.2015.17.3/lwolgensinger

PERSON-CENTERED THERAPY

A. Person-centered psychotherapy was introduced by Carl Rogers and is based on three conditions: unconditional positive regard, empathic understanding, and congruence by the therapist.
1. The following are additional three conditions that are less well-known: psychological contact between the person and the therapist, the person must be in a state incongruence and distressed in some way, and communication of empathic understanding and unconditional positive regard of the therapist to the patient must at least be minimally achieved.

B. People can move toward becoming fully functioning in a growth-promoting environment. Rogers emphasized that the individual's perception of reality is important in understanding their behavior and that the best understanding of a person is that person themselves.

C. Research for person-centered therapy is primarily qualitative and thus does not meet the medical model of evidence. Person-centered psychotherapy was *the* evidence-based treatment early in Rogers's career.

REFERENCE AND BIBLIOGRAPHY

Joseph, S., & Murphy, D. (2013). Person-centered approach, positive psychology, and relational helping: Building bridges. *Journal of Humanistic Psychology, 53*(1), 26–51. https://doi.org/10.1177/0022167812436426

SPECIAL POPULATION CONSIDERATIONS

PEDIATRICS

A. Developmental considerations influence what the child can understand and include understanding the developmental level of reasoning, perspective, language, and social emotional regulation.
B. Family involvement has a critical place in the treatment of the child, and it is important to note that this does not mean that the family is the focus of treatment.
C. A multisystematic approach may be necessary and interventions are aimed at various interactive systems with the child. There are many systems that promote a child's development; these can include things like family, school, peers, and the community. Engaging a child in therapy requires the understanding of the intersections of these systems.
D. Evidence-based treatment considerations with children and adolescents may differ for each child and their situation.
   1. Specific evidence-based interventions include CBT, interpersonal psychotherapy, EMDR, behavioral parent training, family therapy, and TF-CBT, among others.
   2. It is important to identify the underlying constructs that influence the mental health of the child. ACE studies demonstrate the link of these adverse experiences to future development of psychopathology and medical issues and should be assessed before deciding on the specific therapeutic approach for the child and their family.
   3. Other therapies for children that have evidence behind them include acceptance and commitment therapy (ACT), DBT, parent–child interaction therapy, and play therapy. It is important for the APRN to obtain specific training and certification in dealing with children.

OLDER ADULTS

A. The American Psychological Association (2024) notes that Medicare reimbursement affects the ability of older adults to find a therapist. The higher prevalence of dementia and medical disorders in this population requires assessment to determine which evidence-based practice approach might be the most efficacious.
B. Sleep disorders respond to CBT and depression in older adults with intact cognition and can also respond well to psychodynamic, cognitive, and behavioral therapies.
C. Memory retraining and cognitive training may be efficacious in slowing cognitive decline.
D. Life review and reminiscence therapy may produce higher life satisfaction and treat depression.
E. Therapies may need to be adapted for working with older adults but NOT because they are older according to the American Psychological Association (2022). A therapist should take into account contextual effects like living in a retirement community or long-term healthcare settings.
   1. Cohort effects, generational groups are particularly useful (e.g., Greatest Generation: 1901–1924; Silent: 1925–1945; Baby Boomer: 1946–1965; Generation X: 1965–1980; Millennial: 1980–2000).
F. There are challenges with working with older adults who are physically ill and those with death and dying issues.
G. Caregivers to the older adult will also need therapeutic support.
H. The therapist must keep in mind physical limitations, as well as hearing issues and vision difficulties, and adapt the process to include an appropriate therapeutic technique.
I. Positive mental attitudes, participation in social activities, lifestyle management, social support, cognitive engagement, self-care enhancement, spiritual support, and exercise appear to have a protective factor on cognitive and physical decline in older adults.
J. Successful aging includes positive mental aging, wisdom, resilience, and a sense of personal control and empowerment with decisional control. Life preferences and issues with the aging adult provide a context for level of care. Most older adults prefer to "age in place" in their own homes, and should they consider a residential move, the APRN should be aware that these are major transitions.
K. Care should be taken to assess substance use, gambling, and suicidal risk in this population.

REFERENCES AND BIBLIOGRAPHY

American Psychological Association. (2024, February). *APA guidelines for psychological practice with older adults.* Author. https://www.apa.org/practice/guidelines/guidelines-psychological-practice-older-adults.pdf

Delaney, K. R. D., DeSocio, J., & Carbray, J. A. (2022). Psychotherapy with children. In K. Wheeler (Ed.), *Psychotherapy for the advanced practice psychiatric nurse: A how-to guide for evidence-based practice* (3rd ed., pp. 749–778). Springer Publishing Company.

Felitti, V. J., Anda, R. F., Nordenberg, D., Williamson, D. F., Spitz, A. M., Edwards, V., Koss, M. P., & Marks, J. S. (1998). Relationship of childhood abuse and household dysfunction to many of the leading causes of death in adults. The Adverse Childhood Experiences (ACE) study. *American Journal of Preventive Medicine, 14*(4), 245–258. https://doi.org/10.1016/s0749-3797(98)00017-8

Stevens, G. L., Kauss, M. J., & Hjartardottir, K. L. (2022). Psychotherapy with older adults. In K. Wheeler (Ed.), *Psychotherapy for the advanced practice registered nurse: A how-to guide for evidence-based practice* (3rd ed., pp. 823–865). Springer Publishing Company.

DOCUMENTATION

A. Chart documentation, which is reminiscent of the old narrative style—**s**ubjective and **o**bjective data, **a**ssessment and diagnosis, and **p**lan (SOAP)—has been replaced by a more standardized format of chief complaint, history of present illness, review of systems, past psychiatric history, mental status exam, and diagnostic formulation that arrives at a treatment plan.
B. There are a number of electronic medical record systems that may aid in the documentation, and in fact the Centers for Medicare & Medicaid services (CMS) has outlined documentation guidelines for the provision and reimbursement of mental health services.
C. Clinicians should be aware of their individual state's program rules and should reflect the requirements reflecting medical necessity and justify the treatment and clinical rationale. The documentation should be complete, concise, and accurate, with a notation regarding the face-to-face time spent

with the patient. It must be legible, signed, dated, and kept for review if an audit is done.

D. It is important for the APRN to become familiar with Current Procedural Terminology billing for psychiatric services. Much of them are time-based, but are not reflective of the complexity inherent in psychotherapy. Billing must be accompanied by correct coding to be processed.

E. Self-auditing rules that the CMS recommends for behavioral health include the following:

1. There should be a solid medical record documentation policy that covers federal and state Medicaid regulations.
2. Use a standard medical audit tool that covers documentation and coding standards.
3. Have a staff member who understands documentation and coding review a random sample of charts periodically.
4. Do not audit your own charts. Most people can read their own writing and understand the meaning of abbreviations or other areas that may not actually be in the chart. Having someone else do it will remove bias.
5. Use self-audit to improve the compliance of the practitioner and identify any problem areas.

REFERENCES AND BIBLIOGRAPHY

Moller, M., & Mraz, S. (2022). Reimbursement and documentation. In K. Wheeler (Ed.), *Psychotherapy for the advanced practice registered nurse: A how-to guide for evidence-based practice* (3rd ed., pp. 869–910). Springer Publishing Company.

Centers for Medicare & Medicaid Services. (2024, September 10). *CMS cross cutting initiative: Behavioral health.* https://www.cms.gov/files/document/cms-behavioral-health-stategy.pdf

CONCLUSION

Psychotherapy can add great depth to the APRN's practice and requires lifelong learning and skill development. To practice effectively, they should pursue specific certification in a therapy technique and have supervision from another qualified professional. There is abundant research that supports the use of this therapeutic tool, with or without psychopharmacologic management, to improve long-lasting outcomes for patients. They should be aware that there is no "one-size-fits-all" psychotherapy and it might be prudent to obtain training in several approaches, along with supervision.

II DIAGNOSIS-SPECIFIC PROCEDURES AND PATIENT TREATMENT PLANNING

9 ANXIETY DISORDERS

Brenda Marshall and Nhat Nguyen

INTRODUCTION

This chapter examines disorders that bring disabling symptoms of anxiety to individuals' activities of daily living. Despite anxiety disorders being the most common form of mental illness in the United States, it was not until 1980 that the American Psychiatric Association first identified anxiety as a separate, official disorder. Those who had anxiety disorders prior to that were treated for stress, or a bad case of "nerves."

Historically, those with anxiety disorders, many of which are discussed in this chapter, were misunderstood, mistreated, and usually left untreated to wrestle alone with their symptoms. Finally, in the 1990s, anxiety began to be treated with medication specific for anxiety as well as with some antidepressants. Anxiety disorders present specific challenges to the healthcare provider, not the least of which is understanding the debilitating impact of these symptoms and empowering the patient to be an active, engaged part of the treatment plan.

ANXIETY

Anxiety, as defined by the American Psychiatric Association, includes feelings of tension, excessive worries, and a sense of apprehension and dread, which impact a person's activities of daily living more days than not for at least 6 months. Anxiety should not be confused with stress, which allows a person to continue to perform, although it might be at the very border of their capacity; unlike anxiety, stress could be a result of either positive or negative events. Sometimes, anxiety can be protective, especially when the associated worry can be resolved by a behavioral response, such as the anxiety related to a test, which can be alleviated by studying. In those situations, anxiety is part of the normal fear response, which often motivates behaviors to mitigate or escape from dangerous situations. The physiologic response to a fear stimulus, in the person without pathology, includes alterations in perception, changes in brain and endocrine chemicals, and the autonomic activation of the central nervous system (CNS). The body systems return to homeostasis when that threat stimulus is gone. When, however, the sense of dread has no reasonable activator, a dysregulation of this fear response occurs. When this occurs, the level of alarm far surpasses the situation. The response, which can include hyperarousal, vigilance, panic, avoidance behaviors, and escape behaviors, is debilitating.

Anxiety is an umbrella diagnosis, affecting all age groups, all nationalities, and all genders, with multiple specific forms including generalized anxiety disorder (GAD), obsessive-compulsive disorder (OCD), acute stress disorder (ASD), posttraumatic stress disorder (PTSD), social anxiety disorder, specific phobias, separation anxiety disorder, and illness anxiety disorder (IAD). Anxiety disorders are the most common psychiatric diagnosis. The National Institute of Mental Health (NIMH) reports that about 19% of American adults have an anxiety disorder. In the ages between 18 and 29 years, the prevalence is 22.3%, and increases to 31.9% in adolescents (13–18 years of age). Risk factors are especially important when assessing a pediatric or adolescent patient for an anxiety disorder, including adverse childhood experiences (ACEs), behavioral inhibition, and other social risk factors. Anxiety is often comorbid with depression, as almost 50% of those who have depression are also diagnosed with an anxiety disorder.

DEFINITION

When a person's level of anxiety has become persistent, intrusive, and difficult to control so that activities of daily living are affected, the normal reaction of anxiety has possibly elevated to GAD.

Anxiety Disorders Classification

The *Diagnostic and Statistical Manual of Mental Disorders*, Fifth Edition (*DSM-5*; American Psychiatric Association, 2013), and the *International Classification of Diseases*, 11th Revision (*ICD-11*; World Health Organization [WHO], 2019a) diagnostic criteria (anxiety or fear-related disorders) identify the presence of prominent, uncontrollable tension, apprehension, and/or worry that impact activities of daily living on a majority of days during a period of at least 6 months as criteria for GAD.

INCIDENCE

A. The NIMH estimates that about one-third of American adults experience anxiety in their lifetime (Figure 9.1).

PREDISPOSING FACTORS

A. There are multiple predisposing or risk factors for anxiety disorders, including:
1. Low self-esteem
2. Family history of major depressive disorder (MDD)
3. Female sex assigned at birth
4. ACEs, childhood sexual abuse
5. White race
6. Disturbed family environment
7. Perinatal stress
8. Perceived discrimination

COMMON COMPLAINTS

A. Physical complaints
1. Nausea
2. Difficulty breathing
3. Sweating
4. Fatigue
5. Trembling
6. Heart racing
7. Lightheadedness

B. Psychological complaints
1. Feeling detached
2. Feeling "keyed up" and unable to relax

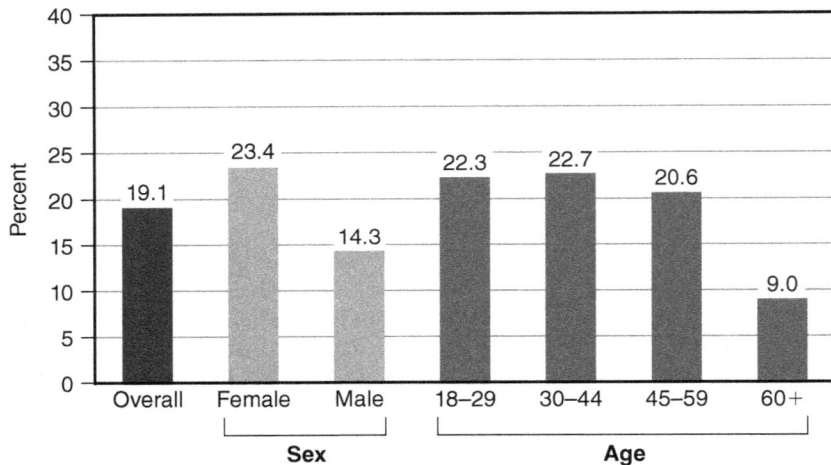

FIGURE 9.1 Past year prevalence of any anxiety disorder among U.S. adults, 2001 to 2003.

Source: National Institute of Mental Health. (n.d.). *Any anxiety disorder*. U.S. Department of Health and Human Services. https://www.nimh.nih.gov/health/statistics/any-anxiety-disorder; Data from National Comorbidity Survey Replication (NCS-R).

COMMON COMPLAINTS
A. Constant irritability
B. Excessive worry even in the absence of a clear threat
C. Fear of loss of control (environment, self, situation)
D. Unrelenting sense of apprehension
E. Sleep disturbances

C. PHYSIOLOGIC SYMPTOMS
A. Autonomic symptoms
  1. Increased heart rate/pounding heart, palpitations
  2. Trembling or shaking
  3. Dry mouth not related to another medical condition or medications
  4. Sweating
B. Chest and abdominal symptoms
  1. Chest pain/discomfort
  2. Closing of throat, experience of a choking sensation
  3. Nausea, upset stomach, general abdominal distress
  4. Difficulty breathing
C. Brain and mind symptoms
  1. Derealization: sensation that things are not real
  2. Depersonalization: feeling that the self is absent/not there
  3. Dizziness, unsteady gait, lightheadedness
  4. Apprehension of loss of control
  5. Apprehension of death
  6. Apprehension of passing out and/or "going insane"
D. Tension affecting connective tissue and musculoskeletal system
  1. Muscle pains and aches
  2. Tingling feelings, restlessness, inability to relax
  3. Difficulty swallowing
  4. Sensation of internal activity, feeling "hyper" and jumpy
E. Generalized/nonspecific symptoms
  1. Generalized numbness
  2. Volatile body temperature: hot flushes, cold, chilly feeling
  3. Overreaction to unexpected events or experiences
  4. Inability to focus or recall things, or suddenly forgetting current dialogue
  5. Persistent irritability
  6. Insomnia, difficulty going to sleep and staying asleep
  7. General exhaustion

PATHOPHYSIOLOGY
A. The etiology of anxiety is considered multifactorial.
B. In the normal adaptive model, fear will activate the amygdala, which then activates the prefrontal cortex. The higher executive functioning of the ventral/medial prefrontal cortex then mediates the response to the stress by acting directly on the amygdala to reduce its activation. In the pathologic model, however, neither the hippocampus nor the prefrontal cortex is successful in mediating the hyperactivation of the amygdala, resulting in the signs and symptoms of anxiety.
C. Family history, environmental factors, neurobiology, and substance use contribute to the etiology of anxiety disorders (interaction of biopsychosocial factors).
  1. Family history: Genetics have been identified as a component in the etiology of anxiety/panic disorder but not in GAD.
  2. Environmental factors: Family dynamics and parental psychopathology have been implicated in the etiology of anxiety disorders. Those with a history of trauma are at higher risk for anxiety disorders.
  3. Neurobiology: The limbic system (the insular cortex and cingulate cortex, hippocampus, amygdala, septal area, and hypothalamus) may have some disruption in balance leading to the development of anxiety.
  4. Substance use: Certain substances, like cocaine, increase the stress hormones. The presence of substance use disorder (SUD) is a risk factor for anxiety disorder and vice versa, with high rates of co-occurring SUD and anxiety.
  5. Racial discrimination: Racism is the categorization of people based on phenotypes that make one set of people subservient to another within a society or political system. Those who are having the lived experience of racism encounter multiple, persistent, daily microaggressions. This can lead to, and predict, the development of multiple anxiety-related disorders.

PHYSICAL EXAMINATION

A. For all anxiety disorders, a full review of systems and a physical exam should be conducted. The exam should be done by the psychiatric specialist, or the patient can be referred to the primary care provider for a full workup to rule out medical conditions that might activate these symptoms.
  1. Vital signs
  2. Height, weight, body mass index (BMI)
  3. Assessment of the patient's general constitution
  4. Appearance

B. Specific diagnostic tests for all anxiety disorders to establish any differential diagnosis include the following:
  1. Thyroid function tests
  2. Urine drug screen
  3. EKG
      a. A baseline EKG is recommended before starting some psychotropic medications.

Psychometric Tools

A. There are multiple psychometric tools for evaluating anxiety. The following are free assessments available online. Specific surveys and tools are listed for each disorder:
  1. *DSM-5* (American Psychiatric Association, 2013) Cross-Cutting Measure
      a. Can be accessed online at www.psychiatry.org/getmedia/e0b4b299-95b3-407b-b8c2-caa871ca218d/APA-DSM5TR-Level1MeasureAdult.pdf
  2. *DSM-5* (American Psychiatric Association, 2013) Level 2 Anxiety Tool
      a. Can be accessed online at www.psychiatry.org/getmedia/f284f967-ed9e-4754-99fc-b32765b1c4a0/APA-DSM5TR-Level2AnxietyAdult.pdf

REFERENCES AND BIBLIOGRAPHY

American Psychiatric Association. (2013). *Diagnostic and statistical manual of mental disorders* (5th ed.). https://doi.org/10.1176/appi.books.9780890425596

American Psychological Association. (2012). *Fact sheet: Health disparities and stress*. https://www.apa.org/topics/racism-bias-discrimination/health-disparities-stress

Mental Health America. (2022). *Quick facts and statistics about mental health*. https://mhanational.org/mentalhealthfacts

National Alliance on Mental Illness. (2023). *Mental health by the numbers*. https://nami.org/mhstats?gclid=Cj0KCQiA7bucBhCeARIsAIOwr-_mryPgVr3hp8Lz9-i-aijtm5GJWQeY_Q8IM0faz9Dl722oo2Q2TFAaAjFGEALw_wcB

World Health Organization. (2019a). Anxiety or fear-related disorders. *International statistical classification of diseases* (11th rev.). https://icd.who.int/browse/2024-01/mms/en#1336943699

World Health Organization. (2019b). *International statistical classification of diseases* (11th rev.). https://icd.who.int

DISSOCIATIVE DISORDERS

A. Dissociative neurologic symptom disorder
B. Dissociative amnesia
C. Trance disorder
D. Possession trance disorder
E. Dissociative identity disorder
F. Partial dissociative identity disorder
G. Depersonalization–derealization disorder

DEFINITION

A. Dissociative disorders are conditions characterized by a disruption of thoughts and memories in which the individual is unable to connect feelings, surroundings, memories, thoughts, behaviors, and their identity. Dissociative disorders usually start after a traumatic experience, with symptoms ranging from memory loss to the development of disconnected identities, depending on the specific type of dissociative disorder. Stress can worsen the symptoms.

DISSOCIATIVE IDENTITY DISORDER

Definition

An individual has the experience of more than one identity, and these identities function independently of each other. The identities are autonomous with their own behaviors, memories, and possibly even languages. When the patient switches identities, signs of an altered state might include, but not be limited to, eye blinking, posture changes, and eye rolling.

A. Formerly known as *multiple personality disorder*
  1. Two or more personality states exist.
  2. Some cultures see this as "possession."

B. Disruption in autobiographical memory
  1. Unable to remember everyday experiences and events (amnesia)
  2. Subconscious attempt to avoid difficult memories or traumas
  3. May have experienced ACEs

C. Affect, behavior, memory, perceptions, consciousness, and sensory motor functions possibly involved
  1. Intrusive thoughts and behaviors
  2. Inability to control mental functioning
  3. Fragmentation, depersonalization, and derealization: positive symptoms of dissociative disorders
  4. Negative symptoms: include amnesia
  5. Patients often first seen due to attempts of suicide or engaging in nonsuicidal self-injury (NSSI)

INCIDENCE

A. The prevalence of dissociative identity disorder is estimated to be approximately 1% in community-based studies.
  1. More than 85% of patients diagnosed with dissociative identity disorder have a history of childhood trauma.
  2. The prevalence of dissociative identity disorder is higher among patients receiving mental healthcare, but with wide variation.

B. This disorder is observed in 12% to 13% of the psychiatric population.
  1. Females are more likely to present with dissociative identity disorder (5:1–9:1).
  2. Lifetime prevalence is 1.5% globally, similar to that of schizophrenia.

PATHOGENESIS

A. Trauma model
  1. Based on a stress-diathesis model
      a. Occurs in individuals with a predisposition to the illness (i.e., the diathesis)
      b. Patients who have experienced a significant "stress" (e.g., a life event or environmental factor)

PREDISPOSING FACTORS

A. Person has inborn tendency to dissociate (i.e., "dissociativity").

B. Primary stressors may include sexual abuse, physical abuse, or other severe trauma occurring during childhood.
  1. Dissociativity is a common stressor.
      a. Dissociativity can be common without experiencing mental illness and presents as an ability to be totally absorbed and detached from distraction.

b. When related to trauma, the detachment is maladaptive, including symptoms of freezing, tonic immobility, passivity, hypoarousal, and analgesia.

2. Genetic and biological factors may influence the possibility of a dissociative reaction to stressful environments.

a. A possible link between levels of dissociation and genes associated with dopamine metabolism, neuronal growth and repair, glucocorticoid response to trauma, and serotonin transport has been identified.

b. Healthy twin pairs drawn from the general population suggested a moderate to substantial genetic component to variation in dissociativity.

COMMON COMPLAINTS

A. Complaints of unaccountable or lost time, blackout spells, inability to recall information, or gaps in childhood memories
B. Presence of two or more identities/personality states
C. Rapid mood changes
D. Obsessive-compulsive personality traits
E. Use of first-person plural ("we/us") or third-person plural or singular ("he/him," "she/her," "they/them") in speech (Note: Many persons use they/them pronouns routinely.)

SUBJECTIVE REPORTS

A. Assess onset, course, and history of symptoms; evaluate ACEs.
B. Assess coping mechanisms and social functioning.
C. Assess for suicidal ideation and NSSI.
D. Assess for co-occurring SUDs.
E. Conduct a mental status exam.

PHYSICAL EXAMINATION

A. The practitioner should perform a physical examination or refer the patient to a primary care provider to rule out medical causes of the symptoms.
B. Obtain a complete medical history, including onset of symptoms.
C. Conduct a mental evaluation.

DIAGNOSTIC TESTS AND SCREENING

A. Longitudinal assessments over time are the gold standard.
B. Scales specifically for dissociative identity disorder include the following:
  1. Structured Interview for *DSM-5* Dissociative Disorders (SCID-D-R)
  2. Dissociative Disorders Interview Schedule (DDIS)
  3. Dissociative Experiences Scale
     a. Consists of 28 items
     b. Evaluates outside information related to imagination depersonalization, amnesia, and derealization
  4. Dissociation Questionnaire
     a. Consists of 63 items
     b. Measures identity fragmentation and confusion, loss of control, amnesia, and absorption
  5. Difficulties in Emotion Regulation Scale (DERS)
     a. A 36-item scale of subjective questions
     b. Investigates challenges in goal direction, impulsivity, situational responses, and emotional self-regulation

DIFFERENTIAL DIAGNOSIS

A. Anxiety disorders
B. Psychotic disorders
C. PTSD
D. Affective disorders
E. Any factitious, imitative, and/or malingered dissociative disorders
F. Neurologic/seizure disorders
G. Conversion disorder
H. MDD
I. Somatic symptom disorders
J. Neurocognitive disorders
K. Other dissociative disorders

PLAN

A. Identify and treat/reduce the intrusive, disruptive symptoms of dissociative identity disorder.
B. Establish safety and stabilization for the patient, and mitigate risk of suicide and self-injury.
  1. More than 70% of patients diagnosed with dissociative identity disorder have attempted to die by suicide.
  2. Self-injurious behavior is common with these patients.
C. Assist patient in identifying methods for integration as well as recovery/rehabilitation.

TREATMENT

A. Psychopharmacology: should target reported symptoms as well as take into account co-occurring mental health conditions
  1. Antidepressants
     a. Fluoxetine (prozac), sertraline (zoloft), and duloxetine (cymbalta): selective serotonin reuptake inhibitors (SSRIs) that may help with associated depressive symptoms
     b. Bupropion (Wellbutrin)
     c. Tricyclic antidepressants (Doxepin)
  2. Antipsychotic medications: reduce associated nightmares, disorders, frequency of alternate personality transitions, and intrusive symptoms, as well as the dissociative symptoms
     a. Aripiprazole (Abilify)
     b. Olanzapine (Zyprexa)
     c. Risperidone (Risperdal)
  3. Beta-blockers (clonidine): reduce hyperarousal and anxiety and stabilize mood
  4. Anticonvulsants: may stabilize moods
  5. Alpha-1 adrenergic receptor antagonist (Prazosin): treats PTSD-associated nightmares
  6. Benzodiazepines (use with caution due to high risk of dependence/addiction)
B. Psychotherapy
  1. Eye movement desensitization and reprocessing (EMDR)
  2. Cognitive behavioral therapy (CBT)
  3. Dialectical behavioral therapy (DBT)
  4. Hypnotherapy to reduce flashbacks
C. Complementary and alternative/adjunctive therapies
  1. Group therapy
  2. Family therapy
  3. Self-help groups
  4. Occupational therapy

PATIENT TEACHING

A. Explain all medications to the patient, including any interactions that will occur with food or drink.
B. Discuss the importance of ongoing therapy due to the chronicity of the disorder.
C. Provide the patient with the 988 crisis/suicide prevention hotline number.

FOLLOW-UP

A. Follow-up should be weekly for the first 3 months, then monthly.

B. Depending on the severity and the healthcare provider's judgment, the follow-up can be modified to occur more frequently.

CONSULTATION AND REFERRAL
A. Refer to psychiatric specialist (psychiatrist, psychiatric pharmacist) for consultation related to best practice in medication management.
B. A certified psychotherapist with experience in providing trauma-informed care and therapies should be consulted to begin or continue with the patient in psychotherapy.
C. Referrals to substance use professional or other medical specialties should be made in cases where comorbid medical issues are discovered.

INDIVIDUAL CONSIDERATIONS

Pediatrics and Adolescents
A. Transient episodes of dissociation are common and normative in childhood, decreasing as the child ages.
  1. Childhood abuse and other ACEs increase the risk of dissociative identity disorder in adulthood.
  2. Dissociation is a survival mechanism used by traumatized children and may take on the form of amnesia, derealization, depersonalization, and identity confusion.
  3. Signs and symptoms of dissociation in children include memory of a trauma, but no emotional response; behaviors that are not appropriate but no understanding of why the behavior is surfacing; and somatic illnesses like stomachaches, but without anxiety or any other evident cause.

B. There has been an increase in incidence of teens seeking help for dissociative identity disorder after self-diagnosis. Misdiagnosis of the changes in a teen's personality can be as MDD, bipolar disorder, or attention deficit hyperactivity disorder.
  1. Teens, like adults, with dissociative identity disorder have distinct personalities that are dramatically different from each other and can include differences in gender identification, speech, language, and age.
  2. These changes are not related to use of any substance, nor subsequent to any altered state of consciousness during or after a religious/spiritual ceremony.

Transgender Individuals
A. Gender incongruence (*ICD-11*; WHO, 2019) is a sexual health classification that indicates a marked incongruence between assigned gender and experienced gender.
B. Being transgender is not a risk factor for dissociative identity disorder; however, childhood trauma is a risk factor, and all patients should be screened for past abuse.

Veterans and Minority/Underrepresented Individuals
A. These patients are at higher risk for dissociative symptoms due to experiences in adulthood. These symptoms should not be confused with dissociative disorder. It is childhood abuse that is the greatest risk factor for developing dissociative disorder.

Geriatrics/Older Adults
A. Diagnosis of dissociative identity disorder is rare in older adults. Patients must be evaluated for neurocognitive disorders that may produce dissociative-like symptoms.

Families/Significant Others
A. Concerned family members and significant others may want to consider:
  1. Learning about dissociative identity disorder and other dissociative disorders
  2. Listening to the loved one and offering support
  3. Staying connected with support services
  4. Addressing suicidal and self-harming behaviors and ideations
  5. Engaging in self-care

RESOURCES
A. American Psychiatric Association: www.psychiatry.org/patients-families/dissociative-disorders/expert-q-and-a
B. Support Sheet for Dissociative Disorders: www.isst-d.org/wp-content/uploads/2022/03/2022-Support-Sheet-Supporting-a-Loved-One.pdf

REFERENCES AND BIBLIOGRAPHY
Atilan Fedai, Ü., & Asoğlu, M. (2022). Analysis of demographic and clinical characteristics of patients with dissociative identity disorder. *Neuropsychiatric Disease and Treatment, 18,* 3035–3044. https://doi.org/10.2147/NDT.S386648

Foote, B. (2024, August). *Dissociative identity disorder: Epidemiology, pathogenesis, clinical manifestations, course, assessment, and diagnosis.* UpToDate. https://www.uptodate.com/contents/dissociative-identity-disorder-epidemiology-pathogenesis-clinical-manifestations-course-assessment-and-diagnosis

World Health Organization. (2019). *International statistical classification of diseases* (11th rev.). https://icd.who.int

GENERALIZED ANXIETY DISORDER

DEFINITION
A. Generalized anxiety disorder (GAD) presents with complaints of persistent worry that is in excess of what is reasonable. The worrying is uncontrollable and irrational.
B. The apprehension is experienced often, occurring more days in the week than not and persisting for at least 6 months. The *DSM-5* (American Psychiatric Association, 2013) specific criteria for GAD are listed under anxiety disorders. The *ICD-11* (WHO, 2019) correlates anxiety with fear-related disorders, which reflect specific cognitions that are helpful in differentiating the associated conditions.
C. The worry may be accompanied by physical signs and symptoms that include:
  1. Fatigue
  2. Restlessness
  3. Irritability
  4. Inability to concentrate
  5. Disturbances in sleeping patterns
  6. Unrelenting muscle tension

D. The worrying feelings and accompanying physical symptoms are not explained by a different psychological/psychiatric disorder, including but not limited to:
  1. Worry about having panic attacks in panic disorder
  2. Contamination or other obsessions in OCD
  3. Separation from attachment figures in separation anxiety disorder
  4. Reminders of traumatic events in PTSD
  5. Delusional beliefs in schizophrenia or delusional disorder

E. The signs and symptoms are not attributable to the physiologic effects of a substance, including but not limited to:
  1. Prescribed medication
  2. Polypharmacy
  3. Illegal drug use

F. The signs and symptoms are not attributable to the physiologic effect of a medical condition, including but not limited to:
  1. Hyperthyroidism
  2. Traumatic brain injury

INCIDENCE
A. 5% to 7% of adults in the United States will experience GAD in their lifetime.
B. 3.1% of Americans are affected by GAD, with less than half (43.2%) being treated for it.

PATHOGENESIS
A. The exact pathogenesis of GAD is not fully known.
B. The pathogenesis of GAD involves the neurologic structures of the brain as well as genetics.
C. Common pathways identified in GAD include the serotonin systems and the noradrenergic system.

PREDISPOSING FACTORS
A. There are multiple predisposing or risk factors for anxiety disorders, including low self-esteem, family history of MDD, female sex assigned at birth, ACEs, childhood sexual abuse, White race, and disturbed family environment.
B. Perinatal stress is also a predisposing factor.
C. Perceived discrimination is another predisposing factor.

COMMON COMPLAINTS
A. See Table 9.1.

SUBJECTIVE REPORTS
A. Assess onset, course, and history of symptoms.
B. Assess coping mechanisms and social functioning.
C. Assess suicidal ideation.
D. Conduct a mental status exam.

PHYSICAL EXAMINATION
A. The practitioner should perform a physical examination or refer the patient to a primary care provider to rule out medical causes of the symptoms.
B. Obtain a complete medical history, including onset of symptoms.
C. Perform a mental evaluation.

TABLE 9.1 COMMON COMPLAINTS IN GENERALIZED ANXIETY DISORDER

Possible Psychological Symptoms	Possible Physical Signs
Persistent, uncontrollable worry	Feeling twitchy or trembly
Difficulty concentrating	Unable to sleep, fatigue
Indecisiveness that leads to dread or paralyzing concern of making a wrong choice	Nervousness
Belief that situations and events, which are not threatening, are menacing or very hazardous	Irritability
Unable to relax or let go of worry	Muscle tensions, muscle aches
Always seeing the worst possible outcomes, leading to overthinking common plans or solutions	Gastrointestinal symptoms, nausea, diarrhea, irritable bowel syndrome

D. Suggestions for the exam can be found in the "Physical Examination" and "Psychometric Tools" sections for all anxiety disorders earlier in this chapter.

DIAGNOSTIC TESTS AND SCREENING
A. There are no laboratory tests for GAD.
B. Screening tools include the following:
  1. Level 1 *DSM-5* (American Psychiatric Association, 2013) Cross-Cutting Symptoms Measures for Adults and Youth
  2. Level 2 *DSM-5* (American Psychiatric Association, 2013) Cross-Cutting Symptom Measures: Anxiety (Patient-Reported Outcomes Measurement Information System [PROMIS]) for Adults and Youth
  3. Generalized Anxiety Disorder-7 (GAD-7)
  4. Generalized Anxiety Disorder Severity Scale (GADSS)
  5. Hamilton Anxiety Rating Scale (HARS)
  6. *DSM-5* (American Psychiatric Association, 2013) Level 2 Anxiety Tool, which can be found online and used for free at www.psychiatry.org/getmedia/f284f967-ed9e-4754-99fc-b32765b1c4a0/APA-DSM5TR-Level2AnxietyAdult.pdf

DIFFERENTIAL DIAGNOSIS
A. Hyperthyroidism
B. Substances abuse disorders
C. Pheochromocytoma
D. Panic disorders

PLAN
A. Identification and treatment/reduction of the disruptive symptoms of anxiety
B. Psychopharmacology
  1. SSRIs or serotonin and norepinephrine reuptake inhibitors (SNRIs): first line
  2. Anxiolytics
     a. Buspirone: if the patient cannot tolerate SSRI or SNRI due to its adverse effects
     b. Antihistamines such as hydroxyzine, but be cautious in the older adult population due to anticholinergic adverse effect
  3. Benzodiazepines: in case of emergency or in the context of panic disorder, but only short term due to quick development of tolerance
  4. Pharmacologic treatment to be combined with psychotherapy
C. Psychotherapy
  1. CBT
  2. DBT
D. Complementary and alternative medicine
  1. Acupuncture
  2. Supplements (magnesium 400 mg)
  3. Acupressure
  4. Aromatherapy
  5. Meditation

GENERAL TREATMENT AND INTERVENTIONS
A. General treatment is focused on reducing the patient's dysregulating level of anxiety. A combination of treatments may be needed (psychopharmacology, milieu therapy, and psychotherapy) to support patient recovery.
B. Listening to the patient's needs and worries will allow the patient to express what is required. It also increases trust between the healthcare provider and the patient.

COMMON MEDICATIONS
A. SSRI: fluoxetine, sertraline, escitalopram
B. SNRI: venlafaxine, duloxetine, sibutramine

C. Buspirone
D. Hydroxyzine
E. Benzodiazepines: lorazepam, alprazolam, diazepam
F. Atypical antidepressants: mirtazapine, trazodone, bupropion

PATIENT TEACHING
A. Explain all medications to the patient, including any interactions that will occur with food or drink.
B. Discuss the need for the patient to continue taking all prescribed medications as prescribed and to alert the healthcare provider of any unwanted side effects.
C. Engage the patient to agree to notify the healthcare provider of any over-the-counter (OTC) medications that are being taken.
D. Provide patient with the 988 suicide prevention hotline number.

FOLLOW-UP
A. Follow-up should be weekly for the first 3 months, then monthly.
B. Depending on the severity and the healthcare provider's judgment, the follow-up can be modified for more frequent follow-up.

CONSULTATION AND REFERRAL
A. Refer to a psychiatric specialist (psychiatrist, psychiatric pharmacist) for consultation related to best practices in medication management.
B. A certified psychotherapist should be consulted to begin or continue with the patient in psychotherapy.
C. Referrals to endocrinology, substance use professional, or other medical specialties should be made in cases where medical issues are discovered during the initial history and medical workup.

INDIVIDUAL CONSIDERATIONS

Pediatrics and Adolescents
A. Due to the pandemic and other natural disasters, anxiety in youth has risen substantially.
B. Youth may demonstrate excessive fears and phobia-like anxiety that need to be addressed.
C. Use simple language and include supportive individuals identified by the youth.
D. Assess for suicidality. Provide the 988 suicide prevention service for text or phone call.

Transgender Individuals
A. Youth with gender dysphoria have increased prevalence of comorbid mental health challenges, including social anxiety.
B. No formal guidelines have been identified for treatment of anxiety in transgender persons.
C. CBT has been the effective standard treatment for social anxiety that uses a gender-affirming approach.
D. Refer to a certified psychotherapist.
   1. Assess the existing support system.
   2. Approach using nonbiased methods.
   3. Ask for their pronouns before initiating any conversation.
   4. Establish therapeutic rapport to build trust relationship.

Veterans
A. The most prevalent anxiety disorders in veterans are social anxiety, GAD, panic attacks, PTSD, and specific phobias.
B. CBT and exposure therapy have been identified as effective in veterans.

Minority/Underrepresented Individuals
A. Include social workers in the care.
   1. Reach out for community resources.
   2. Some cultures may consider mental health a taboo subject; a nonjudgmental approach should be used.
   3. All persons should have equal treatment regardless of their immigration status.

Geriatrics/Older Adults
A. Fears and concerns are a natural part of aging.
B. Approach the older adult with respect and a calm, reassuring demeanor.
C. Encourage engagement in social activities when possible.
D. Be aware of other conditions and medications that could increase symptoms of anxiety.

Families/Significant Others
A. Patients' rights must be primary in working with adults with GAD.
   1. Assess relationships.
   2. Identify support systems.
   3. Recognize protective factors.
   4. Examine for any risk factors.
      a. Assess for domestic violence.
B. Psychoeducation for the family includes destigmatizing the diagnosis, the medications, and the therapy.

RESOURCES
A. American Academy of Child and Adolescent Psychiatry: www.aacap.org/AACAP/Families_and_Youth/Resource_Centers/Anxiety_Disorder_Resource_Center/Home.aspx
B. Anxiety and Depression Association of America: https://adaa.org/find-help/support/community-resources
C. Veterans Association: 877-4AID-VET; 1-855-VA-WOMEN

REFERENCES AND BIBLIOGRAPHY
American Psychiatric Association. (2013). *Diagnostic and statistical manual of mental disorders* (5th ed.). https://doi.org/10.1176/appi.books.9780890425596

Blanco, C., Rubio, J., Wall, M., Wang, S., Jiu, C. J., & Kendler, K. S. (2014). Risk factors for anxiety disorders: Common and specific effects in a national sample. *Depression and Anxiety, 31*(9), 756–764. https://doi.org/10.1002/da.22247

Greene, A., Bailey, C., & Neumeister, A. (2013). A biopsychosocial approach to anxiety. In S. M. Stahl & B. A. Moore (Eds.), *Anxiety disorders: A guide for integrating psychopharmacology and psychotherapy* (pp. 25–50). Routledge.

MacIntyre, M. M., Zare, M., & Williams, M. T. (2023). Anxiety-related disorders in the context of racism. *Current Psychiatry Reports, 25*(2), 31–43. https://doi.org/10.1007/s11920-022-01408-2

Radez, J., Reardon, T., Creswell, C., Orchard, F., & Waite, P. (2022). Adolescents' perceived barriers and facilitators to seeking and accessing professional help for anxiety and depressive disorders: A qualitative interview study. *European Child & Adolescent Psychiatry, 31*, 891–907. https://doi.org/10.1007/s00787-020-01707-0

Santomauro, D., & COVID-19 Mental Disorders Collaborators. (2021). Global prevalence and burden of depressive and anxiety disorders in 204 countries and territories in 2020 due to the COVID-19 pandemic. *Lancet. 398*(10312), 1700–1712. https://doi.org/10.1016/S0140-6736(21)02143-7

World Health Organization. (2019). *International statistical classification of diseases* (11th rev.). https://icd.who.int

ILLNESS ANXIETY DISORDER

DEFINITION
A. Illness anxiety disorder (IAD; previously called *hypochondriasis*) is a psychiatric disorder defined by unnecessary worry about, or preoccupation with, having or developing a serious

medical condition. People with IAD usually present with anxiety or fear of developing or having a serious medical illness despite normal physical examination and laboratory testing results. Actual somatic symptoms are either missing or mild. This is a chronic and relapsing condition. There are generally two types: (a) care-seeking type and (b) care-avoidant type.

INCIDENCE
A. The estimated prevalence of IAD in the medical outpatient environment is about 0.75%.
B. In the general population, IAD is about 0.1%.
C. IAD is common in adolescents, with no gender preponderance, and it typically worsens with age.
D. IAD is more common in persons who are not employed or who have a lower level of education.

PATHOGENESIS
A. The exact etiology of IAD is unknown.
B. Comorbidities with anxiety disorders include GAD, panic disorder, and OCD.
C. 66% of those with IAD present with at least one comorbid psychiatric disorder, with cluster C personality disorders more common.
D. IAD usually begins in early or middle adulthood and worsens with age.
  1. In the older individual, the preoccupation might focus on memory loss.
E. The condition is affected by multiple risk factors.
  1. Family history of anxiety disorders
  2. Serious illness in childhood
  3. Underlying anxiety disorders
  4. Excessive amount of time spent on the internet reviewing diseases

PREDISPOSING FACTORS
A. Threat of a major illness that proves to be not as serious as believed
B. Experiencing a serious childhood illness or having a significant other with a serious illness during the patient's childhood
C. Temperament of a worrier, coming from a family that is preoccupied with health issues
D. Experiencing a time of major life stress
E. ACEs
F. Anxiety disorders, panic disorder
G. Sleep disorder: insomnia

COMMON COMPLAINTS
A. Excessive worry/preoccupation about developing a life-threatening or debilitating disease
B. Mild or absent somatic symptoms; excessive anxiety related to medical conditions experienced by family members possibly also a risk factor
C. Easy to alarm related to personal health; maintains an excessive level of fear about failing health
D. Obsessive health-related behaviors such as examining self for signs of illness or maladaptive avoidance of healthcare professionals and institutions
E. Condition persisting for at least 6 months
F. No different psychiatric disorder that would explain the preoccupation with the illness

PHYSICAL EXAMINATION
A. Perform a physical examination or refer the patient to a primary care provider to rule out medical causes of the symptoms.
B. Assess onset, course, and history of symptoms.
C. Include assessment on coping mechanisms and social functioning.
D. Assess suicidal ideation.
E. Conduct a mental status exam.

DIAGNOSTIC TESTS AND SCREENING
A. There are no diagnostic tests for IAD.
B. Screening tools include the following:
  1. The Short Health Anxiety Inventory (SHAI) is an 18-item survey used to assess health anxiety independent of physical health status. The items assess worry about personal health, awareness of bodily sensations and/or changes, and the feared consequences of having an illness.
  2. The Whiteley Index (WI) is a 14-item test for three dimensions: disease phobia, somatic preoccupation, and disease conviction.

DIFFERENTIAL DIAGNOSIS
A. Other medical conditions, including neurologic or endocrine conditions, occult malignancies, or other conditions involving multiple organs
B. Adjustment disorder/nonpathologic health anxiety
C. Anxiety disorders
D. OCD and related disorders
E. MDD
F. Body dysmorphic disorder
G. Conversion disorders
H. Somatic symptom disorder
I. Psychotic disorders: schizophrenia and delusional disorder

PLAN
A. Focus treatment to help the patient deal with the health anxieties they are experiencing.
B. Establish therapeutic alliance.
  1. Acknowledge the patient's fears.
  2. Avoid overuse of the medical system's diagnostic testing once IAD is established.

General Treatment and Interventions
A. Psychotherapy
  1. Psychotherapy is the gold standard as it can address the behavior of repeated, excessive body checking for signs of illness.
  2. CBT includes education related to normal somatic sensations as well as normal variations.
  3. Other therapies to consider are mindfulness-based cognitive therapy, exposure therapy, group therapies, and acceptance and commitment therapy.
B. Psychopharmacology
  1. Pharmacologic drugs are the second-line treatment for IAD.
  2. SSRIs and SNRIs are proven to be effective in IAD.

COMMON MEDICATIONS
A. SSRIs: fluoxetine (Prozac, Reconcile), sertraline (Zoloft), paroxetine (Paxil, Pexeva), escitalopram (Lexapro), fluvoxamine, vilazodone
B. SNRIs: venlafaxine (Effexor, Effexor XR), duloxetine (Cymbalta), desvenlafaxine (Pristiq), levomilnacipran (Fetzima)

PATIENT TEACHING
A. Patient education is the gold standard for IAD treatment. Empathetically validate the concerns of the patient while reassuring and educating them about normal body functions. ▶

B. Provide patient with the 988 crisis/suicide prevention hotline number.
C. Encourage regular physical activity and other activities such as breathing exercises, meditation, or yoga.
D. Suggest support groups and explore eligibility for a service animal.
E. Advise establishing a sleep hygiene routine.

FOLLOW-UP
A. Patients who are able to follow up with their primary healthcare provider may not overuse the ED or other medical facilities.
   1. Schedule regular appointments that are not contingent on the presence of symptoms.
   2. Validate the patient experience.
B. Collaboration between the psychiatric care provider and the primary care provider can support patient recovery and reduce unnecessary burden on the healthcare system.
C. Follow-up by a psychiatric team is as clinically indicated.

CONSULTATION AND REFERRAL
A. Referral to psychiatric professionals with routine follow-up with primary care provider
B. Psychotherapist

INDIVIDUAL CONSIDERATIONS

Pediatrics and Adolescents
A. Use simple language and include supportive individuals identified by the youth.
B. Assess for ACEs and past or present/ongoing physical or sexual abuse.
C. Assess for suicidality. Provide the 988 suicide prevention service for text or phone call.

Transgender Individuals
A. Transgender persons are more likely to experience psychological, physical, and sexual violence than cisgender individuals.
B. Sexual assault is a risk factor for IAD.
C. The transgender population has increased prevalence of comorbid mental health challenges, including social anxiety, and require expert treatment from medical personnel with knowledge of, and empathy for, their life experiences.
D. Refer to certified psychotherapist who uses a gender-affirming approach.
E. Ask for their preferred pronouns before initiating any conversation.
F. IAD also stands for International Asexuality Day, a coordinated worldwide campaign to support sexual/gender freedom.

Veterans
A. The most prevalent anxiety disorders in veterans are social anxiety, GAD, panic attacks, PTSD, and specific phobias.
B. CBT is effective in veterans.

Minority/Underrepresented Individuals
A. The disparity in healthcare delivery to minority/underrepresented individuals can make treating IAD in this population difficult.
B. Include social workers in the care.
   1. Reach out for community resources.
   2. Some cultures may consider mental health a taboo subject; a nonjudgmental approach should be used.
   3. All persons should have equal treatment regardless of their immigration status.

Geriatrics/Older Adults
A. Fears and concerns are a natural part of aging, fears of illness and memory loss included. Demonstrate empathy for the patient's lived experiences while avoiding unnecessary treatments, medications, or investigations.
B. Approach the older adult with respect and a calm, reassuring demeanor.
C. Encourage engagement in social activities when possible.

Families/Significant Others
A. Assess relationships and willingness of family/significant others to respect the lived experiences and fears of the patient.
B. Identify support systems.
C. Recognize protective factors.
D. Examine for any risk factors.
E. Assess for domestic violence.
F. Psychoeducation for the family includes destigmatizing the diagnosis, the medications, and the therapy.

RESOURCES
A. National Alliance on Mental Illness: www.nami.org/About-Mental-Illness/Mental-Health-Conditions/Anxiety-Disorders

REFERENCES AND BIBLIOGRAPHY
French, J. H., & Hameed, S. (2023, July 16). Illness anxiety disorder. StatPearls Publishing. https://www.ncbi.nlm.nih.gov/books/NBK554399
Salkovskis, P. M., Rimes, K. A., Warwick, H. M. C., & Clark, D. M. (2002). The health anxiety inventory: Development and validation of scales for the measurement of health anxiety and hypochondriasis. *Psychological Medicine, 32*(5), 843–853. PMID: 12171378.

MEDICATION-INDUCED ANXIETY DISORDER

DEFINITION
A. Substance/medication-induced anxiety disorder is when symptoms of anxiety or panic disorder are a direct result of taking a substance/medication. Symptoms start shortly after or during the use of the specific substance/medication or during withdrawal. The symptoms must be directly related to the substance/medication used.

INCIDENCE
A. Medication-induced anxiety disorder has a 12-month prevalence of 0.002%.
B. Approximately 17.7% of respondents with an SUD in the past 12 months also met the criteria for an independent (i.e., not attributed to withdrawal or intoxication) anxiety disorder, and 15% of those with any anxiety disorder in the past 12 months had at least one co-occurring SUD.

PREDISPOSING FACTORS
A. Use of a substance
   1. Alcohol
   2. Caffeine
   3. Cannabis
   4. Sedatives
   5. Phencyclidine
   6. Other hallucinogen
   7. Inhalant
   8. Opioid

9. Sedative-hypnotic or anxiolytic
10. Amphetamine or other stimulant
11. Cocaine
12. Other or unknown substance

COMMON COMPLAINTS

A. Recurring and unexpected panic attacks—a surge of intense fear or anxiety that goes together with certain physical symptoms
   1. Heart palpitations
   2. Sweating
   3. Shaking or trembling
   4. Feeling short of breath or unable to breathe
   5. Chest pain
   6. Nausea or abdominal pain
   7. Feeling dizzy, lightheadedness, or fainting

OTHER SIGNS AND SYMPTOMS

A. Feelings of apprehension or dread
B. Trouble concentrating
C. Feeling tense and jumpy
D. Anticipating the worst
E. Restlessness
F. Pounding heart

SUBJECTIVE REPORTS

A. Assess onset, course, and history of symptoms.
   1. Is the onset of panic or anxiety occurring in association with intoxication with alcohol, caffeine, cannabis, phencyclidine, other hallucinogens, inhalants, or stimulants?
   2. Is the occurrence of panic or anxiety associated with withdrawal from alcohol, opioids, sedatives, hypnotics, anxiolytics, or stimulants (including cocaine)?
   3. Has the patient ingested medications that can cause anxiety symptoms, including anesthetics, analgesics, sympathomimetics, bronchodilators (e.g., theophylline), anticholinergics, insulin, thyroid replacement medications, oral contraceptives, antihistamines, antiparkinsonian medications, corticosteroids, antihypertensives, cardiovascular medications, anticonvulsants, lithium, antipsychotics, and antidepressants?
   4. Was the patient exposed to any heavy metals and toxins that could also cause panic or anxiety symptoms, including organophosphate insecticide, nerve gases, carbon monoxide, carbon dioxide, and volatile substances (e.g., gasoline, paint)?
B. Assess suicidal ideation or past suicide attempts.
C. Conduct a mental status exam.

PHYSICAL EXAMINATION

A. Observation of symptoms during abstinence over time
B. Screening of patients presenting at primary care, substance use, or psychiatric treatment settings
C. Routine urine drug screening

DIFFERENTIAL DIAGNOSIS

A. GAD not due to substance use or another medical condition
B. Delirium
C. Panic disorder
D. Substance use withdrawal

PLAN

A. The symptoms should be remedied when the medication is stopped.
B. Implement mindfulness-based relapse prevention.

PATIENT TEACHING

A. Assess the patient's knowledge of medications that are prescribed as well as those that are taken recreationally.
B. Evaluate the patient's understanding of environmental hazards that could cause the symptoms of panic and anxiety.

FOLLOW-UP

A. Once the symptoms are resolved, there is no need for follow-up.
B. If the symptoms do not resolve, explore other possible causes.

CONSULTATION AND REFERRAL

A. If the patient has a co-occurring SUD or comorbid medical condition that requires follow-up, appropriate referrals can be made.

INDIVIDUAL CONSIDERATIONS

A. With the older adult patient, assess their ability to take medications properly and their knowledge of the side effects.
B. Remind patients and family members to keep all substances out of the reach of children.

REFERENCE AND BIBLIOGRAPHY

Brady, K. T., Haynes, L. F., Hartwell, K. J., & Killeen, T. K. (2013). Substance use disorders and anxiety: A treatment challenge for social workers. *Social Work in Public Health, 28*(3–4), 407–423. https://doi.org/10.1080/19371918.2013.774675

OBSESSIVE-COMPULSIVE DISORDER

DEFINITION

A. Obsessive-compulsive disorder (OCD) is a long-lasting disorder in which a person has uncontrollable and recurring thoughts, engages in repetitive behaviors (compulsions), or both. People with OCD have time-consuming symptoms that can cause significant distress or interfere with daily life.

INCIDENCE

A. See Figure 9.2.

PATHOGENESIS

A. The pathophysiology of OCD is overly persistent and uncontrolled neural activity in the sympathetic nervous system, possibly due to a dopamine–serotonin imbalance. Evidence of OCD symptoms from drugs, brain injury, and infection is consistent with disturbed basal ganglia regulation as the pathophysiology of OCD.

   B. Obsessions are intrusive or unwanted repetitive or persistent thoughts, images, or urges that cause marked distress or anxiety. Obsessions often involve content that is odd, irrational, or of a seemingly magical nature (e.g., harm will come if the closet is not arranged in a specific order). Individuals with OCD attempt to ignore, suppress, or neutralize these thoughts, often with another thought or behavior (compulsion).

   C. Compulsions (or rituals) involve repetitive behaviors (e.g., washing, checking) or mental acts (e.g., counting, repeating words silently) that an individual feels driven to perform to reduce the distress triggered by an obsession or according to rules that must be applied rigidly.

PREDISPOSING FACTORS

A. OCD appears to be more common in individuals with some psychiatric disorders than in the general population.
B. These disorders include the following:
   1. Anxiety disorders

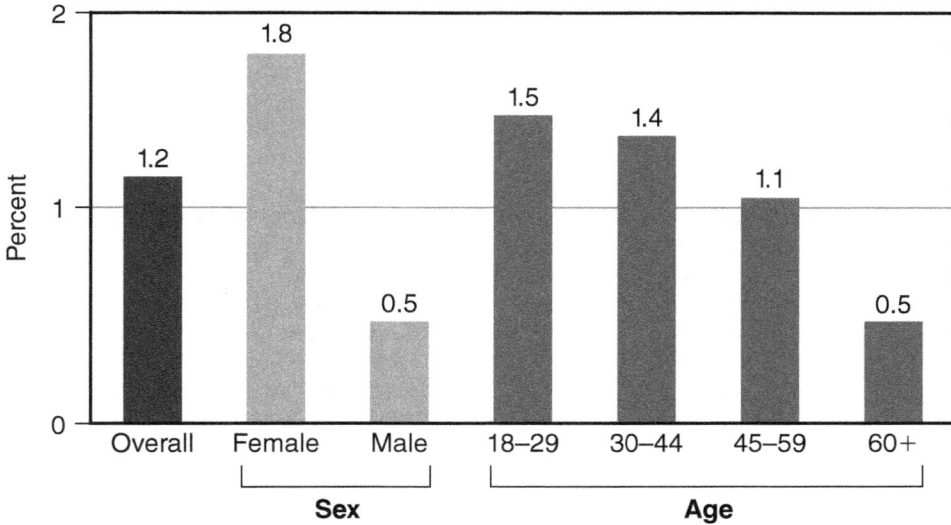

FIGURE 9.2 Past year prevalence of obsessive-compulsive disorder among U.S. adults, 2001 to 2003.

Source: National Institute of Mental Health. (n.d.). *Obsessive-compulsive disorder (OCD)*. U.S. Department of Health and Human Services. https://www.nimh.nih.gov/health/statistics/obsessive-compulsive-disorder-ocd; Data from National Comorbidity Survey Replication (NCS-R).

2. Mood disorders
3. Obsessive-compulsive personality disorder
4. Tic disorders
5. Genetic factors
6. Stress/trauma

COMMON COMPLAINTS
A. Patient has inability to control obsessive or compulsive behaviors and/or thoughts.
B. Obsessive-compulsive behaviors are not pleasurable but they provide temporary relief from the anxiety.
C. Obsessions might revolve around a theme like fear of contamination, or needing things to be very orderly, or worry about loss of control of one's behavior.
D. Complaints about compulsion symptoms might include having skin that has been washed so frequently it is raw, or the inability to leave the house without rechecking the lights/stove/door multiple times.

SUBJECTIVE REPORTS
A. Excessive worries, as in GAD
B. Preoccupation with appearance, as in body dysmorphic disorder
C. Difficulty discarding or parting with possessions, as in hoarding disorder
D. Hairpulling, as in trichotillomania (hairpulling disorder)
E. Skin picking, as in excoriation (skin picking) disorder
F. Stereotypies, as in stereotypic movement disorder
G. Ritualized eating behavior, as in eating disorders
H. Preoccupation with substances or gambling, as in substance-related and addictive disorders
I. Preoccupation with having an illness, as in IAD
J. Sexual urges or fantasies, as in paraphilic disorders
K. Impulses, as in disruptive, impulse control, and conduct disorders
L. Guilty ruminations, as in MDD
M. Thought insertion or delusional preoccupations, as in schizophrenia spectrum and other psychotic disorders
N. Repetitive patterns of behavior, as in autism spectrum disorder

PHYSICAL EXAMINATION
A. Perform a physical examination or refer the patient to a primary care provider to rule out medical causes of the symptoms.
    1. Obtain a complete medical history, including onset of symptoms.
    2. Assess course and history of symptoms.
    3. Assess coping mechanisms and social functioning.
B. Assess suicidal ideation.
C. Conduct a mental status exam.

DIAGNOSTIC TESTS AND SCREENING
A. There is currently no lab or other diagnostic test for OCD.
B. Screening scales include the following:
    1. Yale-Brown Obsessive Compulsive Scale (Y-BOCS)
    2. Leyton Obsessional Inventory Short Form (30 items)
    3. Obsessive Intrusions Inventory (OII): a questionnaire examining intrusive thoughts, images, and impulses

DIFFERENTIAL DIAGNOSIS
A. Anxiety disorders
B. Specific phobia
C. Hoarding disorder
D. MDD

PLAN
A. Medication management
    1. Tricyclic antidepressant
        a. Clomipramine (Anafranil)
    2. SSRIs
        a. Fluoxetine
        b. Fluvoxamine
        c. Paroxetine
        d. Sertraline
        e. Citalopram
        f. Escitalopram
B. Psychotherapy
    1. CBT
    2. Exposure and response prevention therapy

PATIENT TEACHING

A. Explain the benefit of the combination of medication and psychotherapy.
B. Educate patient on medication management.
  1. Explain all medications to the patient and any interactions that will occur with food or drink.
  2. Discuss the need for the patient to continue taking all prescribed medications as prescribed and to alert the healthcare provider of any unwanted side effects.
  3. Engage the patient to agree to notify the healthcare provider of any OTC medications that are being taken.
C. Provide patient with the 988 suicide prevention hotline number.

FOLLOW-UP

A. Follow-up should be weekly for the first 3 months, then monthly.

CONSULTATION AND REFERRAL

A. Refer to psychiatric specialist (psychiatrist, psychiatric pharmacist) for consultation related to best practice in medication management.
B. A certified psychotherapist with experience in providing trauma-informed care and therapies should be consulted to begin or continue with the patient in psychotherapy.
C. Referrals to substance use professional or other medical specialties should be made in cases where comorbid medical issues are discovered.

INDIVIDUAL CONSIDERATIONS

Pediatrics and Adolescents

A. Patient exhibits diminished ability to articulate concerns.
  1. These patients lack ability to recognize that obsessions are not normal.
  2. Obsessions might be inferred by parents who observe the rituals.
  3. Hoarding is seen in about 25% of youth with OCD, who collect items that are not usual for their age and become upset if they are discarded
B. Adolescents might have tensions that focus on sexual, moral, and religious ideas.
  1. Confessing and apologizing for ritualistic behaviors
  2. Contamination obsessions related to disgust
C. Greater family involvement increases OCD symptoms and functional impairment.

Transgender Individuals

A. People with transgender OCD (TOCD) worry that their thoughts might be a sign of a desire to transition their gender presentation. This is reflected in their discomfort and intolerance for uncertainty, which heightens their anxiety.
  1. TOCD is not gender dysphoria.
  2. Compulsive behaviors include emotional checking, memory review, researching, and reassurance seeking.
B. Exposure and response prevention is recommended for all patients with OCD and also those with TOCD.
C. Find therapists who specialize in treating TOCD.

Veterans

A. Exposure and response prevention therapy is the psychotherapeutic treatment for OCD in veterans.
B. Assessment of PTSD for veterans is imperative.
  1. If the veteran has co-occurring PTSD, exposure and response prevention therapy has been demonstrated to be adversely influenced by the PTSD.
  2. Examine the differential diagnosis between OCD and PTSD in veterans at www.mirecc.va.gov/visn16/docs/ocd-and-ptsd-fact-sheet.pdf.

Minority/Underrepresented Individuals

A. Minorities face many barriers to treatment for OCD. Only 20% of minority patients receive specialized mental health treatment for OCD.
  1. Cultural factors may contribute to a higher prevalence of magical/superstitious OCD subtype.
  2. Assess for religious affiliation and cultural beliefs/norms that may present as OCD rituals.

Geriatrics/Older Adults

A. Integrating behavior activation, family involvement, and CBT supports better outcomes for exposure and response prevention therapy of OCD in the older population.
B. Older persons with dementia present difficulties to the caregiver. Exposure and response prevention therapy coupled with mindfulness and medications can be helpful to this population.

Families/Significant Others

A. Assist family members in modifying their expectations and recognize small improvements.
B. Help family members find support to allow them to create supportive environments.
C. Support family members in identifying modes of self-care.

RESOURCES

A. International OCD Foundation: Conference series: https://iocdf.org/programs/conferences/?gclid=EAIaIQobChMIycb8xLa9ggMVkEZHAR3jxAETEAAYASAAEgJLMPD_BwE
B. National Alliance on Mental Illness: Obsessive-compulsive disorder: www.nami.org/about-mental-illness/mental-health-conditions/obsessive-compulsive-disorder

REFERENCES AND BIBLIOGRAPHY

Geller, D. A., Homayoun, S., & Johnson, G. (2021). Developmental considerations in obsessive compulsive disorder: Comparing pediatric and adult-onset cases. *Frontiers in Psychiatry, 12,* 678538. https://doi.org/10.3389/fpsyt.2021.678538

National Institute of Mental Health. (n.d.). *Obsessive-compulsive disorder.* U.S. Department of Health and Human Services. https://www.nimh.nih.gov/health/topics/obsessive-compulsive-disorder-ocd

Richter, M. A., Cox, B. J., & Direnfeld, D. M. (1994). A comparison of three assessment instruments for obsessive-compulsive symptoms. *Journal of Behavior Therapy and Experimental Psychiatry, 25*(2), 143–147. https://doi.org/10.1016/0005-7916(94)90007-8

Szechtman, H., Shivji, S., & Woody, E. Z. (2014). Pathophysiology of obsessive-compulsive disorder: Insights from normal function and neurotoxic effects of drugs, infection, and brain injury. In R. M. Kostrzewa (Ed.), *Handbook of neurotoxicity* (pp. 1–23). Springer Publishing Company. https://link.springer.com/referenceworkentry/10.1007/978-1-4614-5836-4_118

Pittenger, C. (n.d.). *Obsessive-compulsive disorder in adults: Epidemiology, clinical features, and diagnosis.* UpToDate. https://www.uptodate.com/contents/obsessive-compulsive-disorder-in-adults-epidemiology-clinical-features-and-diagnosis

PANIC DISORDER

DEFINITION

A. Panic disorder is an anxiety disorder characterized by unexpected and repeated episodes of intense fear accompanied by

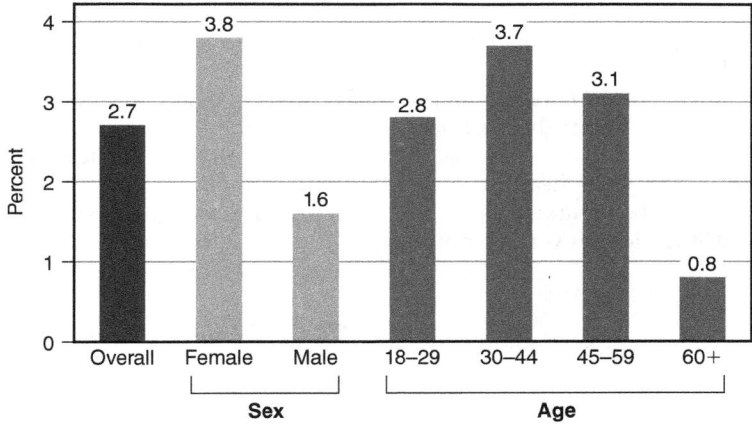

FIGURE 9.3 Past year prevalence of panic disorder among U.S. adults, 2001 to 2003.

Source: National Institute of Mental Health. (n.d.). *Panic disorder.* U.S. Department of Health and Human Services. https://www.nimh.nih.gov/health/statistics/panic-disorder; Data from National Comorbidity Survey Replication (NCS-R).

physical symptoms that may include chest pain, heart palpitations, shortness of breath, dizziness, or abdominal distress. These episodes occur "out of the blue," not in conjunction with a known fear or stressor.

INCIDENCE
A. See Figure 9.3.

PATHOGENESIS
A. CNS neurotransmitters and peptides underlie the physical systems.
  1. Limbic and frontal brain regions demonstrate increased flow and receptor activity.
  2. Dysfunction of the amygdala is prominent.
  3. There is a high correlation between medical illness and panic disorder.
  4. Theoretical basis for the pathogenesis of panic disorder include the following:
     a. Neurochemical mechanisms inhibit serotonin malfunction, causing increased serotonin to activate the fear network model in the autonomic nervous system.
     b. Endogenous opioids deficiency activates the patient's level of separation anxiety, thereby increasing the sense and awareness of suffocation.

PREDISPOSING FACTORS
A. Family history of panic attacks or panic disorder
B. Major life stress, such as the death or serious illness of a loved one
C. Traumatic event, such as sexual assault or a serious accident
D. Major life changes, such as a divorce or the addition of a baby
E. Smoking or excessive caffeine intake
F. History of childhood physical or sexual abuse

COMMON COMPLAINTS
A. Chest pain
B. Palpitations
C. Dyspnea
D. Diaphoresis
E. Tremors
F. Choking sensation
G. Nausea
H. Chills
I. Paresthesia
J. Feelings of depersonalization

SUBJECTIVE REPORTS
A. Assess onset, course, and history of symptoms.
B. Assess coping mechanisms and social functioning.
C. Assess suicidal ideation.
D. Conduct a mental status exam.

PHYSICAL EXAMINATION
A. Perform a physical examination or refer the patient to a primary care provider to rule out medical causes of the symptoms.
B. Obtain a complete medical history, including onset of symptoms.
C. Perform a mental status exam.
D. Suggestions for the exam can be found in the "Physical Examination" and "Psychometric Tools" sections for all anxiety disorders earlier in this chapter.

DIAGNOSTIC TESTS AND SCREENING
A. Presently, there are no lab tests specific to panic disorder.
  1. Indiana University has developed a blood test to measure levels of a person's anxiety and risk. This test is still in the development stage and not yet validated.
B. Screening tools include the following:
  1. Panic Disorder Severity Scale (PDSS)
  2. Panic Disorder Screener (PADIS)

DIFFERENTIAL DIAGNOSIS
A. Anxiety disorders
B. Substance-induced anxiety
C. Specific phobia
D. PTSD

PLAN
A. Identify psychopharmacologic intervention.
B. Identify psychotherapeutic interventions.
C. Include supportive resources for patient and family/significant others as indicated.

COMMON MEDICATIONS
A. Antidepressants and benzodiazepines
B. SSRIs
C. Gabapentin and mirtazapine

PATIENT TEACHING
A. Explain all medications to the patient, including any interactions that will occur with food or drink.
B. Discuss the need for the patient to continue taking all prescribed medications as prescribed and to alert the healthcare provider of any unwanted side effects.
C. Engage the patient to agree to notify the healthcare provider of any OTC medications that are being taken.
D. Provide the patient with the 988 suicide prevention hotline number.

FOLLOW-UP
A. Follow-up should be weekly for the first 3 months, then monthly.
B. Depending on the severity and the healthcare provider's judgment, the follow-up can occur more frequently.

CONSULTATION AND REFERRAL
A. Refer to or consult with a psychiatric specialist (psychiatrist, psychiatric pharmacist) for consultation related to best practice in medication management.
B. A certified psychotherapist should be consulted to begin or continue with the patient in psychotherapy.
C. Referrals to endocrinology, substance use professional, or other medical specialties should be made in cases where medical issues are discovered during the initial history and medical workup.

INDIVIDUAL CONSIDERATIONS

Pediatrics and Adolescents
A. Due to the pandemic and other natural disasters, anxiety in youth has risen substantially.
B. Youth may demonstrate excessive fears and phobia-like anxiety that needs to be addressed.
C. Use simple language and include supportive individuals identified by the youth.
D. Assess for suicidality. Provide the 988 suicide prevention service for text or phone call.

Transgender Individuals
A. Youth with gender dysphoria have increased prevalence of comorbid mental health challenges, including social anxiety.
B. No formal guidelines have been identified for treatment of anxiety in transgender persons.
C. CBT has been an effective standard treatment for social anxiety that uses a gender-affirming approach.
D. Refer to a certified psychotherapist versed in transgender issues.
   1. Assess existing support system.
   2. Approach using nonbiased methods.
   3. Ask for their pronouns before initiating any conversation.
   4. Establish therapeutic rapport to build trust relationship.

Veterans
A. The most prevalent anxiety disorders in veterans are social anxiety, GAD, panic attacks, PTSD, and specific phobias.
B. CBT is effective in veterans.

Minority/Underrepresented Individuals
A. Include social workers in care.
   1. Reach out for community resources
   2. Some cultures may consider mental health a taboo subject; a nonjudgmental approach should be used.
   3. All persons should have equal treatment regardless of their immigration status.

Geriatrics/Older Adults
A. Fears and concerns are a natural part of aging.
B. Approach the older adult with respect and a calm, reassuring demeanor.
C. Encourage engagement in social activities when possible.
D. Be aware of other conditions and medications that could increase their symptoms of anxiety.

Families/Significant Others
A. Patients' rights must be primary in working with adults with panic disorder.
   1. Assess relationships.
   2. Identify support systems.
   3. Recognize protective factors.
   4. Examine for any risk factors.
      a. Assess for domestic violence.
B. Psychoeducation for the family includes destigmatizing the diagnosis, the medications, and the therapy.

RESOURCES
A. Anxiety and Depression Association of America provides webinars and videos: https://adaa.org/understanding-anxiety/panic-disorder/resources
B. Panic Disorder: Answers to Your Most Important Questions: www.apa.org/topics/anxiety/panic-disorder
C. Panic Attacks and Panic Disorder: www.anxiety.org/panic-disorder-panic-attacks

REFERENCES AND BIBLIOGRAPHY
Cackovic, C., Nazir, S., & Marwaha, R. (2023, August 6). *Panic disorder*. StatPearls Publishing. https://www.ncbi.nlm.nih.gov/books/NBK430973

National Institute of Mental Health. (n.d.). *Panic disorder*. U.S. Department of Health and Human Services. https://www.nimh.nih.gov/health/statistics/panic-disorder

PHOBIAS

DEFINITION
A. A phobia is an uncontrollable, irrational, and lasting fear of a certain object, situation, or activity. The fear can be so overwhelming that a person may go to great lengths to avoid the source of this fear. One response can be a panic attack. This is a sudden, intense fear that lasts for several minutes. It happens when there is no real danger.
B. Three main groups of phobias have been identified:
   1. Specific or simple phobias, which usually focuses on objects and is the most common type of phobia
   2. Social phobia, which occurs in situations that are public and can be very anxiety-provoking
   3. Agoraphobia, which is fear of public places or situations
      a. Agoraphobia with panic disorder
      b. Agoraphobia without panic disorder

INCIDENCE
A. See Figure 9.4.

PATHOGENESIS
A. The exact etiology of specific phobias is not known. However, some theories suggest that specific phobias may develop due to an association of a specific object or situation with emotions such as fear and panic. Two theories have been proposed to show this pairing.

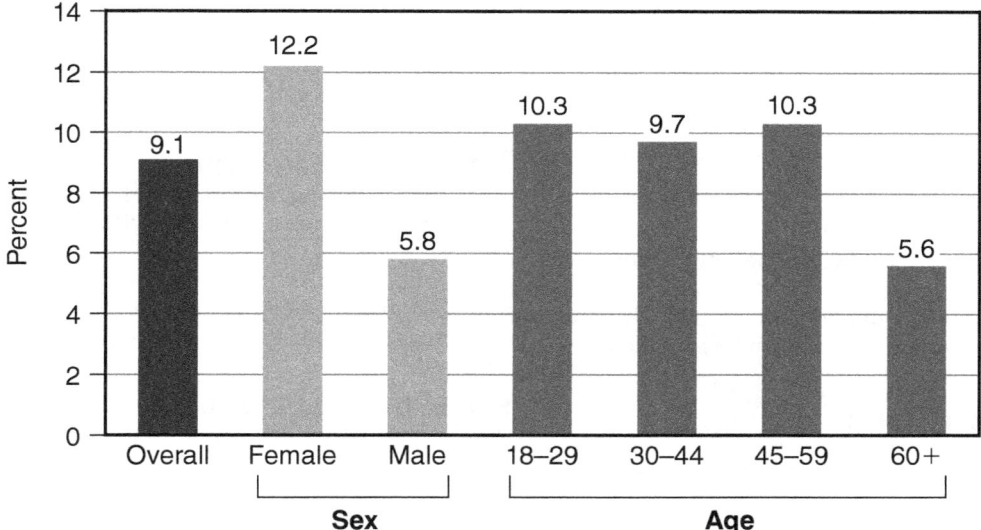

FIGURE 9.4 Past year prevalence of specific phobia among U.S. adults.

Source: National Institute of Mental Health. (n.d.). *Specific phobia.* U.S. Department of Health and Human Services. https://www.nimh.nih.gov/health/statistics/specific-phobia; Data from National Comorbidity Survey Replication (NCS-R).

B. The most common theory—classical conditioning model—postulates that a phobia precipitates when an event that provokes fear or anxiety is paired with a neutral event. An example of this would be in which a specific event such as driving is paired with an emotional experience such as an accident. As a result, the person is susceptible to a chronic emotional association between driving and anxiety. Although a person may not experience a panic attack or meet the criteria for a panic disorder, they may develop a fear that is expressed as having a specific phobia.

C. Another mechanism of association is through modeling, in which a person observes a reaction in another person and internalizes that other person's fears or warnings about the dangers of a specific object or situation.

PREDISPOSING FACTORS
A. Bad or adverse experiences
B. Genetics or learned behavior
C. Brain function and structure

COMMON COMPLAINTS
A. Feeling unsteady, dizziness, lightheadedness, or fainting
B. Feeling of choking
C. Pounding heart, palpitations, or accelerated heart rate
D. Chest pain or tightness in the chest
E. Sweating
F. Hot or cold flushes
G. Shortness of breath or a smothering sensation
H. Nausea, vomiting, or diarrhea

SUBJECTIVE REPORTS
A. Assess onset, course, and history of symptoms.
B. Assess coping mechanisms and social functioning.
C. Assess suicidal ideation.

PHYSICAL EXAMINATION
A. Perform a physical examination or refer the patient to a primary care provider to rule out medical causes of the symptoms.
B. Obtain a complete medical history, including onset of symptoms.

C. Conduct a mental status exam.
D. Note marked fear or anxiety regarding a specific object or situation, often including the following features:
  1. The specific object or situation almost always provokes immediate fear or anxiety.
  2. Children may express fear or anxiety by crying, tantrums, freezing, or clinging.
  3. The phobic object or situation is actively and persistently avoided for 6 months or more.
  4. The fear or anxiety experienced is out of proportion to the actual danger posed by the specific object or situation.
  5. Notable, clinical distress or impairment in social, occupational, or other important areas of functioning is evident.
  6. The symptoms cannot be explained by another psychiatric disorder such OCD, PTSD, separation anxiety disorder, or social anxiety disorder.

DIAGNOSTIC TESTS AND SCREENING
A. There are no lab tests that test for phobias.
B. The Social Phobia Inventory (SPIN) can be used to screen patients for the disorder.

DIFFERENTIAL DIAGNOSIS
A. Angina
B. Asthma
C. Congestive heart failure
D. Mitral valve prolapse
E. Pulmonary embolism
F. SUD
G. Other mental health disorders associated with panic attacks

PLAN

General Treatment and Interventions
A. Exposure therapy is the most common effective treatment.

PATIENT TEACHING
A. Educate patient on medication management.
  1. Explain all medications to the patient, including any interactions that will occur with food or drink.

2. Discuss the need for the patient to continue taking all prescribed medications as prescribed and to alert the healthcare provider of any unwanted side effects.
3. Engage the patient to agree to notify the healthcare provider of any OTC medications that are being taken.

B. Provide patient with the 988 suicide prevention hotline number.

FOLLOW-UP
A. Follow-up should be weekly for the first 3 months, then monthly.
B. Specific follow-up will depend on the severity and the healthcare provider's judgment and can be modified to occur more frequently.

CONSULTATION AND REFERRAL
A. Refer to a psychiatric specialist (psychiatrist, psychiatric pharmacist) for consultation related to best practice in medication management.
B. A certified psychotherapist should be consulted to begin or continue with the patient in psychotherapy.
C. Referrals to endocrinology, substance use professional, or other medical specialties should be made in cases where medical issues are discovered during the initial history and medical workup.

INDIVIDUAL CONSIDERATIONS

Pediatrics and Adolescents
A. Due to the pandemic and other natural disasters, anxiety in youth has risen substantially.
1. Youth may demonstrate excessive fears and phobia-like anxiety that need to be addressed.
2. CBT and exposure therapy have been demonstrated to be effective in youth.

B. Use simple language and include supportive individuals identified by the youth.
C. Assess for suicidality. Provide the 988 suicide prevention service for text or phone call.

Transgender Individuals
A. Youth with gender dysphoria have increased prevalence of comorbid mental health challenges, including phobias.
B. No formal guidelines have been identified for treatment of anxiety disorders in transgender persons.
C. Exposure therapy, which employs a gender-affirming approach, has been the effective standard treatment for phobias.
D. Refer to a certified psychotherapist.
1. Assess the existing support system.
2. Approach using nonbiased methods.
3. Ask for the patient's preferred pronouns before initiating any conversation.
4. Establish therapeutic rapport to build trust relationship.

Veterans
A. The most prevalent anxiety disorders in veterans are social anxiety, GAD, panic attacks, PTSD, and specific phobias.
B. CBT has been demonstrated to be effective in veterans.

Minority/Underrepresented Individuals
A. Include social workers in the care.
1. Reach out for community resources.

2. Some cultures may consider mental health a taboo subject; a nonjudgmental approach should be used.
3. All persons should have equal treatment regardless of their immigration status.

Geriatrics/Older Adults
A. Fears and concerns are a natural part of aging.
B. Approach the older adult with respect and a calm, reassuring demeanor.
C. Encourage engagement in social activities when possible.
D. Be aware of other conditions and medications that could increase their symptoms of anxiety.

Families/Significant Others
A. Patients' rights must be primary in working with individuals experiencing phobias.
1. Assess relationships.
2. Identify support systems.
3. Recognize protective factors.
4. Examine for any risk factors.
   a. Assess for domestic violence.

B. Psychoeducation for the family includes destigmatizing the diagnosis, the medications, and the therapy.

RESOURCES
A. 988 Suicide & Crisis Lifeline: https://988lifeline.org/
B. National Alliance on Mental Illness: www.nami.org

REFERENCES AND BIBLIOGRAPHY
Johns Hopkins Medicine. (n.d.). *What is a phobia?* https://www.hopkinsmedicine.org/health/conditions-and-diseases/phobias#:~:text=A%20phobia%20is%20an%20uncontrollable,can%20be%20a%20panic%20attack

Samra, C. K., & Abdijadid, S. (2024, August 12). *Specific phobia*. StatPearls Publishing. https://www.ncbi.nlm.nih.gov/books/NBK499923/

POSTTRAUMATIC STRESS DISORDER

DEFINITION
A. The American Psychiatric Association defines *PTSD* as a disorder experienced by a person who is exposed to an event (real or threatened) that is traumatizing, multiple ongoing traumatizing events, or circumstances. These experiential exposures make the individual fear for their life or safety, or the lives or safety of their loved ones.
B. PTSD is also known as *combat fatigue* and *shell shock* as it is common in veterans in the field.
C. PTSD can result from experiencing (virtually or in present reality) accidents, natural disasters, terrorism, sexual assault/rape, historical trauma (slavery/Holocaust), bullying, and intimate partner violence.
D. This response involves multiple systems, impacts the individual's activities of daily living, and can affect the mental, social, emotional, and physical sense of well-being.

INCIDENCE
A. PTSD affects 3.5% of adults in the United States. One in 11 Americans will be diagnosed with PTSD in their lifetime.
B. It occurs in all ethnicities and cultures and at any age.
1. Women are twice as likely to experience PTSD; however, more men (60%) have exposure to trauma than women (50%), according to the Department of Veterans Affairs.

2. The prevalence in adolescents (13–18 years of age) is 8%.
3. Latinx/Hispanic Americans, African/Black Americans, and Native Americans/Native Alaskans have higher incidence of PTSD than non-Hispanic White Americans.

PATHOGENESIS
A. Changes in the functioning of neurohormones and neurotransmitters
B. Changes in levels of glutamate (increased), serotonin (decreased), gamma-aminobutyric acid (GABA; decreased), neuropeptide Y (decreased), and other endogenous opioids
C. Reduction in hippocampal size
D. Overreactive amygdala

PREDISPOSING FACTORS
A. Sex assigned at birth: more prevalent in women
B. ACEs
C. Comorbid, preexisting psychiatric illnesses
D. Psychosocial factors: lack of support, low socioeconomic status, and low level of education
E. Exposure to a stressor

COMMON COMPLAINTS
A. Reexperiencing the original traumatic event, situation, or experience
B. Recurrent and intrusive thoughts related to the traumatic event
C. Racing heart, increased blood pressure

OTHER SIGNS AND SYMPTOMS
A. Engaging in persistent avoidance of any thought, experience, person, or situation that can activate the memory of the event
B. Thought distortions, negative self-beliefs (e.g., "I'm bad")
C. Ongoing negative emotional state that can include fear, anger, shame, or guilt
D. Social isolation or withdrawal

Possible Psychological Symptoms of Posttraumatic Stress Disorder
A. Recurrent thoughts of the event(s) arousing a fear response and hypervigilance
B. Unprovoked irritability, sense of being unsafe
C. Sudden intrusive memory or thought associated with the event(s)
D. Mood alterations
E. Self-blame for the event that caused the PTSD
F. Flashbacks and other intrusive thoughts that intensify the feeling that the event is or will be happening again

Possible Physical Signs of Posttraumatic Stress Disorder
A. Increased heart rate, increased blood pressure, exaggerated startle response, reduced interest in activities of daily living that were previously enjoyed
B. Aggressive behaviors, feeling detached or estranged from others
C. Inability to concentrate, dissociation, sleep disturbances, inability to enjoy positive emotional responses
D. Poor memory, dissociative amnesia
E. Self-destructive behaviors, suicidal ideations, reckless behaviors
F. Nervousness, hypervigilance, reenactment of the event (children with ACEs), nightmares, dissociative reactions

SUBJECTIVE DATA
A. Assess onset, course, and history of symptoms.
B. Assess coping mechanisms and social functioning.
C. Assess suicidal ideation.
D. Conduct a mental status exam.

PHYSICAL EXAMINATION
A. Perform a physical examination or refer the patient to a primary care provider to rule out medical causes of the symptoms.
B. Obtain a complete medical history, including onset of symptoms.
C. Perform mental status exam.
D. Suggestions for the exam can be found in the "Physical Examination" and "Psychometric Tools" sections for all anxiety disorders earlier in this chapter.

DIAGNOSTIC TESTS AND SCREENING
A. Structured clinical interview
 1. Clinician-Administered PTSD Scale (CAPS-5)
 2. Structured Clinical Interview for *DSM-5* (SCID-5)
B. Self-report questionnaires
 1. PTSD Checklist (PCL-5)

DIFFERENTIAL DIAGNOSIS
A. Anxiety
B. Panic disorder
C. Depression
D. Phobias

PLAN
A. Identification and treatment/reduction of the PTSD activators, engagement in symptom reduction, and assistance with reengaging in activities of daily living
B. Psychopharmacology
 1. SSRI or SNRI: first line
   a. Sertraline and paroxetine: only medications currently approved by the U.S. Food and Drug Administration (FDA) for PTSD
    i. Also strong evidence for fluoxetine (Prozac) and venlafaxine (Effexor) through Veterans Affairs research
    ii. Department of Veterans Affairs/Department of Defense Clinical Practice Guidelines: www.healthquality.va.gov/guidelines/MH/ptsd
   b. Exception made for adverse side effects on an individual basis
 2. Alpha- and beta-blockers
   a. Prazosin (alpha-blocker) for PTSD-related nightmares
   b. Propranolol (beta-adrenergic receptor blocker) to reduce tachycardia and sweating
 3. Anxiolytics
   a. Buspirone may reduce anxiety from PTSD without sedation or addiction.
   b. Antihistamine such as hydroxyzine can be used to treat insomnia in PTSD.
   c. Pharmacologic treatment should be combined with psychotherapy.
 4. 3,4-Methylenedioxymethamphetamine (MDMA): phase III trials to treat PTSD
   a. Short-term MDMA therapy is now in clinical trials with FDA.
   b. When combined with psychotherapy, MDMA has been successful in treating signs and symptoms of PTSD.

C. Psychotherapy
1. Individual trauma-focused psychotherapy
    a. Prolonged exposure (PE), cognitive processing therapy (CPT), and EMDR
    b. Somatic experiencing therapies (e.g., sensory motor psychotherapy)
2. Psychotherapy with sufficient evidence for PTSD symptom reduction
    a. Cognitive therapy, written exposure therapy (WET), and present-centered therapy (PCT)
3. Group therapy
    a. Trauma-focused group therapy
    b. Group therapy to address comorbid conditions (e.g., Seeking Safety [SS] for PTSD and comorbid SUD).
D. Complementary and alternative medicine
1. Yoga
2. Meditation and breathing exercises
3. Supplements (magnesium 400 mg) and traditional Chinese herbal medicines
4. Tai chi
5. Biofeedback
6. Acupuncture

GENERAL TREATMENT AND INTERVENTIONS
A. Medications: SSRIs, SNRIs, and alpha- and beta-blockers (see previous "Plan" section)
B. Psychotherapy: individual and group

PATIENT TEACHING
A. Explain all medications to the patient, including any interactions that will occur with food or drink and the need to avoid or limit alcohol intake.
B. Discuss the need for the patient to continue taking all prescribed medications as prescribed and to alert the healthcare provider of any unwanted side effects.
C. Engage the patient to agree to notify the healthcare provider of any OTC medications that are being taken.
D. Provide patient with the 988 suicide prevention hotline number.
E. Encourage regular physical activity and other activities such as as breathing exercises, meditation, or yoga.
F. Suggest support groups and explore eligibility for a service animal.
G. Advise establishing a sleep hygiene routine.
H. Provide resource links to the National Center for PTSD at www.ptsd.va.gov and the NIMH at www.nimh.nih.gov.

FOLLOW-UP
A. Follow-up should be weekly for the first 3 months, then monthly.
B. Review symptoms and support systems with each medication management visit.

CONSULTATION AND REFERRAL
A. Refer to psychiatric specialist (psychiatrist, psychiatric pharmacist) for consultation related to best practices in medication management.
B. A certified psychotherapist with experience in providing trauma-informed care and therapies should be consulted to begin or continue with the patient in psychotherapy.
C. Referrals to substance use professional or other medical specialties should be made in cases where comorbid medical issues are discovered.

INDIVIDUAL CONSIDERATIONS

Pediatric and Adolescent Patients
A. In the post-COVID-19 world and due to ongoing climate change-related events:
1. Assess for suicidality. Provide 988 suicide hotline number.
2. Assess for NSSI or eating disorders.
3. Due to the pandemic and other natural disasters, trauma and stress responses in youth have risen substantially.
4. Youth may demonstrate excessive fears and phobia-like anxiety that need to be addressed.
5. Use simple language and include supportive individuals identified by the youth.

Veterans
A. The most prevalent group experiencing signs and symptoms of PTSD
1. Assess female and male veterans and enlisted troops for PTSD from sexual abuse.
2. Assess all veterans of minority and underrepresented groups for ethnic-related trauma.

Minority/Underrepresented Individuals
A. Belonging to a minority group does not increase the chances of PTSD, unless that person has experienced a traumatic event.
1. The lifetime prevalence rate of PTSD is highest among African Americans (8.7%) compared with Hispanic and White Americans (7.0% and 7.4%, respectively) and Asian Americans (4.0%).
B. Include social workers early in the care: Assess all for ACEs.
1. Identify the risk factors for PTSD (child maltreatment, domestic violence, war-related events, unexpected death, witnessing violence or death).
2. Reach out for community resources that have meaning for the patient.
3. Some cultures may consider mental health a taboo subject; a nonjudgmental, culturally sensitive approach should be used.
4. Understand the traumatic impact of undocumented immigrant status, trauma during the migration experience, and the border-crossing experiences of the newly arriving migrants.

Geriatrics/Older Adult Patients
A. PTSD can increase with age, and earlier traumas may become more challenging to deal with as coping mechanisms fail to adequately deal with some memories.
1. Early unresolved trauma where avoidance or substance use was the coping strategy and has become less available
2. Unresolved military trauma or domestic abuse
3. Ongoing trauma such as loss of income, change in role, loss of loved ones, increased health problems and treatments, and possible elder abuse situations

Families/Significant Others
A. Patients' rights must be primary in working with adults with PTSD. In some cases, the perpetrator of the trauma may be a family member or close associate.

1. The patient is the healthcare provider's partner. Establishing safety with the patient will inform the healthcare provider as to the inclusion of family members and significant others.
    a. Assess relationships. Provide patient bill of rights to all patients.
    b. Identify support systems with the patient.
    c. Recognize protective factors; include the patient in identification of resiliencies and past effective coping strategies.
    d. Examine for any risk factors.
        i. Assess for past domestic violence and/or trauma.
        ii. Assess for ongoing personal violence or trauma.

B. Psychoeducation for the family with the patient involved includes recognition of worsening symptoms, referral systems, suicide hotline (988), destigmatizing the diagnosis, and identification of family support mechanisms and therapies.

RESOURCES
A. Give an Hour (for veterans and their families): https://giveanhour.org/military
B. National Center for PTSD: www.ptsd.va.gov
C. PTSD Coach App: https://mobile.va.gov/app/ptsd-coach
D. Understanding PTSD and PTSD Treatment: www.ptsd.va.gov/understand_tx/index.asp

REFERENCES AND BIBLIOGRAPHY
American Psychiatric Association. (2023). *What is posttraumatic stress disorder (PTSD)?* https://www.psychiatry.org/patients-families/ptsd/what-is-ptsd

Brom, D., Stokar, Y., Lawi, C., Nuriel-Porat, V., Ziv, Y., Lerner, K., & Ross, G. (2017). Somatic experiencing for posttraumatic stress disorder: A randomized controlled outcome study. *Journal of Traumatic Stress, 30*(3), 304–312. https://doi.org/10.1002/jts.22189

Brown, K. (2023, May 23). *Legalizing MDMA for PTSD treatment: Phase 3 clinical trial results*. Psychiatrist.com. https://www.psychiatrist.com/news/legalizing-mdma-for-ptsd-treatment-phase-3-clinical-trial-results

Held, R. F., Santos, S., Marki, M., & Helmer, D. (2016). Veteran perceptions, interest, and use of complementary and alternative medicine. *Federal Practitioner, 33*(9), 41–47. PMID: 30930617.

Mann, S. K., & Marwaha, R. (2024, February 25). *Posttraumatic stress disorder*. StatPearls Publishing. https://www.ncbi.nlm.nih.gov/books/NBK559129

Roberts, A. L., Gilman, S. E., Breslau, J., Breslau, N., & Koenen, K. C. (2011). Race/ethnic differences in exposure to traumatic events, development of post-traumatic stress disorder, and treatment-seeking for post-traumatic stress disorder in the United States. *Psychological Medicine, 41*(1), 71–83. https://doi.org/10.1017/S0033291710000401

Sloan, D. M., & J. G. Beck. (2016). Group treatment for PTSD. *PTSD Research Quarterly, 27*(2), 1–9. https://www.ptsd.va.gov/publications/rq_docs/V27N2.pdf

U.S. Department of Veterans Affairs. (n.d.). *PTSD: National Center for PTSD*. https://www.ptsd.va.gov/professional/treat/txessentials/overview_therapy.asp

SELECTIVE MUTISM

DEFINITION
A. Selective mutism presents as the inability to initiate speech or to answer others in a conversation. Although it is more common in childhood, it is rare and shows up as a persistent failure to speak in specific contexts where speech is typically expected, despite hearing and speaking in other contexts.

INCIDENCE
A. The prevalence of selective mutism is 0.03% and 1% from clinic and school samples, respectively. It usually starts before the age of 5 years and is more common in young children than in adults.
B. There are no sex or racial/ethnic differences in occurrence.
C. The prevalence of social mutism ranges from 0.47% to 0.76% of the population based on pooled case studies from Western Europe, the United States, and Israel.

PATHOGENESIS
A. The psychopathology, as well as the pathophysiology, is considered to be similar to social anxiety disorder.
B. There are multiple theories based on the etiology of selective mutism.
1. Psychodynamic theory: This theory is based on the concept of unresolved conflict. Underlying oral or anal fixation persists. Mutism represents a coping mechanism for anger and anxiety and a means for punishing parents.
2. Behavior theory: Individuals learn behaviors for manipulating the environment in response to activating events, and develop an adaptive response to sympathetic nervous system arousal that affects behavior, including speech.
3. Social anxiety and phobia: There is an association between selective mutism and excessive social anxiety. Selective mutism falls on the extreme end of the spectrum of social anxiety disorders.
4. Family systems perspective: Intense attachments to parents lead to extreme interdependency and distrust of the outside world.
5. Response to trauma: Association with PTSD is a potential, albeit uncommon, cause. Case studies of children exposed to extreme trauma or abuse reveal mutism as an avoidance reaction to trauma.
6. Dissociative identity disorder: Possessing multiple identities inhibits individual from talking to other people for fear of revealing traumatic conflicts and experiences.

PREDISPOSING FACTORS
A. Children of parents who may have social anxiety disorder or social inhibitions are at risk.
B. Overprotective parenting may be a risk factor for selective mutism.

COMMON COMPLAINTS
A. Persons with selective mutism may avoid direct eye contact.
B. Their behavior might be nervous, uneasy or socially awkward, rude, disinterested, sulky, or clingy.
C. They might appear to be shy and withdrawn, stiff, tense or poorly coordinated, stubborn, or aggressive.
D. Children might be having temper tantrums when they get home from school, or getting angry when questioned by parents.

SUBJECTIVE REPORTS
A. Assess onset, course, and history of symptoms: Is there failure to speak in social situations? Is the mutism interfering with education or activities of daily living? Has the mutism persisted for at least 1 month?
B. Assess coping mechanisms and social functioning: Is the failure to speak due to a lack of knowledge of the language or a communication disorder? Is the patient willing to engage in social situations that do not require speaking?
C. Conduct a mental status exam.

PHYSICAL EXAMINATION
A. Perform a physical examination or refer the patient to a primary care provider to rule out medical causes of the symptoms.
1. Include dental evaluation.

2. Include hearing evaluation.
3. Assess for learning disabilities.

B. Obtain a complete medical history, including onset of symptoms.

C. Psychiatric evaluation includes evaluation for oppositional defiant disorder (ODD), social phobia, social anxiety disorder, and separation anxiety disorder.

DIAGNOSTIC TESTS AND SCREENING

A. There are no laboratory tests for selective mutism.

B. Screening tools include the following:
1. Selective Mutism Questionnaire (SMQ)
2. Anxiety Disorder Interview Schedule for Children
3. Social Anxiety Scale for Children-R

DIFFERENTIAL DIAGNOSIS

A. Communication disorders: language disorder, speech sound disorder, childhood-onset fluency disorder (stuttering), pragmatic (social) communication disorder, expressive language disorder

B. Social anxiety disorder

C. Neurodevelopmental disorders: autism spectrum disorder, intellectual disability, pervasive developmental disorders

D. Psychotic disorders: schizophrenia

E. Transient adaptational shyness in an adjustment disorder

F. Mood disorders

G. Hearing impairment

PLAN

General Treatment and Interventions

A. Psychotherapy
1. CBT: the gold standard for selective mutism
2. Psychodynamic therapy
3. Behavioral therapy
4. Family therapy

B. Skills training
1. Anxiety management skills
2. Communication skills

C. Psychopharmacology
1. SSRIs to relieve anxiety-reducing symptoms in 75% of affected youth

COMMON MEDICATIONS

A. SSRIs
1. Fluvoxamine
2. Fluoxetine

PATIENT TEACHING

A. Work with parents on psychoeducation for selective mutism.

B. Explain that although selective mutism might self-resolve it can take months for benefits to be seen.

FOLLOW-UP

A. As clinically indicated

CONSULTATION AND REFERRAL

A. Multidimensional assessment
1. Psychotherapist, psychologist, psychiatric APRN with experience in treating youths with selective mutism
2. Parents and teachers
3. Health professionals such as audiologists and speech-language pathologists

INDIVIDUAL CONSIDERATIONS

Pediatrics and Adolescents

A. Selective mutism usually affects children between 3 and 6 years old.

B. Due to the pandemic and other natural disasters, anxiety and anxiety disorders in youth have risen substantially.

C. Youth may demonstrate excessive fears and phobia-like anxiety that need to be addressed.

D. Use simple language and include supportive individuals identified by the youth.

E. Assess for suicidality. Provide the 988 crisis/suicide prevention service for text or phone call.

Minority/Underrepresented Individuals

A. Assess if microaggressions or bullying due to minority status or racism is affecting the child's ability to engage verbally in social situations.

B. Include social workers in care.
1. Reach out for community resources.
2. Some cultures may consider mental health as taboo subject; a nonjudgmental approach should be used.
3. All persons should have equal treatment regardless of their immigration status.

Families/Significant Others

A. Psychoeducation for the family includes destigmatizing the diagnosis, the medications, and the therapy.

RESOURCES

A. Selective Mutism Association: www.selectivemutism.org

REFERENCE AND BIBLIOGRAPHY

Wong, P. (2010). Selective mutism: A review of etiology, comorbidities, and treatment. *Psychiatry (Edgmont)*, 7(3), 23–31. PMID: 20436772.

SEPARATION ANXIETY

DEFINITION

A. Separation anxiety disorder is excessive anxiety demonstrated as fear, distress, avoidance of separation situations, and impaired adaptive functioning when separated from a parental figure.

B. Children diagnosed with separation anxiety disorder are often preoccupied with the potential harm or negative events associated with the separation, such as illness, car accidents, or kidnapping.
1. They usually experience persistent nightmares in which these events occur.
2. Sleep disturbance may be associated with separation anxiety disorder.
3. These patients may be reluctant to participate in daily activities, such as going to school, socializing with friends, or getting out of bed.
4. Severe cases may have tantrums, tearfulness, and difficulty concentrating.

INCIDENCE

A. Separation anxiety disorder is seen more widely in persons younger than 12 years, but can occur at any age. It is equally identified in males and females.

B. Separation anxiety disorder has a prevalence of 4% in children and adolescents. However, this number decreases from childhood to adolescence.

C. The incidence of separation anxiety disorder is higher in females than in males.
D. Lower socioeconomic status and lower education level are also associated with separation anxiety disorder.

PATHOGENESIS
A. The etiology of separation anxiety disorder is unknown, but it is assumed that genetics may play a role in the disorder.
B. Pathophysiology: The amygdala is classically associated with provoking a fear response when stimulated. The amygdala and other fear-related neurocircuitry may share a similar neuroanatomy to anxiety neurocircuitry. The amygdala and its connections to the frontal cortex (perirhinal cortex, ventrolateral prefrontal cortex, anterior insula) have received the most attention.
  1. As the amygdala is part of the limbic system, other limbic system structures likely contribute to the development of anxiety, with a specific interest in the hippocampus as it plays an integral role in fear learning and extinction.
  2. Functional MRI (fMRI) studies have found that hypofunction of the prefrontal cortex and anterior cingulate cortex is associated with emotional dysregulation and cognitive dysfunction in those with anxiety.
  3. The activation of fear neurocircuitry, with presumed anxiety neurocircuitry overlap, involves the release of various neurochemicals that lead to sympathetic stimulation.
C. Classically characterized as a "fight-or-flight" reaction, the sympathetic response evolved to be adaptive and a prompt behavioral response to avoid actual or perceived danger.
  1. When conditioned to overactivate, the sympathetic response can lead to pathologic anxiety demonstrated even when exposure to threat is low or should be low.
  2. The neurochemicals involved in producing a fight-or-flight response are many and include norepinephrine, epinephrine, cortisol, neurosteroids, and vasopressin.
  3. Dopamine likely has a modulatory role in producing anxiety-like behavior.

PREDISPOSING FACTORS
A. Life stressors
  1. Recent death of a loved one or pet
  2. Divorce
  3. Parental absence or SUD
  4. Moving from one home to another: changing cities, states, or countries
  5. Foster care
B. Temperament
  1. Some personality types are more anxious than others.
  2. Children with anxiety are more likely to experience separation anxiety disorder.
C. Family history
  1. Overprotective family/parents
  2. Family members with anxiety disorders
D. Environmental issues
  1. Trauma of a disaster that involves separation

COMMON COMPLAINTS
A. Excessive anxiety when there is a separation from the individual to whom the patient is attached
B. Distress when separation occurs
C. Persistent worry about losing major attachment figures
D. Unwillingness to go anywhere or do anything without the attachment figures
E. Fear of abduction
F. Nightmares
G. Bedwetting

OTHER SIGNS AND SYMPTOMS
A. Panic attacks
B. Nausea and vomiting
C. Chest pain
D. Trouble breathing
E. Dizziness

SUBJECTIVE REPORTS
A. Assess onset, course, and history of symptoms.
  1. For children, the symptoms are present for at least 4 weeks and cause impairment to normal activities of daily living.
  2. For adults, symptoms must be present for 6 or more months, causing impairment to activities of daily living, and cannot be explained by another diagnosis.
B. Assess coping mechanisms and social functioning.
C. Assess for risk of self-harm or suicidal ideation.
D. Conduct a mental status exam.

PHYSICAL EXAMINATION
A. The practitioner should perform a physical examination or refer the patient to a primary care provider to rule out medical causes of the symptoms.
B. Obtain a complete medical history, including onset of symptoms.
C. Separation anxiety disorder-specific psychiatric evaluation should include the following:
  1. Assessment of history of trauma
  2. Obtaining developmental and social history
  3. Behavior
      a. How does the patient's behavior change when united/separated from the caregiver?
      b. Does the patient have anxious behaviors like constant movement, shaking, and/or small tremors?
      c. Are clinging behaviors present?
  4. Speech
      a. Is the patient's tone frightened when talking about separation from caregiver?
      b. Does the patient seek permission to speak from the caregiver?
  5. Impulse control
      a. Is the patient impulsive?
  6. Insight
      a. For the adult, assess insight and assist them in understanding that the behaviors they are engaging in are maladaptive. For the child, insight will probably be poor.

DIAGNOSTIC TESTS AND SCREENING
A. Separation Anxiety Avoidance Inventory (SAAI)
B. Children's Separation Anxiety Scale (CSAS)
C. Youth Anxiety Measure (YAM)
D. Anxiety Disorder Interview Schedule (ADIS)
E. Pediatric Anxiety Rating Scale (PARS)

DIFFERENTIAL DIAGNOSIS
A. Another anxiety disorder
  1. GAD
  2. Social anxiety disorder
  3. IAD
  4. PTSD

B. In children
1. Conduct disorder
2. ODD
C. Mood disorders
D. Psychotic disorders
E. Personality disorder
F. Agoraphobia or other specific phobias

PLAN
A. Identification and reduction of anxiety associated with separation
B. Involvement of caregivers/family in therapy where possible
C. Psychotherapy
1. CBT
2. DBT for adults
3. Family therapy
4. Group therapy
D. Psychopharmacology
1. Treat the anxiety.
    a. SSRIs
        i. Fluoxetine: the only FDA-approved SSRI for use in children younger than 12 years
        ii. Sertraline (Zoloft)
    b. SNRI for adults
        i. Venlafaxine SR
    c. Benzodiazepines
        i. Limited, short-term role only for alleviation of overwhelming anxiety

General Treatment and Interventions
A. Relaxation exercises
B. Mindfulness
C. Stress reduction through music therapy

PATIENT TEACHING
A. Include family in education on the development of separation anxiety disorder, assisting the level of insight into potential experiences, like fear of significant losses, that can increase anxiety.
B. Engage patients in learning mindful breathing techniques.

FOLLOW-UP
A. Assess and work with the team to determine the best strategy for follow-up appointments.

CONSULTATION AND REFERRAL
A. Refer to psychiatric specialist (psychiatrist, psychiatric pharmacist) for consultation related to best practice in medication management.
B. A certified psychotherapist with experience in pediatric therapies as well as providing trauma-informed care and therapies should be consulted to begin or continue with the patient in psychotherapy.
C. Referrals to substance use professional or other medical specialties should be made in cases where comorbid medical issues are discovered.

INDIVIDUAL CONSIDERATIONS
A. Separation anxiety disorder does not impact any special population. It is the intense fear of separation from a person who is a caregiver or who is loved. Careful consideration to the dynamics of the home can provide important information about the patient's expression of anxiety.

RESOURCES
A. National Alliance on Mental Illness: https://nami.org/Home
B. American Academy of Child and Adolescent Psychiatry Anxiety Disorders Resource Center: www.aacap.org/AACAP/Families_and_Youth/Resource_Centers/Anxiety_Disorder_Resource_Center/Home.aspx

REFERENCE AND BIBLIOGRAPHY
Feriante, J., Torrico, T. J., & Bernstein, B. (2023, February 26). *Separation anxiety disorder*. StatPearls Publishing. https://www.ncbi.nlm.nih.gov/books/NBK560793

SOCIAL ANXIETY DISORDER

DEFINITION
A. Social anxiety disorder is a common type of anxiety disorder. A person with social anxiety disorder feels symptoms of anxiety or fear in situations where they may be scrutinized, evaluated, or judged by others, such as speaking in public, meeting new people, dating, being on a job interview, answering a question in class, or having to talk to a cashier in a store. Doing everyday things, such as eating or drinking in front of others or using a public restroom, may also cause anxiety or fear due to concerns about being humiliated, judged, and rejected.

INCIDENCE
A. Second most common anxiety disorder
B. Affects over 15 million adults in the United States (Figure 9.5)

PATHOGENESIS
A. Overreaction of the autonomic nervous system, promoting performance-type social anxiety
1. Tachycardia, pounding heart
2. Sweating
B. Neurotransmitter system activation
1. Patient has increased level of serotonin, dopamine, and glutamate.
2. Patient has increased activity of paralimbic and limbic circuitry.
3. Some toddler temperaments along with maternal stress may increase the likelihood of developing a social anxiety disorder later in life.

PREDISPOSING FACTORS
A. Family history
1. ACEs: family trauma, abuse, unresolved ongoing conflict
2. Exposure to teasing, bullying, rejection, or humiliation, either at home or in other social situations
3. Typically begins in late adolescence (teenage years)
B. Temperament
1. Timid individuals who fear new situations
2. Withdrawn or restrained individuals
C. Life changes and social demands
1. Changes in work situations or social situations that require the individual to reach out to those with whom they are not already familiar
2. Public speaking engagements, including presentations for work, that can activate the symptoms for the first time
D. Apparent disease or disorder that can draw attention
1. Facial disfigurement or other visible physical alteration
2. Parkinson disease or other movement disorders

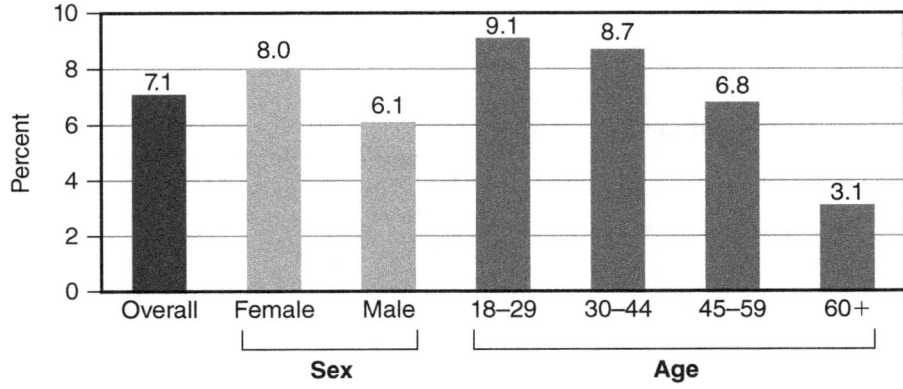

FIGURE 9.5 Past year prevalence of social anxiety disorder among U.S. adults, 2001 to 2003.

Source: National Institute of Mental Health. (n.d.). *Social anxiety disorder.* U.S. Department of Health and Human Services. https://www.nimh.nih.gov/health/statistics/social-anxiety-disorder; Data from National Comorbidity Survey Replication (NCS-R).

COMMON COMPLAINTS
A. Patient might state the following:
  1. "My heart starts pounding when I have to speak, I am afraid people will be judging me."
  2. "I can't control how much I sweat so I feel humiliated when I have to be so public."
  3. "I hate having to speak with strangers, I get so anxious, I know they will know."
  4. "I am so afraid that people will notice that I am trembling (I am sweating, my voice is shaking)."
  5. "I just can't speak in public" or "I hate being the center of attention!"
  6. "I know that nothing is going to go well. I always fail in social situations."

SUBJECTIVE REPORTS
A. Assess onset, course, and history of symptoms.
B. Assess coping mechanisms and social functioning.
C. Assess suicidal ideation.
D. Conduct a mental status exam.

PHYSICAL EXAM
A. Perform a physical examination or refer the patient to a primary care provider to rule out the medical causes of the symptoms.
  1. Obtain a complete medical history, including onset of symptoms.
  2. Perform mental status exam.
  3. Suggestions for the exam can be found in the "Physical Examination" and "Psychometric Tools" sections for all anxiety disorders earlier in this chapter.

DIAGNOSTIC TESTS AND SCREENING
A. There is no specific medical test for social anxiety disorder.
B. Validated screening tools include the following:
  1. Liebowitz Social Anxiety Scale (LSAS): free for practitioners and researchers
  2. Social Phobia Inventory (SPIN)
  3. Brief Social Phobia Scale (BSPS)

DIFFERENTIAL DIAGNOSIS
A. Anxiety
B. Panic disorder
C. Depression
D. Phobias

PLAN

General Treatment and Interventions
A. CBT: first-line intervention
B. Antidepressants, such as SSRIs and SNRIs
C. Beta-blockers
D. Antianxiety medications, such as benzodiazepines

COMMON MEDICATIONS
A. Paroxetine (Paxil) or sertraline (Zoloft)
B. Venlafaxine (Effexor XR)
C. Propranolol
D. Lorazepam, alprazolam, diazepam

PATIENT TEACHING
A. Educate patient on medication management.
  1. Explain all medications to the patient, including any interactions that will occur with food or drink and the need to avoid or limit alcohol intake.
  2. Discuss the need for the patient to continue taking all prescribed medications as prescribed and to alert the healthcare provider of any unwanted side effects.
  3. Engage the patient to agree to notify the healthcare provider of any OTC medications that are being taken.
B. Provide patient with the 988 crisis/suicide prevention hotline number.
C. Encourage regular physical activity and other activities such as breathing exercises, meditation, or yoga.
D. Suggest support groups and explore eligibility for a service animal.
E. Advise establishing a sleep hygiene routine.
F. Provide resource links to the National Center for PTSD at www.ptsd.va.gov and the NIMH at www.nimh.nih.gov.

FOLLOW-UP
A. Follow-up should be weekly for the first 3 months, then monthly.
B. Review symptoms and support systems with each medication management visit.

CONSULTATION AND REFERRAL
A. Refer to psychiatric specialist (psychiatrist, psychiatric pharmacist) for consultation related to best practice in medication management.

B. A certified psychotherapist with experience in providing trauma-informed care and therapies should be consulted to begin or continue with the patient in psychotherapy.
C. Referrals to substance use professional or other medical specialties should be made in cases where comorbid medical issues are discovered.

INDIVIDUAL CONSIDERATIONS

Youth
A. Due to the pandemic and other natural disasters, trauma and stress responses in youth have risen substantially.
B. Youth may demonstrate excessive fears and phobia-like anxiety that need to be addressed.
C. Use simple language and include supportive individuals identified by the youth.

Veterans
A. Social anxiety is often correlated with PTSD.
B. Social anxiety is listed in federal regulations; patients may be able to qualify for disability benefits.
   1. For more information, see https://veteranshelpgroup.com/social-anxiety-va-benefits.

Minority/Underrepresented Individuals
A. Increased exposure to trauma and stress makes all anxiety disorders more common in minority populations.
B. Include social workers early in the care; assess all for ACEs.
   1. Reach out for community resources that have meaning for the patient.
   2. Some cultures may consider mental health a taboo subject; a nonjudgmental, culturally sensitive approach should be used.
   3. Understand the traumatic impact of undocumented immigrant status, trauma during the migration experience, and the border-crossing experiences of the newly arriving migrants.

Geriatrics/Older Adults
A. Early unresolved trauma where avoidance or substance use was the coping strategy and has become less available
B. Unresolved military trauma or domestic abuse
C. Ongoing trauma such as loss of income, change in role, loss of loved ones, increased health problems and treatments, and possible elder abuse situations

Families/Significant Others
A. The patient is the healthcare provider's partner. Establishing safety with the patient will inform the healthcare provider as to the inclusion of family members and significant others.
   1. Assess relationships. Provide patient bill of rights to all patients.
   2. Identify support systems with the patient.
B. Recognize protective factors; include the patient in identification of resiliencies and past effective coping strategies.
C. Examine for any risk factors.
   1. Assess for past domestic violence and/or trauma.
   2. Assess for ongoing personal violence or trauma.
D. Psychoeducation for the family with the patient involved includes recognition of worsening symptoms, referral systems, suicide hotline (988), destigmatizing the diagnosis, and identification of family support mechanisms and therapies.

RESOURCES
A. Digital Shareables for Professionals: www.nimh.nih.gov/get-involved/digital-shareables/shareable-resources-on-anxiety-disorders
B. Social Anxiety Self-Help Guide: www.nhsinform.scot/illnesses-and-conditions/mental-health/mental-health-self-help-guides/social-anxiety-self-help-guide
C. Anxiety and Depression Association of America: https://adaa.org/understanding-anxiety/social-anxiety-disorder

REFERENCES AND BIBLIOGRAPHY
National Institute of Mental Health. (n.d.). *Social anxiety disorder: More than just shyness*. https://www.nimh.nih.gov/health/publications/social-anxiety-disorder-more-than-just-shyness

Rose, G. M., & Tadi, P. (2022, October 25). *Social anxiety disorder*. StatPearls Publishing. https://www.ncbi.nlm.nih.gov/books/NBK555890

10 FEEDING AND EATING DISORDERS

Kim K. Johnson

INTRODUCTION

Feeding and eating disorders (FEDs) are a group of important disorders affecting individuals across the life span. They encompass various conditions such as anorexia nervosa (AN), binge eating disorder (BED), and bulimia nervosa (BN), as well as feeding disorders (FDs), avoidant/restrictive food intake disorder (ARFID), pica and rumination disorders, other specified feeding and eating disorder (OSFED), and unspecified feeding and eating disorder (UFED). These disorders are categorized based on observed symptoms, as outlined in the *International Classification of Diseases*, 11th Revision (*ICD-11*; World Health Organization [WHO], 2019), and the American Psychiatric Association's *Diagnostic and Statistical Manual of Mental Disorders*, Fifth Edition, Text Revision (*DSM-5-TR*; 2022). The *DSM-5* (5th ed.; American Psychiatric Association, 2013) first integrated FDs into the broader classification of eating disorders (EDs), aiming to provide a more comprehensive and updated framework for diagnosing mental health conditions, including those related to eating behaviors. While FDs have gained more recognition in recent years, the volume of research is smaller than that of EDs.

The prevalence of FEDs—especially BEDs—is rising and has caused significant problems due to the associated comorbidities of metabolic syndrome, diabetes mellitus, and cardiac complications. Patients with AN have the highest mortality rates of any psychological disorder. Early intervention and a holistic, collaborative approach are emphasized for the best treatment outcomes. Patients with ED usually present to primary care outpatient clinics, urgent care centers, and gastroenterology clinics, and may only see psychiatrists and APRNs after referral. Diagnosis and management of these patients are challenging. Psychotherapy continues to be the mainstay of treatment. Unfortunately, the lack of trained therapists and the unwillingness of patients with ED to be truthful about their symptoms prevent diagnosis and referral. Reluctance by patients with ED to see a therapist puts a significant burden on APRNs to treat these patients to the best of their abilities.

While appetite is controlled by the hypothalamus, environment, culture, and stress play a role in mind-sets regarding food. Food availability, the smell of food, social interactions, and social media greatly influence how much is eaten and when and what foods are consumed. When anxiety and stress are present, food may be used in a dysfunctional manner, resulting in severe EDs that can be life-threatening. Psychiatric comorbidities include depression, personality disorders, substance use disorders, posttraumatic stress disorder (PTSD), and anxiety. Treatment for EDs focuses on normalizing eating patterns and addressing the issues raised by the illness. Early intervention and a holistic, collaborative approach are emphasized for the best treatment outcomes.

Distinguishing between different ED diagnoses poses practical challenges as there is significant overlap among patients assigned these classifications. Additionally, subtle shifts in a patient's overall behavior can lead to a transition from an anorexia: binge eating type of diagnosis to BN. It is common for individuals with FDs or EDs to traverse various FED diagnoses as their behaviors evolve over time.

DEFINITIONS OF FEEDING AND EATING DISORDERS

FEDs are behavioral conditions characterized by severe persistent disturbances in eating behavior and associated distressing thoughts and emotions that may lead to significant impairments in physical health, psychological well-being, and overall functioning. They involve deviations from normal eating patterns that are not better accounted for by other health conditions and are not developmentally appropriate or culturally sanctioned.

EDs involve body image concerns and, often, co-occurring psychological disorders and medical complications. It should be noted that obesity is not considered a mental disorder, although it may be a risk factor for EDs.

DEFINITIONS OF FEEDING DISORDERS

FDs typically involve difficulties related to food consumption as opposed to body image concerns. Challenges with accepting a variety of foods, sensory issues, and aversions are characteristic. They include pica, rumination, and ARFID. FDs are more commonly observed in children, although they can occur in individuals of any age.

Pica

Pica involves the persistent eating of nonnutritive, nonfood substances over a duration of at least 1 month. Pica is often more prevalent in children. This behavior is not developmentally appropriate and is not part of widely accepted cultural or social norms. Pica in adults may be linked to certain medical conditions such as nutritional deficiencies (e.g., iron, zinc), pregnancy, mental health disorders, developmental disorders, or neurologic conditions.

Rumination Disorder

Rumination disorder is characterized by the repeated regurgitation of food, which may be rechewed, reswallowed, or spit out. While it can occur in individuals of any age, rumination disorder is more commonly observed in infants, children, and individuals with intellectual or developmental disabilities.

Avoidant/Restrictive Food Intake Disorder

ARFID is characterized by significant weight loss, nutritional deficiency, dependence on nutritional supplements, or marked interference with psychosocial functioning due to persistent failure to meet appropriate caloric and/or nutritional needs, but without weight or shape concerns. Individuals with ARFID can have other sensory aversions to food due to food textures, temperatures, colors, or smells. ARFID can include extremely selective eating, disrupted appetite cues, lack of interest in food, sensory processing difficulties, or anxiety regarding the consequences of eating (e.g., illness, vomiting, choking).

DEFINITIONS OF EATING DISORDERS
EDs are a group of mental health conditions characterized by persistent disturbances in eating behavior and attitudes and preoccupation with food, weight, and body image. These disorders often have serious physical and psychological consequences and can significantly impact a person's health and overall well-being. In adolescents and adults, EDs present in three primary classic clinical presentations: AN, BN, and BED.

Anorexia Nervosa
AN is a reversible, biologically based disorder characterized by restriction of energy intake leading to significantly low body weight in the context of age, sex, developmental trajectory, and health status, and associated with a disturbance of body image, intense fear of gaining weight, lack of recognition of the seriousness of the illness, and/or behaviors that interfere with weight gain. Two subtypes are distinguished: restricting type and binge eating/purging type.

Bulimia Nervosa
BN is characterized by binge eating (eating a large amount of food in a relatively short period of time associated with a sense of loss of control over eating) followed by purging or other compensatory behavior (e.g., self-induced vomiting, laxative or diuretic abuse, insulin misuse, excessive exercise, fasting, diet pills) once a week or more, on average, for at least 3 months. Self-evaluation is unduly influenced by body shape and weight. For individuals who are underweight, the diagnosis of AN binge eating/purging subtype overrides the diagnosis of BN.

Binge Eating Disorders
Binge eating involves eating a large amount of food in a relatively short period of time (associated with a sense of loss of control over eating) in the absence of compensatory behavior, at least once a week for 3 months or more. Binge eating episodes are associated with eating rapidly, regardless of hunger, until extreme fullness, and/or are associated with depression, shame, or guilt.

Other Specified Feeding and Eating Disorder
OSFED is an ED that does not meet the full criteria for one of the previously mentioned categories but involves specific disordered eating behaviors such as restricting intake, purging, and/or binge eating as key features. Atypical AN, for example, is a common type of OSFED characterized by all the features of AN in an individual whose weight remains above a minimum weight for age despite significant weight loss.

Unspecified Feeding and Eating Disorder
UFED is a preliminary diagnosis used when ED behaviors are present; however, there is insufficient information to make a firm diagnosis.

INCIDENCE AND PREVALENCE OF FEEDING AND EATING DISORDERS

Since most people with FEDs never seek formal treatment for their disorder and are therefore undiagnosed, it is difficult to research. Incidence refers to the number of people who first develop an ED during a specific period (usually 1 year). Prevalence refers to the total number of people who have an ED during a specific period.

A. Thirty million people in the United States have an FED.
B. When Stice et al. (2013) followed a group of 496 adolescent girls for 8 years until they were 20, they found that 5.2% of the girls met the *DSM-5* (American Psychiatric Association, 2013) criteria for anorexia, bulimia, or BED. When the researchers included nonspecific ED symptoms, they found that a total of 13.2% of the girls had suffered from a *DSM-5* ED by age 20 years.
C. Approximately 95% of persons with an ED are 12 to 25 years old. EDs typically begin in adolescence or early adulthood. Anorexia and bulimia rarely begin before the age of puberty; 90% of cases are diagnosed before the age of 20, whereas fewer than 10% of all cases occur before the age of 10.
D. Although 90% of patients with an ED are female, the incidence of diagnosed EDs in males is increasing, with more research being done on males with EDs.
E. Incidence is increasing in Black, Indigenous, and people of color (BIPOC) and LGBTQ+ communities, with more research being done on these populations.
F. EDs affect at least 9% of the population worldwide. Of the U.S. population, 9%, or 28.8 million Americans, will have an ED in their lifetime. Less than 6% of people with EDs are medically diagnosed as "underweight." Some studies have found that White adults have a higher lifelong prevalence of EDs, including AN, BN, and BED, compared with other ethnic groups.

INCIDENCE OF FEEDING DISORDERS

A. Less is known about the epidemiology of FDs than EDs. Their prevalence is challenging to determine due to underreporting and variation in diagnostic criteria. FDs are more commonly reported in certain populations such as individuals with intellectual disabilities, autism spectrum disorder, and certain medical conditions.
B. 1% to 5% of all hospital admissions are for failure to thrive, a condition that is correlated with FDs. Prevalence numbers range widely from 5% to 20% of children in the normal population being diagnosed with FDs.
C. Children of all backgrounds can have an FD.
D. Groups of children who are more likely to be diagnosed with an FD include premature infants, children with failure to thrive, children with autism, and children with various genetic syndromes.
E. The prevalence of FDs in children with disabilities ranges from 40% to 80%.

  1. Pica: The prevalence of pica can vary depending on the population studied and the criteria used for diagnosis. It is most commonly observed in children, pregnant people, and individuals with developmental disabilities. In children, pica is often considered developmentally normal up to a certain age, as exploration through oral stimulation is a common part of early childhood. However, when this behavior persists beyond age-appropriate levels, it may be considered a disorder. Between 4% and 26% of institutionalized individuals are believed to have pica.
  2. Rumination disorder: Rumination disorder is a relatively rare ED. The exact incidence of rumination disorder is not well-established as research on the prevalence of rumination disorder is limited. It may be underdiagnosed or misdiagnosed due to lack of awareness among healthcare professionals. Rumination is developmentally normal

in infants 3 to 12 months of age and typically resolves on its own. However, when rumination persists beyond infancy and becomes a more chronic issue, it may be diagnosed as a disorder. The limited European data available on prevalence suggest that the disorder may occur in approximately 1% to 2% of grade-school-age children.

3. ARFID: ARFID is a relatively newly recognized ED. It can occur in both children and adults. It is more prevalent in early childhood but can persist beyond this age group. It is not driven by concerns about weight or body image. Specific prevalence rates for ARFID may vary depending on the population studied and the diagnostic criteria used, but it is less common than other AN or BN. As awareness among healthcare professionals has increased, more research has been conducted to better determine its prevalence. A 2023 Australian study of 5,072 adolescents between 11 and 19 years of age found that 1.98% of adolescents had possible ARFID. In a group of adolescents with EDs receiving treatment at a specialized clinic, 14% met the criteria for ARFID. People with an ARFID diagnosis are more likely to be young boys.

INCIDENCE OF EATING DISORDERS

A. The incidence of AN is estimated to be 0.3% to 1% in females and lower among males. It often begins in adolescence. Up to 20% of people with chronic AN will die if their illness is not treated. 13% of patients report at least one suicide attempt, 29% report recent suicidal ideation, and 26% of attempters reported multiple attempts.

B. The incidence of BN is higher than that of AN, ranging from 1% to 3% among females. It can affect males as well. BN affects 4 to 6 out of 200 females in the United States. AN is much less common, with a lifetime prevalence of 1 out of 200 females in the United States.

C. BED is considered the most common ED. The incidence is estimated to be 1% to 3% of the general population, both males and females. Research estimates that:

1. 28.4% of people with current BED are receiving treatment for their disorder.
2. 43.6% of people with BED at some point in their lives will receive treatment.
3. Approximately 40% of those with BED are male.
4. Three out of ten individuals looking for weight loss treatments show signs of BED.

PATHOGENESIS

A. Genetic, neurobiological, cognitive, psychosocial, and environmental factors contribute to the development of EDs, as well as personality characteristics, interpersonal pressures, and cultural pressures.

B. Fear of obesity, intense fear of gaining weight, and erroneous self-perception of weight and body shape drive the desire to restrict, binge, and purge food. In our culture, children as young as 5 years have knowledge about weight control and dieting.

C. Biological factors set the stage for the development of EDs. Gene variations responsible for serotonin transport and monoamine oxidase enzyme activity are noted in EDs.

D. Epigenetic studies show methylation of genes associated with stress response, regulation of nutritional intake, and impulsivity or craving behaviors.

E. Individuals who have engaged in dieting with little to no weight loss are in danger of purging behaviors as their metabolic rates have decreased from frequent food restriction.

F. The development of an ED is associated with the following factors:

1. Neurobiological factors: Impaired transport of serotonin, which contributes to the sensation of satiety and fullness, may increase dopamine, causing an increase in sensitivity, motivation, and desire to seek rewards despite risks.

   a. Tryptophan, an amino acid essential to serotonin levels, is available only through diet. Individuals with EDs show significantly lower levels of circulating serotonin and tryptophan (the precursor necessary to synthesize serotonin). Because serotonin supports satiety, the decreased levels of serotonin metabolism predispose individuals to EDs. Declines in tryptophan may relieve anxiety symptoms and increase dysphoria, a reward for calorie restriction in AN. The cycle of temporary relief followed by the dysphoria of starvation sets up a positive feedback loop that reinforces regulation in food. Antidepressants that boost serotonin do not improve mood for those with AN until they have returned to 90% of their optimal weight. This may be caused by a lack of tryptophan caused by food restriction.

   b. In BN, abnormalities in dopamine circulating pathways cause decreased satisfaction after eating, resulting in bingeing and purging. Endorphin levels are found to be reduced in individuals with BN and correlate with higher levels of depression. In some purging individuals, endorphin levels become elevated after vomiting, resulting in a feeling of well-being.

2. Neuroendocrine changes: AN is associated with significant neuroendocrine disturbances, such as disruptions in the hypothalamic–pituitary–gonadal axis, which can lead to amenorrhea in females.

3. Gut–brain connection: Hunger and satiety are controlled by two areas in the hypothalamus: the lateral hypothalamus, which tells us when to begin eating; and the ventromedial nuclei, which indicate when to stop eating. The gastrointestinal tract only controls short-term eating by feeling satisfied. Microbiota homeostasis is being researched as an essential need for a healthy communication network between the gut and the brain.

4. There is evidence that repeated dieting alters gut flora and causes inflammation, which can lead to immune responses that contribute to the pathophysiology of EDs. Future studies on nutritional rehabilitation are an important focus for EDs.

5. Intake of macronutrients can significantly improve the nutritional imbalance in the gut. Therapeutic strategies proposed include fecal microbiota transplantation, prebiotics, and probiotics to correct balance alterations.

G. Psychological factors: Distorted body image and low self-esteem are common psychological factors in EDs. Cultural pressures emphasizing thinness, as well as societal ideals of beauty, can contribute to the development of unrealistic body standards.

H. Cognitive factors: The egosyntonic nature of EDs means that the individuals who suffer from them value the disorder. Although they know their actions are potentially harmful, they believe the benefits outweigh the harm. The tendency toward obsessive, perfectionistic, and anxious temperament reflects a need to control and achieve the unrealistic ideal of thinness.

1. AN: Patients struggle with emotional identification apart from weight, emotional regulation, and processing. Many exhibit poor tolerance and control in response to distress.

2. **BN:** Patients often exhibit attachment problems with friends, family, and intimate partners. As with AN, those with BN evaluate themselves based on shape and weight. They rigidly view being overweight negatively and exhibit black-and-white thinking, overgeneralization, and errors in attribution.

3. **BED:** Individuals exhibit high impulsivity and may experience an addictive response to certain foods. Foods high in sugar, fat, and carbohydrates are exceptionally addictive.

I. Environmental factors: Trauma, abuse, or stressful life events may play a role. Social and cultural pressures to be thin, unrealistic images, and comparisons on social media promote the development of emotional eating.

1. Viewing and comparing beautifully edited pictures (e.g., "filters") can be isolating or damaging and contribute to body image concerns and harmful behaviors. Poorer body image is associated with uploading more photos or spending more time on social media.
2. Particularly, young children and adolescents with existing concerns about their bodies use social media to look for positive or negative feedback on appearance.
3. Stereotyping or discrimination based on an individual's weight is common and perpetuates the cycle of restriction, bingeing, and purging.
4. A history of food insecurity with insufficient food is associated with BED.
5. Additionally, activities such as sports, ballet, and gymnastics may contribute to EDs.

PREDISPOSING FACTORS

A. Genetic factors: Positive family history of biological relatives with disordered eating and/or mental disorders increases the risk of an individual developing the disorder. EDs are more commonly seen when a first-degree relative has an ED (up to two times the increase of those reported).

B. Parental and familial mental illness is associated with psychopathology in offspring, establishing that children with first-degree relatives with psychiatric disorders are at higher risk of developing psychopathology themselves.

C. Family dynamics that highly value appearance, weight, and dieting: Dysfunctional family communication patterns may play a role.

D. Personality traits of perfectionism, low self-worth, anxiety, or impulsivity, or a history of abuse, may increase the risk.

E. Childhood experiences of being teased, bullied, or criticized about weight or body shape may contribute to body image issues and disordered eating. Early dieting may also be a factor.

F. Environmental influence includes societal idealization about weight and body shape.

G. Parenting style and stress: Household stress and parental discord may contribute to anxiety and personality traits that are risk factors for an ED. Still, parenting style has been discounted as a primary cause of EDs.

1. An early emphasis on success with external rewards may lead to overly high expectations and perfectionism.
2. Children may feel more successful with something they can control, such as regulating their eating and appearance.

H. Sexual assault or abuse is a risk factor for BN but has not been associated with AN.

I. Biological factors for EDs, with twin studies suggesting a genetic link: Weight stigma, weight-related bullying, cultural fixation on the "thin ideal," and the concept that smaller bodies are inherently better are all prominent risk factors that aggravate the likelihood of developing an ED.

J. Individual preoccupation with weight: The individual fits the risk profile for EDs, including having a history of dieting, being picky eaters as children, participating in athletics where a lean body build is valued, and having an occupation that values slimness. Individuals who participate in elite-level competitions or in a sport where a lean body build is prized are predisposed to developing EDs.

K. Biological influences include the following:
1. Gut–brain nutritional deficiencies
2. Biochemical disturbances of serotonin neurotransmitter pathways also implicated in the development of EDs

L. Psychological influences include the following:
1. Positive feedback loop that reinforces restriction in food
2. Rigidity, ritualism, separation, and individuation conflicts
3. Major depression, distorted body image, internal and external locus of control or self-identity, and history of abuse
4. Feelings of ineffectiveness, self-esteem being contingent upon weight, difficulty with decision-making, impulsivity, and emotional dysregulation

M. Neurocognitive profiles associated with EDs include the following:
1. Involve alterations in attention, visuospatial ability, memory, social cognition, and executive functions
2. Observed during active illness, serve as both risk and protective factors, influenced by genetic predisposition and the drive for high educational achievement and perfectionism also common in EDs

N. Environmental influences include the following:
1. Social stigma and societal pressure linked to higher body mass index (BMI) contribute to significant social stigma and isolation in individuals with overweight or obesity, leading to feelings of marginalization and shame. Negative attitudes toward obesity correlate with higher levels of depression and eating pathology.
2. Social media exerts significant influence, promoting unrealistic body ideals and standards of attractiveness, particularly affecting adolescents and young adults. Exposure to these standards can lead to poor body image and increase the risk of EDs.
3. Expectations related to physical attractiveness strongly correlate with career success, especially among young women. Discriminatory practices against those with obesity are observed in some modern businesses.
4. First-degree relatives with EDs may exhibit behaviors such as differential facial emotion processing and the use of negatively expressed emotions during mealtime. First-degree relatives without EDs tend to make more positive eating comments at mealtimes.

COMMON COMPLAINTS AND CHARACTERISTICS

Historically, FEDs have been diagnosed more frequently in females from adolescence to young adulthood, but the frequency of young males developing the disorder is being studied. The onset of an FED can be associated with a stressful life event, such as going off to college or missing school due to a pandemic.

A. Malnutrition can cause a dangerously low heart rate or abnormal heart rhythm, causing dizziness, heart arrhythmias, and even death.

B. Excessive dieting, restriction, or purging may cause the stomach and intestines to work slower, leading to pain, constipation, and bloating.

C. Purging via vomiting can cause teeth enamel to erode due to contact with stomach bile.

D. Females may stop having periods, which weakens bones. Males may develop low levels of testosterone.

E. Individuals with EDs have more irritability, mood changes, and difficulty focusing. Children may have delayed puberty or slow growth. APRNs should note individuals who present for evaluation who have the following alterations related to mood, weight, or eating or exercise patterns:

1. patient reports a weight of less than 85% of their ideal body weight, or weight loss of 15% of the ideal body weight.
2. Low body weight is not sufficient to assess malnutrition in patients with EDs because malnutrition occurs at all weights. In some EDs, patients may be close to or above their ideal body weight. This is common in those diagnosed with bulimia marked by binging and purging.
3. The percentage or magnitude of body weight loss, also called *weight suppression*, is a more important indicator of the severity of illness in AN.
4. Patient is preoccupied with body image.
   a. Spends excessive time looking in the mirror, makes negative comments about their physical appearance, and insists that they are overweight
   b. Preoccupied with certain celebrities and models, compares themselves unfavorably, or wears baggy clothing to hide their body shape
   c. Disruptions in eating patterns
      i. Stops eating with their family, dislikes previously enjoyed foods, is preoccupied with counting calories and fat grams, drinks excessive amounts of water and caffeine to suppress appetite, eats noticeably smaller portions, or refuses to eat
      ii. Binges on certain foods and goes to the bathroom immediately after meals (presumably to vomit what they just ate)
      iii. Develops eating rituals such as chewing for long periods before swallowing, cutting food into small portions, moving food around on the plate, or hiding food to dispose of later
   d. Preoccupation with nutritional content
      i. Classifies foods as "good" or "bad," "healthy" or "unhealthy," "safe" or "unsafe"
      ii. Constantly searches for organic, low-fat, or diet foods, frequently visiting websites focused on nutrition
      iii. Suddenly declares they are vegetarian or vegan
   e. Changes in exercise patterns
      i. Becomes preoccupied with physical fitness
      ii. Spends hours exercising in a ritualistic way
      iii. Misses important events due to working out
      iv. Talks excessively about the number of calories they have burned
      v. Becomes upset if their exercise routine is disrupted
   f. Mood fluctuations
      i. Signs of irritability, depression, and anxiety
      ii. Stops socializing and loses interest in previously enjoyed activities

SUBJECTIVE DATA

A. APRNs should be diligent when asking questions regarding eating habits to identify those with symptoms of EDs quickly. Questions such as "Have you had any concerns about your eating behaviors or your relationship with food?" "Are there times when you eat more rapidly than usual or eat alone because of embarrassment about others seeing how much or how you eat?" "Does your weight fluctuate?" and "Do you eat more when you are stressed or anxious?" may allow APRNs to openly discuss symptoms with their patients. If patients make statements such as "I'm on a diet but can't seem to lose weight" or "I stay up late after my spouse goes to sleep" (which can be a time when binge eating occurs), it may necessitate further questioning.

B. Information to be gathered by the APRN includes the following:

1. Patient's perception of the issue
2. Eating habits and dietary recall
3. History of dieting
4. Methods of weight control (restricting, purging, exercising)
5. Value attached to specific shape or weight
6. Interpersonal and social functioning
7. Difficulty with impulsivity and compulsivity
8. Family and interpersonal relationships (frequently troublesome and chaotic, with lack of nurturing)
9. Failure to disclose symptoms and secrecy surrounding eating (may pose particular challenges to providing professional help)
10. Reports from family and friends regarding purging, including vomiting, taking laxatives or diuretics, excessive exercise, weight changes, dizziness, anemia, loss of periods, tooth enamel erosion, and bingeing on large portions of food
11. History of hostility or competitive behaviors

PHYSICAL EXAMINATION

A. APRNs should note physical signs such as lanugo hair, tooth enamel erosion from vomiting, parotid gland swelling, and such symptoms as gastroesophageal reflux and amenorrhea as indicators to explore.

B. APRNs must remain alert for disordered eating, especially in female athletes and patients with diabetes. Treatment requires a multidisciplinary team, including a primary care practitioner, nutritionist, mental health professionals, and specialists in gastroenterology, cardiology, and so on, depending on need. The role of the APRN is to determine the need for hospitalization and to manage medical complications (e.g., arrhythmias, refeeding syndrome, osteoporosis, electrolyte abnormalities such as hypokalemia). Severe medical complications are often associated with AN, BN, and ARFID.

1. Vital signs
   a. Of particular importance are hypothermia, bradycardia, hypotension, and orthostatic changes in pulse and blood pressure. These are common indicators of AN.
2. Weight less than 75% of ideal body weight or BMI less than 15, or rapid massive weight loss

3. Severe malnutrition
4. Unstable vital signs, such as temperature lower than 35.5°C (95.9°F) and low irregular heart rate of less than 45 beats per minute
5. Abnormal heart rhythm or heart failure
6. Systolic blood pressure level lower than 80 mmHg and loss of consciousness due to hypotension
7. Orthostatic change in pulse higher than 20 beats per minute
8. Orthostatic change in blood pressure greater than 10 mmHg
9. Consult with an adolescent medicine specialist highly recommended for adolescents with these vital signs
10. Height and weight
    a. Patients with AN can have a body weight less than 85% of the expected average weight. However, body weight less than 75% or BMI less than 16 meets hospitalization criteria. BMI is not designed for children and adolescents younger than 18 years; other charts are required for younger individuals.
    b. Most patients with BN maintain a weight within the normal range or slightly higher.
    c. Patients who have BED typically have BMIs in the overweight or obese category.
11. Integumentary
    a. The skin, hair, and nails undergo changes with EDs and can provide useful information about its severity.
        i. Fine, downy hair (lanugo) on the face and back
        ii. Jaundice, pale cool extremities, and poor skin turgor
        iii. Calluses or scars on hands from self-induced vomiting (Russell's sign)
12. Head, neck, mouth, and throat
    a. Sialadenitis, or enlargement of the parotid glands, is caused by the glands being forced to produce excess amounts of saliva. Glands swell with chronic purging. Enlarged glands are caused by dehydration and the body's attempt to contain the body's fluids. Enlargement occurs between 2 and 6 days after a purging episode.
    b. Assess for dental erosion and caries, which may be caused by induced vomiting.
13. Cardiovascular system
    a. Assess for irregular and/or low heart rate. Bradycardia can lead to dizziness, fainting, fatigue, and lack of energy. A slowed heart rate may also lead to hypotension. The healthcare provider must differentiate between a low heart rate due to physical fitness and bradycardia due to malnutrition. Patients with ED may try to deflect the cause of their low heart rate by saying they exercise and have an "athletic heart." Patients with malnutrition have a low resting heart rate but exhibit tachycardia (elevated heart rate) with minimal activity.
    b. Assess for mitral valve prolapse, chest pain, and palpitations. Structural heart disease occurs in patients with EDs, attributable to wasting of the cardiac muscle, resulting in decreased left ventricular mass and cardiac output. Reduced cardiac function is associated with the degree and duration of malnutrition. Patients with AN are more likely to have mitral valve prolapse, which can be seen in a minority of patients, causing chest pain and heart palpitations.
    c. Assess for peripheral edema caused by postprandial hypoglycemia. Edema is most common in individuals who abuse laxatives or diuretics and self-induce vomiting once they stop purging. Purging results in water loss, which prompts the body to release antidiuretic hormones, which signal the body to hold on to as much water and minerals as possible. Water retention and edema are usually in the extremities.
14. Fluid and electrolyte balance
    a. Acidosis and alkalosis
    b. Abnormal blood glucose caused by either starvation or bingeing on foods high in calories
    c. Electrolyte imbalances depending on the method of purging (laxatives, diuretics, vomiting)
15. Musculoskeletal system
    a. Muscle weakness and wasting
    b. Decreased energy
    c. Loss of bone density and possible osteoporosis
16. Gastrointestinal system
    a. Constipation due to dehydration
    b. Diarrhea due to laxative use
    c. Abdominal cramping
    d. Esophageal tears or gastric rupture from bulimia
17. Reproductive status
    a. Assess for amenorrhea caused by restrictive dieting. Menstruation stops due to inadequate fuel to support the menstrual process.
    b. Menstrual irregularities should prompt the healthcare provider to inquire about eating abnormalities.
18. Mental status
    a. Low self-esteem, impulsivity, and difficulty with interpersonal relationships
    b. Depressed mood and irritability
    c. Social withdrawal
    d. Cognitive distortions
        i. Overgeneralizations: "Other people don't like me because I'm fat."
        ii. "All or nothing" thinking: "If I eat dessert, I'll gain 50 pounds."
        iii. Catastrophizing: "My life is over if I gain weight."
        iv. Personalization: "When I walk down the hallway, I know everyone is looking at me."
        v. Emotional reasoning: "I look bad because I'm bloated."
        vi. Guilt or shame due to binge eating behavior
        vii. Fear of gaining weight
        viii. Interpreting their image in the mirror as severely overweight
        ix. High interest in preparing food but not eating
        x. Exhibiting the need for an intense physical regimen
        xi. Obsessive-compulsive features related to food, such as collecting recipes, hoarding food, and having concerns about eating in public

DIAGNOSTIC TESTS AND SCREENING

SCREENING
A. Individuals suffering from EDs use primary health services most frequently; therefore, APRNs in primary care, urgent care, and standing clinics should screen for EDs with the first suspicion of symptoms.

B. Many primary care providers inadequately identify individuals with EDs because they do not associate electrolyte imbalances with emotional difficulties. They may have several other constraints in providing care, such as a lack of time to treat this pervasive illness.

C. Potential harms of screening questionnaires include false-positive screening results that lead to unnecessary referrals (and associated time and financial costs), treatment, labeling, anxiety, and stigma. Pharmacologic interventions may result in adverse events such as dry mouth, headache, insomnia, paresthesia, and taste perversion (topiramate) or insomnia, nausea, and tremor (selective serotonin reuptake inhibitors [SSRIs]). Psychological interventions are likely to have minimal harms.

D. Individuals to screen for possible identification of an ED include those who are underweight compared with age norms, those who have sustained rapid weight loss, those who are disproportionately concerned about their weight or are dieting when underweight, those with menstrual disturbances, those with unexplained gastrointestinal symptoms, and those who present with the physical signs of malnutrition or repeated vomiting.

E. EDs are also more common in those who have other mental health problems. Those with type 1 diabetes who have poor treatment adherence should be screened. In children, poor growth or a sudden change in eating habits can be indicators of an FED. Physicians rate themselves highly competent in recognizing FEDs but seldom screen for them.

F. APRNs must be particularly attuned to signs and symptoms of FEDs, ask about eating behaviors, and administer a screening tool, as patients seldom disclose this disorder.

G. Annual health supervision examinations and sports physicals are ideal screening opportunities. In addition to weight, height, and BMI measurements, a screening tool such as the SCOFF questionnaire (Morgan et al., 1999) is valid for adults and may be an appropriate approach for children and adolescents. The SCOFF questionnaire is an easy screening tool for EDs designed for use by professionals when the presenting symptoms suggest an ED. It consists of five questions that focus on key areas related to eating behaviors and attitudes: inducing purging, controlling food intake, rapid weight loss, body image concerns, and preoccupation with food. The SCOFF questions are designed to clarify suspicion that an ED might exist rather than to make a diagnosis. Questions can be delivered either verbally or in written form. The SCOFF is a highly efficient tool for the detection of EDs, and its use is highly recommended. This questionnaire is easily accessible online for personal use; to view the complete questionnaire, visit www.bmj.com/content/319/7223/1467.

H. Two further questions are shown to indicate a high sensitivity and specificity for BN. The following questions indicate a need for further questioning and discussion regarding BN:
1. Are you satisfied with your eating patterns?
2. Do you ever eat in secret?

I. Other surveys that may be used to diagnose and determine the severity of symptoms include the following:
1. Eating Disorder Inventory
2. Body Attitude Test
3. Diagnostic Survey for Eating Disorders
4. Eating Disorder Inventory 3 (EDI-3)

DIAGNOSTIC TESTS

A. Labs can be valuable in assessing the physical health of individuals with FEDs. However, it is important to note that the selection of specific tests may vary based on the individual's symptoms, medical history, and the type of ED. The following are some basic lab tests that will help in the evaluation of a patient with FED:
1. Complete blood count may provide information regarding anemia and nutritional deficiencies. Anemia and leukopenia are caused by a diet consistently low in iron, folate, and vitamin B_{12}.
2. Serum electrolytes: Purging behaviors can lead to electrolyte imbalances, which can cause arrhythmia and other serious consequences caused by disordered acid–base balance, such as an increase in blood bicarbonate (metabolic alkalosis) related to self-induced vomiting and a decrease in blood bicarbonate (metabolic acidosis) related to laxative use. Nutritional status and hydration should be checked. Vomiting and diuretic misuse may also cause hyponatremia; hypokalemia; hypoalbuminemia caused by direct loss of potassium, protein, and sodium due to purging; hypophosphatemia; and hypomagnesemia (malnutrition).
3. Liver function tests: Check for malnutrition and altered nutritional intake. Transaminases increase with purging. Elevated liver enzymes may be caused by refeeding syndrome or persistent malnutrition.
4. Serum prealbumin: 15 mg/dL is the best marker of malnutrition.
5. Kidney function test: Perform kidney function test especially in cases where dehydration or electrolyte imbalances may impact renal health.
6. Bone health markers: Restrictive behaviors can impact bone health (e.g., osteoporosis, fractures).
7. Thyroid function test: Thyroid dysfunction may follow disordered eating patterns.
8. Serum amylase and serum lipase may increase with purging behaviors.
9. Blood glucose: Abnormal blood glucose is caused by either starvation or bingeing on foods high in calories.
10. Lipid panel: Elevated cholesterol from bingeing on high-fat foods, or a total cholesterol of less than 160 mg/dL, is a marker of malnutrition.
11. Nutrient levels: In cases of severe malnutrition, assessing specific nutrient levels (e.g., iron, vitamin B_{12}, folate) may be important.
12. Hormone levels: Assess for abnormal thyroid, estrogen, estradiol, progesterone, and testosterone function; decreased estrogen in females who have AN; and decreased testosterone in males who have AN.
13. Cortisol levels: Stress and malnutrition can impact cortisol levels.
14. Urine analysis: Increased urine specific gravity and elevated ketones and blood urea nitrogen (BUN) due to dehydration may be seen.

B. Diagnostics
1. EKG: Sinus bradycardia is commonly associated with AN and severe malnutrition. It can result from a decrease in metabolic rate and reduced cardiac output. Electrolyte imbalances, such as QT prolongation, hypokalemia, and hypomagnesemia, can contribute to arrhythmias resulting from purging behaviors. These can increase the risk of life-threatening ventricular arrhythmias, myocardial ischemia, or other cardiac issues. ST-segment changes, atrial fibrillation or flutter, and low voltage can occur in severe cases of malnutrition.
2. Bone densitometry: This test is recommended for adults after 2 years or children after 1 year of being underweight, or earlier if there is bone pain or fracture, due to risk of osteopenia or osteoporosis.

DIFFERENTIAL DIAGNOSIS

A. FEDs must be differentiated from other diseases. Many medical and psychiatric conditions can mimic the symptoms of EDs and can cause chronic restriction of food, nausea, vomiting, binge eating, or amenorrhea, which may result in severe weight changes. However, patients with these conditions do not fear gaining weight or have a preoccupation with body shape or weight. It is important to rule out underlying medical and other psychiatric conditions such as mood disorders before diagnosing FED.

   1. Medical issues that can mimic an ED include, but are not limited to, esophageal achalasia, malignancy, inflammatory bowel disease, immunodeficiency, hypothyroidism or hyperthyroidism, malabsorption, chronic infections, adrenal insufficiency, diabetes, celiac, HIV, and tuberculosis. Disturbed eating may be present in some neurologic and medical conditions, but patients with these conditions do not fear gaining weight or have a preoccupation with body shape or weight.

   2. Patients with ED should be given only one ED diagnosis. The healthcare provider must consider whether food restriction is associated with purging, a fear of gaining weight, or preoccupation with body shape or weight.

B. Psychiatric differentials include the following:

   1. Anorexia: Disorders that present with anorexia and cachexia include medical conditions such as malignancies, brain tumors, and other neurologic disorders such as Kleine–Levin syndrome, as well as gastrointestinal disease and endocrine disorders such as adrenal insufficiency, pituitary prolactinoma, diabetes mellitus, hyperthyroidism, and AIDS. BN and other EDs may share similarities but not meet all diagnostic criteria.

   2. Major depressive disorder (MDD): Severe weight loss may also present in MDD and other mood disorders; however, these patients do not have a desire for weight loss or have an intense fear of weight gain. MDD is often comorbid with FEDs.

   3. Schizophrenia: Patients with schizophrenia may exhibit odd eating behaviors and occasional weight loss due to paranoia but rarely demonstrate body image disturbance or an intense fear of gaining weight.

   4. Substance use disorders: Patients with substance use may exhibit low body weight or have a reduced appetite based on the drug they use (e.g., alcohol, cocaine, methamphetamine) but rarely demonstrate body image disturbance or an intense fear of gaining weight or a distortion in perception of body shape or weight.

   5. Anxiety disorders, such as obsessive-compulsive disorder, body dysmorphic disorder, and social anxiety disorder, can overlap with FEDs, specifically embarrassment or fear of eating in public, obsessions and compulsions related to food, and preoccupation with a specific defect in the body (e.g., "my feet are too big"). If the patient has social fears not related to food, such as fear of speaking in public, fear of being in crowds, obsessions related to contamination, or a distorted embarrassment of a body part, further evaluation to determine a comorbid disorder or if a FED is the appropriate diagnosis should be conducted.

   6. Borderline personality disorder: Patients with borderline personality disorder often have impulsive behaviors such as binge eating. If criteria for both disorders are present, both diagnoses should be given.

C. FED differentials include the following:

   1. AN differential diagnoses that present with cachexia include medical conditions such as brain tumors; other neurologic disorders such as Kleine–Levin syndrome; gastrointestinal disease; and endocrine disorders and complications such as adrenal insufficiency, pituitary prolactinoma, diabetes mellitus, hyperthyroidism, malignancies, and AIDS. BN and other EDs may share similarities but not meet all diagnostic criteria.

   2. BN: Medical conditions like brain tumors and central nervous system conditions can mimic BN symptoms. The binge–purge subtype of AN and borderline personality disorder may exhibit binge eating behavior. BED differentiates from BN by the absence of compensatory behaviors. Other psychiatric disorders, including MDD and borderline personality disorder, may present similarly to BN.

   3. BED: Differential diagnosis includes BN, anxiety disorder, mood disorder, Kleine–Levin syndrome, and borderline personality disorder. BED lacks compensatory weight loss behaviors, distinguishing it from BN. Overvaluation of body weight and shape and psychiatric comorbidity are key features. Mood disorders may feature increased appetite and weight gain, but binges are not associated with loss of control. The key is that episodes occur at least weekly for 3 months.

   4. Pica: Differential diagnosis for pica includes AN, factitious disorder, and nonsuicidal self-injury. In AN, ingesting nonnutritive substances is an attempt to control appetite. Factitious disorder involves ingesting nonfood substances to create physical symptoms, while nonsuicidal self-injury may involve swallowing harmful objects for attention or as negative coping.

   5. Rumination disorder: Rumination disorder can occur with other medical or psychiatric conditions, especially anxiety disorders, AN, and pediatric BN. Medical conditions include esophagitis, gastroesophageal reflux disease (GERD), hypercalcemia, pediatric adrenal insufficiency (Addison disease), pediatric hypertrophic pyloric stenosis, peptic ulcer disease, Sandifer syndrome, small bowel obstruction, and type 1 diabetes mellitus. Diagnosis is appropriate when symptoms require additional attention.

   6. ARFID: Loss of appetite, a nonspecific symptom, can be seen in various medical and psychiatric disorders. Children with certain neurologic or neuromuscular disorders might experience feeding difficulties due to problems in the innervation of oropharyngeal muscles, hypotonia, or swallowing issues. Medical conditions such as gastrointestinal disorders, food allergies, intolerances, and cancer may also cause loss of appetite. Psychiatric disorders may cause food avoidance or restriction, such as reactive attachment disorder, autism spectrum disorder, anxiety disorders, AN, obsessive-compulsive disorder, mood disorders, schizophrenia, and factitious disorder. Anxiety disorders are a common comorbidity.

MEDICAL COMORBIDITIES

A. High medical comorbidity rates are observed in individuals with FEDs. FEDs may serve as maladaptive coping mechanisms for managing emotional pain or stress, further intertwining psychological and physical elements. Medical comorbidities contribute to increased FED symptom severity, maintenance of some FED behaviors, reduced functioning, and poorer treatment outcomes. Early identification and management of medical comorbidities in patients with an ED improves response to treatment and overall outcomes.

B. Medical comorbidities that complicate FEDs include the following:
1. Nutritional deficiencies
   a. Malnutrition is a common consequence of many EDs, leading to deficiencies in essential nutrients such as vitamins and minerals. This can result in a range of health issues, including fatigue, weakness, and impaired immune function.
   b. FEDs can result in growth faltering (failure to thrive) and stunted growth in children.
2. GERD
   a. Individuals with BED or BN may experience frequent episodes of overeating followed by purging, which can contribute to GERD.
   b. Restriction of food intake in AN can lead to digestive issues, including constipation.
3. Cardiovascular complications
   a. Electrolyte imbalances: Purging behaviors, such as vomiting or laxative use, can lead to electrolyte imbalances, affecting the heart's rhythm and potentially leading to cardiac complications.
   b. Bradycardia: An abnormally slow heart rate is commonly associated with AN.
   c. Other associated cardiovascular complications include heart failure, hypertension, and shortness of breath.
4. Endocrine disorders
   a. Amenorrhea: Irregular or absent menstrual periods are common in individuals with AN and may also occur in other EDs.
   b. Hormonal imbalances: Disruptions in hormones, including those related to the thyroid and reproductive system, may occur.
   c. Other associated endocrine disorders include type 2 diabetes, metabolic syndrome, and obesity.
5. Bone health issues
   a. Osteopenia and osteoporosis may occur.
   b. Inadequate nutrition, especially insufficient calcium and vitamin D intake, can lead to reduced bone density and an increased risk of fractures.
6. Dental problems
   a. Dental problems include tooth decay from frequent vomiting associated with BN, which exposes the teeth to stomach acid, increasing the risk of dental problems such as enamel erosion and cavities.
7. Neurologic complications
   a. Seizures: Electrolyte imbalances and malnutrition in severe cases of EDs may contribute to the development of seizures.
   b. Neuropathy: Nerve damage may occur due to nutritional deficiencies.
8. Complications in pregnancy
   a. For individuals with EDs who become pregnant, there may be an increased risk of complications, including preterm birth, low birth weight, and developmental issues for the fetus.
9. Compromised immune function
   a. Malnutrition can weaken the immune system, making individuals more susceptible to infections and illnesses.
10. Psychiatric comorbidities
    a. EDs often coexist with other psychiatric conditions such as depression, anxiety disorders, and obsessive-compulsive disorder, as well as sleep disturbances.
    b. Some EDs, such as night eating syndrome, involve consuming a significant portion of daily food intake during nighttime hours, potentially disrupting normal sleep–wake cycles.
    c. Emotional distress: Pain, sleep disturbances, and functional impairment can contribute to emotional distress, exacerbating the psychological aspects of EDs.
11. Pain
    a. Bingeing and purging behaviors such as BN may occur, and patient may experience abdominal pain due to frequent vomiting or laxative use.
    b. Other pain syndromes include neck and shoulder pain, low back pain, and chronic muscular pain in men.
    c. Musculoskeletal pain and headaches related to fibromyalgia and irritable bowel syndrome have also been noted as medical comorbidities.
    d. Malnutrition can lead to muscle wasting, weakness, and general bodily discomfort.
    e. Reduced bone density may result in bone pain and increase the risk of fractures.
12. Functional impairments
    a. Inadequate energy intake can result in physical weakness, fatigue, and overall functional impairment.
    b. Individuals with severe EDs, particularly AN, may engage in excessive exercise, contributing to physical exhaustion and impairment.
13. Cognitive impairment
    a. Poor nutrition affects cognitive function, potentially leading to difficulties in concentration, memory, and decision-making, impacting daily functioning.

COMPLICATIONS WITH DIAGNOSES

A. Before making a diagnosis, APRNs must understand the patient's culture and psychopathology; how they handle stress, anxiety, and challenging situations; and how these affect the presenting symptoms. Secretive thoughts and behaviors of patients with EDs can impact the formation, maintenance, and diagnosis of an ED.

B. The nature of eating disordered behaviors changes over time. Because of this, psychopathology researchers are considering changing the current state of clearly defined ED categories to a spectrum or transdiagnostic approach as they recognize that boundaries between distinct psychiatric disorders do not cleanly map to complex configurations of human experience.

C. Patients with EDs often attempt to keep their thoughts and behaviors a secret from others. They describe several reasons for not revealing food restriction, purging, or excessive exercise to others:
1. Lack of awareness of or insight into the problem
2. Being concerned about judgment from others
3. Being concerned that others will try to stop them (e.g., telling someone would mean that they would "lose" the ED or that they would be made to "get fat")
4. Avoiding hurting those they love
   a. Facing their issues means "admitting" to a problem, and they are not prepared to change their behavior. There may be a variety of ways individuals hide EDs, including wearing loose clothes to conceal weight loss, destroying and throwing away food, or eating in secrecy or inconspicuously. Some have elaborate ways of making it look like they have eaten or hiding evidence of bingeing: "I used to go to extreme lengths to

make it look like I'd eaten. I would chop the food up and dip it around in the ketchup on the plate and leave a few crumbs and stuff, so it was convincing."

b. Individuals in recovery from EDs believe that family members must be aware of the secrecy, emphasizing that hiding behavior from family was not something they chose to do but felt they had to do. Some individuals with EDs worry about how others would react and try to protect them from getting upset. Many feel they must be the "perfect child" and not let their parents down. They might arrange school counseling and doctor appointments outside the primary provider, so parents do not find out. Some are embarrassed and worried that if others found out, they would ridicule them for "not being thin enough to have an eating disorder." Individuals feel the ED belongs to them, and they do not want to let others control it.

c. Individuals with bulimia may find it easy to purge without others realizing it at home, school, and work.
   i. When others challenge them about their behavior, they feel pushed to be more secretive. Some feel compelled to keep their illness secret, have a "catalog of excuses," and describe how, after years of having the ED, "lying comes naturally" or family "believe what they want to." Some convince their family and doctors that their weight loss is due to a physical cause, not self-induced. Those treated in the hospital say spending time with others with EDs has taught them lots of "tricks of the trade" for hiding their ED. Often patients with EDs feel angry that medical professionals do not see through their excuses because they should realize that secrecy is part of the illness. As individuals start to feel better, they feel less need to be secretive. Being able to have open, nonjudgmental, and trusting relationships with family and therapists can help tackle secrecy in EDs.

DIAGNOSTIC CRITERIA

EDs in adults present in three primary classic clinical presentations: AN, BN, and BED. Many cases seen in clinical practice are difficult to diagnose and distinguish until a clear picture of the patient's symptomology can be matched to the correct diagnosis. Diagnosis may take several visits for healthcare provider–patient trust-building and patient disclosure of symptoms. Specialist treatment experts characterize EDs primarily as pathologic disturbances of attitudes and behaviors related to food. Food may be used in a dysfunctional manner to relieve anxiety and stress. When individuals view their bodies as barriers to emotional growth (e.g., "I'm too fat to do…"), emotional conflict develops. Psychosomatic symptoms manifest when individuals feel their bodies are problematic, and as a result initiate dysfunctional behaviors to resolve the issue.

ANOREXIA NERVOSA

Individuals with AN have persistent food intake restriction, leading to significantly low body weight based on age, sex, development, and physical health.

A. Signs and symptoms
   1. Consistent extremely restrictive eating, emaciation
   2. Lethargy fatigue
   3. Body image distortion with intense fear of gaining weight, manifesting in behaviors designed to prevent weight gain
   4. Lack of awareness of the seriousness of low body weight
   5. Unwillingness to maintain a healthy weight or relentless pursuit of thinness
   6. Osteopenia or osteoporosis
   7. Anemia, muscle wasting
   8. Dry brittle skin, lanugo
   9. Dehydration, constipation
   10. Bradypnea, hypotension, bradycardia, arrhythmias
   11. Amenorrhea, infertility

B. Other factors to consider
   1. Three consecutive missed menstrual cycles may strengthen the diagnosis but are not required to diagnose AN.
   2. AN does not require a specific degree of weight loss, but guidelines indicate the individual should demonstrate at least 15% less than average/ideal body weight.
   3. Typically, treatment requires restoration to 90% of the average body weight.
   4. There are two subtypes of AN: restricting type and binge purging type. In the restricting type of AN, the patient loses weight through food restriction and/or exercise. In the binge purging type, the patient loses weight by vomiting or using laxatives after eating.
   5. Risk factors for anorexia include obsessional traits in childhood, growing up in a culture or setting where thinness is valued, and having a first-degree biological relative with an ED. There is also an increased risk for individuals who have a first-degree relative with bipolar and depressive disorders.
   6. AN has the highest rate of death of any psychiatric illness.
   7. Suicide risk is elevated in AN. A comprehensive evaluation of individuals with AN should include an assessment of suicide-related ideation and a history of suicide attempts.
   8. In cases with AN, suicide attempters were older, had a more prolonged illness duration, weighed less, had more often used drugs and alcohol, and tended to be more obsessive than nonattempters.
   9. Determination of the severity of AN in an individual may be assisted by evaluation of BMI.
      a. Mild: BMI of 17 kg/m^2 or higher
      b. Moderate: BMI of 16 to 16.99 kg/m^2
      c. Severe: BMI of 15 to 15.99 kg/m^2
      d. Extreme: BMI of less than 15 kg/m^2
   10. Individuals with AN may be considered in *partial* remission if their weight is improved but they still fear gaining weight or have a disturbed body images. *Full* remission occurs when the individual no longer has any signs or symptoms of AN.

BULIMIA NERVOSA

BN is recurrent, uncontrolled binge eating of an abnormally large amount of food in a short period of time, followed by compensatory behaviors and a sense of lack of control over eating during episodes.

A. Individuals with BN engage in repeated episodes of binge eating (at least once per week over the course of a month). Inappropriate compensatory behaviors (purging) typically follow excessive eating to prevent weight gain (e.g., self-induced vomiting; misuse of laxatives, enemas, diuretics, or other medications; fasting; excessive exercise) to rid the body of the excess calories.

B. Self-evaluation is unduly influenced by weight and body shape. Patient may check body weight repeatedly or exhibit ▶

avoidant behaviors such as refusing to have mirrors in the home or to purchase clothing of certain sizing.
C. Due to being mostly normal weight or even having weight gain, the patient does not meet the criteria for AN.
D. Binging and inappropriate compensatory behavior both occur on average at least once per week for 3 months and are not accompanied by weight loss. There may be significant impairment in personal, family, social, educational, occupational, or other areas of functioning. BN is a significant disturbance in the individual's perception of body shape and weight.
E. Individuals who binge may eat more rapidly than usual, feel that they cannot stop eating or control how much they eat, and often eat until they become uncomfortable or are in pain. Some individuals describe a dissociative feeling during or following binge eating episodes. They often eat alone due to a sense of shame, and may feel guilt and disgust, which negatively impact self-worth.
F. Binge eating appears to be characterized by adding excessive food rather than craving certain foods, such as carbohydrates. Attempts to conceal bingeing are influenced by the individual's shame of excessive eating and occur in secrecy or as inconspicuously as possible.
G. Signs and symptoms of bulimia include the following:
1. Food hoarding
2. Excessive exercising or fasting to burn calories
3. Using the bathroom during or immediately following meals
4. Russell's sign, which include scars on fingers or knuckles from repeated instances of self-induced vomiting that causes irritation, calluses, or scars on knuckles or on the back of hands
5. Chronically inflamed and sore throat
6. Swollen salivary glands in the neck and jaw area
7. Dental issues, such as worn tooth enamel, tooth sensitivity, and tooth decay as a result of exposure to stomach acid
8. Gastrointestinal issues like reflux, GERD, persistent hoarseness, and dysphagia
9. Intestinal distress and irritation from laxative abuse
10. Weakness, severe dehydration from purging of fluids
11. Electrolyte imbalance (too low or too high levels of sodium, calcium, potassium, and other minerals), which can lead to stroke or heart attack
12. Social withdrawal, dysphoria, and/or anxiety

H. Severity of BN may be determined based on the number of episodes of inappropriate compensatory behavior per week: mild (1–3 episodes), moderate (4–7 episodes), severe (8–13 episodes), or extreme (14 or more episodes).
I. Negative triggers to bingeing include interpersonal stressors, dietary restraints, negative feelings, or comments related to body weight, body shape, and food. Binge eating may lessen negative emotions associated with food in the immediate time frame, but harsh and negative self-evaluation and dysphoria develop long term.
1. Vomiting is the most common method of purging, with immediate relief of the physical discomfort from overeating and reduction of the fear of gaining weight.
2. Ways to induce vomiting include using fingers or instruments such as a toothbrush to stimulate the gag reflex. Those who purge using vomiting become adept at inducing vomiting and eventually can vomit at will.

J. Individuals with bulimia who misuse enemas rarely use these as the sole compensatory method.
K. Other compensatory strategies include using thyroid hormone to speed up metabolism or misusing insulin to affect the metabolism of food for those with diabetes mellitus.
L. Individuals with bulimia may fast for a day before bingeing to prevent weight gain. Exercise as a compensatory method is determined as excessive when it significantly interferes with meaningful activities or occurs at inappropriate times or settings, or when the individual continues to exercise despite injury or medical complications.
M. Risk factors for developing bulimia include the following:
1. Genetic and biological factors
   a. Family history of EDs or mental health issues
   b. Abnormalities in brain chemicals and neurotransmitters that regulate mood and appetite
2. History
   a. Trauma or childhood sexual or physical abuse, low self-esteem, perfectionism, body dissatisfaction, childhood obesity, early puberty, childhood anxiety disorders
   b. Past or current social anxiety disorder
3. Societal factors
   a. Pressure for thinness or an idealized body shape
   b. Participation in activities or sports that emphasize weight and appearance or peer pressure with focus on weight and body image
4. Personality factors
   a. Impulsivity, alexithymia, perfectionism
   b. Body image distortion
5. Stressful life events
   a. Moving, starting college, job changes, academic pressures
   b. Relationship problems
6. Dieting and weight control behaviors
   a. History of restrictive dieting
   b. Engaging in extreme weight control measures
7. Co-occurring mental health disorders
   a. Severe psychiatric comorbidities, which predict a worse long-term outcome of bulimia
   b. Personality disorder, anxiety, depression, mood disorder, substance use disorders, and PTSD
8. Severe role impairment and elevated suicide risk
   a. Patients who present with bulimia should be evaluated for social impairment, suicidality, and previous suicide attempts.
9. History of suicide attempts more prevalent among binge eating/purging EDs and BN than in the other subgroups
   a. In cases of BN, attempters present with more psychiatric symptoms and had more frequently been sexually abused.

N. Individuals with BN may be considered in *partial* remission if they no longer meet all of the criteria for BN. *Full* remission occurs when the individual no longer has any signs or symptoms of BN.

BINGE EATING DISORDER

A. BED often begins in the late teens or early 20s, although it has been reported in both young children and older adults.
B. Individuals with BED repeatedly eat large quantities of food over a short period (less than 2 hours) without the compensatory behaviors (e.g., purging, fasting, using medications, excessive exercise) associated with BN.

C. Excessive food consumption occurs at least once per week for 3 months. Patients with BED feel a lack of control during the eating episode (i.e., they cannot stop eating or control how much they eat).
D. Three of the following behaviors must be present to diagnose BED:
  1. Eating more rapidly than usual
  2. Eating until uncomfortably full
  3. Eating large amounts of food even when not hungry or eating alone due to embarrassment of the quantity of food consumed
E. Individuals who binge-eat will typically feel distressed, disgusted, depressed, or guilty after overeating. Binge eating is not associated with weight loss and most likely causes weight gain.
F. Severity of BED may be determined based on the number of episodes of binge eating per week: mild (1–3 episodes), moderate (4–7 episodes), severe (8–13 episodes), or extreme (14 or more episodes).
G. Weight gain associated with binge eating increases the patient's risk for other disorders related to obesity, such as diabetes mellitus, hypertension, and cancer.
H. Binge eating occurs in individuals with average weight, overweight, or obesity, and those with BED are not typically underweight as with AN. Those with the disorder consume more calories and have a more significant functional impairment, lower quality of life, distress, and psychiatric comorbidities. Loss of control of eating or episodic bingeing may precede another ED.
I. Risk factors identified are adverse childhood experiences, parental depression, vulnerability to obesity, and repeated exposure to negative comments about shape, weight, and eating.
J. Compared with individuals with other psychiatric disorders, those with BED report more childhood obesity and more exposure to negative comments about shape, weight, and eating. BED affects males and females of all ages but most commonly occurs in adults 46 to 55 years of age. BED appears to run in families and has genetic influences.
K. Individuals with BED may be considered in *partial* remission if they no longer meet all of the criteria for BED. *Full* remission occurs when the individual no longer has any signs or symptoms of BED.

FEEDING DISORDERS

FDs are characterized by extreme food selectivity (beyond pickiness) by type (e.g., excluding more than one food group from the child's diet); by texture (e.g., eat only smooth or crunchy foods); or by brand, shape, or color. Some children develop feeding problems due to a medical condition such as reflux or a severe illness. FDs are characterized by extreme food selectivity (beyond pickiness) and by type (excluding those with oral motor skills who have difficulty chewing and swallowing, which restricts their diet). What separates FDs from pickiness is that children with FDs tend to not eat in situations outside of their home due to their extreme selectivity.

FDs are best diagnosed by a team of professionals including APRNs, gastroenterologists, registered dietitians, pediatric psychologists, child/adolescent psychiatric-mental health advanced practice nurses (PMHAPNs), occupational therapists, and speech therapists. These professionals should have specialized training in FDs. They will evaluate medical concerns, oral motor skills, swallowing skills, nutritional concerns, and behavioral concerns associated with mealtimes. Children having problems in two or more areas should be seen by a feeding team.

Avoidant/Restrictive Food Intake Disorders

A. ARFID is a feeding disturbance characterized by avoidance, aversion, or restriction of food or certain foods through oral intake, causing a persistent failure to meet nutritional needs.
B. Food restriction is based on avoiding certain foods due to sensitivity to appearance, color, smell, texture, temperature, and taste. Food avoidance may represent a conditioned negative response such as choking, trauma involving the gastrointestinal tract (e.g., endoscopy), or vomiting caused by a physical condition (emetophobia).
C. For ARFID to be diagnosed in adults, significant weight loss, nutritional deficiency, interference with psychosocial functioning, or malnutrition must be present. Adult patients with ARFID may have had a food aversion as a child that continues into adulthood. When patients with ARFID are not getting their daily nutrients, physical complications may necessitate enteral feeding.
D. Psychosocial functioning is significantly affected, leading to negative impacts on personal life, relationships, employment, and other areas.
E. Determination of nutritional insufficiency is based on clinical presentation, including dietary intake, physical assessment, and lab testing. Malnutrition symptomology caused by food restriction is similar to that seen in AN, with symptoms such as hypothermia, bradycardia, and anemia.
F. Individuals with heightened sensory sensitivities associated with autism show similar behavior.
G. The risk of ARFID is associated with anxiety disorders, mood disorders, autism spectrum disorder, obsessive-compulsive disorder, and attention deficit hyperactivity disorder (ADHD). Familial anxiety and a first-degree relative with an ED are contributing risk factors. Gastrointestinal conditions, GERD, vomiting, esophageal stricture, and various medical problems and procedures increase the risk of ARFID.
H. ARFID is equally common in males and females. Pregnancy sensory sensitivities can occur but are not extreme, and most do not present with malnutrition.
I. Diagnosis of ARFID should exclude eating disturbances caused by lack of available food types; by cultural practices; or by AN, BN, or other conditions, including mental health disorders and substance use.
J. Remission occurs when the patient no longer exhibits any signs or symptoms of ARFID.

Rumination Disorder

A. Rumination disorder (also called *rumination-regurgitation disorder*) is a rare syndrome characterized by undigested food being returned to the mouth and then rechewed, reswallowed, or spat out.
B. This behavior occurs often over several weeks in individuals 2 years of age or older. It is not caused by other medical conditions that lead to regurgitation or nausea/vomiting.
C. Additional features include intentional regurgitation for anxiety relief, shame, and reluctance to seek treatment. The disorder may persist, with variations in prevalence and presentation across developmental stages, cultures, and age groups. It is crucial to differentiate rumination disorder from infant rumination syndrome, self-induced vomiting in EDs or cultural practices, and psychogenic vomiting. Regurgitation is volitional and intentional in rumination disorder.
D. The individual will repeatedly regurgitate their food effortlessly and painlessly, caused by voluntary muscle relaxation

of the diaphragm similar to the belching reflex. The learned habit causes food, rather than gas, to come back up.
E. Regurgitation of food may be diagnosed after 1 month of continued regurgitation.
F. Frequent regurgitation often diminishes spontaneously but may become habitual, resulting in severe malnutrition and death. Rumination behaviors can begin at any age, but in adults they occur more frequently among people with intellectual disabilities. In these cases, clinical attention is needed.
G. Rumination disorder can have an episodic course or occur continuously until treated. In infants as well as in older individuals with intellectual developmental disorder or other neurodevelopmental disorders, the regurgitation and rumination behavior appears to have a self-soothing or self-stimulating function, similar to that of other repetitive motor behaviors such as head banging.
H. There is substantial risk of choking in children.
I. Rumination disorder should not be diagnosed in infants. Similar phenomena in infants should be diagnosed as infant rumination syndrome in the grouping of functional digestive disorders of infants, toddlers, or children in the *ICD-11* (WHO, 2019). When this occurs in infants, it can potentially be fatal.
J. It is often misdiagnosed as gastroparesis or GERD.
K. Individuals with rumination disorder often experience shame and embarrassment about the behavior and try to keep the behavior a secret because they recognize it as socially unacceptable.
L. Individuals with rumination disorder are often reluctant to seek treatment. The disorder may persist for a long time if left untreated.
M. The disorder may be chronic, continuous, or episodic, brought on by stress or anxiety.
N. Medication does not effectively treat rumination syndrome, and the patient must relearn to digest food properly using diaphragmatic breathing training. A behavioral psychologist can conduct diaphragmatic breathing training.
O. Remission occurs when the patient no longer exhibits any signs or symptoms of rumination disorder.

Pica
A. Pica is the persistent eating of nonfood substances over at least 1 month that is not a manifestation of a nutritional deficiency or other medical condition.
B. Eating nonfood items may interfere with eating nutritious foods and can be dangerous. Objects that cannot be digested, such as stones, hair, or paper clips, can cause intestinal damage. Bacteria or parasites in soil can infect individuals who eat dirt or clay (geophagia). Patients can also contract illnesses from eating feces, which may contain parasites or other bacteria. Eating paint can cause lead poisoning.
C. Pica is more common in children than in adults. When the disorder occurs in adults, it tends to be associated with intellectual disabilities, autism spectrum disorder, schizophrenia, anemia, sickle cell disease, or pregnancy.
D. Pica may include eating items such as hair (trichophagia), laundry starch, soap, cloth, string, chalk, talcum powder, paint, pebbles, ash, starch, or ice. It also includes food ingredients like large quantities of salt or flour.
E. Pica may manifest during pregnancy when cravings lead to the ingestion of nonnutritive substances that pose potential medical risks. The course of the disorder can be protracted, resulting in medical emergencies (e.g., intestinal obstruction, acute weight loss, poisoning).
F. Remission occurs when the patient no longer exhibits any signs or symptoms of pica.

Unspecified Feeding or Eating Disorder
A. UFED is a general category used when symptoms of an FED are present but do not meet the criteria for specific FEDs, and there may be insufficient information for a more specific diagnosis.

Other Specified Feeding or Eating Disorders
A. OSFED is designated when the full criteria for other eating disorders are not met or insufficient information is known. This category includes atypical AN, subthreshold BN, and BED, among others. OSFED is a specified category for cases that have distinct features not fitting into other categories. This category applies to presentations in which symptoms characteristic of an FED that cause clinically significant distress or impairment in social, occupational, or other important areas of functioning predominate but do not meet the full criteria for any of the disorders in the FED diagnostic class. In addition, the symptoms are not explained by another disorder or by a cultural practice and are not developmentally appropriate. The OSFED category is used in situations in which the clinician chooses to communicate the specific reason that the presentation does not meet the criteria for any specific FED. This is done by recording "other specified feeding or eating disorder" followed by the specific reason (e.g., "bulimia nervosa of low frequency"). Examples of presentations that can be specified using the "other specified" designation include the following:
  1. Atypical AN: All of the criteria for AN are met, except that despite significant weight loss the individual's weight is within or above the normal range. Individuals with atypical AN may experience many of the physiologic complications associated with AN.
  2. BN (of low frequency and/or limited duration): All of the criteria for BN are met, except that the binge eating and inappropriate compensatory behaviors occur, on average, less than once a week and/or for less than 3 months.
  3. BED (of low frequency and/or limited duration): All of the criteria for BED are met, except that the binge eating occurs, on average, less than once a week and/or for less than 3 months.
  4. Purging disorder: Patient exhibits recurrent purging behavior to influence weight or shape (e.g., self-induced vomiting; misuse of laxatives, diuretics, or other medications) in the absence of binge eating.
  5. Night eating syndrome: Patient exhibits recurrent episodes of night eating, as manifested by eating after awakening from sleep or by excessive food consumption after the evening meal. There is awareness and recall of the eating. The night eating is not better explained by external influences such as changes in the individual's sleep–wake cycle or by local social norms. The night eating causes significant distress and/or impairment in functioning. The disordered pattern of eating is not better explained by BED or another mental disorder, including substance use, and is not attributable to another medical condition or to an effect of medication.

COMORBIDITIES
High medical comorbidity rates are observed in individuals with FEDs. Medical comorbidities contribute to increased FED symptom severity, maintenance of some FED behaviors,

functioning impairment, and treatment outcomes. The relationship between FEDs and conditions like chronic pain, fibromyalgia, and irritable bowel syndrome is complex and not straightforward. While FEDs can have various physical and psychological effects, it is important to note that specific causal links between these disorders are not well-established. However, some indirect connections may exist: Pain conditions include headaches, neck and shoulder pain, low back pain, and chronic muscular pain in men. Fibromyalgia and irritable bowel syndrome have also been noted as medical comorbidities. Early identification and management of medical comorbidities in patients with an FED improves response to treatment and overall outcomes. Medical comorbidities that complicate FEDs include the following:

A. AN
1. Psychiatric comorbidities: depression, anxiety disorders (especially obsessive-compulsive disorder), personality disorders (such as borderline personality disorder), sleep issues due to hormonal dysregulation
2. Medical comorbidities: osteoporosis; electrolyte imbalances; cardiovascular complications, including arrhythmias and heart failure; gastrointestinal problems; amenorrhea

B. BN
1. Psychiatric comorbidities: depression, anxiety disorders, substance use, personality disorders; sleep issues due to electrolyte imbalances
2. Medical comorbidities: electrolyte imbalances, arrhythmias and heart failure, gastrointestinal issues, dental problems (due to repeated vomiting)

C. BED
1. Psychiatric comorbidities: depression, anxiety disorders, ADHD, substance use, mood disorders, night eating behaviors that contribute to sleep issues
2. Medical comorbidities: gastrointestinal problems, type 2 diabetes, cardiovascular issues, hypertension, obesity, dyslipidemia, metabolic syndrome, sleep apnea

D. ARFID
1. Psychiatric comorbidities: anxiety disorders, obsessive-compulsive disorder, ADHD, autism spectrum disorder; sleep issues due to anxiety
2. Medical comorbidities: nutrient deficiencies, failure to thrive, weight loss, gastrointestinal issues

E. Pica
1. Psychiatric comorbidities: intellectual disabilities, autism spectrum disorder, obsessive-compulsive disorder
2. Medical comorbidities: nutrient deficiencies, gastrointestinal complications (due to ingestion of nonfood items)

F. Rumination disorder
1. Psychiatric comorbidities: anxiety disorders, mood disorders
2. Medical comorbidities: dental issues, malnutrition, gastrointestinal problems

PLAN

Early intervention and treatment prevents serious psychological and health consequences. If left untreated, EDs tend to become more severe and less receptive to treatment. An ED is not a conscious choice. People with EDs are often reluctant to seek help as they do not understand the severity of their illness. Early intervention saves lives. It includes screening and education. In many cases, EDs can be prevented by targeting at-risk groups. The Body Project by the National Eating Disorders Association is an example of an ED prevention program for high school and college-age people.

Treatment plans should be individualized based on the specific needs and characteristics of each person. A collaborative approach involving healthcare professionals, therapists, dietitians, and family members is often the most effective way to address the complex nature of FEDs. Early intervention is key to improved outcomes.

INITIAL STABILIZATION

A. Effective family-based treatment has gained prominence, emphasizing weight restoration, healthy eating, reducing blame, and empowering caregivers. However, the initial assessment of individuals with EDs involves determining medical stability, with hospitalization considered based on the following criteria:
1. Body weight is below 75% of the ideal weight.
2. Temperature falls below 35.5°C (95.9°F).
3. Heart rate is less than 45 beats per minute.
4. Systolic blood pressure is below 80 mmHg.
5. Orthostatic change in pulse exceeds 20 beats per minute.
6. Orthostatic change in blood pressure is greater than 10 mmHg.
7. Severe electrolyte imbalances are present.

B. Immediate treatment goals for all individuals with EDs include medical stabilization, nutritional rehabilitation for weight restoration, addressing nutrient deficiencies, managing refeeding, and interrupting purging/compensatory behaviors. Additional psychological and therapeutic goals are addressed as appropriate. Initial stabilization involves the following:
1. Managing acute and chronic medical conditions, including acute medical stabilization when necessary
2. Achieving spontaneous (not hormonally induced) resumption of menses and/or return of normal gonadal hormone levels (testosterone or estrogen)
3. Addressing appropriate electrolyte imbalances
4. Resuming growth and/or pubertal progression as needed

C. Refeeding syndrome, a potentially fatal complication of malnutrition, occurs when fluids, electrolytes, and carbohydrates are reintroduced too rapidly to patients with severe malnutrition. Key considerations include the following:
1. Consider slow repletion of calories, typically at 1,000 kcal/d, with frequent monitoring of electrolyte levels through blood tests, as well as intravenous infusions based on body weight to replace electrolytes as needed.
2. Electrolyte level shifts may lead to serious complications such as seizures, heart failure, and coma.
3. Individuals with malnutrition are at risk, and symptoms typically manifest around 4 days into the refeeding process. Edema, peripheral edema, congestive heart failure, ileus, anasarca, lanugo hair, double vision, confusion, swallowing problems, nausea, vomiting, fatigue, muscle weakness, and death are potential outcomes.
4. Intravenous infusion therapy may not be suitable for individuals with impaired kidney function, hypocalcemia, or hypercalcemia. Fluid reintroduction may require careful monitoring, and those at risk of heart complications may need continuous heart monitoring.

MEDICAL INSTABILITY

A. Patients may require inpatient admission.

1. Nutritional rehabilitation (via oral, enteral, or parenteral nutrition) can evoke distressing feelings in patients; psychosocial support, empathy, and compassion are crucial for effective treatment.
2. Hospital care may occur in medical or psychiatric facilities, depending on the severity of physical symptoms and the unit's experience in managing malnutrition.
3. Inpatient care is recommended for patients with very low weight, rapid weight loss, medical complications, and psychiatric instability, including suicidality.
4. Caloric prescription initiation varies; patients at risk for refeeding syndrome need lower initial caloric intake and slow gradual increases. Begin with 1,000 kcal/d. Management may require intensive care and clinicians experienced in handling this complication.

B. Otherwise, treatment for low-weight patients may begin with caloric prescriptions of 1,500 to 1,800 kcal/d, increasing by 400 kcal/d every 48 to 72 hours if tolerated, aiming for consistent weight change.

C. Vitamin and mineral supplementation, including thiamine, should be considered.

D. Dietary assessment by a skilled dietitian/nutritionist is essential for identifying deficiencies and developing optimal plans.

E. Oral feeding is preferable for weight restoration; if not possible, enteral feeding is preferred. Total parenteral nutrition is rarely necessary and carries increased risk, which introduces ethical considerations.
1. Patients with nasogastric or intravenous methods are at higher risk for refeeding syndrome; immediate attention is needed for specific symptoms, and management may require intensive care and a physician experienced in handling this complication.
2. Patients with nasogastric or intravenous methods are at higher risk for refeeding syndrome.

GENERAL TREATMENTS AND INTERVENTIONS

A. Following initial stabilization, ongoing evidence-based treatment is delivered by a multidisciplinary team of healthcare professionals, including psychotherapy, nutrition education, medical monitoring, and medication. Weight restoration alone is not sufficient for a full recovery because distorted body image and other ED thoughts and behaviors, psychological and psychiatric comorbidities, and any social or functional impairments must be addressed in outpatient treatment. Family members should be included in ED treatment whenever possible and above all for minors.

B. Goals of outpatient treatment for FEDs are comprehensive, aiming to address both the physical and the psychological aspects of the disorder. Treatment goals will vary based on the specific type of FED and individual needs; however, some common objectives include the following:
1. Nutritional rehabilitation
   a. Nutritional counseling and education are crucial to address malnutrition and normalize eating patterns. This will likely involve working with dietitians or nutritionists. The goals include the following:
      i. Weight restoration
      ii. Restoration of meal patterns that promote health and social connections
      iii. Broadening of food repertoire and macronutrient balance
2. Normalization of eating behavior
   a. Establishment of regular and balanced eating behaviors to restore healthy weight
   b. Cessation of restrictive, binge eating, and/or purging behaviors
   c. Elimination of disordered or ritualistic eating behaviors
   d. Eating without overconcern about foods and elimination of fears around eating
3. Medical stabilization
   a. Manage and resolve medical complications and comorbidities such as electrolyte, cardiac, and nutritional irregularities.
4. Medical monitoring
   a. Regularly assess physical health, address complications, and manage any medical issues related to the ED.
5. Psychosocial stabilization
   a. Evaluation and treatment of any comorbid psychological diagnoses
   b. Reestablishment of appropriate social engagement
   c. Improvement in psychological symptoms associated with ED
   d. Improved body image
6. Family intervention
   a. Trust family concerns for safety of the patient.
   b. Diffuse blame by helping families understand that they did not cause the illness, nor did the individual with the ED choose to have it.
      i. Recognition facilitates acceptance of the diagnosis, referral, and treatment.
      ii. Undue stigma associated with having the disorder is minimized.
   c. Empower caregivers, which has a positive impact on treatment outcomes.
      i. Keep families fully informed and engaged at all stages of treatment.
      ii. Self-care for caregivers is necessary.
   d. Provide resources and support.

C. Build trust, withhold judgment, and create a safe environment for the patient to disclose information. Frequently assess for psychiatric comorbidities, including depression, anxiety disorders, and substance use disorders. Carefully monitor for safety, suicidal behaviors, self-injury, and self-loathing.

D. ED specialists, often with backgrounds in psychiatry or adolescent medicine, should ideally be involved but may not be available in some locations. Treatment should include a nutrition specialist to help select calorie-rich foods. In those who are in school, involving school counselors is necessary. Most states require special accommodations, such as snack breaks in class or allowances for missed school, to allow equal educational opportunities for students with medical disabilities such as EDs. Treatment success may be dependent on developing a therapeutic alliance with the patient, involvement of the patient's family, and close collaboration within the treatment team.

Patient-Centered Care

A. The healthcare provider should perform a self-assessment regarding frustration toward the patient's eating behaviors, the belief that the disorder is self-imposed, or the need to nurture rather than provide treatment for the patient.

B. Develop and maintain a trusting relationship through consistency and therapeutic communication. This will help diminish secrecy over time.

C. Provide a positive, supportive approach to promote the patient's self-esteem and positive self-image.
D. Encourage patient decision-making and participation in the plan of care to allow for a sense of control.
E. Establish realistic goals for weight loss or gain.
F. Arrange for the patient to receive the following:
   1. Individual cognitive behavioral therapies (CBTs)
   2. Group and family therapy to assist in resolving personal issues contributing to the ED
G. Suggest cognitive reframing.
H. Advise relaxation techniques and mindfulness.
   1. Journal writing
   2. Desensitization exercises
I. Provide a highly structured milieu in an acute care setting for patients requiring intensive therapy, monitoring of intake and output, and exercise level.
J. Monitor the patient's vital signs, intake and output, and weight (2–3 lb per week gain is medically acceptable).
K. Reward the patient for positive behaviors (completing meals or consuming a set number of calories).
L. Teach and encourage self-care activities.
M. Work with a dietitian to provide nutrition education to include correcting misinformation regarding food, meal planning, and food selection.

THERAPIES USED TO TREAT EATING DISORDERS

A. Nutrition counseling
   1. Expectation is to gain 2 to 3 lb per week.
   2. Goals focus on reestablishing healthy eating habits.
   3. Supplement diet with vitamins and minerals.
   4. Dietitian may share a meal with patient to view eating habits.
B. CBT or cognitive behavioral therapy for eating disorders (CBT-ED)
   1. Leading evidence-based treatment to change cognitive distortions
   2. Changes core psychopathology of EDs, the overevaluation of shape and weight, which is cognitive in nature
C. Interpersonal psychotherapy
   1. Strongly supported evidence-based treatment for BN and BED
   2. Brief treatment that addresses the social and interpersonal context in which the disorder begins and is maintained
D. Dialectical behavioral therapy
   1. Defines emotional dysregulation as a central problem with BN
   2. Therapy based on emotional regulation skills and authenticating patient's self-worth
E. Family therapy
   1. Potentially crucial to recovery
   2. Provides support for caregivers
   3. Relieves caregiver strain
   4. To be strongly considered with children and adolescents
F. Behavior modification in patient
   1. Uses rewards and reinforcements to help patients obtain normal weight and eating habits
   2. Directly supervises refeeding

COMMON MEDICATIONS

A. Treatment for EDs includes normalizing eating patterns and therapy to help cognitive bias surrounding food, weight, eating, and body image. In some cases, psychotropic medication can make recovery more successful (Table 10.1). As therapy reveals psychiatric comorbidities, medication may increasingly become important to address symptoms. Pharmacotherapy is useful in specific contexts, especially for co-occurring conditions, but not as a stand-alone treatment. Proceed with caution in this population due to potential for biochemical alterations, especially in patients with malnutrition. Primary care providers can be key players in treatment success.
   1. Antidepressants, including SSRIs, may help mitigate symptoms of depression and suicidal ideation in patients with AN.
   2. Topiramate has been associated with significant improvements in both binge and purge symptoms for BN.
   3. Lisdexamfetamine has shown promise in reducing compulsive behaviors of BED.
   4. Olanzapine has been shown to significantly increase the rate of weight increase over time (although there are not enough data on adolescents). However, olanzapine, as well as other psychotropics that cause weight gain, may affect compliance and intensify the cycle of dietary restriction, binging, and purging.
   5. Drugs excreted by the kidney, such as lithium, should be avoided because of risk of toxicity due to recurrent dehydration and electrolyte disturbances.
   6. Caution use of tricyclics, some neuroleptics, and other psychotropics that can prolong QTc intervals because they can cause fatal arrhythmias. Regular EKGs are advised.
   7. Bupropion is contraindicated in BN due to risk of seizure.
   8. Semaglutide has been approved for chronic weight management under certain binge eating conditions, but its use in EDs is more complex and nuanced and potentially risky. More data are needed here.
B. If psychotropic medications are attempted, the APRN or psychiatrist typically needs to supervise this administration, including medication titration and changes to prevent discontinuation syndrome or serotonin syndrome.
C. In patients with BN, studies have suggested that SSRIs may be beneficial in decreasing the frequency of binge eating and purging. Thus, the addition of an SSRI might be considered for patients who are not responding to an initial trial of psychotherapy and for patients with major depression or another comorbid disorder responsive to antidepressant medications.

PATIENT TEACHING

A. Effective patient teaching should cover the following:
   1. Understanding the disorder: Educate the patient about the psychological and physical impacts of EDs.
   2. Course of treatment will combine psychotherapy, nutrition counseling, and medication.
   3. Nutritional education: Provide information on balanced diets and the risks of malnutrition.
   4. Medication education, including side effect precautions and expected time for response: Instruct the patient to notify the healthcare provider if side effects occur.
   5. Managing triggers: Help identify and cope with triggers for disordered eating.
   6. Relapse prevention: Teach how to recognize and prevent relapse signs.
   7. Support system: Encourage building a supportive network and educate family and friends.
   8. Treatment adherence: Stress the importance of following treatment plans and attending therapy.

TABLE 10.1 COMMON MEDICATIONS IN EATING DISORDER TREATMENT

Medication	Usage	Age 10–18 Years (Youth)	Age 19–65 Years (Adult)	Age 66–74 Years (Older Adult)	Age 85–99 Years (Oldest Old + Centenarians)
Generic: cyproheptadine Trade: Periactin	Anorexia nervosa	Refer to Chapter 20, "Special Considerations for Childhood and Adolescent Populations," or PDR. Indication for usage: allergic rhinitis and urticaria	Average dose: 8 mg orally four times a day; start 2 mg orally four times a day, then increase to maintenance dose over 3 weeks Max dose: 32 mg/d	Refer to Chapter 21, "Aging and Older Adult Populations," or PDR.	Refer to Chapter 21, "Aging and Older Adult Populations," or PDR.
Generic: fluoxetine Trade: Prozac	Bulimia nervosa	Refer to Chapter 20, "Special Considerations for Childhood and Adolescent Populations," or PDR. Indication for usage: various psychiatric illnesses: cataplexy and insomnia	Average dose: 60 mg orally once daily in the morning; may titrate dose to 60 mg/d over several days; taper dose gradually to discontinue	Refer to Chapter 21, "Aging and Older Adult Populations," or PDR.	Refer to Chapter 21, "Aging and Older Adult Populations," or PDR.
Generic: sertraline Trade: Zoloft	Bulimia nervosa	Refer to Chapter 20, "Special Considerations for Childhood and Adolescent Populations," or PDR. Indication for usage: various psychiatric illnesses: cataplexy and insomnia	Average dose: 50–200 mg orally once daily in the morning	Refer to Chapter 21, "Aging and Older Adult Populations," or PDR.	Refer to Chapter 21, "Aging and Older Adult Populations," or PDR.
Generic: phenelzine Trade: Nardil	Bulimia nervosa	Refer to Chapter 20, "Special Considerations for Childhood and Adolescent Populations," or PDR. Indications and dosing not applicable to this drug	Average dose: 15 mg orally three times a day; start 15 mg three times a day, titrate to effect Max: 90 mg/d; taper dose gradually to discontinue	Refer to Chapter 21, "Aging and Older Adult Populations," or PDR.	Refer to Chapter 21, "Aging and Older Adult Populations," or PDR.
Generic: lisdexamfetamine Trade: Vyvanse	Binge eating disorder, moderate to severe	Refer to Chapter 20, "Special Considerations for Childhood and Adolescent Populations," or PDR. Indication for usage: ADHD; approved for BED	Average dose: 50–70 mg orally once daily in the morning; start 30 mg orally once daily in the morning, increase by 20 mg/d each week Max: 70 mg/d; taper dose gradually to discontinue if prolonged use	Refer to Chapter 21, "Aging and Older Adult Populations," or PDR.	Refer to Chapter 21, "Aging and Older Adult Populations," or PDR.

ADHD, attention deficit hyperactivity disorder; BED, binge eating disorder; PDR, Physician's Desk Reference.

9. Body image issues: Work on strategies to improve body image and self-esteem.
10. Healthy coping mechanisms: Teach coping strategies for emotions and stress without relying on disordered eating.
11. Monitoring of physical health: Highlight the need for regular medical checkups due to potential health consequences.
12. Long-term management: Emphasize the chronic nature of EDs and the need for ongoing care and self-management.

B. Patient should understand that if complications occur with treatment, hospitalization may be needed, including intravenous electrolyte supplementation, and monitoring of cardiac function, vital signs, and labs.

FOLLOW-UP

A. Clinical changes and the level of risk in mental and physical health should be monitored throughout treatment. Changes in ED symptoms (including behaviors, cognitions, and physical symptoms) should be monitored weekly during treatment. This provides important information about the progress and likely effectiveness of any intervention. It is commonly done using brief self-report measures that should be regularly discussed with patients. In some cases, physical and/or mental health risks may increase (e.g., continued weight loss in AN). This is why it is important to monitor levels of risk so that treatment can be reviewed and changed as required.

B. Assist patient in maintaining regularly scheduled outpatient therapy appointments and taking medication as prescribed.
C. Assist patient in developing and implementing a maintenance plan related to weight management.
D. Encourage patient and family participation in a support group.
E. Encourage the patient to see a registered dietitian for nutritional and dietary guidance periodically.

CONSULTATION AND REFERRALS

A. High rates of EDs occur among marginalized populations, including individuals from minority racial and ethnic backgrounds, sexual and gender minority individuals, and individuals experiencing homelessness and/or food insecurity. As severity and treatment resistance increase with illness duration, timely intervention is key. However, recovery from EDs is possible and common—even many years after the initial diagnosis.
B. Intensity of monitoring and treatment, and the need for acute intervention, may change over time.
C. No current U.S. Preventive Services Task Force (USPSTF) recommendation exists regarding screening for EDs in adolescents and adults; there is an ongoing USPSTF research plan to answer questions.
   1. Malnutrition requires urgent attention. Malnutrition can occur with disordered eating behaviors regardless of weight.
   2. Individuals with restrictive eating behaviors, binge eating, or purging require an immediate comprehensive assessment and intervention.
D. Urgent psychosocial evaluation is crucial when suicidality or self-harm is evident.
E. Patients with AN often experience suicidal ideation, with 20% of deaths of patients with AN attributed to suicide.
F. Common comorbidities include mood, anxiety disorders, and obsessive-compulsive disorder, with substance use disorders more prevalent in the binge eating/purging subtype.
G. Diagnosing comorbidities can be challenging due to symptom overlap, and SSRIs may be less effective in low-weight patients.
H. Weight gain is associated with improved comorbid symptoms.
I. Cardiovascular abnormalities are common in low-weight patients with AN, and caution is advised with medications having adverse cardiac effects. If comorbid symptoms persist after weight restoration, evidence-based interventions and specialist consultation are recommended.

INDIVIDUAL CONSIDERATIONS

A. Researchers have found that dieting may increase the risk of EDs in populations that are forced to maintain a thin body shape. Studies of eating behavior and attitudes in athletes and models found abnormal eating behaviors, such as fasting and purging, to be very common.
B. Frequent findings of populations forced to maintain low weights or maintain thin body shapes include the following:
   1. Amenorrhea
   2. Osteoporosis
   3. Disordered eating
C. Unintentional insufficient caloric intake can occur in adolescent athletes. Any increase in training volume, coupled with inadequate knowledge of proper nutrition, can result in energy output to food imbalance. Those caring for athletes' health need to monitor their caloric intake and provide appropriate nutritional counseling.

PEDIATRICS

A. Early identification and treatment of FEDs are crucial as they can significantly impact physical health, growth, development, and emotional well-being. Treatment typically involves a multidisciplinary approach, including medical, nutritional, and psychological interventions:
   1. All six primary FEDs are recognized in the pediatric population.
   2. With the high prevalence of these disorders in children and adolescents, it is critical that APRNs recognize these disorders and connect children and families with available treatments. Older teens often have difficulty with perfection, dieting, EDs, and body image that can take their toll in adulthood. See Chapter 20, "Special Considerations for Childhood and Adolescent Populations," for further information on the pediatric population.

PREGNANCY AND INFERTILITY

A. FEDs can have significant impact on pregnancy and fertility. Management of EDs during pregnancy requires an early detection and multidisciplinary approach, focusing on the physical health of both the patient and the developing fetus, as well as psychological support. EDs are prevalent among females, with a prevalence of 0.5% to 1% of those of reproductive age and a lifetime prevalence of 0.9% for AN and 1.5% for BN. BED may affect up to 3.5%.
   1. Fertility issues: Disorders like anorexia and bulimia can lead to hormonal imbalances, affecting menstrual cycles and ovulation, thereby reducing fertility. Patients with irregular or absent periods often assume that they cannot conceive. This can lead to inadequate use of contraception and the risk of unplanned pregnancies.
   2. Pregnancy complications: Women with a history of or presently active FEDs have a higher risk of complications such as miscarriage, premature labor and birth, intrauterine growth restriction, and small-for-gestational age or low birth weight infant. Severe malnutrition during critical periods of fetal development can impact brain development.
   3. Nutritional deficiencies: EDs can result in deficiencies in key nutrients essential for fetal development. Conversely, pica can be caused by nutritional deficiencies. Pregnancy cravings and aversions can lead to dysfunctional eating.
   4. Gestational diabetes risk: Bulimia and BED may increase the risk of gestational diabetes, which in turn can influence eating behaviors.
   5. Psychological impact: EDs can exacerbate stress, anxiety, and depression during pregnancy, impacting both the patient and the fetus.
   6. Postpartum concerns: There is an increased risk of postpartum depression and difficulties in bonding with the newborn.
   7. Menstruation and return of fertility can be delayed in up to 30% of those with AN who regain normal weight.
   8. Patients with a history of an ED have a higher rate of miscarriage, small-for-gestational age infants, low birth weight infants, and infants with microcephaly, intrauterine growth restriction, and premature labor.

GERIATRICS

A. Reduced appetite and intake is common in older adults due to diminished sense of smell and taste, dental problems, and medication side effects. FEDs are unlikely to begin in later years but may continue from earlier history. Older adults may develop FEDs as a result of underlying medical problems or fear of a medical condition, such as heart attack or stroke.
B. FEDs may present as a protest against being placed in a nursing home, change in body image, loss of control, depression, or loneliness.
C. FEDs occur in older adults and should be included in the differential diagnosis for unexplained weight loss. See Chapter 21, "Aging and Older Adult Populations," for further information.

LGBTQ POPULATION

A. Very few studies have reached a clear conclusion as to whether being transgender increases the risk of developing disordered eating, possibly due to the low reported prevalence rate of transgender people in society.
B. Studies investigating EDs among the gay and lesbian population have reached more firm conclusions, with more EDs among gay men compared with straight men but not compared with lesbian women. Femininity has been hypothesized as a possible risk factor for the development of EDs, more so than sexual orientation, with masculinity as a protective factor; however, this requires further study. Refer to Chapter 19, "Special Considerations for the LGBTQ+ Population," for further information.

RESOURCES

FOR PATIENTS AND FAMILIES

A. Alliance for Eating Disorders Awareness (The Alliance) is a nonprofit organization providing programs and activities aimed at outreach, education, and early intervention for all EDs. The Alliance has an interactive referral site (https://findedhelp.com). The organization seeks volunteers to join committees, volunteer, and intern. They also accept donations and support for fundraisers. The Alliance's helpline is 1-866-662-1235.
B. Families Empowered and Supporting Treatment of Eating Disorders (F.E.A.S.T.) serves families by providing information and mutual support, promoting evidence-based treatment, and advocating for research and education. F.E.A.S.T provides international support resources via its website (www.feast-ed.org). Around the Dinner Table is F.E.A.S.T.'s online support forum for parents of patients with ED from all around the world. It is moderated 24 hours a day, 6 days a week (www.feast-ed.org/forum).
C. National Association for Males with Eating Disorders (N.A.M.E.D.) offers information and resources to support this underrepresented population and their families, including boys and men. N.A.M.E.D. is the only organization in the United States exclusively dedicated to representing and providing support to males with EDs. They provide access to collective expertise and promote the development of effective clinical intervention and research in this population.
D. National Association of Anorexia Nervosa and Associated Disorders (ANAD) is committed to providing free peer support services to anyone struggling with an ED. Their Eating Disorders Helpline is toll-free: 1-888-375-7767. They offer phone and text help and referral for treatment; email hello@anad.org.
E. National Eating Disorders Association (NEDA) raises awareness, builds communities of support and recovery, funds research, and provides resources. In 2018, NEDA merged with the Binge Eating Disorder Association (BEDA). The association's national toll-free confidential hotline (1-800-931-2237) is staffed daily by trained volunteers who provide information, support, and referrals to treatment. They also offer 24/7 crisis support via text (text "NEDA" to 741741).
F. Project HEAL funds resources and treatment costs that insurance does not cover. Project HEAL has a peer support program called Communities of Healing, which offers one-on-one mentors and a weekly support group. Visit www.theprojectheal.org to apply for support, donate, or learn about services.

FOR PROFESSIONALS

A. The Academy for Eating Disorders is a leading professional association that provides global access to knowledge, research, and best treatment practice for EDs. The guidelines for the medical management of EDs are an important resource for all professionals. Their website (www.aedweb.org/resources/professional-resources) offers continuing education/continuing medical education, current research studies, scholarships, online referrals, a member directory, webinars, and an online community.

REFERENCES AND BIBLIOGRAPHY

Academy for Eating Disorders. (n.d.). *Resources.* https://community.aedweb.org/resources/about-eating-disorders

American Association of Psychiatric Pharmacists. (n.d.). *Treatment guidelines: Eating disorders.* https://aapp.org/faq/457957/treatment-guidelines-eating-disorders

American Psychiatric Association. (2013). *Diagnostic and statistical manual of mental disorders* (5th ed.). https://doi.org/10.1176/appi.books.9780890425596

American Psychiatric Association. (2022). *Diagnostic and statistical manual of mental disorders* (5th ed., text rev.). https://doi.org/10.1176/appi.books.9780890425787

Claudino, A. M., Pike, K. M., Hay, P., Keeley, J. W., Evans, S. C., Rebello, T. J., Bryant-Waugh, R., Dai, Y., Zhao, M., Matsumoto, C., Herscovici, C. R., Mellor-Marsá, B., Stona, A.-C., Kogan, C. S., Andrews, H. F., Monteleone, P., Pilon, D. J., Thiels, C., Sharan, P., … Reed, G. M. (2019). The classification of feeding and eating disorders in the *ICD-11*: Results of a field study comparing proposed *ICD-11* guidelines with existing *ICD-10* guidelines. *BMC Medicine, 17*(1), 93. https://bmcmedicine.biomedcentral.com/articles/10.1186/s12916-019-1327-4

Deloitte Access Economics. (2020, June). *Social and economic cost of eating disorders in the United States of America: Report for the Strategic Training Initiative for the Prevention of Eating Disorders and the Academy for Eating Disorders.* https://www.hsph.harvard.edu/striped/report-economic-costs-of-eating-disorders

Ganie, M. A., Vasudevan, V., Wani, I. A., Baba, M. S., Arif, T., & Rashid, A. (2019). Epidemiology, pathogenesis, genetics & management of polycystic ovary syndrome in India. *Indian Journal of Medical Research, 150*(4), 333–344. https://doi.org/10.4103/ijmr.ijmr_1937_17

Han, R., Bian, Q., & Chen, H. (2022). Effectiveness of olanzapine in the treatment of anorexia nervosa: A systematic review and meta-analysis. *Brain and Behavior, 12*(2), e2498. https://doi.org/10.1002/brb3.2498

Harrington, B. C., Jimerson, M., Haxton, C., & Jimerson, D. C. (2015). Initial evaluation, diagnosis, and treatment of anorexia nervosa and bulimia nervosa. *American Family Physician, 91*(1), 46–52. PMID: 25591200.

Hilbert, A., Petroff, D., Herpertz, S., Pietrowsky, R., Tuschen-Caffier, B., Vocks, S., & Schmidt, R. (2019). Meta-analysis of the efficacy of psychological and medical treatments for binge-eating disorder. *Journal of Consulting and Clinical Psychology, 87*(1), 91–105. https://doi.org/10.1037/ccp0000358

Hodel, M. A., Hoff, P., Irwin, S. A., Biller-Andorno, N., Riese, F., & Trachsel, M. (2019). Attitudes toward assisted suicide requests in the context of severe and persistent mental illness: A survey of psychiatrists in Switzerland. *Palliative and Supportive Care, 17*(6), 621–627. https://doi.org/10.1017/s1478951519000233

Khalifa, I., & Goldman, R. D. (2019). Anorexia nervosa requiring admission in adolescents. *Canadian Family Physician, 65*(2), 107–108. PMID: 30765357.

Klein, D. A., Sylvester, J. E., & Schvey, N. A. (2021). Eating disorders in primary care: Diagnosis and management. *American Family Physician, 103*(1), 22–23. PMID: 33382560.

Morgan, J. F., Reid, F., & Lacey, J. H. (1999). The SCOFF questionnaire: assessment of a new screening tool for eating disorders. *BMJ, 319*, 1467. https://doi.org/10.1136/bmj.319.7223.1467

National Institute for Health and Care Excellence. (2020, December 16). *Eating disorders: Recognition and treatment.* NICE Guideline No. 69. https://www.ncbi.nlm.nih.gov/books/NBK568394

Nationwide Children's Hospital. (n.d.). *Feeding disorders.* https://www.nationwidechildrens.org/conditions/feeding-disorders

Resmark, G., Herpertz, S., Herpertz-Dahlmann, B., & Zeeck, A. (2019). Treatment of anorexia nervosa—new evidence-based guidelines. *Journal of Clinical Medicine, 8*(2), 153. https://doi.org/10.3390/jcm8020153

Stice, E., Marti, C. N., & Rohde, P. (2013). Prevalence, incidence, impairment, and course of the proposed *DSM-5* eating disorder diagnoses in an 8-year prospective community study of young women. *Journal of Abnormal Psychology, 122*(2), 445–457. https://doi.org/10.1037/a0030679

Stice, E., Marti, C. N., Shaw, H., & Jaconis, M. (2009). An 8-year longitudinal study of the natural history of threshold, subthreshold, and partial eating disorders from a community sample of adolescents. *Journal of Abnormal Psychology, 118*(3), 587–597. https://doi.org/10.1037/a0016481

Tusaie, K., & Fitzpatrick, J. J. (Eds.). (2022). *Advanced practice psychiatric nursing: Integrating psychotherapy, psychopharmacology, and complementary and alternative approaches across the life span* (3rd. ed.). Springer Publishing Company.

Vandergriendt, C. (2020, January 6). *Everything you should know about refeeding syndrome.* Healthline. https://www.healthline.com/health/refeeding-syndrome

World Health Organization. (2019). *International statistical classification of diseases* (11th rev.). https://icd.who.int

11 MOOD DISORDERS, DEPRESSION DISORDERS, AND BIPOLAR DISORDERS

Shaquita Starks

INTRODUCTION

Mood disorders are pervasive emotional disturbances that impact a significant portion of the population. These disorders can bear significant burden on a person's life and influence their emotional well-being, behavior, perception, interaction with others, and functioning in all areas of life. A person's mood is their emotional state or overall mindset in relation to how they feel. This chapter provides a description and background of each mood disorder, assessment and evidence-based treatment option, and suggestions for follow-up and patient education. An overview of the myriad factors that induce or mimic symptoms of these disorders is provided.

BIPOLAR DISORDERS

DEFINITION

A. Bipolar disorder is a chronic disorder characterized by recurrent, dramatic, and debilitating deviations in mood (elevated, irritable, or depressed) and changes in sleep, activity level, and energy associated with physical, behavioral, and cognitive symptoms that impact an individual's daily functioning in all areas of their life.
B. Mood associated with bipolar disorders entails a combination of depressive, hypomanic, and manic states, and is associated with poor psychiatric outcomes.
C. Bipolar disorder is characterized as type I or type II.
  1. Bipolar type I is characterized by having at least one manic episode (an abnormally expansive and elevated or irritable mood for greater than 1 week) in one's lifetime, with episodes of depression and mania.
  2. Bipolar type II is associated with having at least one hypomanic episode (of 4 days or less) with no history of mania.
  3. Depressive episodes are common and sometimes dominate symptomatology in both disorders.

INCIDENCE

A. Bipolar disorder impacts nearly 3% of U.S. adults and adolescents. In adults, bipolar disorders are experienced equally among cisgender females and cisgender males; however, prevalence is higher among cisgender female adolescents than cisgender adolescent males.
B. Bipolar disorders usually have their onset in early adulthood (ages 18–20 years).
C. People with these disorders are more likely to attempt suicide and are about 20 times more likely to die by suicide compared with the general population.

PATHOGENESIS

A. Pathogenesis is largely unknown, but thought to be familial, related to gene–environmental interactions and life stressors. The gene–environmental interactions, mediated by epigenetic changes, lead to neuronal modifications that change brain circuitry (e.g., frontotemporal grey matter loss, dysfunctional emotional processing) and behaviorally and systemically impact the body, causing cognitive and psychosocial impairments.
B. Chronic stressors and adverse life events may precipitate the disorder, as well as childhood neglect and sexual or physical abuse.

PREDISPOSING FACTORS

A. Being a cisgender female or having a first-degree relative with bipolar disorder increases an individual's risk threefold. Having a family history of other mental health disorders, such as obsessive-compulsive disorder (OCD), schizophrenia, attention deficit hyperactivity disorder (ADHD), depression, panic, or anxiety, also increases one's risk of developing the disorder.
B. Bipolar disorder also has biological and psychosocial implications. Significant life stressors (e.g., incarceration of family member, family history of suicides) can cause neuronal loss and changes in neurotransmitter levels and synaptic signaling.
C. Persons with personality disorders, such as borderline personality disorder, OCD, or histrionic personality disorder, are likely to have bipolar disorder. Biological factors include elevated inflammatory markers; chronic stress; monoamine and hormone dysregulation; and neurodegeneration of the thalamus, basal ganglia, and periventricular region of the brain. Bipolar disorders have a high genetic association, especially bipolar I. If one parent has the disorder, their offspring's chance of acquiring bipolar disorder ranges from 10% to 25%.

COMMON COMPLAINTS

A. Patients do not often seek help during manic phases but may present during the depressed phase with complaints of fatigue, racing thoughts, increased appetite, agitation, sadness, sleep disturbances, suicidal ideation and behaviors, and hopelessness.
B. Patients may experience other common symptoms related to depression, such as recurrent thoughts of suicide, psychomotor retardation or agitation, anhedonia, and poor decision-making.

OTHER SIGNS AND SYMPTOMS

A. Mania: decreased need for sleep, elevated self-esteem, impulsive or risky behavior, psychomotor agitation, restlessness, inattentiveness, psychosis
B. Depression: emptiness, low energy, anhedonia, unexpected weight loss or gain within the last 30 days, hypersomnia or insomnia, inattentiveness, suicidal ideation or behavior

SUBJECTIVE DATA

A. Review family history, substance use history, presence of chronic conditions, medication history, trauma or adverse childhood experiences, presence of other mental health disorders, and medical history.
B. Investigation of past medical history may reveal multiple hospitalizations and suicide attempts/ideation.
C. Family history may include incarceration, suicide, substance use disorder, depression, OCD, ADHD, general anxiety disorder (GAD), depression, and panic disorder.
D. Social history may reveal a history of trauma or neglect, drug and alcohol use, recurrent job loss, risky sexual behaviors, poor interpersonal relationships, and suicide attempts.

PHYSICAL EXAMINATION

A. Variations in presentations among people with bipolar disorder who are mood-dependent
  1. Depressed phase
     a. General appearance/behavior: psychomotor retardation, low energy, mood-congruent grooming, avolition, tearfulness, depressed posture, downcast eyes, unexplained weight loss or gain
     b. Mood/affect: dysphoric/depressed, tearful, sad
     c. Speech: soft, slow, low in volume, minimal in quantity
     d. Thought content and process: general negative ruminations and thought
     e. Perception: mood-congruent delusions (guilt)
     f. Cognition: impaired thinking and memory; usually oriented to time, person, place
     g. Judgment and insight: overstated symptoms
     h. Reliability: overemphasized treatment failures and negative symptoms
  2. Euphoric phase
     a. General appearance/behavior: hyperkinetic, erratic, restless, unpredictable, agitated, aggressive, assaultive or threatening, mood-congruent grooming, intrusive
     b. Mood and affect: irritable, elevated, labile, unnaturally happy, euphoric, delusional, expansive
     c. Speech: pressured, rapid, difficult to interrupt, flight of ideas, excessive, talkative
     d. Thought content and process: distractable, poor concentration, illogical/flight of ideas
     e. Perceptions: mood-congruent delusions (wealth, special ability, power); hallucinations possible depending on severity
     f. Judgment and insight: limited and impaired
     g. Cognition: delirium possible depending on severity
     h. Reliability: may be an unreliable historian

DIAGNOSTIC TESTS AND SCREENING

A. Evaluation for bipolar disorders is mostly subjective, relying on patient narrative, healthcare provider observation, and validated screening tools such as the Mood Disorder Questionnaire (MDQ) and the Bipolar Spectrum Diagnostic Scale (BSDS). Routine evaluation to rule out medical causes is necessary.
B. Labs such as a lipid panel, liver function test (LFT), complete blood count (CBC), comprehensive metabolic panel (CMP), fasting glucose urinalysis, thyroid panels, serum alcohol levels, sexually transmitted infection (STI) testing, urine drug screen, and other toxicology screenings, along with a physical examination, can be conducted to rule out medical or substance use etiology.
C. If patients present with new-onset psychosis, they may need MRI, EEG, hepatitis C screening, syphilis screening, and urine screening for heavy metals.

DIFFERENTIAL DIAGNOSES

A. Other psychiatric disorders: schizophrenia, personality disorders, major depressive disorder (MDD), substance- or medication-induced bipolar and related disorder, cyclothymic disorder, schizoaffective disorder, ADHD, disruptive mood dysregulation disorder, personality disorders (borderline personality disorder), others
B. Endocrine/metabolic: adrenal disorders, Wernicke encephalopathy, vitamin B_{12} deficiency, Wilson disease, obstructive sleep apnea, pituitary and thyroid diseases, hypercalcemia, hemochromatosis, Cushing disease
C. Autoimmune: systemic lupus erythematosus, vascular disorders
D. Neurologic/cognitive: normal pressure hydrocephalus, traumatic brain injury (TBI), frontotemporal dementia, Alzheimer disease, hemorrhagic stroke, ischemic stroke, delirium, Huntington disease, Parkinson disease, complex partial seizures, migraine, multiple sclerosis, Wilson disease, encephalitis, stroke, cerebrovascular accident (CVA)
E. Infectious: tertiary syphilis, HIV, tuberculosis (TB), herpes simplex encephalitis, influenza
F. Malignancy: cerebral tumors, paraneoplastic limbic encephalitis
G. Medications, substance use/other toxins: serotonin syndrome, withdrawal from drugs of abuse or alcohol, opioid use disorder, cocaine, hallucinogens, amphetamine intoxication, chemotherapy, carbon monoxide poisoning, levodopa, cimetidine, corticosteroids, interferon, hydralazine, captopril, bromocriptine, venlafaxine, methylphenidate, baclofen, isoniazid, disulfiram, trazodone
H. Other: deficiency of B vitamins (thiamine, folate, vitamin B_{12}, niacin)

PLAN

A. Acute plan goals entail ensuring the safety of the patient and others and most often necessitate hospital admission. Parenterally delivered antipsychotics and anxiolytics can be used to manage bipolar symptoms in acute situations.
B. A combination of oral medications and therapies can be used to manage patients' symptoms in outpatient settings.

GENERAL TREATMENTS AND INTERVENTIONS

A. Medications are the first choice for treatment of bipolar disorders (Table 11.1).
B. For patients who cannot tolerate medication, who have a life-threatening psychosis, or who need a rapid response, electroconvulsive therapy (ECT) can be used.
C. For patients taking lithium, kidney function should be assessed before treatment and at least annually. Avoid valproate in pregnancy due to risk of neural tube defects.
D. Cognitive behavioral therapy (CBT) and interpersonal therapy may be helpful nonpharmacologic treatments for the disorder.

PATIENT TEACHING

A. Teach patients that bipolar disorder is a lifelong, chronic mental health issue that requires long-term management. Therefore, it is crucial to teach the importance of medication adherence.
B. Teach the patient and family the signs and symptoms of mania and hypomania.

TABLE 11.1 COMMON MEDICATIONS FOR THE TREATMENT OF BIPOLAR DISORDERS

Medication	Usage	Aged 10–18 Years (Youth)	Aged 19–65 Years (Adult)	Aged 66–74 Years (Older Adult)	Aged 85–99 Years (Oldest Old + Centenarians)
Generic: lithium Trade: Eskalith	FDA-approved for mania, acute and mixed, and bipolar maintenance *Narrow therapeutic range; note signs of toxicity such as tremor, ataxia, sedation, diarrhea, vomiting.*	Refer to Chapter 20, "Special Considerations for Childhood and Adolescent Populations."	Average dose: 300–1,200 mg Dose adjusted according to plasma lithium levels; recommended levels for depression 0.6–1.0 mEq/L; mania 1.0–1.5 mEq/L; maintenance 0.7–1.0 mEq/L	Refer to Chapter 21, "Aging and Older Adult Populations."	Refer to Chapter 21, "Aging and Older Adult Populations."
Generic: quetiapine Trade: Seroquel, Seroquel XR	FDA-approved for acute mania in adults, bipolar maintenance, and bipolar depression May increase risk for diabetes/dyslipidemia and may cause diabetic ketoacidosis in patients with diabetes	Refer to Chapter 20, "Special Considerations for Childhood and Adolescent Populations."	Average dose for bipolar mania: 400–800 mg/d Average dose for bipolar depression: 300 mg/d In some patients, may require more than 800–1,200 mg/d for mania	Refer to Chapter 21, "Aging and Older Adult Populations."	Refer to Chapter 21, "Aging and Older Adult Populations."
Generic: aripiprazole Trade: Abilify	Used for maintenance, mania, and as adjunct for depression with an antidepressant	Refer to Chapter 20, "Special Considerations for Childhood and Adolescent Populations."	Average dose for mania 15–30 mg/d	Refer to Chapter 21, "Aging and Older Adult Populations."	Refer to Chapter 21, "Aging and Older Adult Populations."
Generic: olanzapine Trade: Zyprexa, Symbyax (olanzapine-fluoxetine)	FDA-approved for acute mania/mixed mania, bipolar maintenance, acute agitation associated with bipolar I, and bipolar depression, along with fluoxetine	Refer to Chapter 20, "Special Considerations for Childhood and Adolescent Populations."	Average dose: 10–20 mg/d (intramuscular or oral) and 6–12 mg olanzapine/25–50 mg fluoxetine combination Max dose: 20 mg/d Olanzapine/fluoxetine combination max dose: 18 mg/75 mg	Refer to Chapter 21, "Aging and Older Adult Populations."	Refer to Chapter 21, "Aging and Older Adult Populations."
Generic: valproate Trade: Depakene, Depakote, Depakote ER, Depacon, Stavzor	FDA-approved for treatment of acute mania and mixed episodes; bipolar maintenance	Refer to Chapter 20, "Special Considerations for Childhood and Adolescent Populations."	Average dose: 1,200–1,500 mg/d Max dose: 60 mg/kg/d	Refer to Chapter 21, "Aging and Older Adult Populations."	Refer to Chapter 21, "Aging and Older Adult Populations."
Generic: lamotrigine Trade: Lamictal	Maintenance of bipolar I *Life-threatening rash with high dose and rapid dose escalation; discontinue at the first sign of serious rash.*	Refer to Chapter 20, "Special Considerations for Childhood and Adolescent Populations."	Average dose: 100–200 mg/d Start weeks 1–2, 25 mg/d; weeks 3–4, 50 mg/d; week 5, 100 mg/d; week 6, 200 mg/d Max dose: 200 mg	Refer to Chapter 21, "Aging and Older Adult Populations."	Refer to Chapter 21, "Aging and Older Adult Populations."
Generic: NA Trade: Latuda (lurasidone)	FDA-approved for adjunct treatment of bipolar depression *Take with food at a minimum of 350 calories for optimal absorption.*	Refer to Chapter 20, "Special Considerations for Childhood and Adolescent Populations."	Average dose: 20–80 mg/d for bipolar depression; may increase to 120 mg/d if needed	Refer to Chapter 21, "Aging and Older Adult Populations."	Refer to Chapter 21, "Aging and Older Adult Populations."

(continued)

TABLE 11.1 COMMON MEDICATIONS FOR THE TREATMENT OF BIPOLAR DISORDERS (CONTINUED)

Medication	Usage	Aged 10–18 Years (Youth)	Aged 19–65 Years (Adult)	Aged 66–74 Years (Older Adult)	Aged 85–99 Years (Oldest Old + Centenarians)
Generic: asenapine Trade: Saphris	Used for bipolar mania as monotherapy or adjunct	Refer to Chapter 20, "Special Considerations for Childhood and Adolescent Populations."	Average dose: 10–20 mg/d sublingually	Refer to Chapter 21, "Aging and Older Adult Populations."	Refer to Chapter 21, "Aging and Older Adult Populations."
Generic: carbamazepine Trade: Equetro	Use to treat acute or mixed mania; off-label use for bipolar maintenance *Avoid in pregnancy.*	Refer to Chapter 20, "Special Considerations for Childhood and Adolescent Populations."	Average dose: 200–1,200 mg/d Max dose: 1,200 mg	Refer to Chapter 21, "Aging and Older Adult Populations."	Refer to Chapter 21, "Aging and Older Adult Populations."
Generic: NA Trade: Vraylar	Use to treat acute or mixed mania and depressed phase	Refer to Chapter 20, "Special Considerations for Childhood and Adolescent Populations."	Average dose: mania 3–6 mg/d Depression 1.5–3 mg/d	Refer to Chapter 21, "Aging and Older Adult Populations."	Refer to Chapter 21, "Aging and Older Adult Populations."
Generic: ziprasidone Trade: Geodon	FDA-approved for treating acute/mixed mania and bipolar maintenance (oral) *Recommend taking with food to double bioavailability*	Refer to Chapter 20, "Special Considerations for Childhood and Adolescent Populations."	Average dose: 80–160 mg/d in divided doses orally	Refer to Chapter 21, "Aging and Older Adult Populations."	Refer to Chapter 21, "Aging and Older Adult Populations."
Generic: NA Trade: Caplyta (lumateperone)	FDA-approved for bipolar depression	Refer to Chapter 20, "Special Considerations for Childhood and Adolescent Populations."	Average dose: 42 mg/d	Refer to Chapter 21, "Aging and Older Adult Populations."	Refer to Chapter 21, "Aging and Older Adult Populations."
Generic: risperidone Trade: Risperdal	FDA-approved for acute/mixed mania and bipolar maintenance	Refer to Chapter 20, "Special Considerations for Childhood and Adolescent Populations."	Average dose: 2–8 mg/d	Refer to Chapter 21, "Aging and Older Adult Populations."	Refer to Chapter 21, "Aging and Older Adult Populations."
Generic: NA Trade: Lybalvi (olanzapine/samidorphan)	FDA-approved for treating acute mania/mixed mania and bipolar I maintenance *Patient should be opioid-free for 7–14 days before starting.*	Refer to Chapter 20, "Special Considerations for Childhood and Adolescent Populations."	Average dose: 5 mg/10 mg to 20 mg/10 mg (olanzapine/samidorphan)	Refer to Chapter 21, "Aging and Older Adult Populations."	Refer to Chapter 21, "Aging and Older Adult Populations."

FDA, U.S. Food and Drug Administration.

FOLLOW-UP

A. Frequent follow-up is important not only to monitor patient symptoms but also to screen for medical comorbidities that may occur due to treatment.

B. The prognosis is usually poor in those with bipolar I disorder due to substance use, depression, and psychotic features.

   1. About 50% of people diagnosed with bipolar I have a second episode within 2 years of the first occurrence.

C. Individuals with bipolar disorder also have exponential risk for suicide attempts, so constant screening for suicidal risk is essential.

D. Medical comorbidities are common in persons with bipolar disorder due to the adverse effects of antipsychotics, mood stabilizers, and anticonvulsants, as well as lifestyle factors (e.g., smoking, alcohol use, limited physical activity, poor dietary habits).

E. It is important to screen for metabolic disorders because people with bipolar disorders have a higher mortality rate than the general population.

CONSULTATION AND REFERRALS

A. Bipolar disorder is best managed with interdisciplinary teams (social workers, psychologists, therapists, nurse

practitioners, nurses, pharmacists, physicians, and physician assistants). Consultation with individual primary care providers is important due to the risk of metabolic disorders and cardiovascular mortality.
B. Therapists may help patients develop appropriate coping skills to manage the range of symptoms they have and may also provide support to family members.

INDIVIDUAL CONSIDERATIONS

Pediatrics
A. Refer to Chapter 20, "Special Considerations for Childhood and Adolescent Populations."

Pregnancy
A. Treatment of bipolar disorder in pregnancy requires consideration of the risks and benefits of using mood stabilizers, which are mostly teratogenic (carbamazepine and valproate). Lithium may also cause congenital heart disease in children exposed in utero. If lithium is used, careful monitoring of its level is suggested.
B. When considering treatment for pregnant people with bipolar disorder, the well-being of the fetus and the pregnant person must be assessed.

Geriatrics
A. Refer to Chapter 21, "Aging and Older Adult Populations."

Partners/Family
A. Support and education of family are essential. The family should be taught warning signs of exacerbation and understand when a higher level of care is necessary.

RESOURCES
A. Bipolar disorder (National Institute of Mental Health): www.nimh.nih.gov/health/topics/bipolar-disorder
B. Bipolar disorders: A review (*American Family Physician*): www.aafp.org/pubs/afp/issues/2012/0301/p483.html
C. Treatment guidelines for bipolar disorder in adults (International College of Neuro-Psychopharmacology): https://academic.oup.com/ijnp/article/20/2/180/2667726
D. Diagnosing and treating bipolar spectrum disorders (American Psychological Association): www.apa.org/monitor/2022/01/ce-bipolar-spectrum

REFERENCES AND BIBLIOGRAPHY
American Psychiatric Association. (2013). *Diagnostic and statistical manual of mental disorders* (5th ed.). https://doi.org/10.1176/appi.books.9780890425596

Chiang, K. J., Tsai, J. C., Liu, D., Lin, C. H., Chiu, H. L., & Chou, K. R. (2017). Efficacy of cognitive-behavioral therapy in patients with bipolar disorder: A meta-analysis of randomized controlled trials. *PloS One, 12*(5), e0176849. https://doi.org/10.1371/journal.pone.0176849

First, M. B. (2014). *DSM-5 handbook of differential diagnosis*. American Psychiatric Association Publishing.

Vieta, E., Berk, M., Schulze, T. G., Carvalho, A. F., Suppes, T., Calabrese, J. R., Gao, K., Miskowiak, K. W., & Grande, I. (2018). Bipolar disorders. *Nature Reviews Disease Primers, 4*(1), Article 18008. https://doi.org/10.1038/nrdp.2018.8

Yonkers, K. A., Vigod, S., & Ross, L. E. (2011). Diagnosis, pathophysiology, and management of mood disorders in pregnant and postpartum women. *Obstetrics & Gynecology, 117*(4), 961–977. https://doi.org/10.1097/AOG.0b013e31821187a7

CYCLOTHYMIC DISORDER

DEFINITION
A. Cyclothymia is a mood disorder characterized by mood dysregulation and emotional reactivity present for at least 2 years that impacts functioning in all areas of life. While the disorder shares diagnostic criteria with bipolar disorder (e.g., hypomania, depressive symptoms) and MDD, the full criteria for the other disorders are not met and cyclothymia has an earlier onset.
B. To meet the diagnostic criteria, the stability of mood cannot exceed 2 months or be related to another medical or psychiatric illness.

INCIDENCE
A. Cyclothymia is rare, with a lifetime prevalence of about 1%, and equally impacts cisgender males and cisgender females.

PATHOGENESIS
A. Cyclothymia shares symptoms with other mental health disorders but, of note, is a neurodevelopmental disorder. The frontal lobe, limbic system, and amygdala are thought to have dysfunction as evidenced by the emotional dysregulation and hyperreactivity associated with the disorder.
B. Exposure to adverse life events and genetic/environmental interactions may also predispose individuals to the disorder.

PREDISPOSING FACTORS
A. Family history of bipolar disorder

COMMON COMPLAINTS
A. Patients may present with vague symptoms such as insomnia, fatigue, poor motivation, daily mood shifts, and periods of euthymia.

OTHER SIGNS AND SYMPTOMS
A. Some patients with cyclothymia somaticize symptoms and complain of issues such as headaches, chest pain, weight loss, and hair loss. They may also have suicidal ideation and behavior.
B. Other reported symptoms may include panic, anxiety, racing thoughts, irritability, anger or aggression, sleep disturbances, and feelings of despair.

PHYSICAL EXAMINATION
A. The patient may present with emotional lability and hypercreativity. They may also have evidence of self-harm or self-mutilation.
B. They exhibit irritable mood and affect, are hopeless and helpless, or are depressed, with anhedonia in a depressed state. Individuals may also experience hypomania (i.e., racing thoughts, hyperactivity, pressured speech, grandiosity, and impulsivity).

DIAGNOSTIC TESTS AND SCREENING
A. Patients require screening and evaluation for medical issues.
B. Helpful laboratory tests to consider are CMP, CBC, thyroid panel, folate, vitamin B_{12}, drug toxicology, ammonia, urinalysis (UA), and brain imaging.
C. Validated questionnaires may also help, such as Temperament Evaluation of Memphis, Pisa, Paris and San Diego–Autoquestionnaire Version (TEMPS-A).

DIFFERENTIAL DIAGNOSES

A. Other psychiatric disorders: bipolar disorders with rapid cycling, borderline personality disorder, bipolar and related disorder due to another medical condition, dysthymia, ADHD, GAD, posttraumatic stress disorder (PTSD), postpartum depression (PPD), substance/medication-induced bipolar and related disorder
B. Medication: captopril, hydralazine, levodopa, steroids, bromocriptine, monoamine oxidase inhibitors (MAOIs), cimetidine, isoniazid, baclofen
C. Endocrine: thyroid disorders, Cushing disease
D. Neurologic: dementia, Huntington chorea, complex partial seizures, TBI, Wilson disease, stroke, multiple sclerosis, neoplasm, migraine
E. Immunologic: systemic lupus erythematosus
F. Substance use disorder: opioids, alcohol use disorder
G. Other: vitamin deficiencies such as folate, thiamin, and vitamin B_{12}

PLAN

A. General treatments and interventions are similar to bipolar disorder because there are no medications approved by the U.S. Food and Drug Administration (FDA).
B. Start with a low dose and slow titration.
C. Medications to consider include valproate, lithium, quetiapine, carbamazepine, and lamotrigine. CBT can also be used.
D. For common medications, see treatment for bipolar disorder.

PATIENT TEACHING

A. Educate patients about symptoms, treatment options, coping skills, and adherence to alleviate symptoms. Safety planning is also important to reduce the risk of suicide. Medication side effects and adverse effects should also be reviewed.
B. If female patients are taking carbamazepine or valproate and become pregnant, they need to be informed of possible congenital malformations.

FOLLOW-UP

A. Frequent follow-up is suggested due to suicide risk when rapid mood cycling occurs.

CONSULTATION AND REFERRALS

A. Refer to ED for suicidality or danger to self and others; may be best managed with interdisciplinary teams (social workers, psychologists, therapists, nurse practitioners, nurses, pharmacists, physicians, and physician assistants).
B. Therapists may help patients develop appropriate coping skills to manage the range of symptoms they have and may also provide support to family members.

INDIVIDUAL CONSIDERATIONS

Pediatrics
A. Refer to Chapter 20, "Special Considerations for Childhood and Adolescent Populations."

Pregnancy
A. Avoid the use of valproate and carbamazepine.

Geriatrics
A. Refer to Chapter 21, "Aging and Older Adult Populations."

Partners/Family
A. Aberrant behaviors may be observed, such as excessive gambling, repeated job loss, financial problems, and relationship problems that may lead to multiple divorces.
B. Mood shifts may impact relationships. Support groups may be helpful.

RESOURCE

A. Cyclothymic disorder: A critical review (*Clinical Psychology Review*): https://pubmed.ncbi.nlm.nih.gov/22459786

REFERENCES AND BIBLIOGRAPHY

American Psychiatric Association. (2013). *Diagnostic and statistical manual of mental disorders* (5th ed.). https://doi.org/10.1176/appi.books.9780890425596
First, M. B. (2014). DSM-5 *handbook of differential diagnosis*. American Psychiatric Association Publishing.
Perugia, G., Hantouche, E., & Vannucchi, G. (2017). Diagnosis and treatment of cyclothymia: The "Primacy" of temperament. *Current Neuropharmacology, 15*(3), 372–379. https://doi.org/10.2174/1570159X14666160616120157
Van Meter, A. R., Youngstrom, E. A., & Findling, R. L. (2012). Cyclothymic disorder: A critical review. *Clinical Psychology Review, 32*(4), 229–243. https://doi.org/10.1016/j.cpr.2012.02.001

MAJOR DEPRESSIVE DISORDER

DEFINITION

A. MDD is characterized by the presence of a depressed mood, anhedonia, sleep and appetite disturbances, cognitive impairment, and guilt or low self-worth for at least 2 consecutive weeks.
B. The presentation of MDD symptoms is variable and appears to occur along a spectrum, but in all cases at least a depressed mood distinct from a previous state of being and a loss of interest must be present to suspect the disorder.
C. The disorder can be classified by severity (i.e., mild, moderate, severe) or specified by subtype (e.g., with anxious distress, psychotic features).

INCIDENCE

A. Major depression is the most common mental health and mood disorder in the United States, with about 8.4% and 17% of U.S. adults and adolescents, respectively, reporting at least one episode annually.
B. Major depression impacts cisgender females more than cisgender males.
C. MDD can occur at any age, but the mean age is 20 years.

PATHOGENESIS

A. Pathogenesis is unknown, but structural and hormonal changes are thought to influence the development of MDD, alongside several theories.
B. Cognitive theory suggests that cognitive distortions in susceptible individuals lead to depression. The monoamine deficiency theory suggests that monoamines (e.g., serotonin, dopamine, norepinephrine) are inadequate within the brain.
  1. Serotonin, synthesized from the amino acid tryptophan, regulates mood, anxiety, appetite, sleep, body temperature, and gastrointestinal functioning. About 90% of serotonin originates in the gastrointestinal tract, and the rest is generated in the brain.
  2. Dopamine, synthesized from the amino acid tyrosine, creates feelings of motivation, drive, pleasure, reward, enjoyment of food and sex, drugs, learning, motor control, and executive functioning.
  3. Norepinephrine, also synthesized from tyrosine, regulates feelings of alertness, attention, and concentration;

increases blood pressure; elevates mood; and can increase anxiety. Gamma-aminobutyric acid (GABA), the inhibitory neurotransmitter, and glycine and glutamate, the excitatory neurotransmitters, also play a role in depression. People with depression have been reported to have deficient GABA levels in plasma, cerebrospinal fluid (CSF), and the brain.
C. Growth and thyroid abnormalities play a role, as well as trauma and adverse childhood experiences.
D. Psychosocial stress may lead to increased levels of inflammatory markers that impact pathways within the brain, reducing neurotrophic support, altered glutamate activity, and oxidative stress.
E. Structural causes are thought to be related to decreased hippocampal volume, which contributes to problems with executive functioning and memory and cortical thinning in the frontal regions of the brain. Dysregulation of the hypothalamic–pituitary–adrenal (HPA) axis decreases levels of brain-derived neurotrophic factor (BDNF), heightens amygdala activation, and disturbs the default mode network.

PREDISPOSING FACTORS
A. A combination of factors contribute to the development of MDD, including psychosocial, genetic, biological, and environmental factors.
B. Female sex assigned at birth, middle age, Indigenous American ethnicity, low income, and disability are social risk factors for MDD.
C. Individuals are more likely to experience MDD if they have a first-degree relative with the disorder. The presence of a chronic medical illness (e.g., diabetes, stroke, thyroid disorders), chronic pain, substance or alcohol use, domestic abuse, and major life changes are also risk factors.
D. Adverse childhood experiences increase the risk of developing the disorder by causing structural changes in the cerebral cortex.
E. Recently, a national focus on social determinants of health (SDOH) has been paramount as scientists have learned that an individual's zip code carries more significance than their genetic code. The conditions in which people are born, live, play, work, worship, and age impact their exposure to adversity, access to care, and other issues that can impact one's quality of life.
F. Experiencing a lifetime of adversity; trauma; and a lack of adequate finances, housing, education, social networks, and supportive neighborhood infrastructure can leave people feeling hopeless, over time leading to MDD.
G. People with chronic conditions, such as diabetes mellitus type 2, obesity, and cardiovascular disease, are likely to experience depression.
H. Other risk factors include low folate levels, COVID-19 leading to MDD, high consumption of social media, and low birth weight.

COMMON COMPLAINTS
A. Patients rarely present to clinicians soliciting treatment for depression. Rather, they or others notice a change in demeanor, behavior, level of interest, or activity.
B. Fatigue, generalized pain, insomnia, and lack of motivation are common complaints that cause people to seek care, but these symptoms may be overlooked as symptoms of depression without careful screening.
C. A key complaint of MDD is anhedonia. Knowledge of patients' hobbies and social interests is important to determine during initial assessment so that clinicians can monitor subtle changes in mood and activity. When people discontinue engaging in activities that bring joy into their lives, MDD should be considered.

OTHER SIGNS AND SYMPTOMS
A. Individuals with depression may exhibit a combination of psychological and somatic symptoms.
   1. Somatic symptoms include chronic pain (e.g., head, back, neck, joint, abdominal), nausea/indigestion and other gastrointestinal symptoms, low libido, anorgasmia and sexual dysfunction, fatigue, dyspnea, dizziness, and chest palpitations. Other symptoms, such weight gain or weight loss, insomnia or excessive sleeping, psychomotor retardation, and physical and mental fatigue, may be present.
   2. Psychological symptoms include sadness; hopelessness; anger; irritability; low motivation; loss of interest; guilt; worthlessness; problems with planning, problem-solving, concentration, focus, or recalling information; and suicidal ideation or behavior.

SUBJECTIVE DATA
A. Depression can impact individuals' functioning in every part of their life, including work, relationships, and social life. Hygiene and self-care may be compromised. People seeking treatment are likely to report symptoms that may be mistaken for a physical health condition.
B. Individuals presenting with symptoms of MDD may also report first-degree family members with a history of depression and a family history of mood disorders, suicide, or substance use disorders.
C. Subjective data to consider include recent loss, abuse, difficult interpersonal relationship, and family estrangement. These individuals may also report a history of medications that induce depressive symptoms; use of alcohol, smoking, or ingestion of other substances; or a history of depressive episodes or hospitalizations, pain, or medical conditions associated with depression.

PHYSICAL EXAMINATION
A. The diagnosis of MDD is based on an interview, to obtain subjective history, and the mental status and physical examination.
B. The diagnostic interview provides a description of the history of the present symptoms, including temporal factors and information about personal medical history and medications, psychiatric and substance use history, family history, and social history. Cultural formulation should also be executed because one's religion, culture, and ethnic background may influence the presentation of symptoms.
C. The healthcare provider may also survey the patient's affect, demeanor, movement, speech, memory, thought content and process, insight, judgment, and risk for suicide to corroborate with subjective complaints.
D. Patients often present with a flat, restricted, or dysphoric affect and psychomotor agitation and retardation. Individuals may report unexplained weight changes or poor appetite and may also report suicidal thoughts and plans.
E. Additional information may be obtained from family and friends when warranted. A physical examination can be performed to rule out medical causes of symptoms.

DIAGNOSTIC TESTS AND SCREENING
A. Screening and testing for MDD are mostly subjective, relying on patient narrative, healthcare provider observation, and validated screening tools such as the Patient Health

Questionnaire (PHQ)-9, PHQ-2, Geriatric Depression Scale, and Hamilton Depression Rating Scale (HAM-D).
B. Routine labs, such as vitamin D, free thyroxine (T4), thyroid-stimulating hormone (TSH), UA, toxicology screenings, CMP, CBC, vitamin B_{12}, cortisol levels, and HIV testing, can be done to rule out other causes of depression.
C. Urine pregnancy and STI testing may be warranted in some cases.

DIFFERENTIAL DIAGNOSES

A. Other psychiatric disorders: adjustment disorder, substance/medication-induced depressive disorder, bipolar disorders, persistent depressive disorder (PDD), premenstrual dysphoric disorder (PMDD), disruptive mood dysregulation disorder, schizophrenia spectrum disorders, schizoaffective disorder, neurocognitive disorder, adjustment disorder with depressed mood, bereavement, nonpathologic periods of sadness, eating disorders, or anxiety disorders
B. Endocrine: adrenal and thyroid disorders, diabetes mellitus, hypogonadism, polycystic ovary syndrome (PCOS)
C. Respiratory: sleep apnea, chronic obstructive pulmonary disease (COPD)
D. Neurologic/immunologic: Alzheimer disease, multiple sclerosis, CVA, seizure disorders, Parkinson disease, delirium, Huntington disease, TBI, subdural hematoma, central nervous system (CNS) tumor, lupus, rheumatoid arthritis
E. Hematologic/oncologic: malignancies, anemias
F. Infectious disease: syphilis or HIV, hepatitis B or C, TB, urinary tract infection (UTI)
G. Metabolic: iron, thiamin, folate, vitamins B_6, B_{12}, or D deficiency; hyponatremia or hypercalcemia; uremia; heavy metal poisoning; hepatic or metabolic encephalopathy
H. Drugs/medications: misuse or use of hypnotics, sedatives, anticonvulsants, steroids, antihypertensives, antibiotics, and steroids; also, chemotherapy drugs, propranolol, interferon-alpha, interleukin-2, progestin-containing contraceptive implants, isotretinoin, and acamprosate

PLAN

A. There are several evidence-based medical treatments and therapies to treat MDD.
B. Remission with medications may take 3 to 6 months to achieve.
C. Medications should be continued for about 1 year once remission is achieved. Patients may stop treatment when symptoms improve, so it is important to educate patients about adherence recommendations.

GENERAL TREATMENTS AND INTERVENTIONS

A. Treatment is based on the severity of symptoms.
B. All patients in imminent danger of harming self or others or experiencing severe functional limitations or psychosis should be considered for hospital admission immediately.
C. A combination of psychotherapy and medication provides the fastest road to remission of symptoms.
  1. The recommended initial treatment for mildtomoderate MDD is psychotherapy (e.g., CBT, mindfulness-based therapy, interpersonal and psychodynamic therapy).
  2. While psychotherapy is the recommended treatment for mild MDD, many individuals are treated with medications. FDA-approved medications used for MDD include selective serotonin reuptake inhibitors (SSRIs), serotonin and norepinephrine reuptake inhibitors (SNRIs), atypical antidepressants, serotonin modulators, tricyclic antidepressants (TCAs), MAOIs, and augmenting agents, including mood stabilizers and antipsychotics (Table 11.2).
  3. Treatment should be initiated with an SSRI or SNRI before other classes of antidepressants are used. All forms ▶

TABLE 11.2 COMMON MEDICATIONS FOR TREATMENT OF MAJOR DEPRESSIVE DISORDER

Medication	Usage	Aged 10–18 Years (Youth)	Aged 19–65 Years (Adult)	Aged 66–74 Years (Older Adult)	Aged 85–99 Years (Oldest Old + Centenarians)
Generic: bupropion Trade: Wellbutrin XL, Wellbutrin SR, Forfivo XL, Aplenzin, Zyban	FDA-approved for MDD, seasonal affective disorder, nicotine addiction **WARNING:** Lowers seizure threshold, may increase blood pressure	Refer to Chapter 20, "Special Considerations for Childhood and Adolescent Populations," or *PDR*. It is often used for ADD and smoking cessation in youth.	Bupropion: 225–450 mg three times a day; SR: 200–450 mg twice a day; XL: 150 mg–450 mg four times a day Max dose: 450 mg/d	Refer to Chapter 21, "Aging and Older Adult Populations," or *PDR*.	Refer to Chapter 21, "Aging and Older Adult Populations," or *PDR*.
Generic: amitriptyline Trade: Elavil	FDA-approved for depression **WARNING:** Can increase QTc interval at toxic doses	Refer to Chapter 20, "Special Considerations for Childhood and Adolescent Populations." It is not recommended for use under 12 years of age.	Average dose: 50–150 mg/d; initial dose 25 mg/d at bedtime, increase by 25 mg every 3–7 days Max dose: 300 mg/d	Baseline EKG is recommended over 50 years of age. Refer to Chapter 21, "Aging and Older Adult Populations."	Baseline EKG is recommended over 50 years of age. Refer to Chapter 21, "Aging and Older Adult Populations."

(continued)

TABLE 11.2 COMMON MEDICATIONS FOR TREATMENT OF MAJOR DEPRESSIVE DISORDER (CONTINUED)

Medication	Usage	Aged 10–18 Years (Youth)	Aged 19–65 Years (Adult)	Aged 66–74 Years (Older Adult)	Aged 85–99 Years (Oldest Old + Centenarians)
Generic: citalopram Trade: Celexa	FDA-approved for depression **WARNING:** Caution using doses greater than 40 mg/d in individuals with heart disease	Refer to Chapter 20, "Special Considerations for Childhood and Adolescent Populations."	Average dose: 20–40 mg/d Max dose: 40 mg/d Max dose for over 60 years of age: 20 mg/d	Avoid dosages over 20 mg/d for 60 years of age and up. Refer to Chapter 21, "Aging and Older Adult Populations."	Refer to Chapter 21, "Aging and Older Adult Populations."
Generic: desvenlafaxine Trade: Pristiq	FDA-approved for MDD	Refer to Chapter 20, "Special Considerations for Childhood and Adolescent Populations."	Average dose: 50 mg/d Max dose: 100 mg/d	Refer to Chapter 21, "Aging and Older Adult Populations."	Refer to Chapter 21, "Aging and Older Adult Populations."
Generic: duloxetine Trade: Cymbalta	FDA-approved for MDD, fibromyalgia, diabetic neuropathy, chronic musculoskeletal pain	Refer to Chapter 20, "Special Considerations for Childhood and Adolescent Populations."	Average dose: 40–60 mg once or twice daily Max dose: 120 mg/d	Refer to Chapter 21, "Aging and Older Adult Populations."	Refer to Chapter 21, "Aging and Older Adult Populations."
Generic: escitalopram Trade: Lexapro	FDA-approved for MDD	It is approved for adolescents 12–17 years of age. Refer to Chapter 20, "Special Considerations for Childhood and Adolescent Populations."	Average dose: 10–20 mg/d Max dose: 20 mg	Refer to Chapter 21, "Aging and Older Adult Populations."	Refer to Chapter 21, "Aging and Older Adult Populations."
Generic: NA Trade: Spravato (esketamine)	FDA-approved for MDD with acute suicidality and treatment-resistant depression **WARNING:** Only available through restricted program under REMS; may raise blood pressure or heart disease	Not approved	Give nasal spray with antidepressant Average dose: weeks 1–4, 84 mg twice per week; after 4 weeks, reevaluate for need to continue	Refer to Chapter 21, "Aging and Older Adult Populations."	Refer to Chapter 21, "Aging and Older Adult Populations."
Generic: fluoxetine Trade: Prozac, Sarafem, Prozac weekly	FDA-approved for MDD, bulimia, panic, treatment-resistant depression	Refer to Chapter 20, "Special Considerations for Childhood and Adolescent Populations." It is FDA-approved for 8 years of age and older.	Average dose: 20–80 mg/d Max dose: 80 mg/d	Refer to Chapter 21, "Aging and Older Adult Populations."	Refer to Chapter 21, "Aging and Older Adult Populations."
Generic: mirtazapine Trade: Remeron	FDA-approved for MDD **WARNING:** May cause photosensitivity and may increase cholesterol	Refer to Chapter 20, "Special Considerations for Childhood and Adolescent Populations."	Average dose: 15–45 mg at bedtime Max dose: 45 mg/d	Refer to Chapter 21, "Aging and Older Adult Populations."	Refer to Chapter 21, "Aging and Older Adult Populations."

(continued)

TABLE 11.2 COMMON MEDICATIONS FOR TREATMENT OF MAJOR DEPRESSIVE DISORDER (*CONTINUED*)

Medication	Usage	Aged 10–18 Years (Youth)	Aged 19–65 Years (Adult)	Aged 66–74 Years (Older Adult)	Aged 85–99 Years (Oldest Old + Centenarians)
Generic: nefazodone Trade: Dutonin	FDA-approved for depression **WARNING:** Hepatotoxicity, sometimes requiring liver transplantation	Refer to Chapter 20, "Special Considerations for Childhood and Adolescent Populations."	Average dose: 300–600 mg/d Max dose: 300 mg twice daily	Refer to Chapter 21, "Aging and Older Adult Populations." Start at half adult dose.	Refer to Chapter 21, "Aging and Older Adult Populations." Start at half adult dose.
Generic: nortriptyline Trade: Pamelor	FDA-approved for MDD **WARNING:** Can increase QTc interval at toxic doses	Refer to Chapter 20, "Special Considerations for Childhood and Adolescent Populations." It is not recommended under 12 years of age.	Average dose: 75–150 mg/d once daily or on 4 divided days Max dose: 150 mg/d	Refer to Chapter 21, "Aging and Older Adult Populations." Baseline EKG is recommended for more than 50 years.	Refer to Chapter 21, "Aging and Older Adult Populations."
Generic: paroxetine Trade: Paxil, Paxil CR	FDA-approved for MDD, OCD, social anxiety, PTSD, vasomotor symptoms	Refer to Chapter 20, "Special Considerations for Childhood and Adolescent Populations."	Average dose: 20–50 mg/d (CR 25–62.5 mg/d) Max dose: 50 mg/d (CR 62.5 mg/d)	Refer to Chapter 21, "Aging and Older Adult Populations." There is risk of SIADH.	Refer to Chapter 21, "Aging and Older Adult Populations." There is risk of SIADH.
Generic: sertraline Trade: Zoloft	FDA-approved for MDD, panic disorder, PTSD, social phobia	Refer to Chapter 20, "Special Considerations for Childhood and Adolescent Populations." It is FDA-approved for OCD 6 years and up.	Average dose: 50–200 mg/d Max dose: 200 mg/d	Refer to Chapter 21, "Aging and Older Adult Populations."	Refer to Chapter 21, "Aging and Older Adult Populations."
Generic: trazodone Trade: Desyrel	FDA-approved for depression	Refer to Chapter 20, "Special Considerations for Childhood and Adolescent Populations."	Average dose: 150–600 mg Max dose: 400 mg/day outpatient; 600 mg/d inpatient	Refer to Chapter 21, "Aging and Older Adult Populations."	Refer to Chapter 21, "Aging and Older Adult Populations."
Generic: venlafaxine Trade: Effexor, Effexor XR	FDA-approved for depression and anxiety disorders	Refer to Chapter 20, "Special Considerations for Childhood and Adolescent Populations."	Average dose: 75–225 mg/d (XR) or twice to three times daily (IR) Max dose: 375mg/d	Refer to Chapter 21, "Aging and Older Adult Populations."	Refer to Chapter 21, "Aging and Older Adult Populations."
Generic: vilazodone Trade: Viibryd	FDA-approved for MDD	Refer to Chapter 20, "Special Considerations for Childhood and Adolescent Populations."	Average dose: 20 mg/d Max dose: 40 mg/d	Refer to Chapter 21, "Aging and Older Adult Populations."	Refer to Chapter 21, "Aging and Older Adult Populations."
Generic: NA Trade: Trintellix (vortioxetine)	FDA-approved for MDD	Refer to Chapter 20, "Special Considerations for Childhood and Adolescent Populations."	Average dose: 10 mg/d Max dose: 20 mg/d	Refer to Chapter 21, "Aging and Older Adult Populations."	Refer to Chapter 21, "Aging and Older Adult Populations."

(continued)

TABLE 11.2 COMMON MEDICATIONS FOR TREATMENT OF MAJOR DEPRESSIVE DISORDER (CONTINUED)

Medication	Usage	Aged 10–18 Years (Youth)	Aged 19–65 Years (Adult)	Aged 66–74 Years (Older Adult)	Aged 85–99 Years (Oldest Old + Centenarians)
Generic: NA Trade: Auvelity	**WARNING:** Dextromethorphan may cause dizziness.	Refer to Chapter 20, "Special Considerations for Childhood and Adolescent Populations."	Average dose: 90 mg/210 mg/d Initial dose: 45 mg/105 mg	Refer to Chapter 21, "Aging and Older Adult Populations."	Refer to Chapter 21, "Aging and Older Adult Populations."
Generic: selegiline (oral only) Trade: Emsam, Eldepryl	FDA-approved for MDD **WARNING:** Risk for hypertensive crisis with high tyramine diet and oral administration of medication; risk with transdermal application present with doses 9 mg/12 mg or 24 hours or more	Refer to Chapter 20, "Special Considerations for Childhood and Adolescent Populations."	Average dose: transdermal 6 mg/24 hr to 12 mg/24 hr; oral 30–60 mg/d	Refer to Chapter 21, "Aging and Older Adult Populations."	Refer to Chapter 21, "Aging and Older Adult Populations."
Generic: NA Trade: Zulresso	Endogenous hormone FDA-approved for postpartum depression	NA	Continuous IV infusion over 60 hours, titrated as follows: 0–4 hours: 30 mcg/kg/hr 4–24 hours: 60 mcg/kg/hr 24–52 hours: 90 mcg/kg/hr (may also administer 60 mcg/kg/hr for those who do not tolerate 90-mcg dose) 52–56 hours: 60 mcg/kg/hr 56–60 hours: 30 mcg/kg/hr	NA	NA

ADD, attention deficit disorder; FDA, U.S. Food and Drug Administration; IV, intravenous; MDD, major depressive disorder; OCD, obsessive-compulsive disorder; PDR, Physician's Desk Reference; PTSD, posttraumatic stress disorder; REMS, risk evaluation and mitigation strategy; SIADH, syndrome of inappropriate secretion of antidiuretic hormone.

of psychotherapy have comparable effects, so the APRN and the patient can decide on the appropriate type of therapy. For treatment-resistant depression, some stimulants may be used, as well as esketamine. Other therapies for moderatetosevere MDD include ECT and transcranial magnetic stimulation (TMS).

PATIENT TEACHING
A. Education about treatment options and adherence is necessary since there is stigma associated with the disorder.
B. Individuals may be reluctant to get treatment without the understanding that MDD is a chronic, debilitating disorder that worsens and complicates one's ability to care for themselves.
C. Safety planning is also important to reduce the risk of suicide.

FOLLOW-UP
A. Prognosis of MDD is variable, being favorable for those with mild episodes who adhere to medication or recommended treatment, do not have psychosis, and have a good support system.
B. The prognosis is poor in those with other psychiatric disorders, including personality disorders, or those who acquire MDD at late stages in life.
C. Left untreated, depression can last indefinitely, but usually lasts from 6 months to a year, with a climbing recurrence rate after the first episode.
D. About 35% of patients have an increasing risk of recurrence with each episode of MDD. A small percentage (10% or less) may develop bipolar disorder, where about 15% die by suicide.
E. Follow-up is patient-specific and based on remission of symptoms, but occurs during the initial stages every 4 to 6 weeks, with increasing visit intervals as symptoms improve. Care of a person with MDD is lifelong and ongoing, with careful evaluation of suicide risk at every visit.

CONSULTATION AND REFERRALS
A. If the patient has failed to respond to two or more trials of medication for at least 3 months, the patient must be referred for a higher level of care.
B. Referral is also warranted if the suicide risk is high or if the patient is experiencing psychotic features.

C. Additional reasons for referral include homicidal ideation, plan, or intent; suicidal plan and intent; inability to care for self; and need for detox from substances.

INDIVIDUAL CONSIDERATIONS

Pediatrics
A. Refer to Chapter 20, "Special Considerations for Childhood and Adolescent Populations."

Pregnancy
A. PPD occurs during the first 12 months after delivery and is suggested to be related to a rapid decline in sex hormones, estrogen, and progesterone during the postpartum period.
B. The incidence of PPD is between 7% and 20% in postpartum people. Risk factors for PPD include a family history of PPD or other mood and anxiety disorders.
  1. The Edinburgh Postnatal Depression Scale can be used to screen for PPD and standard screening tools and tests (see screening tools).
  2. Other diagnoses that may be considered with mood changes after pregnancy include postpartum psychosis, thyroid disease, and bipolar disorder.
  3. Only one treatment, brexanolone (Zulresso), is FDA-approved for the treatment of PPD, but SSRIs (e.g., sertraline, paroxetine) should be considered first line, especially for breastfeeding patients.
  4. Patients who do not respond to treatment after 6 weeks should be referred for psychiatric consult.

Geriatrics
A. Refer to Chapter 21, "Aging and Older Adult Populations."

Partners/Family
A. Depression not only impacts the individual but also the family. Family members may not understand the severity of depression or understand how to manage patient symptoms such as irritability and avolition.
B. Some researchers have found that family arguments increase when a family member is depressed, so family intervention is necessary to support the patient and their family.
C. Individuals and families supporting an individual with depression, including PPD, may experience marital and family discord.
D. With PPD, finances may also be impacted if the patient cannot return to work due to depression. Because depression may impact the family, clinicians may consider screening for family functioning and discord during routine visits.

RESOURCES
A. Statistics (National Institute of Mental Health): www.nimh.nih.gov/health/statistics
B. Recurrent depressive disorder (*International Classification of Diseases, 10th Revision*): https://icd.who.int/browse10/2019/en#F33

REFERENCES AND BIBLIOGRAPHY
American Psychiatric Association. (2013). *Diagnostic and statistical manual of mental disorders* (5th ed.). https://doi.org/10.1176/appi.books.9780890425596
First, M. B. (2014). *DSM-5 handbook of differential diagnosis.* American Psychiatric Association Publishing.
Otte, C., Gold, S. M., Penninx, B. W., Pariante, C. M., Etkin, A., Fava, M., Mohr, D. C., & Schatzberg, A. F. (2016). Major depressive disorder. *Nature Reviews Disease Primers, 2,* Article 16065. https://doi.org/10.1038/nrdp.2016.65
Qaseem, A. F., Barry, M. J., & Kansagara, D. (2016). Nonpharmacologic versus pharmacologic treatment of adult patients with major depressive disorder: A clinical practice guideline from the American College of Physicians. *Annals of Internal Medicine, 164*(5), 350–359. https://doi.org/10.7326/M15-2570
Siu, A. L., & the U.S. Preventive Services Task Force. (2016). Screening for depression in adults: US preventive services task force recommendation statement. *JAMA, 315*(4), 380–387. https://doi.org/10.1001/jama.2015.18392
Wong, J. J., Frost, N. D., Timko, C., Heinz, A. J., & Cronkite, R. (2020). Depression and family arguments: Disentangling reciprocal effects for women and men. *Family Practice, 37*(1), 49–55. https://doi.org/10.1093/fampra/cmz048

PERSISTENT DEPRESSIVE DISORDER (DYSTHYMIA)

DEFINITION
A. Persistent depressive disorder (PDD) is characterized by a depressed state that is more long-lasting and less severe than MDD. The definition of PDD has evolved over time from a personality state to a mild chronic depression occurring most of the day, for more days than not, for more than 2 years in adults.
B. Mood can be irritable instead of depressed in children and adolescents for 1 year, with the absence of symptoms for no more than 2 months. The disorder can be classified by severity (i.e., mild, moderate, severe) and may also include two or more symptoms, such as appetite and sleep disturbances, fatigue, low self-esteem, concentration difficulties, and hopelessness.

INCIDENCE
A. PDD impacts 1.5% of U.S. adults and is more prevalent in cisgender females than in cisgender males.

PATHOGENESIS
A. The underlying cause of PDD is unknown. It may be related to monoamine deficiency, inflammation, decreased BDNF, and structural and functional changes in the brain (e.g., increased activation of the amygdala, HPA axis dysregulation). The frontal cortex and hippocampus show a volume reduction in individuals with PDD.
B. While dopamine, GABA, epinephrine, and glutamate have been implicated, serotonin is often the target neurotransmitter in pharmacologic treatment.

PREDISPOSING FACTORS
A. Similar to MDD, the cause of PDD is unknown, but it is thought to be attributed to a combination of factors, including psychosocial, genetic, biological, and environmental.
B. Psychosocial factors include substance use, childhood maltreatment and neglect, traumatic events such as car crashes, bereavement, family history of depressive disorders, and financial insecurity.
C. Individuals with TBI are also at risk for PDD.

COMMON COMPLAINTS
A. Patients with PDD do not often complain of a depressed mood but may present with physical complaints such as sleep disturbances, pain, chronic fatigue, irritable bowel syndrome, and other unexplained symptoms.
B. The onset of these symptoms, in most cases, occurs after a psychosocially stressful major life event.

OTHER SIGNS AND SYMPTOMS
A. Individuals with PDD may have the same symptoms as those with MDD.

B. In addition to an irritable or depressed mood, individuals may have two of the following types of symptoms: appetitive (undereating or overeating), weight loss or gain, sleep disturbances (insomnia or hypersomnia), fatigue (low energy), low self-esteem, sexual dysfunction, hopelessness, and poor concentration and decision-making.

SUBJECTIVE DATA

A. Individuals with PDD may have a history of fibromyalgia and chronic fatigue syndrome, personality disorders, substance use disorder, MDD, obesity, and severe illnesses such as cancer, dementia, cardiovascular disease, and physical disabilities.
B. Because individuals with PDD have many unexplained but bothersome symptoms, they may have evidence of excessive medical visits within a year.
C. Although patients may present for numerous medical visits, they tend to exhibit poor adherence behavior regarding treatment recommendations.
D. Suicide risk screening, past medical history, and family history are also important. Individuals impacted by PDD have early onset of depression associated with a family history of depression and may have a history of significant loss, interpersonal conflict, abuse, or financial problems.

PHYSICAL EXAMINATION

A. The diagnosis of PDD is based on an interview, to obtain subjective history, and the mental status and physical examination. The interview provides a description of the history of the present symptoms, including temporal factors and information about personal medical history and medications, psychiatric and substance use history, family history, and social history.
B. Cultural formulation should also be executed because one's religion, culture, and ethnic background may influence the presentation of symptoms.
C. The APRN surveys the patient's affect, demeanor and movement, speech, memory, thought content and process, insight, judgment, and risk for suicide to corroborate with subjective complaints.
D. When performing the physical examination, it is also important to note general appearance and behavior, noting grooming, signs of fatigue, or weight changes; and the neurologic system, evaluating for deep tendon reflexes to assess for thyroid problems or cognitive difficulties such as memory and concentration.
E. Additional information may be obtained from family and friends when warranted. A physical examination can be performed to rule out medical causes of symptoms.

DIAGNOSTIC TESTS AND SCREENING

A. Diagnosis is based on clinical history and physical examination, and validated screening tools such as the PHQ-9 and the Cornell Dysthymia Rating Scale may be used.
B. A suicide risk assessment should be conducted at baseline and upon follow-up.
   1. The Suicide Assessment Five-Step Evaluation and Triage (SAFE-T) and the Ask Suicide-Screening Questions (ASQ) can be used to assess suicide risk.
C. Helpful laboratory tests include CMP, UA and urine toxicology screening, thyroid function test, CBC, vitamin B_{12}, HIV testing, and cortisol levels.

DIFFERENTIAL DIAGNOSES

A. Other mental health disorders: GAD, somatoform disorder, MDD, adjustment disorder, chronic psychotic disorders (schizophrenia, delusional disorder, schizoaffective disorder), substance/medication-induced depressive disorder, bipolar disorders, cyclothymic disorder, personality disorder
B. Endocrine: Cushing disease or hypothyroidism

PLAN

A. There are several evidence-based medical treatments and therapies for treating depression. Remission with medications may take 3 to 6 months to achieve. Medications should be continued for about 1 year once remission is achieved.
B. Patients may stop treatment when symptoms improve, so it is important to educate patients about adherence recommendations.

GENERAL TREATMENTS AND INTERVENTIONS

A. Treatment is based on the severity of symptoms. All patients in imminent danger of harming self or others or who are experiencing severe illnesses and functional limitations or psychosis should be considered for hospital admission immediately.
B. Group physical activity should be an initial recommendation in persons with mildtomoderate symptoms, including about an hour of activity three times weekly for about 3 months.
C. Medication can be administered if the duration of the individual's symptoms is greater than 2 years or if they have a past history of moderatetosevere depression and unremitting symptoms.

COMMON MEDICATIONS

A. All medications used to treat MDD can be used to treat PDD.
B. SSRIs are associated with lower discontinuation rates than SNRIs and TCAs (Table 11.3).
C. Paroxetine has been specifically recommended in combination with problem-solving therapy for PDD; however, caution is to be taken when prescribing to older adults due to its anticholinergic side effect.
D. If there is a concern with prescribing to older adults, SSRIs such as sertraline and escitalopram are recommended. Sertraline and imipramine improve psychosocial outcomes.

PATIENT TEACHING

A. Medications may take about 4 to 6 weeks for an initial response, and an additional 4 weeks may be necessary to notice improvement of symptoms.
B. Patients should also be educated about the black box warning for antidepressants, including increased risk of suicidal thinking within the first 1 to 2 months in individuals 18 to 24 years of age.
C. Education about the side effects of the medications and reporting of adverse effects if prescribed is also important.

FOLLOW-UP

A. Prognosis is poor, with more than half of individuals with PDD experiencing functional disability and elevated suicide risks.
B. Ongoing follow-up is necessary in individuals with PDD because the length of treatment time is indefinite.
C. At onset of medications, patient follow-up can occur every 4 to 6 weeks until stable and then adjusted according to patients' symptom severity and response to medication.
D. Using the PHQ-9 to monitor symptoms may help with this determination.

TABLE 11.3 COMMON MEDICATIONS FOR THE TREATMENT OF PERSISTENT DEPRESSIVE DISORDER

Medication	Usage	Aged 10–18 Years (Youth)	Aged 19–65 Years (Adult)	Aged 66–74 Years (Older Adult)	Aged 85–99 Years (Oldest Old + Centenarians)
Generic: escitalopram Trade: Lexapro	FDA-approved for MDD	Refer to Chapter 20, "Special Considerations for Childhood and Adolescent Populations."	Average dose: 10–20 mg/d Max dose: 20 mg/d	Refer to Chapter 21, "Aging and Older Adult Populations."	Refer to Chapter 21, "Aging and Older Adult Populations."
Generic: paroxetine Trade: Paxil, Paxil CR	FDA-approved for MDD, OCD, social anxiety, PTSD, vasomotor symptoms	Refer to Chapter 20, "Special Considerations for Childhood and Adolescent Populations."	Average dose: 20–50 mg/d (CR 25–62.5 mg/d) Max dose: 50 mg/d (CR 62.5 mg/d)	Refer to Chapter 21, "Aging and Older Adult Populations." There is risk of SIADH.	Refer to Chapter 21, "Aging and Older Adult Populations." There is risk of SIADH.
Generic: sertraline Trade: Zoloft	FDA-approved for MDD, panic disorder, PTSD, social phobia	Refer to Chapter 20, "Special Considerations for Childhood and Adolescent Populations."	Average dose: 50–200 mg/d Max dose: 200 mg/d	Refer to Chapter 21, "Aging and Older Adult Populations."	Refer to Chapter 21, "Aging and Older Adult Populations."
Generic: imipramine Trade: Tofranil	FDA-approved for depression, including treatment resistance	Refer to Chapter 20, "Special Considerations for Childhood and Adolescent Populations."	Average dose: 50–150 mg/d Max dose: 300 mg/d	Refer to Chapter 21, "Aging and Older Adult Populations."	Refer to Chapter 21, "Aging and Older Adult Populations."

FDA, U.S. Food and Drug Administration; MDD, major depressive disorder; OCD, obsessive-compulsive disorder; PDD, persistent depressive disorder; PTSD, posttraumatic stress disorder; SIADH, syndrome of inappropriate secretion of antidiuretic hormone.

CONSULTATIONS AND REFERRALS
A. Refer to ED if the patient is at risk of harming self or others.
B. If the patient fails to respond to two or more trials of medication for at least 3 months, the patient must be referred to a higher level of care.
C. A referral is also warranted if suicide risk is high or if the patient is experiencing psychotic features.
D. Additional reasons for referral include homicidal ideation, plan, or intent; suicidal plan and intent; inability to care for self; and need for detox from substances.

INDIVIDUAL CONSIDERATIONS

Pediatrics
A. Refer to Chapter 20, "Special Considerations for Childhood and Adolescent Populations."

Geriatrics
A. Refer to Chapter 21, "Aging and Older Adult Populations."

Partners/Family
A. Depression not only impacts the individual but also the family. Family members may not understand the severity of depression nor understand how to manage patient symptoms such as irritability and avolition.
B. Clinicians may consider screening for family functioning and discord during routine visits.
C. Provide educational material to family members, partners, and friends. It is also important to assess the needs of caregivers and refer them to local support groups as needed because their loved one's symptoms can have a significant impact on their life.

RESOURCES
A. Practice guideline for the assessment and treatment of patients with suicidal behaviors (*American Journal of Psychiatry*): https://pubmed.ncbi.nlm.nih.gov/14649920
B. Suicide assessment five-step evaluation and triage for clinicians (Substance Abuse and Mental Health Services Administration): https://store.samhsa.gov/product/SAFE-T-Pocket-Card-Suicide-Assessment-Five-Step-Evaluation-and-Triage-for-Clinicians/sma09-4432
C. American Psychological Association clinical practice guideline for the treatment of depression across three age cohorts: www.apa.org/depression-guideline/guideline.pdf
D. Ask Suicide-Screening Questions (ASQ) toolkit (National Institute of Mental Health): www.nimh.nih.gov/research/research-conducted-at-nimh/asq-toolkit-materials

REFERENCES AND BIBLIOGRAPHY
American Psychiatric Association. (2013). *Diagnostic and statistical manual of mental disorders* (5th ed.). https://doi.org/10.1176/appi.books.9780890425596
First, M. B. (2014). *DSM-5 handbook of differential diagnosis*. American Psychiatric Association Publishing.
Gilbody, S., Richards D, Brealey, S., & Hewitt, C. (2007). Screening for depression in medical settings with the Patient Health Questionnaire (PHQ): A diagnostic meta-analysis. *Journal of General Internal Medicine, 22*(11), 1596–1602. https://doi.org/10.1007/s11606-007-0333-y

Hellerstein, D. J., Batchelder, S. T., Lee, A., & Borisovskaya, M. (2002). Rating dysthymia: An assessment of the construct and content validity of the Cornell Dysthymia Rating Scale. *Journal of Affective Disorders, 71*(1–3), 85–96. https://doi.org/10.1016/s0165-0327(01)00371-8

Kocsis, J. H., Zisook, S., Davidson, J., Shelton, R., Yonkers, K., Hellerstein, D. J., Rosenbaum, J., & Halbreich, U. (1997). Double-blind comparison of sertraline, imipramine, and placebo in the treatment of dysthymia: Psychosocial outcomes. *The American Journal of Psychiatry, 154*(3), 390–395. https://doi.org/10.1176/ajp.154.3.390

Maurer, D. M. (2012). Screening for depression. *American Family Physician, 85*(2), 139–144. https://www.ncbi.nlm.nih.gov/pubmed/22335214

von Wolff, A., Holzel, L. P., Westphal, A., Harter, M., & Kriston, L. (2013). Selective serotonin reuptake inhibitors and tricyclic antidepressants in the acute treatment of chronic depression and dysthymia: A systematic review and meta-analysis. *Journal of Affective Disorders, 144*(1–2), 7–15. https://doi.org/10.1016/j.jad.2012.06.007

PREMENSTRUAL DYSPHORIC DISORDER

DEFINITION
A. Premenstrual dysphoric disorder (PMDD), known as a severe and debilitating form of premenstrual syndrome (PMS), is characterized by the presence of anxiety symptoms or mood changes (e.g., irritability, anger, depression, hopelessness) and physical health nuances such as headache, breast tenderness, abdominal distension, changes in appetite, and sleep disturbances that impact functioning in all areas of life for 1 to 2 weeks before a menstrual cycle.
B. PMDD usually occurs during the luteal phase of a patient's menstrual cycle and resolves with menstruation, but it may occur during the ovulatory stage in some.

INCIDENCE
A. PMDD impacts about 3% to 9% of menstruating patients.
B. In the United States, patients with PMDD experience about 6 days of severe symptoms per cycle, totaling about 8 years of disability, during menstrual cycles.

PATHOGENESIS
A. Changing levels of sex steroids (e.g., progesterone, estrogen, allopregnanolone) that accompany an ovulatory menstrual cycle are understood to trigger PMDD.
B. Scientists speculate that patients who experience PMDD have heightened sensitivity to cyclic variations in these sex steroids, making them more susceptible to drastic shifts in mood and behavior and their debilitating somatic symptoms.
  1. There is conflicting evidence as to whether a decline in progesterone during either the luteal phase or the ovulatory phase is the culprit since management with this hormone does not remit symptoms. Some scientists propose that allopregnanolone, a metabolite of progesterone, fluctuates during the menstrual cycle, causing diminished functional sensitivity of GABA type A (GABA-A) receptor agonists (i.e., cause of hallmark symptoms of PMDD, such as irritability, mood lability, and anxiety).
  2. Peaks in estrogen before ovulation may trigger symptoms of PMDD, but as with progesterone there is debate about the cause and timing of symptoms.
C. The neurotransmitters GABA, beta endorphins, serotonin, and glutamate may also contribute to PMDD symptomatology. Sex steroids affect the transmission of serotonin.
  1. Abnormalities in serotonin transmission can occur with tryptophan-free diets, serotonin receptor agonists (e.g., sumatriptan, flibanserin) that cause PMDD symptoms, or administration of SSRI before menstruation that diminishes symptoms.
  2. Patients with PMDD have an altered responsiveness of the GABA-A receptor compared with those without the disorder and increased sensitivity to cyclic fluctuations of glutamate. Lower levels of beta endorphins during the luteal and follicular phases are present and suggest a dysregulation of the hypothalamic–pituitary–gonadal axis. Thus, the stress response in patients with PMDD is distorted, resulting in altered physiologic symptoms and perceived stress.

PREDISPOSING FACTORS
A. Obesity; current or past history of cigarette smoking; history of trauma, domestic violence, physical or sexual abuse, or stressful event in the past year; White race; and anxiety disorders are risk factors for developing PMDD.
B. Family history of MDD or PPD, intimate partner violence, and high potassium intake are also risk factors.

COMMON COMPLAINTS
A. Patients with PMDD may report changes in mood, cognitive functioning, and sleep patterns, while also experiencing abdominal bloating and cramps, fatigue, breast fullness and tenderness, nausea, swelling in extremities, and joint and muscle aches a week before menstruation starts.
B. Patients may also complain of acne flares related to their cycles.

OTHER SIGNS AND SYMPTOMS
A. Patients with PMDD may experience symptoms such as headaches, weight gain, bloating, labile affect, irritability, anger, anxiety, hopelessness, depressed mood, anhedonia, fatigue/lethargy, food cravings, overeating, concentration difficulties, and a sense of overwhelm.

SUBJECTIVE DATA
A. Diagnosis of PMDD is based on an interview to obtain a subjective history. PMDD is cyclic, but can impair the patient's functioning in every part of their life, such as work, relationships, and social life.
B. Symptoms may last from a few days to 2 weeks and may intensify anywhere between 2 and 6 days before menses.
C. Patients seeking treatment are likely to report debilitating physical symptoms such as headaches or breast tenderness, as well as anger and irritability. These symptoms must be present for at least two consecutive cycles, have a temporal relationship with the menstrual cycle, and not characterize the symptomatology of any other mental health disorder.
D. Patients with PMDD may also have a history of GAD, PTSD, PPD, or MDD, or report a family history of MDD and PPD.
E. Social history may reveal physical or sexual abuse and trauma or a history of substance use.

PHYSICAL EXAMINATION
A. The diagnosis of PMDD is based on an interview, to obtain subjective history, and the mental status and physical examination. The interview provides a description of the history of the present symptoms, including temporal factors and information about personal medical history and medications, psychiatric and substance use history, family history, and social history.
B. Cultural formulation should also be executed because one's religion, culture, and ethnic background may influence the presentation of symptoms.

C. The healthcare provider surveys the patient's affect, demeanor and movement, speech, memory, thought content and process, insight, judgment, and risk for suicide to corroborate with subjective complaints. Additional information may be obtained from family and friends when warranted.

D. A physical examination can be performed to rule out medical causes of symptoms. When performing the physical examination, it is also important to note general appearance and behavior, noting grooming and signs of fatigue or weight changes. The patient's skin needs to be assessed for acne lesions, and their abdomen and extremities should be assessed for bloating and swelling.

DIAGNOSTIC TESTS AND SCREENING

A. Screening and testing for PMDD are mostly subjective, relying on patient narrative, healthcare provider observation, and validated screening tools such as the Premenstrual Symptoms Screening Tool (PSST) and the Calendar of Premenstrual Experiences (COPE).

B. Visual Analog Scale (VAS), Daily Record of Severity of Problems (DRSP), and the Patient-Reported Outcomes Measurement Information System (PROMIS) may be used.
  1. If using the DRSP, patients must record daily symptoms over two cycles.

C. Routine labs to check triiodothyronine (T3), free T4, and TSH can be done to rule out thyroid disease.

DIFFERENTIAL DIAGNOSES

A. Other mental health disorders such as MDD, GAD, substance/medication-induced depressive disorder, depressive disorder due to another medical condition, PDD, depression that may worsen during the luteal phase but persist throughout the cycle, chronic fatigue syndrome

B. Endocrine: thyroid disease

C. Reproductive: mastalgia, PMS, dysmenorrhea, exogenous progestogen-induced premenstrual disorder, endometriosis, chronic pelvic pain

D. Neurologic: migraines

E. Gastrointestinal: irritable bowel syndrome

F. Musculoskeletal: rheumatologic disorders, connective tissue disorders

PLAN

A. Pharmacologic and nonpharmacologic options are available for treatment of PMDD.

B. Treatment targets the potential cause of symptoms (e.g., mood related to monoamine deficiency or ovulatory hormone cyclicity).

C. Nonpharmacologic options include CBT.
  1. Patients may also be encouraged to keep a log or diary to record the timing and characteristics of symptoms.

D. Three SSRIs are FDA-approved for treatment of PMDD (Table 11.4), but other antidepressants such as citalopram, clomipramine, desvenlafaxine, escitalopram, and venlafaxine are used off-label to treat the disorder.

E. Sertraline may be helpful in reducing anger and irritability.

F. Antipsychotics such as quetiapine may be used along with an SSRI in patients who do not respond to monotherapy.

G. Hormones and oral contraceptives (with and without drospirenone) may be used to suppress ovulation.

H. Adjunct therapy with alprazolam and buspirone may help reduce anxiety and irritability in some patients.

PATIENT TEACHING

A. Educate patients about symptoms, treatment options, coping skills, and adherence to alleviate symptoms.

B. Safety planning is also important to reduce the risk of suicide.

C. Medication side effects and adverse effects should also be reviewed. If patients are taking SSRIs and become pregnant, they need to be informed of possible congenital malformations.

TABLE 11.4 COMMON MEDICATIONS FOR THE TREATMENT OF PREMENSTRUAL DYSPHORIC DISORDER

Medication	Usage	Aged 10–18 Years (Youth)	Aged 19–65 Years (Adult)	Aged 66–74 Years (Older Adult)	Aged 85–99 Years (Oldest Old + Centenarians)
Generic: fluoxetine Trade: Prozac, Prozac Weekly, Sarafem	FDA-approved for PMDD	Refer to Chapter 20, "Special Considerations for Childhood and Adolescent Populations," or PDR.	Average dose: 20 mg/d Max dose: 20 mg/d	NA	NA
Generic: paroxetine Trade: Paxil, Paxil CR	FDA-approved for PMDD	Refer to the Chapter 20, "Special Considerations for Childhood and Adolescent Populations," or PDR.	Average dose: 12.5 mg/d CR; administered as a single dose in the morning; may be taken daily or only during the luteal phase of cycle Max dose: 25 mg/d	NA	NA
Generic: sertraline Trade: Zoloft	FDA-approved for PMDD	Refer to Chapter 20, "Special Considerations for Childhood and Adolescent Populations."	Average dose: 50–150 mg/d; initial 50 mg/d can be dosed through the menstrual cycle up to 150 mg/d or limit to luteal phase up to 100 mg/d Max dose: 150 mg/d	NA	NA

FDA, U.S. Food and Drug Administration; NA, not applicable; PDR, Physician's Desk Reference; PMDD, premenstrual dysphoric disorder.

FOLLOW-UP
A. The initial visit should occur 4 weeks after starting medication and then may vary depending on the patient's symptoms and response to medication.

CONSULTATIONS AND REFERRALS
B. If in a psychiatric setting, the patient may need a referral or coordination with primary care provider or gynecologist and may need to be referred to a therapist to help with coping skills to deal with dysphoria or anxious behavior.

INDIVIDUAL CONSIDERATIONS

Partners/Family
A. The family may experience interpersonal conflicts due to affect instability. Teach families the cause and symptoms of PMDD to preserve family dynamics and to empower family members.

RESOURCES
A. PMS and PMDD (*American Family Physician*): www.aafp.org/pubs/afp/issues/2016/0801/p236.html
B. PMDD (Office on Women's Health): www.womenshealth.gov/menstrual-cycle/premenstrual-syndrome/premenstrual-dysphoric-disorder-pmdd

REFERENCES AND BIBLIOGRAPHY
American Psychiatric Association. (2013). *Diagnostic and statistical manual of mental disorders* (5th ed.). https://doi.org/10.1176/appi.books.9780890425596

First, M. B. (2014). DSM-5 *handbook of differential diagnosis*. American Psychiatric Association Publishing.

Lanza di Scalea, T., & Pearlstein, T. (2019). Premenstrual dysphoric disorder. *Medical Clinics of North America, 103*(4), 613–628. https://doi.org/10.1016/j.mcna.2019.02.007

Pearlstein, T. (2016). Treatment of premenstrual dysphoric disorder: Therapeutic challenges. *Expert Review of Clinical Pharmacology, 9*(4), 493–496. https://doi.org/10.1586/17512433.2016.1142371

Yonkers, K. A., Kornstein, S. G., Gueorguieva, R., Merry, B., Van Steenburgh, K., & Altemus, M. (2015). Symptom-onset dosing of sertraline for the treatment of premenstrual dysphoric disorder: A randomized clinical trial. *JAMA Psychiatry, 72*(10), 1037–1044. https://doi.org/10.1001/jamapsychiatry.2015.1472

SUBSTANCE-INDUCED BIPOLAR AND RELATED DISORDERS

DEFINITION
A. *Substance-induced bipolar and related disorders* refers to the presence of manic or depressive symptoms due to medications or substances of abuse.
B. The symptoms of the mood disorder may appear during use, with intoxication, or during withdrawal.

PATHOGENESIS
A. Cerebral structures such as the frontal cortex, hippocampus, nucleus accumbens, amygdala, and hypothalamus undergo changes due to drug ingestion.
B. Alterations in dopaminergic, corticotropin-releasing factor, and serotonergic activity occur.

PREDISPOSING FACTORS
A. Genetic factors increase the diathesis for developing substance-induced bipolar and related disorders.
B. Heavy alcohol use or cannabis, cocaine, or opioid use may precipitate pathologic affective states.
C. Medications used for treating medical disorders (e.g., digoxin, seizure medication, corticosteroids, interferon) may also cause symptoms.

COMMON COMPLAINTS
A. Feelings of guilt, depressed mood, insomnia, suicidal ideation and behavior, decreased libido, avolition, irritability, helplessness, distractibility, psychomotor retardation, impulsivity, insomnia

OTHER SIGNS AND SYMPTOMS
A. Grandiosity, pressured speech, increased energy, distractibility

SUBJECTIVE DATA
A. When evaluating people with this diagnosis, the affective symptoms will have a temporal relationship with ingestion of the substance, with symptoms resolving when the medication is removed.
B. It is important to ask about family history to determine if the person has any first-degree relatives with the disorder, investigate prior or current use of illicit substances, review past medical history for presence of condition requiring use of drugs known to alter mood, and review psychiatric history to rule out other mental health disorders.

PHYSICAL EXAMINATION
A. The patient may present with emotional lability and hypercreativity. They may also have evidence of self-harm or self-mutilation.
B. The patient may have irritable mood and affect, hopeless and helpless, depressed, or with anhedonia in a depressed state. The patient may also appear "antsy" or restless and exhibit pressured speech, grandiosity, and impulsivity.

DIAGNOSTIC TESTS AND SCREENING
A. Substance-induced bipolar and related disorders will follow the diagnostic criteria used to evaluate bipolar disorders.
B. Labs and imaging can also be used to rule out medical causes of symptoms. Urine drug screen, toxicology, CMP, CBC, and creatine phosphokinase can be used to rule out rhabdomyolysis.

DIFFERENTIAL DIAGNOSES
A. Bipolar disorder type I or II
B. Substance use disorder comorbid with bipolar disorder

PLAN
A. Remove the medication or substance eliciting symptoms, and provide familial support and psychotherapy.
B. Treatment with a medication may be necessary and should be determined on a case-by-case basis.
C. Supportive care and safety should be instituted while the person is experiencing any range of symptoms.
D. Suicide assessment and prevention is also important because the most prevalent complication of the disorder is suicide.
E. Care may also differ depending on the setting. In the outpatient setting, patient safety is of utmost concern; proper transport to the ED or psychiatric hospital is necessary.

GENERAL TREATMENTS AND INTERVENTIONS
A. See "Bipolar Disorders."

PATIENT TEACHING
A. Avoid use of medication or substance. Support groups such as Alcoholics Anonymous or Narcotics Anonymous may be considered. Limit use of tobacco and caffeine and consume a balanced diet.

B. Discuss any use of medications, substances, or supplements with the healthcare provider before use.

FOLLOW-UP
A. Prognosis of substance-induced bipolar and related disorders is promising as mood symptoms dissipate after the substance or medication is removed.
B. If the induction of symptoms is caused by illicit drugs, then abstinence from the substance is necessary to prevent the recurrence of symptoms. Social support from family networks and therapies can be effective.
C. Patient environment that supports the use of illicit substances may worsen the prognosis.

CONSULTATION AND REFERRALS
A. Referral for medical assistant treatment or substance use treatment may be necessary; may refer to anonymous support groups.
B. Consultation with the patient's primary care provider is important due to the risk for chronic health conditions. Therapists may help patients develop appropriate coping skills to manage the range of symptoms they have and may also provide support to family members.

INDIVIDUAL CONSIDERATIONS
Pediatrics
A. Refer to Chapter 20, "Special Considerations for Childhood and Adolescent Populations."

Pregnancy
A. Treatment of bipolar disorder in pregnancy requires consideration of the risks and benefits of using mood stabilizers that are mostly teratogenic (carbamazepine and valproate).
B. Lithium may also cause congenital heart disease in children exposed in utero. If lithium is used, careful monitoring of these levels is suggested. When considering treatment for pregnant patients with bipolar disorder, the well-being of the fetus and the patient must be assessed.

Geriatrics
A. Refer to Chapter 21, "Aging and Older Adult Populations."

Partners/Family
A. Condition may impact the family. Provide educational material to family members, partners, and friends.
B. It is also important to assess the needs of caregivers and refer them to local support groups as needed because their loved one's symptoms can have a significant impact on their life.

REFERENCES AND BIBLIOGRAPHY
American Psychiatric Association. (2013). *Diagnostic and statistical manual of mental disorders* (5th ed.). https://doi.org/10.1176/appi.books.9780890425596

First, M. B. (2014). DSM-5 *handbook of differential diagnosis*. American Psychiatric Association Publishing.

Khan, M. A., & Akella, S. (2009). Cannabis-induced bipolar disorder with psychotic features: A case report. *Psychiatry (Edgmont), 6*(12), 44–48. https://www.ncbi.nlm.nih.gov/pubmed/20104292

Price, A. L., & Marzani-Nissen, G. R. (2012). Bipolar disorders: A review. *American Family Physician, 85*(5), 483–493. https://www.ncbi.nlm.nih.gov/pubmed/22534227

12 PERINATAL MENTAL HEALTH

Barbara Caldwell and Mamilda Robinson

INTRODUCTION

This chapter presents the following perinatal mood disorders: mood disorders (anxiety and depression) during pregnancy, postpartum depression, and postpartum psychosis. We also address substance use during pregnancy and in the postpartum period. As an APRN, the assessment, management, and ongoing evaluation of pregnant patients with psychiatric problems during the perinatal period are complex and high risk due to the need to be accountable for the mother's physical and mental health and the health of the developing fetus. *Perinatal mental illness* refers to psychiatric disorders that are prevalent during pregnancy and as long as 1 year after delivery.

OPIOID USE DISORDER DURING PRENATAL AND POSTNATAL PERIOD

Substance use disorder (SUD) is characterized by a group of cognitive, behavioral, and physiologic symptoms that signify an individual's continued use of a substance despite significant substance-related problems. One of the most important SUDs in female patients during the childbearing years is opioid use disorder (OUD). OUD during pregnancy is a complicated illness because it has negative outcomes for the mother, the fetus, and the baby. SUD is recognized to be a chronic disease with expected lapses.

Pregnant and postpartum patients with OUD are encouraged to keep trying, through pharmacotherapy and behavioral interventions, not abstinence, to reach the goal of ending substance use. Treatment involving therapy and medication-assisted treatment (MAT) and recovery using methadone or buprenorphine is included in a comprehensive care model that has been recommended for use during pregnancy. Even though the mother is in treatment during the prenatal period, the fetus and the neonate are at significant risk for poor fetal growth and neonatal abstinence syndrome (NAS), respectively.

DEFINITION
A. Perinatal OUD in pregnancy is a serious medical condition whereby the pregnant woman uses or is addicted to opioids such as prescription painkillers (e.g., oxycodone, hydrocodone), heroin, or synthetics such as fentanyl. It causes physical dependence and can lead to withdrawal symptoms if they try to stop suddenly. Opioids bind to opioid receptors in the brain and other parts of the body, leading to various effects including pain relief and euphoria. The substance crosses the placenta and has been associated with poor infant outcomes, such as neonatal opioid withdrawal syndrome (NOWS), preterm birth, poor fetal growth, and stillbirth.

INCIDENCE
A. Data from the National Survey on Drug Use and Health (Center for Behavioral Health Statistics and Quality, 2017) indicate that approximately 285,000 pregnant women (12.6%) used alcohol or illicit drugs in the past 30 days.
B. According to the Centers for Disease Control and Prevention (CDC; Ko et al., 2020) analysis of survey data in 34 jurisdictions, 6.6% of women reported prescription opioid use during pregnancy. Among these women, 21.2% reported misuse (a source other than a healthcare provider or a reason for use other than pain), 27.1% wanted or needed to cut down or stop using, and 31.9% reported not receiving healthcare provider counseling about how use could affect an infant. In this same study, it was noted that 1 in 15 (6.6%) respondents self-reported using prescription opioid pain relievers during pregnancy.
C. "Among women who used prescription opioids, 88.8% reported using the opioids for pain reasons, 14.4% for reasons other than pain, and 4.9% for other/undetermined reasons. In particular, prescription opioids were used to relieve pain from an injury, condition, or surgery that occurred before (22.2%) or during (63.8%) pregnancy or during an unstated time frame (11.7%). Commonly reported reasons for use other than pain were to help sleep (7.9%) and relieve tension or stress (7.7%)" (Ko et al., 2020, p. 899). This has implications for prescribers to be alert to pregnancy possibilities and to find alternative strategies, rather than the use of opioids, to alleviate the stress and poor sleep that childbearing and pregnant women are experiencing.
D. A study conducted by Heil et al. (2011) found that among women with OUD, unintended pregnancy rates are significantly higher than the general obstetrical population. Almost 9 in every 10 pregnancies were unintended (86%), with comparable percentages mistimed (34%), unwanted (27%), and ambivalent (26%). It is reasonable in this environment for healthcare providers to anticipate that more women will conceive while maintained on buprenorphine-naloxone and they will require thoughtful counseling on how best to treat their OUD in these circumstances.

PATHOGENESIS
A. Opioid use can be present before, during, or after pregnancy. Life stress places childbearing patients at risk of substance use, and therefore understanding the patient's background stressors and coping strategies will provide a foundation to treatment.
B. Individuals with substance use problems are known to have adverse childhood events (ACEs) and psychological traumas that have precipitated the use of substances to cope with their stressors.
C. A thorough understanding of the pathogenesis of substance use is important to provide effective assessment, interventions, and recovery strategies.
D. The concept of allostasis is the process by which a state of internal, physiologic equilibrium is maintained by an organism in response to actual or perceived environmental and psychological stressors. When an individual is repeatedly challenged, the stress can lead to allostatic load, which is a chronic deviation from normal functioning and leads to a pathologic state. Knowledge of the underlying pathophysiology of addiction is fundamental to healthcare practitioners. *Drug addiction* can be defined as a compulsion to seek and take ▶

a drug, loss of control in limiting intake, and the emergence of a negative state when access to the drug is prevented.

E. The neurobiological basis of addiction consists of a three-stage cycle, each corresponding to different brain regions or neurocircuitry. With chronic drug exposure, the three stages feed into each other, become more intense, and ultimately lead to addiction. Simply put, it is a vicious cycle of use → abuse → tolerance → dependence → craving → withdrawal → continued use or relapse.

1. Binge/intoxication stage
   a. Functional domain: incentive salience/habits
   b. Brain region: basal ganglia
   c. This stage is characterized by the consumption of a mind-altering substance and the intense "high" pleasure associated with it. The basal ganglia play a crucial role in the formation of habits and the experience of reward. Over time, the substance use becomes more about seeking this reward (incentive salience) rather than the pleasure of the substance itself. This leads to habit formation, where the use of the substance becomes more automatic. Excessive drug-taking behaviors in the binge/intoxication stages drive an allostatic-like process that generates the withdrawal/negative affect stage and the preoccupation/anticipation stage.
2. Withdrawal/negative affect stage
   a. Functional domain: negative emotional states
   b. Brain region: amygdala
   c. During this stage, the absence of the substance leads to withdrawal symptoms, which can be both physical and psychological. The amygdala, a region involved in processing emotions, becomes more active, contributing to negative emotional states like anxiety, irritability, and depression. The negative emotional state can be defined as irritability, physical pain, emotional pain, malaise, dysphoria, alexithymia, and loss of motivation for natural rewards. Additionally, pain in addiction and withdrawal from opioids (and alcohol) can lower pain thresholds and exacerbate pain with heightened pain perception, and so pain is one of the main triggers of relapse. These negative feelings create a strong motivation to alleviate them through further substance use.
3. Preoccupation/anticipation stage
   a. Functional domain: executive function
   b. Brain region: prefrontal cortex
   c. This stage involves the cognitive processes related to thinking about the substance. The prefrontal cortex, which is responsible for executive functions such as decision-making, planning, and self-control, becomes engaged. In addiction, there is a decreased functioning in this area, leading to poor decision-making and increased focus on obtaining and using the substance. This stage is often associated with craving and planning the next opportunity for substance use.

F. Given that the childbearing and pregnant patient is surrounded by stressful environments, this cycle can be difficult to ameliorate unless the underlying problems are addressed. According to Ko, D'Angelo, Haight, and colleagues (2020), the main reason for opioid use in pregnant women is pain. Coping with chronic pain and experiencing stress can trigger drug-seeking to gain relief. Paradoxically, in the presence of tolerance from prolonged use, opioids enhance pain perception (hyperalgesia) and hypersensitivity to emotional distress (hyperkatifeia), prompting relief through further opiate use, thus continuing the cycle.

G. In general, before prescribing opioids to their patients, healthcare providers should ensure that opioids are appropriately indicated; discuss the risks and benefits of opioid use and review treatment goals; and take a thorough history of substance use and review the Prescription Drug Monitoring Program to determine whether patients have received prior opioid prescriptions.

H. For chronic pain, practice goals include strategies to avoid or minimize the use of opioids for pain management, highlighting alternative pain therapies such as nonpharmacologic (e.g., exercise, physical therapy, behavioral approaches) and nonopioid pharmacologic treatments.

Impact of Opioids on Pregnant Woman, Fetus, and Neonate

A. Untreated substance use in pregnancy places the mother, fetus, and neonate at high risk for significant complications, including miscarriage, preterm labor, opioid overdose, placental abruption, preeclampsia, and cardiac arrest. They are also 4.6 times more likely to die during hospitalization.

B. Significant barriers exist for these pregnant patients to access appropriate OUD care. Fewer MAT providers will serve pregnant patients with OUDs. Additionally, pregnant patients with OUDs may have limited access to prenatal care, face increased stigma and discrimination, and face possible mandatory child welfare involvement with potential removal of children from the home.

C. They may carry sexually transmitted diseases (STDs), abuse other drugs, smoke cigarettes, drink alcohol, and/or have a history or presence of intimate partner violence or psychological abuse.

D. The developing fetus is at risk of intrauterine growth retardation, preterm birth, and birth defects depending on the drugs taken by the pregnant mother.

E. The neonate is at risk of intrauterine growth restriction; small-for-gestational age (SGA); low birth weight; NAS, or more specifically NOWS; long-term developmental and neurocognitive delays; and behavioral issues, among others.

1. NAS or NOWS requires the infant to be hospitalized, sometimes in the neonatal intensive care unit (NICU), for a minimum of 4 to 7 days to monitor disturbances in autonomic, gastrointestinal (GI), and central nervous system as they withdraw from opioids. The neonate can be treated with oral methadone or morphine at a required dosage to eliminate symptoms of withdrawal.

COMMON COMPLAINTS

A. Common complaints can be viewed as those general discomforts or complications arising from the pregnancy itself and those relative to opioid use. This section deals with the latter.

B. A common reason for substance use in pregnancy is pain associated with bodily changes exacerbated by hyperalgesia, hyperkatifeia, and physical demands on the individual.

C. GI complaints may be more pronounced, such as heartburn and indigestion. Constipation is a common side effect of opioids and diarrhea in withdrawal.

D. Substance use does co-occur with other psychiatric disorders and can be the patient's maladaptive strategy for symptom reduction of depression, anxiety, poor sleep, or chronic pain.

E. Other complaints to explore are those associated with interpersonal violence, psychological trauma, stress, depression, and anxiety, and a range of mental health and psychosocial and other social determinants of health (SDOH) issues.

OTHER SIGNS AND SYMPTOMS

A. Substance craving and withdrawal symptoms in the absence of opioid
B. Inadequate weight gain due to poor nutrition or opioid-related GI issues
C. Gestational hypertension or preeclampsia more commonly seen in pregnant women with OUD
D. Abdominal pain possibly related to pregnancy complications or signs of withdrawal
E. Anemia and other nutritional deficiencies
F. Signs of use, including evidence of track marks, abscesses, and infections at the injection site
G. Signs of intoxication, including drowsiness or "nodding off," constricted pupils, slow breathing, impaired coordination, or cognition
H. Signs of overdose, including pinpoint pupils (miosis), gurgling, flaccid limp, muscles, pale skin, clammy or blue skin, bradycardia, loss of consciousness, and respiratory depression or arrest

SUBJECTIVE DATA

A. The patient may be having difficulty accessing care or adhering to treatment plan due to logistical barriers.
B. In the assessment of pregnant women who may have OUD, it is critically important to remember that the woman may be anxious, fearful, and ambivalent about coming for services and sharing their stories with a stranger.
C. Patients need to feel safe and reassured that there is help available to them, but talking about the problems will be a way to ensure that the right services are included. Shame and stigma are very much active with pregnant substance-using women, so an atmosphere of respect and openness should be incorporated into the overall assessment and treatment process.

PHYSICAL EXAMINATION

A. Take a thorough history of substance use and consult the Prescription Drug Monitoring Program to confirm other prescribed potential drugs of abuse.
B. In patients with OUD prior to pregnancy, multiple body systems may be impacted.
C. Table 12.1 outlines an in-depth review of the medical problems that are associated with opioid use, especially for women with longer term use.

DIAGNOSTIC TESTS AND SCREENING

A. Early universal first-visit screening as part of a comprehensive care, brief intervention (such as engaging the patient in a short conversation, providing feedback and advice), and referral for treatment of pregnant women with opioid use and OUD improve maternal and infant outcomes.
  1. Refer if positive. This includes fetal ultrasound and maternal blood testing. This screening process can help determine the risk of the fetus having certain birth defects. Second trimester prenatal screening may include several blood tests for multiple markers.
B. The CDC recommends that all pregnant women get tested at first prenatal visit for HIV, hepatitis B virus (HBV), hepatitis C virus (HCV), and syphilis and other STDs during each pregnancy and repeated in the last trimester and at the time of delivery depending on the risk factors.
C. Other laboratory testing in patients with possible SUD include the following:
  1. Urine toxicology screen for opioids and illicit drugs used in the community that includes confirmatory testing
  2. Urine screen for alcohol that includes confirmatory testing

TABLE 12.1 BODY SYSTEMS IMPACTED BY OPIOID USE

Body System	Medical Problem
Cardiovascular	From injecting drugs: endocarditis (infection in the lining or valves of the heart that can cause fever, chills, and fatigue), septic thrombophlebitis (redness and inflammation of veins and arteries)
Endocrine and metabolic	Opioids: osteopenia (back pain, stooped posture, and easily fractured bones), hypogonadism (reduced sex drive, erectile dysfunction, absence of menstruation, mood swings, irritability, infertility)
Hematologic	From injecting drugs: hematologic consequences of liver disease from hepatitis C, hepatitis C-related cryoglobulinemia, and purpura (bruising and bleeding easily, fatigue, poor appetite, yellow discoloration of the skin and eyes, itchy skin and distended abdomen, dark-colored urine)
Hepatic	From injecting drugs: hepatitis B, C, and D; infectious and toxic hepatitis and hepatocellular cancer (joint pain, fever, nausea, vomiting, clay-colored stools and all the symptoms noted in hematologic section)
Infectious	Opioids: pneumonia, sexually transmitted infections From injecting drugs: endocarditis (infection in heart and valves), cellulitis (infection of the skin), pneumonia, thrombophlebitis (inflammation of veins and arteries), aneurysm (rupture of artery), septic arthritis (pain and swelling of joints), osteomyelitis (inflammation in the legs, arms, or spine with redness), epidural and brain infections, soft tissue infections, tetanus, HIV, botulism (from open skin infections and contaminated food)
Renal	Opioids: acute renal failure, hematuria From injecting drugs: inflammation of the kidneys, glomerulonephritis, amyloidosis (protein buildup in the kidneys)
Nutritional	Protein malnutrition
Pulmonary	Opioids: respiratory depression/failure; bronchospasm; sleep apnea, wheezing during respirations From injecting drugs: pulmonary hypertension
Gastrointestinal	Opioids: constipation, bowel obstruction, nausea

3. Liver enzymes and serum bilirubin test to detect liver disease
4. Serum creatinine levels test to detect silent renal disease

D. Screening instruments for identification of SUDs include the following:
1. The Substance Use Risk Profile-Pregnancy Scale (SURP-P) and the 4Ps Plus (**P**arent, **P**artner, **P**ast, **P**resent Pregnancy) are ideal universal screening tests. The SURP-P contains only three items, and scoring is very simple. This is particularly useful because busy clinicians do not have time to administer separate questionnaires that would screen for a variety of substances individually. Given the brevity of the screener, it can be readministered on multiple occasions with minimal burden to the patient or the clinician.
2. The 4Ps can be found at https://nortonhealthcareprovider.com/news/using-the-t-ace-and-4ps-substance-abuse-screening-tools-with-pregnant-women and has the following questions:
   a. Parents: Did any of your parents have a problem with alcohol or other drug use?
   b. Partner: Does your partner have a problem with alcohol or drug use?
   c. Past: In the past, have you had difficulties in your life because of alcohol or other drugs, including prescription medications?
   d. Present: In the past month, have you drunk any alcohol or used other drugs?
   e. Scoring: Any "yes" should trigger further questions.
      i. Document a "yes" to each question individually.
      ii. Document a "negative" if all answers are "no."
   f. The 4Ps Plus includes additional questions about depression and domestic violence.
3. The National Institute on Drug Abuse (NIDA) Quick Screen and CRAFFT (**C**ar, **R**elax, **A**lone, **F**orget, **F**riends, **T**rouble; for women 26 years or younger) are also validated tools.
4. Screen for co-occurring mental health conditions. A waiting room questionnaire such as the Patient Health Questionnaire-9 (PHQ-9) is ideal.
5. Screen for posttraumatic stress disorder (PTSD) using the PTSD Checklist for the *DSM-5* (PCL-5).
6. For partner violence, the STaT (Intimate Partner Violence Screening Tool) can be helpful (Paranjape & Liebschutz, 2003).
7. For eating disorders commonly co-occurring with SUD, the use of the SCOFF Questionnaire can help screen for these disorders (see Chapter 10, "Feeding and Eating Disorders").

DIFFERENTIAL DIAGNOSIS

A. Other SUDs often overlap with OUDs.
B. Psychiatric illnesses such as depression, anxiety, PTSD, bipolar disorder, and personality disorders can co-occur with substance use.
C. Differential diagnosis also includes chronic pain conditions such as fibromyalgia and chronic back or pelvic pain.
D. It is important for the nurse practitioner (NP) to take a history of the relationship between the patient's psychiatric symptoms and periods of abstinence and periods of use. In addition, the NP should determine if the patient meets the *Diagnostic and Statistical Manual of Mental Disorders*, Fifth Edition (*DSM-5*; American Psychiatric Association, 2013) criteria for OUD and other psychiatric diagnoses.
E. There are several medical complications of opioid use in pregnancy.

1. GI disorders such as gastritis, hepatitis, and pancreatitis may be related to SUD, or symptoms may mimic withdrawal symptoms.
2. Cholestasis of pregnancy is not unique to pregnant patients with OUD; however, there is an association between cholestasis of pregnancy and chronic liver diseases such as HCV and nonalcoholic liver cirrhosis.
   a. Diagnosed by pathognomonic itching of the palms and soles, elevated bile acids, and elevated hepatic function testing
   b. Associated with negative pregnancy outcomes of stillbirth if delivery is not done by 37 weeks due to cardiotoxic effects resulting in fatal arrhythmia
3. Soft tissue infections (e.g., cellulitis and abscesses) can occur due to contaminated needles.
   a. Cellulitis is characterized by skin erythema, edema, and warmth, with or without purulence.
   b. Infective endocarditis (IE) is a complication of intravenous (IV) opioid drug use with infection and damage to the tricuspid, aortic, and mitral valves in the heart.
4. Additional problems are pneumonia, pulmonary septic emboli, and mycotic aneurysms of the pulmonary artery, which should prompt evaluation with echocardiogram.

PLAN

A. The most significant morbidity associated with OUD and pregnancy is overdose. From 2018 to 2021, the mortality ratio more than tripled among pregnant and postpartum women aged 35 to 44 years. The highest overdose rate was at 7 to 12 months postpartum. Opioid overdose is more likely to occur in women who use sedatives, inject illicit opioids of unknown potency and purity, have co-occurring pulmonary disease, or have sleep apnea.

B. Motivational interviewing (MI) is an evidence-based method that helps guide the patient's own thinking through the stages of the transtheoretical model of change. It can assist the NP in determining where the individual is in thinking about change related to their opioid use, why treatment is necessary, and the benefits it brings to the patient and their family. MI describes the process of change as a cycle of six stages: precontemplation, contemplation, preparation, action, maintenance, and termination. It is important to match the intervention with the stage and remain flexible as these stages are not linear.
1. The NP should acknowledge the problems, any ambivalence the patient may have about starting treatment, and the treatment process.
2. The NP should make efforts to understand past treatment failures and the negative events that occurred so that those areas can be addressed during current treatment and efforts made to change in response to what was shared.
3. Intake of an individual considering treatment for OUD should be the beginning of a strong therapeutic relationship. The NP can start by encouraging a focus on motivation to change. Research is clear that the intake clinician can be responsible for verbal or nonverbal communication, including the tone of their voice that sets a negative tone to the interaction.

C. Key concepts: Maintain a positive, strengths-based, nonjudgmental approach with a shared decision-making approach.
1. Show consistent unconditional positive regard for the patient.
2. Be empathetic and encouraging, promoting empowerment.
3. Engage with open questions, active listening, and good eye contact.

4. Clarify the session's purpose, ensure confidentiality, and encourage questions.
5. Prevent the recurrence of past negative treatment experiences.
6. Offer specific support and address patient concerns.

D. Due to the high rate of unintended pregnancies among opioid-using women, postpartum family planning counseling is critical.

E. NPs should consider the following recommendations when a pregnant patient is diagnosed with OUD:
1. Discuss the risks and benefits of buprenorphine or methadone. Note the lack of consensus on developmental risks from intrauterine exposure to buprenorphine or methadone and assure minimal risk of birth defects and neurodevelopmental impact.
2. Highlight the necessity of pharmacotherapy for fetal health in reducing relapse and overdose risks.
3. Discuss the possibility of NAS and prepare the patient for the infant's NICU care due to opioid or MAT exposure.
4. Teach the patient about NAS diagnosis, management, and consequences.
5. Review ways to optimize the health of the fetus, such as healthy nutrition and prenatal vitamins. Offer support for tobacco cessation and other SUD during pregnancy.
6. Discuss early pediatric care after delivery and hospital discharge.
7. Breastfeeding should be encouraged in women who are stable on their opioid agonists, who are not using illicit drugs, and who have no other contraindications, such as HIV infection. Women should be counseled about the need to suspend breastfeeding in the event of a relapse.
8. Suggest nonpharmacologic interventions for the neonate to reduce NAS symptoms during and after discharge, such as rooming-in and skin-to-skin contact, soothing measures such as swaddling, and baby carriers and slings.

F. Pregnant patients need to demonstrate the following characteristics to enroll in an MAT program:
1. Able to make their own decision to enter an MAT program
2. Psychiatrically stable, in control of behaviors, and can commit to taking MAT as prescribed, along with behavioral counseling and support services
3. Willing to taper or stop current use of alcohol and other drugs of abuse

G. The pregnant patient should be counseled on the following areas as part of the action plan:
1. Discuss the side effects of MAT during the first weeks: somnolence, insomnia, weight gain, sexual dysfunction, constipation, or mental fog.
2. Discuss the protracted withdrawal symptoms that can occur during MAT: anxiety, hostility, irritability, depression, mood instability, fatigue, insomnia, problems concentrating, reduced libido, and physical complaints; the NP should have strategies to address some of these issues with nonpharmacologic treatments, such as exercise, sleep hygiene, massage, and so forth.
3. MAT initiation protocols can be found at www.samhsa.gov/sites/default/files/quick-start-guide.pdf
4. Use the Clinical Opioid Withdrawal Scale (COWS) for monitoring.
5. Discuss diversion, overdose, and close monitoring for overmedication.
6. Review the "Patient Teaching" section for other areas of interventions.

> **EMERGENCY PLAN**
> Naloxone to reverse overdose. Training can be found here:
> **PrescribeToPrevent.org**

GENERAL TREATMENT AND INTERVENTIONS

A. To achieve positive pregnancy outcomes, gender sensitivity and cultural humility should be practiced within an environment of trauma-informed care delivery.

B. Treatment considerations should reflect assessments and interventions conducted in the patient's preferred language, with sensitivity to the patient's level of ethnic identity, including acculturation level, and reflect the patient's cultural lens.

COMMON MEDICATIONS

A. MAT is the standard of care for pregnant patients with OUD. The overall goal is to minimize serious complications of opioid use during pregnancy, reducing the risk of relapse and improving outcomes. Opioid agonist pharmacotherapy is safer during pregnancy than continued use or medically supervised withdrawal because withdrawal is associated with high relapse rates, with worse outcomes. More research is needed to assess the safety (particularly regarding maternal relapse), efficacy, and long-term outcomes of medically supervised withdrawal.

B. Individualized pharmacotherapy is coupled with counseling, behavioral therapy, and group therapy.

C. Table 12.2 outlines the common drugs used in treatment of OUD during pregnancy and postpartum.

D. Results from a systematic review and meta-analysis indicate that pregnancy outcomes for patients using either buprenorphine-naloxone, buprenorphine monotherapy, or methadone are generally comparable. However, buprenorphine-naloxone carries a lower risk of abuse or diversion due to its lower street value and abuse deterrent properties compared with buprenorphine alone. While methadone is effective, its requirement for daily supervised administration can be challenging to pregnant and new mothers due to time constraints.

E. Historically, buprenorphine-naloxone was preferred during pregnancy (due to concerns about naloxone's safety), with a switch to buprenorphine monotherapy or methadone postpartum to manage increased stress and reduce risk of relapse. However, current understanding suggests maintaining a consistent MAT approach throughout pregnancy and postpartum is beneficial, avoiding the risks and barriers associated with changing medications. Rather than running the risks of interrupting MAT or increasing the barriers to treatment, healthcare providers should use this information to reassure women who have been exposed to buprenorphine-naloxone. Consideration of switching MAT to buprenorphine alone should be based on individual circumstances and not simply a blanket recommendation.

F. Naloxone should be on hand in the home and in the medical facility.

PATIENT TEACHING

A. Support family planning services, which include preconception services, pregnancy intention screening, and contraceptive counseling, to prevent unintended pregnancy by increasing access to the full range of contraceptive methods, including long-acting reversible contraception (e.g., intrauterine devices and implants).

TABLE 12.2 METHADONE AND BUPRENORPHINE DRUGS

Type of Drug	Actions	Maternal Side Effects	Adverse Reactions	Dosage/Administration	Regulations on Administration
Methadone					
Schedule II synthetic opioid	Acts as a potent agonist at the mu-opioid receptor; metabolized by CYP450 pathways, CYP2B6, and CYP3A4 in the liver; blocks NMDA receptors and monoaminergic reuptake transporters; suppresses withdrawal symptoms, blocks euphoria, and reduces cravings; has a long half-life (25–52 hours)	Constipation, nausea/vomiting; diaphoresis, sedation/respiratory depression, decreased libido; prolonged QT interval	Respiratory depression and prolonged QT cardiac interval (torsade de pointes); interacts with antivirals	Starting doses 20–30 mg/d and gradually increase in 5–10 mg; in a study, the mean initial maintenance dose was 69 mg (range 8–160 mg); mean dose at delivery was 93 mg (12–185 mg); due to physiologic changes of pregnancy (increased volume and renal clearance)	Only SAMHSA-certified opioid treatment centers permitted to dispense methadone for daily administration
Buprenorphine					
	Schedule III mixed opioid receptor agonist–antagonist; as a partial mu-opioid agonist; able to displace and antagonize full mu-agonists such as morphine, leading to acute withdrawal; long half-life (24–48 hours); metabolized and eliminated in the urine and feces; in moderate liver impairment, the half-life of buprenorphine is increased by 35%; has ceiling effect for pain relief and respiratory suppression—safe risk from overdose	Headache, anxiety, constipation, perspiration, fluid retention in lower limbs, urinary hesitancy, and sleep disturbances	Concomitant use of CNS depressants, alcohol, sedatives, hypnotics, or anxiolytic medications due to respiratory depression	Poor oral availability; administered sublingually or with oral tablet; typical dosage is 8–16 mg daily with a maximum dose of 24 mg	Require additional training but waiver has been removed; has a high rate of diversion and misuse

CNS, central nervous system; NMDA, N-methyl-D-aspartate; SAMHSA, Substance Abuse and Mental Health Services Administration.

B. MAT is considered the standard of care for pregnant women with OUD. If both the counseling and prescribing are done together by the same practitioner, these areas should be reviewed:

1. Emphasize the importance of prenatal care to monitor the health of the mother and the fetus and manage complications if they arise. Stress the importance of MAT adherence and the danger of opioid withdrawal during pregnancy (i.e., harm to fetus and risk of relapse).
2. Discuss the likelihood of NAS or NOWS, what to expect, symptoms, and management, and reassure the mother that it is treatable.
3. Stress the need for mental health support: Ongoing trauma-informed group and/or individual counseling and therapy to address the OUD or SUD, triggers, and relapse prevention, and its impact on self, baby, and family should be integrated into sessions. MI, cognitive behavioral therapy (CBT), and contingency management are effective strategies, as is the support of 12-Step and SMART Recovery groups. Provide guidance on building a strong support network, including family, sober friends, and peer support groups.
4. Advise about healthy lifestyle choices: good nutrition, exercise, and avoidance of harmful substances. MI, CBT, and contingency management are effective strategies, as is support of recovery groups such as 12-Step.
5. Provide strategies as to how to manage pain safely, both emotional and physical pain.
6. Prenatal, preparation for labor and delivery, and parenting classes should be included in the counseling sessions or outside classes available in the community. Learning what to expect and how to manage enormous changes has been shown to reduce fear and anxiety, improve coping skills, reduce pain, and promote healthy lifestyles and attachments.
7. Pain management and medication can also be explored with the anesthesiologist or the obstetrician (OB)/certified nurse midwife (CNM).
8. Prepare for breastfeeding if possible. Methadone and buprenorphine, with or without naloxone, are all regarded as safe for use during breastfeeding. The benefits of breastfeeding include fostering mother–baby bonding, providing nutritional and immune benefits to the infant, and potentially reducing the severity and duration of NAS in babies exposed to opioids in utero. If the mother is using other substances (like alcohol, benzodiazepines, or illicit drugs), breastfeeding might not be safe.
9. Stress the importance of continuing MAT and aftercare, including mental health support, after childbirth to reduce the risk of relapse.
10. Legal and social services: Inform about legal rights and available social services and the importance of engaging with these resources as needed. Discuss the possibility of child protective services involvement and how this might work in their favor by providing access to more resources, adding additional support and motivation to the mother's recovery.

FOLLOW-UP

A. Follow-up care is the linchpin to long-term recovery. Due to the complex and chronic nature of the disorder and the risk to the mother, the fetus, the neonate, and the entire family, continuous care is essential. It provides an opportunity to coordinate between the OB provider, addiction specialists, psychiatric-mental health providers, and pediatricians.
B. Regular consistent comprehensive care allows for continual monitoring and management of physical and mental health of the mother. The risk of relapse is high, so close contact and support of multidisciplinary team improve outcomes.
C. Ensure MAT adherence and address any barriers to treatment.
D. Regular follow-up ensures prenatal care adherence and early detection of complications.
E. Follow-up visits can screen for early signs of emerging mental health issues and can adjust treatments accordingly.
F. Follow-up appointments provide opportunities for education on nutrition, self and baby care, and lifestyle adjustments to support recovery and parenting.
G. Follow-up visits may offer opportunities to connect with others and access community resources for housing and social support. Reducing isolation reduces the risk of relapse.
H. Regular nonjudgmental contact with trusted professionals improves adherence to treatment recommendations.

RECOMMENDATIONS

A. The CDC and the American College of Obstetricians and Gynecologists (ACOG) indicate that clinicians and patients thoroughly address and carefully weigh risks and benefits when considering initiation of opioid therapy for chronic pain during pregnancy.
B. Opioids, if indicated, should be prescribed only after consideration of alternative pain management therapies.

Primary Prevention

A. Strategies to prevent the incidence of NAS center on responsible opioid prescribing and access to preconception care and family planning services. The *CDC Guideline for Prescribing Opioids for Chronic Pain* (Dowell et al., 2016) recommends that clinicians address the unique sensitivities of prescribing opioid medications to pregnant and nonpregnant patients of reproductive age.
B. Recommendations include discussing how long-term opioid use might affect current and future pregnancies and how patients of reproductive age with a need for long-term opioid use can avoid unintended pregnancy.

CONSULTATION, REFERRALS, AND RESOURCES

A. Given the unique needs of pregnant patients with an OUD, healthcare providers will need to consider modifying some elements of prenatal care (e.g., expanded sexually transmitted infection [STI] testing, additional ultrasound examinations to assess fetal weight if there is concern for fetal growth abnormalities, and consultations with various types of healthcare providers) in order to meet the clinical needs of the patient's particular situation.
B. Two national initiatives encourage clinicians to practice responsible prescribing and help patients of reproductive age optimize their health before pregnancy.
  1. The CDC's Treating for Two: Safer Medication Use in Pregnancy initiative encourages evidence-based prescribing practices and informed decision-making specifically for pregnant women and for nonpregnant women of reproductive age.
  2. The National Preconception Health and Health Care Initiative provides educational resources to clinicians and their patients, and coordinates outreach and social media campaigns related to improving preconception health, including reducing substance use and treating SUDs before pregnancy.

C. The Substance Abuse and Mental Health Services Administration (SAMHSA) offers clinical materials to assess patients' readiness to change and to end their substance use. Use MI to identify and support positive changes to all health behaviors, starting with the riskiest ones.
  1. Substance Abuse and Mental Health Services Administration. *A Collaborative Approach to the Treatment of Pregnant Women with Opioid Use Disorders.* HHS Publication No. (SMA) 16-4978. Substance Abuse and Mental Health Services Administration, 2016. Available at store.samhsa.gov.

D. Refer to the ACOG for information on opioid use and opioid use disorder during pregnancy (www.acog.org/clinical/clinical-guidance/committee-opinion/articles/2017/08/opioid-use-and-opioid-use-disorder-in-pregnancy).

REFERENCES AND BIBLIOGRAPHY

American Psychiatric Association. (2013). *Diagnostic and statistical manual of mental disorders* (5th ed.). https://doi.org/10.1176/appi.books.9780890425596

Center for Behavioral Health Statistics and Quality. (2017, September 7). *Results from the 2016 national survey on drug use and health.* Substance Abuse and Mental Health Services Administration.

Cerdá, M., & Krawczyk, N. (2020). Pregnancy and access to treatment for opioid use disorder. *JAMA Network Open*, 3(8), e2013899. https://doi.org/10.1001/jamanetworkopen.2020.13899

Cohen, S. P., Christo, P. J., Wang, S., Chen, L., Stojanovic, M. P., Shields, C. H., Brummett, C., & Mao, J. (2008). The effect of opioid dose and treatment duration on the perception of a painful standardized clinical stimulus. *Regional Anesthesia and Pain Medicine*, 33(3), 199–206. PMID: 18433669.

Coleman-Cowger, V. H., Oga, E. A., Peters, E. N., Trocin, K. E., Koszowski, B., & Mark, K. (2019). Accuracy of three screening tools for prenatal substance use. *Obstetrics and Gynecology*, 133(5), 952–961. https://doi.org/10.1097/AOG.0000000000003230

Dowell, D., Haegerich, T. M., & Chou, R. (2016, April 19). CDC guideline for prescribing opioids for chronic pain—United States, 2016. (2016). *JAMA*, 315(15), 1624–1645. https://doi.org/10.1001/jama.2016.1464

Gavin, L., Moskosky, S., Carter, M., Curtis, K., Glass, E., Godfrey, E., Marcell, A., Mautone-Smith, N., Pazol, K., Tepper, N., Zapata, L., & Centers for Disease Control and Prevention. (2014, April 25). Providing quality family planning services: Recommendations of CDC and the U.S. Office of Population Affairs. *MMWR Recommendations and Reports*, 63(RR04), 1–54. https://www.cdc.gov/mmwr/preview/mmwrhtml/rr6304a1.htm?s

Han, B., Compton, W. M., Einstein, E. B., Elder, E., & Volkow, N. D. (2024). Pregnancy and postpartum drug overdose deaths in the US before and during the COVID-19 pandemic. *JAMA Psychiatry*, 81(3), 270–283. https://doi.org/10.1001/jamapsychiatry.2023.4523

Heil, S. H., Jones, H. E., Arria, A., Kaltenbach, K., Coyle, M., Fischer, G., Stine, S., Selby, P., & Martin, P. R. (2011). Unintended pregnancy in opioid-abusing women. *Journal of Substance Abuse Treatment*, 40(2), 199–202. https://doi.org/10.1016/j.jsat.2010.08.011

Ko, J. Y., D'Angelo, D. V., Haight, S. C., Morrow, B., Cox, S., von Essen, B. S., Strahan, A. E., Harrison, L., Tevendale, H. D., Warner, L., Kroelinger, C. D., & Barfield, W. D. (2020, July 17). Vital signs: Prescription opioid pain reliever use during pregnancy—34 U.S. jurisdictions, 2019. *Morbidity and Mortality Weekly Report*, 69(28), 897–903. http://doi.org/10.15585/mmwr.mm6928a1

Ko, J. Y., Wolicki, S., Barfield, W. D., Patrick, S. W., Broussard, C. S., Yonkers, K. A., Naimon, R., & Iskander, J. (2017, March 10). CDC grand rounds: Public health strategies to prevent neonatal abstinence syndrome. *Morbidity and Mortality Weekly Report*, 66(9), 242–245. http://doi.org/10.15585/mmwr.mm6609a2

Koob, G. F. (2020). Neurobiology of opioid addiction: Opponent process, hyperkatifeia, and negative reinforcement. *Biological Psychiatry, 87*(1), 44–53. https://doi.org/10.1016/j.biopsych.2019.05.023

Koob, G. F., & Schulkin, J. (2019). Addiction and stress: An allostatic view. *Neuroscience and Biobehavioral Reviews, 106,* 245–262. https://doi.org/10.016/j.neubiorev.2018.09.008

Johnson, A. J., & Jones, C. W. (2018). Opioid use disorders and pregnancy. *Obstetrics and Gynecology Clinics of North America, 45*(2), 201–216. https://doi.org/10.1016/j.ogc.2018.01.008

Liebling, E., Yedinak, J., Green, T., Hadland, S., Clark, M., & Marshall, B. (2016). Access to substance use treatment among young adults who use prescription opioids non-medically. *Substance Abuse Treatment, Prevention, and Policy, 11*(1), Article 38. https://doi.org/10.1186/s13011-016-0082-1

Link, H. M., Jones, H., Miller, L., Kaltenbach, K., & Seligman, N. (2020). Buprenorphine-naloxone use in pregnancy: A systematic review and metanalysis. *American Journal of Obstetrics & Gynecology MFM, 2*(3), 100179. https://doi.org/10.1016/j.ajogmf.2020.100179

Martin, D. S. (2020, October 30). *Using the T-ACE and 4P's substance abuse screening tools with pregnant women.* Norton Healthcare. https://nortonhealthcareprovider.com/news/using-the-t-ace-and-4ps-substance-abuse-screening-tools-with-pregnant-women

Morgan, J. F., Reid, F., & Lacey, J. H. (2000). The SCOFF questionnaire: A new screening tool for eating disorders. *The Western Journal of Medicine, 172*(3), 164–165. https://doi.org/10.1136/ewjm.172.3.164

Ondersma, S. J., Chang, G., Blake-Lamb, T., Gilstad-Hayden, K., Orav, J., Beatty, J. R., Goyert, G. L., & Yonkers, K. A. (2019). Accuracy of five self-report screening instruments for substance use in pregnancy. *Addiction, 114*(9), 1683–1693. https://doi.org/10.1111/add.14651

Paranjape, A., & Liebschutz, J. (2003). STaT: A three-question screen for intimate partner violence. *Journal of Women's Health, 12*(3), 233–239. https://doi.org/10.1089/154099903321667573

Paranjape, A., Rask, K., & Liebschutz, J. (2006). Utility of STaT for the identification of recent intimate partner violence. *Journal of the National Medical Association, 98*(10), 1663–1669. PMID: 17052059.

Patrick, S. W., Dudley, J., Martin, P. R., Harrell, F. E., Warren, M. D., Hartmann, K. E., Ely, E. W., Grijalva, C. G., & Cooper, W. O. (2015). Prescription opioid epidemic and infant outcomes. *Pediatrics, 135*(5), 842–850. https://doi.org/10.1542/peds.2014-3299

Prasad, M., & Jones, M. (2019). Medical complications of opioid use disorder in pregnancy. *Seminars in Perinatology, 43*(3), 162–167. https://doi.org/10.1053/j.semperi.2019.01.005

Rodriguez, C. E., & Klie, K. A. (2019). Pharmacological treatment of opioid use disorder in pregnancy. *Seminars in Perinatology, 43*(3), 141–148. https://doi.org/10.1053/j.semperi.2019.01.003

Substance Abuse and Mental Health Services Administration. (2018, January). *Clinical guidance for treating pregnant and parenting women with opioid use disorder and their infants* (Report No. SMA18-5054). U.S. Department of Health and Human Services. https://store.samhsa.gov/product/clinical-guidance-treating-pregnant-and-parenting-women-opioid-use-disorder-and-their

Substance Abuse and Mental Health Services Administration. (2021). *Addressing the specific needs of women for treatment of substance use disorders.* Advisory. (Publication No. PEP20-06-04-002). U.S. Department of Health and Human Services. https://store.samhsa.gov/sites/default/files/pep20-06-04-002.pdf

Towers, C. V., Katz, E., Weitz, B., & Visconti, K. (2020). Use of naltrexone in treating opioid use disorder in pregnancy. *American Journal of Obstetrics and Gynecology, 222*(1), 83.e1–83. e8. https://doi.org/10.1016/j.ajog.2019.07.037

Verbiest, S., McClain, E., & Woodward, S. (2016). Advancing preconception health in the United States: Strategies for change. *Upsala Journal of Medical Sciences, 121*(4), 222–226. https://doi.org/10.1080/03009734.2016.1204395

Whiteman, V. E., Salemi, J. L., Mogos, M. F., Cain, M. A., Aliyu, M. H., & Salihu, H. M. (2014). Maternal opioid drug use during pregnancy and its impact on perinatal morbidity, mortality, and the costs of medical care in the United States. *Journal of Pregnancy, 2014*(1), Article 906723. https://doi.org/10.1155/2014/906723

Zhao, L., Cheng, C., & Bouchard, L. (2020). Medication-assisted treatment for opioid use disorder in pregnancy: Practical applications and clinical impact. *Obstetrical & Gynecological Survey, 75*(3), 175–189. https://doi.org/10.1097/OGX.0000000000000744

PERINATAL MOOD DISORDERS

Perinatal depression occurs in approximately 6% to 30% of female patients. Because of the high risk that perinatal depression poses to the mother and developing fetus, the treatment of mild to moderate depression needs to be assessed and discussed with the significant other and other team members. The American Psychiatric Association and the American Congress of Obstetrics and Gynecology (ACOG) both recommend that either psychotherapy or antidepressant medication be utilized for first-line treatment of mild to moderate perinatal depression. Further, a strong focus on attachment and bonding and supportive interventions will assist in positive parenting outcomes post pregnancy. Recent research indicates that the father of the developing fetus experiences similar mental health issues as the mother and should be included in the assessment and intervention process.

Research indicates that childbearing females have higher rates of mood disorders than males. Females have 1.5- to 3-fold higher rate than males beginning in early adolescence and at greater risk for ongoing mood problems during pregnancy. Unfortunately, lack of assessment and treatment leads to adverse pregnancy outcomes for both the mental health of the mother and psychosocial and developmental progression of the infant.

Untreated mental illness during the perinatal period is associated with a range of common neurodevelopmental disorders in the offspring. These maternal states, such as depression and stress, are associated with inflammation in pregnancy that can influence the fetal inflammatory pathway, epigenetic changes that increase the expression of abnormal neurodevelopmental pathways, and behavioral outcomes in childhood such as autism and attention deficit hyperactivity disorder (ADHD). Further, depression in the perinatal period is associated with poor mother–infant bonding and attachment.

DEFINITION

A. The psychological and physical stress of pregnancy contributes an additional burden to the patient.

B. The core symptoms of depression are changes in mood, affect, sleep, hygiene, appetite, cognition, and activity. According to the *Diagnostic and Statistical Manual of Mental Disorders*, Fifth Edition, Text Revision (*DSM-5-TR*; American Psychiatric Association, 2022b), five or more symptoms present during the same 2-week period and at least one symptom, either (a) depressed mood or (b) loss of interest or pleasure, with emphasis on significant change in previous functioning and clinical significance of these symptoms.

C. Pregnant women may also have anxiety and panic symptoms, which are risk factors for postpartum depression. These symptoms can range from mild to severe.

D. More serious symptoms include mood episodes with psychotic features during the postpartum period that is most associated with infanticide. The psychotic symptoms are related to command hallucinations to harm their infant during the postpartum period.

INCIDENCE

A. According to the World Health Organization (2023), depression is a common illness worldwide, with an estimated 3.8% of the population affected, including 5% among adults. One in ten women in developed countries have perinatal depression and one in five women have perinatal depression in developing countries.

B. Mood disorders can be present during pregnancy or during the postpartum period, but approximately 50% of postpartum depressed episodes begin prior to delivery.

   1. Major depressive disorder (MDD) can develop during the perinatal period and is associated with the onset of mood symptoms that occur during pregnancy or in the 4 weeks to 12 months that follow delivery.
   2. Anxiety problems co-occur with depressed symptoms; it is likely that both these disorders will be present during pregnancy and in the first year postpartum.

      a. Peripartum anxiety disorders are prevalent, with one in five women in a typical sample meeting diagnostic criteria for at least one disorder.

      b. Prenatal anxiety is noted to be a strong predictor of postpartum depression. Antenatal depression is significantly associated with preterm birth and low birth weight, with higher risk among women of lower socioeconomic status.

      c. Postpartum anxiety is even more prevalent than postpartum depression and often underdiagnosed. Another study found the incidence of postnatal anxiety was 17.1%, surpassing the incidence of postpartum depression at 4.8%.

   3. Depressive symptoms affect between 10% and 20% of pregnant patients and new mothers, and the nonchildbearing parent can experience problems as well. In 2011, 9% of pregnant women and 10% of postpartum women met the criteria for MDD. One in seven women are impacted by perinatal and postnatal depression with either major or minor depressive episodes. The prevalence is higher in females of low income; additionally, the prevalence in the United States is higher among Black and Hispanic females than among White females. Women with bipolar disorder and depression are at greater risk of psychiatric hospitalization, particularly women with bipolar affective disorder and those with past histories of MDD. The risk of maternal suicide is significantly elevated among patients with perinatal depression, and maternal suicides account for up to 20% of all postpartum deaths, making it one of the leading causes of maternal mortality in the perinatal period. Untreated postpartum psychosis is associated with an estimated 4% chance of infanticide and a 5% risk of suicide.

PATHOGENESIS

A. A combination of genetics, environment, and epigenetics appears to interact during a time when the body is experiencing substantial stress.

B. During pregnancy, reproductive steroids (estrogen and progesterone) are increased, cortisol is elevated, and the hypothalamic–pituitary–adrenal (HPA) axis is activated.

   1. Reproductive steroids regulate all aspects of neural function implicated in the development of depression and most of the neurotransmitters, including serotonin, dopamine, norepinephrine, glutamate, and gamma-aminobutyric acid (GABA).
   2. Deficiencies in these neurotransmitters, in turn, are also responsible for change in mood and development of depression.
   3. Stress from pregnancy can alter the HPA axis and sensitize the limbic system.

C. Inflammation has been implicated in the development of depression. There is increasing evidence that environmental and lifestyle factors, including obesity, unhealthy diet, psychosocial stress, physical inactivity, disturbed sleep, and exposure to toxicants like smoke and pollution, collectively known as the *exposome*, contribute to systematic chronic inflammation (SCI). Parental SCI and disease risk may be transmitted to their offspring via a "DNA inflammatory signature" through epigenetic alterations, resulting in increased risk of inflammatory diseases in the next generation. The inflammatory states can lead to depression and fatigue.

BOX 12.1 RISK FACTORS FOR PERINATAL DEPRESSION

Abuse during childhood, adverse childhood experiences
Antenatal and/or childbirth complications
Autoimmune disease
Body image negativity
Chronic physical illness: ongoing chronic infection, diabetes, preeclampsia
Domestic violence
Exosome: environmental and individual exposures (e.g., smoking, diet)
Family or personal history of mood disorders
Insufficient emotional/social support
Life stress or recent adverse events
Lower socioeconomic factors
Maternal age
Maternal anxiety
Perinatal loss, grief
Poor coping skills, low resilience
Single status
Unintended pregnancy
Unrealistic expectations of baby and postpartum

PREDISPOSING FACTORS

A. Several risk factors are identified in Box 12.1.

B. The attachment (bonding) of the mother to the infant is at risk with perinatal depression. Risk factors associated with impaired mother–infant bonding include advanced maternal age, history of depression, low social support, and Beck Depression Inventory scores above 20. These factors should alert the NP to assess for depression in postpartum mothers.

COMMON COMPLAINTS

A. Each pregnancy is different and experienced by each patient in a unique way. Common perinatal complaints include hormonally induced mood swings, emotional sensitivity and lability, as well as heightened anxiety about the pregnancy, childbirth, and impending parenthood.

B. Obsessive-compulsive symptoms, such as obsessive fears about the baby's health or intrusive thoughts, may also occur.

C. The "baby blues" affect up to 80% of mothers, involving mood swings, sadness, irritability, and anxiety, usually peaking around the fourth day and resolving by the tenth day after childbirth. Postpartum anxiety often centers around excessive worries about the baby's health and irrational fears. Some of the more general signs of perinatal depression are listed in Box 12.2.

OTHER SIGNS AND SYMPTOMS

A. Pregnancy can be a risk factor for depression, particularly in those with a history of mood disorders. Pregnant women may have panic attacks and postpartum obsessive-compulsive

BOX 12.2 COMMON COMPLAINTS DURING PREGNANCY

- Abnormal appetite, weight changes, or both Difficulty concentrating, remembering, or making decisions
- Aches or pains, headaches, cramps, or digestive problems that do not have a clear physical cause or do not ease even with treatment
- Difficulty sleeping (even when the baby is sleeping), awakening early in the morning, or oversleeping
- Fatigue or abnormal decrease in energy
- Feelings of guilt, worthlessness, hopelessness, or helplessness
- Feeling restless or having trouble sitting still
- Irritability
- Loss of interest or pleasure in hobbies and activities
- Persistent doubts about the ability to care for the new baby
- Persistent sad, anxious, or "empty" mood
- Trouble bonding or forming an emotional attachment with the neonate

disorder (OCD), which involves intrusive, repetitive thoughts (often about harm coming to the baby) and compulsive behaviors aimed at reducing anxiety.

B. Postpartum depression, a more severe form of mood disturbance, can involve prolonged periods of intense sadness, despair, loss of interest in activities, feelings of worthlessness or guilt, changes in appetite and sleep, and sometimes thoughts of harming oneself or the baby.

C. A rare but serious condition, postpartum psychosis typically develops within the first 2 weeks postpartum. Symptoms include delusions, hallucinations, severe mood swings, and confusion. It is a medical emergency requiring immediate attention.

D. The NP should perform a thorough assessment of the thoughts and feelings the mother has about the fetus and what they imagined having a newborn would be like.

E. Thoughts about death, suicide, or harming oneself or the baby must be evaluated in detail.

F. Fantasies of aggression, violence, or other distorted thinking must be evaluated and followed during the counseling sessions. These are red flags for postpartum psychosis where the infant may be at risk of harm.

G. Depression that is not adequately treated is a risk factor for infanticide and maternal suicide.

SUBJECTIVE DATA

A. Chronic conditions may develop during the perinatal period and may contribute to depressed mood. Examples include the following:

 1. Patients may experience back pain and joint pain exacerbated by the pregnancy.
 2. Poor sleep quality is a major determinant of depressed mood and a focus of intervention by the NP. Sleep apnea will also contribute to depressed mood and can be evaluated using the Sleep Apnea Index.
 3. Patients may develop anxiety as a result of coping with perinatal changes. Pregnant patients may struggle with coping with psychological and physical changes and feel that the pregnancy is a burden.

B. Many patients with perinatal depression and anxiety have problems with decision-making and have issues with memory and concentration.

C. Isolating oneself from family or friends is considered a risk factor for depressed mood and should be evaluated.

PHYSICAL EXAMINATION

A. Patient history should focus on obtaining a detailed family and personal history of any past depression, anxiety, mood, suicidal gestures, SUD, or other behavioral health issues during the developmental timeline, as well as what types of treatments, medication, and psychotherapy, were initiated, for what time frame, and the type of outcome.

B. In collaboration with the patient's OB provider, a complete physical examination should be performed with review of systems with attention to cardiovascular signs that may mask as anxiety, neurologic system including mental status examination (MSE), and evaluation of the cranial nerves.

DIAGNOSTIC TESTS AND SCREENING

A. Laboratory workup should be reviewed or performed to identify any underlying medical condition that may be contributing to or exacerbating dysphoric mood.

 1. Laboratory workup includes toxicology; serum and urine tests; thyroid panel; complete blood count (CBC); vitamin D, vitamin B_{12}, and folic acid tests; chemistry panel; hemoglobin A1c (HbA1c), liver, and kidney function tests; lipid panel; and EKG.
 2. Current lab tests will ensure that baseline data are available if and when psychotropic medication is prescribed.

B. Diagnostic screening is an effective method to identify and inform early interventions for perinatal depression. Integrate into prenatal and postpartum visits.

 1. The ACOG Committee on Obstetric Practice recommends that universal screening for depression and anxiety be done at least once during the perinatal period.
 2. Screen for SUDs at first visit and initiate any positive findings for referral to appropriate behavioral health practitioners if necessary.

C. The following screening tools provide clear guidelines for actions based on cut scores, as specified in the *DSM-5* (American Psychiatric Association, 2013). Be aware that screening tools do not confirm a full diagnosis.

 1. Edinburgh Postnatal Depression Scale (EPDS): The EPDS consists of only 10 items and is easy to administer. An EPDS depression screening score of 10 or higher is a positive screening for depression and indicates the patient may be experiencing a depressive illness of varying severity. Severity is based on the number of criterion symptoms, the severity of those symptoms, and the impact the symptoms are having on the patient's capacity to function in daily activities.
 2. Other screening instruments: Other screening instruments include the Patient Health Questionnaire-9 (PHQ-9), the Beck Depression Inventory, the Center for Epidemiologic Studies Depression Scale, and the Zung Self-Rating Depression Scale; however, the sensitivity and the specificity for perinatal depression are diminished and the number of items is greater.
 3. SUD screening: The Modified NIDA Quick Screen can screen for SUD.
 4. Sleep evaluation: Sleep is a modifiable risk factor for emotional distress that plays a pivotal role in postpartum adjustment. Given the potential negative implications of disrupted sleep in the perinatal period, interventions such as review of sleep hygiene and cognitive behavioral sleep interventions should be considered to address sleep problems during pregnancy.

D. Comprehensive decision tools: Decision aids enhance the impact of early identification, intervention, monitoring, and ▶

TABLE 12.3 EDINBURGH POSTNATAL DEPRESSION SCALE SCORING AND ACTION PLAN

EPDS Score	0–4 Points	5–9 Points	10–12 Points	13–20 Points
Interpretation of score	Negative for depression	Increased risk for depression	Mild to moderate depression	Moderate to severe depression
Treatment	None	Increased attention to self-care	Referral to mental health services for counseling with CBT or interpersonal therapy and consideration for medication management. Ancillary actions such as yoga, massage, and ongoing daily exercise under clinician's instructions	Referral to mental health services for counseling and medication management. If suicidal or psychotic, emergency admission if cannot be handled in home setting
Education	Perinatal depressive symptoms	Increased self-care with attention to specific issues related to reduction of stress, improved coping, increased social support, increased activity and improved sleep hygiene	Counseling for depression with CBT or interpersonal therapy and ways to improve mood; sleep evaluation; suicide evaluation and ongoing follow-up; discussion on use of psychopharmacology and risks and benefits	Work with partner or family member for course of action plan to hospitalize or manage in home setting; increase weekly contact with patient if at home with more frequent counseling sessions either in person or by telehealth until more stable
Screening and follow-up	Routine screening	Routine screening again during pregnancy	Follow-up weekly either for counseling or medication management	Follow-up on at least a twice-per-week basis if at home and ongoing intensive counseling with CBT or interpersonal therapy

CBT, cognitive behavioral therapy; EPDS, Edinburgh Postnatal Depression Scale.
Source: Latendresse, G., Elmore, C., & Deneris, A. (2017). Selective serotonin reuptake inhibitors as first-line antidepressant therapy for perinatal depression. *Journal of Midwifery Women's Health, 62*(3), 317–328. https://doi.org/10.1111/jmwh.12607.

follow-up, and should continue throughout the prenatal and postpartum period.
1. The Massachusetts Child Psychiatry Access Program (MCPAP) for Moms offers a free downloadable Obstetric Provider Toolkit (see "Resources"). This tool was created to assist perinatal (obstetric and pediatric) care providers in preventing, identifying, and treating perinatal mood, anxiety, and SUDs. The toolkit contains evidence-based point-of-care algorithms for intervention and follow-up care.
2. As with all diagnostic instruments, the NP should conduct a clinical assessment to ensure that the score is associated with the level of symptoms present.
3. Table 12.3 provides clear guidelines for actions based on the scores on the EPDS and the severity of MDD.

DIFFERENTIAL DIAGNOSIS

A. Changes in mood, appetite, activity, sleep, and cognition occur during pregnancy. Given the prevalence of mood and anxiety disorders occurring during young adulthood, experiencing these symptoms during pregnancy requires further evaluation. Anxiety normally co-occurs with depression and should be evaluated with depressive symptoms.

B. Conduct a comprehensive assessment for differential diagnosis.
1. Diagnostic screening and assessment along with exploration of the patient's psychosocial, family, and developmental history can reveal traumatic abuse, neglect, violence, or other events that may contribute to increased symptomatology.
2. Stigma around mental illness may hinder assessment, requiring trust to ensure a thorough evaluation and differentiation of anxiety and depression, adjustment disorders, sleep disorders, bipolar disorders, SUDs, posttraumatic stress disorders (PTSD), and psychotic disorders.
3. Medical differentials and co-occurring disorders such as medication side effects, infections, anemia, as well as thyroid, autoimmune, and chronic pain disorders can mimic psychiatric disorders.
4. Bipolar disorder should be screened using tools such as the Mood Disorder Questionnaire to identify manic and hypomanic episodes. A positive screen suggesting impairment warrants further investigation.
5. SUDs: Distinguishing between substance-induced symptoms and underlying psychiatric disorders should include substance use screening, physical examinations, laboratory tests, and collateral information from multiple sources. Differential diagnoses may include withdrawal syndromes, maternal mental health conditions, medical complications, and social factors.
6. A complete review of suicidal thinking and behaviors is critical during both perinatal and postnatal periods and should be a collaborative effort among healthcare providers.
7. Close collaboration between NPs, CNMs, obstetricians, psychiatrists, neonatologists, and social workers is crucial for accurate diagnosis and effective management, ensuring the well-being of both the mother and the fetus/infant.

PLAN

A. The following are the key concepts recommended by Reist et al. (2022), the American Psychiatric Association (n.d.), and Lewis et al. (2019).

    1. Standardized screening and diagnostic instruments inform plan for counseling, psychopharmacology, and other treatment options that may be prescribed during the perinatal period.

    2. Interdisciplinary collaboration between the NP, patient, obstetrician, and pediatrician is considered an evidence-based practice and ensures accurate differential diagnosis and treatment planning.

B. Once a comprehensive psychiatric assessment and evaluation are completed, the results are shared with the patient and the collaborative team.

    1. Safety plans must be instituted and a designated clinician who is responsible for the overall management of any suicidal thinking and behaviors over the course of the pregnancy and postpartum period must be ensured. Plans include suicide and/or intimate violence plans as needed.

    2. Decisions on psychotropic medication during pregnancy should involve the care team, the patient, and their partner in consideration of the patient's medication history and the safety for the fetus. Continuous assessment is necessary to monitor for symptom escalation if medication is declined.

    3. Plan for evidence-based behavioral interventions to treat the perinatal population (e.g., interpersonal therapy, CBT, or mindfulness-based cognitive therapy) should be discussed as a first option with the patient.

C. The collaborative team, including the patient, should be involved in decision-making on the use of psychotropic medication during pregnancy. If a patient decides not to take a medication with a moderate symptom profile, *ongoing* assessment for a worsening condition should be completed by a behavioral health clinician to ensure symptoms do not worsen.

    1. The collaborative team and the patient will need to be involved in decision-making on psychotropic medication. If the patient has a past history of taking psychotropic medication with good results, the medication should be considered first choice as long as it is identified as safe for the fetus.

GENERAL TREATMENTS AND INTERVENTIONS

A. The American Psychiatric Association and the ACOG both recommend that psychotherapy and antidepressant medication be utilized for first-line treatment of mild to moderate perinatal depression.

B. According to van Niel and Payne (2020), the use of individual psychotherapy can be effective in treating perinatal depression without medication. Other modalities include the following:

    1. Dialectical behavioral therapy (DBT), cognitive behavioral therapy (CBT), interpersonal psychotherapy (IPT), family-focused therapy, and support services to include the partner and family living at home

    2. Lifestyle modifications (e.g., sleep hygiene, stress management, mindfulness meditation, yoga, regular exercise, healthy diet)

C. Pharmacotherapy: Risk ratio should be discussed with the patient and the partner. For some patients, taking medication is more effective for the mother's health and the child's development than not taking medication.

COMMON MEDICATIONS

A. Perinatal depression has serious complications, especially if it is moderate to severe, including apathy, poor nutrition, poor compliance with prenatal care, lack of self-care, and increased alcohol and drug use. These complications often worsen, increasing risk of preterm birth, postpartum depression, bonding difficulties with the infant, and parenting challenges.

B. Placental passage of antidepressants varies greatly among individuals for each specific drug. There is not a consistent correlation between antidepressants with higher rates of placental transfer and those linked to perinatal antidepressant syndrome (PNAS).

C. Prescribers should be aware of the U.S. Food and Drug Administration's (FDA's) Pregnancy and Lactation Labeling Rule (PLLR). In 1975, the FDA provided guidelines to drug companies for labeling medications with regard to their safety during pregnancy.

    1. This system of classification used five risk categories (A, B, C, D, and X) based on data derived from human and animal studies, but was widely criticized due to being misleading.

    2. The FDA proposed a newly designed system on June 30, 2015. The PLLR abolishes the letter categories and instead includes a more comprehensive information in narrative form, discussing the potential risks and benefits to the mother and the fetus and how these risks may change during pregnancy and lactation.

    3. Companies are required to remove the pregnancy letter categories from the labeling for all prescription drugs and must now revise the labeling with updated information.

    4. Medications approved before June 30, 2001 are not yet covered by the PLLR.

D. The use of apps like ePocrates and NbN3 can facilitate rational prescribing for pregnant and lactating individuals and shared decision-making.

    1. According to the Guttmacher Institute (2019), 45% of all pregnancies are unplanned; therefore, when any woman of childbearing age is prescribed a psychotropic medication, the safety of the medication for possible pregnancy should be taken into consideration and discussed with the patient.

    2. Drugs that may increase pregnancy complications, neonatal complications, or neurodevelopmental problems should be weighed. According to Lusskin et al. (2018), for patients who are already on a medication, the decision will be guided by the individual and family history and by the reproductive safety data at the time of the review. Medication studies have produced discrepant results due to study methodology and failure to control for confounders. Decisions on which drug to prescribe are based on past history and current research findings.

    3. The following is a summary of the literature:

        a. Selective serotonin reuptake inhibitors (SSRIs) and their metabolites cross the placenta in the second and third trimesters.

        b. The greatest risk of teratogenicity is primarily during the first trimester, but this has not been validated by randomized controlled trials (RCTs).

        c. Fluoxetine is associated with a possible risk of craniosynostosis, ventricular septal defect, and cardiac malformations, but other database studies claimed no association.

        d. Sertraline may have potential association with anencephaly, omphalocele, limb reduction defects and ▶

anal atresia, and atrial septal defects, yet other database studies claimed no association.

  e. Paroxetine is more frequently associated with birth defects, including right ventricular outflow defects, when used in the first trimester. Overall risk is still low and findings are not conclusive.

  f. There is a small increase in the risk of cardiac malformations associated with intrauterine exposure to methylphenidate but not to amphetamines. This information is important when weighing the risks and benefits of alternative treatment strategies for ADHD in women of reproductive age and during early pregnancy.

4. Table 12.4 summarizes the medications, dosing, and specific considerations for use during the perinatal, postnatal, and breastfeeding time frames.

5. Patients are encouraged to enroll in the National Pregnancy Registry for Psychiatric Medications at 1-866-961-2388 or www.womensmentalhealth.org.

PATIENT TEACHING

A. The pregnant patient and their partner should be informed that the healthcare provider should be notified immediately of any changes occurring in the patient's mental state.

B. The risk of suicidal thinking and behaviors must be communicated during the perinatal and postnatal period.

C. The risk of maternal suicide and infanticide with the administration of an SSRI in particular needs to be discussed and an action plan in place.

D. The patient and their partner should be informed of the SSRI's side effects and adverse reactions, including serotonin syndrome and discontinuation syndrome in the mother as well as neonatal adaptation syndrome (NAS). The patient should be counseled on attending their scheduled appointments for monitoring of their medication and on attending their counseling sessions on a regular basis.

E. If attending counseling sessions is a burden, online meetings can be interspersed with in-person sessions.

F. Mothers and their partners should be counseled on what to expect in each trimester and deal with the fears and anxiety that come with parenthood.

G. Other resources should be made available to them to expand their insight and knowledge on how parenthood will impact them. Widely available, prenatal, childbirth, parenting, and lactation prep classes can be most valuable in learning what to expect and the social support and connections made.

FOLLOW-UP

A. Follow-up appointments involving shared decision-making provide opportunities for reinforcing healthy coping strategies, recognizing warning signs and identifying worsening symptoms, and reinforcing emergency plans as appropriate. These visits ensure that physical, emotional, psychological, and family and social health issues continue to be addressed and supported as the new family moves toward full integration of their new member.

B. Follow-up can improve long-term health outcomes for individuals and their children. Addressing these issues early and often, with referrals as needed, can prevent chronic mental health conditions, reduce the risk for the mother and the infant, and promote healthier family dynamics.

CONSULTATION AND REFERRALS

A. It is important for the NP to recognize the limits of their expertise and the scope of their practice, and not hesitate to seek consultation or refer patients when it is in the best interest of the patient's care. Multidisciplinary collaboration, especially with the patient's OB provider, yields the best outcome. Referral or consultation is warranted depending on the following:

  1. The severity of the symptoms (e.g., severe depression, psychosis or mania, suicidal or homicidal ideation)
  2. Lack or inadequate response to treatment
  3. Co-occurring disorders such as SUDs
  4. Bipolar disorder, schizophrenia, eating disorders, which may require specialized treatment
  5. Diagnostic uncertainty in complex cases or multiple comorbidities
  6. Anytime there are legal, ethical, or risk management issues
  7. Patient preference for second opinion or alternative approach
  8. High-risk populations such as maternal age, preexisting or current medical conditions, pregnancy complications, recurrent pregnancy loss, lifestyle factors, or fetal concerns
  9. Whenever the patient's need outpaces the NP's expertise

B. If in the best interest of the patient to promote maternal and child health, it is imperative that we harness the perinatal period and perinatal care setting as an opportunity to screen, diagnose, and treat depression.

INDIVIDUAL CONSIDERATIONS

A. No two pregnancies are alike, even within the same carrier. Because of the unique challenges, assessment, treatment plans, monitoring, and follow-up should be tailored to the needs, preferences, and unique circumstances of the individual and their family. Care that is holistic and flexible—and delivered within the framework of a collaborative team with the family as central—optimizes outcomes.

RESOURCES

A. Patients should be given pamphlets from various resources listed below and explained how to use the information. The following are excellent resources available online for use during and after pregnancy:

  1. World Health Organization. *Thinking Healthy: A Manual for Psychosocial Management of Perinatal Depression* (WHO generic field-trial version 1.0). Geneva, WHO, 2015.
  2. MotherToBaby provides up to date information on the risks of medications (not just psychiatric), chemicals, herbal products, illicit drugs, and diseases during pregnancy and while breastfeeding.
  3. The National Institutes of Health (NIH) LactMed database has information on chemicals and drugs that breastfeeding mothers may be exposed to, including levels and possible adverse effects on nursing infants.
  4. Massachusetts Child Psychiatry Access Program (MCPAP) for Moms. (2019). *Assessment and management of perinatal mood and anxiety disorders.* www.mcpapformoms.org/Docs/AdultProviderToolkit_2019.pdf.
  5. MGH Center for Women's Mental Health's Reproductive Psychiatry Resource and Information Center provides a range of current information including discussion of new research findings on women's mental health and how to inform clinical practice.
  6. Download a copy of the EPDS online at www.cope.org.au/wp-content/uploads/2018/02/EPDS-Questionnaire.pdf.

TABLE 12.4 MEDICATIONS FOR PERINATAL DEPRESSION

Generic Name	Brand Name	Dosage Range	Notes
SSRIs			Implications for perinatal and postnatal period; risk of ASD with SSRIs is controversial; exposure to SSRIs may be associated with other developmental outcomes such as language, growth, and motor development
Sertraline	Zoloft	50–200 mg and increase by 25 or 50 mg; for very anxious patients increase by 12.5 mg	Due to half-life, small amounts are found in breastmilk (Kimmel et al., 2018); serotonin syndrome after completion of breastfeeding
Fluoxetine	Prozac	20–80 mg; can increase by 10 to 20 mg	Longer half-life; greater amounts in breastmilk; adverse effects possible; some case reports of colic, fussiness, drowsiness, poor suck reflex, sedation, and hypotonia
Citalopram	Celexa	20–40 mg increase by 10 or 20 mg	U.S. Food and Drug Administration Drug Safety Communication that greater than 40 mg can result in a life-threatening heart arrhythmia; some case reports of newborn drowsiness, fussiness, poor suck reflex, hypertonia, and hypotonia
Escitalopram	Lexapro	10–20 mg and increase by 5 or 10 mg	Some case reports of newborn somnolence, decreased feeding, and weight loss
Paroxetine	Paxil, Brisdelle	10–60 mg; increase by 10 or 20 mg	Data demonstrated an increase in cardiovascular malformation in infants, leading to a 2005 warning; case reports of irritability and feeding problems
Fluvoxamine	Luvox	25–150 mg increase by 25 mg	Used for treatment of obsessive-compulsive disorder
SNRIs			
Venlafaxine	Effexor, Effexor XR	37.5–375.0 mg; can increase by 37.5 mg	Older and more data available; cardiac anomalies
Duloxetine	Cymbalta	20–120 mg; can increase by 20 mg	
Milnacipran	Savella	100 mg twice a day; can increase by 12.5, 25, and 50 mg	No studies currently available on use during pregnancy
Bupropion	Wellbutrin SR, Wellbutrin XL, Zyban	150–450 mg; can increase by 150 mg; SR twice a day dosing	Cannot exceed 450 mg owing to increased risk of seizure in those with seizure disorder or those with a purging behavior; can be used for smoking cessation; can be helpful with ADHD; cardiac defects such as ventricular septal defect
Mirtazapine	Remeron	15–45 mg; can increase by 7.5 and 15 mg	Antiemetic effects in addition to antidepressant and antianxiety effects; can improve sleep at lower dosages
Mood stabilizers			
Lamotrigine	Lamictal	Can start at 25 mg and increase by 25 mg every 2 weeks	Need close monitoring for Stevens–Johnson Syndrome; not associated with increased risk of congenital malformations
Lithium		Can be increased by 150 mg, 300 mg; therapeutic blood levels 0.4–0.8 for depression; augmentation 0.8–1.2 for mood stabilization	Associated with cardiac malformations and must be weighed against risk of the illness itself
Atypical antipsychotics	Ability, Seroquel, Zyprexa, Risperdal, Geodon, Latuda, Invega		

ADHD, attention deficit hyperactivity disorder; ASD, autism spectrum disorder; SNRI, serotonin and norepinephrine reuptake inhibitor; SSRI, selective serotonin reuptake inhibitor.

7. Local chapters of Postpartum Support International offers support including a patient warm lines, peer support groups, and referral resources (website: www.postpartum.net; phone: 1-800-944-4773).

REFERENCES AND BIBLIOGRAPHY

American Psychiatric Association. (n.d.). *Learn about the collaborative care model.* https://www.psychiatry.org/psychiatrists/practice/professional-interests/integrated-care/learn

American Psychiatric Association. (2013). *Diagnostic and statistical manual of mental disorders* (5th ed.). https://doi.org/10.1176/appi.books.9780890425596

American Psychiatric Association. (2020, December). *Position statement on screening and treatment of mood and anxiety disorders during pregnancy and postpartum.* https://www.psychiatry.org/File%20Library/About-APA/Organization-Documents-Policies/Policies/Position-Pregnancy-Postpartum-Mood-Anxiety-Disorders.pdf

American Psychiatric Association. (2022a). *Desk reference to the diagnostic criteria from DSM-5-TR.* American Psychiatric Association Publishing.

American Psychiatric Association. (2022b). *Diagnostic and statistical manual of mental disorders* (5th ed., text rev.). https://doi.org/10.1176/appi.books.9780890425787

Badr, L. K., Ayvazian, N., Lameh, S., & Charafeddine, L. (2018). Is the effect of postpartum depression on mother-infant bonding universal? *Infant Behavior & Development, 51,* 15–23. https://doi.org/10.1016/j.infbeh.2018.02.003

Byatt, N., Levin, L. L., Ziedonis, D., Moore Simas, T. A., & Allison, J. (2015). Enhancing participation in depression care in outpatient perinatal care settings: A systematic review. *Obstetrics and Gynecology, 126*(5), 1048–1058. https://doi.org/10.1097/AOG.0000000000001067

Ewing, G., Tatarchuk, Y., Appleby, D., Schwartz, N., & Kim, D. (2015). Placental transfer of antidepressant medications: Implications for postnatal adaptation syndrome. *Clinical Pharmacokinetics, 54*(4), 359–370. https://doi.org/10.1007/s40262-014-0233-3

Fairbrother, N., Janssen, P., Antony, M. M., Tucker, E., & Young, A. H. (2016). Perinatal anxiety disorder prevalence and incidence. *Journal of Affective Disorders, 200,* 148–155. https://doi.org/10.1016/j.jad.2015.12.082

Fawcett, E. J., Fairbrother, N., Cox, M. L., White, I. R., & Fawcett, J. M. (2019). The prevalence of anxiety disorders during pregnancy and the postpartum period: A multivariate bayesian meta-analysis. *The Journal of Clinical Psychiatry, 80*(4). Article 18r12527. https://doi.org/10.4088/jcp.18r12527

Friedman, S. H., & Sorrentino, R. (2012). Commentary: Postpartum psychosis, infanticide, and insanity—implications for forensic psychiatry. *Journal of the American Academy of Psychiatry and the Law, 40*(3), 326–332. https://jaapl.org/content/40/3/326

Furman, D., Campisi, J., Verdin, E., Carrera-Bastos, P., Targ, S., Franceschi, C., Ferrucci, L., Gilroy, D. W., Fasano, A., Miller, G. W., Miller, A. H., Mantovani, A., Weyand, C. M., Barzilai, N., Goronzy, J. J., Rando, T. A., Effros, R. B., Lucia, A., Kleinstreuer, N., & Slavich, G. M. (2019). Chronic inflammation in the etiology of disease across the life span. *Nature Medicine, 25,* 1822–1832. https://doi.org/10.1038/s41591-019-0675-0

Guintivano, J., Manuck, T., & Meltzer-Brody, S. (2018). Predictors of postpartum depression: A comprehensive review of the last decade of evidence. *Clinical Obstetrics and Gynecology, 61*(3), 591–603. https://doi.org/10.1097/GRF.0000000000000368

Guttmacher Institute. (2019, January). *Unintended pregnancy in the United States.* https://www.guttmacher.org/fact-sheet/unintended-pregnancy-united-states

Han, V. X., Patel, S., Jones, H. F., Nielsen, T. C., Mohammad, S. S., Hofer, M. J., Gold, W., Brilot, F., Lain, S. J., Nassar, N., & Dale, R. C. (2021). Maternal acute and chronic inflammation in pregnancy is associated with common neurodevelopmental disorders: A systematic review. *Translational Psychiatry, 11,* Article 71, 1–12. https://doi.org/10.1038/s41398-021-01198-w

Huybrechts, K. F., Bröms, G., Christensen, L. B., Einarsdóttir, K., Engeland, A., Furu, K., Gissler, M., Hernandez-Diaz, S., Karlsson, P., Karlstad, Ø., Kieler, H., Lahesmaa-Korpinen, A. M., Mogun, H., Nørgaard, M., Reutfors, J., Sørensen, H. T., Zoega, H., & Bateman, B. T. (2018). Association between methylphenidate and amphetamine use in pregnancy and risk of congenital malformations: A cohort study from the international pregnancy safety study consortium. *JAMA Psychiatry, 75*(2), 167–175. https://doi.org/10.1001/jamapsychiatry.2017.3644

Kimmel, M. C., Cox, E., Schiller, C., Gettes, E., & Meltzer-Brody, S. (2018). Pharmacologic treatment of perinatal depression. *Obstetrics Gynecology Clinics of North America, 45*(3), 419–440. https://doi.org/10.1016/j.ogc2018.04.007

Lee, C. H., & Giuliani, F. (2019). The role of inflammation in depression and fatigue. *Frontiers in Immunology, 10,* 1696. https://doi.org/10.3389/fimmu.2019.01696

Lewis, C. C., Boyd, M., Puspitasari, A., Navarro, E., Howard, J., Kassab, H., Hoffman, M., Scott, K., Lyon, A., Douglas, S., Simon, G., & Kroenke, K. (2019). Implementing measurement-based care in behavioral health: A review. *JAMA Psychiatry, 76*(3), 324–335. https://doi.org/10.1001/jamapsychiatry.2018.3329

Lim, G. (2021). Perinatal depression. *Current Opinion in Anesthesiology, 34*(3), 233–237. https://doi.org/10.1097/ACO.0000000000000998

Lusskin, S. I., Khan, S. J., Ernst, C., Habib, S., Fersh, M. E. & Albertini, E. S. (2018). Pharmacotherapy for perinatal depression. *Clinical Obstetrics and Gynecology, 61*(3), 544–561. https://doi.org/10.1097/GRF.0000000000000365

Meltzer-Brody, S. (2011) New insights into perinatal depression: Pathogenesis and treatment during pregnancy and postpartum. *Dialogues in Clinical Neuroscience, 13*(1), 89–100. https://doi.org/10.31887/DCNS.2011.13.1/smbrody

Meltzer-Brody, S., Larsen, J. T., Petersen, L., Guintivano, J., Di Florio, A., Miller, W. C., Sullivan, P. F., & Munk-Olsen, T. (2018). Adverse life events increase risk for postpartum psychiatric episodes: A population-based epidemiologic study. *Depression and Anxiety, 35*(2), 160–167. https://doi.org/10.1002/da.22697

Pao, C., Guintivano, J., Santos, H., & Meltzer-Brody, S. (2019). Postpartum depression and social support in a racially and ethnically diverse population of women. *Archives of Women's Mental Health, 22*(1), 105–114. https://doi.org/10.1007/s00737-018-0882-6

Payne, J. L. (2017, June). Psychopharmacology in pregnancy and breastfeeding. *Psychiatric Clinics of North America, 40*(2), 217–238. https://doi.org/10.1016/j.psc.2017.01.001

Reist, C., Petiwala, I., Latimer, J., Raffaelli, S. B., Chiang, M., Eisenberg, D., & Campbell, S. (2022, December 30). Collaborative mental health care: A narrative review. *Medicine, 101*(52), Article e32554. https://doi.org/10.1097/MD.0000000000032554

Samara, M. T., Levine, S. Z., & Leucht, S. (2023). Linkage of young mania rating scale to clinical global impression scale to enhance utility in clinical practice and research trials. *Pharmacopsychiatry, 56*(1), 18–24. https://doi.org/10.1055/a-1841-6672

Van Niel, M. S., & Payne, J. L. (2020). Perinatal depression: A review. *Cleveland Clinic Journal of Medicine, 87*(5), 273–277. https://doi.org/10.3949/ccjm.87a.19054

van Heyningen, T., Honikman, S., Tomlinson, M., Field, S., & Myer, L. (2018). Comparison of mental health screening tools for detecting antenatal depression and anxiety disorders in South African women. *PLoS ONE, 13*(4), e0193697. https://doi.org/10.1371/journal.pone.0193697

Yonkers, K. A., Ramin, S. M., Rush, A. J., Navarrete, C. A., Carmody, T., March, D., Heartwell, S. F., & Leveno, K. J. (2001). Onset and persistence of postpartum depression in an inner-city maternal health clinic system. *The American Journal of Psychiatry, 158*(11), 1856–1863. https://doi.org/10.1176/appi.ajp.158.11.1856

Yonkers, K. A., Wisner, K. L., Stewart, D. E., Oberlander, T. F., Dell, D. L., Stotland, N., Ramin, S., Chaudron, L., & Lockwood, C. (2009). The management of depression during pregnancy: A report from the American Psychiatric Association and the American College of Obstetricians and Gynecologists. *Obstetrics and Gynecology, 114*(3), 703–713. https://doi.org/10.1097/AOG.0b013e3181ba0632

Zayas, L. H., Cunningham, M., McKee, M. D., & Jankowski, K. R. B. (2002). Depression and negative life events among pregnant African-American and Hispanic women. *Womens' Health Issues, 12*(1), 16–22. https://doi.org/10.1016/s1049-3867(01)00138.4

POSTPARTUM DEPRESSION

The delivery of the baby is usually a joyful event for the mother. If the mother is experiencing any depressed symptoms prior to delivery, the symptoms can exacerbate and lead to postpartum depression. Unfortunately, postpartum depression is underdiagnosed and undertreated, leading to negative outcomes for the mother, the baby, and the family system. As noted in the "Perinatal Mood Disorders" section, patients in the childbearing period are at higher risk of depression and may already be depressed at the time of conception.

DEFINITION

A. Postpartum depression (PPD) is a type of mood disorder associated with childbirth that can affect both sexes. Typically, it affects mothers within the postpartum period (the first 12 months after giving birth), although it can start earlier—during pregnancy or just following childbirth. The American Psychiatric Association specifies that PPD is a type of major depressive disorder that begins during the peripartum period (pregnancy through the 4 weeks after giving birth; American Psychiatric Association, 2013).

INCIDENCE

A. PPD most commonly occurs within 6 weeks after childbirth. It occurs in about 6.5% to 20% of women, more commonly in adolescent females, mothers who deliver premature infants, and women living in urban areas. African American and Hispanic mothers reported the onset of symptoms within 2 weeks of delivery, unlike White mothers, who reported the onset of symptoms later, according to one study.
B. In a predominately Latinx sample, one in five mothers (20.4%) screened positive for depressive symptoms.
C. The prevalence and incidence are considered underestimated due to differences in screening measures, socioeconomic status, cultural norms, social support, and perceptions of mental health and associated stigma.
D. The rate of PPD is as high as 40% in the early postpartum period among patients with premature infants. Sustained depression during pregnancy is associated with small-for-gestational age, lower birth weight, ongoing infant illness/disability, and perceived lack of social support.
E. Paternal PPD is also a major issue that needs to be addressed, with an incidence ranging from 4% to 25% in community samples.
   1. A strong predictor of paternal postpartum depression is maternal postpartum depression.
   2. Risk factors for fathers are a family history of depression, poverty, and hormonal changes.
   3. Fathers may present with symptoms such as irritability, withdrawal, and depressed mood.

PATHOGENESIS

A. The pathogenesis of postpartum depression is currently unknown. It has been hypothesized that genetics, hormonal, psychological, and social life stressors play a role in its development. The interrelationship between stress, environment, neurotransmitters, neuroendocrine, and inflammation is posited in the pathogenesis of depression in the postpartum period. Further research is still needed to fully uncover the underlying mechanisms of action.
   1. Allostatic load
      a. Allostatic load measures the cumulative impact of chronic stress and is associated with adverse health outcomes. In a study by Adynski et al. (2019), interpersonal violence was a statistically significant risk factor for stress, depression, and anxiety symptoms over the first year postpartum. Furthermore, using SDOH and allostatic load score, significant risk factors included low-income level, nativity, and perceived food security.
      b. Receiving food stamps was a significant protective factor for stress symptoms.
   2. Hormones
      a. Reproductive hormones are important in altering emotional processing, arousal, cognition, and motivation, and regulate thyroid function, lactating hormones (oxytocin), the immune system, the HPA axis, and genetic expression.
      b. The pathogenesis of PPD is similar to perinatal depression; however, because there is a precipitous drop in reproductive hormones immediately after delivery, it has been postulated that concentration changes can account for the affective dysregulation, especially among those with genetic susceptibility.
      c. The brain is impacted by metabolites of steroid hormones known as *neuroactive steroids*. The neuroactive metabolite of progesterone, allopregnanolone (ALLO), exerts anxiolytic and antidepressant effects that are thought to be mediated, at least in part, by the ability to potentiate $GABA_A$ receptors. These neuroactive steroids are postulated to reduce the risk of depression.
   3. Neurotransmitters
      a. GABA is noted to play an inverse role with depressive symptoms in the postpartum period. GABA is a major inhibitory neurotransmitter in the brain.
      b. Serotonin is associated with reduced depressive symptoms, and dopamine in animal studies is associated with improved maternal behavior and reduced depressed behaviors.
      c. Glutamate, an excitatory neurotransmitter, is noted to increase depressive symptoms in animal studies.
   4. Inflammation
      a. Conflicting and limited numbers of reports on inflammatory changes associated with PPD make it difficult to determine whether there is a role for neuroinflammation in the underlying neurobiology of postpartum depression.
   5. Environmental factors
      a. Environmental factors, such as adverse life events, have a role in the development of PPD.
B. Other areas associated with PPD include sudden decrease in β-endorphin levels postdelivery, low omega-3 levels, and lower vitamin D levels, but have yet to be fully researched.

PREDISPOSING FACTORS

A. The two strongest risk factors for PPD are prenatal depression and current abuse.
B. Additional common risk factors include unfavorable SDOH factors, high life stress, lack of social support, current or past abuse, prior depression, marital or partner dissatisfaction, adverse life events during pregnancy such as marital conflict, immigration issues, lack of social support, employment issues, and limited financial support.
C. Being a first-time mother, along with very young or old maternal age, complications of pregnancy for the mother, and newborn health issues contribute to the anxiety and worry associated with health problems. Admission to the NICU can trigger postpartum depression in both the mother and the father. Research has identified that 40% to 45% of mothers and fathers who were screened were positive for depression and anxiety.

COMMON COMPLAINTS

A. The baby blues can cross over to PPD in mothers after delivery. Normal baby blues can include episodic sadness, ▶

BOX 12.3 COMMON COMPLAINTS IN POSTPARTUM DEPRESSION

Compulsive behaviors
Feelings of hopelessness and worthlessness, or sadness
Feeling overwhelmed
Intrusive thoughts
Isolation of self
Maladaptive behaviors in caring for the infant (attend well-baby clinic, place infant on back to sleep)
Mood lability
Problems with bonding with and caring for infant
Sadness with ongoing tearfulness
Problems with self-care
Sleeping issues

feelings of being overwhelmed, and crying, and are usually limited to 2 weeks after delivery.

B. In contrast, PPD is intense and pervasive in the overall maternal functioning. Major depressive disorder criteria based on the *DSM-5* (American Psychiatric Association, 2013) are found in the "Perinatal Mood Disorders" section. Some signs of postpartum depression are included in Box 12.3. They may include anhedonia, change in eating pattern, sleep disturbances, persistent worry and anxiety, sense of worthlessness, self-blame, irritability, agitation, mood swings, sadness, crying bouts, feeling worthless, or guilty.

OTHER SIGNS AND SYMPTOMS

A. Signs and symptoms include racing, scary thoughts; fear of being left alone with the baby; misery; disinterest in the baby, family, and friends; and difficulty with memory, concentrating, or decision-making. Worsening or severe symptoms and thoughts of self-harm or harming the baby indicate an urgent need for immediate evaluation and intervention.

SUBJECTIVE DATA

A. Suicide is the leading cause of death in postnatal women, and 3% of postnatal women have suicidal ideation. Women with PPD may be significantly depressed and have impaired functioning associated with inability to care for self and the infant. When asked about the baby, they may respond with a lack of interest in the newborn and their care. There may also be feelings of obsessive thoughts over the neonate.

PHYSICAL EXAMINATION

A. Physical examination should be conducted postpartum by the OB provider. In addition to vitals, review of systems, and follow-up on pregnancy complications, contraception and sexual health should be addressed. It is important to note physical symptoms that may be associated with dysphoria, such as disordered sleep apart from the baby's schedule, not feeling rested, fatigue, pain from delivery or cesarean section, back pain, changes in appetite, and other somatic symptoms such as GI symptoms that do not have clear medical cause. This may indicate that the mother may be unable to share their depressed and fearful feelings.

DIAGNOSTIC TESTS AND SCREENING

A. Testing and screening for PPD utilizes many of the same tools as in perinatal screening. Use of the EPDS is considered the gold standard for brief screening. Utilizing comprehensive algorithms and decision tools such as the MCPAP is optimal with a complete psychiatric evaluation.

B. It has been noted that in a large-scale screen for depression, 22.6% of screen-positive women had bipolar disorder. The Mood Disorder Questionnaire is an important screening tool during the postpartum period.

DIFFERENTIAL DIAGNOSIS

A. It is important to rule out postpartum psychosis and bipolar disorder.

   1. The incidence of first-lifetime postpartum psychosis from population-based psychiatric admissions can range from 0.25 to 0.6 per 1,000 births.

      a. Postpartum psychosis is considered a psychiatric emergency and requires immediate psychiatric evaluation.
      b. Symptoms of postpartum psychosis include insomnia, mood changes, and irritability, and can be accompanied by mania, depression, or a mixed state.
      c. It is associated with delirium-like appearance, with cognitive symptoms such as hallucinations, delusions, disorientation, confusion, derealization, and depersonalization.
      d. Delusions of altruistic homicide (often associated with maternal suicide) to "save them both from a fate worse than death" may occur and are an important exploration within the clinical psychiatric examination.
      e. Postpartum psychosis is associated with an increased risk of both suicide and infanticide.

   2. The postpartum period is also a high-risk period for relapse among patients with ongoing psychiatric illness, in particular bipolar disorder.

      a. Pregnant patients with bipolar disorder are more likely to experience a puerperal psychiatric admission compared with women with other psychiatric diagnoses.
      b. Bipolar disorder during pregnancy can occur when medication is tapered. There is consistent literature that associates bipolar disorder and postpartum psychosis with circadian rhythm disruption due to severe sleep deprivation that can develop predelivery or in the postpartum period.

B. Psychiatric problems should be screened, but medical problems should also be explored as possible underlying causes of psychosis (e.g., infections such as mastitis, endometritis, cystitis, perinatal blood loss, substance use withdrawal, and endocrine and autoimmune diseases).

   1. Thyroid autoimmune problems (e.g., hypoparathyroidism) should be explored.

   2. Anti-N-methyl-D-aspartate receptor (NMDAR) encephalitis is a relatively common autoimmune encephalitis characterized by complex neuropsychiatric features and the presence of immunoglobulin G (IgG) antibodies against the NMDA receptors in the central nervous system (CNS). It is the best known and likely the most common type of immune-mediated limbic encephalitis. Variable positive and negative psychiatric symptoms, such as visual or auditory hallucination, acute schizoaffective episodes, depression, mania, and addictive or eating disorders, can appear rapidly within days to weeks in these patients with no prior psychiatric diagnosis. The onset occurs fairly quickly in contrast to the slow progression noted in primary psychiatric diseases.

   3. Metabolism alterations such as late-onset inborn errors of metabolism can cause postpartum psychosis.

BOX 12.4 POSTPARTUM PSYCHOSIS SYMPTOMS

Agitation
Apathy or disconnect from one's baby and other things one cares about
Bursts of energy or heightened sex drive
Delusions
Feeling confused or disoriented
Hallucinations
Insomnia
Irritability
Paranoia or feeling suspicious
Sudden shifts in moods (sometimes similar to bipolar disorder)
Thoughts and/or attempts to harm oneself or one's baby

Postpartum Depression Versus Postpartum Psychosis

A. PPD symptoms should meet most of the criteria for a major depressive disorder but with a few caveats.
   1. Timing of onset: It occurs in the postpartum period and may extend to the first year after delivery, but may begin during pregnancy.
   2. Context and triggers: PPD is associated with physical, hormonal, and emotional changes that accompany pregnancy and childbirth.
   3. Symptoms: Symptoms may include intense worries about the baby, apathy toward the baby, and difficulties in bonding.

B. Postpartum mood episodes with psychotic features appear to occur more commonly in primiparous women and those with a prior postpartum mood episode. Postpartum patients who have a prior history of depressive or bipolar disorder and those with family history of bipolar disorder have higher risk for postpartum psychosis.
   1. The incidence of first-time onset of postpartum psychosis from studies of psychiatric admissions can vary from 0.25 to 0.6 per 1,000 births.
   2. The relative risk for a first onset of affective psychosis is 23 times greater in the 4 weeks after delivery compared with any other time in a woman's life.
   3. The onset is between 3 and 10 days after birth.

C. Just like the baby blues and PPD, the symptoms of postpartum psychosis typically begin within the first few days to the first few weeks after birth (Box 12.4).

Postpartum Anxiety

A. Because depression and anxiety frequently co-occur, assessment for postpartum anxiety is important (Box 12.5). Becoming a new parent is accompanied by normal worry. Feelings of being overwhelmed can be present but not on an ongoing basis. In addition to postpartum anxiety,

BOX 12.5 SIGNS AND SYMPTOMS OF POSTPARTUM ANXIETY

Constant fear or worry that cannot be eased
Feelings of numbness and tingling
Feelings of impending doom or fearing terrible things are going to happen to you or your baby
Heart palpitations
Hyperventilation/shortness of breath
Panic attacks
Racing thoughts
Shaking or trembling

obsessive-compulsive disorder or posttraumatic stress disorder should be assessed. Screening instruments that are available are the Zung Self-Rating Anxiety Scale or the General Anxiety Disorder Scale (GAD) and Primary Care PTSD Screen for *DSM-5* (PC-PTSD-5). Further clinical interview can determine if the patient meets the criteria for these disorders.

B. New mothers and their partners should be reassured that the feelings are transitory; however, if they persist or seriously impact normal functioning, further assessment is necessary.

PLAN

A. A comprehensive and multidisciplinary team approach is advised for effective overall management for the seriousness and immediacy of postpartum depression and psychosis.
B. For PPD without psychosis, both psychiatric and psychosocial interventions will be necessary.
C. Both pharmacologic and counseling should be integrated into the treatment action plan.
D. The overall goal in postpartum psychosis is twofold: reduce psychotic and other psychiatric symptoms, and support the mother's self-esteem and confidence in mothering, improve social and family functioning, and ensure infant health and emotional development.
E. Psychiatric hospitalization will be necessary for evaluation, safety assessment, and treatment.
F. The NP must ensure that family members are engaged in treatment, especially given the seriousness of potential harm to the mother and the baby.
G. The use of lithium is the first drug of choice and should have a target blood level of 0.6 to 0.8 for the first 6 to 9 months. Patient education is vital.
H. Electroconvulsive therapy (ECT) can be considered with catatonic features if necessary.
I. Avoid use of any antidepressant for PPD with psychotic features due to the risk of increasing mood lability.
J. Psychosocial factors can interact to increase the symptoms of PPD. In a study of Latinx women, over one-third (36.7%) reported one or more psychosocial issues during the perinatal period and postnatal period. Screening for multiple risk factors rather than just one can help clinicians tailor interventions for the successful management of psychosocial issues such as lack of social support, interpersonal violence, substance use, socioeconomic issues such as financial problems for formula, or not having the home prepared for the baby, which may contribute to depressed mood.
K. The use of a visiting nurse can be a tremendous resource and should be recommended.

GENERAL TREATMENTS AND INTERVENTIONS

A. There are numerous psychological interventions for PPD available. Many postpartum patients prefer psychological to pharmacologic interventions, but in more moderate to severe cases the use of both is warranted. Interventions for PPD include CBT, interpersonal therapy (IPT), behavioral activation (BA; or aerobic exercise), and internet-based CBT. In addition, literature indicates that CBT is effective in the treatment of PPD.
B. For CBT, a focus on the dysfunctional patterns of cognition with the postpartum mother to identify, evaluate and modify these belief patterns is key. The focus is varied from working on becoming a new mother, parenting skills, their thoughts and relationship with the new infant, and getting the social support they need to carry out their new role.
C. Interpersonal therapy has strong evidence as an effective intervention for PPD.

1. The underlying theory focuses on three areas: loss, role dispute, or in the case of PPD a role transition.
2. Therapy is time-limited to about 12 sessions and addresses the mother's ability to assert their needs and wishes in interpersonal encounters, validate their feelings of being overwhelmed in their new role, support the expression of their fears and anxieties, and encourage taking appropriate control.
3. Part of this process requires effectively coping with changes to the new marital dynamics and family issues.

D. Internet-based interventions can include methods to increase activity, improve coping skills, cognitive restructuring, problem-solving skills, and assertiveness training skills. Issues such as sleep hygiene for both the mother and the baby can significantly improve depression symptoms with improved sleep patterns. It is vital to assess sleep quality in new mothers and provide interventions or support as needed. This can include education on sleep hygiene, strategies for sharing nighttime infant care responsibilities, and when necessary clinical interventions to address more severe sleep disturbances. Recognizing and addressing sleep issues is a crucial step in both the prevention and treatment of PPD.

E. A self-help program, MumMoodBooster, has 12 modules and has been found to be effective.
1. The results demonstrated that self-help CBT and BA were more effective for PPD, relative to control conditions. A systematic review of the effectiveness of CBT in treating and preventing perinatal depression reported an overall effect size of 0.65 (95% CI 0.54 to 0.76, $p < .001$), indicating that participants who received CBT exhibited significantly greater reductions in depressive symptoms relative to those observed in control conditions.

F. Light- to moderate-intensity aerobic exercise improves mild to moderate depressive symptoms and increases the likelihood that mild to moderate depression will resolve.

G. Fathers' involvement in the care of their newborns in the NICU was significantly associated with fewer symptoms of PPD among mothers. Targeted interventions to promote fathers' involvement in the NICU can mitigate the symptoms of PPD among mothers of newborns in the NICU.

COMMON MEDICATIONS

A. Pharmacologic interventions are commonly used and can be particularly advantageous over psychological interventions, especially for patients who have not responded to psychological treatments and those with more severe symptoms or suicidal tendencies. Selective serotonin reuptake inhibitors (SSRIs) are first-line medications. SSRIs are outlined in the "Perinatal Mood Disorders" section, but in the postpartum period breastfeeding is an important consideration for medication management. The risk to the infant is based on the following areas:
1. Medications taken by the mother are metabolized in an immature liver of the infant.
2. Preterm or premature infants have immature hydration and immature renal function.
3. The half-life of the antidepressant medication can impact drug levels in the infant; use of sertraline is recommended due to short half-life.
4. All SSRIs pass in small amounts into the breastmilk, with rare instances of adverse events in healthy full-term infants.
5. Bupropion should be avoided due to case reports of infant seizures.
6. Tricyclic antidepressants are to be avoided due to greater entry to breastmilk.

B. A new intervention, brexanolone, an intravenous form of allopregnanolone, a positive allosteric modulator of GABA receptor, is found to have a significant and meaningful reduction in depression scores in women treated with the drug postpartum. The side effects to date are minor dizziness and somnolence. It has been noted that it requires a 60-hour infusion in a hospital setting.

Medications for Postpartum Psychosis

A. The overall treatment goals are to promote sleep, target psychosis, and stabilize mood.
B. Medications are selected to address these three areas:
1. Short-term benzodiazepines
2. Antipsychotics
3. Lithium
    a. Lithium is noted to be an effective monotherapy for postpartum psychosis and maintenance treatment.
    b. Postpartum lithium exposure was not associated with any of the predefined pregnancy complications or delivery outcomes.
    c. Lithium exposure during the first trimester was associated with an increased risk of major malformations.
    d. An increased risk for neonatal readmission within 28 days of birth was seen in the lithium-exposed group compared with the reference group.

PATIENT TEACHING

A. Postpartum education for postpartum depression or anxiety should include treatment options, and if the depression or anxiety is serious enough to impact overall functioning, collaboration with the healthcare team, including the pediatrician, is warranted.
B. An in-depth discussion on the use of psychotropic medication is necessary, and mothers and partners should be given a written handout or the site for their education on the impact of medications on their breastfeeding infant.
C. Sleep hygiene for the mother and the father is vitally important. Equally important is helping the mother with the sleep habits of their infant.
D. The pediatrician should be involved in effective collaborative care to improve outcomes.
E. There are important adjustments that the mother needs to be informed about. These should include how to deal with the lack of sleep, fatigue associated with PPD, and change in the relationship with their partner.
F. Mothers need support and guidance on how to deal with their own self-care, work responsibilities, and clinical mood changes. Mothers who have an infant admitted to the NICU will need the support and counseling to cope with this scary and frightening event. These areas should be addressed during the counseling process. Family members should be included to assist the mother in the care of themselves and their infant, relieving the mother of duties to sleep, and to understand what to look for should the mother's symptoms of depression or mania become worse.
G. Additional interventions can be discussed for improving depression symptoms, such as meditation, relaxation techniques, movement, massage therapy, and eye movement desensitization and reprocessing (EMDR) therapy, which can be used to treat psychological trauma. ECT is an option for PPD in specific, severe cases, including rapid deterioration or extreme symptoms or high risk of suicide.

BOX 12.6 PARTNER ISSUES ASSOCIATED WITH A NEW BABY IN THE HOME

A change in relationship between the two parents; lack of intimacy and/or attention
A new baby to help care for
Complete disruption of the past environment
Difficulty in forming a bond or attachment with the new baby
Feelings of being unsure how to help, especially if their partner is breastfeeding
Feelings of financial pressure
"Loss" of a portion of their partner as they also become a new parent

H. For the partner, it is also a difficult time and they may struggle as well (Box 12.6).

FOLLOW-UP

A. Ongoing assessment is recommended especially for at-risk patients, as well as monitoring for change in mental status as often as needed. Follow-up with the mother and their partner is critical so as to stay current with the status of the mother's symptoms and progress during treatment.

CONSULTATION AND REFERRALS

A. Consultation and referral for psychiatric services must be considered a high priority for the NP due to the associated complications that can occur during the postnatal period.
B. Follow-up should also include the OB/CNM and pediatrician to ensure that they are observing and reporting any negative changes.

RESOURCES

Please see "Resources" in the "Perinatal Mood Disorders" section.

A. MumMoodBooster, online cognitive behavioral therapy for women with postnatal depression, is available here: www.mummoodbooster.com/public
B. PC-PTSD-5 scale: This measure was developed by staff at the U.S. Department of Veterans Affairs' National Center for PTSD and is in the public domain and not copyrighted (Prins et al., 2015). Download the PC-PTSD-5 here: www.ptsd.va.gov/professional/assessment/screens/pc-ptsd.asp

REFERENCES AND BIBLIOGRAPHY

Adynski, H., Zimmer, C., Thorp Jr, J., & Santos Jr, H. P. (2019). Predictors of psychological distress in low-income mothers over the first postpartum year. *Research in Nursing & Health*, 42(3), 205–216. https://doi.org/10.1002/nur.21943

American Psychiatric Association. (2013). *Diagnostic and statistical manual of mental disorders* (5th ed.). https://doi.org/10.1176/appi.books.9780890425596

Berkink, V., Rasgon, N., & Wisner, K. L. (2016). Postpartum psychosis: Madness, mania, and melancholia in motherhood. *The American Journal of Psychiatry*, 173(12), 1179–1188. https://doi.org/10.1176/appi.ajp.2016.16040454

Berkink, V., Burgerhout, K. M., Koorengevel, K. M., Kamperman, A. M., Hoogendijk, W. J., Lambregtse-van den Berg, M. P., & Kushner, S. A. (2015). Treatment of psychosis and mania in the postpartum period. *The American Journal of Psychiatry*, 172(2), 115–123. https://doi.org/10.1176/appi.ajp.2014.13121652

Bright, K. S., Charrois, E. M., Mughal, M. K., Wajid, A., McNeil, D., Stuart, S., Hayden, K. A., & Kingston, D. (2020). Interpersonal psychotherapy to reduce psychological distress in perinatal women: A systematic review. *International Journal of Environmental Research and Public Health*, 17(22), 8421. https://doi.org/10.3390/ijerph17228421

Connelly, C. D., Hazen, A. L., Baker-Ericzén, M. J., Landsverk, J., & Horwitz, S. M. (2013). Is screening for depression in the perinatal period enough? The co-occurrence of depression, substance abuse, and intimate partner violence in culturally diverse pregnant women. *Journal of Women's Health*, 22(10), 844–852. https://doi.org/10.1089/jwh.2012.4121

Couto, T. C., Brancaglion, M. Y., Alvim-Soares, A., Moreira, L., Garcia, F. D., Nicolato, R., Aguiar, R. A., Leite, H. V., & Corrêa, H. (2015). Postpartum depression: A systematic review of the genetics involved. *World Journal of Psychiatry*, 5(1), 103. https://doi.org/10.5498/wjp.v5.i1.103

Davanzo, R., Copertino, M., De Cunto, A., Minen, F., & Amaddeo, A. (2011). Antidepressant drugs and breastfeeding: A review of the literature. *Breastfeeding Medicine: The Official Journal of the Academy of Breastfeeding Medicine*, 6(2), 89–98. https://doi.org/10.1089/bfm.2010.0019

Gavin, N. I., Gaynes, B. N., Lohr, K. N., Meltzer-Brody, S., Gartlehner, G., & Swinson, T. (2005). Perinatal depression: A systematic review of prevalence and incidence. *Obstetrics & Gynecology*, 106(5 Pt. 1), 1071–1083. https://doi.org/10.1097/01.AOG.0000183597.31630.db

Gueron-Sela, N., Shahar, G., Volkovich, E., & Tikotzky, L. (2021). Prenatal maternal sleep and trajectories of postpartum depression and anxiety symptoms. *Journal of Sleep Research*, 30(4), e13258. https://doi.org/10.1111/jsr.13258

Grunberg, V. A., Geller, P. A., Hoffman, C., Njoroge, W., Ahmed, A., & Patterson, C. A. (2022). Parental mental health screening in the NICU: A psychosocial team initiative. *Journal of Perinatology*, 42(3), 401–409. https://doi.org/10.1038/s41372-021-01217-0

Heron, J., Gilbert, N., Dolman, C., Shah, S., Beare, I., Dearden, S., Muckelroy, N., Jones, I., & Ives, J. (2012). Information and support needs during recovery from postpartum psychosis. *Archives Women Mental Health*, 15(3), 155–165. https://doi.org/10.1007/s00737-012-0267-1

Huang, L., Zhao, Y., Qiang, C., & Fan, B. (2018). Is cognitive behavioral therapy a better choice for women with postnatal depression? A systematic review and meta-analysis. *PloS One*, 13(10), e0205243. https://doi.org/10.1371/journal.pone.0205243

Jones, I., Chandra, P. S., Dazzan, P., & Howard, L. M. (2014). Bipolar disorder, affective psychosis, and schizophrenia in pregnancy and the post-partum period. *Lancet*, 384(9956), 1789–1799. https://doi.org/10.1016/S0140-6736(14)61278-2

Kim, T. H. M., Delahunty-Pike, A., & Campbell-Yeo, M. (2020). Effect of fathers' Presence and involvement in newborn care in the NICU on mothers' symptoms of postpartum depression. *Journal of Obstetric, Gynecologic, and Neonatal Nursing*, 49(5), 452–463. https://doi.org/10.1016/j.jogn.2020.05.007

Kroska, E. B., & Stowe, Z. N. (2020). Postpartum depression: Identification and treatment in the clinic setting. *Obstetrics and Gynecology Clinics of North America*, 47(3), 409–419. https://doi.org/10.1016/j.ogc.2020.05.001

Lewis, K. J., Foster, R. G., & Jones, I. R. (2016). Is sleep disruption a trigger for postpartum psychosis? *British Journal of Psychiatry*, 208(5), 409–411. https://doi.org/10.1192/bjp.bp.115.166314

Lueth, A. J., Allshouse, A. A., Blue, N. M., Grobman, W. A., Levine, L. D., Simhan, H. N., Kim, J. K., Johnson, J., Wilson, F. A., Murtaugh, M., Silver, R. M., & National Institutes of Health (NIH), Eunice Kennedy Shriver National Institute of Child Health and Human Development (NICHD), Nulliparous Pregnancy Outcomes Study: Monitoring Mothers-to-Be (nuMoM2b), and National Heart, Lung, and Blood Institute (NHLBI) nuMoM2b Heart Health Study (nuMoM2b-HHS). (2022). Allostatic load and adverse pregnancy outcomes. *Obstetrics and Gynecology*, 140(6), 974–982. https://doi.org/10.1097/AOG.0000000000004971

Lin, P. Z., Xue, J. M., Yang, B., Li, M., & Cao, F. L. (2018). Effectiveness of self-help psychological interventions for treating and preventing postpartum depression: A meta-analysis. *Archives of Women's Mental Health*, 21(5), 491–503. https://doi.org/10.1007/s00737-018-0835-0

Lindahl, V., Pearson, J. L., & Colpe, L. (2005). Prevalence of suicidality during pregnancy and the postpartum. *Archives of Women's Mental Health*, 8(2), 77–87. https://doi.org/10.1007/s00737-005-0080-1

Markowitz, J. C., & Weissman, M. M. (2004). Interpersonal psychotherapy: Principles and applications. *World Psychiatry : Official Journal of the World Psychiatric Association*, 3(3), 136–139. PMID: 16633477.

Milgrom, J., Danaher, B. G., Gemmill, A. W., Holt, C., Seeley, J. R., Tyler, M. S., Ross, J., & Erickson, J. (2016). Internet cognitive behavioral therapy for women with postnatal depression: A randomized controlled trial of MumMoodBooster. *Journal of Medical Internet Research*, 18(3), e54. https://doi.org/10.2196/jmir.4993

McCurdy, A. P., Boulé, N. G., Sivak, A., & Davenport, M. H. (2017). Effects of exercise on mild-to-moderate depressive symptoms in the postpartum period: A meta-analysis. *Obstetrics and Gynecology, 129*(6), 1087–1097. https://doi.org/10.1097/AOG.0000000000002053

Mughal, S., Azhar, Y., & Siddiqui, W. (2024, August 12). *Postpartum depression*. StatPearls Publishing. https://www.ncbi.nlm.nih.gov/books/NBK519070/#:~:text=Postpartum%20depression%20most%20commonly%20occurs

Munk-Olsen, T., Liu, X., Viktorin, A., Brown, H. K., Di Florio, A., D'Onofrio, B. M., Gomes, T., Howard, L. M., Khalifeh, H., Krohn, H., Larsson, H., Lichtenstein, P., Taylor, C. L., Van Kamp, I., Wesseloo, R., Meltzer-Brody, S., Vigod, S. N., & Bergink, V. (2018). Maternal and infant outcomes associated with lithium use in pregnancy: An international collaborative meta-analysis of six cohort studies. *Lancet, 5*(8), 644–652. https://doi.org/10.1016/S2215-0366(18)30180-9

Munk-Olsen, T., Laursen, T. M., Pedersen, C. B., Mors, O., & Mortensen, P. B. (2006). New parents and mental disorders: A population-based register study. *JAMA, 296*(21), 2582–2589. https://doi.org/10.1001/jama.296.21.2582

Parsons, C. E., Young, K. S., Rochat, T. J., Kringelbach, M. L., & Stein A. (2012). Postnatal depression and its effects on child development: A review of evidence from low- and middle-income countries. *British Medical Bulletin, 101*(1), 57–79. https://doi.org/10.1093/bmb/ldr047

Payne, J. L., & Maguire, J. (2019). Pathophysiological mechanisms implicated in postpartum depression. *Frontiers in Neuroendocrinology, 52*, 165–180. https://doi.org/10.1016/j.yfrne.2018.12.001

Prins, A., Bovin, M. J., Kimerling, R., Kaloupek, D. G., Marx, B. P., Pless Kaiser, A., & Schnurr, P. P. (2015). *The Primary Care PTSD Screen for DSM-5 (PC-PTSD-5)*. National Center for PTSD, U.S. Department of Veterans Affairs. https://www.ptsd.va.gov/professional/assessment/screens/pc-ptsd.asp

Rafferty, J., Mattson, G., Earls, M. F., Yogman, M. W., Gambon, T. B., Lavin, A., Wissow, L. S., & Committee on Psychosocial Aspects of Child and Family Health. (2019). Incorporating recognition and management of perinatal depression into pediatric practice. *Pediatrics, 143*(1), e20183260. https://doi.org/10.1542/peds.2018-3260

Resnick, P. J. (1969). Child murder by parents: a psychiatric review of filicide. *The American Journal of Psychiatry, 126*(3), 325–334. https://doi.org/10.1176/ajp.126.3.325

Righetti-Veltema, M., Conne-Perréard, E., Bousquet, A., & Manzano, J. (2002). Postpartum depression and mother-infant relationship at 3 months old. *Journal of Affective Disorders, 70*(3), 291–306. https://doi.org/10.1016/s0165-0327(01)00367-6

Samanta, D., & Lui, F. (2023, July 17). *Anti-NMDA receptor encephalitis*. StatPearls Publishing. https://www.ncbi.nlm.nih.gov/books/NBK551672

Scarff, J. R. (2019). Postpartum depression in men. *Innovations in Clinical Neuroscience, 16*(5–6), 11–14. PMID: 31440396.

Schiller, C. E., Meltzer-Brody, S., & Rubinow, D. R. (2015). The role of reproductive hormones in postpartum depression. *CNS Spectrums, 20*(1), 48–59. https://doi.org/10.1017/S1092852914000480

Schüle, C., Nothdurfter, C., & Rupprecht, R. (2014). The role of allopregnanolone in depression and anxiety. *Progress in Neurobiology, 113*, 79–87. https://doi.org/10.1016/j.pneurobio.2013.09.003

Shorey, S., Chee, C. Y. I., Ng, E. D., Chan, Y. H., Tam, W. W. S., & Chong, Y. S. (2018). Prevalence and incidence of postpartum depression among healthy mothers: A systematic review and meta-analysis. *Journal of Psychiatric Research, 104*, 235–248. https://doi.org/10.1016/j.jpsychires.2018.08.001

Shovers, S., Bachman, S., Popek, L., & Turchi, R. (2021). Maternal postpartum depression: Risk factors, impacts, and interventions for the NICU and beyond. *Current Opinion in Pediatrics, 33*(3), 331–341. https://doi.org/10.1097/MOP.0000000000001011

Sockol L. E. (2015). A systematic review of the efficacy of cognitive behavioral therapy for treating and preventing perinatal depression. *Journal of Affective Disorders, 177*, 7–21. https://doi.org/10.1016/j.jad.2015.01.052

Sockol L. E. (2018). A systematic review and meta-analysis of interpersonal psychotherapy for perinatal women. *Journal of Affective Disorders, 232*, 316–328. https://doi.org/10.1016/j.jad.2018.01.018

Stadtlander, L. (2015). Paternal postpartum depression. *International Journal of Childbirth Education, 30*(2), 11–13.

Stein, A., Pearson, R. M., Goodman, S. H., Rapa, E., Rahman, A., McCallum, M., Howard, L. M., & Pariante, C. M. (2014). Effects of perinatal mental disorders on the fetus and child. *Lancet, 384*(9956), 1800–1819. https://doi.org/10.1016/S0140-6736(14)61277-0

Stewart, D. E., & Vigod, S. N. (2019). Postpartum depression: Pathophysiology, treatment, and emerging therapeutics. *Annual Review of Medicine, 70*, 183–196. https://doi.org/10.1146/annurev-med-041217-011106

Vigod, S. N., Villegas, L., Dennis, C. L., & Ross, L. E. (2010). Prevalence and risk factors for postpartum depression among women with preterm and low-birth-weight infants: A systematic review. *BJOG: An International Journal of Obstetrics and Gynaecology, 117*(5), 540–550. https://doi.org/10.1111/j.1471-0528.2009.02493.x

Wisner, K. L., Sit, D. K., McShea, M. C., Rizzo, D. M., Zoretich, R. A., Hughes, C. L., Eng, H. F., Luther, J. F., Wisniewski, S. R., Costantino, M. L., Confer, A. L., Moses-Kolko, E. L., Famy, C. S., & Hanusa, B. H. (2013). Onset timing, thoughts of self-harm, and diagnoses in postpartum women with screen-positive depression findings. *JAMA Psychiatry, 70*(5), 490–498. https://doi.org/10.1001/jamapsychiatry.2013.87

13 PERSONALITY DISORDERS

Alex Cheng

INTRODUCTION

In recent years, there has been a renewed interest in and increased public awareness of behavioral health needs globally. This heightened attention is likely due to the significant impact of the global COVID-19 pandemic on mental health. While there has been more focused research into affective disorders, anxiety disorders, and other psychiatric diagnoses over the years, relatively little research has been directed toward personality disorders. This lack of attention could be due to clinical bias among psychiatric providers regarding the ability to treat personality disorders or the presence of stigma among the general public.

Over the years, personality disorders have remained on the periphery of psychiatric consciousness and research efforts. Yet these disorders, considered to be lifelong and persistent, impose an enormous toll on patients and public health over time. Furthermore, changing definitions of personality disorders by various behavioral health organizations have further complicated matters, with more changes expected with the next editions of the *Diagnostic and Statistical Manual of Mental Disorders* (*DSM*; current edition is the Fifth Edition, Text Revision, American Psychiatric Association, 2022) and the *International Classification of Diseases* (*ICD*; current edition is the 11th Revision, World Health Organization, 2019).

While these changes have generally added more clarity and precision to personality disorder diagnoses based on latest research data, they have also compounded the healthcare provider's dilemma of determining, "Is this a personality disorder or something else?"

The APRN should bear in mind that irrespective of the diagnostic criteria used, personality disorders are characterized by enduring and persistent patterns of thoughts, behaviors, and character traits that deviate from the normative range of the general population, causing significant distress and/or functional deficits for patients. This holds true independent of any primary medical or psychiatric diagnosis. To that end, the gold standard in diagnosing a personality disorder has been, and will always be, in-person patient evaluations. These evaluations include careful history taking, thorough assessment of the patient's psychosocial patterns, and in-room observations to determine if the patient meets the threshold for diagnosis.

Over time, as the APRN becomes more experienced, they may also develop a "gut feeling" about a patient's personality disorder diagnosis. However, it is important to be cautious as this feeling can sometimes be influenced by the APRN's own countertransference toward the patient. Through residency in New York City, the author had the pleasure of training at the Center for Intensive Treatment of Personality Disorders (CITPD), meeting and treating patients with various personality disorders. Discussions with experienced clinicians at the CITPD helped the author identify his own strong, subtle, conscious and unconscious thoughts, behaviors, and feelings toward patients with different personality disorders. This experience served as a learning opportunity for better diagnostic identification, as well as for delivery of improved patient-focused treatment modalities. Many people, including members of the medical community, have the misconception that behavioral health providers cannot be precise and accurate in their diagnosis and treatment because they do not have diagnostic tests or imaging studies available to them; in the author's opinion, a clinician who is finely trained in the art of behavioral health medicine becomes a diagnostic instrument unto themselves that is just as accurate and precise as any tests or studies.

Unless a patient has been previously diagnosed with a personality disorder and given the proper psychoeducation about it, it is rare for them to seek therapeutic interventions with the chief complaint of "I have a personality disorder/problem." This points to another phenomenon concerning personality disorders, namely, the core personality symptoms used for diagnostic criteria are often egosyntonic. Many patients have little to no insight as to the reasons they are experiencing distress, if they experience any distress at all. Generally, higher functioning individuals may experience less distress from their personality pathology as they likely have developed adaptive coping mechanisms to manage or even leverage their personality pathologies in their daily lives. It is crucial to remember that a lack of distress or functional impairment does not necessarily preclude a diagnosis because the severity of personality disorders may wax and wane over time due to various factors, even if the core symptoms remain consistent. Therefore, treatment requires adjustment according to different severity levels.

Treatment options for personality disorders are considered limited compared with other psychiatric diagnoses. There are fewer evidence-based treatments or effective medications for any of the personality disorders discussed in this chapter.

The general guiding treatment principles for the vast majority of patients with personality disorders are the following:

A. Identify comorbid medical and psychiatric illnesses.
B. Focus medication management on improving comorbid psychiatric illnesses.
C. Provide ample psychoeducation to patients about their diagnoses and course of treatment.
D. Provide/refer psychotherapy as the main treatment option for the patient.

For lower functioning patients, involving the patient's family and/or friends in the treatment plan can be useful. As the majority of behavioral health providers are not trained to provide the specialized psychotherapy options discussed in this chapter, it is important for the APRN to establish a network of therapy referrals in their local practicing area. However, some adventurous practitioners may wish to explore further psychotherapy training options.

SPECIFIC PERSONALITY DISORDERS

DEFINITION

A. This umbrella category encompasses all the personality disorders that are discussed in this chapter, namely:
1. Antisocial personality disorder
2. Avoidant personality disorder
3. Borderline personality disorder (BPD)
4. Dependent personality disorder
5. Histrionic personality disorder
6. Narcissistic personality disorder
7. Obsessive-compulsive personality disorder
8. Other specific personality disorders
9. Paranoid personality disorder (PPD)
10. Personality disorder, unspecified
11. Schizoid personality disorder

DIAGNOSTIC CRITERIA

A. There is evidence that the individual's characteristic and enduring patterns of inner experience and behavior deviate markedly as a whole from the culturally expected and accepted range (or "norm"). Such deviation must manifest in more than one of the following areas:
1. Cognition (i.e., ways of perceiving and interpreting things, people and events; forming attitudes and images of self and others)
2. Affectivity (range, intensity, and appropriateness of emotional arousal and response)
3. Control over impulses and need gratification
4. Relating to others and manner of handling interpersonal situations

B. The deviation must manifest itself pervasively as behavior that is inflexible, maladaptive, or otherwise dysfunctional across a broad range of personal and social situations (i.e., not being limited to one specific "triggering" stimulus or situation).

C. There is personal distress, or adverse impact on the social environment, or both, clearly attributable to the behavior.

D. There must be evidence that the deviation is stable and of long duration, having its onset in late childhood or adolescence.

E. The deviation cannot be explained as a manifestation or consequence of other adult mental disorders, although episodic or chronic conditions may coexist or be superimposed on it.

F. Organic brain disease, injury, or dysfunction must be excluded as possible cause of the deviation.

REFERENCE AND BIBLIOGRAPHY

American Psychiatric Association. (2022). *Diagnostic and statistical manual of mental disorders* (5th ed., text rev.). https://doi.org/10.1176/appi.books.9780890425787

World Health Organization. (2016). Disorders of adult personality and behaviour (F60–F69). F60.8: Other specified personality disorders. *International statistical classification of diseases* (10th rev.). https://icd.who.int/browse10/2016/en#/F60-F69

World Health Organization. (2019). *International statistical classification of diseases* (11th rev.). https://icd.who.int

ANTISOCIAL PERSONALITY DISORDER

DEFINITION

A. Diagnostic criteria include the following:
1. The general criteria for personality disorder must be met.
2. At least three of the following must be present:
   a. Callous unconcern for the feelings of others
   b. Gross and persistent attitude of irresponsibility and disregard for social norms, rules, and obligations
   c. Incapacity to maintain enduring relationships, although having no difficulty establishing them
   d. Very low tolerance to frustration and a low threshold for discharge of aggression, including violence
   e. Incapacity to experience guilt or to learn from adverse experience, particularly punishment
   f. Marked proneness to blame others or to offer plausible rationalizations for the behavior, bringing the subject into conflict with society

INCIDENCE AND PREVALENCE

A. Incidence
1. One in four American adults have syndromal antisocial behaviors.
2. The percentage of crimes committed by a person with antisocial behavior is 80% to 90%.

B. Prevalence
1. General population prevalence is between 2% and 3%.
2. However, in male incarcerated population, it could be as high as 60%.

PATHOGENESIS

A. Antisocial personality disorder has multifactorial pathogenesis.

B. There appears to be a significant genetic influence on youth antisocial behaviors, with various twin/adoption studies estimating 38% to 58% being accountable to genetic differences. However, large-scale, genome-wide studies have yet to identify significant genome polymorphisms that influence these behaviors.

C. Imaging studies have identified possible brain areas associated with antisocial personality disorder.
1. Right cerebellar hemisphere, orbital frontal cortex, right thalamic region
2. Anterior cingulate gyrus, prefrontal cortex, hippocampal region containing the amygdala, medial temporal gyrus

PREDISPOSING FACTORS

A. There is a well-documented predisposition to antisocial behaviors and personality disorder among those assigned male at birth, with observed odds ratio for violence between male and female sex of 18.8 and higher.

B. Other factors indicating association with youth antisocial behaviors include the following:
1. Harsh parenting, delinquent peer affiliation
2. Social/economic disadvantages (growing up in poverty or high-crime area)
3. Trauma: childhood abuse

COMMON COMPLAINTS

A. Antisocial personality disorder is a diagnosis that must be established with persistent symptoms starting in childhood or early adolescence.
1. Typical history from that period would include frequent, persistent rule-breaking behaviors and/or overt aggressive behaviors. Rule-breaking behaviors may include theft, vandalism, truancy, swearing, running away, and substance use.
2. Aggressive behaviors may include fire setting, physical fighting, bullying, threatening others, and oppositionality. These antisocial behaviors likely continue into

adulthood, with frequent encounters with law enforcement and legal issues being a common complaint among these patients.
B. Two cardinal features of patients with antisocial personality disorder are a lack of empathy and a lack of shame.
 1. A lack of empathy can be described as an inability to "put oneself in someone else's shoes" as the patient is unable to fathom the feelings of those around them.
 2. A lack of shame is frequently observed when the patient boasts or brags about an unethical act as if it were a great accomplishment. Willing manipulation of others is also frequently observed, where the patient acts in an egosyntonic, deliberate way to use someone for their own goals.

OTHER SIGNS AND SYMPTOMS
A. Poor frustration tolerance and acting out those frustrations can also be observed in patients with antisocial personality disorder. For example, the patient might request a specific medication from the APRN and, when refused, become instantly irate and verbally abusive in the office.
B. Other behaviors that the APRN might observe include commenting on the APRN's performance, complaining about the APRN and/or the system, bragging behaviors, and manipulative behaviors.

SUBJECTIVE DATA
A. Given the patient's lack of empathy and shame, and also the patient's purchase for manipulation, the APRN should try to corroborate any self-reported history, symptoms, or other relevant issues by the patient with a collateral source if possible.

PHYSICAL EXAMINATION
A. The APRN could perform a physical examination or refer the patient to a primary care provider to rule out medical causes of personality changes; however, a physical examination is usually not required.

DIAGNOSTIC TESTS AND SCREENING
A. No diagnostic tests are available; however, the APRN should order appropriate laboratory tests and/or imaging studies to rule out medical causes of personality changes. Urine toxicology can be useful to rule out substance contribution to the illness.
B. The Minnesota Multiphasic Personality Inventory may be used.

DIFFERENTIAL DIAGNOSES
A. Differential diagnoses include the following:
 1. Conduct disorder/oppositional defiant disorder (typically with youth)
 2. Intermittent explosive disorder, other personality disorders such as narcissistic personality disorder and BPD

PLAN
A. Patients with antisocial personality disorder commonly have comorbidities in schizophrenia, affective disorders, anxiety, posttraumatic stress disorder (PTSD), and substance use disorders; therefore, prompt diagnosis and treatment of these separate disorders is essential.
 1. It may be difficult, and perhaps impossible, for the APRN to develop a true therapeutic relationship with patients with antisocial personality disorder.
 2. Supportive, empathic statements by the APRN may be viewed by the patient as nongenuine since the patient lacks empathy and therefore cannot imagine empathy from others around them.
 3. Trying to elicit expression of emotional state may be viewed hostilely by the patient as an attempt to expose their "weakness." Instead, the treatment should focus on any comorbid conditions, as well as treatment rules and boundaries between the APRN and the patient.

GENERAL TREATMENTS AND INTERVENTIONS
A. There are no medications approved by the U.S. Food and Drug Administration (FDA) for the treatment of antisocial personality disorder.
B. Once the diagnosis is identified:
 1. The APRN should share the diagnosis with the patient. A thorough session of psychoeducation should be provided regarding prognosis and treatment options.
 2. Patients with antisocial personality disorder are generally considered to be resistant to psychotherapy.
  a. There is some evidence that schema therapy, contingency management, and dialectical behavioral therapy (DBT) may improve social functioning and/or self-harming behaviors.
  b. Cognitive behavioral therapy (CBT) is sometimes used, but current evidence remains at a low-certainty stage for all psychotherapeutic interventions with this patient population.
C. The APRN's focus is on treatment and management of any comorbid psychiatric conditions that the patient might have.

COMMON MEDICATIONS
A. Medication management should primarily focus on treating comorbid psychiatric conditions as there are no established or FDA-approved medications for symptoms of antisocial personality disorder.
B. Given the commonly reported impulsive and aggressive behaviors in patients with antisocial personality disorder, with at times reported dysphoric mood, an antidepressant may be helpful in addressing these symptoms.
 1. For the same reason, the use of a mood stabilizer may also be helpful.
 2. However, literature review has shown very little evidence that the addition of medications helped with the core symptoms of antisocial personality disorder, with the use of phenytoin being the only medication that showed low-certainty evidence of benefits versus placebo.

FOLLOW-UP
A. APRNs should follow up with patients regularly to assess for severity of the disease over time, as well as for comorbid psychiatric conditions that may require treatment over time.

CONSULTATION AND REFERRALS
A. The patient should be referred for individual psychotherapy, possibly DBT/schema therapy, or CBT for behavioral and cognitive changes.
B. The patient should be referred to a primary care provider for management of other medical comorbidities and general health maintenance.

INDIVIDUAL CONSIDERATIONS

Pediatrics
A. In the patient exhibiting antisocial behaviors, consider conduct disorder or oppositional defiant disorder. Attention deficit hyperactivity disorder (ADHD) is also often comorbid with these disorders.

REFERENCES AND BIBLIOGRAPHY

Burt, S. A. (2022). The genetic, environmental, and cultural forces influencing youth antisocial behavior are tightly intertwined. *Annual Review of Clinical Psychology, 18*, 155–178. https://doi.org/10.1146/annurev-clinpsy-072220-015507

Gibbon, S., Khalifa, N. R., Cheung, N. H., Völlm, B. A., & McCarthy, L. (2020). Psychological interventions for antisocial personality disorder. *The Cochrane Database of Systematic Reviews, 9*(9), Article CD007668. https://doi.org/10.1002/14651858.CD007668.pub3

Khalifa, N. R., Gibbon, S., Völlm, B. A., Cheung, N. H., & McCarthy, L. (2020). Pharmacological interventions for antisocial personality disorder. *The Cochrane Database of Systematic Reviews, 9*(9), Article CD007667. https://doi.org/10.1002/14651858.CD007667.pub3

Moran, P. (1999). The epidemiology of antisocial personality disorder. *Social Psychiatry and Psychiatric Epidemiology, 34*(5), 231–242. https://doi.org/10.1007/s001270050138

Nichita, E. C., & Buckley, P. F. (2020). Comorbidities of antisocial personality disorder. In A. R. Felthous & H. Saß (Eds.), *The Wiley international handbook on psychopathic disorders and the law* (2nd ed., pp. 645–670). Wiley. https://doi.org/10.1002/9781119159322.ch28

Shea, D. C. (2017). *Psychiatric interviewing: The art of understanding* (3rd ed.). Elsevier.

Solmi, M., Dragioti, E., Croatto, G., Radua, J., Borgwardt, S., Carvalho, A. F., Demurtas, J., Mosina, A., Kurotschka, P., Thompson, T., Cortese, S., Shin, J. L., & Fusar-Poli, P. (2021). Risk and protective factors for personality disorders: An umbrella review of published meta-analyses of case-control and cohort studies. *Frontiers in Psychiatry, 12*, 679379. https://doi.org/10.3389/fpsyt.2021.679379

World Health Organization. (2016). Disorders of adult personality and behaviour (F60–F69). F60.8: Other specified personality disorders. *International statistical classification of diseases* (10th rev.). https://icd.who.int/browse10/2016/en#/F60-F69

Zarnowski, O., Ziton, S., Holmberg, R., Musto, S., Riegle, S., Van Antwerp, E., & Santos-Nunez, G. (2021). Functional MRI findings in personality disorders: A review. *Journal of Neuroimaging : Official Journal of the American Society of Neuroimaging, 31*(6), 1049–1066. https://doi.org/10.1111/jon.12924

AVOIDANT PERSONALITY DISORDER

DEFINITION
A. Diagnostic criteria include the following:
  1. The general criteria for personality disorder must be met.
  2. At least four of the following must be present:
     a. Persistent and pervasive feelings of tension and apprehension
     b. Belief that oneself is socially inept, personally unappealing, or inferior to others
     c. Excessive preoccupation with being criticized or rejected in social situations
     d. Unwillingness to get involved with people unless certain of being liked
     e. Restrictions in lifestyle because of need of security
     f. Avoidance of social or occupational activities that involve significant interpersonal contact due to fear of criticism, disapproval, or rejection

INCIDENCE AND PREVALENCE
A. General population prevalence is 1.7%, with estimate of the disorder as a comorbid diagnosis of about 14.7% in psychiatric outpatients.

PATHOGENESIS
A. There is limited research into the etiology of the disorder; however, a population twin study estimated a heritability of 0.64 for symptoms of avoidant personality disorder. Brain areas that are possibly affected in this disorder include the hippocampal and parahippocampal regions, cingulate cortex, the insular region, and the amygdala.

PREDISPOSING FACTORS
A. Risk factors: Studies have suggested a combination of personality factors, including:
  1. Harm avoidance
  2. Negative/adverse childhood experiences
  3. Childhood/adolescent anxiety disorders

B. Negative/adverse childhood experiences can include outright abuse by caretakers, neglect, or parenting styles that lead to an anxious/avoidant attachment style by the child.

COMMON COMPLAINTS
A. Patients with avoidant personality disorder have two main features that are enduring and persistent:
  1. Incredibly low self-regard
  2. Fear of rejection by others

B. When asking patients to describe themselves, the APRN might hear the patient use numerous negative adjectives in various situations and settings. The fear of rejection might be then magnified by the patient's own past experiences of repeated rejections and low self-regard, which then leads to other symptoms of this disorder that are more functional in nature. For example, the patient might report that they have repeatedly avoided social situations at work and in their personal life due to having "anxiety," leading to professional setbacks and lack of intimacy in their lives. This high level of anxiety about social situations, and the resulting depressive symptoms such as anhedonia and being withdrawn, can then further impair the patient, leading to ever-lower functional status.

OTHER SIGNS AND SYMPTOMS
A. Intense anxiety surrounding social situations should be further investigated by the APRN since there are other anxiety disorders, panic disorders, or even personality disorders that can produce this level of anxiety.
B. Even though social anxiety disorder symptoms are similar, avoidant personality disorder anxiety is usually more severe, much more prevalent, and persistent, and it is usually completely egosyntonic, which is again related to low self-regard.
C. Patients with social anxiety disorder usually are higher functioning with full, rich relationships in their lives, as opposed to patients with avoidant personality disorder, in whom the impairment leads to poor functioning overall, and the avoidance extends beyond social functions to avoidance of intimate relationships/friendships.
D. Panic disorder might produce anxiety levels similar to or more severe than avoidant personality disorder; however, fear experienced in panic disorder is usually more about having a panic attack in public and less about being judged as a person, as it is in avoidant personality disorder.

SUBJECTIVE DATA
A. The APRN should carefully rule out other diagnoses that could lead to lower functional status over time, such as recurrent depressive episodes, undertreated anxiety disorders, and other personality disorders.
B. To assess the severity of the patient's impairment from this disorder, the APRN should try to take an extensive psychosocial history because low functional status such as strings of professional/relationship setbacks are the eventual consequences of this disease.

PHYSICAL EXAMINATION
A. The APRN could perform a physical examination or refer the patient to a primary care provider to rule out medical

causes of personality changes; however, a physical examination is usually not required.

DIAGNOSTIC TESTS AND SCREENING
A. No diagnostic tests are available; however, the APRN should order appropriate laboratory tests and/or imaging studies to rule out medical causes of personality changes. Urine toxicology can be useful to rule out substance contribution to the illness.
B. Structured clinical interviews remain the primary means of arriving at the diagnosis.

DIFFERENTIAL DIAGNOSES
A. Differential diagnoses include social anxiety disorder, affective disorders, other anxiety disorders, and other personality disorders such as BPD, schizoid personality disorder, and dependent personality disorder.
B. The most common comorbid psychiatric condition is social anxiety disorder.

PLAN
A. Special consideration should be given to either ruling out or identifying comorbid social anxiety disorder given possible similar presentation of symptoms on the surface.

GENERAL TREATMENTS AND INTERVENTIONS
A. There are no FDA-approved medications for the treatment of avoidant personality disorder.
B. Once the diagnosis is made, share the diagnosis with the patient. A thorough session of psychoeducation should be provided regarding prognosis and treatment options.
C. There is limited research about specific psychotherapy treatment for this disorder. It is suggested that CBT, psychodynamic psychotherapy, and/or schema therapy are effective treatment options.
D. The APRN's focus is on treatment and management of any comorbid psychiatric conditions that the patient might have.

COMMON MEDICATIONS
A. Medication management focuses on treating comorbid psychiatric conditions as there are no established or FDA-approved medications for symptoms of avoidant personality disorder.
B. There are limited data on the efficacy of medications for patients diagnosed with only avoidant personality disorder; however, since social anxiety disorder is commonly comorbid with it, it is sometimes recommended to initiate antidepressant medications such as serotonin or norepinephrine reuptake agents.

FOLLOW-UP
A. APRNs should follow up with patients regularly to assess for severity of the disease over time, as well as for comorbid psychiatric conditions that may require treatment over time.

CONSULTATION AND REFERRALS
A. The patient should be referred to a primary care provider for management of other medical comorbidities and general health maintenance.
B. The patient should be referred to practitioners trained in CBT, psychodynamic psychotherapy, and/or schema therapy. In cases where the disorder is severely impairing the patient's daily functioning, the patient may be referred to a specialized treatment center for personality disorders.

INDIVIDUAL CONSIDERATIONS
Geriatrics
A. Research suggests that severity of symptoms increases with age.

REFERENCES AND BIBLIOGRAPHY
Bangash, A. (2020). Personality disorders in later life: Epidemiology, presentation and management. *British Journal of Psychiatry Advances, 26*(4), 208–18. https://doi.org/10.1192/bja.2020.16
Lampe, L., & Malhi, G. S. (2018). Avoidant personality disorder: Current insights. *Psychology Research and Behaviour Management, 11*, 55–66. https://doi.org/10.2147/PRBM.S121073
Shea, D. C. (2017). *Psychiatric interviewing: The art of understanding* (3rd ed.). Elsevier.
Weinbrecht, A., Schulze, L., Boettcher, J., & Renneberg, B. (2016). Avoidant personality disorder: A current review. *Current Psychiatry Reports, 18*(3), Article 29. https://doi.org/10.1007/s11920-016-0665-6
World Health Organization. (2016). Disorders of adult personality and behaviour (F60–F69). F60.8: Other specified personality disorders. *International statistical classification of diseases* (10th rev.). https://icd.who.int/browse10/2016/en#/F60-F69
Zarnowski, O., Ziton, S., Holmberg, R., Musto, S., Riegle, S., Van Antwerp, E., & Santos-Nunez, G. (2021). Functional MRI findings in personality disorders: A review. *Journal of Neuroimaging: Official Journal of the American Society of Neuroimaging, 31*(6), 1049–1066. https://doi.org/10.1111/jon.12924

BORDERLINE PERSONALITY DISORDER

DEFINITION
A. Diagnostic criteria include the following:
  1. The general criteria for personality disorder must be met.
  2. At least three of the following must be present:
     a. A marked tendency to act unexpectedly and without consideration of the consequences
     b. A marked tendency to quarrelsome behavior and to conflicts with others, especially when impulsive acts are thwarted or criticized
     c. Liability to outbursts of anger or violence, with inability to control the resulting behavioral explosions
     d. Difficulty in maintaining any course of action that offers no immediate reward
     e. Unstable and capricious mood
  3. At least two of the following must be present:
     a. Disturbances in and uncertainty about self-image, aims, and internal preferences (including sexual)
     b. Liability to become involved in intense and unstable relationships, often leading to emotional crises
     c. Excessive efforts to avoid abandonment
     d. Recurrent threats or acts of self-harm
     e. Chronic feelings of emptiness

INCIDENCE AND PREVALENCE
A. General population prevalence is 0.7% to 2.7%.
B. The estimated mean prevalence is 22.4% among hospitalized patients in psychiatric units and 11.8% in outpatient psychiatric settings.

PATHOGENESIS
A. Twin studies have suggested that BPD is approximately 55% heritable. It is most likely multifactorial and heterogeneous.

PREDISPOSING FACTORS
A. BPD may be associated with pronounced amygdala hyperreactivity in response to negative emotional stimuli. ▶

It may be associated with abnormal neuroimaging findings areas related to social cognition, self-functioning, and identity functioning; these areas include the orbitofrontal cortex, medial prefrontal cortex, anterior cingulate cortex, precuneus and posterior cingulate cortex, cortical and subcortical regions of the temporal lobes, and somatosensory cortexes. However, these physiologic findings may be more generally applied to other mood disorders and/or other personality disorders and not specific to BPD.
  B. Environmental factors include the following:
    1. Lower socioeconomic status
    2. Family psychopathology, especially maternal BPD
    3. Parent–child relationship and/or maladaptive parenting
    4. Bullying/rejection by peers
    5. Adverse childhood events (ACEs), such as abuse, maltreatment/neglect, or sexual abuse
  C. Temperamental and personality factors from childhood can also predispose someone to develop BPD. These include the following:
    1. Affective instability
    2. Negative emotionality
    3. Inappropriate anger
    4. Poor emotional control
    5. Impulsivity
    6. Aggression

COMMON COMPLAINTS
  A. Patients often report, separate from any episodic mood symptoms, a persistent feeling of "emptiness" in their mood.
    1. Related to this, patients might also report difficulty in "being by myself," which enhances the feeling of emptiness.
    2. Patients often report a history of relationships and/or friendships typically described as "stormy," with frequent and unstable romantic relationships and friendships that end abruptly, with patient reporting "having to cut people out of my life from time to time."
    3. Also related to this are reports of fear of abandonment, which may be typified by unreasonable fear that romantic partners, friends, or family members will no longer want to be with the patient for various reasons.
  B. Some patients report affective instability as "I feel like I have bipolar" with "a lot of highs and lows" or "a rollercoaster of emotions," but when the APRN investigates further the affective changes fluctuate greatly within minutes or hours instead of days or weeks as required for other psychiatric disorders. Increase in impulsivity can result in a wide range of behaviors; some common reports include unsafe sexual practices, increase in sexual promiscuity, and inappropriate increase in monetary spending.
  C. The most notable cognitive pattern in patients with BPD is dichotomous thinking, commonly known as *black-and-white thinking*, in which patients think about themselves and the world around them in absolute terms. This can apply to many things in the patient's life, so the APRN should listen for a pattern of the patient reporting in absolute terms such as "best," "worst," "greatest," "the most," "highest," or "lowest."
  D. A history of self-injurious behavior, chronic suicidal ideation, and parasuicidal behaviors may also be reported by patients with BPD. When asked about their self-injurious behaviors, the patient commonly explains them as "not really suicidal" and states "I just wanted to have some kind of release," all while undergoing an intense emotional experience.

OTHER SIGNS AND SYMPTOMS
  A. Auditory verbal hallucinations and paranoid, delusional thought content can sometimes present in patients with BPD.
    1. Generally considered to be present during times of elevated emotional duress
    2. Some evidence, however, that psychotic symptoms can be persistent in these patients and may predict a more severe form of the illness
  B. Patients with BPD may also display the following behaviors:
    1. Commenting on the APRN's performance
    2. Complaining about the APRN or the system
    3. Having dramatic behavior or appearance
    4. Being helpless and childlike
    5. Being manipulative

PHYSICAL EXAMINATION
  A. The APRN could perform a physical examination or refer the patient to a primary care provider to rule out medical causes of personality changes; however, a physical examination is usually not required.

DIAGNOSTIC TESTS AND SCREENING
  A. No diagnostic tests are available; however, the APRN should order appropriate laboratory tests and/or imaging studies to rule out medical causes of personality changes. Urine toxicology can be useful to rule out substance contribution to the illness.
  B. Structured clinical interviews remain the primary means of arriving at the diagnosis.
  C. For screening purposes, the Mclean Screening Instrument for BPD, Borderline Personality Questionnaire, and Borderline Personality Features Scale for Children may be used.

DIFFERENTIAL DIAGNOSES
  A. Differential diagnoses include affective disorders, bipolar spectrum disorders, psychotic spectrum disorders, PTSD, and other personality disorders.

PLAN
  A. Patients with BPD commonly have comorbidities in trauma-related and affective disorders; therefore, prompt identification and treatment of these separate but related disorders is essential.
  B. The first priority in addressing the underlying BPD is to identify and treat crisis behaviors.
    1. Suicide attempts
    2. Serious attacks on other people
    3. Self-injurious behaviors
    4. Frequent hospital visits/admissions
    5. Dangerous, high-risk behaviors
  C. Second, patient education about the diagnosis and about evidence-based treatment should be initiated.
    1. Encourage patient to accept treatment options.
    2. Assist in finding therapeutic support in the short term.
  D. Lastly, goals of treatment should be discussed with the patient and a mutually accepted treatment plan should be reached.

GENERAL TREATMENTS AND INTERVENTIONS
  A. There are no FDA-approved medications for the treatment of BPD.
  B. Once the diagnosis is made:
    1. The APRN should share the diagnosis with the patient. A thorough session of psychoeducation should be provided regarding prognosis and treatment options.

2. Psychotherapy remains the main treatment modality for patients with BPD. It has been found to reduce severity of symptoms, self-injurious behaviors, suicidality, and psychosocial dysfunction.
3. Evidence supports two psychotherapy treatment options: DBT and mentalization-based treatment. Transference-focused psychotherapy and schema-focused therapy are also established treatment options; however, they are less studied.

C. The phenomenon of "splitting" is also often observed in patients with BPD, and it can be observed by individual members of the patient's treatment team over time.
1. Splitting happens when a patient, unintentionally, presents different sets of symptoms to different members of the treatment team, thereby "splitting" the treatment focus of the team and, over time, creating dynamics that become unhelpful to the patient's treatment.
2. Therefore, it is usually best for the patient's treatment to have all treatment modalities closely colocated, such as a comprehensive outpatient clinic with individual sessions with therapist/counselor, psychiatric provider, and group therapy.
3. If the APRN is sharing treatment of the patient with outside healthcare providers, frequent collaboration among all healthcare providers is recommended to address the issue of splitting.

D. The APRN should also focus on treatment and management of any comorbid psychiatric conditions that the patient might have.

COMMON MEDICATIONS

A. Medication management should primarily focus on treating comorbid psychiatric conditions as there are no established or FDA-approved medications for symptoms of BPD.

B. There have been studies aimed at finding support for the use of antidepressants, antipsychotic medications, and mood stabilizers for the treatment of BPD; however, thus far, evidence remains weak or conflicting that any medication has sustained treatment effects. Instead, medication treatment for a patient's underlying BPD should primarily focus on regular psychoeducation and avoidance of polypharmacy and prescribing of controlled substances.

C. Some commonly prescribed medications include the following:
1. Lamotrigine for mood stabilization
2. Olanzapine and quetiapine for impulsivity/aggression
3. Antidepressants such as selective serotonin reuptake inhibitors (SSRIs) and serotonin and norepinephrine reuptake inhibitors (SNRIs) for affective/anxiety symptoms

FOLLOW-UP

A. APRNs should follow up with patients regularly to assess for severity of the disease over time, preferably on a weekly or biweekly basis.
1. As a general guideline, if the patient's only treatment provider is the psychiatric APRN, follow-ups should be more frequent while referrals to therapy/groups are made.
2. If the patient is engaging with multiple healthcare providers, then psychiatric follow-up can be less frequent. Whatever the frequency of follow-up, it should be reviewed and specified in the treatment plan agreed upon by both the APRN and the patient.

CONSULTATION AND REFERRALS

A. Refer patients for individual and group psychotherapy, possibly DBT/mentalization therapy for behavioral and cognitive changes.

B. Refer patients to a primary care provider for management of other medical comorbidities and general health maintenance.

INDIVIDUAL CONSIDERATIONS

Pediatrics

A. Patients with BPD often present with symptoms in their childhood or adolescence; the APRN should try to differentiate between age-appropriate behaviors and borderline pathology.

REFERENCES AND BIBLIOGRAPHY

Bohus, M., Stoffers-Winterling, J., Sharp, C., Krause-Utz, A., Schmahl, C., & Lieb, K. (2021). Borderline personality disorder. *Lancet, 398*(10310), 1528–1540. https://doi.org/10.1016/S0140-6736(21)00476-1

Bozzatello, P., Garbarini, C., Rocca, P., & Bellino, S. (2021). Borderline personality disorder: Risk factors and early detection. *Diagnostics (Basel, Switzerland), 11*(11), 2142. https://doi.org/10.3390/diagnostics11112142

Chanen, A. M., Nicol, K., Betts, J. K., & Thompson, K. N. (2020). Diagnosis and treatment of borderline personality disorder in young people. *Current Psychiatry Reports, 22*(5), 25. https://doi.org/10.1007/s11920-020-01144-5

Gartlehner, G., Crotty, K., Kennedy, S., Edlund, M. J., Ali, R., Siddiqui, M., Fortman, R., Wines, R., Persad, E., & Viswanathan, M. (2021). Pharmacological treatments for borderline personality disorder: A systematic review and meta-analysis. *CNS Drugs, 35*(10), 1053–1067. https://doi.org/10.1007/s40263-021-00855-4

Paris, J. (2018). Differential diagnosis of borderline personality disorder. *Psychiatric Clinics of North America, 41*(4), 575–582. https://doi.org/10.1016/j.psc.2018.07.001

Sharp, A. (2022). Personality Disorders. *The New England Journal of Medicine, 387*(10), 916–923. https://doi.org/10.1056/NEJMra2120164

Shea, D. C. (2017). *Psychiatric interviewing: The art of understanding* (3rd ed.). Elsevier.

World Health Organization. (2016). Disorders of adult personality and behaviour (F60–F69). F60.8: Other specified personality disorders. *International statistical classification of diseases* (10th rev.). https://icd.who.int/browse10/2016/en#/F60-F69

DEPENDENT PERSONALITY DISORDER

DEFINITION

A. Diagnostic criteria include the following:
1. The general criteria for personality disorder must be met.
2. At least four of the following must be present:
   a. Encouraging or allowing others to make most of one's important life decisions
   b. Subordination of one's own needs to those of others on whom one is dependent, and undue compliance with their wishes
   c. Unwillingness to make even reasonable demands on the people one depends on
   d. Feeling uncomfortable or helpless when alone due to exaggerated fears of inability to care for oneself
   e. Preoccupation with fears of being left to take care of oneself
   f. Limited capacity to make everyday decisions without an excessive amount of advice and reassurance from others

INCIDENCE AND PREVALENCE

A. General population prevalence is 0.49% to 2%; an estimated prevalence as a comorbid diagnosis is about 10% to

25% in psychiatric inpatient populations and up to 47% in outpatient populations. Some evidence suggests being assigned female at birth is associated with a 40% greater likelihood of being diagnosed with dependent personality disorder compared with being assigned male at birth.

PATHOGENESIS
A. Limited research suggests there is about 30% variability in risk of dependent personality disorder attributable to genetic factors.

PREDISPOSING FACTORS
A. Sociocultural risk factors for dependent personality disorder include parenting styles (being "overprotective" or "authoritarian") and early childhood traumatic experiences such as neglect, abuse, or serious medical illness.

COMMON COMPLAINTS
A. The patient might come to the APRN seeking help for their "anxiety and depression," and upon further exploration the APRN might find that the patient's anxiety is mostly associated with the dependent relationships in their lives.
  1. The patient might report a deep fear of abandonment by the people whom the patient has grown to depend on for physical care (money, housing) and also for validation of self-worth.
  2. However, as opposed to the fear of abandonment in BPD, where the patient develops a seeking–rejecting relationship, the patient with dependent personality disorder is entirely seeking closeness in the relationship.

B. This reported need to depend on someone would become pervasive in the patient's life. It is not uncommon for the patient to make statements of helplessness and dependency, such as:
  1. "My partner is my whole life; I can't live without them."
  2. "My partner makes all the decisions for me."

C. Further investigation of important relationships throughout the patient's life should reveal a pattern of such dependent relationships; the patient might report, "I always have someone, I am never not dating or in a relationship."

D. Once the pattern of dependency has been established, assess the severity to which it impacts the patient's functioning over the years, including:
  1. Assessing for anxiety and affective symptoms related to the dependent relationship
  2. Assessing how the dependent relationships have contributed to poorer psychosocial functioning
  3. Determining whether the patient has significantly altered academic/professional decisions associated with dependent relationships

OTHER SIGNS AND SYMPTOMS
A. Patients' reported intense anxiety is only or mostly associated with fear of abandonment in the dependent relationship.
  1. Patients would also report extreme feelings of low self-regard; thoughts of "being worthless" or inadequacy are quite common.
  2. Patients might also appear helpless and childlike in front of the APRN, essentially trying to develop another dependent relationship with the APRN.

SUBJECTIVE DATA
A. Given that the patient is likely in a dependent, unequal relationship where the patient has little to no agency, the chance for abuse and/or intimate partner violence is higher than in other personality disorders.
  1. Survey for risk factors and assess the patient's safety during evaluations and visits.
  2. Assess suicidality. It is also possible that if the patient suspects the dependent relationship is in jeopardy, the patient might engage in suicidal/self-harming/violent behaviors.

PHYSICAL EXAMINATION
A. Perform a physical examination or refer the patient to a primary care provider to rule out medical causes of personality changes; however, a physical examination is usually not required.

DIAGNOSTIC TESTS AND SCREENING
A. No diagnostic tests are available; however, the APRN should order appropriate laboratory tests and/or imaging studies to rule out medical causes of personality changes. Urine toxicology can be useful to rule out substance contribution to the illness.
B. Structured clinical interviews remain the primary means of arriving at the diagnosis.
C. Some self-reported screening tools may be used, such as the Interpersonal Dependency Inventory and the Dependent Personality Style Scale.

DIFFERENTIAL DIAGNOSES
A. Differential diagnoses include the following:
  1. Anxiety disorders
  2. Affective disorders
  3. Other personality disorders, such as BPD, schizoid personality disorder, or avoidant personality disorder
B. Dependent personality disorder is often comorbid with eating disorder, anxiety disorders, somatization disorders, affective disorders, and substance use disorders.

GENERAL TREATMENTS AND INTERVENTIONS
A. There are currently no FDA-approved medications for the treatment of dependent personality disorder.
B. Once the diagnosis is made, the APRN should share the diagnosis with the patient, and a thorough session of psychoeducation should be provided regarding prognosis and treatment options. There is limited research about specific psychotherapy treatment for this disorder; however, psychodynamic psychotherapy and CBT may be effective.
C. The APRN should also focus on treatment and management of any comorbid psychiatric conditions that the patient might have.

COMMON MEDICATIONS
A. There are very limited data on the efficacy of medications for patients diagnosed with only dependent personality disorder. Medication management should focus on comorbid psychiatric diagnoses.

FOLLOW-UP
A. Follow up with patients regularly to assess for (a) suicidality, (b) severity of the disease over time, and (c) comorbid psychiatric conditions that may require treatment over time.

CONSULTATION AND REFERRALS
A. Refer to a primary care provider for management of other medical comorbidities and general health maintenance.
B. Refer to specialists trained in CBT or psychodynamic psychotherapy.

1. In cases where the disorder is severely impairing the patient's daily functioning, the patient may be referred to a specialized treatment center for personality disorders.

C. If the APRN determines abuse or intimate partner violence is present, report suspected abuse and refer the patient to available domestic violence/intimate partner violence shelters and resources in their location.

REFERENCES AND BIBLIOGRAPHY

Simonelli, A., & Parolin, M. (2017). Dependent personality disorder. In V. Zeigler-Hill & T. K. Shackelford (Eds.), *Encyclopedia of personality and individual differences*. Springer Publishing Company.

Shea, D. C. (2017). *Psychiatric interviewing: The art of understanding* (3rd ed.). Elsevier.

World Health Organization. (2016). Disorders of adult personality and behaviour (F60–F69). F60.8: Other specified personality disorders. *International statistical classification of diseases* (10th rev.). https://icd.who.int/browse10/2016/en#/F60-F69

HISTRIONIC PERSONALITY DISORDER

DEFINITION

A. Diagnostic criteria include the following:
   1. The general criteria for personality disorder must be met.
   2. At least four of the following must be present:
      a. Self-dramatization, theatricality, or exaggerated expression of emotions
      b. Suggestibility, being easily influenced by others or by circumstances
      c. Shallow and labile affectivity
      d. Continually seeking excitement and activities in which the subject is the center of attention
      e. Being inappropriately seductive in appearance or behavior
      f. Being overly concerned with physical attractiveness

INCIDENCE AND PREVALENCE

A. The incidence of histrionic personality disorder is about 1% of the population.
B. General population prevalence is between 0.36% and 3.2%; in the psychiatric population, the prevalence is as high as 6.0%.
C. Some consider the disorder to be more prevalent in patients with female sex assignment at birth; however, evidence remains inconclusive.

PATHOGENESIS

A. Pathogenesis is unclear with limited research, but likely moderate genetic influence with multifactorial and heterogeneous factors.

PREDISPOSING FACTORS

A. Predisposing factors are unclear with limited research; emotional neglect is suggestive of association with the disorder.

COMMON COMPLAINTS

A. Patients with histrionic personality disorder often express themselves in an exaggerated manner. This may be reflected in their appearance, including their accessories, clothes, and styling, and also in their speech patterns and thought content. A typical presentation is a patient who walks into the office with a highly stylized appearance and describes themselves and things around them in a colorful, impressionistic manner lacking in detail. The patient might complain of "anxiety" or uncomfortable feelings in social situations; however, these situations would be specific to when the patient is not the center of attention in some way; often it would be coupled with the use of physical appearance or dramatic behaviors to draw attention to oneself.

B. Interactions with other people are characterized by inappropriate seductive or provocative behaviors, with rapidly changing, shallow expressions of emotion. As such, the patient may describe a pattern of friendships/relationships that the patient considers to be close, but on closer examination lack emotional intimacy.

OTHER SIGNS AND SYMPTOMS

A. Some patients might comment on the APRN's performance, become helpless and childlike, or be manipulative.
B. Patients might display dramatic anger and/or physical fighting, as well as poor empathic abilities.

SUBJECTIVE DATA

A. The symptoms of histrionic personality disorder need to be globally applied in the patient's life, meaning:
   1. The patient with this character pathology should display these traits and behaviors in every aspect of their lives.
   2. In patients whose professional careers involve drawing others' attention to them with dramatic display of their abilities or talents, such as patients employed as performers in the entertainment industry, the APRN will have to consider whether histrionic characteristics are globally applied and/or whether the patient suffers from functional impairment due to these characteristics.

PHYSICAL EXAMINATION

A. The APRN could perform a physical examination or refer the patient to a primary care provider to rule out medical causes of personality changes; however, a physical examination is usually not required.

DIAGNOSTIC TESTS AND SCREENING

A. No diagnostic tests are currently available; however, the APRN should order appropriate laboratory tests and/or imaging studies to rule out medical causes of personality changes. Urine toxicology can be useful to rule out substance contribution to the illness.
B. Structured clinical interviews remain the primary means of arriving at the diagnosis.
C. There are almost no screening tools developed specifically for histrionic personality disorder. The APRN may use the Brief Histrionic Personality Scale for screening, although its validity is unclear.

DIFFERENTIAL DIAGNOSES

A. Differential diagnoses include the following:
   1. Narcissistic personality disorder
   2. BPD
   3. Antisocial personality disorder
   4. Dependent personality disorder
   5. Chronic substance use
   6. Other affective disorders

PLAN

A. Histrionic personality disorder is comorbid with other personality disorders such as narcissistic personality disorder, BPD, and antisocial personality disorder. It is also associated with substance use disorders, as well as ADHD and major depressive disorder. It is also found that among patients ▶

diagnosed with anorexia nervosa or bulimia nervosa, there is a high prevalence of histrionic personality disorder.
B. Prompt diagnosis and treatment of any comorbid psychiatric disorder is an essential first step for the APRN in devising a treatment plan for the patient.
C. Periodic assessment for suicidal behaviors, self-injurious behaviors, and high-risk behaviors should be performed by the APRN to determine if acute interventions are required.

GENERAL TREATMENTS AND INTERVENTIONS
A. There are no FDA-approved medications for the treatment of histrionic personality disorder.
B. Once the diagnosis is made, share the diagnosis with the patient and provide a thorough session of psychoeducation regarding prognosis and treatment options. Psychotherapy remains the main treatment modality for patients with histrionic personality disorder. Schema therapy has been suggested to induce greater functional improvement and symptom reduction compared with treatment-as-usual and clarification-oriented psychotherapy.
C. Impulsive/aggressive behaviors displayed by the patient may benefit from SSRI antidepressants or mood stabilizers, although evidence is unclear.
D. The APRN should also focus on treatment and management of any comorbid psychiatric conditions that the patient might have.

COMMON MEDICATIONS
A. Medication management primarily focuses on treating comorbid psychiatric conditions as there are no established or FDA-approved medications for symptoms of histrionic personality disorder.

FOLLOW-UP
A. Follow up with patients regularly to assess for severity of the disease over time, as well as for comorbid psychiatric conditions that may require treatment over time.

CONSULTATION AND REFERRALS
A. Refer for individual psychotherapy, possibly schema/DBT therapy for behavioral and cognitive changes.
B. Refer to a primary care provider for management of other medical comorbidities and general health maintenance.

INDIVIDUAL CONSIDERATIONS

Pediatrics
A. Histrionic personality disorder is not diagnosed in the pediatric population.

Geriatrics
A. Patients may experience an exacerbation in symptoms due to the reduction in their "sex appeal" as they age, leading to increased difficulty relating to others without trying to attract them. Alternatively, these patients may try to draw attention of others in other ways, such as dramatizing somatic complaints.

REFERENCES AND BIBLIOGRAPHY
Bangash, A. (2020). Personality disorders in later life: Epidemiology, presentation and management. *British Journal of Psychiatry Advances*, 26(4), 208–218. https://doi.org/10.1192/bja.2020.16
Candel, O. S. (2019). A review of the present condition of histrionic personality disorder. *Bulletin of Integrative Psychiatry*, 82(3), 39–44. https://doi.org/10.36219/BPI.2019.03.03
Shea, D. C. (2017). *Psychiatric interviewing: The art of understanding* (3rd ed.). Elsevier.
Stern, D. (2022). Histrionic personality disorder. In F. F. Ferri (Ed.), *Ferri's clinical advisor 2023* (pp. 752.e17–752.e18). Elsevier Health Sciences.
World Health Organization. (2016). Disorders of adult personality and behaviour (F60–F69). F60.8: Other specified personality disorders. *International statistical classification of diseases* (10th rev.). https://icd.who.int/browse10/2016/en#/F60-F69

NARCISSISTIC PERSONALITY DISORDER

DEFINITION
A. Diagnostic criteria include the following:
  1. The general criteria for personality disorder must be met.
  2. At least five of the following must be present:
     a. Has a grandiose sense of self-importance (e.g., exaggerates achievements and talents, expects to be recognized as superior without commensurate achievements)
     b. Preoccupied with fantasies of unlimited success, power, brilliance, beauty, or ideal love
     c. Believes that they are "special" and unique and can only be understood by, or should associate with, other special or high-status people (or institutions)
     d. Requires excessive admiration
     e. Has a sense of entitlement and unreasonable expectations of especially favorable treatment or automatic compliance with their expectations
     f. Interpersonally exploitative and takes advantage of others to achieve their own ends
     g. Has a lack of empathy; is unwilling to recognize or identify with the feelings and needs of others
     h. Often envious of others or believes that others are envious of them
     i. Arrogant, with haughty behaviors or attitudes

INCIDENCE AND PREVALENCE
A. General population prevalence is up to 5.3%, with rates up to 17% in clinical samples.

PATHOGENESIS
A. Twin studies suggest 45% to 80% heritability. Regions in the brain affected by narcissistic traits include the cingulate cortex and the insular region.

PREDISPOSING FACTORS
A. Risk factors include male sex assigned at birth, younger age, and single marital status.

COMMON COMPLAINTS
A. Although the diagnostic criteria would classify these patients into a single, unified diagnosis of narcissistic personality disorder, clinical experience and research have suggested there are variant presentations of the core features of this disorder, with each variant displaying different outward signs and symptoms by patients at different times in their lives, depending on life circumstances and stressors.
B. The "overt" presentation is probably the more easily recognized; the patient would present with the following:
  1. Overt grandiosity
  2. Attention seeking
  3. Entitlement
  4. Arrogance
  5. Little observable anxiety

C. The patient might present as socially charming but oblivious to the needs of others around them. This is in contrast to the "covert" or "depleted" presentation, where the patient appears vulnerable, thin-skinned, inhibited, and hypersensitive to evaluations of others while being chronically envious and comparing themselves with others.
D. The "overt" presentation patient in the office might report to the APRN that the reason they came to the office is not "because of me, it's because of" someone else in their lives that they are having issues with, possibly a spouse or close family member.
   1. The patient would report feeling superior to others around them and feeling entitled to "the next big promotion" or other things in their lives.
   2. The patient might constantly call the APRN's attention to things in their lives that display their extreme high sense of self, such as their "impeccable" academic background, their taste in high-end clothing or jewelry, and their "premium, best" choice of residence in their neighborhood.
E. The "covert" presentation patient in the office might report being "depressed all my life" or chronically anxious, and when being evaluated for affective symptoms might meet the criteria for major depressive episode symptoms. A detailed history, however, would indicate this is not episodic in nature.
F. Patients might further report chronic social isolation due to being easily slighted in social settings by peers and coworkers, "not being appreciated for who I am" at their workplace, and also constantly comparing themselves with others, displaying intense envy for others' success in life.
G. In actuality, most patients would present with a mix of both "overt" and "covert" variants, or their dominant presentation usually changes with life circumstances and stressors. For example, a patient might present with primarily "overt" variant symptoms throughout their 30s, with seemingly stable family life and a string of professional successes, but then gradually switch to a "covert" presentation after being laid off from a high-powered job, having settled for a lesser paying or less prestigious job, and eventually having their marriage end in divorce.

OTHER SIGNS AND SYMPTOMS
A. Given the wide spectrum of presentation between the "overt" and "covert" variants, it is important for the APRN to assess severity not purely based on the functional level of the patient.
   1. As the severity of the illness increases, aggression toward self and others might increase.
   2. Interpersonal functioning starts to deteriorate.
   3. Deficits in moral functioning start to become more problematic.
B. It is quite common for the APRN to feel "excluded" and "talked at" rather than "talked to" during their evaluations and sessions with these patients. As part of this phenomenon, the patient might not appear to respond to what the APRN is saying, could simply not acknowledge a statement/question from the APRN, or could redirect the conversation altogether.
C. Given that high-functioning patients rarely come to the office of their own accord, the APRN might miss the diagnosis during their initial evaluation. However, over time, narcissistic traits and behaviors will start to display themselves, which should prompt the APRN to rethink their differential diagnosis.
   1. Common examples of these revolve around traits such as:
      a. Patients feeling entitled to access to the APRN even though they were late for their appointments
      b. Patients, after not being able to get what they wanted from the APRN, openly questioning the competency of the APRN or clinic staff
         i. For example, the patient might oscillate between over-idealization and devaluation of treatment providers. They may exclaim on the first meeting, "You are the best doctor ever, the only one that really got me!" but when the patient disagrees with the clinical assessment later on in treatment, the patient will become agitated and enraged. It is not unusual for the patient with narcissistic personality disorder to question the healthcare provider's background and qualifications, including education, ethnicity, and place of birth.

SUBJECTIVE DATA
A. The APRN should identify the important relationships in the patient's life and explore how the patient feels and thinks about each of them. Collateral information from family and friends may be needed in this case. Patients with this disorder display poor empathic abilities and at times manipulative behaviors. For the most part, functional level could be considered as inversely equating to severity of the illness.
   1. The APRN should carefully take stock of the patient's past and present functional levels in the patient's professional and personal lives in order to evaluate the current severity of illness.
   2. Establishing a baseline for further evaluations is necessary because the severity of the illness changes due to differing life circumstances and stressors.

PHYSICAL EXAMINATION
A. The APRN could perform a physical examination or refer the patient to a primary care provider to rule out medical causes of personality changes; however, a physical examination is usually not required.

DIAGNOSTIC TESTS AND SCREENING
A. No diagnostic tests are available; however, the APRN should order appropriate laboratory tests and/or imaging studies to rule out medical causes of personality changes. Urine toxicology can be useful to rule out substance contribution to the illness.
B. Structured clinical interviews remain the primary means of arriving at the diagnosis.

DIFFERENTIAL DIAGNOSES
A. Differential diagnoses include mania/hypomania, persistent depressive disorder and other affective disorders, and other personality disorders.
B. Narcissistic personality disorder is frequently comorbid with substance use disorders, bipolar disorder, and other personality disorders. Comorbidity with BPD and antisocial personality disorder usually indicates higher severity of the disease and lower functioning status.

GENERAL TREATMENTS AND INTERVENTIONS
A. There are currently no FDA-approved medications for the treatment of narcissistic personality disorder.

B. Suicidal risk is not well-understood in these patients; however, a depressed state might not necessarily be the reason suicidality develops and worsens.
  1. Suicidal risk should be assessed regularly.
  2. This is especially true if the patient is perceived to be undergoing an acute narcissistic injury, in which a perceived/real injury to the patient's sense of self results in intense shame, defeat, self-loathing, anger, and other intense feelings.
C. Once the diagnosis is made, the APRN should share the diagnosis with the patient.
  1. The APRN should conduct a thorough session of psychoeducation regarding prognosis and treatment options.
  2. There is limited research about specific psychotherapy treatment for this disorder; however, long-term psychodynamic psychotherapy and CBT may be effective.
  3. Patients with comorbid BPD or antisocial personality disorder/traits may benefit from specific therapy modalities in those disorders.
D. The APRN should not take the patient's criticisms personally but rather try to understand it as the patient's maladaptive way of managing their own distress and anxiety arising from the underlying character pathology.
E. The APRN should respond to the patient's entitlement strategically; statements such as "You are entitled to the best care that my team and I can provide" and "You deserve the best care that our hospital can provide" are such examples.
F. The APRN should also focus on treatment and management of any comorbid psychiatric conditions that the patient might have.

COMMON MEDICATIONS
A. There are very limited data on the efficacy of medications for patients diagnosed with only narcissistic personality disorder. Medication management should focus on comorbid psychiatric diagnoses.

FOLLOW-UP
A. APRNs should follow up with patients regularly to assess for severity of the disease over time, as well as for comorbid psychiatric conditions that may require treatment over time.

CONSULTATION AND REFERRALS
A. The patient should be referred to a primary care provider for management of other medical comorbidities and general health maintenance.
B. The patient should be referred to trained professionals in CBT or psychodynamic psychotherapy. In cases where the disorder is severely impairing the patient's daily functioning, the patient may be referred to a specialized treatment center for personality disorders.

INDIVIDUAL CONSIDERATIONS

Geriatrics
A. Research indicates the majority of patients do not improve later in life.

REFERENCES AND BIBLIOGRAPHY
Belcher, R., Taylor, S. T., Bido-Medina, R. O., Kreider, T. R., & Young, J. Q. (2022). Narcissistic personality disorder. In F. F. Ferri (Ed.), *Ferri's clinical advisor 2023* (pp. 1038.e8–1038.e9). Elsevier Health Sciences.
Caligor, E., Levy, K. N., & Yeomans, F. E. (2015). Narcissistic personality disorder: Diagnostic and clinical challenges. *The American Journal of Psychiatry, 172*(5), 415–422. https://doi.org/10.1176/appi.ajp.2014.14060723
Gabbard, G. O. (2022). Narcissism and suicide risk. *Annals of General Psychiatry, 21*(1), Article 3. https://doi.org/10.1186/s12991-022-00380-8
Shea, D. C (2017). *Psychiatric interviewing: The art of understanding* (3rd ed.). Elsevier.
World Health Organization. (2016). Disorders of adult personality and behaviour (F60–F69). F60.8: Other specified personality disorders. *International statistical classification of diseases* (10th rev.). https://icd.who.int/browse10/2016/en#/F60-F69
Zarnowski, O., Ziton, S., Holmberg, R., Musto, S., Riegle, S., Van Antwerp, E., & Santos-Nunez, G. (2021). Functional MRI findings in personality disorders: A review. *Journal of Neuroimaging, 31*(6), 1049–1066. https://doi.org/10.1111/jon.12924

OBSESSIVE-COMPULSIVE PERSONALITY DISORDER

DEFINITION
A. Diagnostic criteria include the following:
  1. The general criteria for personality disorder must be met.
  2. At least four of the following must be present:
    a. Feelings of excessive doubt and caution
    b. Preoccupation with details, rules, lists, order, organization, or schedule
    c. Perfectionism that interferes with task completion
    d. Excessive conscientiousness and scrupulousness
    e. Undue preoccupation with productivity to the exclusion of pleasure and interpersonal relationships
    f. Excessive pedantry and adherence to social conventions
    g. Rigidity and stubbornness
    h. Unreasonable insistence that others submit to exactly their way of doing things or unreasonable reluctance to allow others to do things

INCIDENCE AND PREVALENCE
A. General population prevalence is 3% to 8%, suggesting that obsessive-compulsive personality disorder is the most prevalent personality disorder in the general population.

PATHOGENESIS
A. Pathogenesis is unclear with limited research, likely with moderate genetic influence with multifactorial and heterogeneous factors. It has been suggested that genetics explain approximately 27% of the variance in the disorder.

PREDISPOSING FACTORS
A. Predisposing factors are unclear with limited research; however, parental overcontrol, learned compulsive behavior, and reinforced hyper-responsibility have been suggested to be associated with the disorder.

COMMON COMPLAINTS
A. Given that the symptoms experienced by the patient with obsessive-compulsive personality disorder are mostly ego-syntonic, it is likely the patient would not directly have any complaints relating to themselves, but rather report difficulties with others around the patient and/or paraphrase other people's complaints about the patient.
B. Due to preoccupation with details, the patient might report, "Other people say I often miss the point" or "miss the big picture" of what the patient/group is trying to accomplish.
  1. Extreme perfectionism might also result in tasks/jobs not being completed on time, but patients might report it as "I needed to do it the right way."

2. The patient's sense of perfectionism would also lead to difficulty in delegating tasks to others, insisting that other people "don't know how to do it the right way."
3. The patient's excessive devotion to work could be expressed in terms of actual hours of work or it might come at the expense of underdeveloped friendships/relationships.
4. The patient's inflexibility will be displayed in multiple areas, including work and personal life, but will also be present in the patient's moral principles in terms of an overdeveloped sense of justice, similar to dichotomous or black-and-white thinking.

OTHER SIGNS AND SYMPTOMS
A. The patient might present for treatment of intense "anxiety" upon further evaluation, and the APRN may find that the patient does indeed have high anxiety, but it is primarily associated with the above-reported symptoms. For example, the patient could say, "I feel really anxious when I can't finish doing things at work, or projects at home," but on further clarification the anxiety may be more related to having to "perfect" what may seem acceptable to most people.

SUBJECTIVE DATA
A. Patients with obsessive-compulsive personality disorder are generally considered to be higher functioning than those with other personality disorders; the APRN may find that these patients have successful careers and fulfilling personal lives.
B. Patients with this disorder may not necessarily view the above symptoms as detrimental to their well-being or professional success. The APRN should explore further if symptoms are actively disrupting/interfering with the patients' lives and their relationships with other people.

PHYSICAL EXAMINATION
A. The APRN could perform a physical examination or refer the patient to a primary care provider to rule out medical causes of personality changes; however, a physical examination is usually not required.

DIAGNOSTIC TESTS AND SCREENING
A. A commonly used screening test is the Yale-Brown Obsessive Compulsive Scale (Y-BOCS).
  1. Identifies the patient's obsessions and compulsions
  2. Establishes a timeline for the current symptoms
  3. Quantifies the intrusiveness of the symptoms on the patient's activities of daily living
B. No diagnostic tests are available; however, the APRN should order appropriate laboratory tests and/or imaging studies to rule out medical causes of personality changes.
C. Urine toxicology can be useful to rule out substance contribution to the illness.
D. Structured clinical interviews remain the primary means of arriving at the diagnosis.

DIFFERENTIAL DIAGNOSES
A. Differential diagnoses include obsessive-compulsive disorder, autism spectrum disorder, anxiety disorder, and other affective disorders.
B. Common psychiatric comorbid diagnoses include obsessive-compulsive disorder, eating disorders, anxiety disorders, panic disorder, social phobia, and substance use disorder.

PLAN
A. Special consideration should be given to either ruling out or identifying comorbid obsessive-compulsive disorder given possible similar presentation of symptoms on the surface.
  1. In obsessive-compulsive personality disorders, the patient's symptoms are mostly egosyntonic.
  2. This differs from obsessive-compulsive disorder in which the symptoms are mostly egodystonic to the patient.

GENERAL TREATMENTS AND INTERVENTIONS
A. There are no FDA-approved medications for the treatment of obsessive-compulsive personality disorder.
B. Once the diagnosis is made, the APRN should share the diagnosis with the patient, and a thorough session of psychoeducation should be provided regarding prognosis and treatment options. There is limited research about specific psychotherapy treatment for this disorder, but uncontrolled treatment trials seem to indicate that psychodynamic psychotherapy, CBT, and/or DBT could be helpful to the patient.
C. The APRN should also focus on treatment and management of any comorbid psychiatric conditions that the patient might have.

COMMON MEDICATIONS
A. Medication management should primarily focus on treating comorbid psychiatric conditions as there are no established or FDA-approved medications for symptoms of obsessive-compulsive personality disorder.
B. Preliminary evidence from two randomized controlled studies suggests that citalopram and fluvoxamine might have fair efficacy.

FOLLOW-UP
A. APRNs should follow up with patients regularly to assess for severity of the disease over time, as well as for comorbid psychiatric conditions that may require treatment over time.

CONSULTATION AND REFERRALS
A. The patient should be referred to a primary care provider for management of other medical comorbidities and general health maintenance.
B. The patient should be referred to psychodynamic psychotherapy, CBT, and/or DBT. In cases where the disorder is severely impairing the patient's daily functioning, the patient may be referred to a specialized treatment center for personality disorders.

INDIVIDUAL CONSIDERATIONS

Teens With Obsessive-Compulsive Disorder Versus Obsessive-Compulsive Personality Disorder
A. Having uncertainties in thoughts, especially with LGBTQ+ teens, related to sexuality, sexual identities, body changes, questions of religion and morality, and shifts in personal responsibilities
B. Possibly appearing to excessively go over homework, focusing on mental and academic rituals
C. Teen included as a partner in treatment and tools for recovery, with treatments including:
  1. Mindfulness training
  2. CBT
  3. Exposure with response prevention

Geriatrics
A. There is some evidence to suggest that this disorder might worsen over time or manifest later in life.

REFERENCES AND BIBLIOGRAPHY

Finch, E. F., Choi-Kain, L. W., Iliakis, E. A., Eisen, J. L., & Pinto, A. (2021). Good psychiatric management for obsessive–compulsive personality disorder. *Current Behavioral Neuroscience Reports, 8*, 160–171. https://link.springer.com/article/10.1007/s40473-021-00239-4

Gecaite-Stonciene, J., Williams, T., Lochner, C., Hoffman, J., & Stein, D. J. (2022). Efficacy and tolerability of pharmacotherapy for obsessive-compulsive personality disorder: A systematic review of randomized controlled trials. *Expert Opinion on Pharmacotherapy, 23*(11), 1351–1358. https://doi.org/10.1080/14656566.2022.2100695

Marincowitz, C., Lochner, C., & Stein, D. J. (2022). The neurobiology of obsessive-compulsive personality disorder: A systematic review. *CNS Spectrums, 27*(6), 1–12. https://doi.org/10.1017/S1092852921000754

Shea, D. C. (2017). *Psychiatric interviewing: The art of understanding* (3rd ed.). Elsevier.

World Health Organization. (2016). Disorders of adult personality and behaviour (F60–F69). F60.8: Other specified personality disorders. *International statistical classification of diseases* (10th rev.). https://icd.who.int/browse10/2016/en#/F60-F69

OTHER SPECIFIC PERSONALITY DISORDERS

DEFINITION

A. Applicable to and inclusive of the following:
  1. Eccentric personality disorder
  2. Haltlose type personality disorder
  3. Immature personality disorder
  4. Passive–aggressive personality disorder
  5. Psychoneurotic personality disorder
  6. Self-defeating personality disorder

B. Diagnostic criteria include the following:
  1. The general criteria for personality disorder must be met.
  2. Patients exhibit a personality disorder characterized by an indirect resistance to demands for adequate social and occupational performance; anger and opposition to authority and the expectations of others are expressed covertly by obstructionism, procrastination, stubbornness, dawdling, forgetfulness, and intentional inefficiency.

INCIDENCE AND PREVALENCE

A. The illness is poorly defined/researched with unknown prevalence.

PATHOGENESIS

A. The illness is poorly defined/researched with unclear pathogenesis.

PREDISPOSING FACTORS

A. The illness is poorly defined/researched with unclear risk factors.

COMMON COMPLAINTS

A. With regard to haltlose personality disorder, some commonly described features include:
  1. Living in the present only with no interest in the future and no hold in the past
  2. Possibly being at the mercy of the environment and easily persuaded
  3. Possibly exhibiting sociopathic traits with no sincere sense of remorse and inability to learn from experience
  4. Possibly exhibiting histrionic traits with pleasant but superficial affect

B. With regard to immature personality disorder, the patient may:
  1. Exhibit frequently irresponsible behaviors
  2. Be often unable to fulfill their obligations
  3. Be prone to act before thinking
  4. Have labile affect and mood swings
  5. Have emotional and behavioral levels that are inappropriate and unstable for their age group and cultural/educational levels, as well as fleeting remorse or guilt

C. Patients with passive–aggressive personality disorder may exhibit the following symptoms:
  1. Procrastinates and postpones completing routine tasks that need to be done, especially those that others seek to have completed
  2. Protests, without justification, that others make unreasonable demands of them
  3. Becomes sulky, irritable, or argumentative when asked to do something they do not want to do
  4. Unreasonably criticizes or scorns people in positions of authority
  5. Works deliberately slowly or does a poor job on tasks that they really do not want to do
  6. Obstructs the efforts of others by failing to do their share of the work
  7. Avoids obligations by claiming to have forgotten

D. According to the definitions that were proposed to *DSM-III-R* (American Psychiatric Association, 1987) for further review, a patient with self-defeating personality disorder may exhibit the following features:
  1. Chooses people and situations that lead to disappointment, failure, or mistreatment even when better options are clearly available
  2. Rejects or makes ineffective attempts of others to help them
  3. Following positive personal events (e.g., new achievement), responds with depression, guilt, or a behavior that produces pain (e.g., an accident)
  4. Incites angry or rejecting responses from others and then feels hurt, defeated, or humiliated (e.g., makes fun of spouse in public, provoking an angry retort, then feels devastated)
  5. Rejects opportunities for pleasure or is reluctant to acknowledge enjoying themselves (despite having adequate social skills and the capacity for pleasure)
  6. Fails to accomplish tasks crucial to their personal objectives despite having demonstrated ability to do so (e.g., helps fellow students write papers, but is unable to write their own)
  7. Uninterested in or rejects people who consistently treat them well
  8. Engages in excessive self-sacrifice that is unsolicited by the intended recipients of the sacrifice
  9. May often avoid or undermine pleasurable experiences

E. This disorder was entirely excluded from *DSM-IV* (American Psychiatric Association, 1994) and all subsequent publications.

F. Little research or clinical information can be found directly for eccentric personality disorder and psychoneurotic personality disorder.

PHYSICAL EXAMINATION

A. The APRN could perform a physical examination or refer the patient to a primary care provider to rule out medical causes of personality changes; however, a physical examination is usually not required.

DIAGNOSTIC TESTS AND SCREENING
A. No diagnostic tests are available; however, the APRN should order appropriate laboratory tests and/or imaging studies to rule out medical causes of personality changes. Urine toxicology can be useful to rule out substance contribution to the illness.
B. Structured clinical interviews remain the primary means of arriving at the diagnosis.

DIFFERENTIAL DIAGNOSES
A. Differential diagnoses include other personality disorders, affective disorders, anxiety disorders, substance use disorder, and medical etiologies affecting personality changes.

GENERAL TREATMENTS AND INTERVENTIONS
A. There are currently no FDA-approved medications for the treatment of other specific personality disorders.
B. Once the diagnosis is made, the APRN should share the diagnosis with the patient, and a thorough session of psychoeducation should be provided regarding prognosis and treatment options.
  1. There is limited research about specific psychotherapy treatment for this disorder; however, long-term psychodynamic psychotherapy may be effective.
  2. Patients with comorbid BPD or antisocial personality disorder/traits may benefit from specific therapy modalities in those disorders.
C. The APRN should also focus on treatment and management of any comorbid psychiatric conditions that the patient might have.

COMMON MEDICATIONS
A. There are very limited data on the efficacy of medications for patients diagnosed with only other specific personality disorders. Medication management should focus on comorbid psychiatric diagnoses.

FOLLOW-UP
A. APRNs should follow up with patients regularly to assess for severity of the disease over time, as well as for comorbid psychiatric conditions that may require treatment over time.

CONSULTATION AND REFERRALS
A. The patient should be referred to a primary care provider for management of other medical comorbidities and general health maintenance.
B. The patient should be referred to CBT or psychodynamic psychotherapy. In cases where the disorder is severely impairing the patient's daily functioning, the patient may be referred to a specialized treatment center for personality disorders.

REFERENCES AND BIBLIOGRAPHY
Almeida, F., Ribeiro, P., & Moreira, D. (2019). Immature personality disorder: Contribution to the definition of this personality. *Clinical Neuroscience & Neurological Research International Journal*, 2(2), 180013. https://academicstrive.com/CNNRIJ/CNNRIJ180013.pdf
American Psychiatric Association. (1987). *Diagnostic and statistical manual of mental disorders* (3rd ed., text rev.).
American Psychiatric Association. (1994). *Diagnostic and statistical manual of mental disorders* (4th ed.).
Gama Marques, J. (2019). Pharmacogenetic testing for the guidance of psychiatric treatment of a schizoaffective patient with haltlose personality disorder. *CNS Spectrums*, 24(2), 227–228. https://doi.org/10.1017/S1092852917000669
World Health Organization. (2016). Disorders of adult personality and behaviour (F60–F69). F60.8: Other specified personality disorders. *International statistical classification of diseases* (10th rev.). https://icd.who.int/browse10/2016/en#/F60-F69

PARANOID PERSONALITY DISORDER

DEFINITION
A. Diagnostic criteria include the following:
  1. The general criteria for personality disorder must be met.
  2. At least four of the following must be present:
     a. Excessive sensitivity to setbacks and rebuffs
     b. Tendency to bear grudges persistently (e.g., inability to forgive insults, injuries, or slights)
     c. Suspiciousness and a pervasive tendency to distort experience by misconstruing the neutral or friendly actions of others as hostile or contemptuous
     d. Combative and tenacious sense of personal rights out of keeping with the actual situation
     e. Recurrent suspicions, without justification, regarding sexual fidelity of spouse or sexual partner
     f. Persistent self-referential attitude, associated particularly with excessive self-importance
     g. Preoccupation with unsubstantiated "conspiratorial" explanations of events around the subject or in the world at large

INCIDENCE AND PREVALENCE
A. General population prevalence is between 1.21% and 4.4%; however, in clinical settings, it can be as high as 25%. Prevalence is also thought to be higher in men and in cultural minorities.

PATHOGENESIS
A. Paranoid personality disorder has multifactorial pathogenesis.
B. Genetic studies appear to show some relationship between PPD and schizophrenia; however, the link appears stronger to delusional disorder and affective disorders.

PREDISPOSING FACTORS
A. Predisposing factors include childhood trauma, both physical and sexual. There may be a relationship between degree of trauma and severity of PPD symptoms in adulthood.
B. Patients with brain trauma may have a likelihood of developing PPD ranging between 8.3% and 26%; PPD may be the second most common personality disorder following a traumatic brain injury.

COMMON COMPLAINTS
A. Patients often experience what is described as "personalized bias," which is a phenomenon in which patients perceive common occurrences around them to be specifically for or against them.
B. Patients also experience a high degree of "suspiciousness and hostility," with the two traits positively correlated with each other. Common complaints in this area can include "People are out to get me," or "People are always talking about me behind my back" or "plotting against me."
C. Doubts about the loyalty of friends are often found, while similar doubts in a loved one are not as prevalent.

OTHER SIGNS AND SYMPTOMS
A. Patients also experience difficulty in social activities and settings, and they typically have trouble sustaining romantic relationships. Reality testing is often mostly intact; however, the somewhat plausible paranoid thoughts about romantic partners and/or friends keep the patients from being able to trust in others.

B. Dramatic anger against others may sometimes be observed in these patients and at times accompanied by actual physical violence.

SUBJECTIVE DATA
A. Given the general mistrust patients have about everyone around them, the APRN should take care during the evaluations to attempt to establish therapeutic rapport first, rather than trying to "correct" patients' cognitive distortions, which are often egosyntonic.
    1. Often, validating the patient's feelings, such as anxiety, anger, and depressed mood, while asking them to clarify the circumstances leading to those feelings will enhance the relationship with the patient.
    2. Reflection and validation can allow for the development of more insight into the patient's cognitive distortions.
B. A comprehensive history of possible childhood trauma and brain injuries should be obtained by the APRN because they are risk factors for PPD diagnosis and possible severity of symptoms.
C. Symptoms of PPD may become more severe if the patient experiences sensory impairment, such as hearing loss or visual impairment.

PHYSICAL EXAMINATION
A. The APRN could perform a physical examination or refer the patient to a primary care provider to rule out medical causes of personality changes; however, a physical examination is usually not required.

DIAGNOSTIC TESTS AND SCREENING
A. No diagnostic tests are available; however, the APRN should order appropriate laboratory tests and/or imaging studies to rule out medical causes of personality changes. Urine toxicology can be useful to rule out substance contribution to the illness.
B. Screening tools include the Paranoid Personality Disorder Features Questionnaire and the Ambiguous Intentions Hostility Questionnaire; however, they are not widely used.

DIFFERENTIAL DIAGNOSES
A. Differential diagnoses include the following:
    1. Schizophrenia or other psychotic spectrum disorders
    2. Affective disorders with psychosis
    3. Delusional disorder
    4. PTSD
    5. Other personality disorders
B. An estimated 75% of patients with PPD have a comorbid personality disorder, with avoidant personality disorder, BPD, and narcissistic personality disorder being the most common.

PLAN
A. Foster a supportive environment and establish therapeutic rapport with the patient; given the patient's general mistrust of others, this first step alone could prove therapeutic to the patient.
B. Rule out psychotic symptoms that may be due to other psychotic disorders, bipolar disorder, affective disorders with psychosis, and/or substance use disorder. Establish if there are any comorbid psychiatric disorders that should be concurrently treated alongside PPD. Obtaining collateral information from the patient's loved ones may be helpful in this regard.

GENERAL TREATMENTS AND INTERVENTIONS
A. There are currently no FDA-approved medications for the treatment of PPD.
B. Once the diagnosis is made, the APRN should share the diagnosis with the patient and provide a thorough session of psychoeducation regarding prognosis and treatment options.
    1. Research regarding PPD-specific psychotherapy treatment options is currently very limited. That said, CBT, psychodynamic therapy, and interpersonal psychotherapy may be valid approaches to treatment.
C. The APRN should focus on treatment and management of any comorbid psychiatric conditions that the patient might have.

COMMON MEDICATIONS
A. The primary focus of medication management should be on treating comorbid psychiatric conditions. Currently, there are no established or FDA-approved medications for symptoms of PPD.
B. APRNs may consider using antipsychotic medications given that PPD's paranoia borders with psychotic symptoms. However, there is little evidence to suggest this is an effective way to treat non–psychosis-based paranoia. The only likely clinically justified use of antipsychotic medication is the patient's overt aggression toward others. The use of a mood stabilizer can also be considered in those cases. In this regard, the healthcare provider is using medications for symptom management, not treatment of the diagnosis.
C. If the patient continues to experience overt anxiety or affective symptoms resulting from exacerbation of PPD, despite other comorbid psychiatric conditions having been properly addressed by the APRN, antidepressant medications may be considered.

FOLLOW-UP
A. APRNs should follow up with patients regularly to assess for severity of PPD over time, as well as for comorbid psychiatric conditions that may require treatment.

CONSULTATION AND REFERRALS
A. The patient should be referred for individual psychotherapy and perhaps group-based therapy.
    1. Trauma-based therapy may be more helpful if the patient has a history of childhood trauma.
    2. If the patient has a history of traumatic brain injury or suspected other brain injuries, referral to a neurologist should be made.
B. The patient should be referred to a primary care provider for ongoing management of other medical comorbidities and general health maintenance.

INDIVIDUAL CONSIDERATIONS

Geriatrics
A. When being admitted to a long-term care facility, the older patient may complain of being "held against my will." In this way, the patient's paranoia may become more pronounced.

REFERENCES AND BIBLIOGRAPHY
Bangash, A. (2020). Personality disorders in later life: Epidemiology, presentation and management. *British Journal of Psychiatry Advances, 26*(4), 208–18. https://doi.org/10.1192/bja.2020.16

Blais, M. A., Smallwood, P., Groves, J. E., Rivas-Vazquez, R. A., & Hopwood, C. J. (2016). Personality and personality disorders. In T. A. Stern (Ed.), *Massachusetts general hospital comprehensive clinical psychiatry* (2nd ed., pp. 433–444.e5). Elsevier. https://www.clinicalkey.com/#!/content/book/3-s2.0-B9780323295079000391

Lee, R. (2017). Mistrustful and misunderstood: A review of paranoid personality disorder. *Current Behavioral Neuroscience Reports*, 4(2), 151–165. https://doi.org/10.1007/s40473-017-0116-7

Lewis, K. C., & Ridenour, J. M. (2020). Paranoid personality disorder. In V. Zeigler-Hill & T. K. Shackelford (Eds.), *Encyclopedia of personality and individual differences* (2nd ed., pp. 3413–3421). Springer Publishing Company. https://doi.org/10.1007/978-3-319-24612-3_615

Shea, D. C. (2017). *Psychiatric interviewing: The art of understanding* (3rd ed.). Elsevier.

World Health Organization. (2016). Disorders of adult personality and behaviour (F60–F69). F60.8: Other specified personality disorders. *International statistical classification of diseases* (10th rev.). https://icd.who.int/browse10/2016/en#/F60-F69

PERSONALITY DISORDER, UNSPECIFIED

DEFINITION
A. Diagnostic criteria include the following:
  1. The general criteria for personality disorder must be met.
  2. The patient does not meet the criteria for other personality disorders.

INCIDENCE AND PREVALENCE
A. General population prevalence is suggested to be between 3% and 6%.

PATHOGENESIS
A. The illness is poorly defined/researched with unclear pathogenesis.

PREDISPOSING FACTORS
A. The illness is poorly defined/researched with unclear risk factors.

COMMON COMPLAINTS
A. Patients would commonly exhibit a combination of character traits, signs, and symptoms, and a history resembling a mix of other defined personality disorders discussed in this chapter, but would not meet the full criteria for diagnosis for any of them.

SUBJECTIVE DATA
A. Since patients might have signs and symptoms across various defined personality disorders, collateral information may be necessary to fully rule out a more specific personality disorder.

PHYSICAL EXAMINATION
A. The APRN could perform a physical examination or refer the patient to a primary care provider to rule out medical causes of personality changes; however, a physical examination is usually not required.

DIAGNOSTIC TESTS AND SCREENING
A. No diagnostic tests are available; however, the APRN should order appropriate laboratory tests and/or imaging studies to rule out medical causes of personality changes. Urine toxicology can be useful to rule out substance contribution to the illness.
B. Structured clinical interviews remain the primary means of arriving at the diagnosis.

DIFFERENTIAL DIAGNOSES
A. Differential diagnoses include other personality disorders, affective disorders, anxiety disorders, substance use disorder, and medical etiologies affecting personality changes.

GENERAL TREATMENTS AND INTERVENTIONS
A. There are currently no FDA-approved medications for the treatment of personality disorder, unspecified.
B. Once the diagnosis is made, the APRN should share the diagnosis with the patient and a thorough session of psychoeducation should be provided regarding prognosis and treatment options. There is limited research about specific psychotherapy treatment for this disorder; however, long-term psychodynamic psychotherapy may be effective.
C. The APRN should also focus on treatment and management of any comorbid psychiatric conditions that the patient might have.

COMMON MEDICATIONS
A. There are very limited data on the efficacy of medications for patients diagnosed with only personality disorder, unspecified.
B. Medication management should focus on comorbid psychiatric diagnoses.

FOLLOW-UP
A. APRNs should follow up with patients regularly to assess for severity of the disease over time, as well as for comorbid psychiatric conditions that may require treatment over time.

CONSULTATION AND REFERRALS
A. The patient should be referred to a primary care provider for management of other medical comorbidities and general health maintenance.
B. The patient should be referred to specialists trained in CBT or psychodynamic psychotherapy. In cases where the disorder is severely impairing the patient's daily functioning, the patient may be referred to a specialized treatment center for personality disorders.

REFERENCES AND BIBLIOGRAPHY
Verhuel, R., & Widiger, T. A. (2004). A meta-analysis of the prevalence and usage of the Personality Disorder Not Otherwise Specified (PDNOS) diagnosis. *Journal of Personality Disorders*, 18(4), 309–319. https://doi.org/10.1521/pedi.18.4.309.40350

World Health Organization. (2016). Disorders of adult personality and behaviour (F60–F69). F60.8: Other specified personality disorders. *International statistical classification of diseases* (10th rev.). https://icd.who.int/browse10/2016/en#/F60-F69

SCHIZOID PERSONALITY DISORDER

DEFINITION
A. Diagnostic criteria include the following:
  1. The general criteria for personality disorder must be met.
  2. At least four of the following criteria must be present:
     a. Pleasure provided by few, if any, activities
     b. Emotional coldness, detachment, or flattened affectivity
     c. Limited capacity to express warm, tender feelings or anger toward others
     d. Indifferent to either praise or criticism from others
     e. Little interest in having sexual experiences with another person (taking age into account)
     f. Almost always chooses solitary activities
     g. Excessive preoccupation with fantasy and introspection
     h. Neither desires, nor has, any close friends or confiding relationships (or has only one)
     i. Marked insensitivity to prevailing social norms and conventions; if these are not followed, it is unintentional

INCIDENCE AND PREVALENCE
A. General population prevalence is less than 1%, with no observed difference in frequency between males and females.

PATHOGENESIS
A. Schizoid personality disorder has multifactorial pathogenesis.
B. Twin studies using self-report questionnaires have estimated heritability to be around 30%. It is unclear how much environmental factors contribute to the etiology of the disease.

PREDISPOSING FACTORS
A. The illness is poorly defined/researched with unclear risk factors.

COMMON COMPLAINTS
A. The patient may not actually have many complaints relating to the diagnosis.
   1. In fact, given that many of the pathologies are ego syntonic in nature, these patients rarely present to APRNs of their own volition.
   2. The times patients do present to the APRN's office are often prompted by family members or loved ones and/or in relation to comorbid psychiatric conditions.

OTHER SIGNS AND SYMPTOMS
A. Isolation is a cardinal feature of this disorder, where the patient maintains few to no close relationships/friendships.
B. Patients often present with blunted affect, muted emotional responses, and little desire for sexual activity with a partner.
C. If the patient is employed, the occupation is often one that requires little to no human interaction.

SUBJECTIVE DATA
A. Given the fact a patient with this diagnosis would have few complaints of their own, it is therefore important for the APRN to obtain collateral information from people around the patient to gather more history and to confirm the diagnosis.

PHYSICAL EXAMINATION
A. The APRN could perform a physical examination or refer the patient to a primary care provider to rule out medical causes of personality changes; however, a physical examination is usually not required.

DIAGNOSTIC TESTS AND SCREENING
A. No diagnostic tests are available; however, the APRN should order appropriate laboratory tests and/or imaging studies to rule out medical causes of personality changes. Urine toxicology can be useful to rule out substance contribution to the illness.
B. Structured clinical interviews remain the primary means of arriving at the diagnosis.

DIFFERENTIAL DIAGNOSES
A. Differential diagnoses include schizophrenia or other psychotic spectrum disorders, autism spectrum disorder, affective disorders, schizotypal disorder, other personality disorders such as PPD, avoidant personality disorder, and obsessive-compulsive personality disorder.
B. It is important to note the historical comparison between schizoid personality disorder and schizotypal disorder as both share multiple similar symptoms and signs and have been described together in the past, along with schizophrenia, as being along a similar spectrum of psychotic symptoms.
   1. Although historically schizotypal disorder was considered part of personality disorder diagnoses, in the 10th revision of the *ICD* (ICD-10; World Health Organization, 1990), schizotypal disorder is not classified as such and instead is part of psychotic disorders.
   2. Schizotypal disorder can be distinguished by the patient's characteristic "magical" or eccentric thinking processes.
   3. Patients with PPD are often resentful toward people and can express overt anger, as opposed to the aloofness of schizoid personality disorder. In patients with avoidant personality disorder, social isolation is characterized by a fear of rejection by others, whereas patients with schizoid personality disorder would express indifference to such rejection/acceptance by others.

PLAN
A. Rule out the existence of other psychiatric disorders.
   1. Establish if there are any comorbid psychiatric disorders that should be concurrently treated alongside schizoid personality disorder.
   2. Obtaining collateral information from the patient's loved ones is likely important in this regard.
B. Given the egosyntonic nature of the patient's symptoms, the patient may see little reason to continue to follow up with the APRN.
C. Patient and family education is important in continuing treatment, especially to impress upon the family the pervasive and chronic nature of the disease.
   1. Family education is probably the most likely way the patient will continue to receive positive support going forward.
   2. Familial understanding of the disease process/prognosis can temper frustrations in seeming lack of clinical progress in the patient, creating a more supportive environment.

GENERAL TREATMENTS AND INTERVENTIONS
A. There are no FDA-approved medications for the treatment of schizoid personality disorder.
B. Once the diagnosis is made, the APRN should share the diagnosis with the patient, and a thorough session of psychoeducation should be provided regarding prognosis and treatment options.
C. There has been very little research into specific psychotherapy treatment options; however, some studies have suggested psychotherapy can help improve the isolation experienced by the patients.
D. Focus on symptom treatment and management of any comorbid psychiatric conditions that the patient might have.

COMMON MEDICATIONS
A. Medication management should primarily focus on treating comorbid psychiatric conditions as there are no established or FDA-approved medications for symptoms of schizoid personality disorder.
B. By definition of the disease, the patient experiences few emotional fluctuations, is usually not aggressive, and has few to no psychotic symptoms. Therefore, the patient lacks any traditional targets of psychotropic medications, and addition of them is unlikely to be helpful.

FOLLOW-UP
A. APRNs should regularly follow up with patients to assess severity of the disease over time, as well as identify any other comorbid psychiatric conditions that may require treatment over time.

CONSULTATION AND REFERRALS

A. Patient referrals can be made for individual psychotherapy, possibly CBT. Behavioral changes to decrease social isolation would be the primary goal.

B. Patient referral to a primary care provider for management of other medical comorbidities and general health maintenance is appropriate.

INDIVIDUAL CONSIDERATIONS

Geriatrics

A. Patients can become more eccentric and withdrawn in later life. Given the patient's desire for social isolation, a long-term facility or hospital setting where the patient will need to share personal spaces may be painful for them, prompting them to leave the setting as soon as possible.

REFERENCES AND BIBLIOGRAPHY

Bangash, A. (2020). Personality disorders in later life: Epidemiology, presentation and management. *British Journal of Psychiatry Advances, 26*(4), 208–18. https://doi.org/10.1192/bja.2020.16

Fariba, K. A., Madhanagopal, N., & Gupta, V. (2024, March 1). *Schizoid personality disorder*. StatPearls Publishing. https://www.ncbi.nlm.nih.gov/books/NBK559234

World Health Organization. (2019). *International statistical classification of diseases and related health problems* (10th rev). https://icd.who.int/browse10/2019/en

World Health Organization. (2016). Disorders of adult personality and behaviour (F60–F69). F60.8: Other specified personality disorders. *International statistical classification of diseases* (10th rev.). https://icd.who.int/browse10/2016/en#/F60-F69

14 SLEEP–WAKE DISORDERS

Rosa Landinez

INTRODUCTION

Sleep is a fundamental part of being human. Sleep restores the human body, aids in human cell division and regeneration, and creates the environment for necessary homeostasis. Humans spend approximately 30% of their lifetime sleeping. For individuals who suffer from sleep disorders, loss of adequate sleep creates a detrimental cascade of problems. These problems lead to reduced life expectancy, increased medical and psychological issues, and diminished overall quality of life. Early intervention is critical as, left untreated, sleep disorders have been associated with the development of other chronic health issues such as heart disease and diabetes. By completing thorough sleep disorder assessments, patient treatment can be initiated as soon as possible. When a diagnosis is made, treatment of sleep disorders can be initiated, leading to recovery and an improved sleep prognosis for the patient.

AN OVERVIEW OF SLEEP DISORDERS

DEFINITION

A. A sleep disorder is any ongoing pattern of disruption to a person's sleep, which may affect the amount, quality, and timing of sleep, as well as impact activities of daily living.
  1. Sleep problems can present in all age and socio demographic groups.
     a. Difficulty falling asleep is more common in late adolescence and young adulthood.
     b. Difficulty remaining asleep is more common with middle age and older adults.
B. The biological process of sleep is complex and involves functions of the brain, heart, lung, metabolic, and musculoskeletal system.
  1. Brain: The glymphatic system (GS) is activated during deep sleep and serves as a brain waste management system, clearing detritus from the brain and refreshing brain functions. Disruption of the GS may be associated with disorders causing neurodegeneration (e.g., Alzheimer disease).
  2. Heart: During light sleep, the heart, lung, and biological processes slow, which results in lower temperature and reduced heart and breathing rates. During rapid eye movement (REM) sleep, biological functions (e.g., heart and lung rates) mimic the dream content of the individual (e.g., faster if running or scared and slower for soothing and content).
  3. Metabolic: The metabolic processes during sleep are shown to decrease by 5% or greater in all areas except for glucose and antioxidant capacity, which can increase by 50%.
  4. Musculoskeletal: Sleep and muscle growth and recovery are linked via the metabolism of glucose, the secretion of hormones (e.g., testosterone), and reduction in inflammation (e.g., antioxidation).
C. Sleep disorders are significantly related to medical comorbidities, onset of disease, and mental health illness.
D. Sleep disruption can occur during any of the periods of sleep, including while awake and getting ready for sleep, during REM sleep, or during non-rapid eye movement (NREM) sleep.

PREDISPOSING FACTORS

A. Risk factors for sleep disorders may be social, physical, and behavioral, and can include the following:
  1. Physical pain, chronic pain, headaches
  2. Sleep apnea and other medical conditions (e.g., obesity)
  3. Depression, anxiety, mania, hypomania, and other psychiatric disorders
  4. Environmental issues preventing sleep (e.g., noise, light)
  5. Behavioral and lifestyle factors (e.g., smoking, inactivity, alcohol consumption)

COMMON COMPLAINTS

A. Sleep disorder symptoms are divided into episodic, persistent, and recurrent, and include the following:
  1. Excessive tiredness during the day, lack of concentration
  2. Diminished social functioning
  3. Frequent naps
  4. Risky behaviors from a lack of restorative sleep, such as those that impact driving or using machinery at work

DIAGNOSTIC TESTS AND SCREENING

A. Patient screening and conducting a complete, comprehensive assessments of patients' sleep abnormalities and sleep disorders are always indicated if sleep disorder is being considered. The use of sleep screening data can help identify differential diagnoses.
B. Screening also supports the development of appropriate treatment plans.
C. Tests for sleep disorders include the following:
  1. Polysomnography (PSG): PSG requires an overnight at a sleep center. The stay is monitored by a sleep technician and includes monitoring of EEG, EKG, oxygen (O_2) levels, muscle movement, and eye and extremity movements.
  2. Overnight oximetry: This test requires overnight use of pulse oximetry probe; it can be done at home or at a medical center.
  3. Titration study: This test is frequently done during the PSG. The patient begins with a continuous positive airway pressure (CPAP) machine on low levels of pressure. Pressure is increased to determine the level of pressure required for deterring sleep apnea.
  4. Multiple sleep latency testing (MSLT): MSLT is a nap study that is similar to PSG. A person is given multiple opportunities to nap every 2 hours over a 10-hour period following PSG to assess daytime sleepiness.
  5. Actigraphy: Wristwatch device is used to assess circadian rhythms and sleep–wake cycles. Data obtained are usually correlated with a sleep diary.

6. Sleep diary: The patient records bedtime and waketimes over a period of weeks. The patient may be required to record intake of caffeine, alcohol, or medications.
7. Home study: At-home technologies that record breathing rates, pulse O_2, heart rate, abdominal movement, and chest movements are used, although not as accurate as PSG.

CLASSIFICATION OF SLEEP DISORDERS

Diagnostic Classification

A. Sleep disorders are divided into seven diagnostic categories according to the *International Classification of Sleep Disorders, Third Edition, Text Revision* (*ICSD-3-TR*; American Academy of Sleep Medicine [AASM], 2023). The classification of sleep disorders is based on the symptomatology reported by the patient.
B. The following are the six categories of sleep disorders:
1. Insomnia
2. Sleep-associated breathing disorders
3. Central disorders of hypersomnolence
4. Circadian rhythm sleep–wake disorders
5. Parasomnia
6. Sleep-related movement disorders
7. Other sleep disorders

C. The diagnostic categories can be further subdivided into transient, short-term, and chronic.
1. Transient sleep disorder: This type of sleep disorder is related to a specific change in the circadian rhythm, such as jet lag or an unexpected temporary change in the work schedule.
   a. It can also be associated with psychological issues such as anxiety, increased stress, and poor coping skills.
   b. It can last a few days up to 1 week.
   c. A study of aircrew members indicated that approximately 67% reported different effects of jet lag, such as feeling tired and exhausted. They also noted that their internal clock constantly attempted to change to time zones and had difficulties regulating their normal sleep.
2. Short-term sleep disorder: This type of sleep disorder is related to trauma, changes in medical conditions, grief, and break in relationships.
   a. It can last several weeks or months; however, it can be resolved with treatment.
   b. A systematic review of research data and articles demonstrates an association between grief and sleep disturbance—the importance of early assessment and treatment made a difference in resolving the sleep disorder.
3. Chronic sleep disorders: These are sleep disturbances that have not been resolved in several months or years, and that can be debilitating to the individual suffering from them.
   a. Chronic sleep disorders can be associated with psychological or mental health issues, chronic medical conditions, uncontrolled pain, and physical discomfort.
   b. This sleep disorder must be treated to prevent further medical or psychological deterioration.

Sleep Cycles

A. The classification of sleep disorders is based on the length of time the patient has experienced issues with sleep interruption.

B. Other aspects to consider in this classification include the following:
1. Timing of sleep cycles
2. Onset of sleep
3. Duration of sleep
4. Efficiency of sleep
5. Number of times the individual wakes through the night

Sleep Stages

A. Sleep is divided into five stages: wake, N1, N2, N3, and REM.
1. The N1 to N3 stages are NREM sleep.
   a. Literature often discusses three stages of sleep as wake, NREM, and REM sleep.
2. The first stage of sleep is the initial presentation and may last 15 to 30 minutes.
   a. The person feels tired and begins to feel drowsy, and the body and muscles start to relax.
   b. The person's head begins to nod, and there is the sensation of falling asleep and the inability to keep eyes open.
3. The NREM stage can last from 30 to 80 minutes with periods of deep sleep.
   a. An individual begins complete relaxation, has difficulty with arousal, begins eye movements, and decreases body temperature and heart rate.
   b. Some parasomnias may be evident (e.g., sleep talking, sleepwalking, and vivid dreams). This NREM stage accounts for approximately 75% of the total sleep time.
   c. NREM is subdivided into three stages from N1 to N3 with various periods of arousal, and people spend most of their sleep time during N2.
   d. Individuals may complete approximately four to five cycles per night. Each sleep cycle can take between 60 minutes and 120 minutes and constitute NREM and REM.
4. The final stage of sleep is REM, which occurs approximately 90 minutes after sleep onset.
   a. This stage includes a dreaming stage, with intense eye movement and more activity in brain waves.
   b. There is easy arousal as the individual is not in a deep sleep, but reports of drowsiness and not being awake are common.

GENERAL CLINICAL PRESENTATION OF SLEEP DISORDERS

A. To diagnose sleep disorders, the clinician must include a careful review of the information collected from the patient's history. The following are two essential components:
1. The patient has issues falling asleep or staying asleep.
2. The patient reports difficulties with daytime functioning (work, home, school, and other activities).

B. Other important items to consider include irritability, mood changes, excessive daytime sleepiness, inattention, fatigue, decreased concentration, and proclivity to accidents (e.g., falling asleep while driving).

C. Sleep disorders may be considered a disability that interferes with essential daily activities.
1. The Social Security Administration (SSA) does not specifically identify sleep disorders as disabilities.
2. To qualify for SSA, the patient must provide evidence that the sleep disorder directly affects their ability for employment.

D. Sleep disorders hinder individuals from having a good quality of life and may lead to poor health outcomes and difficulties with treatment. Sleep disorders disrupt normal processes, increase mortality rate, increase levels of stress, and reduce functional abilities.

INCIDENCE

A. The incidence of sleep disorders in the United States is estimated at 35% to 50%, or 70 million people.
B. The incidence of sleep disorders increases in individuals who also have a mental health diagnosis.
   1. Approximately 40% to 50% of persons with a mental health challenge also complain of insomnia.
   2. Stress is a bidirectional variable with sleep disorders. Those with more stress commonly have fewer hours of sleep.
C. Healthy sleep is noted when individuals fall asleep with ease, do not fully wake up during the night, do not wake up too early, and feel refreshed after waking.
   1. Healthy sleep is vital to medical and physical health.
   2. Healthy sleep regulates vital human processes such as maintaining balance and regulating hormones (endocrine system), metabolism, and mood.

SLEEP PATTERNS AND SLEEP DISORDERS IN VARIOUS AGE GROUPS

A. Sleep disorders increase across age groups, with those 18 and younger in the lowest risk category and older adults (more than 65 years) at the highest risk.
B. Of persons over 65 years of age, 50% to 60% experience a sleep disorder including but not limited to sleep apnea, restless legs syndrome (RLS), and REM sleep behavior disorder.
C. Common complaints among older adults with a sleep disorder include the following:
   1. Feeling tired and sleepy during the day
   2. Impact of comorbid medical conditions and psychological problems such as depression and anxiety
   3. A decline in functioning
D. Note that many older adults interpret their sleep difficulties as part of the normal aging process and may underreport sleep disturbances to their healthcare provider.
E. Among children, the presentation of sleep disorders differs.
   1. The most common complaints by parents and caregivers are hyperactivity, irritability, and conduct disorders.
   2. The root cause of sleep disorders varies depending on the specific condition. For children and young adults, it may be related to behavioral health issues.
F. Females experience insomnia and RLS more often than males; conversely, males experience obstructive sleep apnea (OSA) more frequently than females at a ratio of 2:1.

PATHOGENESIS

A. The mechanisms of sleep disorders depend on the type of sleep disorder. The cause of sleep disorders, such as insomnia, can be related to stress, anxiety, chronic pain, or environmental factors including noise, light, or extreme temperature.
B. For sleep disorders associated with disordered breathing, the most common causes are obstruction of the upper airway, obesity, respiratory issues causing gaps in normal breathing patterns, and sleep apnea.
C. For conditions related to hypersomnolence, such as narcolepsy, sleep disorders are related to dysregulation in the central nervous system.
D. For sleep–wake disorders, the circadian rhythm is not aligned with the internal circadian rhythm during instances of jet lag disorders and night shift work.
E. The remaining types of sleep disorders are related to other medical conditions including psychiatric diagnoses and terminal illnesses.
   1. People diagnosed with a psychiatric disorder commonly have a sleep disorder.
      a. Practitioners should be vigilant to observe for any interference of a sleep disorder with the effectiveness of psychiatric treatment.
      b. Psychopharmacologic treatments may result in sleep interference and lead to poor adherence, increased risk of relapse, and other mental health setbacks.
      c. Impact may also be observed in behavioral response to treatment.
   2. There is a significant correlation between sleep disorders and psychiatric conditions among the older adults, where they may experience anxiety, depression, posttraumatic stress disorder (PTSD), and cognitive decline.
   3. Relationship between sleep disorders and psychiatric diagnoses may manifest interchangeably—individuals with psychiatric diagnoses may report co-occurring symptoms of sleep disorders and individuals with sleep disorders may report signs of psychiatric symptoms.
   4. Evidence suggests that similar mechanisms of action are shared by both psychiatric disorders and sleep disorders, enhancing the opportunity to optimize patient treatments to improve outcomes.

PREDISPOSING FACTORS

A. Age and sex appear to be predisposing factors for sleep disorders. Sleep disorders are more prevalent among females during pregnancy, menopause, and menses.
B. Sleep disorders are more prevalent among those with chronic illnesses such as arthritis, fibromyalgia, Alzheimer disease, obesity, pain, respiratory issues, menopause, chronic fatigue disorders, and substance use disorders.
C. Psychiatric illnesses such as depression and anxiety are also predisposing factors of sleep disorders. Some psychiatric medications may interfere with regular sleep cycles.
D. Specific patient behaviors may impact sleep, including the following:
   1. Excessive consumption of caffeinated beverages and alcohol, use of nicotine, and cigarette smoking
   2. Engaging in stimulating activities before going to bed
E. Environmental factors such as noise, room temperature, and light can also interfere with sleep.

COMMON COMPLAINTS

A. Common complaints are usually reported during primary care visits and may include chronic fatigue, excessive daytime sleepiness, decreased concentration, impaired daytime functioning, exhaustion, irritability, moodiness, insomnia, hypersomnia, urinary frequency, heartburn, premenstrual syndrome, and peri-/postmenopausal diaphoresis.

OTHER SIGNS AND SYMPTOMS

A. Patients also report increased pain, dysregulated body temperature, elevated heart rate related to anxiety, excessive worry related to stress, poor performance at work, tension headaches, migraines, gastrointestinal issues such as constipation and diarrhea, and safety concerns related to worries of falling asleep while operating machinery driving and during extended work hours.

SUBJECTIVE DATA

A. Detailed information should be recorded during the initial patient encounter related to sleep patterns and habits.
   1. Record patient medical history, psychiatric history, past and present, a comprehensive list of medications including all over-the-counter (OTC), complete demographic information, daily routine, exercise, work schedule, and type of work.
   2. A detailed history of sleep symptoms includes a sleep log, how long it takes to fall asleep, how many hours one sleeps, how many times one wakes up from sleep, if patient can fall asleep again, excessive daytime sleepiness, daily exercise, and intervals of time taking naps or siesta during the day.

PHYSICAL EXAMINATION

A. The physical examination includes a complete review of systems and a mental status exam.
   1. Screen for medical comorbidities.
   2. Establish baseline body mass index (BMI).
   3. Record any sexual dysfunction.
   4. Note cognitive impairments or changes in cognitive functioning.

DIAGNOSTIC TESTS AND SCREENING

A. Medical history: The nurse practitioner should screen for medical comorbidities such as hypertension, diabetes, OSA, and substance use (alcohol, stimulants, sedatives, benzodiazepines, and painkillers), and any OTC medicines.
B. Complete medical evaluation through a physical exam.
C. Sleep disorders are usually diagnosed by obtaining a comprehensive medical history and reviewing sleep diary from the patient.
D. Complete and review a 2-week sleep diary (Table 14.1).
E. Complete a psychiatric evaluation.
F. Obtain a detailed history of sleep hygiene and bedtime rituals.
G. Conduct PSG and other sleep studies.
   1. Epworth Sleepiness Scale: The Epworth Sleepiness Scale is an eight-item questionnaire that helps assess daytime sleepiness. The final score ranges from 0 to 24 points; if the final score exceeds 10, further evaluation should be done. This is a self-administered questionnaire.
   2. Fatigue Severity Scale. The Fatigue Severity Scale is a nine-item assessment tool that can help distinguish between degree of sleepiness and fatigue.
   3. Insomnia Severity Scale. This tool is helpful in monitoring insomnia severity.
H. Laboratory tests include arterial blood gas (ABG), thyroid functioning test, drug and alcohol screening, iron studies, ferritin levels, and cerebrospinal fluid (CSF), as well as MSLT.

DIFFERENTIAL DIAGNOSES

A. The differential diagnoses can be generated based on the initial presentation, chief complaint, and patient information obtained from the intake assessment. Differentials may include the following:
   1. Akathisia
   2. Neuropathy
   3. PTSD and trauma
   4. Depression
   5. Anxiety
   6. Bipolar disorder
   7. Schizophrenia
   8. Substance use disorder
   9. Opioid abuse
   10. Stimulant abuse
   11. Alcoholism
   12. Alzheimer dementia
   13. Attention deficit hyperactivity disorder (ADHD)
   14. Neurocognitive disorders
   15. Other psychiatric disorders
   16. Neurovascular disease
   17. Chronic obstructive pulmonary disease (COPD)

TABLE 14.1 SLEEP DIARY/LOG

	Day 1	Day 2	Day 3	Day 4	Day 5	Day 6	Day 7
Day of the Week							
Did you use any sleep hygiene skills before going to bed? Which one?	Yes No Which one?						
Did you take any sleep aid?	Yes No Which one?						
At what time did you go to bed?							
How long did it take you to fall asleep?							
What is the number of times you woke up during the night?							
If you woke up during the night, how long were you awake?							
At what time did you wake up?							
At what time did you get up from bed?							
Other: Is there anything else you want to include in this diary related to your sleep?							

18. Gastroesophageal reflux disease (GERD)
19. Osteoarthritis
20. Hyperthyroidism
21. Terminal illness and palliative care
22. Caffeine

GENERAL TREATMENT PLAN

A. The treatment plan will describe the actions, protocols, and steps to help the patient resolve a sleep disorder and address their concern of lack of sleep.
B. Create a list of elements that should be considered for the treatment and management of the patient's sleep disorder. The following elements should be included in the care plan:
  1. Information about the disease process
  2. Steps to diagnose and treat
  3. Summary of patient process and outcome goals
  4. Identification of treatment options
  5. Specific implementation plans
  6. Schedule for ongoing monitoring and evaluation of patient progress

C. Keep abreast of novel treatments and alternative treatment modalities as the care plan may be tailored to reflect each patient's unique treatment plan.
D. The treatment plan should be tailored to the individual patient and the type of sleep disorder.
  1. Consider the patient's sex, age, medical comorbidities, and other factors.
  2. The initial treatment plan begins with discussing the nonpharmacologic and pharmacologic treatment options with the patient to increase adherence to a plan that fits their lifestyle.
  3. Include patient education on the risks and benefits of each diagnostic and treatment option.

E. Sleep hygiene: The APRN should help the patient prepare a daily schedule with set specific times to go to bed and wake up, while avoiding alcohol, stimulants, caffeine, large quantities of liquids, or heavy meals 2 hours before bedtime. The patient should abstain from daytime naps. This daily schedule is to include weekends and holidays (Table 14.2).
  1. The patient should only go to bed when feeling sleepy and should make the room as quiet as possible, with appropriate sleep lighting.
  2. If the patient is unable to fall asleep after 20 minutes in bed, the patient should follow additional treatment options discussed in the treatment plan.

TABLE 14.2 NONPHARMACOLOGIC RECOMMENDATIONS FOR TREATMENT OF SLEEP DISORDERS

Treatment Recommendation	Objective	Instructions for Clinician
2-week sleep diary—14 days straight, including weekends	• To track the patient's sleep patterns and baseline, and remind about sleep hygiene strategies	• Carefully review this report paying attention to patterns, discrepancies, and behaviors noted and reported. • Instruct the parents to record any nighttime awakenings.
Psychoeducation	• Provide concise information on sleep, the importance of sleep, signs, and symptoms of sleep disorders, and what to report	• Review the recommended number of hours appropriate to age. • Review the importance of regular sleep time and sleep behaviors.
Sleep hygiene	• To promote good sleeping habits, such as maintaining the bedroom for sleep • Going to bed only when feeling sleepy and ready to fall asleep	• Discuss the importance of daily activities such as exercise and stimulation and avoid extraneous exercise before going to bed. • Teach patients to avoid caffeinated drinks, alcohol, or large quantities of fluids and liquids before bed. • Educate on the importance of voiding before going to bed. • Discuss the importance of sleep in development. • Discuss the importance of a consistent sleep schedule on weekends and holidays. • For children: Establish a consistent bed schedule (sleep and wake-up time) to decrease bedtime resistance. • Discuss decreased stimulation, such as environmental factors (light, noise, and room temperature) and blue light equipment, before going to bed. • Avoid using electronics or having them within reach at nighttime. • Discuss the importance of maintaining a night light in the room and near the bathroom to prevent falls, especially for older adults and for children.
Sleep restriction	• To help with sleep continuity in restorative processes and efficiency of sleeping hours	• Discuss the importance of limiting daytime naps. • Educate on how good sleep hygiene helps with restful sleep.
Relaxation, mindfulness, and/or deep-breathing exercises	• To help the patient with techniques to relax before going to bed	• Discuss the patient's preferences and include them in the treatment plan. Psychoeducation is key.
Use of cognitive behavioral therapy skills	• To help the patient identify automatic thoughts that might interfere with restful sleep	• Include cognitive behavioral therapy in the treatment plan and sleep diaries. The clinician should discuss it with the patient during follow-up visits.

3. If the patient reports a condition that is outside of the scope of the treatment plan, the APRN will initiate referrals to specialists as applicable.

F. Psychoeducation is provided to patients and significant others, where indicated, and includes the following:
1. Stimulus control
2. Relaxation training
3. Examining the association of sleep with thoughts, feelings, behaviors, attitudes, and nutrition with the patients
4. Teaching ways of reporting symptoms that will be manageable for the patient
5. Explanation of all the treatment modalities and approaches to help alleviate or resolve the symptoms
6. Allowing space for the patient to ask questions, repeat what they have learned, and clarify any misunderstandings

G. This is a unique opportunity to help the patient prepare a sleep schedule.
1. Include goals and actions or behaviors the patient can engage in to attain those sleep goals.
2. Treat the patient as a partner and provide a menu of intervention choices from which the patient can choose.

GENERAL BEHAVIORAL SUGGESTIONS FOR AMELIORATION OF SYMPTOMS

A. Providing the patient with suggested behavioral changes will increase their sense of self-efficacy in recovery from some of the symptoms of sleep disorders.
1. Suggest use of eyeshades or sleep masks.
2. Consider different types of earplugs that will be comfortable for the patient.
3. Establish a routine of sleep hygiene: reducing stimulation an hour prior to bedtime, removing electronic devices from the bedroom, reading before sleep, listening to calm music, meditation, and breathing exercises.

B. Specialized treatment plans: A variety of specialized treatment plans are available to help the APRN address the patient's sleep disorders concerns.
1. Sleep restriction therapy: The goal of sleep restriction therapy is to maximize the effectiveness of sleep. The APRN should discuss with the patient that the time spent in bed should be an interval for sleep and sex only. The patient should be discouraged from taking naps during the day and delaying sleep at night.
   a. Special considerations should be proposed if the patient takes naps during the day. Naps should be no longer than 30 minutes. The preparation of a sleep schedule is to include the total number of sleep hours, which may include activities where the patient may take short breaks.
2. Stimulus control therapy: The APRN should discuss behavioral modification strategies to increase the establishment of healthy sleep habits. The patient should avoid going to bed too early, limiting the use of electronics in bed (e.g., night table lamps, cellular telephones, laptop computers, portable radios, or any additional device that might distract the patient). The patient requires reinforcement of the importance of sleep and how environmental stimuli may interfere with normal sleep.
3. Relaxation therapy: The APRN should educate the patient on relaxation techniques to improve readiness for sleep. Relaxation therapies include deep-breathing exercises, yoga, mindfulness, aromatherapy, visualization, guided imagery, and stress relief music.

COMMON MEDICATIONS

A. Various classes of medications are used to treat sleep–wake disorders, including histamine type 1 receptor blockers, benzodiazepines, sedative-hypnotics, melatonin receptor agonists, dopamine agonists, opiates, orexin receptor antagonists, stimulants, and vitamin supplements (Table 14.3).

B. In some cases, OTCs and antidepressants are common medications for insomnia.

PATIENT TEACHING

A. Educate the patient on sleep, including the stages, and emphasize the importance of sleep in everyday life.

B. Untreated sleep disorders can be detrimental and debilitating if left untreated. The APRN should prepare a treatment plan, including the patient on every step.

TABLE 14.3 PHARMACOTHERAPY FOR TREATMENT OF SLEEP DISORDERS

Medication/Indication	Aged 10–18 Years (Youth)	Aged 19–65 Years (Adult)	Aged 66–74 Years (Older Adult)	Aged 85–99 Years (Oldest Old + Centenarians)
Drug class: hypnotic, sedative benzodiazepines (lorazepam [Ativan], clonazepam [Klonopin], temazepam [Restoril]) Used to treat insomnia, parasomnias **WARNING:** Highly addictive; should attempt other class of medications first. Use with caution in the geriatric population. Long-acting benzodiazepines should not be used in older adults as they increase the risk of fall and daytime sedation. ***Avoid in patients with OSA or chronic COPD.***	Refer to Chapter 20, "Special Considerations for Childhood and Adolescent Populations," or PDR. Often used for anxiety and panic disorder in youth; safety not established in children under 12 years old; not recommended in children	Ativan: Average dose 2–6 mg/d in divided doses Initial dose 2–3 mg/d larger dose at bedtime **CAUTION:** Pregnancy and breastfeeding, category D; not generally recommended; can be found in mother's milk if breastfeeding	Refer to Chapter 21, "Aging and Older Adult Populations," or PDR. Ativan: 1–2 mg in divided doses; larger dose at bedtime	Refer to Chapter 21, "Aging and Older Adult Populations," or PDR. **CAUTION:** Benzodiazepines increase the risk of fall and daytime sedation.

(continued)

TABLE 14.3 PHARMACOTHERAPY FOR TREATMENT OF SLEEP DISORDERS (CONTINUED)

Medication/Indication	Aged 10–18 Years (Youth)	Aged 19–65 Years (Adult)	Aged 66–74 Years (Older Adult)	Aged 85–99 Years (Oldest Old + Centenarians)
Drug class: nonbenzodiazepine hypnotic; "Z" drugs (zolpidem [Ambien], intermezzo [Ambien CR], eszopiclone [Lunesta]) Used to treat insomnia **WARNING:** Highly addictive. Medication can be given on an empty stomach and with reported rapid onset.	Close monitoring recommended; should receive lower doses; hallucinations reported in children 6–17 years old Short-term treatment of insomnia	Ambien: Average dose 10 mg at bedtime for 7–10 days (immediate-release) 12.5 mg/d at bedtime (controlled-release)	Use with caution in older adults Initial dose 5 mg (immediate-release), 6.25 mg controlled-release and 1.75 mg intermezzo May have increased risk of falls and confusion	Refer to Chapter 21, "Aging and Older Adult Populations," or PDR. Medication should be prescribed with caution to older adults and patients with history of substance use.
Drug class: melatonin receptor agonists (ramelteon [Rozerem]) Approved by the FDA for insomnia, parasomnias, and circadian rhythm sleep disorders Not habit-forming; minimal reports of side effects; Sustained-release melatonin Low to no residual drowsiness	Safety and efficacy not established in this population Refer to Chapter 20, "Special Considerations for Childhood and Adolescent Populations," or PDR.	Rozerem: Usual dose is 8 mg **CAUTION:** Pregnancy and breastfeeding, category C, and might be secreted in breastmilk	No medication adjustment necessary Increased absorption and plasma drug concentration	Refer to Chapter 21, "Aging and Older Adult Populations," or PDR. Melatonin agonists increase plasma drug concentration.
Drug class: selective H1 antagonists (doxepin [Sinequan, Silenor]) Used to treat insomnia (difficulty with sleep maintenance—Silenor only) Not habit-forming	Safety and efficacy not established in this population Not recommended for use in children less than 12 years	Sinequan/Silenor: Usual dose is 3–6 mg at bedtime, MDD 6 mg Baseline EKG for more than 50 years **CAUTION:** In pregnancy and breastfeeding, category C, and might be secreted in breastmilk	Recommended dose 3 mg Helps with improving quality of sleep and reducing the number of nighttime awakenings	Refer to Chapter 21, "Aging and Older Adult Populations," or PDR.
Drug class: orexin receptor antagonist (suvorexant [Belsomra], daridorexant [Quviviq]) To help with Insomnia by suppressing the wake drive; approved by the FDA in 2022 **CONTRAINDICATION:** Medication is contraindicated in narcolepsy.	Belsomra initial recommended dose 10 mg; however, refer to the pediatric PDR; medication comes in 5-mg tablets as well; for use in children more than 10 years	For adults: more than 19 years Belsomra initial dose 10 mg taken 30 minutes before bedtime; MDD 20 mg; should delay taking it after a full meal **CAUTION:** Pregnancy	Use with caution in this population and refer to Chapter 21, "Aging and Older Adult Populations," or PDR. Reports of hangover feeling due to long half-life; medication promotes wakefulness	Use with caution in this population and refer to Chapter 21, "Aging and Older Adult Populations," or PDR.
Drug class: tricyclic antidepressant, SNRI, antihistamine (mirtazapine [Remeron], doxepin [Sinequan, Silenor], trazodone [Desyrel]) Used to treat depression, insomnia (off-label), parasomnias, and OSA **WARNING:** May have drug–drug interactions. Medication should not be given to patients recovering from MI and with history of QT prolongation.	Not recommended for children less than 12 years	Doxepin: 3–6 mg should be taken 30 minutes before going to bed and at least 3 hours after last meal **CAUTION:** Not recommended for use during pregnancy	Recommended dose 3 mg for older adults Baseline EKG for patients over age 50	Refer to Chapter 21, "Aging and Older Adult Populations," or PDR. The clinician should review the risks vs. the benefits of starting this medication in the older adult population.

(continued)

TABLE 14.3 PHARMACOTHERAPY FOR TREATMENT OF SLEEP DISORDERS (*CONTINUED*)

Medication/Indication	Aged 10–18 Years (Youth)	Aged 19–65 Years (Adult)	Aged 66–74 Years (Older Adult)	Aged 85–99 Years (Oldest Old + Centenarians)
Drug class: nonselective antihistamines/anticholinergic agents (diphenhydramine [Benadryl]) Used to treat occasional sleeplessness	Not recommended for children less than 12 years	Average dose 50 mg **WARNING:** Medication contraindicated in women who are breastfeeding.	Lower dose may be appropriate as older adult patients tolerate it better **WARNING:** Due to anticholinergic effect, medication may not be appropriate for this population.	Refer to Chapter 21, "Aging and Older Adult Populations," or *PDR*.
Drug class: wake-promoting (armodafinil [Nuvigil], modafinil [Provigil]) Stimulants used to treat insomnia by reducing excessive daytime sleepiness and promoting wakefulness; indicated for patients with OSA and for treatment of narcolepsy	Refer to Chapter 20, "Special Considerations for Childhood and Adolescent Populations," or *PDR*. Not recommended for patients less than 16 years	Provigil: 200 mg standard dose given in the morning For excessive sleepiness, may need higher doses up to 800 mg/d In patients with daytime sleepiness, lower doses 50–200 mg **WARNING:** Medication is not FDA-approved and should be discontinued prior to anticipated pregnancy.	Not recommended for use in patients with history of left ventricular hypertrophy, chest pain, arrhythmias, or recent MI Clearance reduced in older adult patients	Use with caution in older adults and refer to Chapter 21, "Aging and Older Adult Populations," or *PDR*.
Drug class: stimulants (methylphenidate [focalin and focalin XR], sodium oxybate, amphetamine salts) Used to treat hypersomnia/narcolepsy In children and adolescents: used for treatment of ADHD and treatment-resistant depression	Refer to Chapter 20, "Special Considerations for Childhood and Adolescent Populations," or *PDR*. Should not be used in children less than 6 years An EKG recommended prior to starting treatment; monitoring of height and weight of the patient **WARNING:** There is high potential for abuse.	Average dose 2.5–10 mg twice a day **CAUTION:** Use with caution in patients with history of hypertension, hyperthyroidism, or substance use disorders Should not be given in conjunction with MAOI Not approved for use in pregnancy	Should not be given if the patient has history of glaucoma, cardiac abnormalities, or an allergy to methylphenidate. In older adults, lower doses more effective and better tolerated	Refer to Chapter 21, "Aging and Older Adult Populations," or *PDR*.
Drug class: dopamine agonists (pramipexole [Mirapex], ropinirole [Requip], rotigotine patch [Neupro]) Used to treat restless legs syndrome	Refer to Chapter 20, "Special Considerations for Childhood and Adolescent Populations," or *PDR*.	Requip: Initial dose 0.25 mg given 1–3 hours before bedtime; medication should be titrated slowly after 2 days to 0.5 mg and after 7 days to 1 mg; medication should not be discontinued abruptly	Same dosage as for adults; increased monitoring for side effects	Refer to Chapter 21, "Aging and Older Adult Populations," or *PDR*.

(*continued*)

TABLE 14.3 PHARMACOTHERAPY FOR TREATMENT OF SLEEP DISORDERS (CONTINUED)

Medication/Indication	Aged 10–18 Years (Youth)	Aged 19–65 Years (Adult)	Aged 66–74 Years (Older Adult)	Aged 85–99 Years (Oldest Old + Centenarians)
Drug class: central nervous system agent (carbidopa/levodopa [Sinemet]) Used to treat restless legs syndrome	Refer to Chapter 20, "Special Considerations for Childhood and Adolescent Populations," or *PDR*.	Starting dose 25 mg/100 mg taken at bedtime or when awaking from sleep due to restless legs syndrome MDD no more than 200 mg due to risk of augmentation	Refer to Chapter 21, "Aging and Older Adult Populations," or *PDR*.	Refer to Chapter 21, "Aging and Older Adult Populations," or *PDR*.
Drug class: antiepileptic/alpha 2 delta calcium channel blocker (gabapentin [Neurontin], enacarbil, pregabalin [Lyrica], clonidine) Used as off-label treatment for restless legs syndrome	Refer to Chapter 20, "Special Considerations for Childhood and Adolescent Populations," or *PDR*.	Gabapentin: 100–300 mg 1 hour prior to bedtime; dosage can be titrated to a maximum of 2.4 g	Initial dose 100 mg; for medication adjustment, refer to Chapter 21, "Aging and Older Adult Populations," or *PDR*.	Refer to Chapter 21, "Aging and Older Adult Populations," or *PDR*.
Drug class: opioids (naloxone, XR oxycodone) Used to treat chronic or severe restless legs syndrome **WARNING:** There is high potential for abuse.	Not recommended or approved in this population	Not a first-line treatment option; a proof of specific protocols completed before initiating therapy with these medications	Refer to Chapter 21, "Aging and Older Adult Populations," or *PDR*.	Refer to Chapter 21, "Aging and Older Adult Populations," or *PDR*.
Nutritional supplements (ferrous gluconate, magnesium oxide, ascorbic acid [vitamin C]) Used to treat restless legs syndrome	Refer to Chapter 20, "Special Considerations for Childhood and Adolescent Populations," or *PDR*.	Refer to the adult *PDR*. Ferrous sulfate starting dose of 325 mg + 100 mg to 200 mg of vitamin C at bedtime; patient to take a full glass of liquid to assist with absorption	Refer to Chapter 21, "Aging and Older Adult Populations," or *PDR*.	Refer to Chapter 21, "Aging and Older Adult Populations," or *PDR*.

ADHD, attention deficit hyperactivity disorder; COPD, chronic obstructive pulmonary disease; FDA, U.S. Food and Drug Administration; MAOI, monoamine oxidase inhibitors; MDD, major depressive disorder; MI, myocardial infarction; OSA, obstructive sleep apnea; *PDR*, Physician's Desk Reference; RLS, restless legs syndrome; SNRI, serotonin and norepinephrine reuptake inhibitors; XR, extended-release.

C. Educate on the importance of comprehensive treatment, including psychotherapy, alternative therapy, nonpharmacologic treatment, behavioral modification, and pharmacologic treatment.
D. Ensure adherence to treatment recommendations, including behavioral modification and nonpharmacologic and pharmacologic treatments, if applicable or prescribed.
E. Discuss potential drug–drug interactions with OTC agents.
F. Discuss potential medication and treatment side effects, what to look for, and how to report to the APRN.
G. Discuss the risks versus the benefits of treatment alternatives and recommendations.
H. Discuss sleep diaries and control environmental factors such as noise, light, temperature, and activities.
I. The APRN should discuss the importance of exercise, a healthy diet, and general physical activity.
J. Stress the importance of sleep hygiene.
K. Patients should avoid alcohol and mixing alcohol with medications.

FOLLOW-UP
A. Schedule a follow up with the patient 2 weeks after beginning treatment. If the patient was prescribed medications specific to treat sleep disorders, the APRN should review any medication side effects, compare baseline assessment with the current presentation, and discuss a revised treatment plan.
B. The APRN should also monitor for any psychological or physical changes and refer to additional specialists if applicable.

CONSULTATION AND REFERRALS
A. The APRN should consult with an interdisciplinary team and make appropriate referrals to therapy, additional medical providers, outpatient treatment centers, or programs.

INDIVIDUAL CONSIDERATIONS
Pediatrics
A. For restoring adequate sleep in the pediatric population, the APRN should be aware of the current guidelines, including sleep hygiene, recommendations on the total number of hours by age, and psychoeducation (Table 14.4).

Pregnancy
A. The APRN should be mindful of special sleep conditions that commonly afflict pregnant patients.

TABLE 14.4 CURRENT RECOMMENDATIONS FOR THE TOTAL NUMBER OF HOURS OF SLEEP BY AGE

Age Group	Sleep Recommended Daily
Newborn (0–3 months)	14 to 17 hours
Infant (4–12 months)	12 to 16 hours (including naps)
Toddler (1–2 years)	11 to 14 hours (including naps)
Preschool (3–5 years)	10 to 13 hours (including naps)
School age (6–12 years)	9 to 12 hours
Teen (13–17 years)	8 to 10 hours
Adult (18–60 years)	7 or more hours
Adult (61–64 years)	7 to 9 hours
Adult (65 years and old)	7 to 8 hours

Source: Centers for Disease Control and Prevention. (2024, May 15). *About sleep.* U.S. Department of Health and Human Services. https://www.cdc.gov/sleep/about/index.html

B. As the pregnancy progresses between the second and third trimester of gestation, patients may report snoring and OSA related to weight gain and postnasal drip causing them to awaken and disrupt their sleep cycle.

C. It is also essential to be vigilant of pregnant patients with sleep disorders since possible oxygen obstruction to the fetus may increase the risk of preeclampsia, cesarean section, and hypertension.

Geriatrics

A. Older adults complain more frequently about lack of sleep or restorative sleep than any other population.

B. Educating older adult patients on the risks of untreated sleep disorders is essential.

C. Lack of sleep interferes with their quality of life, increases medical deterioration, increases mood dysregulation, increases pain, decreases concentration, increases risk of falls and injury, increases morbidity, and decreases ability to lead an independent life.

Partners/Family

A. The APRN should educate caretakers and family members about the importance of being vigilant and reporting any acute changes in sleep habits.

B. Partners and family are and should be the ally in maintaining surveillance and promoting healthy sleep hygiene. They should be considered during the preparation and implementation of a treatment care plan.

SUMMARY

The prognosis of a person suffering from a sleep disorder varies depending on the cause, type of sleep disorder, and treatment. Lack of restful sleep can be detrimental to the well-being of patients diagnosed with a sleep disorder. It can lead to loss of independence among the older adults and increased mortality due to fatigue-induced accidents (e.g., falling asleep while driving). Sleep disorders among adults can also lead to decreased wages due to poor performance and worsening depression, anxiety, and overall satisfaction with life.

Older adults who obtain an adequate amount of sleep present with less cognitive decline when compared with those who do not. Conversely, older adults who have sleep disorders experience worsening cognitive ability. The functions of good sleep help with the renewal of brain cells, the synthesis of proteins, and cognitive restoration.

RESOURCES

A. World Health Organization. (2023). *ICD-10-CM diagnosis code F51.9: Sleep disorder not due to a substance or known physiological condition, unspecified.* ICD10Data. https://www.icd10data.com/ICD10CM/Codes/F01-F99/F50-F59/F51-/F51.9

B. American Academy of Sleep Medicine. (n.d.). *Practice guidelines.* American Academy of Sleep Medicine. https://aasm.org/clinical-resources/practice-standards/practice-guidelines

C. Centers for Disease Control and Prevention. (n.d.). *About sleep.* U.S. Department of Health and Human Services. https://www.cdc.gov/sleep/about/index.html

D. Centers for Disease Control and Prevention. (n.d.). *Sleep resources.* U.S. Department of Health and Human Services. https://www.cdc.gov/sleep/resources

E. Sleep Foundation. (n.d.). *Sleep Foundation.* https://www.sleepfoundation.org

F. Suni, E. (2022, April 12). *Sleep diary.* Sleep Foundation. https://www.sleepfoundation.org/sleep-diary

REFERENCES AND BIBLIOGRAPHY

American Academy of Sleep Medicine. (2023). *International classification of sleep disorders* (3rd ed., text rev.). https://aasm.org/clinical-resources/international-classification-sleep-disorders

Amir, A., Masterson, R. M., Halim, A., & Nava, A. (2022). Restless leg syndrome: Pathophysiology, diagnostic criteria, and treatment. *Pain Medicine, 23*(5), 1032–1035. https://doi.org/10.1093/pm/pnab253

Chance Nicholson, W., & Pfeiffer, K. (2021). Sleep disorders and mood, anxiety, and post-traumatic stress disorders. *Nursing Clinics of North America, 56*(2), 229–247. https://doi.org/10.1016/j.cnur.2021.02.003

Deshpande, P., Salcedo, B., & Haq, C. (2022). Common sleep disorders in children. *American Academy of Family Physicians, 105*(2), 168–176. PMID: 35166510.

Dunphy, L. M. H. (2004). *Management guidelines for nurse practitioners working with adults* (2nd ed.). F.A. Davis.

Gauld, C., Lopez, R., Morin, C., Geoffroy, P. A., Maquet, J., Desvergnes, P., McGonigal, A., Dauvilliers, Y., Philip, P., Dumas, G., & Micoulaud-Franchi, J. (2022). Symptom network analysis of the sleep disorders diagnostic criteria based on the clinical text of the ICSD-3. *Journal of Sleep Research, 31*(1), Article e13435. https://doi.org/10.1111/jsr.13435

Guiu, G., Monin, J., Perrier, E., & Manen, O. (2022). Travel health study in commercial aircrew members. *Travel Medicine and Infectious Disease, 45*, 102209. https://doi.org/10.1016/j.tmaid.2021.102209

Karna, B., Sankari, A., & Tatikonda, G. (2023, June 11). *Sleep disorder.* StatPearls Publishing. https://www.ncbi.nlm.nih.gov/books/NBK560720

Kennedy, K. E. R., Onyeonwu, C., Nowakowski, S., Hale, L., Branas, C. C., Killgore, W. D. S., Wills, C. C. A., & Grandner, M. A. (2022). Menstrual regularity and bleeding is associated with sleep duration, sleep quality and fatigue in a community sample. *Journal of Sleep Research, 31*(1), Article e13434. https://doi.org/10.1111/jsr.13434

Kim, E. S., Hershner, S. D., & Strecher, V. J. (2015). Purpose in life and incidence of sleep disturbances. *Journal of Behavioral Medicine, 38*(3), 590–597. https://doi.org/10.1007/s10865-015-9635-4

Lancel, M., Stroebe, M., & Eisma, M. C. (2020). Sleep disturbances in bereavement: A systematic review. *Sleep Medicine Reviews, 53*, 101331. https://doi.org/10.1016/j.smrv.2020.101331

Marques, D. R., & de Azevedo, M. H. P. (2018). Potentialities of network analysis for sleep medicine. *Journal of Psychosomatic Research, 111*, 89–90. https://doi.org/10.1016/j.jpsychores.2018.05.019

Pavlova, M., & Latreille, V. (2019). Sleep disorders. *The American Journal of Medicine, 132*(3), 292–299. https://doi.org/10.1016/j.amjmed.2018.09.021

Porwal, A., Yadav, Y. C., Pathak, K., & Yadav, R. (2021). An update on assessment, therapeutic management, and patents on insomnia. *BioMed Research International, 2021*(1), 1–19. https://doi.org/10.1155/2021/6068952

Smith, M. G., Cordoza, M., & Basner, M. (2022). Environmental noise and effects on sleep: An update to the WHO systematic review and meta-analysis. *Environmental Health Perspectives, 130*(7), Article 76001. https://doi.org/10.1289/ehp10197

Stahl, S. M., Muntner, N., & Grady, M. M. (2014). *Prescriber's guide: Stahl's essential psychopharmacology* (5th ed.). Cambridge University Press.

Suni, E., & Truong, K. (2023, September 26). *100+ Sleep statistics*. Sleep Foundation. https://www.sleepfoundation.org/how-sleep-works/sleep-facts-statistics

Traupman, E. K., & Dixon, M. A. (2022). Cognitive-behavioral therapy for insomnia for primary care: Review of components and application for residents in primary care. *The International Journal of Psychiatry in Medicine, 57*(5), 423–433. https://doi.org/10.1177/00912174221112466

Voysey, Z. J., Barker, R. A., & Lazar, A. S. (2020). The treatment of sleep dysfunction in neurodegenerative disorders. *Neurotherapeutics, 18*(1), 202–216. https://doi.org/10.1007/s13311-020-00959-7

Zakhari, R. (2020). *The psychiatric-mental health nurse practitioner certification review manual*. Springer Publishing Company.

CIRCADIAN RHYTHM SLEEP–WAKE DISORDERS

DEFINITION
A. Circadian rhythm is a natural process that regulates physiologic processes, including sleep. It is like an internal clock that determines sleep and wake cycles.
B. In the case of circadian rhythm sleep–wake disorders, it is related to an abnormality that causes a dysregulation of the internal clock in response to conflicting signals between the body and the environment. There is a disruption of the homeostasis of the restorative sleep process.
C. Circadian rhythm sleep–wake disorders are characterized by a delay at the start of sleep, which results in fewer hours of sleep. Sleep onset and wake-up times are dysregulated, which can interfere with normal daily functioning.
D. The circadian rhythm is divided into 24 hours with two intervals allotted for the body to be awake and other hours for the body to be asleep, coinciding with the day and night cycle. The internal clock is typically synchronized with environmental cues, such as daylight for being awake and dark light for time to be asleep.
E. For children and adults, circadian rhythm sleep–wake disorders are equally prevalent.
F. There is a close relationship between a circadian rhythm sleep disorder diagnosis and mental illness.
  1. It is associated with anxiety and psychotic disorders, although it is important to note the relationship does not imply causality.
G. The most common circadian rhythm sleep–wake disorder is jet lag. Jet lag is when the body attempts to adjust the internal clock to the environment (day-light or dark-light) after changes in time zones.

INCIDENCE
A. There is a genetic component to this sleep disorder, and evidence suggests that approximately 40% of individuals with a genetic predisposition and family history of circadian rhythm sleep–wake sleep disorder suffer from the same disorder.
B. Age and sex are additional factors that influence the circadian sleep–wake disorder.
  1. Adolescent boys have a 12% higher incidence of sleep–wake cycle disorders than other adults in the general population.
  2. Due to the phenomenon of social jet lag—in which patients do not get enough sleep as a result of electronic and internet activity late into the night—adolescents and young adults may have a diagnosis of circadian rhythm sleep disorder.
  3. Referred to as *night owls*, young adults and adolescents experience fluctuations in their sleep cycle as they wake up early to attend school or college, causing further problems.
  4. Many young adults and adolescents may have comorbid psychiatric conditions with the sleep disorder. Due to physiologic and environmental components, 62% of young adults diagnosed with bipolar disorder also report issues with circadian rhythm sleep disorders.
C. Another at-risk population for this sleep disorder is shift workers, with a 10% to 38% prevalence of circadian rhythm sleep disorders.

PATHOGENESIS
A. The process of the circadian rhythm is located in the suprachiasmatic nucleus in the hypothalamus and serves as the body's regulator of circadian rhythms. It regulates vital processes such as metabolism, body temperature, sleep–wake cycles, and cardiac rhythm. The pineal gland is another essential element that contributes to sleep by producing melatonin, which aids in the onset of sleep.

PREDISPOSING FACTORS
A. Psychiatric diagnosis of anxiety or psychosis is a predisposing factor in children and adolescents. There is evidence to support that a biological component, as well as a social component, might predispose patients to circadian rhythm sleep disorders.
B. Shift work, especially when sudden changes in shifts from nighttime to daytime, may be a predisposing factor.
C. Exposure to frequent environmental stimuli changes, such as increased noise level and bright light, is also a predisposing factor.
D. Presence of a neurodegenerative disease (e.g., Alzheimer disease) and diagnosis of autism are also factors.

COMMON COMPLAINTS
A. Behavioral dysregulation
B. Cognitive impairment and impaired attention
C. Drowsiness during the daytime hours
D. Lower school performance in children and adolescents
E. Increased risky behaviors and compromised safety (more car crashes) and history of accidents
F. Erratic sleep–wake cycle

OTHER SIGNS AND SYMPTOMS
A. Increased aggression
B. Addiction
C. Shift work
D. More alert in the evening and lethargic during the day
E. History of self-medication with OTCs or sleeping aids
F. History of snoring or other sleep disorders
G. Medical conditions such as congestive heart failure (CHF), COPD, and thyroid issues

SUBJECTIVE DATA
A. Patient has a diagnosis of insomnia or hypersomnia. Some individuals are misdiagnosed if this information is not obtained during history taking.

PHYSICAL EXAMINATION
A. Complete review of systems, including vital signs.
B. Ask about sleep habits, sleep hygiene, and duration of symptoms.
C. Review all medications, including prescribed and OTCs.
D. Identify risk factors during intake history.
E. Calculate the BMI.
F. Perform a neurologic exam.

DIAGNOSTIC TESTS AND SCREENING
A. Sleep logs for a 2-week period in children, adolescents, and adults
B. Screening questionnaires such as the Children's Sleep Habits Questionnaire
C. Sleep actigraphy (wristband)
D. Salivary and urine melatonin analysis
E. MSLT to measure degree of sleepiness
F. Overnight PSG
G. Epworth Sleepiness Scale

DIFFERENTIAL DIAGNOSES
A. Shift work syndrome
B. Jet lag syndrome
C. Insomnia
D. Advanced sleep-phase syndrome
E. Irregular sleep–wake rhythm
F. Mood disorder
G. Anxiety disorder
H. Substance use disorder
I. Autism spectrum disorder
J. Neurologic conditions such as Alzheimer disease

PLAN
A. Review sleep diaries and discuss treatment options.
B. Educate on signs and symptoms of circadian rhythm sleep disorders and the consequences of not addressing the problem.
C. Order laboratory tests and actigraphy if appropriate to age.

GENERAL TREATMENT AND INTERVENTIONS
A. Sleep hygiene
B. Exposure to bright natural light during the day and decreasing light exposure at nighttime
C. Regular sleep schedule
D. Behavioral modification
E. Minimizing exposure to blue light technology
F. Chronotherapy

COMMON MEDICATIONS
A. Pharmacologic interventions include benzodiazepines, nonbenzodiazepine hypnotics, orexin receptor antagonists, and melatonin receptor agonists (see Table 14.3).

PATIENT TEACHING
A. Sleep diary for 2 weeks, including weekends (see Table 14.1)
B. Sleep hygiene (see Table 14.2)
C. Avoidance of switching sleep schedules

FOLLOW-UP
A. After the initial evaluation, the APRN should see the patient in 2 weeks to review laboratory results and progress.
B. Discuss the treatment plan, make adjustments as needed, and provide psychoeducation on sleep hygiene.

CONSULTATION AND REFERRALS
A. Consultation and referrals to the patient's pediatrician, primary care provider, neurologist, or endocrinologist if applicable
B. Consultation with a pulmonologist
C. Referrals to sleep specialists for sleep studies
D. Referral to a psychotherapist

INDIVIDUAL CONSIDERATIONS

Pediatrics
A. Educate on the importance of maintaining a sleep schedule. Discuss the impact of social media, use of technology at nighttime, and decreased exposure to natural light, which affects the chronicity of the circadian rhythm clock. Discuss the school schedule related to the total number of hours the child sleeps. Encourage more outdoor physical activities.

Pregnancy
A. Pregnancy is a unique period in which patients undergo many hormonal changes, affecting their circadian rhythm and leading to sleep disorders.
B. The patient should be educated on the signs and symptoms of the sleep disorder and what to report to the APRN.
C. Treatment is tailored to address complaints and should be started as soon as possible.

Geriatrics
A. Educate on the signs and symptoms. Older adult patients usually report going to bed early and waking up very early, have periods of alertness in the morning, and can function most of the morning hours. They usually keep a set sleep schedule, which is essential. Circadian rhythm disorder might present more frequently in older adults with a comorbidity, such as a diagnosis of depression and in treatment for depression.
   1. Older adults are at high risk of being diagnosed with a circadian rhythm sleep disorder due to medical and psychiatric comorbidities.
   2. Educate on the importance of maintaining a sleep schedule, and avoid watching television late at night or switching their sleeping cycles.
   3. Educate on problems related to polypharmacy.

Partners/Family
A. Education on the importance of sleep hygiene
B. Increased exposure to natural daylight and exercise
C. Decreased use of blue light devices at night

RESOURCE
A. Centers for Disease Control and Prevention. (n.d.). *Circadian rhythms*. National Institute for Occupational Safety and Health. https://www.cdc.gov/niosh/work-hour-training-for-nurses/longhours/mod2/13.html

REFERENCES AND BIBLIOGRAPHY
Arns, M., Kooij, J. S., & Coogan, A. N. (2021). Review: Identification and management of circadian rhythm sleep disorders as a transdiagnostic feature in child and adolescent psychiatry. *Journal of the American Academy of Child and Adolescent Psychiatry*, 60(9), 1085–1095. https://doi.org/10.1016/j.jaac.2020.12.035

Cataletto, M. E. (2022, July 26). *Sleeplessness and circadian rhythm disorder*. Medscape. https://emedicine.medscape.com/article/1188944-overview

Deshpande, P., Salcedo, B., & Haq, C. (2022). Common sleep disorders in children. *American Academy of Family Physicians*, 105(2), 168–176. PMID: 35166510.

Moretti, P., Menculini, G., & Gonfia, L. (2022). Sleep disorders in pregnancy. In D. Larrivee (Ed.), *Sleep medicine and the evolution of contemporary sleep pharmacotherapy* (Chapter 9). IntechOpen. https://doi.org/10.5772/intechopen.100300

Pavlova, M., & Latreille, V. (2019). Sleep disorders. *The American Journal of Medicine, 132*(3), 292–299. https://doi.org/10.1016/j.amjmed.2018.09.021

Zakhari, R. (2020). *The psychiatric-mental health nurse practitioner certification review manual*. Springer Publishing Company.

Zisapel, N. (2018). New perspectives on the role of melatonin in human sleep, circadian rhythms and their regulation. *British Journal of Pharmacology, 175*(16), 3190–3199. https://doi.org/10.1111/bph.14116

INSOMNIA

DEFINITION

A. The patient complains on an ongoing basis of an inability to fall asleep and maintain sleep, or awakening often during the night.
B. Subclasses of insomnia were defined in 2014 by the *International Classification of Sleep Disorders*, Third Edition (*ICSD-3*; AASM, 2014).
  1. Short-term: Symptoms are present for less than 3 months.
  2. Chronic: Symptoms are present for at least 3 days per week for more than 3 consecutive months.
     a. Correlates highly with psychiatric disorders such as depression
C. Insomnia can lead to functional impairment, medical complications, and psychological deterioration, and compromise personal safety.
D. AASM is the authority that prepares the *ICSD-3*, which clinicians use to diagnose sleep disorders.
  1. The three criteria for diagnosis of insomnia include those that should be present for at least 3 days per week over at least 3 consecutive months:
     a. The patient has difficulty initiating or maintaining sleep.
     b. The patient has adequate opportunity and circumstances to sleep, typically 6 to 8 hours per night, but fails to achieve restorative sleep.
     c. The patient is less able to function during the day due to lack of restorative sleep.
E. Insomnia is also subdivided into transient cases that can self-resolve, such as jet lag, situational cases of shift work, during temporary increases of stress levels, and during periods of grief.

PATHOGENESIS

A. Insomnia is a sleep disorder related to hyperarousal or increased somatic, cognitive, peripheral, and cortical activation.
  1. Hyperarousal is confirmed by variability in vital signs and/or by completing an EEG.
  2. Situational insomnia can self-resolve once the individual adjusts to the time zone and the jet lag resolves.
B. Difficulty falling asleep and staying asleep despite completing at least 7 hours of sleep and waking up too early are reported by patients with insomnia.
C. It is believed that common contributors to insomnia are genetic, cognitive, emotional, and psychological.
D. Researchers have demonstrated causality between specific medical symptoms of fatigue and low energy with insomnia. Untreated insomnia may lead to chronic medical and psychiatric issues, declining cognition, and reduced attention.

PREDISPOSING FACTORS

A. Predisposing factors for insomnia are characteristics of sleep conditions that affect restful sleep.
B. Age, sex, and psychological, medical, and environmental conditions have been identified as predisposing factors.
C. Hormonal imbalances and mania in bipolar disorder may also be predisposing factors.
D. Psychological factors include anxiety, stress, depression, and unresolved grief.
E. Environmental factors include noise, pets disturbing the sleeping surface, light, and room temperature.
F. The APRN should consider the patient's age and sex as they can influence treatment options.
G. The most common complaint among individuals diagnosed with anxiety is difficulty initiating sleep, leading to insomnia and reports of feeling tired and lack of restorative sleep the next day.
H. Other predisposing factors include pregnancy, menopause, chronic pain, infections, endocrine issues, urinary frequency, use of alcohol, prescribed hypnotics, diuretics, amphetamines, cannabis, steroids, OTCs used for weight loss, antihistamines, and caffeine.

COMMON COMPLAINTS

A. Common complaints are daytime sleepiness, decreased concentration and attention, fatigue, changes in mood, irritability, increased anxiety, and lethargy.
B. Other complaints include excessive diaphoresis, water retention, inability to control body temperature, restlessness, and inability to stay asleep.
C. Some individuals also report headaches upon waking up, excessive grogginess, and mood swings.

OTHER SIGNS AND SYMPTOMS

A. Inability to function during the daytime
B. Aggression and irritability
C. Binge eating where individual uses the time when they cannot sleep to eat
D. Prone to having accidents while operating equipment at work or while driving a vehicle
E. Decreased energy
F. Vital signs lability
G. Sexual dysfunction
H. Lack of motivation or involvement

SUBJECTIVE DATA

A. Need for sleep appropriate for age (Table 14.4)
B. Sex
C. Medical comorbidities or physiologic problems (issues with normal breathing)
D. Type of work
E. Sleep diary (see Table 14.1)
F. Sleep hygiene characteristics and period of time the patient has experienced insomnia
G. Any episodes of daytime sleepiness
H. Ability to function during the day
I. Psychiatric diagnosis (stress, anxiety, depression)
J. Medical history and diagnoses
K. Problems with chronic pain
L. Changes in the sleeping environment
M. Use of alcohol and caffeine
N. Daily and timing of exercise
O. List of all medications, including OTCs, vitamins, and herbal products

P. Diet and nutritional assessment
Q. Presence of grief and depression and impact of family issues and recent losses
R. Memory or concentration problems
S. For females, should inquire about hormonal changes (e.g., pregnancy, menopause, and menses)

PHYSICAL EXAMINATION
A. Complete a physical exam, including a thorough history and the patient's chief complaint.
B. Screen for medical problems (e.g., diabetes, hypertension, endocrine issues, chronic pain, and cancer).
C. Complete a psychiatric evaluation, including a history of psychiatric diagnoses and treatment.
D. Obtain vital signs, including BMI.
E. Complete a sleep history, including sleep hygiene, with a 2-week sleep diary (see Table 14.1).
F. Use the reference manual *ICSD-3*.
G. Assess substance use (i.e., cannabis, alcohol, caffeine, amphetamines, hallucinogens, and OTCs).

DIAGNOSTIC TESTS AND SCREENING
A. Complete blood count (CBC) and ABG analysis
B. Thyroid function tests (TFTs)
C. Drug and alcohol screening
D. Urinalysis if urinary tract infection (UTI) is suspected
E. Iron studies
F. EEG
G. Sleep diary
   1. A sleep diary is a structured 24-hour record of times of sleep and awakenings (Table 14.1). This record should be completed by the patient for several days and reviewed by the APRN. The sleep diary aids in preparing a treatment plan.
H. Epworth Sleepiness Scale
   1. This is a tool/questionnaire used to measure daytime sleepiness. The scores range from 0 to 24, and a score of more than 10 indicates sleep disorder in the individual.
I. Actigraphy
   1. Actigraphy is a tool, usually a wristband, that measures movement. The individual wears it for at least 1 week and then returns to the clinician for a reading.
J. Athens Insomnia Scale
   1. This questionnaire uses the criteria from the *ICSD-3* and features eight parameters divided into two: Parameters 1 to 5 are related to night sleep, and parameters 6 to 8 are related to daytime dysfunction. It is similar to a sleep diary, but the patient is guided to answer the parameters.
K. PSG:
   1. PSG is a test performed in a laboratory setting and is used to diagnose various sleep disorders, including chronic insomnia and REM sleep disorders.
L. MSLT
   1. Used to diagnose insomnia, MSLT measures the time it takes to fall asleep after bed.

DIFFERENTIAL DIAGNOSES
A. Sleep apnea
B. RLS/limb movement disorder
C. Neuropathy
D. Chronic pain
E. Chronic medical condition
F. Anxiety, PTSD, depression, ADHD
G. Medication-induced insomnia
H. Alcohol or substance use disorder
I. Menopause and pregnancy
J. Neurologic disorder
K. Chronic stress disorder

PLAN
A. Review results from laboratory and sleep studies if available and applicable.
B. Identify the cause of insomnia.
C. Discuss the treatment plan and identify objectives.
D. Initiate treatment to target sleep disturbance.
E. Educate the patient on sleep hygiene.
F. Implement sleep diaries and daily structured plans.
G. Review behavioral and environmental changes.
H. Discuss nonpharmacologic treatment modalities, including cognitive behavioral therapy (CBT) for insomnia.
I. Involve the patient, family, and supportive individuals in the treatment plan and implementation.

GENERAL TREATMENT AND INTERVENTIONS
A. A treatment plan should be developed according to the patient's age, sex, and objectives to alleviate insomnia.
B. Consider CBT for insomnia.
C. Consider behavioral modification and sleep hygiene.
D. Provide nonpharmacologic interventions (Table 14.2).
E. Provide bright light exposure therapy to shift sleeping pattern.
F. Initiate pharmacologic treatment.

COMMON MEDICATIONS
A. The most common pharmacologic treatment are orexin antagonists, nonbenzodiazepines or "Z" drugs, benzodiazepines, selective histamine H1 antagonists, nonselective antihistamines, melatonin receptor agonists, antipsychotics, antidepressants, and anticonvulsants.
B. Table 14.3 summarizes the common medications for insomnia.

PATIENT TEACHING
A. The treatment plans should be prepared to attain individual patient goals. The treatment objectives should be identified after a thorough evaluation and assessment of the symptoms reported by the patient.
B. The clinician should discuss sleep hygiene, reduction of environmental sleep disturbances, the importance of structured activities, and adherence to recommendations.
C. Discuss with the patient the importance of restorative sleep.
D. Implement sleep diaries for 2 weeks and follow-up discussion with the clinician.
E. Recommend nonpharmacologic interventions, including sleep restriction, stress reduction techniques, and the benefits of CBT for insomnia.

FOLLOW-UP
A. The initial follow-up should be 2 weeks after the initiation of treatment. The goal is to review sleep diaries, progress, and symptomatology in order to update the treatment care plan.
B. If treatment is favorable and the patient is reporting sleep improvement, it is recommended to schedule a second follow-up in 4 weeks.
C. If treatment results are unfavorable, it is recommended to schedule a second follow-up visit 1 week later and then evaluate for further follow-up.
D. Continue psychoeducation, including the risks versus the benefits of treatment plan.

E. If the patient has medical comorbidities, the clinician should consult with the patient's primary care provider and provide updates.

CONSULTATION AND REFERRALS
A. Consultation with psychologists and or psychotherapists
B. Consultation with neurologists if there is evidence of a neurologic problem
C. Referral to sleep study

INDIVIDUAL CONSIDERATIONS

Pediatrics
A. The prevalence of sleep disturbances in children is approximately 10% to 30%.
B. It is believed that sleep disorders, specifically insomnia in children, are due to parents' lack of enforcement in sleep hygiene habits and schedules and exposure to blue light from technological devices.
C. Parents should be educated on the regular sleep parameters and the recommended number of sleep hours depending on the child's age (see Table 14.4).
  1. The key to pediatric and adolescent restorative sleep is a supportive sleep environment where the child is not exposed to environmental distractions and is going to bed at routine times.
  2. Parents should ascertain that their children's physiologic needs have been met before putting their children to bed.
  3. Review Chapter 20, "Special Considerations for Childhood and Adolescent Populations," for specifics.

Pregnancy
A. During the third trimester of pregnancy, most patients report diaphoresis, uncomfortableness with body positioning at night, and general discomfort related to hormonal changes.
B. There are reports of insomnia increasing as the pregnancy develops.
C. The APRN should educate on nonpharmacologic alternatives such as mindfulness, decreasing environmental distractors, and changing body positions while in bed.

Geriatrics
A. The older adult population reports the highest rate of insomnia, with approximately 65% of adults over 65 years of age reporting insomnia symptoms and having started treatment for the sleep disorder.
B. The reports and diagnosis of insomnia are unrelated to a normal aging process, which is important for the nurse practitioner to identify before initiating any treatment.
C. Older adults may complain about sleep fragmentation due to chronic medical conditions or medication side effects.
D. The APRN should review all the medications the patient is taking and check for potential drug–drug interactions that may cause toxicity. Many older adult individuals also have urinary frequency due to an infection or medication that interferes with their restorative sleep.
E. An empathic approach is key to helping and treating older adults. The APRN should validate the reported symptoms, provide psychoeducation, and monitor closely for any acute changes in mood, behavior, and cognition. A general recommendation for the older adult population is to start slowly with any treatment intervention and establish clear guidelines for follow-up.

Partners/Family
A. The support of partners, parents, and family is critical to the successful treatment of insomnia.
B. The APRN should educate and communicate the treatment plan to all potential and actual parties involved in the care of the individual during office visits.
C. The discussion and inclusion of partners and family in the preparation of treatment plans are pivotal to the success of the treatment plan.
D. Partners and family are key to the success of the treatment plan. The APRN should educate on what insomnia is, the signs and symptoms, and the treatment modalities to the partners and family, if applicable.

RESOURCES
A. Centers for Disease Control and Prevention. (n.d.). *Epworth Sleepiness Scale* [PDF]. National Institute for Occupational Safety and Health. https://www.cdc.gov/niosh/work-hour-training-for-nurses/longhours/mod2/epworth-P.pdf
B. Health in Aging. (2018, June 1). *How severe is insomnia in people 80-years-old and older?* Health in Aging Blog. https://www.healthinaging.org/blog/how-severe-is-insomnia-in-people-80-years-old-and-older
C. Dopheide, J. A. (2020). Insomnia overview: Epidemiology, pathophysiology, diagnosis and monitoring, and nonpharmacologic therapy. *The American Journal of Managed Care, 26*(Suppl. 4), S76–S84. https://doi.org/10.37765/ajmc.2020.42769

REFERENCES AND BIBLIOGRAPHY
American Academy of Sleep Medicine. (n.d.). *Sleep education: Children.* Accessed September 4, 2022. https://sleepeducation.org/category/children

American Academy of Sleep Medicine. (2014). *International classification of sleep disorders* (3rd ed.). American Academy of Sleep Medicine.

Calhoun, S. L., Fernandez-Mendoza, J., Vgontzas, A. N., Liao, D., & Bixler, E. O. (2014). Prevalence of insomnia symptoms in a general population sample of young children and preadolescents: Gender effects. *Sleep Medicine, 15*(1), 91–95. https://doi.org/10.1016/j.sleep.2013.08.787

Dopheide, J. A. (2020). Insomnia overview: Epidemiology, pathophysiology, diagnosis and monitoring, and nonpharmacologic therapy. *The American Journal of Managed Care, 26*(Suppl. 4), S76–S84. https://doi.org/10.37765/ajmc.2020.42769

Dunphy, L. M. H. (2004). *Management guidelines for nurse practitioners working with adults* (2nd ed.). F.A. Davis.

Gauld, C., Lopez, R., Morin, C., Geoffroy, P. A., Maquet, J., Desvergnes, P., McGonigal, A., Dauvilliers, Y., Philip, P., Dumas, G., & Micoulaud-Franchi, J. (2022). Symptom network analysis of the sleep disorders diagnostic criteria based on the clinical text of the *ICSD-3*. *Journal of Sleep Research, 31*(1). https://doi.org/10.1111/jsr.13435

Karna, B., Sankari, A., & Tatikonda, G. (2023, June 11). *Sleep disorder.* StatPearls Publishing. https://www.ncbi.nlm.nih.gov/books/NBK560720

Kyle, S. D., Hurry, M. E. D., Emsley, R., Marsden, A., Omlin, X., Juss, A., Spiegelhalder, K., Bisdounis, L., Luik, A. I., Espie, C. A., & Sexton, C. E. (2020). The effects of digital cognitive behavioral therapy for insomnia on cognitive function: A randomized controlled trial. *Sleep, 43*(9), Article zsaa034. https://doi.org/10.1093/sleep/zsaa034

Lancel, M., Stroebe, M., & Eisma, M. C. (2020). Sleep disturbances in bereavement: A systematic review. *Sleep Medicine Reviews, 53*, 101331. https://doi.org/10.1016/j.smrv.2020.101331

Pacheco, D., & Dimitiu, A. (2023, November 16). *Light therapy for insomnia sufferers.* Sleep Foundation. https://www.sleepfoundation.org/light-therapy

Pavlova, M., & Latreille, V. (2019). Sleep disorders. *The American Journal of Medicine, 132*(3), 292–299. https://doi.org/10.1016/j.amjmed.2018.09.021

Porwal, A., Yadav, Y. C., Pathak, K., & Yadav, R. (2021). An update on assessment, therapeutic management, and patents on insomnia. *BioMed Research International, 2021*(1), Article 6068952. https://doi.org/10.1155/2021/6068952

Qaseem, A., Kansagara, D., Forciea, M. A., Cooke, M., & Denberg, T. D. (2016). Management of chronic insomnia disorder in adults: A clinical practice guideline from the American College of Physicians. *Annals of Internal Medicine*, 165(2), 125–133. https://doi.org/10.7326/m15-2175

Rodriguez, J. C., Dzierzewski, J. M., & Alessi, C. A. (2015). Sleep problems in the elderly. *Medical Clinics of North America*, 99(2), 431–439. https://doi.org/10.1016/j.mcna.2014.11.013

Sailer, C., & Wasner, S. (2022). *Differential diagnosis pocket* (2nd ed.). Borm Bruckmeier Publishing.

Wickwire, E. M., Shaya, F. T., & Scharf, S. M. (2016). Health economics of insomnia treatments: The return on investment for a good night's sleep. *Sleep Medicine Reviews*, 30, 72–82. https://doi.org/10.1016/j.smrv.2015.11.004

Zakhari, R. (2020). *The psychiatric-mental health nurse practitioner certification review manual*. Springer Publishing Company.

NARCOLEPSY

DEFINITION
A. Narcolepsy is a disorder of central hypersomnolence. It is a chronic condition and a neurologic disorder that is characterized by an extreme tendency to fall asleep and is often reported as a sudden attack of sleep by patients. Unlike other sleep disorders, narcolepsy can lead to immediate danger to the patient. Patients with narcolepsy experience immediate REM sleep and potential limb movements. It can be a hereditary condition where the patient experiences decreased CSF levels of orexin-A/hypocretin-1.
B. There are two types of narcolepsy:
  1. NT1: characterized by cataplexy or loss of muscle tone
  2. NT2: characterized without cataplexy

INCIDENCE
A. Narcolepsy is a chronic sleep disorder affecting approximately 44.3 per 100,000 people in the United States and appears to have a similar incidence to hypersomnia, which is reported to be 10.3 per 100,000 persons.
  1. Of patients diagnosed with narcolepsy, 25% currently receive treatment.
  2. Of patients with narcolepsy, 10% will have REM disorders.
B. It is suspected that a large number of people are affected by narcolepsy; however, it has been underreported or not diagnosed.

PATHOGENESIS
A. Although the exact cause of narcolepsy is unknown, there is a relationship in NT1 with decreased levels of orexin A/hypocretin-1, a brain chemical that helps regulate wake cycles and REM sleep.
B. Narcolepsy does affect the regulation of REM necessary for normal sleep and restorative processes.
C. A common genetic association has been found in NT1 patients and their parents who are diagnosed with narcolepsy.

PREDISPOSING FACTORS
A. Diagnosis of dementia
B. Diagnosis of Parkinson disease
C. History of viral infection
D. History of avian flu infection
E. History of head trauma
F. Sarcoidosis
G. Multiple sclerosis
H. Use of substances such as alcohol and amphetamines
I. Family history of narcolepsy
J. History of hallucination/psychosis

COMMON COMPLAINTS
A. Patients report sudden attacks of sleepiness, excessive daytime sleepiness accompanied by loss of muscle tone, sleep paralysis, changes in REM sleep, hallucinations, sudden arousal with confusion, and feelings of drunkenness.

OTHER SIGNS AND SYMPTOMS
A. Sudden sleep attack while performing a task
B. Reports of low mood and irritability
C. Reports of amnesia, cognitive impairment
D. Inability to stay awake during normal hours
E. Hallucinations, vivid dreams

SUBJECTIVE DATA
A. Family history of narcolepsy NT1 or NT2
B. Sleep hygiene characteristics
C. Presence of neurologic diagnosis and other comorbidities

PHYSICAL EXAMINATION
A. Complete review of systems
B. History of a psychiatric disorder and treatment
C. Changes in mood or behavior related to sleep hygiene
D. Complete review of sleep hygiene and habits to include episodes of daily naps, daytime sleepiness, and waking up with confusion
E. Use of alcohol, prescribed medications, and OTCs
F. Review of laboratory values for decreased levels of hypocretin (orexin)

DIAGNOSTIC TESTS AND SCREENING
A. Sleep diary over a 2-week period
B. ABG
C. CSF hypocretin-1 deficiency
D. Drug and alcohol screening
E. Overnight PSG test after ruling out OSA
F. MSLT

DIFFERENTIAL DIAGNOSES
A. Head trauma
B. Encephalopathy
C. Brain tumor
D. Cerebrovascular Insufficiency
E. Primary sleep disorder
F. Brain abscess
G. Epilepsy
H. Sleep apnea
I. Drug-related disorder
J. Periodic limb movement of sleep disorder
K. Multiple sclerosis

PLAN
A. The APRN should communicate with the patient, partners, parents, and other family members as appropriate to discuss the treatment plan.
B. Review laboratory, sleep diary, and other sleep tests results.
C. Educate on the diagnosis and the risks versus the benefits of engaging in treatment.
D. Initiate nonpharmacologic treatment, if applicable.
E. Review medication regimen, if appropriate.
F. Discuss the short-term goals of the treatment plan.

GENERAL TREATMENT AND INTERVENTIONS
A. Discuss nonpharmacologic interventions.
B. Discuss and review complete list of medications, including OTCs.
C. Ask the patient to write down reported symptoms and list questions to ask the healthcare provider. The patient should also be accompanied during the office visit to understand the treatment plan.

COMMON MEDICATIONS
A. Common pharmacologic treatments include modafinil, armodafinil, methylphenidate, amphetamine salts, sodium oxybate, antidepressants (tricyclics, selective serotonin reuptake inhibitors [SSRIs], and serotonin and noradrenaline reuptake inhibitors [SNRIs]), histamine H3 receptor, and pitolisant, recently approved by the Food and Drug Administration (FDA; see Table 14.3).

PATIENT TEACHING
A. Discuss the importance of sleep hygiene and maintaining a regular sleep schedule.
B. Educate on signs, symptoms, and treatment modalities of narcolepsy.
C. Encourage naps during the day of approximately 20 minutes in duration, which will allow the patient to function for 2 to 3 hours.
D. Discuss the importance of an exercise routine 4 to 5 hours before bedtime.
E. Avoid alcohol consumption and self-medication.
F. Communicate with work supervisors, coworkers, schoolteachers, and other family members about the diagnosis of narcolepsy.

FOLLOW-UP
A. Initial follow-up in 2 weeks to review sleep results from laboratory studies, sleep diary, sleep hygiene, and impact of the nonpharmacologic interventions.
B. If patient requires pharmacologic agents such as stimulants, the APRN should monitor blood pressure and evaluate for arrythmias.
C. Review any new presentation of symptoms after initiation of treatment.
D. Obtain collateral from partner, parents, and family if appropriate.
E. Review the initial care plan and update it as needed.
F. Schedule the next visit within 4 weeks after follow-up.

CONSULTATION AND REFERRALS
A. During the follow up process, as appropriate the psychiatric nurse practitioner may initiate referrals and consultation with other specialists. Referrals might include a neurologist, primary care provider, psychologist, therapist, or sleep specialist.

INDIVIDUAL CONSIDERATIONS
Pediatrics
A. Consult with a pediatrician.
B. Educate the child's parents on the signs and symptoms of sleep disorders and narcolepsy.
C. Educate parents on the importance of pediatric sleep hygiene and reporting any concerns to the APRN.
D. Inform schoolteachers and other care providers about the patient's narcolepsy diagnosis.

Pregnancy
A. It is recommended that patients immediately cease pharmacologic treatment for narcolepsy upon confirmation of pregnancy.
B. Pregnant patients diagnosed with narcolepsy will need to discontinue medications for narcolepsy for at least 2 years as pharmacologic agents cross breastmilk and the placenta.
C. Pregnant patients should be carefully monitored for sleep disorders, especially narcolepsy, to promote safety and to prevent injury to the pregnant patient and the fetus.

Geriatrics
A. Educate on the signs and symptoms of sleep disorders and narcolepsy, which are not considered a process of normal aging.
B. Emphasize the avoidance of self-medicating.
C. Encourage behavioral modification to strengthen patients' restorative sleep.

Partners/Family
A. Discuss the importance of providing support to the patient.
B. Educate on signs and symptoms of narcolepsy and what to report to the advanced psychiatric nurse.
C. Discuss safety strategies.
D. Behavioral modification is recommended before initiating pharmacologic treatment.

RESOURCES
A. Narcolepsy Network. (n.d.). *Narcolepsy fast facts*. https://narcolepsynetwork.org/about-narcolepsy/narcolepsy-fast-facts
B. Mayo Clinic Staff. (2023, January 14). *Narcolepsy*. Mayo Clinic. https://www.mayoclinic.org/diseases-conditions/narcolepsy/symptoms-causes/syc-20375497
C. National Institute of Neurological Disorders and Stroke. (n.d.). *Narcolepsy fact sheet*. https://www.ninds.nih.gov/narcolepsy-fact-sheet
D. Project Sleep. (n.d.). *Facts about narcolepsy*. https://project-sleep.com/facts-about-narcolepsy
E. Wake Up Narcolepsy. (n.d.). *What is narcolepsy?* https://www.wakeupnarcolepsy.org/about/what-is-narcolepsy

REFERENCES AND BIBLIOGRAPHY
Acquavella, J., Mehra, R., Bron, M., Suomi, J. M. H., & Hess, G. P. (2020). Prevalence of narcolepsy and other sleep disorders and frequency of diagnostic tests from 2013–2016 in insured patients actively seeking care. *Journal of Clinical Sleep Medicine*, 16(8), 1255–1263. https://doi.org/10.5664/jcsm.8482

Karna, B., Sankari, A., & Tatikonda, G. (2023, June 11). *Sleep disorder*. StatPearls Publishing. https://www.ncbi.nlm.nih.gov/books/NBK560720

Pavlova, M., & Latreille, V. (2019). Sleep disorders. *The American Journal of Medicine*, 132(3), 292–299. https://doi.org/10.1016/j.amjmed.2018.09.021

Scheer, D., Schwartz, S. W., Parr, M., Zgibor, J., Sanchez-Anguiano, A., & Rajaram, L. (2019). Prevalence and incidence of narcolepsy in a US health care claims database, 2008–2010. *Sleep*, 42(7), Article zsz091. https://doi.org/10.1093/sleep/zsz091

PARASOMNIAS

DEFINITION
A. Parasomnias are a group of sleep disorders characterized by unusual behavior and undesirable physical experiences during sleep. These sleep disorders include sleepwalking, vivid dreams,

night terrors, and nightmares. People who suffer from parasomnia may not recall any of the behaviors exhibited during an episode. This is in sharp contrast to other parasomnias where there is evidence of increased motor activity such as punching, kicking, crying, screaming, and sleep eating disorders.

INCIDENCE
A. In children diagnosed with parasomnia, 50% experience lasting effects on their sleep, behavior, normal development, and overall quality of life. A high percentage of parasomnias in children are related to nightmares, with a 40% prevalence rate. Moreover, parasomnias in children increase if the individual has a history of trauma; 75% of children and adolescents report experiencing nightmares more than 3 nights per week after a traumatic loss. This indicates that trauma and bereavement may be risk factors for parasomnias.
B. In children and adolescents, most parasomnias occur during the NREM stage of sleep, resulting in partial amnesia of the parasomnia event. Sleepwalking, nightmares, and confusional arousals are characterized by a child or adolescent resistant to waking up, or partial arousal.
  1. The child or adolescent may be found sleeping in a different place than where they originally went to sleep, or the child or adolescent sitting on the bed screaming.
  2. Parasomnias include nightmares occurring immediately before waking up or during REM sleep. The child or adolescent experiencing nightmares may have a recollection of the dream, causing brief periods of wakefulness.

PATHOGENESIS
A. The pathogenesis of parasomnias has various etiology, including a genetic predisposition, as well as environmental, medical, and psychological factors.
B. Some people may have periods of confusion and amnesia upon waking up after parasomnia activity.
C. Parasomnias may also be considered a dysregulation of slow-wave sleep, affecting the NREM stage as well as the REM stage of sleep. Sleeping aids may worsen parasomnias, such as sleepwalking.

PREDISPOSING FACTORS
A. Family history of parasomnia diagnosis
B. History of substance use
C. History of eating disorders
D. Diagnosis of Parkinson disease, dementia, or multiple system atrophy
E. Diagnosis of ADHD in children and adolescents
F. History of trauma
G. Taking sleeping aids that worsen parasomnias

COMMON COMPLAINTS
A. Reports of vivid dreams, violence during sleep, and sleep talking, including screaming and yelling
B. Reports of nightmares and/or night terrors in children under 12 years of age
C. Exhibits violent behavior during sleep (e.g., punching, kicking, scratching, and biting)

OTHER SIGNS AND SYMPTOMS
A. The person is found sleeping in an area different from when they went to bed.
B. The patient is unable to remember dreams the next day.
C. The patient wakes up feeling tired and physically exhausted.
D. Bed partner/siblings/parents report that the patient appears to be fighting while asleep (e.g., punching, kicking).
E. The patient is seen walking in the dark and appears to be asleep.

SUBJECTIVE DATA
A. A detailed sleep history, including behaviors before, during, and after falling asleep, is especially important for individuals who are reporting parasomnias.

PHYSICAL EXAMINATION
A. A complete review of systems, including a comprehensive history of sleep behaviors, quality of sleep, and sleep hygiene
B. Comprehensive medication review

DIAGNOSTIC TESTS AND SCREENING
A. Nocturnal PSG
B. Comprehensive metabolic panel (CMP), ABG, and thyroid-stimulating hormone (TSH)
C. Sleep diary
D. Actigraphy
E. Drug and alcohol screening

DIFFERENTIAL DIAGNOSES
A. REM sleep behavior disorder
B. Conversion disorder
C. PTSD
D. Parkinson disease
E. Dementia
F. ADHD
G. Other parasomnias
H. Seizure disorder
I. History of substance use disorder, including OTCs
J. Sleep-related eating disorders
K. Night eating syndrome or other eating disorders
L. Bipolar disorder
M. Stimulant abuse disorder

PLAN
A. Review clinical history, results of laboratory work, and sleep diaries, and interview partners/family, parents, teachers, and other healthcare providers.
B. Educate on signs, symptoms, and treatment options.
C. Educate on sleep hygiene.
D. Discuss nonpharmacologic interventions.
E. Discuss safety precautions such as home alarms, motion alarms, locking of doors and windows in the home at night, removing firearms or weapons, and moving the mattress onto the floor to prevent injury in the night.

GENERAL TREATMENT AND INTERVENTIONS
A. Behavioral modification
B. Nonpharmacologic treatment—sleep hygiene (see Table 14.2)
C. Pharmacologic intervention (based on the patient's age and sex)

COMMON MEDICATIONS
A. Pharmacologic treatment of parasomnias includes benzodiazepines, antidepressants, and melatonin (see Table 14.3).

PATIENT TEACHING
A. Sleep hygiene (going to bed at the same time every night, reducing environmental distractions, and avoiding eating large meals or drinking fluids before bed)
B. Use of the bed for sex and sleep only
C. Avoidance of strenuous activity, such as exercise, before bed

FOLLOW-UP

A. The APRN should schedule the first follow-up visit 2 weeks after the initial evaluation. The goal is to review progress, discuss the treatment plan, and adjust the treatment if needed. The patient should be educated on the importance of treatment adherence and report any undesirable side effects or worsening symptoms as soon as possible.
B. Subsequent follow-up visits should initially be scheduled every month and a half for the first 6 months, and thereafter every 3 months is recommended.

CONSULTATION AND REFERRALS

A. The APRN should consult with the patient's primary care provider and other healthcare professionals treating the patient.
B. If appropriate, consult the pharmacist to verify history of medications and any adverse effects or interactions.
C. If appropriate, consult with the patient's parents, teachers, school psychologists, and school nurse.
D. Refer as appropriate for sleep studies, as well as to behavior specialists and psychotherapists.

INDIVIDUAL CONSIDERATIONS

Pediatrics
A. Educate the patients, parents, and other individuals in direct contact or care for the patient on the signs and symptoms of parasomnias. This is due to this population's high prevalence of nightmares and night terrors.
B. Encourage behavioral modification, sleep diaries, and nonpharmacologic interventions before pharmacologic treatment.

Pregnancy
A. Discuss with the obstetrician how the pregnancy is going.
B. Provide psychoeducation and promote sleep hygiene.

Geriatrics
A. The APRN should educate the patient and the family on parasomnias' signs, symptoms, and treatment modalities.
B. Encourage nonpharmacologic interventions before using medications.
C. Older adults are at high risk of accidents, sustaining falls, injuries, and death if diagnosed with a parasomnia sleep disorder. Some older adults might walk out of the house in the middle of the night, become confused, and get hit by a car.

Partners/Family
A. Educate on signs and symptoms of parasomnias and the importance of monitoring and reporting concerns to advanced psychiatric nurse practitioners.
B. Partners/caretakers/family should assist with sleep diaries (children and older adults).
C. Assist with safety measures such as locking all doors and windows at night, removing potential weapons from the house, and installing movement sensors and small night lights.
D. Monitor and dispense medications to the patient.

RESOURCE
A. Bryan, L., & Cotliar, D. (2023, December 8). *Parasomnias*. Sleep Foundation. https://www.sleepfoundation.org/parasomnias

REFERENCES AND BIBLIOGRAPHY
Bryan, L., & Cotliar, D. (2023, December 8). *Parasomnias*. Sleep Foundation. https://www.sleepfoundation.org/parasomnias
Deshpande, P., Salcedo, B., & Haq, C. (2022). Common sleep disorders in children. *American Academy of Family Physicians, 105*(2), 168–176. PMID: 35166510.
Karna, B., Sankari, A., & Tatikonda, G. (2023, June 11). *Sleep disorder*. StatPearls Publishing. https://www.ncbi.nlm.nih.gov/books/NBK560720
Lancel, M., Stroebe, M., & Eisma, M. C. (2020). Sleep disturbances in bereavement: A systematic review. *Sleep Medicine Reviews, 53*, 101331. https://doi.org/10.1016/j.smrv.2020.101331
Pavlova, M., & Latreille, V. (2019). Sleep disorders. *The American Journal of Medicine, 132*(3), 292–299. https://doi.org/10.1016/j.amjmed.2018.09.021

RESTLESS LEGS SYNDROME DISORDER

DEFINITION
A. Restless legs syndrome (RLS) is a sleep disorder characterized by lower extremity movement or the urge to move legs before, during, and after falling asleep. Some individuals also report upper extremities movement in attempts to control and stop the lower extremities.
B. RLS interferes with the patient's quality of life and normal daily functioning and affects their social and psychological aspects.
C. RLS may be associated with an iron deficiency, although may be present in people with normal iron.
D. RLS also affects pregnant patients and patients diagnosed with end-stage renal disease. RLS is reported frequently during office visits. The lack of diagnosis of disrupted sleep associated with RLS may lead to delayed treatment.

INCIDENCE
A. RLS interferes with restorative sleep and affects approximately 13% of the population. The behavior and symptoms are unrelated to other medical conditions, such as leg cramps, edema, myalgia, or arthritis.
B. There is an established relationship with age, where approximately 30% of initial symptoms present before 20 years of age; symptoms worsen and begin disrupting normal sleep after age 50. Approximately 24% of patients have confirmed iron deficiency, 25% of patients receive dialysis, and 26% of pregnant patients in their third trimester get a diagnosis of RLS. A smaller percentage of patients diagnosed with RLS take antiemetic and neuroleptic medications.
C. RLS affects approximately 12% to 35% of the population of children with chronic kidney disease or a psychiatric diagnosis of ADHD.

PATHOGENESIS
A. RLS is a disorder that manifests by a need to move the lower extremities while asleep. It is believed to have several etiologies.
B. Pathogenesis includes iron deficiency, dopaminergic circuitry disruption, genetic components, sex, and age.
C. Iron deficiency can also affect and worsen medical conditions such as fibromyalgia, chronic pain, anemia, and renal failure, leading to increased complaints of RLS symptoms.

PREDISPOSING FACTORS
A. History of sleep disorders related to movement
B. Neurologic conditions, Parkinson disease
C. History of anxiety or mood disorder
D. Prescribed medication side effects
E. Patients with end-stage renal disease and on dialysis
F. Pregnant women in their third trimester of gestation

G. Patients taking antiemetics and neuroleptics
H. Children diagnosed with ADHD
I. People who are frequent blood donors due to depletion of iron
J. Children with family history of RLS

COMMON COMPLAINTS
A. Feelings of restlessness and inability to stay still, especially before, during, and after falling asleep
B. Inability to stay still and the urge to move legs
C. Feelings of discomfort while staying still, but somewhat relieved by movements such as foot tapping and frequent changes in the position of lower extremities
D. Feelings of numbness and/or itchiness
E. In children, may report feelings of ants and tingling and "funny feelings" on their legs

OTHER SIGNS AND SYMPTOMS
A. Feelings of pins and needles in the lower extremities not related to venous stasis, arthritis, or neurologic issues
B. Pain or feelings of numbness while lying down or in children when sitting for long periods of time

SUBJECTIVE DATA
A. History of neurologic conditions that affect movement
B. Diagnosis of anxiety or mood disorder
C. History or diagnosis of diabetes and hypertension

PHYSICAL EXAMINATION
A. Complete review of systems, including vital signs.
B. Obtain a thorough history of symptoms: onset, length of time, and level of functional impairment.
C. Rule out medical etiology (e.g., end-stage renal disease and on dialysis, Parkinson disease, arthritis, diabetes).
D. Determine diagnosis of hypertension.

DIAGNOSTIC TESTS AND SCREENING
A. Laboratory studies to check for iron deficiency
B. CMP, TSH
C. Serum magnesium
D. Methylmalonic acid to check for B_{12} values
E. Homocysteine to rule out folate deficiency
F. Neurology consult
G. Renal function test

DIFFERENTIAL DIAGNOSES
A. Akathisia
B. Neurovascular problems
C. Cardiovascular problems
D. Osteoarthritis
E. Diabetes
F. Substance-induced movement disorder
G. Neuroleptic-induced akathisia
H. Periodic limb movement disorder
I. Leg cramps or positional discomfort

PLAN
A. Address symptoms that interfere with restful sleep and the patient's quality of life.
B. Educate on signs and symptoms and when to report them to the advanced nurse practitioner.
C. Identify goals that the patient wants to accomplish during treatment.

GENERAL TREATMENT AND INTERVENTIONS
A. Suggest other complementary alternative medicine initiatives, such as yoga, exercise, compression devices, massages, and acupuncture.

COMMON MEDICATIONS
A. Pharmacotherapy to treat RLS includes the following:
   1. Dopamine agonists
   2. Opiates
   3. Gabapentin
   4. Benzodiazepines
B. Iron supplements are also recommended if ferritin levels are below 50 (see Table 14.3).

PATIENT TEACHING
A. Explain that early treatment and treatment adherence improve chances of recovery.
B. Provide the patient with the crisis link (988) and explain the function of the resource.
C. Review the need for sleep hygiene and behavioral modification.
D. Educate the patient and other family members/significant others who might be responsible for the patient on the signs, symptoms, and treatment modalities of the patient's specific sleep disorder.
E. Discuss with the patient the importance of reporting undesirable side effects to treatment and worsening symptoms and provide resources.
F. Educate about the risks of self-medication.
G. Review the impact of choice of nourishment per bedtime.
   1. Limit intake of caffeinated drinks before going to bed.
   2. Reduce use of alcohol.
   3. Ensure adequate hydration.
H. Reduce or quit smoking.

FOLLOW-UP
A. Schedule a follow-up visit 2 weeks after initiation of treatment to review effectiveness of intervention and review or update care plan.
B. After the first follow-up visit, follow scheduled visits every 4 to 6 weeks as appropriate.

CONSULTATION AND REFERRALS
A. Provide appropriate consultation with an interdisciplinary team, including but not limited to the patient's primary care provider and age-appropriate specialists.
   1. Women's health provider
   2. Pediatrician
   3. Neurologist
   4. Pulmonary specialist
B. Initiate referrals to psychotherapists and psychologists as appropriate.

INDIVIDUAL CONSIDERATIONS

Pediatrics
A. Discuss psychiatric comorbidities, including ADHD and anxiety.
B. The treatment plan should include input from the patient's pediatrician, parents, and school personnel.

Pregnancy
A. The third trimester of pregnancy is when patients report RLS symptoms. Discuss nonpharmacologic interventions, ▶

including behavioral modifications, and monitor and report undesirable or worsening symptoms.

Geriatrics

A. Older adults are at a higher risk of falls, cognitive impairment, and confusion related to RLS. It is essential to educate on the signs and symptoms and when to report them to the APRN. An emphasis on safety, supportive counseling, and behavioral modifications, including sleep hygiene, is essential for this population.

Partners/Family

A. It is pivotal for the appropriate management of sleep disorders to have an initial comprehensive assessment of the condition and initiate a treatment plan to include the patient and other healthcare providers as needed and applicable.
B. The patient should be educated on the risks versus the benefits of the proposed treatment and monitored closely by the treatment team. Stress the importance of interprofessional collaboration to assist with care coordination, appropriate referrals, consultation, and therapy. The goal is to help the patient improve their quality of life and achieve restful, restorative sleep.

RESOURCES
A. Centers for Disease Control and Prevention. (n.d.). *About sleep.* U.S. Department of Health and Human Services. https://www.cdc.gov/sleep/about/index.html
B. Centers for Disease Control and Prevention. (n.d.). *Sleep resources.* U.S. Department of Health and Human Services. https://www.cdc.gov/sleep/resources/index.html
C. Suni, E., & Truong, K. (2023, September 26). *100+ sleep statistics.* Sleep Foundation. https://www.sleepfoundation.org/how-sleep-works/sleep-facts-statistics

REFERENCES AND BIBLIOGRAPHY
Amir, A., Masterson, R. M., Halim, A., & Nava, A. (2022). Restless leg syndrome: Pathophysiology, diagnostic criteria, and treatment. *Pain Medicine, 23*(5), 1032–1035. https://doi.org/10.1093/pm/pnab253
Centers for Disease Control and Prevention. (n.d.-a). *About sleep.* U.S. Department of Health and Human Services. https://www.cdc.gov/sleep/about/index.html
Centers for Disease Control and Prevention. (n.d.-b). *Sleep resources.* U.S. Department of Health and Human Resources. https://www.cdc.gov/sleep/resources
Chelminiak, L., Sieminski, M., Skrzypek-Czerko, M., & Roszmann, A. (2018). Restless legs syndrome in nursing practice. *The Journal of Neurological and Neurosurgical Nursing, 7*(4), 166–172. https://doi.org/10.15225/PNN.2018.7.4.6
Karna, B., Sankari, A., & Tatikonda, G. (2023, June 11). *Sleep disorder.* StatPearls Publishing. https://www.ncbi.nlm.nih.gov/books/NBK560720
Porwal, A., Yadav, Y. C., Pathak, K., & Yadav, R. (2021). An update on assessment, therapeutic management, and patents on insomnia. *BioMed Research International, 2021*(1), Article 6068952. https://doi.org/10.1155/2021/6068952
Stahl, S. M. (2021). *Stahl's essential psychopharmacology: Neuroscientific basis and practical applications* (5th ed.). Cambridge University Press.
Suni, E., & Truong, K. (2023, September 26). *100+ sleep statistics.* Sleep Foundation. https://www.sleepfoundation.org/how-sleep-works/sleep-facts-statistics
Voysey, Z. J., Barker, R. A., & Lazar, A. S. (2020). The treatment of sleep dysfunction in neurodegenerative disorders. Erratum in: *Neurotherapeutics, 18*(1), 654. https://doi.org/10.1007/s13311-020-00980-w
Zakhari, R. (2020). *The psychiatric-mental health nurse practitioner certification review manual.* Springer Publishing Company.

SLEEP DISORDERED BREATHING/OBSTRUCTIVE SLEEP APNEA

DEFINITION
A. Obstructive sleep apnea (OSA) is a chronic sleep disorder that is caused by an obstruction of the upper airway during sleep. It is associated with snoring and involves a decrease or complete halt in airflow despite an ongoing effort to breath.
B. The etiology is an upper airway obstruction occurring when the muscles relax during sleep, specifically soft muscles and tissue of the upper airway in the back of the throat.
C. Patients with obesity, enlarged uvula, enlarged tonsils, and deformities of the upper airway are at greater risk for OSA.
D. The most common complaints are excessive daytime sleepiness, reports of loud snoring, gasping or shocking sensations, and multiple awakenings from sleep due to shortness of breath.
E. Researchers have found a direct relationship between OSA and fatigue, daytime sleepiness, fear of having shortness of breath, and overall decreased quality of life.
F. OSA may also share pathophysiology with some psychiatric disorders, although OSA may not be causal. OSA can be misdiagnosed as a psychiatric disorder or conduct disorder in children due to the clinical presentation and the parents' reported complaints of mood lability, hyperactivity, and decreased attention.
G. Individuals diagnosed with OSA report somatic complaints such as fatigue, cognitive impairment, and depression.
H. Most patients presenting with OSA at primary care providers report excessive sleepiness and reduced ability to perform at work.

INCIDENCE
A. The prevalence of OSA in the general adult population 30 to 70 years of age is estimated to be between 10% and 32%.
B. OSA is most common in adults, with approximately 25 million people diagnosed annually; however, children can also present with symptoms of OSA at about 2% compared with the percentage of adults.
C. Age is a determinant factor as the incidence of OSA increases to approximately 50% of older adults age 65 and older reporting OSA.
D. Sex also presents a significant risk factor for OSA as males are diagnosed in greater proportion than females. Approximately 20% of females are diagnosed compared with 26% of males.
E. In children, screening criteria are recommended by the American Academy of Pediatrics at different ages of development, starting between 2 and 8 years of age.
  1. A comprehensive evaluation of the adenotonsillar hypertrophy determines airway obstruction leading to OSA.
  2. During these stages of pediatric development, males and females are diagnosed with OSA at the same rate; however, once they become adolescents or reach puberty period, males have a higher prevalence of OSA than females.
  3. Children with physical deformities that compromise the head and neck may be at higher risk of developing OSA.
F. Untreated OSA can be detrimental to the quality of life of individuals and their families. Untreated OSA worsens the prognosis of those with comorbidities, specifically cardiovascular disease, as it increases the risk of hypertension, diabetes, and stroke in males.

1. In children, untreated OSA can affect normal development and growth, causing enuresis and interfering with learning and cognitive processes.

PATHOGENESIS
A. OSA is believed to occur due to an anatomically narrow nasal and oropharynx, preventing the normal flow of air during breathing. Specifically, the patient is believed to stop breathing for approximately 10 seconds due to physical obstruction in the upper airway.
B. Obesity is a common cause of OSA.
C. During an OSA episode, the tongue and throat relax, causing less air to go into the lungs, where the body responds with loud snoring or gasping to breathe.

PREDISPOSING FACTORS
A. The predisposing factors for OSA are sex, age, BMI, size of neck circumference, high blood pressure, excessive daytime sleepiness, reported snoring, reported apnea, poor glycemic control, diabetes, sexual dysfunction, and obesity.
B. Other risk factors include alcohol use and exposure to secondhand smoke, especially in children.

COMMON COMPLAINTS
A. Excessive daytime sleepiness due to sleep deprivation
B. Fatigue
C. Frequent morning headaches
D. Snoring with brief stops to gasp for air while asleep
E. Behavioral dysregulation and irritability
F. Inability to complete tasks with lack of energy during the day
G. Falling asleep while driving
H. Poor work performance
I. Sexual dysfunction
J. Cognitive decline and poor concentration, including in children
K. Enuresis in children

OTHER SIGNS AND SYMPTOMS
A. Mood lability both in children and adults
B. Weight gain/BMI higher than recommended for age and sex
C. GERD
D. Hypertension

SUBJECTIVE DATA
A. Fatigue
B. Inability to function during the day
C. Snoring and occasional lapses in breathing while asleep, as reported by bed partner
D. Frequent headaches, specifically in the morning
E. Memory impairment
F. Changes in mood
G. Weight gain
H. History of sleep disturbance due to medical conditions
I. Female OSA during pregnancy or menopause
J. Anatomic deformity (e.g., deviated septum, enlarged tonsils, enlarged uvula, narrow oropharynx)
K. History of seizure disorders
L. In children, issues with school performance, mood changes, irritability, poor concentration, poor attention, falling asleep in class due to sleep deprivation, and dry mouth

PHYSICAL EXAMINATION
A. Obtain pulmonary workup to rule out COPD or other respiratory problems.
B. Obtain complete history and collateral information from the patient's partner/family/parents.
C. Calculate the BMI of individuals from all populations.
D. For adults, perform a complete review of systems and physical inspection of the head, nose, and throat. Check for any anatomic deformities or signs of infection in the glottis or uvula.
E. For children, perform a complete review of systems and physical inspection of the head, nose and throat, palate, uvula, tonsils (check of hypertrophy), failure to thrive, obesity, any breathing issues, and facial and neck abnormalities, as well as a complete cardiovascular exam.
F. Children and adults should be screened for snoring during sleep.

DIAGNOSTIC TESTS AND SCREENING
A. PSG is the gold standard for diagnosing OSA. It is recommended for adults and children.
B. Use the STOP-BANG questionnaire (four questions [STOP] on **S**noring, **T**iredness during the daytime, **O**bserved apnea, and high blood **P**ressure; and four items [BANG] on physical features: **B**ody mass index >35 kg/m^2, **A**ge >50 years, **N**eck circumference >40 cm, and male **G**ender). The first part is related to signs of apnea, while the second part has questions related to risk factors.
C. EEG is used for definitive diagnosis of apnea. It is recommended for adults and children.
D. Blood studies include ABG, TFTs, serum calcium, CBC, CMP, and drug and alcohol screening.
E. Oximetry is recommended for children.
F. Both adults and children (ages 2–8 years) should be screened for snoring.
G. EKG is recommended for children.
H. Perform MRI, CT, or endoscopy of the upper airway, including the nasal passage.

DIFFERENTIAL DIAGNOSES
A. Mood disorder
B. ADHD
C. PTSD
D. Alcoholism or other substance use disorder
E. Seizures
F. Another sleep disorder, such as circadian rhythm sleep disorder
G. COPD
H. GERD
I. CHF

PLAN
A. The APRN should discuss with the patient and family (if appropriate) the diagnosis, signs and symptoms, as well as treatment options.
B. Prepare a list of goals for the treatment of OSA.
C. Address the importance of safety, mood stability, and control of any medical comorbidities, such as hypertension and diabetes.
D. Identify behavioral changes, including diet, exercise, and use of positive airway pressure (PAP), sleep hygiene, and psychotherapy.

E. For children, discuss close collaboration with the school, pediatrician, and parents.
F. Discuss nonpharmacologic options.
G. Educate on standards of care and treatment appropriate for the patient's age.

GENERAL TREATMENT AND INTERVENTIONS
A. Consider PAP therapy, including nasal CPAP.
B. Consider oral appliances therapy, such as mandibular advancement devices to position the mandible forward to relieve the obstruction. This is often a temporary alternative to using PAP.
C. Encourage dietary and exercise regimen to increase physical activity and promote weight loss.
D. Encourage patient to sleep on their side or in upright position, not in a supine position.
E. Encourage behavioral modification and CBT.
F. Consider surgical interventions to modify the soft palate and the nasal passages: uvulopalatopharyngoplasty, craniofacial reconstruction with advancement of tongue or maxillomandibular bones, and tracheostomy.
G. The first line of treatment for children is adenotonsillectomy. For children with average weight, there is a 70% positive result, in contrast to a 30% success rate for children who are overweight.
H. The second line of treatment for children is PAP. This is indicated for children who continue to experience symptoms of OSA despite having adenotonsillectomy or who did not qualify for the surgery.
I. Avoid alcohol and sedatives 4 to 6 hours before bedtime.
J. Encourage smoking cessation.

COMMON MEDICATIONS
A. The treatment options for OSA are primarily non pharmacologic; however, some researchers recommend that medications be used as a last resort.
   1. In children, nasal corticosteroids and montelukast (Singulair) are prescribed.
   2. In adults, antidepressants, stimulants to reduce sleepiness, inhaled corticosteroids, nasal decongestants, potassium channel blockers, and thyroid replacement therapy agents are options.
B. Details on pharmacologic treatment are available in Table 14.3.

PATIENT TEACHING
A. The APRN should educate the patient and the family on the signs and symptoms of OSA.
B. Implement sleep hygiene.
C. Discuss the importance of eating a balanced diet and exercise.
D. Screen for snoring lapses while asleep.
E. Educate on the risk factors for OSA, such as obesity and other medical conditions.
F. Educate on the negative impact of environmental factors such as exposure to smoking and secondhand smoke.
G. Screen for use of alcohol and substances such as cannabis that might interfere with normal sleep.
H. For children, suggest a structured bed schedule and monitoring of sleep by the parents, specifically snoring.
I. Screen for mood lability, excessive daytime sleepiness, and lack of concentration.

FOLLOW-UP
A. The APRN should schedule the first follow-up visit once all results from sleep studies and laboratory workup are completed. During this visit, the APRN should review all the results, discuss with the patient or parents the recommended treatment, and prepare a treatment plan.
B. Subsequent follow-up visit should occur no more than 4 weeks after initial treatment.
C. Evaluate treatment adherence and effectiveness. Update treatment plan as needed.

CONSULTATION AND REFERRALS
A. Collaborate with a respiratory therapist, cardiologist, and internal medicine specialist as needed.
B. Consult with a sleep medicine specialist for children at high risk of OSA. The child would need an adenotonsillectomy and PSG 2 months after the surgery to evaluate the results of the treatment plan.

INDIVIDUAL CONSIDERATIONS

Pediatrics
A. Although OSA is more common in the adult population, a small percentage of children report OSA. Discuss diet and exercise to prevent obesity. Collaborate with the patient's pediatrician to monitor for signs of apneas and enlargement of the uvula and history of snoring.
B. The first line of treatment is adenotonsillectomy; the success rate depends on the child's weight. Children with a history of snoring should be screened for OSA.

Pregnancy
A. OSA may worsen during pregnancy. Pregnant patients may be at high risk of developing OSA due to hormonal changes, increased body weight, and gestational medical comorbidities like gestational diabetes, preeclampsia, and hypertension.
B. Pregnancy-related OSA may resolve after the delivery; however, the obstetrician must closely monitor any symptoms. Clinicians should screen women using three criteria: age, BMI, and history of hypertension.

Geriatrics
A. Educate patients and their caregivers on the signs and symptoms of OSA. Evidence supports that older adult patients are at higher risk of being diagnosed with OSA due to medical comorbidities, sleep disorders, polypharmacy, and sedentary lifestyles.
B. Educate older adult patients on the benefits of avoiding sedative medications, alcohol consumption, blood pressure control, GERD treatment, and glycemic control.

Partners/Family
A. Partners and family members should be educated on the signs and symptoms of OSA and asked to report symptoms to the APRN. OSA affects the patient suffering from the sleep disorder and interferes with the family's overall quality of life. Family members can be kept awake due to loud snoring or worry that their loved one would stop breathing during sleep.
B. Patients' spouses and others who are close to the patient may be aware that the individual can sleep "anytime anywhere" when in fact sleepiness is one of the potentially morbid symptoms of sleep apnea.

RESOURCE
A. Centers for Disease Control and Prevention. (n.d.). *Sleep facts and stats*. U.S. Department of Health and Human Services. https://www.cdc.gov/sleep/data-research/facts-stats

REFERENCES AND BIBLIOGRAPHY

Arredondo, E., DeLeon, M., Masozera, I., Panahi, L., Udeani, G., Tran, N., Nguyen, C. K., Atphaisit, C., de la Sota, B., Gonzalez, G., Jr., Liou, E., Mayo, Z., Nwosu, J., & Shiver, T. L. (2022). Overview of the role of pharmacological management of obstructive sleep apnea. *Medicina, 58*(2), 225. https://doi.org/10.3390/medicina58020225

Chance Nicholson, W., & Pfeiffer, K. (2021). Sleep disorders and mood, anxiety, and post-traumatic stress disorders. *Nursing Clinics of North America, 56*(2), 229–247. https://doi.org/10.1016/j.cnur.2021.02.003

Deshpande, P., Salcedo, B., & Haq, C. (2022). Common sleep disorders in children. *American Academy of Family Physicians, 105*(2), 168–176. PMID: 35166510.

Dominguez, J. E., Street, L., & Louis, J. (2018). Management of obstructive sleep apnea in pregnancy. *Obstetrics and Gynecology Clinics of North America, 45*(2), 233–247. https://doi.org/10.1016/j.ogc.2018.01.001

Gauld, C., Lopez, R., Morin, C., Geoffroy, P. A., Maquet, J., Desvergnes, P., McGonigal, A., Dauvilliers, Y., Philip, P., Dumas, G., & Micoulaud-Franchi, J. (2022). Symptom network analysis of the sleep disorders diagnostic criteria based on the clinical text of the *ICSD-3*. *Journal of Sleep Research, 31*(1). https://doi.org/10.1111/jsr.13435

Karna, B., Sankari, A., & Tatikonda, G. (2023, June 11). *Sleep disorder*. StatPearls Publishing. https://www.ncbi.nlm.nih.gov/books/NBK560720

Kim, S. W., & Taranto-Montemurro, L. (2019). When do gender differences begin in obstructive sleep apnea patients? *Journal of Thoracic Disease, 11*(S9), S1147–S1149. https://doi.org/10.21037/jtd.2019.04.37

Marques, D. R., & de Azevedo, M. H. P. (2018). Potentialities of network analysis for sleep medicine. *Journal of Psychosomatic Research, 111*, 89–90. https://doi.org/10.1016/j.jpsychores.2018.05.019

Wickramasinghe, H. (2024, May 28). *Obstructive sleep apnea (OSA)*. Medscape. https://emedicine.medscape.com/article/295807-overview

Zakhari, R. (2020). *The psychiatric-mental health nurse practitioner certification review manual*. Springer Publishing Company.

15 SOMATIC SYMPTOM AND RELATED DISORDERS

Nataliya Pilipenko and Kimberly A. Muellers

INTRODUCTION

Formally known as somatoform disorders, somatic symptom and related disorders (SSRDs) pose unique challenges in their diagnosis and treatment. Specifically, SSRDs require that both the patient and the treatment team move away from mind–body dualism and embrace biopsychosocially based conceptualization and treatment planning.

In his seminal 1977 publication, George Engel stated that the biomedical model "assumes that disease is to be fully accounted for by deviations from the norm of measurable biologic (somatic) variables" (1977, p. 130). Thus, the biomedical model requires that medical illnesses are both explained and treated via correction of "disordered somatic (biochemical or neurophysiological) processes" (Engel, 1977, p. 130). While the biomedical model is the cornerstone of evidence-based medicine, it is insufficient in providing culturally informed and patient-centered care, whereby social, psychological, and behavioral dimensions of illness are increasingly recognized and integrated.

Addressing concerns about operationalizability of the biopsychosocial (BPS) model, several groups proposed its adaptations within medical interviewing practices, including the patient-centered interviewing method by Smith and colleagues (2013) and the four habits model by Frankel and Stein (2001). However, in routine clinical care, the "split BPS" model is frequently practiced. Described by McDaniel and colleagues (2004), "split BPS" is a clinical practice whereby biomedical explanations and approaches are exclusively utilized at the start of the medical treatment. When the biomedical approach fails to produce the desired outcome of symptom elimination or reduction, the healthcare provider introduces BPS in shifting the focus from the objective and observable (within the purview of the medical specialist) to the subjective and idiosyncratic. Split approach leads to understandable low patient satisfaction and limited treatment cooperation.

Providing effective care to patients suffering from SSRDs challenges APRNs in approaching health and illness from a BPS perspective both conceptually and practically—with patients, families, and members of the treatment team. Strong knowledge in SSRD diagnosis and treatment is particularly important for APRNs working in medical settings where SSRDs are most frequently identified.

SSRDs include the following conditions: somatic symptom disorder, illness anxiety disorder, conversion disorder, psychological factors affecting other medical conditions, and factitious disorder, as well as other specified somatic symptom and related disorders and unspecified somatic symptom and related disorder. This chapter provides assessment and treatment considerations for each of these SSRD diagnoses.

REFERENCES AND BIBLIOGRAPHY

American Psychiatric Association. (2013). *Diagnostic and statistical manual of mental disorders* (5th ed.). https://doi.org/10.1176/appi.books.9780890425596

Engel, G. L. (1977). The need for a new medical model: A challenge for biomedicine. *Science*, *196*(4286), 129–136. https://doi.org/10.1126/science.847460

Frankel, R. M., & Stein, T. (2001). Getting the most out of the clinical encounter: The four habits model. *The Journal of Medical Practice Management*, *16*(4), 184–191. PMID: 11317576.

McDaniel, S. H., Campbell, T. L., Hepworth, J., & Lorenz, A. (2004). *Family-oriented primary care* (2nd ed.). Springer Publishing Company.

Smith, R. C., Fortin, A. H., Dwamena, F., & Frankel, R. M. (2013). An evidence-based patient-centered method makes the biopsychosocial model scientific. *Patient Education and Counseling*, *91*(3), 265–270. https://doi.org/10.1016/j.pec.2012.12.010

CONVERSION DISORDER: FUNCTIONAL NEUROLOGIC SYMPTOM DISORDER

DEFINITION

A. Diagnostic criteria for functional neurologic symptom disorder (FND) include the following:

   1. Presence of altered *motor control or sensory function symptoms*
   2. Symptom(s) *not compatible* with known medical or neurologic conditions
   3. Symptom(s) *not better explained* by another medical or psychiatric conditions

B. FND diagnostic specifiers include *acute* (less than 6 months in duration) or *persistent* (6 months or more in duration). If FND is associated with a *psychological stressor*, this specifier should be included. Table 15.1 presents specification options for presenting FND symptom(s). Presenting symptoms must be associated with distress and impairment of functioning for the diagnosis to be made.

C. The *International Classification of Diseases, 11th Revision* (*ICD-11*; World Health Organization, 2019), includes FND under both "Mental, Behavioural or Neurodevelopmental Disorders" as well as "Diseases of the Nervous System." Aybek and Perez (2022) note that "this variability within and across classification systems is problematic, as it perpetuates a cartesian dualism and creates coding problems between mental health and neurological disorders" (p. 1).

INCIDENCE

A. Within general medical practice, FND prevalence rates are not well-understood, likely reflecting both diagnostic challenges and narrowing of access to specialists (neurology, psychiatry) who are frequently involved in the diagnostic process.

B. FND accounts for approximately 6% of neurology outpatient contacts and has a putative community incidence rate of 4 to 12 per 100,000 annually. Comorbid neurologic disease occurs in around 10% of cases.

C. FND is common across medical specialties, specifically in clinical neuroscience and physical rehabilitation. FND has been termed psychiatry's *blind spot*.

D. Although functional neurologic disorders can develop at any age, they usually affect young or middle-aged individuals. A recent review by Aybek and Perez (2022) indicates that ▶

motor symptoms (weakness or movement disorders) and seizure-type symptoms are the most common presentations of FND, with the former most prevalent among patients in their 40s and the latter most common among patients in their 30s.

E. It is important for clinicians to keep FND on the differential diagnostic radar as delays in both accurate diagnostics and correct identification of presentation have been noted. For example, Wasserman and Herskovitz (2017) reported that among patients suffering from FND with nonepileptic seizures, delay in diagnosis was greater than 7 years, and fewer than 70% of neurology nurses and only 58% of ED nurses were able to currently differentiate FND presentation from epileptic seizures based on video recordings containing both presentations.

PATHOGENESIS

A. FND is a disorder involving multiple brain networks implicated in a sense of agency, emotion/threat processing, attention, homeostatic balance, interoception, multimodal integration, and cognitive/motor control.

B. The following networks are involved: salience, limbic, dorsal attention, ventral attention, cognitive control, and motor planning, as well as the sensorimotor and temporoparietal junctions.

C. The directionality of FND symptoms and signs of changes in neural circuitry cannot be ascertained based on the current state of research.

PREDISPOSING FACTORS

A. Maladaptive personality traits, a history of trauma, and stress are all risk factors for FND. However, none of these factors are truly pathognomonic of this condition.

B. While females are two to three times more likely to be diagnosed with FND, the etiology of this diagnostic phenomenon is not well-understood.

C. FND may be associated with the presence of known medical conditions. For example, FND with *attacks or seizures* is more common among patients with known diagnosis of epilepsy compared with patients without this diagnosis.

D. FND signs may be present among patients with Parkinson disease and multiple sclerosis.

COMMON COMPLAINTS

A. FND can present with a wide range of symptoms and signs; however, the most common types of FND concern motor and seizure symptoms.

B. See Table 15.1 for FND symptom types.

OTHER SIGNS AND SYMPTOMS

A. La Belle indifference: Clinical presentation characterized by apparent lack of concerns about symptoms and their consequences may be present. It is not a diagnostic indicator for FND and should not be treated as such.

SUBJECTIVE DATA

A. Evaluation of FND should incorporate history of similar symptoms/complaints and temporal association with stress or trauma, in addition to dissociative symptoms including depersonalization, derealization, and/or dissociative amnesia.

B. Gilmour and colleagues (2020) suggest that the following domains are incorporated as part of the interdisciplinary and holistic FND assessment: core symptoms, fatigue, pain, cognitive fog, sleep, symptom beliefs, medication side effects, and psychological and social factors.

C. FND diagnosis can only be supported by demonstrating that clinical signs observed via physical examination are not replicated when testing via alternative methods.

PHYSICAL EXAMINATION

A. The following signs may be common to all FND presentations: variability of the symptom noted between reported history and physical exam, as well as effortful or grimacing expression during the examination when following the examiner's instructions.

B. Table 15.2 outlines the key physical findings that may support FND diagnosis. These are based on a review by Aybek and Perez (2022) of 22 studies of FND motor type (overall specificity 64%–100%, sensitivity 9%–100%, good to excellent interrater reliability) and 27 studies of FND seizure type (overall specificity 11%–100%, sensitivity 9%–96%, excellent interrater reliability).

C. Video electroencephalography (VEEG) can help differentiate FND from epilepsy; however, this method is not always available in clinical practice and specialist referral would be required for diagnostic evaluation.

D. Critically consider evidence of previous medical diagnoses when either FND or somatic symptom disorder (SSD) is included in the differential diagnostic considerations.

E. Due to variability in presentation, a comprehensive review of all symptom tests and observations is outside of the scope of this chapter. See "Resources" for this section for information on practice guidelines and testing.

DIAGNOSTIC TESTS AND SCREENINGS

A. Each patient should receive a physical exam as well as a full diagnostic workup in line with evidence-based recommendations as appropriate for the presenting medical concern(s).

B. Medication reconciliation and review, as well as toxicology report focusing on substances that can be etiologically linked to presenting symptoms, should precede FND diagnosis.

C. Table 15.2 presents information about signs that may be applicable to FND motor and seizure symptoms.

D. Clinicians should avoid overemphasizing a single sign for FND diagnosis as such practice will adversely affect diagnostic specificity.

E. No validated clinical signs are available for dystonia or tics.

TABLE 15.1 FUNCTIONAL NEUROLOGIC SYMPTOM DISORDER SYMPTOM TYPES

Motor symptoms: Weakness, paralysis	Swallowing symptoms: Globus	Abnormal movement: Tremor, dystonia, gait abnormalities	Mixed symptoms: Involve multiple domains of the nervous system
Speech symptoms: Dysphonia, aphonia, dysarthria	Attacks or seizures: Nonepileptic seizures, episodes of unresponsiveness	Anesthesia or sensory: Altered/reduced/absent hearing, vision, skin sensations	Special sensory: Diplopia

TABLE 15.2 PHYSICAL FINDINGS SUPPORTING FUNCTIONAL NEUROLOGIC SYMPTOM DISORDER (FND) DIAGNOSIS

Assessment	Look for:
Gait	• Monoplegic leg dragging • Excessive visible effort • Falling toward support, such as chair nearby, table, wall • Excessive slowness, hesitation, caution • Loss of tone/knee buckling at each step • Noneconomic posture
Hemifacial spasm	• Long contraction (more than 3 seconds) • Tonic deviation of the lip with possible platysma contraction • Absence of "other Babinski sign"—lack of eyebrow elevation on the side of the spasm • Abnormal speech • No chewing movement, no self-biting • Lingual movement without mouth movement
Trunk movement	• Positive sign of asymmetry in strength of the sternocleidomastoid muscle • "Functional Romberg" sign
Cataplexy	• No sudden facial expression change • Facial jerks or grimaces • Lack of postural control • Preserved tendon reflexes
Upper limb weakness	• Discordance or inconsistency in strength during examination • Give-way/collapsing pattern[a] • Drift without pronation • Co-contractions of agonist and antagonist muscles preventing movement of the tested joint
Lower limb weakness	• Discordance or inconsistency in strength during examination • Give-way/collapsing weakness • Hoover sign
Tremor	• Distractibility • Entrainment • Increase in amplitude with weight load on the wrists • Variability in amplitude, frequency, and direction of tremor • "Whack a mole" sign
Seizures	• Duration more than 2 minutes[b] • Ability to recall information during the event • Resistance to passive eye-opening attempts • Asynchronous limb movements[b] • Vocalizations—whispering, stuttering, moaning • Rapid postseizure recovery without postictal confusion

[a]Please note that this is also common among patients with pain-limited weakness.
[b]Caution not to miss status epilepticus.

DIFFERENTIAL DIAGNOSIS

A. FND diagnosis is considered only after relevant neurologic conditions, etiologically connected medical conditions, and substance/medication-induced disorders have been ruled out.
B. Clinical and/or laboratory findings must provide evidence that the neurologic symptoms are incompatible with recognized neurologic or general medical conditions.
C. Diagnosis of FND cannot be made based on the absence of findings of unusual nature of symptoms. It is necessary to demonstrate via clear evidence that presenting symptoms are incompatible with the presenting disease.
D. Symptoms cannot be deliberately produced or feigned as under these circumstances diagnoses of either factitious disorder or malingering (respectively) would be made.
E. Culturally sanctioned practices and rituals need to be considered in order to avoid inappropriate medicalization of culturally bound presentations.
F. The following psychiatric conditions should be ruled out when diagnosing FND:

1. Somatic symptom disorder (SSD): The primary diagnostic focus in SSD is on distress and associated excessive thoughts, feelings, or behaviors, resulting from the presence of a specific physical symptom.
2. Illness anxiety disorder (IAD): Patients suffering from IAD are preoccupied with acquiring a medical condition while minimal or no symptoms of the feared condition are present.
3. Depressive disorders: Depressive disorders may include somatic symptoms (such as leaden paralysis) along with depressed mood or loss of interest and pleasure; however, FND is characterized by focal and prominent somatic symptoms that are incompatible with recognized neurologic or medical conditions.

4. Dissociative disorders: Affect memory and consciousness however do not impact voluntary motor or sensory functioning.

G. Psychiatric-mental health nurse practitioners (PMHNPs) should be aware of conditions that are frequently comorbid with FND. These include anxiety disorders, other SSDs, substance use disorders, and psychotic disorders.

PLAN

Expectation Management

A. Although research notes significant heterogeneity in treatment responses, literature review by Gelauff and Stone (2016) indicates that the overall prognosis of FND is not favorable for either FND with motor symptoms or with seizure symptoms.
B. Quality of life measures tend to remain unchanged or worsen at follow-up.
C. Presence of purely sensory symptoms and younger age are associated with better prognosis.
D. Longer duration of FND symptoms is associated with lack of remission.
E. When discussing FND, it is important to remember that symptoms may be transient or persistent and that shorter symptom duration is a positive prognostic factor.
F. FND treatment plan should be both patient-centered and biopsychosocially grounded.
G. For FND with motor symptoms, physical and occupational therapies are treatments of choice.
H. Psychotherapy approaches may be beneficial across FND subtypes.

General Treatments and Interventions

A. FND treatment should focus on symptom control as well as improved functioning and quality of life rather than complete symptom elimination or resolution. General treatment goals should be discussed upon informing the patient about the FND diagnosis and revisited throughout the treatment.
B. Current expert consensus encourages clear and open patient communication about the FND diagnosis and its management:
  1. Explicitly naming the diagnosis
  2. Demonstrating or outlining how diagnosis was reached, including relevant positive physical examination signs
C. Both patients and treatment teams should be explicitly clear that FND diagnosis was not merely prompted by "all tests are normal." Patients must be apprised of the "rule in" signs and tests that led to FND diagnosis.
D. While some healthcare providers may hesitate to disclose and discuss FND diagnosis directly, evidence indicates that even the act of diagnosis-related discussion can be therapeutic as communication about diagnosis has been linked to symptom improvement.
E. The following five steps are recommended:
  1. Validate symptoms as both real and prevalent.
  2. Provide diagnostic impression via specifically naming FND.
  3. Provide a brief, patient-centered etiologic explanation such as "[when experiencing FND symptoms] your brain becomes overloaded and shuts down."
  4. Inform patient about treatment options. Include information about effectiveness (specifically, what will likely or unlikely work for improved symptom control).
  5. Communicate appropriate optimism about symptom management, with focus on treatment options available to the patient.

F. In line with patient-centered, culturally sensitive practice and to ensure bilateral understanding between the patient and the care team, the following information should be elicited and addressed:
  1. Prior diagnoses: What have you been told about the causes of your symptoms? Do you agree with the explanations that you have been given? Tell me why you do/do not agree? What other questions do you have about these symptoms?
  2. Current symptom understanding: antecedents and maintaining factors: How do you explain your [current] symptoms? In your opinion, what is causing these symptoms? Do you notice anything making these symptoms better/worse? What have you tried for [FND] symptoms? Did anything help?
  3. Patient's illness formulation utilizing *teach-back* following FND diagnosis discussion: We discussed FND diagnosis today. I want to make sure that I explained this diagnosis well. How do you understand this diagnosis? What concerns do you have about this diagnosis? Does this diagnosis "fit" your experience? Tell me why you think so.

COMMON MEDICATIONS

A. Although no specific medications have been identified for FND treatment and symptom management, two important pharmacologic management considerations are relevant.
  1. As FND may be frequently comorbid with other mental health symptoms, patients are often prescribed pharmacologic agents (e.g., selective serotonin reuptake inhibitors [SSRIs]) for treatment of these conditions.
     a. Although clinicians may frequently come across psychiatric medication prescriptions for patients suffering from FND, it is important to consider which comorbid psychiatric condition is being treated with psychopharmacologic agent and the evidence base for the treatment approach since no medications are indicated for direct treatment of FND.
  2. Medication reconciliation is critical. A plan should be developed to discontinue any medications that have been started and may be irrelevant and/or causing harm in the light of the FND diagnosis.
     a. For example, antiepileptic medications in patients with diagnosed FND seizure type should be discontinued when epilepsy/seizure disorders have been ruled out.

PATIENT TEACHING

A. When discussing FND diagnosis and treatment, the use of appropriate terminology is central. Terminology that carries negative judgment and/or can be misleading to the etiologic roots of FND (e.g., *hysteria, pseudoseizures, organic*) should be avoided.
  1. Use of the term *psychogenic* highlights psychiatric aspects of the diagnosis, and patient receptiveness to this label may vary depending on the patient's idiosyncratic illness-related beliefs and interactions with the mental health system.
  2. Using the term *functional* to describe symptoms reflects both symptom variability and possibility of change. Additionally, this term grounds FND in BPS and avoids psychiatric labeling. When discussing this term, however, clinicians may want to highlight that the patient's experience of the symptoms is far from functional.

B. The "General Treatments and Interventions" section outlines the guidelines and specific steps for discussion of FND diagnosis with the patients.
   1. Members of the care team should provide patients with consistent messaging about FND diagnosis and be prepared to revisit conceptualization throughout the treatment to address the patient's concerns and ambivalence.
   2. Agreement with the treatment plan should be reevaluated periodically to ensure ongoing engagement with care.
   3. Patients should be provided with information about FND educational resources as well as testimonials of other patients (see "Resources" section).

C. FND education focuses on "how" and "what" rather than the "why" of the symptoms, reflecting focus on active coping and functional improvement.

D. Patients may be receptive to "hardware/software" analogy of symptoms and illness, which highlights that symptom may persist despite absent or inconsistent findings on tests.

E. Patient teaching requires BPS-grounded FND understanding and conceptualization, as well as patient-centered inquiry and exploration (see "Resources" section).

FOLLOW-UP

A. The following are the two primary domains of FND treatment:
   1. **Physical therapy (PT) with primary focus on motor rehabilitation:** This includes task performance and use of distractions. Additionally, occupational therapy as well as speech-language pathology may be highly relevant.
   2. **Psychotherapy:** While the primary focus of (limited) research is on cognitive behavioral therapy (CBT), mindfulness-based approaches, prolonged exposure, psychodynamic psychotherapy, and dialectical behavior therapy have been utilized for FND treatment.

B. Since FND is frequently accompanied by pain, fatigue, and cognitive difficulties (e.g., "brain fog"), both rehabilitation services and evidence-based psychotherapies can support functional improvement in FDN by targeting these domains.

C. Behavioral approaches can be utilized even when neither PT nor psychotherapy is possible and/or accepted by the patient.
   1. Clinicians can help patients develop self-management "workbook," working with the patient to create a tracking record summarizing the diagnosis (including explanation of symptoms), triggers, coping skills, goals, barriers, and progress toward these goals.
   2. This approach can engage patients in an active role, provide valuable treatment information, and foster active coping.

CONSULTATION AND REFERRALS

A. Close collaboration between different specialties in diagnosis and management of FND is crucial. Initial (prediagnostic) referrals will be dictated by the symptom profile and differential diagnostic considerations and may include neurology, psychiatry/psychology, and physical medicine and rehabilitation (PM&R).

B. Following the establishment of the FND diagnosis, the following referrals should be strongly considered:
   1. PT
   2. Speech-language pathology
   3. Occupational therapy
   4. Psychotherapy

C. Referrals should reflect not merely FND-related needs but also treatment of comorbid conditions.

INDIVIDUAL CONSIDERATIONS

Pediatrics

A. Grattan-Smith and Dale (2016) note that FND symptoms in pediatric populations closely resemble adult presentations and that response to treatment is highly variable.

B. FND appears to be most common in females between the ages of 10 and 14 who are under high academic and other performance pressures.

C. Presentations are typically polysymptomatic and treatments involve both the patient and the family.

D. See Chapter 20, "Special Considerations for Childhood and Adolescent Populations," for additional considerations in working with pediatric patients.

Pregnancy

A. There appears to be paucity of information about FND in pregnancy and postpartum.

B. See Chapter 12, "Perinatal Mental Health," for other recommendations for mental healthcare during pregnancy.

Geriatrics/Older Adults

A. Although research in this patient population is very limited, FND may be common among geriatric patients, particularly in inpatient rehabilitation settings.

B. Corretge and colleagues (2019) report that among 100 patients discharged from geriatric inpatient rehabilitation service, 20% had "suspected or definitive FND" noted, per chart review.

C. Identification of FND among older adult patients may be further complicated by increased prevalence of severe medical comorbidities, polypharmacy, and lack of specialists with appropriate understanding of this population and its needs.

D. For further recommendations on geriatric care, please see Chapter 21, "Aging and Older Adult Populations."

Partners/Family

A. There may be substantial benefits to involving partners/family members in the FND treatment, especially if they are also performing caregiving roles for the patient. However, involvement of anyone other than the patient should not be automatically assumed for adult patients with capacity.

B. Patients should consent to have partners/family involved in their care and be provided with clear information that could affect their decision.
   1. Evaluation of symptoms may involve questions about personal history, including sexual and/or substance use history, which the patient may not wish to disclose to others.
   2. Goals of family/partner involvement should be made clear, while the focus needs to remain on the patient.
   3. Clinicians should be mindful of the complex relationship dynamics, conflicts of interest, hidden agendas, and other complex factors when partners/family become involved.

C. For more information about caregiver issues, see Chapter 35, "Caregiver and End-of-Life Issues."

RESOURCES

Websites

A. Functional Neurological Disorder Society: www.fndsociety.org

B. Functional Neurological Disorder Guide provides educational resources for patients: www.neurosymptoms.org/en

C. Functional Neurological Disorder (FND) Hope provides peer support resources, coping and educational resources: https://fndhope.org

Visual/Video Materials

A. How to explain the diagnosis of FND. Supplemental Material (Video). In Aybek, S., & Perez, D. L. (2022). Diagnosis and management of functional neurological disorder. *British Medical Journal, 376*, o64. https://doi.org/10.1136/bmj.o64
B. Triaging initial treatment recommendations in patients with FND. Supplemental Material (Video). In Aybek, S., & Perez, D. L. (2022). Diagnosis and management of functional neurological disorder. *British Medical Journal, 376*, o64. https://doi.org/10.1136/bmj.o64
C. Carson, A., Lehn, A., Ludwig, L., & Stone, J. (2016). Explaining functional disorders in the neurology clinic: A photo story. *Practical Neurology, 16*(1), 56–61. https://doi-org.ezproxy.cul.columbia.edu/10.1136/practneurol-2015-001242

Practice Guidelines

A. Baslet, G., Bajestan, S. N., Aybek, S., Modirrousta, M. D., Clin Psy, J. P., Cavanna, A., Perez, D. L., Lazarow, S. S., Raynor, G., Voon, V., Ducharme, S., & LaFrance, W. C., Jr. (2021). Evidence-based practice for the clinical assessment of psychogenic nonepileptic seizures: A report from the American Neuropsychiatric Association Committee on Research. *The Journal of Neuropsychiatry and Clinical Neurosciences, 33*(1), 27–42. https://doi.org/10.1176/appi.neuropsych.19120354
B. Perez, D. L., Aybek, S., Popkirov, S., Kozlowska, K., Stephen, C. D., Anderson, J., Shura, R., Ducharme, S., Carson, A., Hallett, M., Nicholson, T. R., Stone, J., LaFrance, W. C. Jr., Voon, V. (2021). A review and expert opinion on the neuropsychiatric assessment of motor functional neurological disorders. *The Journal of Neuropsychiatry and Clinical Neurosciences, 33*(1), 14–26. https://doi.org/10.1176/appi.neuropsych.19120357

REFERENCES AND BIBLIOGRAPHY

Aybek, S., & Perez, D. L. (2022). Diagnosis and management of functional neurological disorder. *British Medical Journal, 376*, o64. https://doi.org/10.1136/bmj.o64

Corretge, M., Chun Ho-Yan, Y., Roscoe, M., & Carson, A. (2019). Functional neurological disorder in geriatric rehabilitation: Incidence, clinical presentations, and impact on discharge. *Journal of Neurology, Neurosurgery, & Psychiatry, 90*(Suppl 2), A21–A22. https://doi.org/10.1136/jnnp-2019-BNPA.45

Duncan, R., Horwood, J., Razvi, S., & Mulhern, S. (2020). Psychogenic nonepileptic seizures that remit when the diagnosis is given: Just good luck? *Epilepsy & Behavior, 102*, 106667. https://doi.org/10.1016/j.yebeh.2019.106667

Gasparini, S., Beghi, E., Ferlazzo, E., Beghi, M., Belcastro, V., Biermann, K. P., Bottini, G., Capovilla, G., Cervellione, R. A., Cianci, V., Coppola, G., Cornaggia, C. M., De Fazio, P., De Masi, S., De Sarro, G., Elia, M., Erba, G., Fusco, L., Gambardella, A., ... Aguglia, U. (2019). Management of psychogenic non-epileptic seizures: A multidisciplinary approach. *European Journal of Neurology, 26*(2), 205–e15. https://doi.org/10.1111/ene.13818

Gelauff, J., & Stone, J. (2016). Prognosis of functional neurologic disorders. *Handbook of Clinical Neurology, 139*, 523–541. https://doi.org/10.1016/B978-0-12-801772-2.00043-6

Gilmour, G. S., Nielsen, G., Teodoro, T., Yogarajah, M., Coebergh, J. A., Dilley, M. D., Martino, D., & Edwards, M. J. (2020). Management of functional neurological disorder. *Journal of Neurology, 267*(7), 2164–2172. https://doi.org/10.1007/s00415-020-09772-w

Grattan-Smith, P. J., & Dale, R. C. (2016). Pediatric functional neurologic symptoms. *Handbook of Clinical Neurology, 139*, 489–498. https://doi.org/10.1016/B978-0-12-801772-2.00040-0

O'Neal, M. A., & Baslet, G. (2018). Treatment for patients with a functional neurological disorder (Conversion Disorder): An integrated approach. *The American Journal of Psychiatry, 175*(4), 307–314. https://doi.org/10.1176/appi.ajp.2017.17040450

Wasserman, D., & Herskovitz, M. (2017). Epileptic vs psychogenic nonepileptic seizures: A video-based survey. *Epilepsy & Behavior, 73*, 42–45. https://doi.org/10.1016/j.yebeh.2017.04.020

World Health Organization. (2019). *International statistical classification of diseases* (11th rev.). https://icd.who.int

FACTITIOUS DISORDER

DEFINITION

A. Diagnostic criteria for factitious disorder (FD) include the following:
  1. Patient exaggerates, fakes, pretends, or induces symptoms of illness (either physical or psychological) or causes injury or disease to themselves or someone else through deceit.
  2. Patient portrays themselves (or someone else) as sick, wounded, or disabled.
  3. Deceptive behavior occurs even in the absence of clear external incentives.
  4. Behavior is not better explained by a psychotic condition (e.g., delusional disorder).
  5. Diagnostic specifiers include single episode or recurrent episodes. FD can be identified in the presence of a preexisting medical condition as long as there is proof of falsified symptoms and signs without any external rewards. Box 15.1 outlines some examples of FD presentations.

B. Factitious disorder imposed on another (FDIA) is diagnosed when the patient falsifies illness or injury in another person and if points 2 to 4 are also met (by the perpetrator). The perpetrator of symptoms, signs, and injury receives the diagnosis of FDIA rather than the victim.

C. Due to the central aspect of concealment and deception, as well as heterogeneity in clinical presentation of FD and FDIA, both conditions are exceptionally challenging to diagnose.

BOX 15.1 EXAMPLES OF FACTITIOUS DISORDER AND FACTITIOUS DISORDER IMPOSED ON ANOTHER

Reporting distress/impairment following an event that did not happen • Example: patient reporting depression and grief following death of a child but patient either did not have children or all children are alive
Manipulating laboratory tests • Example: adding blood or urine to samples
Falsely indicating medical abnormality or altering records to include an illness
Injecting substances to induce abnormal laboratory tests • Example: injecting insulin, self-administering prostaglandin suppositories to elicit labor
Inducing physical injury • Example: cuts, broken bones

D. While the terms *Munchausen syndrome* and *Munchausen syndrome by proxy* are widely used to describe FD and FDIA, respectively, they are not formal diagnostic terms and therefore lack established criteria, leading to further diagnostic confusion. Given the paucity of research, this chapter presents findings based on literature for Munchausen syndrome and Munchausen syndrome by proxy as applicable to FD and FDIA.
E. In their review of FDIA literature (child victims), Abdurrachid and Gama Marques (2022) reported symptom induction as the most common type of falsification behavior, accounting for 74% of FDIA incidents.
   1. Providing false information (20%), simulation (11%), coaching of the child to "play along" (9%), and withholding information (2%) were also reported.
   2. In 15% of cases, multiple types of falsification were noted.
F. Although available literature focuses on children, victims of FDIA can include any vulnerable individual, for example, older adults or patients who are significantly affected by developmental disabilities.

INCIDENCE
A. While the estimated prevalence rate of FD in hospital settings is 1%, the central feature of FD is deception. Therefore, true rates may be impossible to estimate accurately.
B. Jafferany and colleagues (2018) report that up to 5% of all medical encounters may be secondary to FD, while Schreier (2004) estimated that in the United States 1,200 children per year may be victims of FDIA.
C. FD diagnosis appears to be prevalent among females (75%–95%) in their 20s and 30s, with majority (50%–65.7%) having healthcare-related training or employment.
D. Abdurrachid and Gama Marques (2022) reported that over 90% of perpetrators of FDIA were female and 17% were employed in healthcare. With regard to the outcomes of FDIA, the authors noted that in over one-fifth of all reported cases that they reviewed no follow-up was reported. Other outcomes included imprisonment of the perpetrator (14%), death of the victim (12%), treatment of the perpetrator (10%), victim continuing to live with the perpetrator (4%), and suicide of the perpetrator (1%).

PATHOGENESIS
A. FD typically follows an intermittent course and may first emerge following a hospitalization (medical or psychiatric). However, the etiology of both FD and FDIA is unclear.
B. Jafferany and colleagues (2018) noted multiple theories that were proposed to explain FD, including disruption of childhood attachments, intergenerational illness behavior transfer, personal identity and intrapsychic conflicts, and masochistic activity.
C. Associated physiologic findings include abnormal EEG, head injury, central nervous system infections, and frontotemporal cortical atrophy.
D. Barber and Davis (2002) astutely pointed out that it is impossible to fully determine whether symptom production can be fully explained by conscious or unconscious mechanisms. Deception of self and/or others is a complex process, likely best conceptualized as a continuum, rather than a dichotomy. Criminal behavior and the presence of psychopathology when it comes to FDIA can coexist.

PREDISPOSING FACTORS
A. While history of abuse and neglect has been noted in both FD and FDIA, links are nonprognostic.
B. Abdurrachid and Gama Marques (2022) noted that one-third of the FDIA cases were associated with abuse and marital or family conflict.
C. Several authors noted high comorbidity between FD and FDIA, ranging from 10% to 30%.

COMMON COMPLAINTS
A. Both FD and FDIA can present with a wide range of clinical symptoms. However, guidelines proposed by the Royal College of Paediatrics and Child Health (2009) may help identify FDIA. These guidelines appear highly relevant to FD presentation.
   1. Specifically, reported and observed symptoms or signs:
      a. Not explained by any known medical condition(s)
      b. Not explained by testing, procedures, and studies
      c. Exhibits poor response to treatment and/or treatment not tolerated by the patient
      d. Upon resolution, return along with emergence of new symptoms/signs
      e. Observed exclusively under discrete and specific circumstances (e.g., in the presence of a specific caregiver, in care of suspected FDIA)
   2. Additionally:
      a. There is evidence of fabrication, such as conflict between report and biological symptom plausibility, inconsistent/implausible history by report or record review, evidence of alterations to records/results, inexplicable results and findings, and covert video surveillance (CVS) evidence (e.g., observed tampering with syringes, hidden medications).
      b. There is reported suspicion for FDIA and FD based on records, collateral reports, and/or other independent sources.
      c. Life pursuits and activities are restricted significantly beyond the level that known illness or associated impairment would require (e.g., child being removed from school, use of unnecessary assistive devices).
      d. Multiple medical services are sought inappropriately.

OTHER SIGNS AND SYMPTOMS
A. Critical to the FD and FDIA is the absence of evident rewards for the falsification behavior (see "Differential Diagnoses" section).
B. When evaluating FD and FDIA, it is important to be mindful that either of these conditions can coexist with a de facto medical illness. Therefore, careful consideration of clinical symptoms and signs alongside full and appropriate documentation becomes central.

SUBJECTIVE DATA
A. Diagnosis of both FD and FDIA relies on substantive objective evidence of deliberate and deceptive symptom production; therefore, subjective data would be insufficient to make the diagnosis.

PHYSICAL EXAMINATION
A. Physical examination may offer critical insights into the diagnosis of FD and FDIA, including evidence of fabrication, and provide support for incompatibility between the patient's report and the physiologic processes/injuries observed.
B. Evidence of injury induction, tapering with samples (e.g., urine, blood), presence of equipment (e.g., syringes), or medications that are not prescribed or medically indicated should be documented.

C. In the case of FDIA, physical examination can offer evidence of symptom changes when the victim is separated from the suspected perpetrator.

DIAGNOSTIC TESTS AND SCREENINGS

A. Evidence of symptom falsification can be derived from a range of sources (Bass & Wade, 2019), including medical record review, history of present illness obtained via patient interview, direct behavioral observation, collateral information, psychological/neuropsychological testing with symptom validity testing, and CVS.

B. While psychological and neuropsychological testing can help quantify symptoms and can evaluate symptom feigning in addition to overreporting, these tests are developed and utilized largely within the context of forensic work. Appropriateness of these measures in medical settings as well as concerns related to informed consent in testing should be carefully weighed before proceeding, especially in cases of FDIA.

C. While utilization of CVS can provide significant supporting evidence of FD and FDIA, its use is associated with extensive ethical and legal considerations. Use of this method should not be considered nor employed without extensive consultation with the hospital's administration and legal and ethics departments in order to determine appropriateness, scope, and logistics.

DIFFERENTIAL DIAGNOSES

A. The following psychiatric conditions should be ruled out for diagnosis of FD/FDIA:
  1. Malingering: Malingering is characterized by intentional reporting or feigning of symptoms for personal gain (e.g., money, time off work). In FD/FDIA, by contrast, symptoms are ongoing in the absence of obvious external incentives.
  2. Somatic symptom disorder (SSD): While SSD is characterized by significant attention to physical symptoms and treatment seeking, there is no evidence of illness symptoms or signs being deliberately manufactured or falsified.
  3. Functional neurological symptom disorder (FND): In FND, there is an incompatibility between symptoms (involving motor control or sensory function) and recognized medical condition(s). However, symptoms are not falsified.
  4. Primary psychiatric disorders: Conditions like depression, anxiety, or psychotic disorders may present with somatic complaints as part of the clinical picture.
  5. Medical conditions with atypical presentations: Some medical diseases can present in unusual ways that might initially mimic FD, necessitating thorough investigations.
  6. Borderline personality disorder (BPD): While deliberate physical self-harm attempts may be present in BPD, deceptive production of symptoms is not a feature of this condition.

B. Potential differential diagnoses for FDIA include:
  1. Medical abuse of a child or elder: *Medical child or elder abuse* is a more comprehensive term than FDIA as it includes causing sickness in another person as well as harming a child in various ways. The goal of deception should be considered to distinguish FDIA from child or elder abuse. In cases of abuse, lying and deception serve the purpose of self-protection from punishment/liability. If behavior is motivated by the perpetrator's self-protection, FDIA is not considered.

  C. Somatic symptom disorder in child or elder: Children can also experience somatic symptoms influenced by psychological factors, rather than external influences, similar to adults.

  D. Organic medical conditions: These can sometimes be confused with FDIA, especially when caregivers are very attentive or when the child's symptoms are inconsistent or hard to identify.

  E. Malingering by proxy: This is an uncommon occurrence where a caregiver amplifies or invents a child's symptoms for external advantages, like monetary benefits, setting it apart from FDIA where the main goal is to take on the role of a sick person by proxy.

PLAN

A. Concerns about possible presence of FD and FDIA should be raised early as part of team-based care. Supervisors should be notified and involved early to provide appropriate support to both patients and employees.

B. The clinician should be familiar with relevant mandated reporting guidelines for minors and other vulnerable individuals when FDIA is suspected.

C. Jafferany and colleagues (2018) noted that the overall goals of FD treatment are to reduce redundant treatments and associated costs and to minimize risks of adverse reactions to the patient.

General Treatments and Interventions

A. FD/FDIA recovery is rare as patients are very unlikely to be receptive to offered treatments. There is paucity of evidence supporting any FD-related intervention; however, two primary approaches have been used: psychotherapy and confrontation.
  1. Confrontation
     a. Confronting the patient with FD should be nonjudgmental and nonpunitive and incorporate support and follow-up.
     b. Prior to the confrontation, evidence of FD should be collected, collated, and discussed with the facility's legal department, as well as psychiatry (if available) and primary treating physician.
     c. Confrontation should be carried out by a team and not by an individual healthcare provider.
     d. Outcomes should be again discussed with the treatment team and documented.
     e. Although Bass and Wade noted the importance of "face saving" as the key element in the confrontation approach, it is unclear how this can be practically accomplished.
     f. Krahn and colleagues (2003) reported that, among 93 patients hospitalized over 21 years and diagnosed with FD, the majority (76.3%) were confronted about their diagnosis, but only a minority (17.2%) admitted to such behavior, leading the authors to conclude that this approach is largely ineffective.
  2. Psychotherapy
     a. In a 1994 publication, Plassman described psychoanalytic treatment that was offered to 24 patients diagnosed with FD. The proposed treatment consisted of establishing psychotherapy relationships during the inpatient hospitalization and subsequently receiving long-term psychoanalytic treatment. Plassman noted that 50% of patients accepted the treatment. Among ▶

10 patients who engaged in long-term psychoanalysis (up to 4 years per patient), only 3 achieved significant symptom improvements; however, all patients remained in treatment at the time of the publication, with notable termination challenges noted.

B. Evidence supporting time-limited, evidence-based psychotherapeutic approaches is lacking for FD/FDIA.

COMMON MEDICATIONS

A. Evidence supporting use of specific psychopharmacologic agents in FD is lacking, noting however that use of SSRIs, antipsychotics, mood stabilizers, and anxiolytics was described in published case reports, albeit with variable success.

B. Evaluation and management of comorbid psychiatric disorders in FD/FDIA is important for overall care, but the effect of this management on FD/FDIA presentation remains obscure.

PATIENT TEACHING

A. To minimize the possibility of unintentional creation of symptoms, patients with suspected FD should be provided with clear education about their possible illnesses and appropriate management.

1. Possible miscommunications about illness and treatment that the patient may have received from professional and lay sources should be thoroughly assessed and addressed.
2. Evaluate use of complementary and alternative medications (CAM) as a growing body of evidence suggests that CAM is both common and can be associated with harm.

B. Teach-back procedures should be utilized and documented. Written materials should be provided whenever appropriate and confrontation avoided.

FOLLOW-UP

A. Steps regarding surveillance and documentation as described in the previous sections should be anticipated as ongoing.

B. Obtaining and reviewing records (including directly from the hospital system, rather than from the patient), obtaining collateral, and seeking consultation are central to appropriate management of FD/FDIA.

CONSULTATION AND REFERRALS

A. The role of consultations for FD/FDIA management cannot be overemphasized, given high probability of negative consequences of FD/FDIA.

1. Communication within the treatment team should be open, with any observations shared orally and documented.
2. Notifying supervisors and escalating concerns to legal and ethics departments should be expected and timely.
3. Mandated reporting imperatives should be followed.

B. Patients may be referred to psychiatry/psychology, neurology, or any other disciplines that can evaluate presenting medical symptoms and offer insights about treatment strategies.

INDIVIDUAL CONSIDERATIONS

Pediatrics

A. the literature on FDIA primarily focuses on pediatric populations, and it is described elsewhere in this section.

B. It is critically important that PMHNPs are familiar with mandated reporting guidelines for this population.

C. Please see Chapter 20, "Special Considerations for Childhood and Adolescent Populations," for additional considerations in working with pediatric patients.

Pregnancy

A. FD/FDIA in pregnancy is receiving increasing attention as presence of deliberate symptom feigning is becoming more reported by obstetrics and gynecology literature.

1. According to Bérar and colleagues (2021), the most prevalent FD-related complaint is vaginal bleeding with/without associated pain.
2. Feldman and Hamilton (2006) described a case of a patient's self-induction of various labor and delivery events, leading to several cases of fetal demise and child illness, thus raising questions about the appropriateness of FDIA considerations when care of a pregnant patient is considered.

B. See Chapter 12, "Perinatal Mental Health," for other recommendations for mental healthcare during pregnancy.

Geriatrics/Older Adults

A. The impact of FD/FDIA on older adults is largely unknown. Given poor remission rates of FD, it is possible that FD presentation (typically emerging among patients in their 20s and 30s) can in theory persist and remain significant as the patient ages.

B. The true scope of this problem is impossible to ascertain given the current state of literature on FD/FDIA. What appears plausible is that FDIA is poorly detected among older adult patients, reflecting a more global trend in neglecting elder abuse, which is estimated to affect one in six older community-dwelling adults annually.

C. For further recommendations on geriatric care, see Chapter 21, "Aging and Older Adult Populations."

Partners/Family

A. Partners and family can provide valuable information for FD/FDIA. However, the role of significant others in treatment prognosis is unknown. Members of the treatment team should be mindful to follow rules guarding the patient's privacy.

B. Complex dynamics between partners/family and patients should be anticipated.

C. For more information about caregiver issues, see Chapter 35, "Caregiver and End-of-Life Issues."

RESOURCES

Websites

A. U.S. Department of Health and Human Services, Child Welfare Information Gateway, Mandatory Reporters of Child Abuse and Neglect: www.childwelfare.gov/topics/systemwide/laws-policies/statutes/manda

Practice Guidelines

A. American Professional Society on the Abuse of Children. (2017). *Munchausen by proxy: Clinical and case management guidance.* https://docs.wixstatic.com/ugd/4700a8_3a615184374e4210b739f7b75721b567.pdf

B. Royal College of Paediatrics and Child Health. (2009, rev 2012). *Fabricated or induced illness by carers (FII): A practical guide for paediatricians.* www.celcis.org/application/files/5115/5134/8896/Fabricated_or_Induced_Illness_by_Carers_A_Practical_Guide_for_Paediatricians_2009.pdf

REFERENCES AND BIBLIOGRAPHY

Abdurrachid, N., & Gama Marques, J. (2022). Munchausen Syndrome By Proxy (MSBP): A review regarding perpetrators of factitious disorder imposed on another (FDIA). *CNS Spectrums, 27*(1), 16–26. https://doi.org/10.1017/S1092852920001741

Barber, M. A., & Davis, P. M. (2002). Fits, faints, or fatal fantasy? Fabricated seizures and child abuse. *Archives of Disease in Childhood, 86*(4), 230–233. https://doi.org/10.1136/adc.86.4.230.

Bass, C., & Wade, D. T. (2019). Malingering and factitious disorder. *Practical Neurology, 19*(2), 96–105. https://doi.org/10.1136/practneurol-2018-001950

Bérar, A., Bouzillé, G., Jego, P., & Allain, J.-S. (2021). A descriptive, retrospective case series of patients with factitious disorder imposed on self. *BMC Psychiatry, 21*(1), Article 588. https://doi.org/10.1186/s12888-021-03582-8

Feldman, M. D., & Hamilton, J. C. (2006). Serial factitious disorder and Munchausen by proxy in pregnancy. *International Journal of Clinical Practice, 60*(12), 1675–1678. https://doi.org/10.1111/j.1742-1241.2006.00975.x

Jafferany, M., Khalid, Z., McDonald, K. A., & Shelley, A. J. (2018). Psychological aspects of factitious disorder. *The Primary Care Companion for CNS Disorders, 20*(1), 17nr02229. https://doi.org/10.4088/PCC.17nr02229

Krahn, L. E., Li, H., & O'Connor, M. K. (2003). Patients who strive to be ill: Factitious disorder with physical symptoms. *The American Journal of Psychiatry, 160*(6), 1163–1168. https://doi.org/10.1176/appi.ajp.160.6.1163

Plassmann R. (1994). Inpatient and outpatient long-term psychotherapy of patients suffering from factitious disorders. *Psychotherapy and Psychosomatics, 62*(1–2), 96–107. https://doi.org/10.1159/000288910

Rabinerson, D., Kaplan, B., Orvieto, R., & Dekel, A. (2002). Munchausen syndrome in obstetrics and gynecology. *Journal of Psychosomatic Obstetrics and Gynecology, 23*(4), 215–218. https://doi.org/10.3109/01674820209074675

Reich, P., & Gottfried, L. A. (1983). Factitious disorders in a teaching hospital. *Annals of Internal Medicine, 99*(2), 240–247. https://doi.org/10.7326/0003-4819-99-2-240

Schreier, H. (2004). Munchausen by proxy. *Current Problems in Pediatric and Adolescent Health Care, 34*(3), 126–143. https://doi.org/10.1016/j.cppeds.2003.09.003

Yon, Y., Mikton, C. R., Gassoumis, Z. D., & Wilber, K. H. (2017). Elder abuse prevalence in community settings: A systematic review and meta-analysis. *The Lancet Global Health, 5*(2), e147–e156. https://doi.org/10.1016/S2214-109X(17)30006-2

ILLNESS ANXIETY DISORDER

DEFINITION

A. "Hypochondriasis" was recently replaced by two new diagnoses—illness anxiety disorder (IAD) and somatic symptom disorder (SSD)—reflecting an evolution in understanding and diagnosing health-related anxiety disorders over time.

B. IAD is defined by a preoccupation with developing or experiencing a serious medical condition.

C. The core feature of SSD is the presence of one or more somatic symptoms that are distressing or result in significant disruption of daily life, whereas the core feature of IAD is a preoccupation with having or acquiring a serious, undiagnosed medical illness.

D. Criteria for IAD are as follows:

1. Patient is fixated on the possibility of acquiring a health issue.
2. Physical symptoms are either nonexistent or minimal. When there is a possibility of a health issue, the intense concern is disproportionate to the actual risk.
3. Patient has elevated anxiety about health or a tendency to be easily distressed over health matters.
4. Patient engages in excessive health-related actions or inappropriately avoiding medical care.
5. Despite the possibility of changing health worries, the overall duration of symptoms must surpass 3 to 6 months, depending on the diagnostic framework, to qualify for a diagnosis.
6. The symptoms of IAD should not be attributable to another mental health condition.

E. IAD specifiers include the following:

1. Care-seeking type: characterized by significant use of medical care (e.g., medical visits, tests, procedures)
2. Care-avoidant type: when medical care is not utilized even when needed

INCIDENCE

A. Current rates of IAD are not well-understood as estimated prevalence rates are derived from literature about hypochondriasis. An estimated 25% of patients who met previous criteria for hypochondriasis meet the diagnostic criteria for IAD. More recent estimates place the prevalence of IAD as high as 13% of the U.S. adult population. The impact of age, sex and gender, and cultural factors on IAD is not well-understood.

PATHOGENESIS

A. Although the pathogenesis of IAD is not well-understood, it may be precipitated by the experience of major life stressors.

B. Approximately one-third of patients with IAD experience a "transient" form of the condition, which resolves over time and is associated with lower severity and less psychiatric but more medical comorbidity.

C. Newby and colleagues (2017) found that most chronic cases of IAD fluctuate between care-seeking and care-avoidant types over time, with fewer individuals presenting exclusively with one or the other subtype.

PREDISPOSING FACTORS

A. Predisposing factors for IAD may include history of childhood abuse or the experience of serious illness, either by the patient or a family member. There is evidence that this latter risk may be due to early learning and resultant illness-related risk beliefs.

B. IAD may also develop in patients raised by relatively healthy family members who expressed disproportionate concerns about health issues or medical conditions.

C. Underlying anxiety disorders, such as generalized anxiety disorder (GAD), may increase the risk of IAD.

COMMON COMPLAINTS

A. Patients with IAD exhibit anxiety about health that appears disproportionate to actual health conditions and/or health risks.

B. Individuals with this disorder may have difficulty tolerating normal bodily sensations and may interpret these as potentially dangerous to their health.

C. Excessive reading and researching of health information on the internet may result and can also contribute to elevated anxiety about health.

D. Illness anxiety can lead to various behavioral outcomes, including a significant amount of medical care that may not be satisfactory, as some individuals may feel too anxious to seek help. Excessive use of medical care can produce iatrogenic effects, worsening patients' anxiety rather than alleviating it.

OTHER SIGNS AND SYMPTOMS

A. IAD is associated with comorbid psychiatric disorders, most often other anxiety disorders, but also major depressive disorder or personality disorders, which may complicate their presentation.

B. While many individuals experience intrusive thoughts about their health from time to time, individuals who meet the criteria for IAD typically experience these thoughts with greater intensity, leading to greater interference with emotional, cognitive, and behavioral processes.

C. Patients with IAD appraise health risks as severe and high in probability.

SUBJECTIVE DATA

A. IAD is often associated with patterns of care-seeking and/or avoidance behaviors that impact multiple areas of a patient's life.
    1. Patients may experience issues at work due to frequent requests for time off to attend healthcare visits or due to feared illness, and may also be limited in social interactions by these concerns.
B. High utilization of healthcare can lead to financial strain.
C. Patients with IAD might report frequently checking their bodies for signs of illness, and excessive time and concern devoted to this may also interfere with their social and occupational functioning.

PHYSICAL EXAMINATION

A. Physical examination may not provide useful information about IAD, apart from establishing the absence of physiologic signs of illness.
B. Although patients with IAD may request repeated examination and tests, providing these services can worsen health anxiety rather than alleviating it, resulting in iatrogenic effects.

DIAGNOSTIC TESTS AND SCREENINGS

A. The "gold standard" for diagnosis of IAD is assessment by a trained clinician using a validated, structured interview measure, such as the Anxiety Disorders Interview Schedule for *DSM-5* (ADIS-5; Brown & Barlow, 2014; based on the *Diagnostic and Statistical Manual of Mental Disorders*, Fifth Edition [*DSM-5*], American Psychiatric Association, 2013) or the Diagnostic Interview for Anxiety, Mood, and OCD and Related Neuropsychiatric Disorders (DIAMOND; Tolin et al., 2018).
B. A newer structured interview, the Health Preoccupation Diagnostic Interview (Axelsson et al., 2016), has been developed specific to IAD and SSD; however, research on its diagnostic properties is limited.
C. Additionally, symptom screening tools may also be useful in symptom assessment and tracking. The following symptom screeners can be helpful:
    1. Whiteley Index (WI-7)
        a. This scale was developed to assess symptoms of hypochondriasis (older nosology) and may be pertinent to IAD assessment.
        b. The WI-7 contains seven dichotomous items (1, *yes*; 0, *no*), with scores ranging from 0 to 7. The WI-7 has demonstrated good sensitivity and specificity in detecting health anxiety in primary care populations (Fink et al., 1999). The WI-7 includes three subscales: *bodily preoccupation, disease phobia,* and *conviction of the presence of disease.*
        c. Although no validated cutoffs are available for IAD, a score of 1 or higher may indicate presence of health anxiety. Higher scores on the WI-7, particularly on the bodily preoccupation subscale, indicate higher somatic anxiety, indicating need for further assessment.
    2. Illness Attitude Scales (IAS)
        a. The IAS consists of 29 items and 9 subscales. Höfling and Weck (2013) suggest that the bodily preoccupations subscale alone may be sufficient to indicate illness anxiety.
        b. The bodily preoccupations subscale contains three Likert scale items asking patients to rate the frequency at which they experience anxiety about signs and symptoms of possible illness on a 5-point scale (0, *no*; 1, *rarely*; 2, *sometimes*; 3, *often*; 4, *most of the time*). The total score for the subscale ranges from 0 to 15, and a cutoff score of 5.5 was determined to optimize sensitivity and specificity for hypochondriasis and can be used to detect illness anxiety symptoms.
D. It is important to remember that WI-7, IAS, and any other symptom screener cannot be used alone as diagnostic tools for IAD. However, screeners can facilitate symptom assessment and track treatment progress over time.

DIFFERENTIAL DIAGNOSIS

A. The primary characteristic of IAD is the presence of significant anxiety about health when physical symptoms or illness is relatively minor or absent. Transient anxieties that wax and wane with physiologic symptoms do not typically meet the criteria for IAD. Anxiety about health and medical conditions may be a normal response to a new-onset medical condition and should not be pathologized.
B. The following psychiatric conditions should be ruled out when diagnosing IAD:
    1. Nonpsychiatric medical condition: When patients present with prominent health anxiety, the etiologic impact of a medical condition should always be considered first. Medical conditions that are etiologically linked to anxiety presentation (e.g., endocrine, cardiovascular, respiratory, neurologic, metabolic diseases) need to be considered.
    2. Adjustment disorder(s): Adjustment disorder may be diagnosed if following the onset of the medical condition and if the resultant symptoms are clinically significant and disproportionate in comparison to the stressor(s) (American Psychiatric Association, 2013). In cases of IAD, anxiety is exclusively health-focused and does not require a specific event; however, the duration of symptoms should be at least 6 months.
    3. Somatic symptom disorder (SSD): Although historically grouped together, there is sufficient evidence to justify the separation of SSD and IAD into distinct diagnoses. Research suggests that SSD is typically characterized by more severe somatic symptoms, greater impairment in daily functioning, and higher rates of comorbid depressive disorders, GAD, and panic disorder. While there appear to be no significant differences in the levels of health anxiety or illness behavior between patients with SSD and IAD, IAD can be distinguished from SSD based on the presentation of somatic symptoms. IAD should only be considered in individuals with mild or no somatic symptoms who nonetheless experience high levels of anxiety about health-related concerns.
    4. Generalized anxiety disorder (GAD): GAD is characterized by somatic symptoms (e.g., irritability, muscle tension); however, anxiety is not centered on a specific event, activity, or symptom (such as health).
    5. Panic disorder (PD): PD may express elevated health anxiety related to panic attacks, such as fearing that they are experiencing a heart attack or other severe illness. These experiences are distinct from IAD in that the health concerns in PD are typically episodic, occurring in temporal association with panic attacks, while in IAD individuals experience persistent health-related worries. Moreover, anxieties about health in IAD are more salient than any physiologic symptoms that may be present, whereas in

PD anxiety is accompanied by significant somatic symptoms during an attack. Comorbid presence of PD and IAD is also possible as severe illness anxiety may trigger panic attacks in some individuals.

6. Obsessive-compulsive and related disorders: IAD may at times resemble obsessive-compulsive disorder (OCD) as it involves intrusive thoughts about illness, and individuals with IADs often engage in associated compulsive behaviors such as seeking medical care or social support as a strategy for diffusing intrusive health anxieties. However, the nature of health-related thoughts typically differs between the two diagnoses. IAD centers on excessive concern about having an unidentified disease, sometimes resulting in obsessive efforts to seek medical attention for a diagnosis. In OCD, on the other hand, individuals more commonly express concerns about getting a disease in the future, and thus the associated compulsive behaviors, if present, may consist of excessive cleaning or other actions directed at preventing disease.

7. Body dysmorphic disorder (BDD): BDD is characterized by excessive concerns related to a perceived physical defect in their body. By contrast, in IAD, body checking may be present, and it is driven by concerns about medical condition (actual or potential).

8. Major depressive disorder (MDD): MDD can involve medical condition-related rumination and worries. If health-related concerns or ruminations occur only during MDD, IAD should not be diagnosed. However, if excessive health concerns persist after other symptoms of an MDD episode are remitted, a comorbid diagnosis of MDD and IAD may be considered.

9. Psychotic disorders: Psychotic disorders may encompass somatic delusions (i.e., false belief that is held despite the incontrovertible proof or evidence of the contrary).

PLAN
A. Patients with IAD often express dissatisfaction with their medical care as many have faced dismissal or frustration from their medical providers. Building a strong, collaborative relationship with the patient is the first and most crucial step to any treatment of IAD.
B. It is important to assess and examine the meaning of an individual patient's health-related thoughts and anxieties. Evidence from Arnáez and colleagues (2021) suggests that the appraisal of health risks, rather than the frequency of health-related thoughts, is the key source of impairment in IAD. Clinicians can focus on these appraisals as the main target for patient education and intervention, which in combination with building a strong alliance with the patient can lead to favorable outcomes.

General Treatments and Interventions
A. There is growing support for utilization of health-anxiety focused CBT for IAD treatment.
  1. CBT appears more effective than education or supportive counseling alone.
  2. The benefits CBT for IAD appear to be maintained up to 12 months posttreatment and are evident across multiple intervention designs, including internet-administered CBT (iCBT) and CBT incorporating exposure components.
  3. A greater number of sessions of CBT may increase the effect on reductions in health anxiety symptoms, but short intervention programs also produce significant improvements in symptoms, including health anxiety, somatization, psychological distress, and functional impairment.

B. Acceptance and commitment therapy (ACT) and mindfulness-based stress reduction (MBSR) may help patients in developing adaptive skills for coping with illness anxiety, although further research is needed.

COMMON MEDICATIONS
A. Pharmacotherapy is a second-line treatment for IAD.
B. Building patient alliance, providing psychoeducation, and psychotherapeutic approaches should be prioritized before psychopharmacologic interventions are considered.
C. When nonpharmacologic approaches do not sufficiently reduce symptoms, evidence supports the use of selective serotonin reuptake inhibitors (SSRIs) and serotonin and norepinephrine reuptake inhibitors (SNRIs) for IAD treatment.
D. Prescription of antidepressants for IAD should generally be considered as an adjunctive therapy in combination with psychotherapy.
E. Shared decision-making should be practiced, discussing specific agent, duration of treatment, expected outcomes, and potential side effects.

PATIENT TEACHING
A. Educating patients about IAD is both challenging and crucial to effective management of this condition. Newby and colleagues (2017) found that while CBT was most effective in reducing health anxiety symptoms and impairment in IAD, psychoeducation about health anxiety on its own also produced significant improvements in these outcomes.
B. Practitioners must show empathy for their patients' emotional response to health anxiety and validate their concerns without reinforcing excessive care-seeking or care-avoiding behaviors.
C. Educating patients about normal bodily signs and symptoms can be useful but may be misinterpreted as condescending or dismissive unless delivered in a nonjudgmental, empathetic manner.

FOLLOW-UP
A. Because patients with IAD have often seen multiple medical providers in pursuit of a diagnosis, providing effective follow-up is critical to avoid leaving patients feeling abandoned or dismissed.
B. Clinicians should ensure that patients are scheduled for follow-up, ideally with both primary care and psychology.
C. Consistent follow-up in IAD has been shown to reduce care-seeking in other environments such as EDs and allows for more accurate assessment of the course of the disorder, including any new health concerns that emerge that may require new treatment strategies.

CONSULTATION AND REFERRALS
A. Team-based care: Incorporating both medical and mental health specialties is critical to IAD care. Shared treatment goals and alignment in discussion of etiology and maintaining factors are central.
B. BPS model: The role of anxiety and its management in medical care should be discussed early and continue throughout treatment.

INDIVIDUAL CONSIDERATIONS
Pediatrics
A. While the occurrence of IAD in adulthood has been linked to childhood experiences of illness either in the self or a close ▶

family member, limited data exist on the prevalence of IAD emerging during childhood.
B. IAD may commonly emerge in adolescence, with worsening symptoms as the individual enters adulthood.
C. See Chapter 20, "Special Considerations for Childhood and Adolescent Populations," for additional considerations in working with pediatric patients.

Pregnancy

A. Pregnancy may have unique effects on health anxiety for some individuals. It is a period of somatic changes, some of which may be unexpected or new to the patient, and can also be a time of high anxiety about health, as patients worry about risks to both their own bodies and the developing fetus.
B. Some experts have conceptualized pregnancy as a trigger for distinct forms of IAD, referred to as "pregnancy-specific" IAD. Although this is not officially recognized as a separate diagnosis, special consideration may be warranted for people experiencing IAD during pregnancy as stress and anxiety during the perinatal period can have negative effects on the physical and mental health of both the mother and the child.
C. Please refer to Chapter 12, "Perinatal Mental Health," for other recommendations for mental healthcare during pregnancy.

Geriatrics/Older Adults

A. There are limited data on the prevalence of IAD in geriatric populations. Hirsch and colleagues (2012) found that health-related anxiety increases with the burden of medical illness in older adulthood; however, this association has not been tested in samples diagnosed with IAD.
B. Other research suggests that older adults experiencing greater loneliness and generalized anxiety may be more prone to express health anxiety, although these findings focused on the previous diagnosis of hypochondriasis and thus did not distinguish between IAD and SSD.
C. For further recommendations on geriatric care, please see Chapter 21, "Aging and Older Adult Populations."

Partners/Family

A. There is a lack of literature on considerations for partners and family members of individuals with IAD. Based on the known impacts of IAD on social functioning, however, it can be expected that those in close relationship to patients with IAD may experience frustration and concern about their loved one's health anxieties and may be impacted by the effects of IAD on financial, occupational, and other domains.
B. Symptoms of IAD may be associated with insecure attachment, a pattern characterized by interpersonal anxiety and ambivalence, which if present likely affects relationships between individuals with IAD and their partners or families.
C. Those in close relationships to individuals with IAD may require support and empathy for their circumstances, as well as psychoeducation about the condition.
D. For more information about caregiver issues, please see Chapter 35, "Caregiver and End-of-Life Issues."

RESOURCES

Websites

A. Anxiety and Depression Association of America: https://adaa.org/understanding-anxiety/related-illnesses/health-anxiety

B. Centre for Clinical Interventions, Government of Western Australia: www.cci.health.wa.gov.au/Resources/Looking-After-Yourself/Health-Anxiety

REFERENCES AND BIBLIOGRAPHY

Alberts, N., Hadjistavropoulos, H., Sherry, S., & Stewart, S. (2016). Linking illness in parents to health anxiety in offspring: Do beliefs about health play a role? *Behavioral and Cognitive Psychotherapy*, 44(1), 18–29. https://doi.org/10.1017/S1352465814000319

American Psychiatric Association. (2013). *Diagnostic and statistical manual of mental disorders* (5th ed.). https://doi.org/10.1176/appi.books.9780890425596

Arnáez, S., García-Soriano, G., López-Santiago, J., & Belloch, A. (2021). Illness-related intrusive thoughts and illness anxiety disorder. *Psychology and Psychotherapy*, 94(1), 63–80. https://doi.org/10.1111/papt.12267

Axelsson, E., Andersson, E., Ljótsson, B., Wallhed Finn, D., & Hedman, E. (2016). The health preoccupation diagnostic interview: Inter-rater reliability of a structured interview for diagnostic assessment of *DSM-5* somatic symptom disorder and illness anxiety disorder. *Cognitive Behaviour Therapy*, 45(4), 259–269. https://doi.org/10.1080/16506073.2016.1161663

Bailer, J., Kerstnera, T., Witthöft, M., Diener, C., Miera, D., & Rist, F. (2016). Health anxiety and hypochondriasis in the light of *DSM-5*. *Anxiety, Stress, & Coping*, 29(2), 219–239. http://dx.doi.org/10.1080/10615806.2015.1036243

Barnett, M. D., Moore, J. M., & Archuleta, W. P. (2019). A loneliness model of hypochondriasis among older adults: The mediating role of intolerance of uncertainty and anxious symptoms. *Archives of Gerontology and Geriatrics*, 83, 86–90. https://doi.org/10.1016/j.archger.2019.03.027

Brown, T. A., & Barlow, D. (2014). *Anxiety and related disorders interview schedule for DSM–5 (ADIS-5)*. Oxford University Press.

Chappell, A. S. (2018). Toward a lifestyle medicine approach to illness anxiety disorder (formerly hypochondriasis). *American Journal of Lifestyle Medicine*, 12(5), 365–369. https://doi.org/10.1177/1559827618764649

Fink, P., Ewald, H., Jensen, J., Sørensen, L., Engberg, M., Holm, M., & Munk-Jørgensen, P. (1999). Screening for somatization and hypochondriasis in primary care and neurological in-patients: A seven-item scale for hypochondriasis and somatization. *Journal of Psychosomatic Research*, 46(3), 261–273. https://doi.org/10.1016/S0022-3999(98)00092-0

French, J. H., & Hameed, S. (2023, July 16). *Illness anxiety disorder*. StatPearls Publishing. https://www.ncbi.nlm.nih.gov/books/NBK554399

Hedman, E., Axelsson, E., Andersson, E., Lekander, M., & Ljótsson, B. (2016). Exposure-based cognitive-behavioral therapy via the internet and as bibliotherapy for somatic symptom disorder and illness anxiety disorder: Randomised controlled trial. *British Journal of Psychiatry*, 209(5), 407–413. http://dx.doi.org/10.1192/bjp.bp.116.181396

Hirsch, J., Walker, K., Chang, E., & Lyness, J. (2012). Illness burden and symptoms of anxiety in older adults: Optimism and pessimism as moderators. *International Psychogeriatrics*, 24(10), 1614–1621. https://doi.org/10.1017/S1041610212000762

Hoffmann, D., Rask, C., Hedman-Lagerlöf, E., Ljótsson, B., & Frostholm, L. (2018). Development and feasibility testing of Internet-delivered acceptance and commitment therapy for severe health anxiety: Pilot study. *JMIR Mental Health*, 5(2), e28. https://doi.org/10.2196/mental.9198

Höfling, V., & Weck, F. (2013). Assessing bodily preoccupations is sufficient: Clinically effective screening for hypochondriasis. *Journal of Psychosomatic Research*, 75(6), 526–531. https://doi.org/10.1016/j.jpsychores.2013.10.011

Newby, J. M., Hobbs, M. J., Mahoney, A. E. J., Wong, S. K., & Andrews, G. (2017). *DSM-5* illness anxiety disorder and somatic symptom disorder: Comorbidity, correlates, and overlap with *DSM-IV* hypochondriasis. *Journal of Psychosomatic Research*, 101, 31–37. https://doi.org/10.1016/j.jpsychores.2017.07.010

Noyes, R., Stuart, S. P., Langbehn, D. R., Happel, R. L., Longley, S. L. Muller, B. A., & Yagla, S. J. (2003). Test of an interpersonal model of hypochondriasis. *Psychosomatic Medicine*, 65(2), 292–300. https://doi.org/10.1097/01.PSY.0000058377.50240.64

Olatunji, B. O., Kauffman, B. Y., Meltzer, S., Davis, M. L., Smits, J. A. J., & Powers, M. B. (2014). Cognitive-behavioral therapy for hypochondriasis/health anxiety: A meta-analysis of treatment outcome and moderators. *Behaviour Research and Therapy, 58*, 65–74. https://doi.org/10.1016/j.brat.2014.05.002

Rathbone. A. L., & Prescott, J. (2019). Pregnancy-specific health anxiety: Symptom or diagnosis? *British Journal of Midwifery, 27*(5), 288–293. https://doi.org/10.12968/bjom.2019.27.5.288

Scarella, T. M., Boland, R. J., & Barsky, A. J. (2019). Illness anxiety disorder: Psychopathology, epidemiology, clinical characteristics, and treatment. *Psychosomatic Medicine, 81*(5), 398–407. https://doi.org/10.1097/PSY.0000000000000691

Scarella, T. M., Laferton, J. A. C., Ahern, D. K., Fallon, B. A., & Barsky, A. (2016). The relationship of hypochondriasis to anxiety, depressive, and somatoform disorders. *Psychosomatics, 57*(2), 200–207. https://doi.org/10.1016/j.psym.2015.10.006

Sirri, L., Grandi, S., & Fava, G. A. (2008). The illness attitude scales: A clinimetric index for assessing hypochondriacal fears and beliefs. *Psychotherapy and Psychosomatics, 77*(6), 337–350. https://doi.org/10.1159/000151387

Tolin, D. F., Gilliam, C., Wootton, B. M., Bowe, W., Bragdon, L. B., Davis, E., Hannan, S. E., Steinman, S. A., Worden, B., & Hallion, L. S. (2018). Psychometric properties of a structured diagnostic interview for *DSM-5* anxiety, mood, and obsessive-compulsive and related disorders. *Assessment, 25*(1), 3–13. https://doi.org/10.1177/1073191116638410

Weck, F., Bleichhardt, G., & Hiller, W. (2010). Screening for hypochondriasis with the illness attitude scales. *Journal of Personality Assessment, 92*(3), 260–268. https://doi.org/10.1080/00223891003670216

OTHER SPECIFIED/UNSPECIFIED SOMATIC SYMPTOM AND RELATED DISORDERS

OTHER SPECIFIED SOMATIC SYMPTOM AND RELATED DISORDERS

A. Other specified somatic symptom disorders can be applied when the presentation of somatic symptoms that do not meet the full criteria for SSD or IAD yet causes significant distress and/or functional impairment. The following four potential diagnostic options may be appropriate:
  1. Brief somatic symptom disorder (SSD): Diagnostic criteria for SSD are met, but symptom duration is less than 6 months.
  2. Brief illness anxiety disorder (IAD): Diagnostic criteria for IAD are met, but symptom duration is less than 6 months.
  3. Illness anxiety disorder without excessive health-related behaviors: All diagnostic criteria for IAD are met, but there is absence of either excessive behaviors or avoidance (e.g., lack of care-seeking or avoidance).
  4. Pseudocyesis: The patient incorrectly believes that they are pregnant. *Pseudocyesis* is both quite rare and not well-understood, with most evidence originating from individual case studies published in the 1960s to 1990s. Although the causes of pseudocyesis are unknown, it has been noted in patients with comorbid psychotic disorders as well as patients who were eventually diagnosed with "medically explained symptoms," resulting from conditions such as "gallstones, abdominal tumors, hyperprolactinemia, constipation, a tubal cyst, and esophageal achalasia" (Gogia et al., 2022, p. 51). Pseudocyesis is not diagnosed when psychosis is present and the patient is experiencing delusions; however, distinguishing between pseudocyesis and delusions of pregnancy may be challenging.

B. Apart from pseudocyesis, the recommendations for screening, treatment planning, and case management made in the previous sections on SSD and IAD are generally applicable in cases of other specified somatic symptoms and related disorders.

UNSPECIFIED SOMATIC SYMPTOM AND RELATED DISORDERS

A. In cases where patients meet some but not all criteria for an SSD, but where the presentation does not fall under any of the four categories described previously, a label of "unspecified" somatic symptom and related disorder may be appropriate.

B. This diagnosis is used when there is evidence of a somatic disorder without enough evidence to make a specific diagnosis. An "unspecified" diagnosis may be replaced with a more precise medical and/or psychiatric diagnosis as further information is gathered.

REFERENCES AND BIBLIOGRAPHY

American Psychiatric Association. (2013). *Diagnostic and statistical manual of mental disorders* (5th ed.). https://doi.org/10.1176/appi.books.9780890425596

Gogia, S., Grieb, A., Jang, A., Gordon, M. R., & Coverdale, J. (2022). Medical considerations in delusion of pregnancy: A systematic review. *Journal of Psychosomatic Obstetrics & Gynecology, 43*(1), 51–57. https://doi.org/10.1080/0167482X.2020.1779696

Yadav, T., Balhara, Y. P. S., & Kataria, D. K. (2012). Pseudocyesis versus delusion of pregnancy: Differential diagnoses to be kept in mind. *Indian Journal of Psychological Medicine, 34*(1), 82–84. https://doi.org/10.4103/0253-7176.96167

Yeh, Y.-W., Kuo, S.-C., & Chen, C.-Y. (2012). Urinary tract infection complicated by urine retention presenting as pseudocyesis in a schizophrenic patient. *General Hospital Psychiatry, 34*(1), 101.e9–101.e10. https://doi.org/10.1016/j.genhosppsych.2011.06.008

PSYCHOLOGICAL FACTORS AFFECTING OTHER MEDICAL CONDITIONS

DEFINITION

A. This condition is identified by the existence of one or multiple psychological or behavioral factors that negatively impact a medical condition (MC) and its progression, treatment, or result. These elements may worsen the MC, disrupt its treatment, or require further medical care.

B. Diagnostic criteria for psychological factors affecting other medical conditions (PF-AMC) include the following:
  1. Presence of a *medical symptom or an MC*
  2. *Psychological factors/behaviors* negatively affecting the MC in at least one of the following ways:
     a. Close temporal relationship/association *adversely impacting development, course, and recovery*
     b. *Interference* with treatment
     c. Constitute a well-known *health risk* for MC
     d. Negatively impact underlying MC pathophysiology, *causing or worsening symptoms*, leading to need for medical attention

C. Diagnostic specifiers include *mild* (increasing medical risk), *moderate* (exacerbating underlying MC), *severe* (leading to emergency medical care [hospitalization/ED visit]), and *extreme* (leading to life-threatening risk).

D. These behaviors or psychological factors are not better explained by another psychiatric condition and may increase the risk of poor health outcomes, contributing to morbidity and mortality either in the short or long term (Box 15.2).

E. Relevant MCs include but are not limited to chronic illnesses (e.g., diabetes, asthma, kidney disease, cardiac conditions), functional syndromes (e.g., fibromyalgia, irritable bowel syndrome [IBS], migraine), or symptoms of unclear or unknown origin (e.g., dizziness, fatigue).

BOX 15.2 EXAMPLES OF PSYCHOLOGICAL FACTORS AFFECTING OTHER MEDICAL CONDITIONS

- Limited adherence to medication regimen in chronic illness—skipping medications, discontinuing needed medications, inappropriately using medications
- Denying symptoms or illness
- Skipping important procedures and services, for example, not attending follow-up services after hospitalization
- Inactivity/overactivity aggravating chronic pain
- Anxiety aggravating asthma
- Poor diet interfering with diabetes symptom control
- Ignoring symptoms of life-threatening conditions (e.g., chest pain)

INCIDENCE

A. Given the diversity of symptoms and presentations, the incidence of PF-AMC is not possible to assess and can be challenging to determine precisely due to several factors, including variations in diagnostic practices, differences in healthcare systems, and the broad and somewhat subjective nature of the diagnosis.
B. PF-AMC may arise at any point throughout its lifetime, thus mirroring variable prevalence rates of MCs.
C. The Centers for Disease Control and Prevention (CDC, n.d.) notes that chronic illnesses affect six out of ten Americans, while four out of ten are affected by more than one chronic illness.
D. Despite medical advances, chronic illnesses are the leading cause of death and disability, acting as "leading drivers" of the 4.1 trillion annual health costs in the United States (CDC, n.d.).
E. Given the prevalence of chronic illness and the role of behavioral factors in their etiology, maintenance, and poor outcomes, the impact of psychological and behavioral factors on MCs is difficult to underestimate.

PATHOGENESIS

A. Fava and colleagues (2007) proposed basing PF-AMC on the "abnormal illness-behavior" concept proposed early on by Pilowsky (1997). This concept focuses on illness-related perceptions and behaviors that are "maladaptive," although the patient was "provided with opportunities for discussion, negotiation, and clarification, based on adequate assessment of all relevant biological, psychological, social, and cultural factors" (Fava et al., 2007, p. 104).
B. The concept of "abnormal illness-behavior" appears to lack operational definitions for the necessary and sufficient evaluation and patient communication and appears to overlook complex nature of care delivery as well as failures of effective patient-centered communication, which are ever present in medical systems.
C. It is important to avoid conflation between knowledge and behaviors. While knowledge may be a central factor to behavioral change, it is certainly not the only driver of behavioral change.

PREDISPOSING FACTORS

A. Each behavior or psychological factor implicated in PF-AMC presentation is likely to be driven by a complex interplay of internal and external variables. For example, McQuaid and Landier (2018) in their review of factors affecting medication adherence note the following as relevant:
　1. Individual factors: perceived discrimination, depression
　2. Cultural factors: medication beliefs (including historical factors), use of CAM, language barriers
　3. Healthcare system factors: healthcare provider communication, healthcare provider bias

COMMON COMPLAINTS

A. PF-AMC may lead to a range of concerns associated with suboptimal illness management. Concerns may come from the patient, their support network (e.g., family members), or members of the clinical team.

OTHER SIGNS AND SYMPTOMS

A. Quality of life factors and goals of care, specifically those that are not met, can offer insights into PF-AMC; however, as mentioned earlier, presentations can be very highly variable.

SUBJECTIVE DATA

A. Clinical considerations aimed at differentiating between psychological factors and behaviors and culturally sanctioned beliefs and behaviors are critical. There are two primary domains highlighted across research in healthcare that may be helpful to consider when evaluating a patient's MC-related beliefs:
　1. What is the patient's understanding of the relationship between symptoms and underlying illness?
　　a. In many chronic conditions, symptoms are insidious, and the impact of poor control may not be immediately noticed by the patient or habituation may occur.
　　b. For example, a patient may not be aware of high blood sugar levels or high blood pressure, equating lack of perceived symptoms to absence of illness and not engaging in treatment.
　2. What is the patient's understanding of medication management?
　　a. Does the patient understand the role of controller medications (e.g., antihypertensives, inhaled corticosteroids) or instead treats medications as pro re nata basis.
B. An article by Carillo and colleagues (1999) offers great examples of illustrations of how a patient's illness beliefs, informed by culture and a range of other factors, can manifest in clinical settings and offers insights into approaches for improved patient understanding.

PHYSICAL EXAMINATION

A. Not applicable

DIAGNOSTIC TESTS AND SCREENINGS

A. Not applicable

DIFFERENTIAL DIAGNOSIS

A. PF-AMC diagnosis should only be considered when the impact of psychological factors on the MC is clear and clinically significant. It is important to consider the role of cultural norms in illness management and avoid incorrectly labeling a culturally acceptable, nonharmful practice as PF-AMC.
B. PF-AMC should not be diagnosed in cases when a known psychiatric and/or MC accounts for the presentation. This diagnosis is reserved for clinical pictures when psychological or behavioral factors do not meet the criteria for another psychiatric condition.
C. The following psychiatric conditions should be ruled out for the diagnosis of PF-AMC.
　1. Mental disorder due to another medical condition (AMC): If an MC results in the development of psychological or behavioral symptoms (i.e., if the specific MC has a causal mechanism that leads to the development of specific symptoms), then mental disorder due to AMC is a

more appropriate diagnosis. For example, low mood and the resultant inactivity and decreased ability to participate in care can be etiologically caused by a stroke, Huntington disease, Parkinson disease, traumatic brain injury, multiple sclerosis, or systemic lupus erythematosus.
  2. Adjustment disorder: When patients develop a reaction (psychological and/or behavioral) to a new or ongoing MC, adjustment disorder is a more appropriate diagnosis.
  3. Somatic symptom disorder (SSD): The focus of distress in SSD is presence of physical symptom(s); however, these may occur without a diagnosed MC. In PF-AMC, an MC is present and psychological or behavioral factors adversely affect the course or outcome of the MC. Excessive distress or anxiety is not central to PF-AMC diagnosis.
  4. Illness anxiety disorder (IAD): Anxiety about MC development is central to the IAD diagnosis, while symptoms may or may not be present. In contrast, PF-AMC is characterized by a known MC that is negatively affected by psychological or behavioral factors.

PLAN
A. Management of PF-AMC must incorporate a BPS perspective in order to capture and address complex factors that can impact MC management.
B. For any MCs as well as comorbid psychiatric conditions, a full diagnostic assessment needs to be performed in line with current evidence-based practices for the MC in question.
C. Medication reconciliation and evaluation of CAM use are needed to ensure that pertinent illness management components are not overlooked.

General Treatments and Interventions
A. There are several models of medical interviewing that capture the BPS parameters.
  1. Patient-centered interviewing method by Smith and colleagues (2013) and the four habits model by Frankel and Stein (2001) both allow for time-sensitive and patient-centered interviewing based on the BPS model and are open access (please see the "Resources" section for specifics).
  2. Become familiar with these approaches as they allow healthcare providers to build rapport, assess patients' perspectives, evaluate presenting concerns fully, and establish plans in line with a shared agenda.
B. Additionally, Betancourt and colleagues (2002, 2006) offer a culturally informed model that is both brief and practical and allows to evaluate a patient's illness perceptions. Specifically, within the ESFT model:
  1. Explanatory model for health and illness: incorporates questions inquiring about patients' beliefs about illness' causes, timeline, impact on functioning, associated concerns, and treatment preferences
  2. Social and environmental factors: outlines questions about medication access and barriers (price, timeliness, access to assistance)
  3. Fears and concerns: includes questions pertaining to medication-related concerns, side effect concerns, and information that the patient may have already learned about the medication
  4. Therapeutic contracting/treatment: incorporates questions
C. Utilization of the ESFT model for assessment along with validation of patients' perspectives and shared decision-making can pave the way to improved MC management, thus alleviating factors contributing to PF-AMC.

COMMON MEDICATIONS
A. Not applicable

PATIENT TEACHING
A. An important component of PF-AMC management is appropriate communication. Unfortunately, research points toward high prevalence of suboptimal patient communication practices. Talevski and colleagues (2020) note that while patients are increasingly tasked with MC self-management, healthcare providers across various disciplines overestimate their effectiveness as communicators of medical information.
B. Review of literature supports the effectiveness of teach-back across various settings and populations in both improving learning and in addressing illness management metrics.
C. It is important to both acquire teach-back skills and to practice them with all patients. The Institute for Healthcare Advancement (IHA) released an interactive module for learning and practicing teach-back skills. Specifics can be found in the "Resources" section.

FOLLOW-UP
A. Management of PF-AMC is longitudinal.
B. Treatment will need to be individually tailored based on patients' unique circumstances.

CONSULTATION AND REFERRALS
A. A range of referrals may be appropriate; however, to improve outcomes, each healthcare provider or team will need to work with the patient to assess and manage PF-AMC via BPS intervention.
B. A primary care behavioral health (PCBH) model may be particularly beneficial for PF-AMC management. In this model, a behavioral health consultant (BHC) works with the primary care team to provide brief behavioral healthcare interventions to patients suffering from a broad range of psychiatric and/or MCs. The BHC works with both the treatment team and the patient to improve communication as well as illness outcomes. Hunter and colleagues (2014) offer an in-depth explanation of BHC as well as techniques that can be appropriate for improved outcomes in both MC and psychiatric illnesses.

INDIVIDUAL CONSIDERATIONS

Pediatrics
A. Corroboration by the caregiver and/or school may be necessary for PF-AMC diagnosis and management in pediatric populations. It is important to remember that caregivers ultimately make final decisions regarding their children's healthcare.
  1. Arcoleo and colleagues (2020) examined pediatric asthma illness management among Mexican and Puerto Rican children aged 5 to 12 years. Results indicated that when caregivers' asthma illness representations (i.e., beliefs about symptoms, management) agreed with the "professional model" of asthma and its management, this was associated with better pediatric asthma control across a 1-year period.
B. See Chapter 20, "Special Considerations for Childhood and Adolescent Populations," for additional considerations in working with pediatric patients.

Pregnancy
A. Management of PF-AMC in pregnancy may be high-stakes as both patients and fetal health are involved.
B. See Chapter 12, "Perinatal Mental Health," for other recommendations for mental healthcare during pregnancy.

Geriatrics/Older Adults

A. Older adult patients may be at higher risk for PF-AMC as they typically experience greater illness morbidity; however, additional research is needed to improve understanding of unique needs and challenges for this population.
B. For further recommendations on geriatric care, see Chapter 21, "Aging and Older Adult Populations."

Partners/Family

A. Partners and family can influence both PF-AMC as well as its management. Roles of family/caregivers should be assessed and managed proactively. Consider the use of family sessions to address illness management questions and concerns that may be germane.
B. For more information about caregiver issues, please see Chapter 35, "Caregiver and End-of-Life Issues."

RESOURCES

Websites

A. Centers for Disease Control and Prevention: Chronic disease data and surveillance: www.cdc.gov/chronic-disease/data-surveillance/index.html
B. Fortin, A. H., Dwamena, F. C., Frankel, R. M., Lovegrove Lepisto, B., & Smith, R. C. (2019). *Smith's patient-centered interviewing* (4th ed.). McGraw Hill Access Medicine. https://accessmedicine.mhmedical.com/book.aspx?bookID=2446

Visual/Video Materials

A. Institute for Healthcare Advancement (IHA): Always Use Teach Back! https://teachbacktraining.org/teach-back-interactive-learning-module

Practice Guidelines

A. Morrison, J. (2015). *When psychological problems mask medical disorders* (2nd ed). Guildford Press.
B. Hunter, C. L., Goodie, J. L., Oordt, M. S., & Dobmeyer, A. C. (2017). *Integrated behavioral health in primary care: Step-by-step guidance for assessment and intervention* (pp. 55–61). American Psychological Association
C. Smith, R. C., Fortin, A. H., Dwamena, F., & Frankel, R. M. (2013). An evidence-based patient-centered method makes the biopsychosocial model scientific. *Patient Education and Counseling, 91*(3), 265–270. https://doi.org/10.1016/j.pec.2012.12.010

REFERENCES AND BIBLIOGRAPHY

Arcoleo, K., Marsiglia, F., Serebrisky, D., Rodriguez, J., Mcgovern, C., & Feldman, J. (2020). Explanatory model for asthma disparities in Latino children: Results from the Latino childhood asthma project. *Annals of Behavioral Medicine, 54*(4), 223–236. https://doi.org/10.1093/abm/kaz041

Betancourt, J. R. (2006). Cultural competency: Providing quality care to diverse populations. *The Consultant Pharmacist, 21*(12), 988–995. https://doi.org/10.4140/tcp.n.2006.988

Betancourt, J. R., Green, A. R., & Carrillo, J. E. (2002, October). *Cultural competence in health care: Emerging frameworks and practical approaches.* The Commonwealth Fund. https://www.commonwealthfund.org/sites/default/files/documents/___media_files_publications_fund_report_2002_oct_cultural_competence_in_health_care__emerging_frameworks_and_practical_approaches_betancourt_culturalcompetence_576_pdf.pdf

Centers for Disease Control and Prevention. (n.d.). *Chronic disease.* U.S. Department of Health and Human Services. https://www.cdc.gov/chronic-disease/index.html

Carrillo, J. E., Green, A. R., & Betancourt, J. R. (1999). Cross-cultural primary care: A patient-based approach. *Annals of Internal Medicine, 130*(10), 829–834. https://doi.org/10.7326/0003-4819-130-10-199905180-00017

Fava, G. A., Fabbri, S., Sirri, L., & Wise, T. N. (2007). Psychological factors affecting medical condition: A new proposal for *DSM-V*. *Psychosomatics, 48*(2), 103–111. https://doi.org/10.1176/appi.psy.48.2.103

First, M. B., Williams, J. B. W., Karg, R. S., & Spitzer, R. L. (2016). *Structured Clinical Interview for DSM-5 Disorders, Clinician Version (SCID-5-CV).* American Psychiatric Association.

Hunter, C. L., Goodie, J. L., Oordt, M. S., & Dobmeyer, A. C. (2017). *Integrated behavioral health in primary care: Step-by-step guidance for assessment and intervention* (2nd ed.). American Psychological Association

McQuaid, E. L., & Landier, W. (2018). Cultural issues in medication adherence: Disparities and directions. *Journal of General Internal Medicine, 33*(2), 200–206. https://doi.org/10.1007/s11606-017-4199-3

Pilowsky, I. (1997). *Abnormal illness behavior.* Wiley.

Smith, R. C., Fortin, A. H., Dwamena, F., & Frankel, R. M. (2013). An evidence-based patient-centered method makes the biopsychosocial model scientific. *Patient Education and Counselling, 91*(3), 265–270. https://doi.org/10.1016/j.pec.2012.12.010

Talevski, J., Wong Shee, A., Rasmussen, B., Kemp, G., & Beauchamp, A. (2020). Teach-back: A systematic review of implementation and impacts. *PloS one, 15*(4), e0231350. https://doi.org/10.1371/journal.pone.0231350

SOMATIC SYMPTOM DISORDER

DEFINITION

A. Criteria for somatic symptom disorder (SSD) are as follows:
  1. Patient experiences *bodily symptoms* that cause distress or lead to disruption of daily life.
  2. The bodily symptoms and/or related health concerns lead to at least one of the following:
    a. Persistent rumination on bodily symptoms over an extended period
    b. Disproportionate worry and anxiety triggered by physical symptoms
    c. Considerable time and effort devoted to anxiety and actions related to symptoms
B. Although specific symptoms may change over time, total symptom duration must exceed 3 to 6 months to meet the diagnostic criteria depending on classification system.
C. The primary pain specifier is applied when the main concern is pain.
D. The persistent specifier is designated when symptoms last longer than 6 months.
E. Other specifiers for SSD include the following:
  1. Mild: presence of just one of the symptoms noted
  2. Moderate: at least two of the symptoms noted
  3. Severe: at least two of the symptoms noted, along with either numerous bodily symptoms or extremely severe symptoms
F. In medical settings, SSD presentation has been historically linked with the terms *medically unexplained* and *functional symptoms*. However, more recent nosology does not require the symptoms to be unexplained to meet the SSD criteria. The primary focus of the diagnosis is on the patient's response to the physical symptoms of either diagnosed or an undiagnosed medical condition.

INCIDENCE

A. The prevalence of SSD is not well-known. This is in part due to the change in diagnostic criteria from the previous versions of classification systems as well as a focus on "medically unexplained symptoms" without assessment of the symptom-related focus and distress, as currently required for SSD diagnosis.

B. Some research estimates that up to 7% of the general adult population may meet the criteria for SSD, while other researchers have made estimates of SSD prevalence in primary care that range from 5% to 35% of all patients.
C. Changes in terminology and healthcare provider confusion about SSD criteria likely lead to mis- or underdiagnosis.
D. Females tend to present with SSD more often than males, with an estimated female to male ratio of 10:1. However, the etiology behind this discrepancy is not well-understood.

PATHOGENESIS
A. SSD can develop during any stage of the life course. Many patients with somatic symptoms experience chronic waxing and waning of symptoms. Croicu and colleagues (2014) note that approximately 20% to 25% of patients presenting with acute somatic symptoms will develop a chronic somatic condition, while the remainder show improvement over time.

PREDISPOSING FACTORS
A. The etiology of SSD remains unknown and may result from a complex array of causes, which include genetics, epigenetics, neurodevelopmental factors, childhood, family and social environments, learned behavior, personality, and lifestyle.
B. A number of potential risk factors have been identified, including personality traits (e.g., neuroticism); exposure to neglect, abuse, or other adversity during childhood; as well as current or recent stressful life events.
C. Evidence is emerging to suggest that neural networks related to pain, stress, and coping may be impacted by early life adversity, contributing to experiences of somatic pain symptoms in association with psychological stress.
D. None of these factors are truly pathognomonic; however, their role in moderation and causality of SSD symptoms is not well-understood.

COMMON COMPLAINTS
A. Typical SSD complaints belong to one of four categories of somatic symptoms: cardiopulmonary, gastrointestinal, pain-related, or generalized.

OTHER SIGNS AND SYMPTOMS
A. Patients with SSD are often engaged in ongoing and unsuccessful searches for symptom explanations, which can result in feelings of helplessness, frustration, and fear of dismissal by healthcare providers.
B. Presentation with somatic symptoms may also be associated with reinforcing factors that reduce motivation to change.

SUBJECTIVE DATA
A. Patients with fewer symptoms and better premorbid functioning have better SSD prognosis. However, these links are associative rather than algorithmic.
B. Evidence suggests that SSD symptom presentation is influenced by both the psychological stressors as well as cultural context.
  1. Patients suffering from SSD who are seen in primary care were significantly more likely to be experiencing unemployment or occupational impairment. Additionally, patients who experience stigma around psychological symptoms may report somatic symptoms more frequently.

PHYSICAL EXAMINATION
A. No specific medical tests are utilized for SSD diagnostics.

B. Approaching SSD from a purely biomedical model may result in excess medical interventions and testing that can contribute to patients' concerns and delay effective treatments. Additionally, risk–benefit discussion within the scope of shared decision-making and risks of iatrogenic illness should be considered.

DIAGNOSTIC TESTS AND SCREENINGS
A. A diagnosis of SSD is possible via questionnaires, followed by a thorough psychiatric interview. Symptom questionnaires may be valuable as screening tools and for transdiagnostic comparison, while diagnostic interviews are necessary to establish clinically significant FSD diagnoses.
B. Because full comprehensive clinical interviews are lengthy and require appropriate clinical training, patients can be referred for specialty mental health services, Additionally, there are several brief measures to screen for SSD symptoms, monitor progress, and track treatment.
  1. Patient Health Questionnaire 15-Item Subscale (PHQ-15)
     a. The PHQ-15 is the most commonly used screening tool for detection of SSD symptoms. It is a subscale of the larger Patient Health Questionnaire (PHQ), which was developed by Spitzer and colleagues (1999) for primary care use. The PHQ-15 is a self-report screener tool that is well-validated, in open access, and available in multiple languages.
     b. The scale includes 15 items, each item assessing whether the respondent has been "bothered by" a specific physical symptom. Responses are rated on a 3-point Likert scale (from 0, *not at all*, to 2, *bothered a lot*).
     c. Scores for the PHQ-15 range from 0 to 30, with higher scores indicating more severe symptoms. The PHQ-15 cutoffs of 5, 10, and 15 can be utilized as cutoffs for low, medium, and high severity of somatic symptoms, respectively.
     d. To preserve validity and reliability, patients should complete the PHQ-15 independently. However, if the screener is administered to the patient, each item should be read verbatim to the patient.
  2. Somatic Symptom Scale-8 (SSS-8)
     a. The SSS-8 is a newer tool validated for use in the primary care setting. This measure consists of eight items aimed at assessing the extent to which the patient experienced six common somatic complaints (i.e., gastrointestinal distress, back pain, limb or joint pain, headache, chest pain/shortness of breath, dizziness) and two common consequences of somatic symptoms (i.e., fatigue and poor sleep) in the past 7 days.
     b. Items on the SSS-8 are scored on a 5-point scale (from 0, *not at all*, to 4, *very much*), for a total score ranging from 0 to 32.
     c. Scores between 0 and 3 are considered no or minimal symptoms, 4 to 7 as low, 8 to 11 as medium, 12 to 15 as high, and greater than or equal to 16 as very high severity of symptoms.
C. In addition to using screening tools designed for the assessment of SSD symptoms, it may be beneficial to serially administer brief screeners of depression (e.g., Patient Health Questionnaire, nine-item depression screener [PHQ-9]) and anxiety (e.g., Generalized Anxiety Disorder seven-item screener [GAD-7]). Tracking anxiety and depression scores in SSD can serve as an indirect measure of symptom improvement over time.

DIFFERENTIAL DIAGNOSIS

A. It is critical to remember that the core of the SSD diagnosis is the patient's reaction to symptoms rather than the presence of symptoms per se. Thus, differential diagnostic considerations should include the patient's cognitive and emotional response (distress) to somatic symptoms, as well as the associated impairment in functioning.

B. Another challenge in the differential diagnosis of SSD is the high rate of comorbid psychological conditions, particularly anxiety and depression. In a survey of patients with SSD in German primary care practices, Steinbrecher and colleagues (2011) found that 37.1% of patients had a comorbid psychiatric disorder.

C. The clinician should keep in mind that because of both comorbid psychiatric disorders and the fact that undiagnosed SSD will likely result in elevated scores on measures of anxiety and depression, it is critical to establish the cause of the distress rather than only focus on the symptoms. Furthermore, treatment of refractory anxiety and/or depression should raise concerns about overlooked SSD.

Specific Differential Diagnostic Considerations

A. The following diagnoses should be ruled out to diagnose SSD:

1. Panic disorder (PD): Among patients with PD, acute somatic symptoms and health-related anxiety are largely limited to panic episodes, with focus on somatic symptoms of panic (e.g., tachycardia). While patients with PD may report anticipatory anxiety as well as interoceptive and situational avoidance, anxiety is focused on reemergence of panic attacks and fear of the panic symptoms (e.g., fear of dying, fear of having a heart attack).
2. Generalized anxiety disorder (GAD): GAD is characterized by somatic symptoms (e.g., irritability, muscle tension); however, anxiety is not centered on a specific event, activity, or symptom (such as health).
3. Depressive disorders: In depressive disorders, the predominant symptoms are low mood and loss of interest, pleasure, or enjoyment from activities (anhedonia). While somatic symptoms may be present, these symptoms are limited to depressive episodes and are not central to the diagnosis.
4. Illness anxiety disorder (IAD): While there is significant anxiety and distress related to health in IAD, somatic/physical symptoms are either minimal or absent.
5. Functional neurological symptom disorder (FND): FND is characterized by the presence of physical symptoms that are not compatible with known medical or neurologic condition(s). FND is characterized by symptoms believed to originate from psychological causes, with presenting neurologic symptoms (like movement or sensory disruptions) that lack explanation from a neurologic illness. These symptoms may resemble those of neurologic disorders but are not due to structural or electrical issues in the nervous system and may not match known neurologic diseases, as sometimes confirmed by tests.
6. Delusional disorder: SSD should not be diagnosed if patients' beliefs about their somatic symptoms meet the criteria for delusions—false beliefs that are held despite the incontrovertible proof or evidence of the contrary.
7. Body dysmorphic disorder (BDD): While BDD is characterized by excessive concerns related to a perceived physical defect in their body, in SSD, concerns focus on symptoms or illness rather than physical appearance.
8. Obsessive-compulsive disorder (OCD): Excessive concerns and thoughts associated with SSD are less intrusive compared with obsessive thoughts in OCD. SSD does not encompass compulsions, which may be seen in OCD.

B. Consider interactions between SSD and de facto medical diagnosis or condition. While the presence of medically unexplained somatic symptoms is not sufficient for diagnosis, presence of excessive thoughts, feelings, or behaviors associated with a known medical condition that are also associated with distress and impairment should alert to the possibility of SSD comorbidity.

1. It is possible for a patient to meet the criteria for SSD in addition to an identified medical condition as long as the SSD criteria are met for at least 6 months.

PLAN

A. Approach SSD treatment consistently, with awareness of its unique challenges, and from the BPS perspective. Barsky and colleagues (2001) emphasize that SSD is often chronic and resistant to treatment, as symptoms may be maintained by psychological and social contexts.

B. Both practitioners and patients may be reluctant to change the course of treatment to focus on psychological interventions, viewing these as stigmatizing or delegitimizing what they believe to be purely medical problems. This is likely to be the case when the "split BPS" model is used.

C. Given these barriers to initiating and completing treatment for SSD, experts emphasize that building a strong, positive patient–healthcare provider relationship is crucial to successful treatment. Effective clinicians must show support and empathy for the patient's needs, while also avoiding additional prescriptions or tests that may be contraindicated, leading to increased risks of iatrogenic illness and case access consequence.

General Treatments and Intervention

A. The following steps will help provide patient-centered care in line with the BPS model:

1. Use a BPS formulation when initiating treatment.
   a. Effective assessment and treatment in SSD requires attention to biological, psychological, and social elements of the patient's presentation and should avoid a "split" BPS approach, which falls back on psychological and social factors in illness presentation when medical interventions fail to lead to improvements.
2. Combine education about pathophysiology with patient-centered interviewing.
   a. Education is crucial to ensure patient understanding of SSD from the BPS perspective; however, patient-centered interviewing (such as motivational interviewing) is important to incorporate.
3. Maintain professionalism and good clinical practice.
   a. It is essential to approach patients with SSD in a manner that conveys respect and validation for the patient's illness experiences. Evidence-based care should be provided to all patients with SSD.
4. Do not overlook the value of the relationship.
   a. Building rapport and trust between the patient and the members of the care team has been associated with significant symptom reduction in SSD.

Psychotherapy for Somatic Symptom Disorder

A. Multiple randomized controlled trials (RCTs) have tested the effectiveness of cognitive behavioral therapy (CBT) interventions in the treatment of SSD and related conditions. A Cochrane review of treatments for medically unexplained physical symptoms—a medical diagnosis with substantial overlap with SSD—found evidence that CBT can lead to reductions in somatic symptoms compared with usual care or waitlist groups. However, effect sizes were variable and generally small.

B. Other reviews and meta-analyses of RCTs for SSD have similarly found evidence for the effectiveness of CBT in mitigating somatic symptoms, pain intensity, psychological distress, and functional impairment, with improvements lasting for 3 to 12 months posttreatment. However, while some studies suggest that CBT interventions for SSD can reduce healthcare utilization and costs associated with ambulatory medical care, findings have not been consistent.

C. Concerns have been raised about CBT for SSD in medical settings, particularly the primary care setting. Evidence suggests that more and longer sessions may be needed to maximize the effectiveness of CBT treatment. Individual patient presentations, including comorbid mental and physical disorders, may complicate treatment fidelity and effectiveness in the context of real-world care.

COMMON MEDICATIONS

A. Five categories of psychopharmacologic medications can used in the treatment of SSD:
1. Tricyclic antidepressants (TCAs)
2. Selective serotonin reuptake inhibitors (SSRIs)
3. Serotonin and norepinephrine reuptake inhibitors (SNRIs)
4. Atypical antipsychotics
5. Herbs, such as St. John's wort

B. Although all five groups have demonstrated effectiveness, appropriateness may vary depending on the presentation. For example, there is evidence suggesting that SNRIs may be more effective in SSD with predominant pain.

C. While any of these five classes of medications may be considered in the treatment of SSD, there remains insufficient research evidence regarding appropriate dosing and timing, differences between treatments, and long-term effectiveness of pharmacotherapy for SSD.

D. Pharmacotherapy for SSD should follow good practice guidelines of shared decision-making, teach-back, regular follow-up, and symptom reassessment. Finally, it is important to incorporate medication management as a component of BPS-grounded care.

PATIENT TEACHING

A. Education about the BPS model of SSD is crucial to the alignment of patient and clinician expectations for treatment and for the framing of treatment goals.

B. Evidence suggests that a single session of psychoeducation about stress responsiveness, pain pathways, exercise, and diet can produce improvement in somatic symptoms.

C. Providing education on mind–body connection and BPS model/treatment can enhance understanding and engagement with care.

FOLLOW-UP

A. It is prudent to expect that SSD symptoms may require long-standing management.

B. In ongoing care for patients with SSD, the APRN and their colleagues should focus on maintaining good rapport with the individual, communicating empathy, and engaging in active listening.

C. With a strong patient–healthcare provider relationship, individuals with SSD may be more likely to accept and utilize recommended interventions, resulting in more successful symptom reduction.

CONSULTATION AND REFERRALS

A. Involving both physicians and mental health providers in care planning and implementation for patients with SSD is the primary component of success.

B. Providing a consultation letter to the patient's primary care provider (PCP) documenting SSD assessment and diagnosis has shown benefits in reducing patient symptoms and anxieties about symptoms.

C. Despite the potential efficacy of treating SSD in medical settings, limited time, resources, and other priorities may constrain healthcare providers' ability to manage SSD treatment successfully.
  1. Treatment should be interprofessional and BPS-focused from the start. Discuss both the role of mind–body connection as well as the impact of symptoms of emotional well-being and emphasize the importance of coping skills for improved illness management.
  2. Clinicians should directly discuss patients' concerns about mental health referrals with a focus on the goal of providing the patient with the best quality of care within a team-based framework.
  3. By having a behavioral health provider on-site and as part of the patient's care team, integrated primary care approaches may improve attendance to follow-up appointments and effectiveness of treatment for SSD.

D. Referral for psychotherapeutic or psychiatric services can be very beneficial for SSD. Referral to external/internal mental healthcare should be discussed with emphasis on mind–body connection, goals of functional improvement, and distress coping.
  1. The following points should be emphasized:
     a. Experienced physical symptoms are real, and patients will continue to receive thorough and ongoing medical care.
     b. Referral to mental health reflects an understanding that the physical symptoms are complex. Mind and body act together to create and maintain symptoms. Referral to mental health is in line with current understanding of SSD.
     c. Ongoing symptoms (physical symptoms and related anxiety) lead to distress and impairment. Mental health services can provide practical coping skills and techniques that will alleviate distress and promote coping.
     d. The medical team and mental health will work together to help the patient improve quality of life and decrease distress.

INDIVIDUAL CONSIDERATIONS

A. Although prevalence data on SSD are limited, there is evidence that both increased rate and severity of somatic symptoms are associated with female sex and gender.

B. Lower socioeconomic class, preexisting psychological disorders, and history of trauma are also correlated with SSD diagnosis.

Pediatrics

A. The estimated prevalence among pediatric patients is between 5% and 13% among inpatients and up to 33% among outpatients.
B. While many children and adolescents may experience short-term somatic symptoms, others will develop chronic symptoms meeting the criteria for SSD, in which case evidence-based recommendations for the diagnosis and treatment of adults with SSD generally apply.
C. Presentation of SSD may differ between adults and children: A single, prominent somatic symptom is more commonly reported by pediatric patients than adults with SSD.
D. Common pediatric somatic symptoms include abdominal, musculoskeletal, and chest pain, as well as vomiting, dizziness, and fatigue.
E. In screening and treating pediatric patients with somatic symptoms, unique impacts of symptoms on their daily functioning and implications for cognitive and social development should be considered.
  1. Somatic symptoms can necessitate changes in lifestyle, including frequent medical visits and medication use, which interfere with typical activities of childhood and adolescence.
  2. Children experiencing somatic symptoms may have difficulties with school attendance, and their parents' interpretation of and response to their symptoms can greatly impact the child's distress levels.
F. Because of these various situational factors, presentation of pediatric SSD may be complex, and symptoms persisting may indicate that appropriate treatment has not been found.
G. See Chapter 20, "Special Considerations for Childhood and Adolescent Populations," for additional considerations in working with pediatric patients.

Pregnancy

A. The literature on SSD in the context of pregnancy is limited, apart from some evidence that pregnant patients may exhibit somatic symptoms in response to depression and/or anxiety that could be misinterpreted as SSD.
B. See Chapter 12, "Perinatal Mental Health," for other recommendations for mental healthcare during pregnancy.

Geriatrics/Older Adults

A. SSD may be severely underdiagnosed among older adults as their somatic symptoms are often misinterpreted as signs of normal aging. In presentation, older adults may experience greater psychological distress associated with SSD, particularly if their somatic symptoms are medically unexplained.
B. For further recommendations on geriatric care, see Chapter 21, "Aging and Older Adult Populations."

Partners/Family

A. Experiencing somatic symptoms and associated distress can be highly disruptive to patients' daily life, and consequently can also have significant impact on close others such as partners and family members.
B. A partner with SSD often experiences emotional disturbances that can negatively impact dyadic functioning within a couple. However, to date there has been limited research and practical guidelines on supporting caregivers and partners during the treatment of SSD.
C. For more information about caregiver issues, see Chapter 35, "Caregiver and End-of-Life Issues."

RESOURCES

Websites

A. American Psychological Association, Division 12: Chronic or persistent pain: https://div12.org/diagnosis/chronic-or-persistent-pain
B. Patient Health Questionnaire (PHQ) Screeners: www.phqscreeners.com

Visual/Video Materials

A. White, R., Hayes, C., White, S., & Hodson, F. J. (2016). Using social media to challenge unwarranted clinical variation in the treatment of chronic noncancer pain: The "Brainman" story. *Journal of Pain Research, 9*, 701–709. https://doi.org/10.2147/JPR.S115814
B. Brainman. (2014). *Understanding pain in less than 5 minutes.* YouTube. www.youtube.com/watch?v=5KrUL8tOaQs
C. Mosley, L. (2011). *Why things hurt.* Tedx Talks. www.youtube.com/watch?v=gwd-wLdIHjs

Practice Guidelines

A. Johnson, K. K., Bennett, C., & Rochani, H. (2020). Significant improvement of somatic symptom disorder with brief psychoeducational intervention by PMHNP in primary care. *Journal of the American Psychiatric Nurses Association, 28*(2), 171–180. http://doi.org/10.1177/1078390320960524
B. Kurlansik, S. L., & Maffei, M. S. (2016). Somatic symptom disorder. *American Family Physician, 93*(1), 49–54. PMID: 26760840.
C. Somashekar, B., Jainer, A., & Wuntakal, B. (2013). Psychopharmacotherapy of somatic symptoms disorders. *International Review of Psychiatry, 25*(1), 107–115. https://doi.org/10.3109/09540261.2012.729758

REFERENCES AND BIBLIOGRAPHY

Agorastos, A., Pervanidou, P., Chrousos, G. P., & Baker, D. G. (2019). Developmental trajectories of early life stress and trauma: A narrative review on neurobiological aspects beyond stress system dysregulation. *Frontiers in Psychiatry, 10*, 118. https://doi.org/10.3389/fpsyt.2019.00118

Atmaca, M., Sirlier, B., Yildirim, H., & Kayali, A. (2011). Hippocampus and amygdalar volumes in patients with somatization disorder. *Progress in Neuro-Psychopharmacology and Biological Psychiatry, 35*(7), 1699–1703. https://doi.org/10.1016/j.pnpbp.2011.05.016

Barsky, A. J., Ettner, S. L., Horsky, J., & Bates, D. W. (2001, July). Resource utilization of patients with hypochondriacal health anxiety and somatization. *Medical Care, 39*(7), 705–715. https://journals.lww.com/lww-medicalcare/abstract/2001/07000/resource_utilization_of_patients_with.7.aspx

Beck, J. E. (2008). A developmental perspective on functional somatic symptoms. *Journal of Pediatric Psychology, 33*(5), 547–562. https://doi.org/10.1093/jpepsy/jsm113

Carson, A., & Lehn, A. (2016). Epidemiology. In M. Hallett, J. Stone, & A. Carson (Eds.), *Handbook of Clinical Neurology* (Vol. 139; pp. 47–60). Elsevier. https://www.sciencedirect.com/science/article/abs/pii/B9780128017722000059

Creed, F., & Barsky, A. (2004). A systematic review of the epidemiology of somatisation disorder and hypochondriasis. *Journal of Psychosomatic Research, 56*(4), 391–408. PMID: 15094023.

Croicu, C., Chwastiak, L., & Katon, W (2014). Approach to the patient with multiple somatic symptoms. *Medical Clinics of North America, 98*(5), 1079–1095. https://doi.org/10.1016/j.mcna.2014.06.007

D'Souza, R. S., & Hooten, W. M. (2023, March 13). *Somatic syndrome disorders*. StatPearls Publishing. https://www.ncbi.nlm.nih.gov/books/NBK532253

Fava, G. A., Cosci, F., & Sonino, N. (2017). Current psychosomatic practice. *Psychotherapy and Psychosomatics, 86*(1), 13–30. https://doi.org/10.1159/000448856

First, M. B. (2014). *Handbook of differential diagnosis*. American Psychiatric Association Publishing.

Gierk, B., Kohlmann, S., Kroenke, K., Spangenberg, L., Zenger, M., Brähler, E., & Löwe, B. (2014). The Somatic Symptom Scale-8 (SSS-8): A brief measure of somatic symptom burden. *JAMA Internal Medicine, 174*(3), 399–407. https://doi.org/10.1001/jamainternmed.2013.12179

Johnson, K. K., Bennett, C., & Rochani, H. (2020). Significant improvement of somatic symptom disorder with brief psychoeducational intervention by PMHNP in primary care. *Journal of the American Psychiatric Nurses Association, 28*(2), 171–180. http://doi.org/10.1177/1078390320960524

Harris, A. M., Orav, E. J., Bates, D. W., & Barsky, A. J. (2009). Somatization increases disability independent of comorbidity. *Journal of General Internal Medicine, 24*(2), 155–161. https://doi.org/10.1007/s11606-008-0845-0

Kahn, D. (2024, March 27). *Illness anxiety disorder*. Medscape. https://emedicine.medscape.com/article/290955-overview

Kelly, R. H., Russo, J., & Katon, W. (2001). Somatic complaints among pregnant women cared for in obstetrics: Normal pregnancy or depressive and anxiety symptom amplification revisited? *General Hospital Psychiatry, 23*(3), 107–113. https://doi.org/10.1016/S0163-8343(01)00129-3

Kingdon, D., Rowlands, P., & Stein, G. (Eds.). (2024). *Seminars in general adult psychiatry: Vol. 2* (3rd ed.). Royal College of Psychiatrists.

Kroenke, K. (2007). Efficacy of treatment for somatoform disorders: A review of randomized controlled trials. *Psychosomatic Medicine, 69*(9), 881–888. https://doi.org/10.1097/PSY.0b013e31815b00c4

Kroenke, K., Spitzer, R. L., & Williams, J. B. (2002). The PHQ-15: Validity of a new measure for evaluating the severity of somatic symptoms. *Psychosomatic Medicine, 64*(2), 258–266. PMID: 11914441.

Kurlansik, S. L., & Maffei, M. S. (2016). Somatic symptom disorder. *American Family Physician, 93*(1), 49–54A. https://www.aafp.org/pubs/afp/issues/2016/0101/p49.html#

Lanzara, R., Conti, C., Camelio, M., Cannizzaro, P., Lalli, V., Bellomo, R. G., Saggini, R., & Porcelli, P. (2020). Alexithymia and somatization in chronic pain patients: A sequential mediation model. *Frontiers in Psychology, 11*(11), 545881. https://doi.org/10.3389/fpsyg.2020.545881

Liu, J., Gill, N. S., Teodorczuk, A., Li, Z.-J., Sun, J. (2019). The efficacy of cognitive behavioral therapy in somatoform disorders and medically unexplained physical symptoms: A meta-analysis of randomized controlled trials. *Journal of Affective Disorders, 245*(15), 98–112. https://doi.org/10.1016/j.jad.2018.10.114

Malas, N., Donohue, L., Cook, R. J., Leber, S. M., & Kullgren, K. A. (2018). Pediatric somatic symptom and related disorders: Primary care provider perspectives. *Clinical Pediatrics, 57*(4), 377–388. https://doi.org/10.1177/0009922817727467

olde Hartman, T. C., Borghuis, M. S., Lucassen, P. L., van de Laar, F. A., Speckens, A. E., & van Weel, C. (2009). Medically unexplained symptoms, somatization disorder and hypochondriasis: Course and prognosis. A systematic review. *Journal of Psychosomatic Research, 66*(5), 363–377. https://doi.org/10.1016/j.jpsychores.2008.09.018

Oster, C., Morello, A., Venning, A., Redpath, P., & Lawn, S. (2017). The health and wellbeing needs of veterans: A rapid review. *BMC Psychiatry, 17*(1). https://doi.org/10.1186/s12888-017-1547-0

Petersen, M. W., Ørnbøl, E., Dantoft, T. M., & Fink, P. (2021). Assessment of functional somatic disorders in epidemiological research: Self-report questionnaires versus diagnostic interviews. *Journal of Psychosomatic Research, 146*, 110491. https://doi.org/10.1016/j.jpsychores.2021.110491

Pilipenko, N. (2022). Somatic symptom disorder in primary care: A collaborative approach. *Journal of Family Practice, 71*(3), E8–E12. https://doi.org/10.12788/jfp.0384

Scarella, T. M., Boland, R. J., & Barsky, A. J. (2019). Illness anxiety disorder. *Psychosomatic Medicine, 81*(5), 398–407. https://doi.org/10.1097/psy.0000000000000691

Somashekar, B., Jainer, A., & Wuntakal., B. (2013). Psychopharmacotherapy of somatic symptoms disorders. *International Review of Psychiatry, 25*(1), 107–115. https://doi.org/10.3109/09540261.2012.729758

Spitzer, R. L., Kroenke, K., & Williams, J. B. (1999). Validation and utility of a self-report version of PRIME-MD: The PHQ primary care study. Primary care evaluation of mental disorders. Patient health questionnaire. *JAMA, 282*(18), 1737–1744. https://doi.org/10.1001/jama.282.18.1737

Steinbrecher, N., Koerber, S., Frieser, D., & Hiller, W. (2011). The prevalence of medically unexplained symptoms in primary care. *Psychosomatics, 52*, 263–271. https://doi.org/10.1016/j.psym.2011.01.007

van der Horst, H. E., & van Marwijk, H. (2014). Non-pharmacological interventions for somatoform disorders and Medically Unexplained Physical Symptoms (MUPS) in adults. *Cochrane Database of Systematic Reviews, 11*, Article CD011142. https://doi.org/10.1002/14651858.CD011142.pub2

van Dessel, N., den Boe, M., van der Wouden, J. C., Kleinstäuber, M., Leone, S. S., & Terluin, B. (2022). 6C20 Bodily distress disorder. In World Health Organization, *ICD-11 for mortality and morbidity statistics*. https://icd.who.int/browse/2024-01/mms/en#767044268

Yates, W. R., & Xiong, G. L. (Ed.). (2019, April 23). *Somatic symptom disorders*. Medscape. https://emedicine.medscape.com/article/294908-overview

16 SUBSTANCE USE DISORDERS

Rabia Hanif, Jack Spencer, and Brenda Marshall

INTRODUCTION

Despite the persistence of stigmatizing, judgmental, and biased thoughts to the contrary, research has demonstrated that substance use disorders (SUDs) are a category of disease—not a personal failing or weakness. The diseases that fall into this category are many, reflecting the number of substances that result in patterned use, which impacts the individual's social, academic, and employment arenas. There are books that deal only with diagnosis, treatment, and programs for recovery from SUDs. This chapter gives a brief overview of the most common SUDs, with suggestions for best practice when providing treatment to patients with SUDs. References to other resources are listed at the end of the chapter.

> In all cases, the Suicide and Crisis line 988 is available 24/7 and can assist for emotional and substance use support, as is SAMHSA's national helpline 1-800-662-4357 (HELP) and www.FindTreatment.gov.

The American Psychiatric Association shifted the SUD paradigm from an addictive behavior to a disease of substance use and includes all substances from tobacco to opioids. Within each specific drug-related disorder, the clinician is required to identify not only the drug, but also the degree of the disorder (mild to severe), which reflects the number of SUD criteria met. The *Diagnostic and Statistical Manual of Mental Disorders*, Fifth Edition (*DSM-5*; American Psychiatric Association, 2013), has identified 11 criteria that can be used to assess degree: (a) use of the substance in larger amounts or for longer periods of time than the person intended; (b) continued use despite efforts to cut back use or to quit; (c) the individual invests excessive time surrounding the use or recovery from use of the substance; (d) craving the substance; (e) not meeting major personal/professional/academic obligations; (f) inability to stop despite interpersonal and social problems; (g) the person no longer engages in activities and hobbies, or has reduced time spent on them; (h) risk-taking that can be physically hazardous; (i) unable to stop usage despite major physical or psychological problems (e.g., hepatitis C, divorce); (j) increased tolerance, or the need to increase amount of substance to achieve the same level of comfort/relief; and (k) experience of physical withdrawal when substance is not used. After assessing the patient, the severity can be determined by how many criteria exist: no diagnosis; 2 to 3, mild; 4 to 5, moderate; 6+, severe.

USE, MISUSE, AND ABUSE

A. Use: using a substance for the purpose it was intended (medicinal or recreational)
B. Misuse: using a substance for nonintended purposes or inappropriately
C. Abuse: intentional or excessive use that results in physical and/or mental harm to the user

DEFINITION

A. The definition this chapter will use for SUD reflects that of the National Alliance on Mental Illness (NAMI), which states: "an SUD is when a substance or substances results in a clinically significant level of distress" (Marshall & Spencer, 2019, p. 4).

INCIDENCE/PREVALENCE IN THE UNITED STATES

A. 14.5% of Americans over the age of 12 (40.3 million people) had an SUD in 2020 (Lange et al., 2024)
  1. Globally about 39.5 million people have lived experiences of SUD (World Health Organization [WHO], 2021).
B. 18% of nurses demonstrated signs of substance use problems, with almost 7% of those nurses qualifying for an SUD diagnosis (Webster, 2024).
C. The prevalence of SUD is higher in males; however, the adverse physical, medical, and psychiatric consequences are more severe in women (McHugh et al., 2018).
D. Alcohol use by Americans over 18 years of age between 2015 and 2019 was present in all racial/ethnic groups. In all categories from alcohol to sedatives and stimulants, use was highest in two or more races.

Substance Use in Times of Disasters

A. Traumatic events (e.g., natural disasters, pandemics, wars) have significant impact on substance use, with a well-documented rise in substance use during these times. These events also affect the ability of local and federal governments to provide services to persons with SUDs.
  1. Trauma-informed care
    a. Trauma impacts the physical, emotional, and psychological well-being of a person. The following are the principles of trauma-informed care:
      i. Safety and trust
      ii. Empowerment
      iii. Collaboration and mutuality
      iv. Sensitivity and understanding
    b. The following are special populations requiring trauma-informed care:
      i. Abused women and their children
      ii. Veterans
      iii. Survivors of domestic violence
      iv. Persons with a history of adverse childhood experiences (ACEs)
  2. Person-centered care
    a. Respond to the patient and the patient's goals, providing dignity, compassion, and respect for the individual through shared decision-making.
    b. Identify and work with the patient's values and preferences.
    c. Seek and provide coordinated care, support, and treatments.
    d. Support independence and strengths, developing skills for independent living.
    e. Always use person-first language (e.g., a person with diabetes).

Resources During and After a Disaster

A. National Association of State Alcohol and Drug Abuse Directors: https://nasadad.org
B. Substance Abuse and Mental Health Services Administration (SAMHSA): www.samhsa.gov/dtac/disaster-behavioral-health-resources

HARM REDUCTION APPROACHES FOR PEOPLE WHO USE DRUGS

A. Using prevention, risk reduction, and health promotion, this evidence-based approach empowers people who use drugs (PWUD) with alternatives and choices to increase self-reliance.
B. Harm reduction respects the lived experiences of PWUDs and has the goal of preventing death and illnesses resulting from overdose and infection. It is an approach that allows PWUDs to learn about and determine which strategies they want to incorporate into their lives and pathway to recovery. It can also serve as a bridge helping the PWUD access more health services, social services, as well as prevention, treatment, and recovery programs.
C. The following are the six pillars of harm reduction according to the Substance Abuse and Mental Health Services Administration (SAMHSA; www.samhsa.gov/sites/default/files/harm-reduction-framework.pdf):
  1. Led by PWUDs
  2. Embraces the inherent value of people
  3. Commits to deep community engagement and community building
  4. Promotes equity rights and reparative social justice
  5. Offers accessible and noncoercive support
  6. Focuses on any positive change as defined by the person
D. Core practice areas include the following:
  1. Safer practices: education and support on reduction of risk through provision of supplies and materials (i.e., syringe programs)
  2. Safer settings: day centers, access to housing, recovery communities, and public health programs as alternatives to arrest and incarceration
  3. Safer access to healthcare: ensuring nonstigmatizing and person-centered care that is trauma-informed
  4. Safer transition to care: connections and access to harm reduction-informed and trauma-informed care and services
  5. Sustainable workforce and field: provide resources to maintain a skilled workforce and community-based programs
  6. Sustainable infrastructure: building, maintaining, and revitalizing community-led infrastructure to support harm reduction best practice for PWUDs

General Screening for Dependence

A. Leeds Dependence Questionnaire: https://onlinelibrary.wiley.com/doi/pdf/10.1002/9780470693742.app7
B. National Institutes of Health (NIH) access to screening and assessment tools for SUD: https://nida.nih.gov/nidamed-medical-health-professionals/screening-tools-resources/chart-screening-tools

REFERENCES AND BIBLIOGRAPHY

American Psychiatric Association. (2013). *Diagnostic and statistical manual of mental disorders* (5th ed.). https://doi.org/10.1176/appi.books.9780890425596

Lange, R., De Padilla, L., Parker, E., & Holland, K. (2024). *Substance use and substance use disorders*. Centers for disease Control and Prevention. https://wwwnc.cdc.gov/travel/yellowbook/2024/additional-considerations/substance-use

Marshall, B., & Spencer, J. (2019). *Fast facts about substance use disorders: What every nurse, APRN, and PA needs to know*. Springer Publishing Company.

McHugh, R. K., Votaw, V. R., Sugarman, D. E., & Greenfield, S. F. (2018). Sex and gender differences in substance use disorders. *Clinical Psychology Review, 66*, 12–23. https://doi.org/10.1016/j.cpr.2017.10.012

Substance Abuse and Mental Health Services Administration. (2023). *Harm reduction framework*. Center for Substance Abuse Prevention, Substance Abuse and Mental Health Services Administration. https://www.samhsa.gov/find-help/harm-reduction/framework

Webster, A. (2024, May 24). *Drug and alcohol rehab for nurses near you*. American Addiction Centers. https://americanaddictioncenters.org/healthcare-professionals/rehab-for-nurses

World Health Organization. (2023, August 29). *Fact sheets Opioid overdose*. https://www.who.int/news-room/fact-sheets/detail/opioid-overdose

NONPHARMACEUTICAL TREATMENT APPROACHES AND THERAPIES FOR SUBSTANCE USE DISORDERS

CONCEPTUAL FRAMEWORK OF THE BIOPSYCHOSOCIAL MODEL

A. Medical sciences were revolutionized after the proposed concept named the "biopsychosocial model" by George Engel (1977) to study diseases. This model is a valid conceptualization today and provides a broader and deeper understanding of SUDs (Figure 16.1).
B. The following are the 3Ps of SUD:
  1. Precipitating factors: stress, conflict, lack of coping skills, and other emotional/physical/mental stressors
  2. Predisposing factors: some personality traits like neuroticism, history of familial abuse/misuse of substances, and exposure to ACEs including emotional abuse, neglect, and physical and sexual abuse
  3. Protecting/protective factors: strong ties to supportive community, supportive family relationships, and personality traits like conscientiousness, spirituality, and dependability

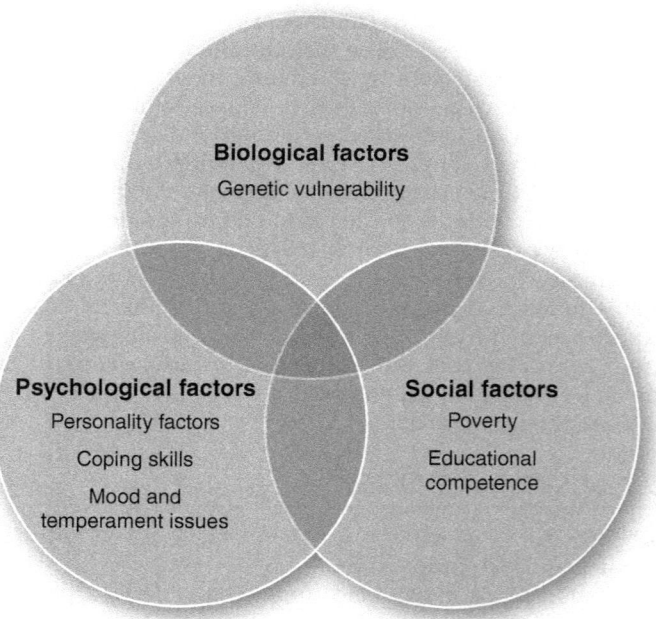

FIGURE 16.1 The biopsychosocial model.

MOTIVATIONAL INTERVIEWING FOR SUBSTANCE USE DISORDERS/ALCOHOL USE DISORDERS

A. Motivational interviewing (MI) is a skill that can be learned gradually and is a guiding tool to resolve ambivalence issues that create resistance.
B. MI is based on person-centered style of counseling.
   1. Ambivalence often brings uncomfortable feelings and emotions, leading people to procrastinate.
   2. It is natural to resist change as a person has to go out of the comfort zone.
   3. MI helps instigate motivation among people who are fighting with ambivalence and help them change in a healthy direction.
C. The following are the OARS skills that clinicians can use during MI counseling:
   1. **O**: Open-ended questions
      a. What brings you here today?
      b. How are you feeling today?
   2. **A**: Affirmations
      a. Instill self-efficacy among patients about the choices they are making or thinking of making related to their perceived obstacles.
   3. **R**: Reflective listening
      a. Reflective listening is the fundamental ingredient to building a healthy bond with the patient.
      b. It provides undivided attention to the content of talk.
      c. Observe associated body language and respond according to the situation.
   4. **S**: Summarization
      a. This skill assists the clinician in keeping focused by summarizing the discussion topic.
      b. This skill aids in shifting the topic when discussion about one aspect is complete or if the patient is resistant to further talk.
D. The following are the key features of the spirit of MI:
   1. Partnership: This is a collaborative approach where the patient and the therapist work jointly to resolve the issue instead of considering the patient as weaker, being they are fully involved in the process of change. The therapist avoids playing being the expert.
   2. Acceptance: This is a unique aspect that itself comprises four essentials, such as respecting the patient's autonomy and considering them worthy. It also talks about accepting the patient's perspective with warmth and believing in their strengths.
   3. Compassion: It is very significant to understand that the patient's needs are the priority and must be met with compassion without any second thought.
   4. Evocation: When a counselor is keenly involved, they must be mindful that the best idea must come through the patient's head, and the therapist focuses on the patient's inner wisdom rather than looking at the deficiencies.
E. Ambivalence: It is normal to feel mixed feelings when change is encountered in life. MI can help the patient in understanding the feelings that may be causing resistance to change.
   1. Common demonstration of patient ambivalence:
      a. Side tracking: This kind of ambivalence can be seen in patients when they try to explain reasons to continue the undesired behaviors (i.e., drug-taking), rather than considering change, and they shift the topic when serious efforts are discussed by changing the focus toward the problem instead of solutions.
      b. Arguing: One of the most commonly seen subtypes of ambivalence is when the discussion about change starts and the patient lists a number of reasons why they cannot consider change.
      c. Interrupting: It provides an insight that the patient is not comfortable discussing change. A frequent interruption from the patient can be considered a resistance to change.
      d. Defensiveness: Like other types of resistance, defensiveness can be observed when a patient thinks that their current behavior is under scrutiny and that their behavior is challenged.

FOUR FUNDAMENTAL PROCESSES OF CHANGE

A. Engaging: The clinician provides a nonjudgmental approach.
   1. Trust building
   2. Readiness for treatment
   3. Discussion of patient's worries openly and without judgment
B. Focusing: Focusing helps prioritize needs.
   1. Narrows down urgent and important issues to be addressed
   2. Assists the patient in gaining insight into important issues and motivation
C. Evoking: Framing open-ended questions provides an overview of readiness for change.
   1. Talks about the intrinsic motivation of the patient
   2. Assists the patient in reflecting on thoughts and feelings
D. Planning: The patient prepares for change.
   1. Assists in identifying potential barriers
   2. Encourages the patient to investigate how to address possible challenges
   3. Done in collaboration with the patient

FOUR PRINCIPLES OF MOTIVATIONAL INTERVIEWING

A. Express empathy: understanding the patient's perspective and acknowledging in a nonjudgmental way, which develops a bond of trust and cooperation
B. Support self-efficacy: fostering the patient's confidence related to their skills and abilities so they can work on themselves
C. Roll with the resistance: utilizing reflection instead of direct confrontation to explore underlying dynamics of the patient's current behaviors
D. Develop the discrepancy: achieved by using an indirect and nonconfrontational approach; motivates the patient by highlighting how their desired values/goals are in conflict with undesirable behaviors

PREPARATORY CHANGE TALK IN MOTIVATIONAL INTERVIEWING

A. Recognizing (mobilizing) change talk: **DARN CAT** (**D**esire to change, **A**bility to change, **R**eason to change, **N**eed for change, **C**ommitment, **A**ction **T**aking steps)
   1. When the patient starts discussing about change more often in their talks, it signifies that change is about to happen.
   2. It identifies when to explore desires, abilities, reasons, needs, commitments, the start of activation, and taking steps.
B. Responding to change talk: **EARS**:
   1. Elaborating
   2. Affirmations
   3. Reflections
   4. Summaries

C. The Importance Ruler: a rating scale, from 0 to 10, in the image of a ruler
   1. Assists the clinician in obtaining insight related to how significant it is for the patient to bring change
      a. For example, the therapist may frame a question like "on a scale of 0 to 10 where do you see the importance of bringing the change."
      b. Based on the patient's reply, the therapist can get further clarification about their confidence in self on a scale of 0 to 10.
      c. It helps identify what is actually preventing progress.
D. The Readiness Ruler: also works on a scale of 0 to 10
   1. Inquires about the willingness and enthusiasm of the patient to make progress
      a. "On a scale of 1 to 10 with 10 being most likely, how confident are you that you can make this change?"
      b. "Why did you say ___?"
   2. Identifies whether the patient feels that change is possible and then discusses the barriers or strengths needed to achieve the change

CHANGE TALK VERSUS SUSTAIN TALK

A. Change talk is about bringing change, as opposed to sustain talk, which is rumination on what is unlikely to change.
B. When evoking change talk, clinicians should consider the following:
   1. Looking forward/backward: The clinician supports the patient's ability to imagine an optimistic future with reference to recovery or relationships. When the patient cannot think of something pleasant in the present moment but remembers having accomplished things in the past, the clinician can use those "wins" to increase the patient's confidence to make change.
   2. Exploring goals and values: When a patient is engaged, it helps to discuss their values and goals. Exploration of these goals and values is helpful in developing rapport and a greater possibility of change talk.
   3. Self-talk: Keeping in view the patient's values discussed, the MI practitioner guides the patient with regard to their goals, whether they are aligned with the practitioner's values or not. This signals the openness of the patient and a chance to reestablish rapport. At times, the patient becomes resistant to discussing more.
   4. Query extremes: These types of questions are unique tools to MI and are applicable when there is diminished or no interest in bringing any change. The therapist asks about the worst and best consequences of bringing any change versus not bringing any change.
      a. "Mr. X, imagine what will happen if you continue to binge-drink for the next 6 months? What is your worst nightmare?"
      b. Or: "Visualize yourself as successfully sustaining recovery for the next 6 months, what will be the best thing you can imagine?"
C. The following are strategies clinicians can use to sustain talk:
   1. Simple reflections: Restate the statement verbatim without posing it as question.
      a. Patient: "I don't think I will be able to quit drinking in near future."
      b. Clinician: "It seems you can't see yourself without drinking right now."
   2. Amplified reflections: In this form of reflection, the therapist further explores the patient's thought behind the process, and without using any sarcasm in the tone an expanded statement that touches deeper level is being used. It helps resolve resistance by opening more doors. It also tabs emotional content about the conversation.
      a. Patient: "I know myself I have done few blunders in the past, but things I am asked to do are weird."
      b. Clinician: "I see it's tough for you to agree with things you don't agree to do."
   3. Double-sided reflections: This type of reflection strategy is used at advanced stages of therapy as it brings two conflicting statements of the patient in session politely to make them understand their reasons for not making progress and to create realization/insight.
      a. Patient: "I can't live without my family!"
      b. Clinician: "I am a bit puzzled here; you have said your family means a lot to you, whereas you value your friend more than your wife and kids and spend more time with them, which poses a threat to your road to recovery."

COGNITIVE BEHAVIORAL THERAPY WITH SUBSTANCE USE DISORDERS

A. Cognitive behavioral therapy (CBT) is an evidence-based intervention that focuses on the relationship among thoughts, emotions, and behaviors.
   1. All three components are interrelated and disturbance in each part impacts the other.
   2. Example: Dysfunctional thinking patterns often lead to unhealthy emotions and ultimately self-defeating coping strategies in the form of behaviors.
B. It is often conceptualized that using addictive substances is a conditioned response to places, people, and other related things.
   1. Abusing drugs often provides a strong reinforcement.
   2. The main aim of CBT is to alter the belief system that grants permission to abuse drugs. This is called *relapse prevention* (Glasner-Edwards, 2015).
C. The following are the aims of CBT in SUDs:
   1. The main aim of CBT is to *identify high-risk situations* that elicit conditioned response in reaction to exposure.
      a. An example is a person visiting the same places and people with whom they used to use drugs.
      b. Coming in contact with the drug paraphernalia increases the likelihood that cravings for drug use will be activated.
   2. CBT helps patients make a list of internal and external triggers and assists them in making healthy choices and learning to adapt new skills, which ultimately promote abstinence.
      a. CBT in SUDs work on the thinking patterns of the patient.
      b. It enables them to work collaboratively and spot unhealthy patterns and replace them with adaptive ones.
D. Clarifying the concept of "schema" in CBT
   1. Schemas are fixed sets of core beliefs that form an individual's perception about self, others, and world.
   2. Schemas are usually shaped by early childhood experiences.
   3. Schemas not only interpret experiences and events but also organize information.
   4. The following are common schemas in persons with SUDs:
      a. Incompetency: These thought patterns perceive oneself as incompetent to deal with real-life challenges ▶

and hassles. Such thoughts about lack of resilience and inadequacy often lead to drug usage.
  b. Shame/flawed: The patient considers themselves inherently flawed, and drug use is needed in order to escape negative emotions.
  c. Emotionally underprivileged: The patient has feelings of emptiness that are "filled" through substance use.
  d. Feelings of entitlement: This refers to a general pattern of impulse control where a person sees that it is their fundamental right to attain immediate gratification.
  e. Unrealistic expectations: Setting high standards by self and others increases stress when they are not achieved.
  f. Powerlessness/subjugation: Inability to meet what are considered perceived obligations (legitimate or illegitimate) increases a sense of hopelessness and lack of control. Using substances eases this feeling of powerlessness.
  g. Desire for validation: Drug use is higher in those who engage in behaviors of approval seeking and rejection avoidance.
  h. Isolation: People with strong feelings of loneliness, feeling of being different, and who are socially disconnected may use substances for relief.
  i. Abandonment: A sense or fear of being left alone is lessened through substance use.

E. Cognitive distortions: beliefs that are false and generalized
  1. These cognitive assumptions have the potential to cause a range of mental health conditions (e.g., depression and anxiety).
  2. Cognitive distortions play a significant role in the development and maintenance of SUDs.
  3. Frequently used cognitive distortions include the following:
   a. All-or-nothing principle: The person considers extreme ways without considering any middle ground. It is also referred to as *black or white* and *polarized thinking*. This kind of thinking brings rigidity in thought processes.
   b. Catastrophizing: The person considers disastrous outcome of a simple or trivial matter. Example: "What if my daughter had a car crash as she is not home from party."
   c. Disqualifying the positives: The person accepts the culpability for all negative consequences by denying the possibility that the person is just as responsible for the good things that occur.
   d. Denial: The person refuses to acknowledge the existence of a problem or behavior.
   e. Emotional reasoning: The person considers emotional experience as factual information: "Since I am feeling this way this must be true."
   f. Personalization: External events are attributed to oneself even without any evidence.
   g. Overgeneralization: A conclusion is derived from a single event.
   h. Mind reading: The person jumps into conclusion without sufficient evidence.
   i. "Should" statements: In this cognitive error, a person puts rigid demands on external environment like "must," "ought to," and "should." So, if things do not go as planned, they get upset quickly.
   j. Control fallacies: This refers to when a person either thinks that they are completely helpless and has zero control over their lives, or that they are the victim of the past, and hence nothing can be changed in their life.

REFERENCES AND BIBLIOGRAPHY

Babor, T. F., Higgins-Biddle, J. C., Saunders, J. B., & Monteiro, M. G. (2001). *The alcohol use disorders identification test: Guidelines for use in primary healthcare* (2nd ed., pp. 1–37). World Health Organization.

Engel, G. L. (1977). The need for a new medical model: A challenge for biomedicine. *Science, 196*(4286), 129–136. https://doi.org/10.1126/science.847460

Erickson, M. (2020). *Alcoholics Anonymous most effective path to alcohol abstinence*. Wu Tsai Neurosciences Institute.

Glasner-Edwards, S., Mooney, L., Ang, A., Garneau, H. C., Hartwell, E. E., Brecht, M. L., & Rawson, R. (2015). Mindfulness based relapse prevention improves stimulant use among adults with major depression and generalized anxiety disorder. *Drug and Alcohol Dependence, 100*(156), e80. https:doi.org/10.1016/j.drugalcdep.2015.07.1135

Humeniuk, R., Henry-Edwards, S., Ali, R., Poznyak, V., & Monteiro, M. G. (2010). *The Alcohol, Smoking and Substance Involvement Screening Test (ASSIST): Manual for use in primary care*. World Health Organization. https://iris.who.int/handle/10665/44320

Klimas, J., Field, C. A., Cullen, W., O'Gorman, C. S., Glynn, L. G., Keenan, E., Saunders, J. A., Bury, G., & Dunne, C. (2011). Psychosocial interventions for problem alcohol use in illicit drug users (Protocol). *Cochrane Database of Systematic Reviews, 7*(8), Article CD009269. https://doi.org/10.1002/14651858.CD009269

Preusse, M., Neuner, F., & Ertl, V. (2020). Effectiveness of psychosocial interventions targeting hazardous and harmful alcohol use and alcohol-related symptoms in low-and middle-income countries: A systematic review. *Frontiers in Psychiatry, 11*, 768. https://doi.org/10.3389/fpsyt.2020.00768

Skinner, H. A. (1982). The drug abuse screening test. *Addictive Behaviors, 7*(4), 363–371. https://doi.org/10.1016/0306-4603(82)90005-3

Webster, L. R., & Webster, R. M. (2005). Predicting aberrant behaviors in opioid-treated patients: Preliminary validation of the opioid risk tool. *Pain Medicine, 6*(6), 432–442. https://doi.org/10.1111/j.1526-4637.2005.00072.x

Wesson, D. R., & Ling, W. (2003). The Clinical Opiate Withdrawal Scale (COWS). *Journal of Psychoactive Drugs, 35*(2), 253–259. https://doi.org/10.1080/02791072.2003.10400007

White, W., Galanter, M., Humphreys, K., & Kelly, J. (2020). "We do recover": Scientific studies on Narcotics Anonymous. *Selected papers of William L. White*. https://www.chestnut.org/resources/d326b538-b4f5-4be8-a9d3-92976b686608/2020-Review-of-Scientific-Studies-on-NA.pdf

SPECIFIC SUBSTANCE USE DISORDERS

ALCOHOL USE DISORDER

DEFINITION

A. Alcohol use disorder (AUD) is a medical condition characterized by inability to limit and control one's intake of alcohol due to an emotional and physical dependence on alcohol.

B. Despite the adverse effects on physical, psychological, and social well-being, there is a continued pattern of misuse that is also associated with a number of other symptoms:
  1. A strong desire (urge/craving) to drink
  2. Experiencing symptoms of withdrawal (e.g., nausea, sweating, anxiety) when not drinking
  3. Spending a great deal of time to either obtain alcohol or manage symptoms related to recovering from the effects of alcohol use
  4. A clear sign of negligence with their chief responsibilities and obligations
  5. Hazardous use, posing a life risk (e.g., driving under the influence of alcohol)

C. Overall, a period of 12 months is required with a minimum of two symptoms to meet the diagnostic criteria.

D. Severity is based on the number of symptoms:
  1. Two to three symptoms: mild AUD
  2. Four to five symptoms: moderate AUD
  3. Six or more symptoms: severe AUD

16: SUBSTANCE USE DISORDERS

INCIDENCE
A. The prevalence of AUD continues to rise despite availability of interventions. One of the attributable reasons is the lack of screening in primary healthcare (Carvalho et al., 2019).
B. AUD is one of the most prevalent disorders on a global scale, especially among upper- and upper-middle-income countries.
   1. A study conducted on a nationally representative sample concluded that around 11.2% of the participants confirm alcohol use in their last 12-month history, of whom 29.9% were categorized as high-risk users and 49.4% were actually diagnosed with AUD per the *DSM-5* criteria (American Psychiatric Association, 2013; Grant et al., 2017).
   2. These data also compare alcohol consumption patterns among adults in the time periods: from 2001 to 2002 and from 2012 to 2013.
      a. Overall alcohol use went from 64.5% (2001–2002) to 72.7% (2012–2013).
      b. High-risk drinking went from 9.7% (2001–2002) to 12.6% (2012–2013).
      c. AUD went from 8.5% (2001–2002) to 12.7% (2012–2013).
   3. Another study underscores the increase in alcohol-attributable diseases by reporting a modeled projected morbidity and mortality rate from 2019 to 2040, which suggests an increase from 8.23/100,000 persons to 15.2/100,000 persons and an increase in attributable mortality from liver diseases of approximately 1,003,400 (Julien et al., 2020).

DIAGNOSTIC TESTS AND SCREENING
A. For patients presenting with suspected alcohol withdrawal, the following may inform diagnosis and treatment:
   1. Symptoms and observations
      a. Autonomic overactivity: Is there excessive sweating or a heart rate exceeding 100 beats per minute?
      b. Tremors: Have you noticed any shaking in your hands?
      c. Sleep disturbances: Are you experiencing difficulties with sleeping?
      d. Nausea and vomiting: Have you had any episodes of feeling sick or vomiting?
      e. Hallucinations or misinterpretations: Have you experienced any brief visual, tactile, or auditory disturbances?
      f. Restlessness or excessive movement: Do you feel restless or find yourself moving excessively?
      g. Emotional state: How would you describe your current level of anxiety or distress?
      h. Seizure history: Have you ever had a grand mal seizure in the past?
   2. Alcohol usage background
      a. Quantity: What amount of alcohol does the patient typically consume on a regular basis?
      b. Frequency: How often does the patient drink alcohol (e.g., daily, weekly)?
      c. Duration: How long has the patient been consuming alcohol?
      d. Last drink: When was the patient's most recent instance of alcohol consumption?
   3. Substance use beyond alcohol
      a. Do you consume any substances other than alcohol (e.g., illicit drugs or prescription medications)?
      b. When was your most recent use of these other substances?
   4. Social support
      a. Are there family members or friends who are aware of your situation and can offer support?
      b. Are you open to receiving assistance for your alcohol use disorder?

GENERAL TREATMENTS AND INTERVENTIONS
Pharmacologic Treatment
A. Treating withdrawal: In choosing to treat alcohol use withdrawal, always take into consideration the patient's preference, the patient's general health status, and the treatment setting (Table 16.1).
B. Promoting abstinence: Several medications are approved by the U.S. Food and Drug Administration (FDA) to support abstinence and recovery for patients after achieving medically assisted withdrawal (Table 16.2):
   1. Acamprosate (Campral) and naltrexone (Revia) reduce alcohol use and increase abstinence. Disulfiram (Antabuse) is a risk reduction agent due to the negative side effects when taken with alcohol.
   2. Topiramate (Topamax) and gabapentin (both anticonvulsants) may reduce alcohol ingestion, but this needs more studies. Antidepressants (sertraline and fluoxetine) treat depression, which might reduce alcohol use.
   3. Consider the following dosing strategies:
      a. Symptom-triggered strategy: benzodiazepines—monitor with the Clinical Institute Withdrawal Assessment for Alcohol–Revised (CIWA-Ar); patient receives medication when withdrawal symptoms are present
      b. Fixed dosing strategy: allows achievement and maintenance of the therapeutic level of medication in the patient

TABLE 16.1 BENZODIAZEPINES TO TREAT ALCOHOL USE WITHDRAWAL

Medication	Time to Onset/Elimination of Half-Life	Route of Administration	Initial Dose
Diazepam	20–25 hours/1–5 minutes IV	IV, PO	10–20 mg IV or PO
Chlordiazepoxide	24–48 hours/2–3 hours PO	PO	50–100 mg PO
Lorazepam	5–20 minutes IV/10–20 hours	IV, PO	2–4 mg IV or PO
Oxazepam	2–3 hours/3–21 hours	PO	15–30 mg PO

IV, intravenously; PO, orally.

TABLE 16.2 DRUGS USED TO SUPPORT ABSTINENCE AND RECOVERY IN ALCOHOL USE DISORDER

Medication	Mechanism of Action	Precautions	Side Effects	Dosing
Naltrexone Revia Vivitrol depot formulation	Opioid antagonist prevents endogenous and exogenous opioids from mu receptor binding.	Can precipitate withdrawals in persons with opioid dependence Not for those with acute hepatitis or hepatic failure or with an allergy to naltrexone	Sedation, nausea, and dizziness	Naltrexone 50 mg PO QD Vivitrol 380 mg IM every 4 weeks
Disulfiram Antabuse	Medication inhibits the enzyme that metabolizes acetaldehyde.	Contraindicated in patients with cerebrovascular accident, psychosis, allergy to disulfiram, or those taking metronidazole, amprenavir, ritonavir, and sertraline USE ONLY AS adjunct to support and psychotherapy.	Negative effects caused by buildup of acetaldehyde, which makes it therapeutic	500 mg PO or less QD for 1–2 weeks Maintenance 125 mg PO or 250 mg PO or 500 mg PO per day
Acamprosate (Campral)	Medication may increase GABA transmission, thereby suppressing excitatory glutamate neurotransmission.	Possible suicidality so use with precaution with persons with psychiatric diagnosis Allergy or renal impairment	Diarrhea, nausea, anxiety, and depression	Dispensed in 333 tablets 666 mg TID or 333 mg TID for patients with some renal impairment

GABA, gamma-aminobutyric acid; IM, intramuscularly; PO, orally; QD, once daily; TID, three times daily.
Source: Adapted from Marshall, B., & Spencer, J. (2019). *Fast facts about substance use disorders: What every nurse, APRN, and PA needs to know.* Springer Publishing Company.

c. Dosing: flat, fixed dosing, rather than body-sized dosing
d. Disposition: absorption, distribution, metabolism, and excretion (ADME)

Psychosocial Interventions for Alcohol Use Disorders

A. Klimas et al. (2011) concluded that valid and robust causal inference cannot be established due to lack of randomized controlled trials on reducing alcohol consumption.
B. Preusse et al. (2020) conducted a systemic review to understand the effectiveness of psychosocial interventions aimed at reducing alcohol consumption and recommended no intervention is superior to the other.
C. Nadkarni et al. (2023), using a meta review of psychological interventions for AUD, identified some common strategies.
   1. A range of interventions were studied, including MI, CBT, couples behavioral therapy, brief interventions, contingency management, family therapies, anonymous groups, 12-step facilitation, and community reinforcement therapies.
   2. It was concluded that the effectiveness of interventions was contingent upon the assessment strategies, utilization of personalized feedback, discussion about the assigned tasks, and problem-focused strategies, with a prime focus on relapse prevention and goal setting for future life ahead.
D. Alcoholics Anonymous (AA): AA is a peer-led support group that can help with AUD.
   1. Free to join, meets online and in person, and provides sponsorship to new members
   2. Abstinence-focused
   3. Cost-effective, with global presence
   4. With established efficacy when compared with other therapies, according to several studies, despite enormous criticism (Erickson, 2020)
   5. Based on 12 steps, which facilitate counseling
E. 12-Step facilitation therapy: The 12-step facilitation therapy focuses on personal spiritual journey, provides guidance on discovering oneself, and allows cooperation and support.
   1. The following are the 12 guiding principles: (a–b) personal acknowledgment of being powerless and that there is a presence of higher power; (c) willingness to submit oneself to higher power and to take guidance from superior power; (d–e) being truthful to self for past mistakes and taking responsibility for their wrongdoings due to alcohol; (f–g) willingness to improve, with the belief that a higher power will grant strength to overcome character shortcomings; (h–j) in this step, the follower is asked to jot down a list of harms that were caused and take responsible actions to undo harms directly if possible and their focus must remain on continued self-reflection; and (k–l) as a result of this spiritual awakening and actions, the person seeks solace through prayers and meditation and building a connection with higher power.
F. Family therapies: According to the SAMHSA (2020) SUD treatment and family therapy guide, family involvement in the treatment of alcohol disorder remains an instrumental intervention to attain recovery. Effective utilization of each intervention is based on individual needs, complexities, strengths, and willingness of the patient to involve their family.
   1. Family behavioral therapy (FBT): FBT focuses mainly on maladaptive behavioral patterns.
   2. Multidimensional family therapy (MDFT): MDFT is an integrative therapy with multiple aspects of family, community, peer, and other factors that affect an individual.
   3. Multisystems therapy (MST): MST is a very intensive therapy that focuses on multiple layers of the system that negatively impact on individual's life.
   4. Brief strategic family therapy (BSFT): BSFT is a time-limited structured therapy that mainly focuses on communication patterns.

G. Contingency management: Contingency management (CM) approaches are grounded on the principles of operant conditioning and focuses on anticipated outcomes by use of rewards and incentives to increase the likelihood of the desired behavior and decrease the likelihood of undesired behaviors.
  1. Techniques for CM:
     a. Use vouchers, behavioral monitoring, goal setting, and clear expectations to promote long-term recovery (Petry, 2011).
     b. A more recent feasibility study on CM has confirmed the efficacious use of automated reinforcement management system to prevent relapse or continuous use of alcohol (Miguel et al., 2023).

H. Alcohol behavioral couples therapy (ABCT): ABCT has its roots in CBT and behavioral couple therapy (BCT; McCrady et al., 2013).
  1. The prime focus of ABCT is to work on the communication pattern, the dynamics of the relationship that has been impacted by AUD, monitoring of alcohol and related drinking behaviors, and the required skills for the partner to improve and support relationship challenges.
  2. Both partners are engaged in therapy and the number of sessions ranges between 12 and 20.

I. CBT
J. MI

COMPLEMENTARY AND ALTERNATIVE MEDICINE IN ALCOHOL USE DISORDER

A. The burden of AUD is steadily increasing each year, prompting a shift toward holistic approaches that incorporate complementary and alternative medicine (CAM) into treatment and recovery management strategies.
  1. Recent literature highlights a growing interest in plant-based treatments for AUD among Ugandan populations, as evidenced by findings from posttreatment interviews (Maling et al., 2023).
  2. Additionally, the role of acupuncture as a CAM modality has been explored in individuals with AUD, demonstrating promising results compared with control groups. This warrants further investigation into its potential implications within the field, with the aim of establishing evidence-based interventions for treating AUD (Shin et al., 2017).
  3. The significance of CAM in addressing AUD is further emphasized by Swiss studies indicating that 25% of the treatment gap for AUD is filled by CAM modalities (Sylvain et al., 2022).

SPECIAL POPULATIONS

Prevalence of Alcohol Use Disorders in Older Adults

A. Older adults are those aged 50 years and older. AUD remains inadequately researched and managed within the older adult demographic. According to Joshi et al. (2021), there is a significant gap in understanding and addressing this issue among older adults. Oslin and Zanjani (2016) reported an estimate of 5.7 million older adults engage in unhealthy use of alcohol, indicating a pressing need for improved management.

B. Stigma and denial often prevent older adults from receiving the necessary evidence-based interventions for AUDs. Implementation of screening measures for older individuals is strongly recommended. Additionally, interventions such as Screening, Brief Intervention, and Referral to Treatment (SBIRT), along with involvement in support groups like AA, can be beneficial (Dibarloto & Jarosinski, 2017).

Prevalence of Alcohol Use Disorders in Youth

A. The use and misuse of alcohol among young individuals remains a significant area of concern.
  1. Brain development continues until early adulthood.
  2. Problematic drinking around this age can have detrimental effects on various aspects of brain development that are crucial to decision-making, planning, and executive function (Hill & O'Brien, 2015).

B. Genetic studies have also investigated families with AUD to understand the genetic contributions to AUD development in the offspring, with the aim of effectively incorporating this knowledge into the treatment of AUDs among youth (Hill & O'Brien, 2015).
  1. A national survey conducted by Ryan et al. (2019) on a sample of 45,000 students from 8th, 10th, and 12th grades revealed a significant decline in AUD prevalence in recent years, contrasting with the spiked trends observed in the 1990s. However, there has been a slight increase in binge drinking within the past 2 weeks, while binge drinking in the past 30 days has decreased.
  2. Studies have indicated that early initiation of drinking poses an equal risk factor for AUD development among African and European Americans, although differing risk factors leading to psychiatric comorbidities were identified between these racial groups. Furthermore, tobacco smoking and social anxiety were identified as common risk factors for alcohol initiation in both racial groups (Sartor et al., 2016).
  3. Another study highlighted subjective responses to alcohol and craving in the daily lives of youths, offering insights into AUD etiology, along with significant gender differences in experiencing AUD symptoms (Treloar & Miranda, 2017).

REFERRAL/RESOURCES

A. Crisis and Suicide Line: 9-8-8
B. National Institute on Alcohol Abuse and Alcoholism: www.niaaa.nih.gov/alcohols-effects-health/niaaa-middle-school/helpful-resources

INDIVIDUAL CONSIDERATIONS

Pregnancy

A. Research suggests that males are more likely to be diagnosed with AUD as compared with females, but this gap seems to be narrowing in recent times.

B. Alcohol addiction in females occurs at a faster rate than males (McCaul et al., 2019).
  1. Pregnant patients are less likely to use alcohol, but even a small amount can bring negative consequences (DeVido et al., 2015).
  2. AUD is one of the hazardous but avoidable conditions that can cause harm to pregnant patients and cognitive impairment to their fetus (Oei, 2020).
  3. One of the preventable neurodevelopmental disorders in children is fetal alcohol spectrum disorder (FASD), and in severe cases a syndrome known as *fetal alcoholic syndrome* (Erng et al., 2020).
  4. Treatment of AUD on special populations (e.g., pregnant women) is still restricted (Kelty et al., 2021).
     a. There are no robust data available that can confirm any safe amount of alcohol use among pregnant patients.
     b. According to Addila et al. (2020), African countries reported lack of education about the harmful effects on

the fetus, depression, unplanned pregnancy, partner's use of alcohol, and being unmarried as common risk factors for alcohol use among pregnant patients.

c. Literature also confirms that socioeconomic status, educational level, depression, and being ethnically Black are common risk factors that make them more prone to binge drinking during pregnancy (Shmulewitz & Hasin, 2019).

REFERENCES AND BIBLIOGRAPHY

American Psychiatric Association. (2013). *Diagnostic and statistical manual of mental disorders* (5th ed.). https://doi.org/10.1176/appi.books.9780890425596

DiBartolo, M. C., & Jarosinski, J. M. (2017). Alcohol use disorder in older adults: Challenges in assessment and treatment. *Issues in Mental Health Nursing, 38*(1), 25–32. https://doi.org/10.1080/01612840.2016.1257076

Han, B., Gfroerer, J. C., Colliver, J. D., & Penne, M. A. (2009). Substance use disorder among older adults in the United States in 2020. *Addiction, 104*(1), 88–96. https://doi.org/10.1111/j.1360-0443.2008.02411.x

Hill, S. Y., & O'Brien, J. (2015). Psychological and neurobiological precursors of alcohol use disorders in high-risk youth. *Current Addiction Reports, 2*(2), 104–113. https://doi.org/10.1007/s40429-015-0051-1

Joshi, P., Duong, K. T., Trevisan, L. A., & Wilkins, K. M. (2021). Evaluation and management of alcohol use disorder among older adults. *Current Geriatrics Reports,* 1–9. https://doi.org/10.1007/s13670-021-00359-5

Klimas, J., Field, C. A., Cullen, W., O'Gorman, C. S., Glynn, L. G., Keenan, E., Saunders, J. A., Bury, G., & Dunne, C. (2011). Psychosocial interventions for problem alcohol use in illicit drug users (Protocol). *Cochrane Database of Systematic Reviews, 7*(8). https://doi.org/10.1002/14651858.CD009269

Maling, S., Kabakyenga, J., Muchunguzi, C., Olet, E. A., & Alele, P. E. (2023). Treatment outcomes of alcohol use disorder by traditional medicine practitioners using plant derivatives in southwestern Uganda: Findings from in-depth interviews. *Frontiers in Psychiatry, 14,* 1185108. https://doi.org/10.3389/fpsyt.2023.1185108

McCrady, B. S., Owens, M. D., & Brovko, J. M. (2013). Couples and family treatment methods. In B. S. McCrady & E. E. Epstein (Eds.), *Addictions: A comprehensive guidebook* (2nd ed., 454–481). Oxford University Press.

Miguel, A. Q., Smith, C. L., Rodin, N. M., Johnson, R. K., McDonell, M. G., & McPherson, S. M. (2023, March). Automated Reinforcement Management System: Feasibility study findings of an app-based contingency management treatment for alcohol use disorder. *Drug and Alcohol Dependence Reports, 6,* 1–5. https://doi.org/10.1016/j.dadr.2023.100140

Nadkarni, A., Massazza, A., Guda, R., Fernandes, L. T., Garg, A., Jolly, M., Andersen, L. S., Bhatia, U., Bogdanov, S., Roberts, B., Tol, W. A., Velleman, R., Moore, Q., & Fuhr, D. (2023, January). Common strategies in empirically supported psychological interventions for alcohol use disorders: A meta-review. *Drug and Alcohol Review, 42*(1), 94–104. https://doi.org/10.1111/dar.13550

Oslin, D. W., & Zanjani, F. (2016). Treatment of unhealthy alcohol use in older adults. In A. Kuerbis, A. Moore, P. Sacco, & F. Zanjani (Eds.), *Alcohol and aging: Clinical and public health perspectives*. Springer Cham. https://doi.org/10.1007/978-3-319-47233-1_12

Petry, N. (2011). *Contingency management for substance abuse treatment*. Routledge.

Ryan, S. A., Kokotailo, P., Camenga, D. R., Patrick, S. W., Plumb, J., Quigley, J., & Walker-Harding, L. (2019). Alcohol use by youth. *Pediatrics, 144*(1). https://doi.org/10.1542/peds.2019-1357

Sartor, C. E., Jackson, K. M., McCutcheon, V. V., Duncan, A. E., Grant, J. D., Werner, K. B., & Bucholz, K. K. (2016). Progression from first drink, first intoxication, and regular drinking to alcohol use disorder: A comparison of African American and European American youth. *Alcoholism: Clinical and Experimental Research, 40*(7), 1515–1523. https://doi.org/10.1111/acer.13113

Shin, N. Y., Lim, Y. J., Yang, C. H., & Kim, C. (2017). Acupuncture for alcohol use disorder: A meta-analysis. *Evidence-Based Complementary and Alternative Medicine, 2017*(1), 7823278. https://doi.org/10.1155/2017/7823278

Substance Abuse and Mental Health Services Administration. (2020). *Substance use disorder treatment and family therapy: Treatment improvement protocol tip 39*. https://store.samhsa.gov/sites/default/files/tip-39-treatment-family-therapy-pep20-02-02-012.pdf

Sylvain, B., Barbara, B., Jean-Michel, G., & Thierry, F. C. (2022). Complementary and alternative medicines in patients with alcohol or tobacco use disorder: Use, expectations and beliefs. *European Journal of Integrative Medicine, 51,* 102115. https://doi.org/10.1016/j.eujim.2022.102115

Treloar, H., & Miranda, R., Jr. (2017). Craving and acute effects of alcohol in youths' daily lives: Associations with alcohol use disorder severity. *Experimental and Clinical Psychopharmacology, 25*(4), 303–313. https://doi.org/10.1037/pha0000133

CANNABIS USE DISORDER AND HALLUCINOGEN USE DISORDER

DEFINITION

A. A diagnosis of cannabis use disorder (CUD) and hallucinogen use disorder (HUD) indicates an inability to stop using these substances despite experiencing health, legal, or social problems. As with the other SUDs, the criteria for CUD and HUD are examined and the level of disorder (mild, moderate, severe) is identified by the number of criteria met.

B. Cannabis continues to become legalized for recreational use in many states, but as of 2024 it remains illegal at the federal level. Both cannabis and a number of hallucinogens (3, 4-methylenedioxy-methamphetamine [MDMA] for posttraumatic stress disorder [PTSD]), psilocybin and ayahuasca for depression or substance use, ibogaine for opioid use disorder) are used for medical interventions.

  1. Crossfade: This occurs when alcohol and cannabis are used together. This increases impairment from the alcohol as well as increases the tetrahydrocannabinol (THC) absorption in the body.

  2. Dabs or cannabis concentrates: Dabs can contain 40% to 90% THC, which is four times higher than THC in cannabis.

  3. Synthetic cannabinoids, cannabis alternatives: These are marketed as less expensive; cannabis alternatives (e.g., K2, Spice) can be life-threatening.

  4. Lacing: Lacing is putting a second or third drug into the primary drug, potentiating the psychotropic effects. Lacing can result in a need for ED treatment.

  a. Signs and symptoms of lacing with cannabis: nausea and vomiting, diarrhea, blood pressure and heart rate changes, derealization, dyspnea, and psychosis

  b. When combined with an opiate: extreme lethargy, confusion, respiratory depression, and bradycardia

C. Hallucinogens:

  1. Common hallucinogens include ketamine, psilocybin (mushrooms), ecstasy (MDMA), and lysergic acid diethylamide (LSD); LSD has the greatest likelihood of long-term damage.

  2. Street names for hallucinogens include blotter, acid, fry, cubes, mind candy, shrooms or mushrooms, special K, X, STP, and XTC.

PREVALENCE

A. Cannabis: Cannabis is the most common drug used in the United States, used by about 18% of American Adults. Of those who use cannabis, about 3% to 4% of 12- to 17-year-olds and 1.5% of those over 18 years of age have CUD. CUD is higher in persons who use cannabis recreationally or for both recreational and nonmedical use. The prevalence of CUD has increased with cannabis legalization (Lapham et al., 2023).

ED visits in states with legalized cannabis use have seen an increase of 54% and hospitalization up by 101%. The National Center for Drug Abuse statistics also reports increased evidence of cannabis in persons who died by suicide, increasing from 7.6% (2006) to 23% (2017).

B. Hallucinogens: 1 in 12, or 8%, 19- to 30-year-olds have reported hallucinogen use (MDMA, mescaline, peyote, psilocybin, LSD, or phencyclidine [PCP]). 1 in 10, or 11%, college students take hallucinogens. It is considered that legalization of cannabis has been a factor in the increase of hallucinogen use (Newport Institute, 2023).

SIGNS AND SYMPTOMS

A. Symptoms of cannabis intoxication:
 1. Euphoria, increased appetite, impaired memory and concentration, relaxation, amotivation
 2. Occasionally, anxiety, panic, and psychosis

B. Symptoms of cannabis withdrawal syndrome:
 1. Start in the first week of abstinence and resolve in a few weeks
 2. Dysphoria, anxiety, depression, restlessness, and irritability
 3. Gastrointestinal (GI) symptoms including nausea and vomiting and decreased appetite

C. Symptoms of hallucinogen intoxication:
 1. Changes in mood, hallucinations, and detachment/dissociation
 2. Anxiety, panic, and transitory psychosis
 3. Persistent psychosis
 4. Suicidal ideation
 5. Hallucinogen persisting perception disorder (HPPD): hallucinations persisting anywhere from days to years, disrupting activities of daily living

GENERAL TREATMENTS AND INTERVENTIONS

A. There are no FDA-approved medications for the treatment of CUD or HUD; clinicians will treat the presenting symptoms.

B. Treatment of HUD: PCP and ketamine are considered substances that can cause dependence. LSD can be less effective for those who use it frequently, indicating that the person develops tolerance. Treatment for HUD is scarce, as are treatment programs that specialize in HUD. Often, patients can be treated in programs focused on co-occurring disorders.

C. Nonpharmacologic treatments include the following (Gates et al., 2016):
 1. Therapy: CBT
 2. MI
 3. CM

INDIVIDUAL CONSIDERATIONS

Pregnancy

A. Cannabis use in pregnancy can result in low birth weight, and is also associated with other adverse birth outcomes such as increased risk of stillbirth, preterm delivery, and long-term brain development issues, resulting in memory, learning, and behavior problems. THC does pass into breastmilk.

B. Use of psychotropic drugs increases the likelihood of neurodevelopmental disorders in children, such as Down syndrome and autism spectrum disorder.

Pediatrics

A. Use of hallucinogens by youth is associated with mental health, impulsivity, and addictive problems.

Older Adults

A. Cannabis use by persons with polypharmacy can interfere with the actions of the prescribed medications or exacerbate other chronic conditions.

REFERENCES AND BIBLIOGRAPHY

Addila, A. E., Bisetegn, T. A., Gete, Y. K., Mengistu, M. Y., & Beyene, G. M. (2020). Alcohol consumption and its associated factors among pregnant women in Sub-Saharan Africa: A systematic review and meta-analysis' as given in the submission system. *Substance Abuse Treatment, Prevention, and Policy, 15*(1), 1–14. https://doi.org/10.1186/s13011-020-00269-3

Bogenschutz, M. P., & Johnson, M. W. (2016). Classic hallucinogens in the treatment of addictions. *Progress in Neuro-Psychopharmacology and Biological Psychiatry, 64*, 250–258. https://doi.org/10.1016/j.pnpbp.2015.03.002

Carvalho, A. F., Heilig, M., Perez, A., Probst, C., & Rehm, J. (2019). Alcohol use disorders. *Lancet, 394*(10200), 781–792. https://doi.org/10.1016/S0140-6736(19)31775-1

Erng, M. N., Smirnov, A., & Reid, N. (2020). Prevention of alcohol-exposed pregnancies and fetal alcohol spectrum disorder among pregnant and postpartum women: a systematic review. *Alcoholism Clinical and Experimental Research, 44*(12), 2431–2448. https://doi.org/10.1111/acer.14489

DeVido, J., Bogunovic, O., & Weiss, R. D. (2015). Alcohol use disorders in pregnancy. *Harvard Review of Psychiatry, 23*(2), 112–121. https://doi.org/10.1097/HRP.0000000000000070

Gates, P. J., Sabioni, P., Copeland, J., Le Foll, B., & Gowing, L. (2016). Psychosocial interventions for cannabis use disorder. *Cochrane Database of Systematic Reviews, 5*, Article CD005336. https://doi.org/10.1002/14651858.CD005336.pub4

Grant, B. F., Chou, S. P., Saha, T. D., Pickering, R. P., Kerridge, B. T., Ruan, W. J., Huang B., Jung J., Zhang H., Fan, A., & Hasin, D. S. (2017). Prevalence of 12-month alcohol use, high-risk drinking, and *DSM-IV* alcohol use disorder in the United States, 2001–2002 to 2012–2013: Results from the national epidemiologic survey on alcohol and related conditions. *JAMA Psychiatry, 74*(9), 911–923. https://doi.org/10.1001/jamapsychiatry.2017.2161

Julien, J., Ayer, T., Bethea, E. D., Tapper, E. B., & Chhatwal, J. (2020). Projected prevalence and mortality associated with alcohol-related liver disease in the USA, 2019–40: A modelling study. *The Lancet Public Health, 5*(6), e316–e323. https://doi.org/10.1016/S2468-2667(20)30062-1

Karnieg, T., & Wang, X. (2018). Cytisine for smoking cessation. *Canadian Medical Association Journal, 190*(19), E596. https://doi.org/10.1503/cmaj.171371

Kelty, E., Terplan, M., Greenland, M., & Preen, D. (2021). Pharmacotherapies for the treatment of alcohol use disorders during pregnancy: Time to reconsider? *Drugs, 81*(7), 739–748. https://doi.org/10.1007/s40265-021-01509-x

Lapham, G. T., Matson, T. E., Bobb, J. F., Luce, C., Oliver, M. M., Hamilton, L. K., & Bradley, K. A. (2023). Prevalence of cannabis use disorder and reasons for use among Adults in a US state where recreational cannabis use is legal. *JAMA Network Open, 6*(8), e2328934. https://doi.org/10.1001/jamanetworkopen.2023.28934

McCaul, M. E., Roach, D., Hasin, D. S., Weisner, C., Chang, G., & Sinha, R. (2019). Alcohol and women: A brief overview. *Alcoholism, Clinical and Experimental Research, 43*(5), 774–779. https://doi.org/10.1111/acer.13985

Newport Institute. (2023). *Hallucinogen use in young adults: New stats and research.* https://www.newportinstitute.com/resources/co-occurring-disorders/young-adult-hallucinogen-use

Oei, J. L. (2020). Alcohol use in pregnancy and its impact on the mother and child. *Addiction, 115*(11), 2148–2163. https://doi.org/10.1111/add.15036

Shmulewitz, D., & Hasin, D. S. (2019). Risk factors for alcohol use among pregnant women, ages 15–44, in the United States, 2002 to 2017. *Preventive Medicine, 124*, 75–83. https://doi.org/10.1016/j.ypmed.2019.04.027

Trivedi, M., Walker, R. Ling, W., Dela Cruz, A., Sharma, G., Carmody, T., Ghitza, U. E., Wahle, A., Kim, M., Shores-Wilson, K., Sparenborg, S., Coffin, P., Schmitz, J., Wiest, K., Bart, G., Sonne, S. C., Wakhlu, S., Rush, A. J., Nunes, E. V., & Shoptaw, S.(2021) Bupropion and naltrexone in methamphetamine use disorder. *The New England Journal of Medicine, 384*(2), 140–151. https://doi.org/10.1056/NEJMoa2020214

UT Southwestern Medical Center. (2023, December 7). *UTSW-led studies are largest ever for stimulant use disorders*. https://www.utsouthwestern.edu/newsroom/articles/year-2023/dec-stimulant-use-disorders.html

Weinstein, A. M., & Gorelick, D. A. (2011). Pharmacological treatment of cannabis dependence. *Current Pharmaceutical Design*, 17(14), 1351–1358. https://doi.org/10.2174/138161211796150846

OPIOID USE DISORDER

DEFINITION
A. Opioid use disorder (OUD) is a medical disorder characterized by the patient experiencing physical and psychological reliance on opioids, which are class 1 prescription drugs. It is the chronic, patterned use of this class of drugs that causes a significant level of distress and impairment in the patient, resulting in the diagnosis of OUD.
B. Specific criteria make up the diagnostic requirement for "harmful pattern of use of opioids" and are listed in the *International Classification of Diseases*, 11th Revision (*ICD-11*; WHO, 2019). These include but are not limited to a pattern that exists for at least 12 months of episodic drug use or monthly when usage is daily or almost daily; health being harmed due to intoxicated behavior; toxic effects on body systems or organs resulting from intoxication or administering the drug through a harmful route; and the inability to cut down on or control usage, despite multiple attempts, resulting in impairments in school, work, or other social domains.
C. Drugs included in this disorder are morphine, oxycodone, hydrocodone, heroin, fentanyl, tramadol, and other similar substances.
  1. Compounds from the poppy plant and also semisynthetic and synthetic compounds
  2. Analgesics and sedatives
  3. Used medicinally for treatment and management of pain
D. Overdose deaths due to opioids result from respiratory arrest. The United States has the highest drug death rate in the world.

INCIDENCE
A. 16 million people worldwide have an opioid dependence.
B. Over 2.1 million people have an opioid dependence in the United States. 80% of first-time heroin users started with misuse of opioids that were prescribed (Marshall & Spencer, 2019).
C. Adolescent use in 2016:
  1. 276,000 had misused pain relievers, with 122,000 meeting the criteria for addiction.
  2. 21,000 had used heroin.
  3. Users between 1999 and 2016 quadrupled.
  4. Prescriptions for benzodiazepines rose by 67% between the 1990s and 2013.
D. Almost 100,000 people (98,268) died from drug overdoses in the United States in 2021.
  1. 7 of 10 preventable opioid overdoses are in males, but the rise in preventable overdoses is rising faster in females (NSC, 2024).
  2. During the pandemic, there was a 41% increase in opioid overdose deaths.
  3. 71% of opioid deaths occur in the 25- to 54-year-old range, but the number of overdose deaths in those 55+ is rapidly increasing.
E. Fentanyl is linked to the large increase in overdose deaths.

SIGNS AND SYMPTOMS
A. Objective signs of opioid intoxication and toxicity include the following:
  1. Decreased respiratory rate is the most notable vital sign abnormality in opioid intoxication and may be the best objective sign to make the diagnosis.
  2. Sedation/impaired mental status is also a sign of opioid intoxication.
  3. Patient reports decreased bowel sounds.
  4. Miosis: Normal pupil size should not rule out a diagnosis of opioid toxicity. Ingestion of meperidine (Demerol) may result in normal pupil size, and ingestion of some sympathomimetics (e.g., amphetamine, cocaine, and ephedrine) as well as some anticholinergic medications makes make pupil size appear normal or large.
B. Signs of opioid withdrawal can begin hours after the last dose.
  1. Symptoms are psychological, emotional, and physiologic.
  2. Withdrawal symptoms are consistent with dependence level.
  3. Signs and symptoms include the following:
     a. Muscle aches
     b. Excessive yawning
     c. Tremors, goosebumps, sweating
     d. Tachycardia, insomnia
     e. Cramping, abdominal pain, vomiting, diarrhea, nausea
     f. Anxiety, discontent, annoyances, short-tempered, restless
C. Patients with OUD in the ED:
  1. Five-point strategy from the U.S. Department of Health and Human Services:
     a. Improve access to recovery services and treatments.
     b. Promote overdose-reversing drugs (Narcan).
     c. Increase public health surveillance and provide support.
     d. Increase research on treating pain and SUDs.
     e. Educate on better pain management practices.
  2. Clinical Opiate Withdrawal Scale (COWS; https://nida.nih.gov/sites/default/files/ClinicalOpiateWithdrawalScale.pdf)
     a. Assesses the common symptoms of withdrawal, with rating from less than 5, *no withdrawal*; 5 to 12, *mild withdrawal*; 13 to 24, *moderate withdrawal*; 25 to 36, *moderate/severe withdrawal*; and greater than 36, *severe*.

DIAGNOSTIC TESTS AND SCREENING
A. Laboratory tests include the following:
  1. Comprehensive metabolic panel
  2. Hepatic function
  3. Complete blood count
  4. Viral hepatitis
  5. Tuberculin skin test (patients have been incarcerated or other risk factors)
  6. Sexually transmitted infections (STIs; for patients at risk)
  7. Drug screening
     a. Urine drug screen (UDS) including fentanyl and buprenorphine; immunoassay test—less accurate
     b. Confirmatory testing—slower, more expensive, more accurate, uses gas chromatography mass spectrometry, used to test questionable UDS results or to verify positive UDS results

B. There are a range of screening tools available to screen for OUD in adult populations of both sexes. These include the following:

 1. Opioid Risk Tool (ORT): ORT was developed by Webster et al. (2005) and is useful in assessing the risk of opioid use among pain-free population. This tool is used in primary care settings and it takes only a minute to administer. A score of 3 or less indicates *low/no risk*, a score of 4 to 7 indicates *moderate risk*, and a score of 8 or higher indicates *higher risk*.
 2. COWS: COWS is mainly used to assess physical dependency on opioids and is used by physicians in outpatient treatment as well as resident patients. It is an 11-item scale that assesses the following: (a) resting pulse rate, (b) GI upset, (c) sweating, (d) tremors, (e) restlessness, (f) yawning, (g) pupil size, (h) anxiety/irritability, (i) bone or joint aches, (j) gooseflesh skin, and (k) running nose and tearing. A score of 5 to 12 indicates mild dependency, 13 to 24 moderate, 25 to 36 moderately severe, and more than 36 severe withdrawal.
 3. Drug Abuse Screening Test (DAST): DAST is a 10-item subjective reporting tool with scores ranging from 0 to 10. It takes only 5 minutes to administer. A score of 0 indicates no reported problems, 1 to 2 low-level problems, 3 to 5, moderate-level problems, 6 to 8 substantial-level problems, and 9 to 10 severe-level problems associated with drug abuse.

GENERAL TREATMENTS AND INTERVENTIONS

Pharmacologic Treatment

A. Key terminology:
 1. Opium: refers to the compound that occurs naturally in the opium poppy, including morphine and codeine
 2. Opioid: any drug, whether natural or synthetic, that acts at any or all three opioid receptors
 3. Opiate: a more specific term referring to a subclass of opioids that contain compounds that occur naturally in the opium poppy
 4. Synthetic/semisynthetic opioid: drugs that contain substances not naturally occurring but having the effect related to the naturally occurring compounds in opiates
 5. Heroin: an opioid processed from morphine, a naturally occurring substance derived from the opium poppy
 6. Endorphins: naturally occurring endogenous peptides that have opioid-like properties, including enkephalins and dynorphins

B. Full opioid agonists include the following:
 1. Morphine
 2. Heroin
 3. Fentanyl
 4. Meperidine
 5. Methadone
 6. Hydromorphone
 7. Oxymorphone
 8. Codeine
 9. Oxycodone
 10. Hydrocodone

C. Opioid agonist–antagonists include the following:
 1. Buprenorphine
 2. Butorphanol
 3. Nalbuphine
 4. Pentazocine

D. Opioid antagonists include the following:
 1. Naloxone
 2. Naltrexone

Clinical Management of Opioid Overdose

A. Airway management
 1. In community settings, rescue ventilations, using mouth barriers when available
 2. Endotracheal tube and bag-mask ventilation with supplemental oxygen

B. Emergency naloxone
 1. In emergencies, administer naloxone, preferably intravenously (IV) for rapid onset, but it may also be administered by the intranasal, subcutaneous (SubQ), or intramuscular (IM) route in a setting where IV naloxone is not available or when the establishment of IV access is delayed.
    a. Adult dosing of naloxone (IV, IM, SubQ): Naloxone is administered initially at 0.4 to 2.0 mg, repeating at 2- to 3-minute intervals until the desired improvement in respiratory function is obtained. If after 10 mg of naloxone is administered and the desired response has not been attained, the diagnosis of opioid toxicity should be reevaluated and an alternative etiology should be considered.
    b. Due to the short half-life of naloxone, repeat doses may need to be administered after 20 to 60 minutes, depending on the duration of the opioid.

Medically Assisted Opioid Withdrawal ("Detox")

A. Withdrawal management using buprenorphine
 1. Although not specifically FDA-approved for this purpose, buprenorphine is an effective opioid agonist for treatment and management of opioid detoxification.
 2. The initiation of buprenorphine for withdrawal follows the same procedure as the initiation (or induction) procedure for maintenance treatment (Table 16.3).
 3. Once withdrawal symptoms are stabilized (usually on 4–16 mg of buprenorphine), the dose can be tapered in decrements of 2 to 4 mg daily. The duration of the taper is individualized based on clinical circumstances, with a duration anywhere from 3 to 30 days.

B. Withdrawal management using methadone
 1. Medically assisted withdrawal using methadone is best accomplished in an inpatient or outpatient setting.
 2. As with buprenorphine, there are many approaches to dosing and tapering. Per the American Society of Addiction Medicine (ASAM) guidelines, the initiation of methadone begins in the range of 20 to 30 mg.

TABLE 16.3 INITIATION OF BUPRENORPHINE FOR OPIOID WITHDRAWAL

	Day 1: Induction	Day 2: Induction	Days 3–7: Stabilization
Buprenorphine[a]	Start with 2 mg or 4 mg, titrate upwards in 2-hour intervals to 8 mg.	A single dose of 16 mg is recommended.	Adjust in increments/decrements of 4 mg or 2 mg.

[a]The buprenorphine/naloxone combination product may be used for induction, keeping the equivalent buprenorphine doses the same based on sublingual Subutex equivalents. Dosage forms will vary for Zubsolv sublingual tablet and Bunavail buccal film. Consult prescribing information for guidance on induction.

3. Once the patient is stabilized, the taper can begin as early as day 2 and is often completed in 6 to 10 days.
4. A brief approach is to taper in decrements of 5 mg/d, assuming a 30-mg starting dose, which can be completed fairly quickly.
5. As with buprenorphine, the tapering schedule should be individualized and adapted to clinical circumstances, such as patient motivation and risk for relapse if tapered too quickly.
6. As the taper progresses, the patient may experience uncomfortable withdrawal symptoms, which may be treated with clonidine and other adjunctive symptom-targeting medications.
7. If the ultimate goal is remission of opioid use, then medically assisted withdrawal alone is not an effective means of achieving that end. For better outcomes, medically assisted withdrawal should generally be used with a treatment plan that includes medication-assisted maintenance and psychosocial treatments.

C. Withdrawal management using nonopioid agents
1. Many unpleasant symptoms of opioid withdrawal result from hyperactivity of the noradrenergic system when opioids are abruptly stopped.
2. The centrally acting alpha-2 adrenergic agonist clonidine (Catapres) has long been used off-label to manage these symptoms.
3. When clonidine is active at alpha-2 adrenergic receptor, the sudden release of norepinephrine is inhibited. This slowing of norepinephrine release helps ameliorate autonomic symptoms such as diaphoresis, "restless legs," GI upset, anxiety, and irritability.
4. The following is a typical clonidine initiation and tapering scheme:
   a. Day 1: If blood pressure is at least 90/60 mmHg and heart rate is at least 60 beats per minute, administer a test dose of clonidine 0.1 mg orally. Reassess after 45 minutes if withdrawal symptoms present (COWS score of greater than 8) and blood pressure and pulse remain within parameters. Administer 0.1 mg every 45 to 60 minutes up to four doses (0.4 mg). Reassess COWS score, blood pressure, and heart rate every 6 hours. For COWS score of 8 to 12, administer 0.1 mg. For COWS score of 12 or higher, administer 0.2 mg; the maximum daily dose is generally 0.8 to 1.2 mg.
   b. Days 2 to 4: Calculate total clonidine dose from day 1 and schedule in equal divided dose three to four times per day through day 4.
   c. Day 5+: Taper in decrements of 0.1 to 0.2 mg/d.
5. Symptom-triggered adjunctive treatments include the following:
   a. Restlessness, anxiety: diphenhydramine, hydroxyzine
   b. Myalgias and arthralgias: nonsteroidal anti-inflammatory drugs (NSAIDs) as tolerated, acetaminophen
   c. Nausea and vomiting: ondansetron, promethazine, prochlorperazine
   d. Diarrhea: loperamide
   e. Abdominal cramping: dicyclomine
   f. Insomnia: trazodone, diphenhydramine, doxepin

Maintenance Treatment
A. Medication-assisted treatment (MAT)
1. The FDA-approved medications for maintenance treatment of OUD are buprenorphine, methadone, and naltrexone.
2. Along with psychosocial interventions in a holistic approach to care, MAT helps support individual recovery.
3. There is no specific time when the medication should be withdrawn. These medications may be taken for months and years, consistent with the standard of care in other chronic medical and psychiatric conditions.
4. Maintenance medications, when used properly and under medical supervision at a safe dose, can help an individual overcome use of an abused opioid, as well as the physical, relational, financial, and legal risks associated with illicit opioid use.
5. See Table 16.4 for treatment selection.

TABLE 16.4 MAINTENANCE MEDICATIONS FOR OPIOID USE DISORDER

	Naltrexone	Buprenorphine	Methadone
Mechanism of action	Opioid receptor antagonist Helps maintain abstinence by blocking mu opioid receptors, thus preventing exogenous opioids from binding at the receptor site, blunting the euphoric and rewarding effects of opioids	Opioid receptor partial agonist Reduces opioid withdrawal symptoms and cravings, diminishes the euphoric and rewarding effects of illicit opioids by cross-tolerance	Opioid receptor full agonist Reduces opioid withdrawal and cravings, diminishes the euphoric and rewarding effects of illicit opioids by cross tolerance
Potentially appropriate patients	• Highly motivated patients • Patients with mild opioid dependence • Patients whose professions prohibit treatment with an opioid agonist • Patients who have already been medically detoxified in a controlled environment (hospitals, correctional facilities)	• Pregnant patients • Patients with prior positive response to buprenorphine • Patients who have demonstrated responsible use and are appropriate for office-based treatment • Patients who do not live close to an OTP • Patients for whom the side effects and drug interactions of methadone are problematic	• Pregnant patients • Patients with prior positive response to methadone • Patients who are appropriate for opioid agonist treatment who cannot afford buprenorphine products • Patients who may benefit from a highly structured outpatient program with supervision of proper use and adherence

OTP, opioid treatment program.

B. Maintenance treatment using buprenorphine/naloxone
1. Buprenorphine, when administered to an opioid-dependent individual, can alleviate the cravings and uncomfortable withdrawal symptoms associated with the discontinuation of full opioid agonists such as heroin, prescription pain medication, and methadone.
2. Because buprenorphine is a partial agonist, it has moderate *intrinsic activity*, meaning that the degree of activation at the mu opioid receptor is not as strong as that of a full agonist. Its lower intrinsic activity produces a *ceiling effect*, meaning that increased doses do not produce an additional effect, thus reducing the potential for abuse and rendering it safer in overdose.
3. What makes buprenorphine unique is that it works as an agonist–antagonist at the mu receptor. In other words, buprenorphine, when active at the mu receptor, partially activates the receptor to the degree that it assuages the effects of opioid withdrawal.
4. It also has a high receptor affinity, meaning that the strength of the bond between buprenorphine and the mu receptor is strong.
5. Buprenorphine's antagonist effects can block the effects of full agonists and can even displace opioids with lower receptor affinity. Thus, administering buprenorphine while a full agonist is active at the receptor can precipitate a withdrawal syndrome.
6. Most buprenorphine products for opioid dependence include naloxone, which when administered by transmucosal route (sublingual, buccal) is absorbed only minimally. The naloxone in the combination buprenorphine/naloxone product is intended as an abuse deterrent because if the product is dissolved and injected, naloxone as an opioid antagonist can precipitate withdrawal.
7. High receptor affinity is also associated with slow *dissociation* (or uncoupling rate) from the mu receptor, resulting in a longer duration of action and reduction in the severity of withdrawal symptoms, making it useful in tapering during opioid detoxification.
8. Buprenorphine/naloxone is available in various transmucosal formulations (Table 16.5), as well as in a buprenorphine-only monthly subcutaneous injection (Sublocade) and in a 6-month subdermal implant (Probuphine).
9. It is available for outpatient office-based treatment without having to present daily at a clinic as with methadone program.

C. Maintenance treatment using methadone
1. Methadone is a long-acting synthetic opioid full agonist that when active at the mu opioid receptor reduces withdrawal effects from opioid abstinence, reduces craving, and blunts the euphoric effects of illicit opioid use.
2. Half-life varies widely from patient to patient, ranging from 8 to 59 hours, with an average of 24 hours.
3. It is the oldest, most frequently used, and most extensively studied medication for OUD worldwide. Methadone has a track record of proven efficacy, and some studies suggest that methadone when used clinically has reduced rates of mortality, HIV seroconversion, and in some studies criminal behavior.

TABLE 16.5 BUPRENORPHINE DELIVERY FORMULATIONS

Product	Route of Administration	Available Dosages
Subutex[a] (buprenorphine) and generic equivalents	Sublingual tablet	2 mg/8 mg
Suboxone[a] (buprenorphine/naloxone) and generic equivalents	Sublingual tablet	2 mg/0.5 mg 8 mg/2 mg
Suboxone (buprenorphine/naloxone)	Sublingual film	2 mg/0.5 mg 4 mg/1 mg 8 mg/2 mg 12 mg/3 mg
Zubsolv (buprenorphine/naloxone)	Sublingual tablet	0.7 mg/0.18 mg 1.4 mg/0.36 mg 2.9 mg/0.71 mg 5.7 mg/1.4 mg 8.6 mg/2.1 mg 11.4 mg/2.9 mg
Bunavail (buprenorphine/naloxone)	Buccal film	2.1 mg/0.3 mg 4.2 mg/0.7 mg 6.3 mg/1 mg
Sublocade	Subcutaneous monthly injection	100 mg/0.5 mL 300 mg/1.5 mL
Brixadi weekly injection	Subcutaneous	8 mg/0.16 mL 16 mg/0.32 mL 34 mg/0.48 mL 32 mg/0.64 mL
Brixadi monthly injection	Subcutaneous	64 mg/0.18 mL 96 mg/0.27 mL 128 mg/0.36 mL

[a]Subutex and Suboxone sublingual tablets have been discontinued in the United States in favor of Suboxone sublingual film.

4. It is regulated as a Schedule II drug in the United States and must be administered by a licensed opioid treatment program (OTP). OTPs must provide adequate medical and psychosocial services either on-site or by referral.
5. It is a proven and reliable MAT for OUD and continues to provide risk reduction and lifesaving benefits to individuals living with OUD. It does have some notable drug class-related side effects, such as sedation, dizziness, diaphoresis, constipation, and sexual dysfunction in men.
6. Some of the potential serious adverse effects of methadone include QTc prolongation and risk of arrhythmias, as well as overdose. (Methadone is a full opioid agonist with no ceiling effect as with buprenorphine.)
7. Multiple drug interactions can occur due to metabolism by CYP450, particularly the isoenzyme 3A4 (some antibiotics, antidepressants, anticonvulsants, antifungals, and antiretrovirals).
8. It is available in a liquid concentrate formulation diluted in juice or water and also in a dispersible tablet.
9. Dosing is individualized and is reliant on the rate of metabolism, individual degree of tolerance to opioids, and overall health.
10. For opioid-tolerant patients, the initial methadone dose is typically 10 to 30 mg. After the first dose, patients should be monitored for 2 to 4 hours for sedation or withdrawal relief. If symptoms improve, they should return the next day for reassessment and possible dose adjustment. Methadone serum levels rise daily until reaching a steady state. Patients experiencing withdrawal relief 4 to 12 hours after dosing may benefit from maintaining the same dose for a few days to stabilize serum levels (SAMHSA, 2021). ASAM recommends dose increases of 5 mg or less every 5 days (Baxter et al., 2013, as cited in SAMHSA, 2021, pp. 3–30), while others suggest 5 to 10 mg every 3 to 4 days (Farrell & Lintzeris, 2014, as cited in SAMHSA, 2021, pp. 3–30).
11. Box 16.1 summarizes some of the basic tenets of methadone dosing.

D. Naltrexone for maintenance treatment
1. Naltrexone is an opioid receptor antagonist that works by blocking mu opioid receptors and preventing exogenous opioids from binding at the receptor.
2. Blocking the mu receptor naloxone blunts the pleasurable and rewarding effects of opioids.
3. Naloxone is FDA-approved for preventing relapse to illicit opioid use; however, initiation must be preceded by a medically supervised withdrawal or 7 to 10 days free of opioids. Naltrexone comes in two formulations: an oral tablet (Revia) and a long-acting monthly injectable (Vivitrol).
4. Oral naltrexone is available in 50-mg tablets, which when administered daily blocks the effects of full opioid agonists at the mu opioid receptor. Oral naltrexone may be administered to an individual dependent upon opioids under these circumstances: (a) ONLY after medically supervised withdrawal and (b) only after 7–10 days of abstinence from opioids. This is to avoid precipitating withdrawal with opioid agonists active at the receptor in the individuals with opioid dependence.
5. Injectable naloxone is a long-acting depot formulation that delivers steady naloxone concentrations and ongoing opioid antagonism for about 1 month. It is available in 380 mg to be administered by IM gluteal injection every 4 weeks. As with the oral formulation of naloxone, the injectable formulation should be administered after 7 to 10 days of being free of opioids to avoid a precipitated withdrawal.

Psychosocial Rehabilitation

A. With all psychosocial interventions, the healthcare provider will be certified in the methodology for therapy delivery. If the APRN does not have training and certification, referral to a specialist (e.g., social worker, psychologist, psychiatrist) is recommended.
1. CBT and mindfulness-based CBT: It is an evidenced-based intervention that focuses on thought processes and role of emotions and behaviors. It helps patients understand the relationship of thoughts, emotions, and behaviors. It further puts emphasis on modification of thought processes, ultimately changing emotional response and behaviors. When CBT is coupled with mindfulness, its efficacy improves. The practice of being aware of surroundings and living in the present moment instead of being preoccupied with the past helps the patient manage their thoughts and their reciprocal effects on emotional outcome and behaviors.
2. Narcotics Anonymous (NA) groups: NA evolved from AA and has its presence throughout the world. Approximately 70,000 meetings are arranged per year. NA groups are free to join, although only people with substance use issues can join. It follows a 12-step program. NA groups provide a strong social support system to its members (White et al., 2020).
3. Motivational enhancement therapies (MET): MET uses MI as a tool to resolve ambivalence issues regarding drug use and helps patients make informed decisions by their own will and develop motivation to change as it prepares them to embrace change.
4. Contingency management (CM): CM has its roots in the behavioral school of thought (Skinner, 1983) that focuses mainly on strengthening the desired behavior through shaping, using the principles of CM rewards and punishment (e.g., vouchers, prizes, star charts), to increase the likelihood of desired behavioral outcome.

Treating Opioid Use Disorder in the Hospital Units

A. Neonatal intensive care unit (NICU)
1. Neonates can be born with opiate dependence if the mother was using opioids during the pregnancy. This is an emergency situation!

B. ED
1. COWs evaluation: diagnosis and treatment plan
2. Planning for recovery and MAT

BOX 16.1 METHADONE DOSING SUMMARY

The initial goal is to reduce opioid withdrawal and craving safely.
- Use the "start low and go slow" approach but increase dose at a rate that minimizes chances of continued illicit drug use, while monitoring for side effects.
- Increase doses gradually over several weeks.
- Assess for sedation at peak serum concentration (2–4 hours after the dose).

The eventual target is an adequate dose that:
- Stops withdrawal symptoms for 24 hours
- Reduces or eliminates craving
- Blunts or blocks euphoria from self-administered illicit opioids

In general, after induction is complete, higher doses are more effective than lower doses.

C. Medical/surgical
  1. Test patients with OUD for hepatitis A, B, and C, as well as for STI, HIV, liver disease, tuberculosis (TB), infections, diabetes, and hypertension.
  2. This population is at higher risk for wound botulism, cellulitis, necrotizing fasciitis, and endocarditis.
  3. Difficult pain management will require pain management referral.

D. Obstetrics
  1. Screening for OUD is part of every OB/GYN assessment; check for use of pain medication as well as misuse and OUD in pregnant women.
  2. OUD during pregnancy exposes the fetus to opioids, as well as to long-term medical, developmental, and other emotional support needs postpartum.
  3. Screening tools include the following:
     a. National Institute on Drug Abuse (NIDA) Quick Screen
     b. CRAFFT (**C**ar, **R**elax, **A**lone, **F**orget, **F**riends, **T**rouble)

E. Geriatrics
  1. Older adults are at high risk of being prescribed opioids. According to the SAMHSA (2016), more than 500,000 Medicare beneficiaries were prescribed opioid.
  2. Assess for impact of opioid use/misuse on respiratory system, level of consciousness, and fall risk.
  3. Explore nonopioid methods of pain reduction.

PATIENT TEACHING

A. Helpful materials for patients at risk for OUD can be found at the U.S. Centers for Disease Control and Prevention (CDC) website www.cdc.gov/overdose-prevention/prevention/preventing-opioid-use-disorder.html.

INDIVIDUAL CONSIDERATIONS

Pediatrics

A. The safety and effectiveness of buprenorphine and methadone in pediatric patients below the age of 18 years have not been established.

Pregnancy

A. The use of MAT during pregnancy requires astute clinical judgment and sharp insight into the risks and benefits of using or not using medications.
B. Some of the risks to evaluate for are the potential adverse effects that repeated exposure to and withdrawal from opioids may have on the mother and the developing fetus.
C. Other associated risks of illicit opioid use during pregnancy are poor nutrition, smoking, and needle sharing. Ideally, MAT would be used in an integrative care environment where OUD, psychiatric services, case management, and prenatal care are offered.
D. Methadone is the accepted standard of care because it has been around longer, and more data are available to support its safety and efficacy.
E. Methadone and buprenorphine can be used as maintenance medications during pregnancy as these medications have better maternal and infant outcomes than no treatment at all. However, neonatal abstinence syndrome (NAS) can occur.
F. The landmark M.O.T.H.E.R. (Maternal Opioid Treatment: Human Experimental Research) study, a double-blind, double-dummy, randomized controlled trial comparing the use of buprenorphine and methadone in pregnancy and subsequent neonatal outcomes, found that in the buprenorphine arm of the study fewer neonates required treatment for NAS, less morphine was required to treat NAS, and fewer number of days of continued hospitalization was required.
G. There is no compelling reason to switch a patient already on methadone to buprenorphine—the switch could be destabilizing. If circumstances determine that buprenorphine is the better option, then the switch should be performed by a skilled clinician, preferably in an inpatient setting and ideally before conception.
H. Naltrexone in pregnancy
  1. The American College of Obstetricians and Gynecologists (ACOG) guidelines note that limited data exist as to the safety of naltrexone during pregnancy. Although there is an excellent response to medically supervised withdrawal in pregnancy, due to the lack of safety for the fetus, there is a need for additional data (Caritis & Venkataramanan, 2020; ACOG Committee on Obstetric Practice, 2017).
  2. It is not recommended to start naltrexone with pregnant women given the risks of precipitated withdrawal and the opioid-free withdrawal period that has to occur before initiation of naltrexone.
  3. Patients already on naltrexone when they become pregnant should collaborate with their healthcare provider for risk versus benefit analysis.

Hospitalized Patients

A. It is essential to continue maintenance treatment in patients who present to the ED or who are admitted to the hospital for an acute medical or psychiatric condition.
B. The clinician should contact the patient's OTP or their buprenorphine provider to verify dose and to arrange a seamless transition of care upon return to community-based treatment after discharge from the hospital.
C. Given the long half-life of methadone, the strong binding affinity and opioid antagonist effects of buprenorphine, and the opioid antagonist effects of naloxone, strategies around pain management in hospitalized patients on maintenance treatment are nuanced and require clinical flexibility and know-how (Table 16.6).

Treating Pain in Patients on Naloxone

A. Since oral naltrexone can block the effects of opioids for up to 72 hours and the long-acting injectable formulation of naloxone (Vivitrol) for up to 4 weeks, pain management in these patients can be tricky. The following are some considerations for pain management with patients on naloxone maintenance treatment:
  1. Nonopioid approaches such as regional anesthesia and injectable NSAIDs are possible options.
  2. The opioid antagonist effects of naloxone can be overcome with higher doses of opioids.
  3. When using higher doses of opioids, patients should be closely monitored for signs and symptoms of opioid overdose, particularly with patients for whom oral naloxone has been discontinued.

Geriatrics

A. Methadone and buprenorphine-containing products should be used with caution in the older population given the increased risk of side effects and adverse drug reactions.

TABLE 16.6 OPIOID AGONIST TREATMENT CONSIDERATIONS FOR HOSPITALIZED PATIENTS

	Buprenorphine	Methadone
Pain	• Continue in hospital, dividing and/or temporarily increasing dose if pain can be managed with buprenorphine. • Continue and add full opioid agonists for additional pain relief. • Discontinue upon hospitalization or prior to anticipated need for pain relief; use opioid full agonists to treat pain and prevent withdrawal; reinitiate after pain crisis is over.	Maintain patient's full usual daily dose barring any contraindications, and add pain medication to the methadone dose as clinically indicated.
Acute withdrawal	Authorized NPs and PAs may legally order buprenorphine without a waiver if an opioid-dependent patient not in treatment is admitted for a medical or psychiatric reason other than OUD, and where an acute opioid withdrawal would complicate the condition for which the patient was admitted.	Authorized NPs and PAs may legally order methadone to patients admitted for reasons other than OUD and where an acute opioid withdrawal would complicate the condition for which the patient was admitted.
Maintenance	Authorized NPs and PAs may order buprenorphine without a waiver for continuation of maintenance treatment during hospitalization where admitted for a reason other than OUD.	Authorized NPs and PAs may legally order methadone for patients already on methadone maintenance if admitted for a reason other than OUD.
Initiation	Authorized NPs and PAs may without a waiver initiate buprenorphine maintenance if arrangements are being made to discharge patient to a waivered prescriber in the community. Any prescription for buprenorphine to be taken outside of the hospital must be written by a waivered prescriber. Nonwaivered prescribers may arrange to have a patient return to the hospital ED for administration of medication for up to 3 days.	Methadone maintenance may be initiated in the hospital if patient can be discharged directly into an OTP program.

NP, nurse practitioner; OTP, opioid treatment program; OUD; opioid use disorder; PA, physician assistant.

Source: Data from Substance Abuse and Mental Health Services Administration. (2018). TIP 63: Medications for opioid use disorder. Author; Title 21 Code of Federal Regulations § 1306.07: Administering or dispensing of narcotic drugs. U.S. Department of Justice and U.S. Food and Drug Administration. https://www.accessdata.fda.gov/scripts/cdrh/cfdocs/cfcfr/cfrsearch.cfm?fr=1306.07.

B. Patients in this age group may tolerate lower doses better and should be monitored for excess sedation and respiratory depression.

C. Due to possible decreased hepatic, renal, and cardiac function, as well as an increased likelihood of medical comorbidities and polypharmacy, buprenorphine should be used cautiously in this population and patients should be monitored frequently for side effects and adverse drug reactions. Product inserts recommend starting at the lower end of the dosing range.

D. The safety and efficacy of naltrexone have not been established. Naltrexone is excreted by the kidney; thus, the risk of adverse reactions may be greater in patients with impaired renal function.

RESOURCES

A. For FDA prescribing information (package inserts): https://dailymed.nlm.nih.gov/dailymed/index.cfm

B. Providers Clinical Support System (PCSS): https://pcssnow.org

C. Federal Guidelines for OTPs: https://store.samhsa.gov/sites/default/files/guidelines-opioid-treatment-pep15-fedguideotp.pdf

D. SAMHSA Clinical Use of Extended-Release Injectable Naltrexone in the Treatment of Opioid Use Disorder: A Brief Guide: https://store.samhsa.gov/product/Clinical-Use-of-Extended-Release-Injectable-Naltrexone-in-the-Treatment-of-Opioid-Use-Disorder-A-Brief-Guide/SMA14-4892R

E. Evaluation and Mitigation Strategies (REMS) for buprenorphine products: www.accessdata.fda.gov/scripts/cder/rems/index.cfm

F. SAMHSA Opioid Overdose Prevention and Response Toolkit: https://store.samhsa.gov/sites/default/files/overdose-prevention-response-kit-pep23-03-00-001.pdf

G. SAMHSA SUD Treatment for People With Co-Occurring Psychiatric Disorders: https://store.samhsa.gov/sites/default/files/pep20-02-01-004.pdf

H. SAMHSA Pharmacologic Guidelines for Treating People With Co-Occurring OUD and Posttraumatic Stress Disorder (PTSD): https://store.samhsa.gov/sites/default/files/sma12-4688.pdf

I. SAMHSA Clinical Drug Testing in Primary Care: https://store.samhsa.gov/sites/default/files/sma12-4668.pdf

J. SAMHSA TIP 63: Mediations for Opioid Use Disorder (free download): https://store.samhsa.gov/product/tip-63-medications-opioid-use-disorder/pep21-02-01-002

REFERENCES AND BIBLIOGRAPHY

American College of Obstetricians and Gynecologists Committee on Obstetric Practice. (2017, August). *Opioid use and opioid use disorder in pregnancy: Committee Opinion no. 711.* American College of Obstetricians and Gynecologists. https://www.acog.org/clinical/clinical-guidance/committee-opinion/articles/2017/08/opioid-use-and-opioid-use-disorder-in-pregnancy

American Society of Addiction Medicine. (2015). *The ASAM national practice guideline for the use of medications in the treatment of addiction involving opioid use.*

BioDelivery Sciences International. (2017). *Bunavail (buprenorphine and naloxone) buccal film: Full prescribing information.* https://bunavail.com/hcp/assets/pdfs/BUNAVAIL_Full_Prescribing_Information.pdf

Brogly, S. B., Saia, K. A., Walley, A. Y., Du, H. M., & Sebastiani, P. (2014). Prenatal buprenorphine versus methadone exposure and neonatal outcomes: Systematic review and meta-analysis. *American Journal of Epidemiology, 180*(7), 673–686. https://doi.org/10.1093/aje/kwu190

Caritis, S. N., & Venkataramanan, R. (2020, January). Naltrexone use in pregnancy: A time for change. *American Journal of Obstetrics and Gynecology, 222*(1), 1–2. https://doi.org/10.1016/j.ajog.2019.08.041

Castells, X., Cunill, R., Pérez-Mañá, C., Vidal, X., & Capellà, D. (2016). Psychostimulant drugs for cocaine dependence. *Cochrane Database of Systematic Reviews, 9*(9), Article CD007380. https://doi.org/10.1002/14651858.CD007380.pub4

Connors, N. J., & Nelson, L. S. (2016). The evolution of recommended naloxone dosing for opioid overdose by medical specialty. *Journal of Medical Toxicology, 12*(3), 276–281. https://doi.org/10.1007/s13181-016-0559-3

Gowing, L., Farrell, M., Ali, R., & White, J. (2016). Alpha$_2$-adrenergic agonists for the management of opioid withdrawal. *Cochrane Database Systematic Reviews, 5*, Article CD002024. https://doi.org/10.1002/14651858.CD002024.pub4

Handford, C., Kahan, M., Srivastava, A., Cirone, S., Sanghera, S., & Palda, V. (2012). *Buprenorphine/naloxone for opioid dependence: Clinical practice guideline.* Centre for Addiction and Mental Health.

Indivior. (n.d.). *Suboxone (buprenorphine and naloxone) sublingual film: Full prescribing information.* https://www.suboxone.com/content/pdfs/prescribing-information.pdf

Ingalsbe, G. S. (2016, February 4). *World Health Organization recommendations for community management of opioid overdose reviewed by ACEP clinical policies committee.* American College of Emergency Physicians. http://www.acepnow.com/world-health-organization-recommendations-for-community-management-of-opioid-overdose

Jones, H. E., Heil, S. H., Baewert, A., Arria, A. M., Kaltenbach, K., Martin, P. R., Coyle, M. G., Selby, P., Stine, S. M., & Fischer, G. (2012). Buprenorphine treatment of opioid-dependent pregnant women: A comprehensive review. *Addiction, 107 Suppl*(1), 5–27. https://doi.org/10.1111/j.1360-0443.2012.04035.x

Marshall, B., & Spencer, J. (2019). *Fast facts about substance use disorders: What every nurse, APRN, and PA needs to know.* Springer Publishing Company.

National Safety Council. (n.d.). *Drug overdoses.* https://injuryfacts.nsc.org/home-and-community/safety-topics/drugoverdoses

Strain, E. (2018). *Opioid use disorder: Pharmacologic management.* UpToDate. https://www.uptodate.com/contents/opioid-use-disorder-pharmacologic-management

Substance Abuse and Mental Health Services Administration. (2021). *TIP 63: Medications for opioid use disorder.* U.S. Department of Health and Human Services. https://store.samhsa.gov/sites/default/files/pep21-02-01-002.pdf

Substance Abuse and Mental Health Services Administration. (2018, January). *Clinical guidance for treating pregnant and parenting women with opioid use disorder and their infants* (Publication No. SMA18-5054). U.S. Department of Health and Human Services. https://store.samhsa.gov/product/clinical-guidance-treating-pregnant-and-parenting-women-opioid-use-disorder-and-their

Substance Abuse and Mental Health Services Administration. (2021, July). *TIP 63: Medications for opioid use disorder.* Publication No. PEP21-02-01-002. U.S. Department of Health and Human Services.

Webster, A. (2024, May 14). *Drug and alcohol rehab for nurses near you.* American Addiction Centers. https://americanaddictioncenters.org/healthcare-professionals/rehab-for-nurses

World Health Organization. (2019). *International statistical classification of diseases* (11th rev.). https://icd.who.int

World Health Organization Alcohol, Drugs, and Addictive Behaviors Guidelines Review Committee. (2014, November 2). *Community management of opioid overdose.* World Health Organization. https://www.who.int/publications/i/item/9789241548816

Yule, A. M., Lyons, R. M., & Wilens, T. E. (2018). Opioid Use Disorders in Adolescents—Updates in Assessment and Management. *Current Pediatrics Reports, 6*(2), 99–106. https://doi.org/10.1007/s40124-018-0161-z

STIMULANT USE DISORDER

DEFINITION

A. *Stimulant use disorder* is defined as the use of stimulants (including amphetamines, both natural and synthetic) and abuse/misuse of prescribed stimulants resulting in behavioral or emotional impairment. The use and behaviors related to stimulants meet the criteria for an SUD. It is categorized from mild to severe based on the number of criteria met.
  1. Prescription stimulants: Adderall, Ritalin, Concerta, modafinil, Dexedrine, Preludin, Fastin, Meridia, and Vyvanse prescribed for ADHD, narcolepsy, obesity, and depression
  2. Street drugs: methamphetamine, cocaine, methcathinone, and other synthetic cathinones, which are referred to as "bath salts"
  3. Street names for stimulants: bennies, black beauties, cat, coke, crank, crystal, flake, ice, molly, pellets, r-ball, skippy, snow, speed, uppers, and vitamin R

B. Stimulants access the brain through the following routes:
  1. Oral: stomach to intestine to bloodstream, mucosa (oral/gums) to bloodstream, then bloodstream to brain
  2. Intranasal (puffing and snorting): nasal mucosa to bloodstream, then bloodstream to brain
  3. Inhalation: igniting the substance to aerosolize, then inhaled into lungs, lungs to bloodstream, bloodstream to brain
  4. Intravenous: injected into bloodstream

PREVALENCE

A. It is estimated that 1.6 billion Americans (over the age of 12) have methamphetamine use disorder (MUD), with an additional 1.4 million with cocaine use disorder.
  1. 5.5 million Americans used cocaine in 2018 (drugabusestatistics.org).
  2. Misuse is greatest in the adolescent and young adult populations.

B. The following are the patterns of misuse:
  1. Bingeing or runs: Amphetamines are used to keep individuals awake, taking them every few hours to maintain a high similar to mania. When the run ends, the individual "crashes" and feels fatigued, depressed, anxious, and can be paranoid, increasing the likelihood of seeking more drugs.
  2. Chronic misuse: Chronic misuse may occur from misuse of prescription drugs or illicit drugs. It presents like psychosis, along with hallucinations.
  3. Short-term experiences: Patient experiences decreased appetite, dry mouth, a sense of euphoria, energized, tachycardia, possible headache, irritability, diarrhea, nausea and vomiting, hospitality, and possibly paranoia.

C. Stimulant withdrawal: This occurs when the cessation of use (either therapeutic or recreational) is abrupt. It may occur in phases—immediate, secondary, and crash.
  1. Immediate (within 24 hours): lethargic, sad, cravings of great intensity
  2. Secondary: physically and mentally tired, depression accompanied by insomnia, can last from days to weeks, but the usual duration is 3 to 5 days
  3. Crash: mood swings and total physical and mental exhaustion

SIGNS AND SYMPTOMS

A. Signs and symptoms of stimulant withdrawal
  1. Muscle aches and pains, anxiety, agitation, and changes in appetite
  2. Headaches, cravings, depression, and hallucinations
  3. Suicidal ideations, mood swings, inability to concentrate, and sleep disturbances
  4. Increased risk for disordered thinking, hallucinations, paranoia, and psychosis

B. Environmental considerations
  1. Reduce stimulation in environment; reduce noise when possible.
  2. Reorient when patient is confused; check level of consciousness.
  3. Assess for hallucinations and remove loose items and clutter from the environment.

GENERAL TREATMENTS AND INTERVENTIONS

A. Pharmacologic

1. There are no FDA-approved medications for the treatment of stimulant use disorder.
2. Topiramate is the first choice for cocaine use disorder.
3. Bupropion with naltrexone (Trivedi et al., 2021), mirtazapine, and psychostimulants are used for MUD.

B. Nonpharmacologic
1. CM and harm reduction
2. MI
3. CBT
4. Mental health counseling and self-help groups

TOBACCO USE DISORDER (NICOTINE DEPENDENCE)

DEFINITION

A. Tobacco use disorder (TUD) is the most common of SUDs, with between 60% and 80% of tobacco users meeting the clinical criteria for drug dependence on nicotine. Any product that delivers nicotine (e.g., vaping, smoking, chewing, transdermal patches, and snuff) contributes to the dependence. However, TUD is specific to the delivery of nicotine through the use of tobacco.

B. Tobacco use is considered the most preventable cause of death in the United States.
1. More than 16 million Americans have a smoking-related disease, which leads to a half million deaths annually.
2. Gen Z, post-millennials, are more likely to begin their smoking experience in adolescence and are targeted by e-cigarette companies (WHO, 2020).

C. TUD and tobacco use impact all body systems.
1. There is not a body system that is immune to the detrimental effects of TUD.
2. Use of tobacco products results in acute and chronic illnesses, disability, and death.
3. Use of tobacco products by smokers increased the severity of COVID-19 by 1.4% and the likelihood of needing ICU care in the hospital by 2.4%.

D. Physical and psychological dependence occurs in TUD.
1. Physical dependence occurs in TUD; without access to the nicotine, the body will have withdrawal symptoms.
2. Psychological dependence is the belief that it is not possible to go through a full day without access to nicotine/cigarettes.

PREVALENCE

A. The prevalence of smoking by Americans has been decreasing since 2001.

B. According to the CDC, around 3 million U.S. students (middle and high school) and 28 million adults in the United States smoke.

SIGNS AND SYMPTOMS

Symptoms and Observations of Use

A. Nicotine is a central nervous system (CNS) stimulant and is absorbed quickly into the blood, increasing dopamine in the brain.

B. Depending on the route of administration, the physical signs and symptoms might be different.
1. Smoking: The patient will smell like cigarettes or might be heavily perfumed to hide the smell. Gum can also be used to cover the odor of cigarette smoke on the breath. Finger discoloration may occur.
2. Patches: Skin irritation may occur.

C. Signs and symptoms of prolonged tobacco use on different systems include the following:
1. Likelihood of increased formation of plaque in blood vessels and developing hypertension
2. Increased frequency of lung infections, chronic obstructive pulmonary disease (COPD), and scarring of lung tissue
3. Increased risk of cancer of the nose, mouth, larynx, throat, and most body systems
4. Impact on autoimmune system, vision, and skeletal and reproductive systems

Symptoms and Observations of Withdrawal After Quitting Nicotine

A. Withdrawal from nicotine is physical, emotional, and cognitive/mental.
1. Cravings to smoke
2. Mood dysregulation: anxiety, depression, sadness
3. Emotional dysregulation: anger, upset, irritability
4. Restlessness
5. Difficulty concentrating
6. Insomnia
7. Increased appetite

B. Positive changes include the following:
1. In the first hour: The heart rate will drop within 20 minutes.
2. Within 12 hours: The carbon monoxide levels in the body return to normal.
3. After 2 to 3 months: Lung function improves and risk of cardiovascular (CV) disease begins to drop. There is also a decrease in coughing and shortness of breath.
4. 1+ year post: Risk of CV disease drops to 0.5 of that of a smoker, stroke risk falls, and within 5 to 15 years is the same as a nonsmoker. Lung cancer risk drops after 10 years, and after 15 years the risk of CV disease is equivalent to a nonsmoker.

DIAGNOSTIC TESTS AND SCREENING

Quick Question Guide

A. When you wake up, how soon do you smoke a cigarette?
B. Of all the cigarettes you smoke during the day, which one would you hate to not be able to smoke?
C. In a normal day, how many cigarettes do you smoke?
D. Is your smoking heaviest after you wake up?
E. If you are sick in bed, do you still smoke?

GENERAL TREATMENTS AND INTERVENTIONS

A. Nicotine replacement therapy (NRT)
1. Replacing the nicotine will reduce the carcinogens that are in cigarettes. The goal is to taper the nicotine to allow the patient to have comfort during withdrawal.
2. There are four available formulations: oral (gum, lozenge), transdermal patches, nasal spray, and inhaler.
   a. Oral: gum and lozenge
      i. Gum: Nicotine is bound to polacrilex. Chewing releases the nicotine. Absorption is through the mucosa in the mouth.
         (1) Dosing: Dosing is 2 and 4 mg per piece of gum and is individualized depending on the level of dependence. The higher the dependence, the higher the dose. The average dose is 9 to 12 pieces of gum; the maximum is 30 pieces

TABLE 16.7 DOSING AND TAPERING SCHEDULE FOR NICOTINE GUM AND NICOTINE LOZENGE

Weeks	Dose
Weeks 1–6	1 dose every 1–2 hours
Weeks 7–9	1 dose every 2–4 hours
Weeks 10–12	1 dose every 4–8 hours

of 2 mg and 20 pieces of 4 mg (see dosing and tapering schedule in Table 16.7).
   (2) Adverse effects: Adverse effects include salivation, GI discomfort/dyspepsia, hiccups, sore jaw, lightheadedness, nausea, vomiting, and irritation of the mouth and throat.
   (3) Patient instructions: Do not chew like chewing gum! Chew the gum a few times, then "park" it so that the nicotine can be absorbed through the oral mucosa. Do not swallow. It can be used every 1 to 2 hours to reduce craving or control withdrawal symptoms. It can be used in combination with a nicotine patch.
   b. Nicotine transdermal system: Nicotine patch allows for gradual release of nicotine into the bloodstream via transdermal route.
      i. Dosing: Available in 21-,14-, and 7-mg strengths. Base dosing on pack usage per day. Suggestion: For patients using more than 10 cigarettes per day, start with 21-mg patch for the first 6 weeks, then decrease to 14-mg patch for 2 weeks and then 7-mg patch for 2 weeks. If less than 10 cigarettes, begin with the 14-mg patch for 6 weeks and decrease to 7 mg for 2 weeks.
      ii. Adverse effects: Adverse effects include site reaction on skin, such as itching, burning, and erythema. Insomnia is also possible.
      iii. Patient information: Collaborate with the patient to establish the best use of the patch for achieving recovery and abstinence from smoking.
   c. Nicotine inhaler: a mouthpiece and cartridge
      i. Dosing: Dosing is 6 to 16 cartridges per day (each cartridge has 10-mg nicotine) for the first 3 months. Taper off over a period of 2 to 3 months (Nicotrol NS Package Insert, 2010).
      ii. Adverse effects: Adverse effects include possible mouth and throat irritation. Coughing is also possible.
      iii. Patient information: When the mouthpiece is fit into the cartridge, the inhaler will release the nicotine vapor. Absorption is through the oral mucosa. Puff on the mouthpiece for a period of 20 minutes, then discard the cartridge.
   d. Nasal spray
      i. Dosing: Dosing is one to two sprays per hour, with a maximum of five sprays in 1 hour. Use a maximum of 40 per day over a 3-month period. Nicotine is absorbed by the nasal mucosa. This produces a rapid rise in nicotine levels, providing more immediate relief from withdrawal symptoms.
      ii. Adverse effects: Adverse effects include irritation in the mouth, throat, and nose. It may cause allergy-like symptoms such as rhinitis, coughing, tearing up, and sneezing.
      iii. Patient information: Explain to the patient the maximum dose and provide information related to side effects.
B. Nonnicotine-containing products
   1. See Table 16.8.
C. Psychotherapeutic approaches
   1. Therapy for cessation of smoking: group therapy
   2. Private counseling with pharmacotherapy
D. CAM
   1. Hypnotherapy
   2. Yoga or mindfulness mediation

REFERRAL/RESOURCES
A. Centers for Disease Control and Prevention: How to Quit Smoking: www.cdc.gov/tobacco/campaign/tips
B. National Cancer Institute: www.cancer.gov/about-cancer/causes-prevention/risk/tobacco/help-quitting-fact-sheet
C. Substance Abuse and Mental Health Services Administration: www.samhsa.gov/find-help/national-helpline

TABLE 16.8 NONNICOTINE-CONTAINING PRODUCTS

Medication	Mechanism of Action	Precautions	Side Effects	Dosing
Bupropion SR Zyban Wellbutrin Forfivo	Antidepressant: reduces urge and irritability; takes 1–2 weeks to reach therapeutic levels	Lowers seizure threshold	Insomnia, dry mouth, agitation	Start 2 weeks before quit date: 150 mg PO QD × 3 days in the morning, then 150 mg PO BID for 7–12 weeks.
Varenicline (Chantix)	Partial agonist at nicotinic receptor; promotes dopamine release, which reduces cravings		Nausea, headache, abnormal dreams, dry mouth, flatulence, sleep disturbances	Start 1 week before quit date. See package insert for daily increases in medication (Chantix Prescribing Information 2016).
Nortriptyline (Pamelor) Second-line	Tricyclic antidepressant	Off-label use for persons who cannot tolerate first-line nicotine drugs	Extensive side effects	
Cystine Second-line	Partial agonist at the alpha–beta nicotinic receptor	Not FDA-approved for smoking cessation	Precaution with arterial hypertension, atherosclerosis, pregnancy, breastfeeding	Medication has complex dosing regimen.[a]

BID, twice daily; FDA, U.S. Food and Drug Administration; PO, orally; QD, once daily
[a]www.ncbi.nlm.nih.gov/pmc/articles/PMC5953578.

INDIVIDUAL CONSIDERATIONS

Pregnancy

A. Those who are pregnant face many risks if smoking or using nicotine during pregnancy.
B. Clinicians can inquire, during the intake interview, about ALL types of tobacco and nicotine products, including cigarette smoking, e-cigarettes, vaping, hookah use, snus, patches, lozenges, and nicotine gum.
C. Advise pregnant patients and those hoping to become pregnant that tobacco use increases the risk of fetal growth restriction, placenta previa, preterm rupture of membranes, low birth weight, perinatal mortality, and decreased thyroid function in the woman.
D. Address psychosocial stressors and alternate means to achieve reduced stress levels.

Pediatrics

A. Smoking often begins in early adolescence, when the youth is at increased risk for nicotine dependence.
B. Behavioral interventions are most effective with youth. Prevention is the key as nicotine addiction usually starts in the teen years, making it a pediatric disease.
C. E-cigarettes may look like common devices (e.g., flash drives) and are often marketed to the youth population. According to the CDC, two-thirds of JUUL users between the ages of 15 and 24 were unaware that the JUUL always contains nicotine.

Smokers of Color

A. Since March 2023, over 170 U.S. communities have banned the sale of flavored tobacco products, including menthol cigarettes; however, a federal ban is still not in place.
B. Antismoking groups have fought to get this ban in place because menthol tobacco products target women, youth, and smokers of color. More than 11% of American adults smoke, but 80% of smokers who are Black, mostly teens, smoke mentholated cigarettes. Elimination of menthol in cigarettes could prevent between 300,000 and 650,000 deaths (mostly among Black Americans) over decades (Perron, 2024). It would reduce the lung cancer gap between Black and White Americans to equal numbers. Educating patients as to this disparity and offering guidance for successful quitting are important during every office visit.

REFERENCES AND BIBLIOGRAPHY

American College of Obstetricians and Gynecologists Committee on Obstetric Practice. (2020, May). *Tobacco and nicotine cessation during pregnancy: Committee Opinion no. 807*. American College of Obstetricians and Gynecologists. https://www.acog.org/clinical/clinical-guidance/committee-opinion/articles/2020/05/tobacco-and-nicotine-cessation-during-pregnancy

Baker, T. B., Breslau, N, Covey, L, & Shiffman, S. (2012). DSM criteria for tobacco use disorder and tobacco withdrawal: A critique and proposed revisions for *DSM-5*. *Addiction*, *107*(2), 263–275. https://doi.org/10.1111/j.1360-0443.2011.03657.x

Curry, S. J., Mermelstein, R. J., & Sporer, A. K. (2009). Therapy for specific problems: Youth tobacco cessation. *Annual Review of Psychology*, *60*, 229–255. https://doi.org/10.1146/annurev.psych.60.110707.163659

Karnieg, T., & Wang, X. (2018). Cytisine for smoking cessation. *Canadian Medical Association Journal*, *190*(19), E596. https://doi.org/10.1503/cmaj.171371

Marshall, B., & Spencer, J. (2019). *Fast facts about substance use disorders: What every nurse, APRN, and PA needs to know*. Springer Publishing Company.

National Institute for Health, National Center for Complementary and Integrative Health. (2021, January). *Complementary health approaches for smoking cessation*. NCCIH Clinical Digest for Health Professionals. https://www.nccih.nih.gov/health/providers/digest/complementary-health-approaches-for-smoking-cessation

Perrone, M. (2024, April 2). *Lawsuit seeks to force ban on menthol cigarettes after months of delays by Biden administration*. Associated Press. https://apnews.com/article/menthol-cigarettes-ban-fda-lawsuit-biden-f1397c032b637c6c2ba44a63b267ea21

World Health Organization. (2020, May 29). *The secret's out: The tobacco industry targets a new generation*. https://who-sandbox.squiz.cloud/en/health-topics/disease-prevention/pages/news/news/2020/5/the-secrets-out-the-tobacco-industry-targets-a-new-generation

NEW AND EMERGING STREET DRUGS: DESIGNER DRUGS

A. Isotonitazene (Nitazene or ISO)
   1. Synthetic opioid: highly potent, high risk of overdose
   2. In powder form, usually mixed into heroin and/or fentanyl
   3. Might be pressed into counterfeit pills and marketed as Dilaudid or oxycodone
B. Xylazine ("Tranq," animal tranquilizer)
   1. Xylazine is often combined with opioids like fentanyl.
   2. It causes severe sedation, difficulty breathing, low blood pressure, bradycardia, and death.
   3. Naloxone will not reverse the effects of xylazine, but should be given in the event that xylazine is used with an opioid. Provide rescue breathing.
   4. Routine toxicology screenings will not identify presence of xylazine. Only xylazine test strips demonstrated efficacy in identifying the presence of xylazine.
C. Phenethylamines
   1. Phenethylamines are psychoactive drugs with stimulant effects.
   2. The 2C series are NBOMes, phenethylamines (PMMA), and benzodifuran (Bromo-Dragonfly).
D. Synthetic cathinones (bath salts)
   1. Made from the khat plant
   2. Can cause life-threatening problems and other health and safety issues
E. Phencyclidine-type substances (novel dissociatives)
   1. Methoxphenidine
   2. Structural features with PCP
   3. Acute toxicity with confusion, tachycardia, hypertension, echolalia, agitation, nystagmus, and amnesia
F. Novel benzodiazepines
   1. Sold as "legal benzodiazepines," "designer benzodiazepines," or "research chemicals"
      a. Diclazepam, flubromazepam, pyrazolam
      b. Very limited information on long- or short-term effects

17 THOUGHT AND PSYCHOTIC DISORDERS

Rosa Landinez and Yovan Gonzalez

INTRODUCTION

Thought disorders are mental problems related to the inability of individuals to write or speak coherently. Thought disorders interfere with how a person expresses their thoughts verbally or in writing. They can manifest as disorganization, incoherence, derailment, and word salad, and signify a mental health disorder. Thought disorders are common in some mental health disorders, such as schizophrenia, psychotic disorders, and mania. They are subdivided into positive and negative thought disorders, distinguishing characteristics of evident symptoms and behaviors. Positive thought disorders have positive symptoms in response to hallucinations or disorganized behaviors. Negative thought disorders exhibit negative symptoms such as mutism and lack of emotional response to stimuli.

Thought disorders are closely related to psychotic disorders as they share symptomatology, diagnostic criteria, and treatment modalities. Psychotic disorders are a group of mental health disorders that affect how the individual's brain and body process thoughts leading to exhibiting certain behaviors in response to stimuli. Psychotic disorders interfere with how individuals behave, think, and communicate with others and their emotional responses. Individuals diagnosed with psychotic disorders have difficulty identifying reality from imaginary situations. People with psychotic disorders cannot discern their thoughts from what they are seeing or experiencing in the outside world. Psychotic disorders can cause cognitive and social dysfunction for a specific time and interfere with typical developmental milestones.

Research from Tor et al. (2017) reported that children and adolescents present with perceptual abnormalities and suspiciousness symptoms and may have comorbid mental conditions such as depression and anxiety. These researchers recommend that the focus should be on prevention, early assessment, and interventions to improve the treatment outcomes for this population. It is essential to provide special attention to this population as their clinical presentation differs from that of adults. Children and adolescents usually go through the processes of brain development, so it is critical to act early and effectively.

Schoer et al. (2019), investigating the differences in the duration of untreated psychosis for racial and ethnic minority groups, reported that minority groups might have a disadvantage in treatment opportunities compared with other populations. The delay in treatment, increasing time of untreated psychosis, leads to poor outcomes. Improved access to early interventions, prevention, assessment, and treatment of racial and ethnic minority groups is pivotal to improving outcomes and reducing healthcare disparity that leads to detrimental psychosocial consequences of psychosis.

THOUGHT DISORDER CLASSIFICATION

The American Psychiatric Association, in the *Diagnostic and Statistical Manual of Mental Disorders*, Fifth Edition (*DSM-5*; American Psychiatric Association, 2013), classifies thought and psychotic disorders into five domains: delusions; hallucinations; disorganized thinking (speech); confusing or abnormal and disorganized behavior, including catatonia; and negative symptoms. The classification of psychotic disorders includes schizophrenia, schizophreniform disorder, schizoaffective disorder, brief psychotic disorder, delusional disorder, substance/medication-induced psychotic disorder, and psychotic disorder due to another medical condition. Each psychotic disorder in this classification must meet at least one of the five established domains and the duration of the symptoms. The initial presentation of psychotic behavior, including symptomatology, assists the clinician with completing a complete assessment, assessing the severity of the illness, and ascertaining the degree of neurologic and cognitive deficiencies. The psychotic symptoms are dysfunctions in perception. Understanding the severity of the person's clinical presentation is critical to assessing the degree of cognitive and neurologic problems.

The reported symptoms can also help the APRN prepare a comprehensive treatment plan for the patient. Early intervention and possible prevention are pivotal to a good prognosis and management of psychosis. Delays in diagnosis and treatment are detrimental to the patient and can have worse consequences.

Hallucinations

A. Hallucinations are perceptions reported by an individual that happen without an external stimulus. Individuals may report seeing things others cannot verify or hearing voices inside their heads having commentary or conversing with them.
B. Some hallucinations might be typical during religious rituals in other cultures and should not be considered abnormal.
C. Hallucinations can be experienced through any/all five senses: olfactory, tactile, visual, auditory, and gustatory.

Delusions

A. Delusions are beliefs and judgments that are false, but are believed despite the provision of demonstrated facts, proof, and other evidence to the contrary.
  1. Persecutory: false belief of being stalked, conspired against by an individual or an organization
  2. Erotomania (De Clerambault syndrome): false belief that a person of interest is in love with the patient, may lead to stalking and rage
  3. Grandiose: false belief of great importance, that the person is extremely talented, rich, or close to someone who is famous or prominent
  4. Jealousy
  5. Somatic: being convinced that there is something wrong with their body/health; can lead to medical consultations, surgeries, and suicide
  6. Mixed
  7. Unspecified

Disorganized Thinking (Speech)
A. An individual's thinking can be inferred by the individual's speech. A person may be unable to sustain a linear conversation, constantly changes topics, or is unable to complete sentences or the sentences are not related to the topic of conversation.
B. To be considered as a sign of a psychotic disorder, disorganized thinking or speech should impair effective communication. It is essential first to consider if the disorganization is related to a language barrier or culture.
C. Disorganized thinking and speech is commonly seen in patients in the prodromal period of schizophrenia.

Grossly Disorganized or Abnormal Motor Behavior (Including Catatonia)
A. Behavior may manifest in different ways, ranging from sudden psychomotor agitation to catatonia or lack of response or reaction to the environment.
B. It can lead to problems and an inability to perform daily activities and overall functioning in the community.
C. Catatonic features range from mutism and stupor to an inability to follow directions.
D. Some individuals might present with echolalia by only repeating everything they are hearing, staring into space for long periods, or grimacing as if they were in front of a mirror.
E. Catatonia can be evident in patients suffering from schizophrenia and other mental health disorders, as well as resulting from a medical condition.

Negative Symptoms
A. The negative symptoms affect most individuals diagnosed with schizophrenia; however, they may also present in other psychotic disorders. The negative symptoms can be evident in the individual's affect, behavior, speech, and thinking.
B. The most common negative symptoms include the following:
   1. Avolition: lack of motivation and goal-directed behaviors
   2. Anhedonia: reduced or absence of the ability to experience pleasure
   3. Alogia: reduction in production of speech and thought
   4. Asociality: decline or inability to engage in social interactions
   5. Affective flattening: difficulty or inability to demonstrate emotions (even when emotions are being experienced)
C. Individuals exhibiting negative symptoms may have a worse prognosis as they may indicate a chronic condition rather than an acute change in behavior. The negative symptoms may go unnoticed until they affect the patient's safety, which may be why they come into contact with the healthcare system.

REFERENCES AND BIBLIOGRAPHY
Albert, N., & Weibell, M. A. (2019). The outcome of early intervention in first episode psychosis. *International Review of Psychiatry, 31*(5–6), 413–424. https://doi.org/10.1080/09540261.2019.1643703
American Psychiatric Association. (2013). *Diagnostic and statistical manual of mental disorders* (5th ed.). https://doi.org/10.1176/appi.books.9780890425596
King, L. M. (2024, August 20). *What is a psychotic disorder?* WebMD. https://www.webmd.com/schizophrenia/guide/mental-health-psychotic-disorders
Lieberman, J. A., & First, M. B. (2018). Psychotic disorders. *New England Journal of Medicine, 379*(3), 270–280. https://doi.org/10.1056/nejmra1801490
Moore, M. (2022, June 16). *All about thought disorder*. PsychCentral. https://psychcentral.com/disorders/thought-disorder
Rivkin, P., & Barta, P. (2017, August 2). *Thought Disorder*. Johns Hopkins Pyschiatry Guide. https://www.hopkinsguides.com/hopkins/view/Johns_Hopkins_Psychiatry_Guide/787025/all/Thought_Disorder
Schoer, N., Huang, C. W., & Anderson, K. K. (2019). Differences in duration of untreated psychosis for racial and ethnic minority groups with first-episode psychosis: An updated systematic review and meta-analysis. *Social Psychiatry and Psychiatric Epidemiology, 54*(10), 1295–1298. https://doi.org/10.1007/s00127-019-01737-3
Tor, J., Dolz, M., Sintes, A., Muñoz, D., Pardo, M., de la Serna, E., Puig, O., Sugranyes, G., & Baeza, I. (2017). Clinical high risk for psychosis in children and adolescents: A systematic review. *European Child & Adolescent Psychiatry, 27*(6), 683–700. https://doi.org/10.1007/s00787-017-1046-3
Zakhari, R. (2020). *The psychiatric-mental health nurse practitioner certification review manual*. Springer Publishing Company.

BRIEF PSYCHOTIC DISORDER

DEFINITION
A. According to the *DSM-5* (American Psychiatric Association, 2013), a brief psychotic disorder is a sudden episode of psychotic behavior lasting at least 1 day and resolving in 1 month. Patients can have a complete remission of that episode but it might occur again in the future.
B. The symptomatology of brief psychotic episodes should include at least one delusion, hallucination, or disorganized speech.
   1. Brief psychotic episodes might be used to diagnose other psychotic disorders if the behavior and symptoms do not resolve within the month of the initial presentation.
C. The presented symptoms would subside, and the patient would return to normal behavior and functioning in less than 1 month. For some individuals, the psychotic symptoms disappear in just a few days.
D. The onset of the psychotic symptoms cannot be a result of other psychotic disorders induced by a medical condition caused by a medication or a result of another psychiatric diagnosis, such as a mood disorder with psychotic features.
E. The APRN should assess for depression, cognitive deficits, and mania symptoms to rule out other psychotic disorders. The APRN should also monitor rapid and frequent changes in the patient's mood, behavior, and affect to prevent safety mishaps due to delusions, hallucinations, or disorganized speech.
F. Individuals having a brief psychotic episode are at a higher risk of having suicidal tendencies, especially during the acute episode.
G. A problematic dilemma reported by Sullivan et al. (2020) and Fusar-Poli et al. (2022) is the incidence of brief psychotic episodes in late adolescence, contrasting with the lack of treatment providers, leading to unmet needs for vulnerable populations such as the one in this study. This is substantiated by Catalan et al. (2020), who also reported on the critical need for early intervention, prevention, and treatment of adolescents suffering from psychosis. In their review, they discussed the benefits of using this approach, including positive outcomes for the patient.
H. Smith et al. (2020), in their research, reported an association between a symptomatic individual with COVID-19 having a brief psychotic episode with symptomatology subsiding after treatment with pharmacotherapy until the psychotic symptoms resolved. Exposure to increased stress levels after the diagnosis and exhibiting psychotic symptoms with hallucinations, paranoid thoughts, and agitation were discussed. These symptoms subsided after a short inpatient admission.

INCIDENCE
A. The National Institute of Mental Health (NIMH) reports that each year in the United States, there are approximately 100,000 new cases of psychosis, with a prevalence of psychosis in the general population of about 3%, while the incidence of brief psychotic disorders is 4 to 10 individuals per 100,000 people each year.
B. The prevalence of first brief psychotic disorders in the United States is approximately 9% of the psychotic disorders diagnosed.
C. Females have a higher prevalence (2:1) of being diagnosed with brief psychotic disorders than males.
D. The diagnosis of brief psychotic disorders can be made in adolescents and young adults, although the onset of symptoms may occur across the life span. The average age of onset is in the 30s.
E. Brief psychotic disorders are also more common in individuals diagnosed with a personality disorder.

PATHOGENESIS
A. The causes of brief psychotic episodes vary. Griswold (2015) discussed the vital role of dopamine in psychosis. The altered neurotransmission in the dopamine and glutamate pathways of the hippocampus, the midbrain, the corpus striatum, and the prefrontal cortex leads to psychotic symptoms. This is supported by the effectiveness of medications that are dopamine receptor antagonists in treating psychotic symptoms.
B. Some brief episodes of psychosis can be attributed to trauma or a stressful event, and other contributing factors can be neurologic, genetic, and environmental.
C. The clinician will need to specify if the onset of the psychotic behavior is related to trauma or a stressful situation. Within 4 weeks postpartum, some women may also present with brief psychotic episodes.

PREDISPOSING FACTORS
A. Preexisting personality disorders and other Axis II pathology, which may predispose individuals to having brief psychotic episodes
B. Has fair prognosis as individuals with this diagnosis can return to normal functioning once the psychotic symptoms subside
C. Significant life stressors
D. Family history of psychotic disorders
E. Acute change in behavior during pregnancy or within 4 weeks postpartum
F. Substance use disorder
G. Exposure to trauma
H. Psychosocial stressors, such as high administrative positions
I. Sociocultural issues including migration and rapid social changes (refugees, COVID-19 lockdown)
J. Delay in getting treatment for psychotic symptoms

COMMON COMPLAINTS
A. Reporting hallucinations, such as seeing, hearing, or feeling something nonexistent
B. Hyperarousal
C. Increased irritability
D. Paranoid thoughts and sudden onset of suspiciousness
E. A sudden decrease in job performance in adults
F. In children, a sudden drop in grades
G. Experiencing problems with concentration and thinking clearly
H. Social withdrawal and increasingly spending time alone
I. Seen talking to themselves
J. Unusual and bizarre ideas, with difficulty expressing thoughts
K. Inability or unwillingness to care for self
L. Having difficulty differentiating reality from fantasy
M. Incongruent behavior
N. Inability to function independently

OTHER SIGNS AND SYMPTOMS
A. Acute onset of paranoia
B. Difficulty sustaining a linear conversation
C. Behavior dysregulation, odd behaviors
D. Delusional thoughts

SUBJECTIVE DATA
A. Complete a review of medications and over-the-counter (OTC) agents to rule out medication-induced psychosis.
B. Determine the presence of risk factors, such as increased stress levels.
C. See "Subjective Data" in the "Schizophrenia" section.

PHYSICAL EXAMINATION
A. See "Physical Examination" in the "Schizophrenia" section.
B. Complete a comprehensive history of presentation (onset of psychosis). Establish that the symptoms have not been present for less than a day or more than 1 month.
C. Identify the presence of at least one positive psychotic symptom (delusion, hallucination, disorganized behavior, or speech).

DIAGNOSTIC TESTS AND SCREENING
A. See "Diagnostic Tests and Screening" in the "Schizophrenia" section.
B. See "Psychometric Tools" in the "Schizoaffective Disorder" section.
C. Conduct thyroid and parathyroid function tests.
D. Conduct urinalysis and urine toxicology to rule out medication-induced psychosis.
E. Conduct EEG, CT, MRI, and PET if appropriate.

DIFFERENTIAL DIAGNOSES
A. Psychosis due to a general medical condition
B. Substance/mediation-induced psychosis
C. Delusional disorder
D. Personality disorder
E. Schizophreniform disorder
F. Schizophrenia
G. Bipolar disorder
H. Other psychotic disorders
I. Depression with psychotic features
J. Dementia
K. Delirium

PLAN

General Treatments and Interventions
A. Consider a multidisciplinary approach to treatment.
B. Interview the patient with their family and the members of the treatment team.
C. Discuss and prepare a safety plan for patients with auditory or visual hallucinations.
D. Discuss the appropriate level of care to meet the basic needs (e.g., food, shelter, hygiene, and safety).

E. If the patient cannot maintain safety in the community, consider inpatient admission for stabilization and medication titration, and complete diagnostic tests. Inpatient admission is recommended in a low-stimulation environment.

F. Discuss pharmacologic and psychotherapy treatment modalities such as cognitive behavioral therapy (CBT). CBT assists the patient with social support, treatment, and group networks. The therapy can be one-to-one or group therapy. The patient learns health and wellness management skills, resilience training, and coping mechanisms.

G. After a review of laboratory results and other tests, discuss treatment options.

H. Provide supportive therapy as needed and close follow-up care if the patient remains in the community, and assist with referrals to care management services.

I. Discuss programs for continued education, employment, housing, social skills training, and vocational and educational counseling.

COMMON MEDICATIONS

A. The first line of treatment for brief psychotic disorders is antipsychotic medications, which help reduce psychotic symptoms. The pharmacotherapy is tailored to the presenting symptoms and considers the age, gender, and history of the patient.

B. See Tables 17.1 and 17.2.

PATIENT TEACHING

A. Educate on the signs and symptoms of psychotic disorders and what to report to the clinician.

B. Educate on the importance of preparing and following a safety plan.

C. Educate on the importance of adherence to the proposed treatment plan, including taking all medications as prescribed and following recommendations from the mental healthcare provider.

D. Educate on nonpharmacologic interventions such as psychotherapy, group therapy, and community involvement.

E. Educate on the risks versus the benefits of taking prescribed medications, including the side effects.

F. Educate on keeping all appointments with the mental healthcare provider.

G. Educate on the importance of sleep hygiene, exercise, and leisure activities to assist with healthcare maintenance.

H. Patients should participate in the treatment planning, including proactively including their treatment goals and keeping them motivated to engage in recovery.

FOLLOW-UP

A. If the patient is treated in the community, the APRN should schedule an initial follow-up visit 2 weeks after the initiation of treatment. This visit is to review/update the treatment plan and monitor the patient's clinical progress.

B. If the patient is discharged from the hospital, the patient should be seen as soon as possible to discuss the treatment plan, review medication and nonpharmacologic treatment, and discuss continued care with the APRN.

C. After the initial follow-up visit, the patient should be seen every 4 to 6 weeks for continued monitoring of symptoms and possible changes or adjustments to the treatment regimen.

CONSULTATION AND REFERRALS

A. The APRN should consult and refer patients appropriately, considering any comorbid medical, substance use, or neurologic conditions.

B. The APRN should initiate referrals to community centers and other agencies that can provide a multimodal treatment option for some patients.

C. The APRN should consult and collaborate with interprofessionals to make a robust treatment for the patient.

D. Consult with a crisis intervention specialist or assertive community treatment (ACT) specialist if the patient needs closer follow-up in the community.

TABLE 17.1 U.S. FOOD AND DRUG ADMINISTRATION-APPROVED CONVENTIONAL ANTIPSYCHOTICS FOR TREATMENT OF PSYCHOTIC DISORDERS

Generic (Trade) Formulations	Maintenance Dose Range by Age/Renal/Hepatic Impairment Dosing	Pharmacokinetics
Chlorpromazine (Thorazine) Tablet: 10 mg, 25 mg, 50 mg, 100 mg, 200 mg Ampoule: 25 mg/mL	**Pediatrics:** Not approved **Adults (more than 18 years):** 200–800 mg/d **Renal impairment:** Use with caution **Hepatic impairment:** Use with caution	CYP450 metabolism: 2d6 Half-life: 8–33 hours Affected by food: No

Fluphenazine (Prolixin)
Tablet: 1 mg, 2.5 mg, 5 mg, 10 mg
Elixir: 2.5 mg/5 mL
Injection immediate-release: 2.5 mg/mL
Decanoate injection: 25 mg/mL
	Pediatrics: Not approved
	Adults (more than 18 years): 1–20 mg/d
	  Immediate-release injection: 1/3–1/2 oral dose
	  Decanoate injection: 12.5–100 mg every 2 weeks
	Renal impairment: Use with caution
	Hepatic impairment: Use with caution
		CYP450 metabolism: 2d6
		Half-life:
		  Oral: 15 hours
		  Injection: 6.8–9.6 days
		Affected by food: No

Haloperidol (Haldol)
Tablet: 0.5 mg, 1 mg, 2 mg, 5 mg, 10 mg, 20 mg
Immediate-release injection: 5 mg/mL
Decanoate injection: 50 mg, 100 mg
	Pediatrics: Not approved
	Adults (18–64): Tablet: 1–40 mg/d
	  Immediate-release injection: 2–5 mg/d
	  Decanoate injection: 10–15x previous daily dose of oral formulation, monthly injection
	Geriatrics (more than 65 years): Use lower doses
	Renal impairment: Use with caution
	Hepatic impairment: Use with caution
		CYP450 metabolism: 2d6 and 3a4
		Half-life:
		  Oral: 12–38 hours
		  Decanoate: 3 weeks
		Affected by food: No

Source: Data from Stahl, S. M. (2020). *Prescriber's guide: Stahl's essential psychopharmacology* (7th ed.). Cambridge University Press.

TABLE 17.2 U.S. FOOD AND DRUG ADMINISTRATION-APPROVED ATYPICAL ANTIPSYCHOTICS FOR TREATMENT OF PSYCHOTIC DISORDERS

Generic (Trade) Formulations	Maintenance Dose Range by Age/Renal/Hepatic Impairment Dosing	Pharmacokinetics
Aripiprazole (Abilify, Abilify Discmelt, Abilify MyCite) Tablet: 2 mg, 5 mg, 10 mg, 15 mg, 20 mg, 30 mg ODT: 10 mg, 15 mg Oral solution: 1 mg/mL	Pediatrics (13–17): 10–20 mg/d Adults (more than 18 years): 15–30 mg/d Renal impairment: No dose adjustment Hepatic impairment: No dose adjustment	CPY450 metabolism: 2D6 and 3A4 Half-life: 75 hours Affected by food: No

Aripiprazole lauroxil (Abilify Maintena, Aristada, Aristada Initio)
Aripiprazole injection (Abilify Maintena): 300 mg, 400 mg
Aripiprazole lauroxil injection (Aristada): 441 mg, 662 mg, 882 mg, 1,064 mg
Aripiprazole lauroxil injection (Aristada Initio): 675 mg injection
	Pediatrics: Not approved
	Adults (more than 18 years):
	  Abilify Maintena: 400 mg monthly
	  Aristada:
	    441 mg, 662 mg, 882 mg monthly
	    882 mg every 6 weeks
	    1,064 mg every 2 months
	  Aristada Initio: 675 mg used as single-dose injection only; to be administered with 30-mg tablet and first dose maintenance injection
	Renal impairment: No dose adjustment
	Hepatic impairment: No dose adjustment
		CPY450 metabolism: 2D6 and 3A4
		Half-life:
		  Abilify Maintena:
		    30 days for 300 mg
		    47 days for 400 mg
		  Aristada: 54–57 days
		Affected by food: No

Brexpiprazole (Rexulti)
Tablets: 0.25 mg, 0.5 mg, 1 mg, 2 mg, 3 mg, 4 mg
	Pediatrics (13–17): 2–4 mg/d
	Adults (18–64): Schizophrenia: 2–4 mg/d
	Geriatrics (more than 65 years): Max 3 mg/d
	Renal impairment: Max 3 mg/d
	Hepatic impairment: Max 3 mg/d
		CPY450 metabolism: 2D6 and 3A4
		Half-life:
		  Brexpiprazole: 91 hours
		  Metabolite DM-3411: 86 hours

Cariprazine (Vraylar)
Capsules: 1.5 mg, 3 mg, 4.5 mg, 6 mg
	Pediatrics: Not approved
	Adults (more than 18 years): Schizophrenia: 1.5–6 mg
	Renal impairment: Not recommended for severe impairment
	Hepatic impairment: Not recommended for severe impairment
		CPY450 metabolism: 3a4
		Half-life:
		  Cariprazine: 2–4 days
		  DDCAR: 1–3 weeks

Clozapine (Clozaril, Versacloz, Fazaclo) Tablet: 12.5 mg, 25 mg, 50 mg, 100 mg, 200 mg Orally disintegrating tablet: 12.5 mg, 25 mg, 50 mg, 100 mg, 150 mg, 200 mg Oral suspension: 50 mg/mL	Pediatrics: Not approved Adults (more than 18 years): 300–450 mg Renal impairment: Use with caution Hepatic impairment: Use with caution	CPY450 metabolism: 1a2, 2d6 (minor), 3a4 (minor) Half-life: 5–16 hours Affected by food: No
Iloperidone (Fanapt) Tablet: 1 mg, 2 mg, 4 mg, 6 mg, 8 mg, 10 mg, 12 mg	Pediatrics: Not approved Adults (more than 18 years): 12–24 mg/d Renal impairment: No adjustment Hepatic impairment: Not recommended	CPY450 metabolism: 2d6 and 3a4 Half-life: 18–33 hours Affected by food: No
Lumateperone (Caplyta) Capsule: 42 mg	Pediatrics: Not approved Adults (more than 18 years): 42 mg/d Renal impairment: No adjustment Hepatic impairment: Not recommended for moderate to severe impairment	CPY450 metabolism: 3a4 and 1a2 Half-life: 18 hours Affected by food: Yes

Lurasidone (Latuda)
Tablet: 20 mg, 40 mg, 60 mg, 80 mg, 120 mg
	Pediatrics (13–17): 40–80 mg
	Adults (more than 18 years): 40–80 mg
	Renal impairment: Moderate to severe impairment start with 20 mg/d, max of 80 mg/d
	Hepatic impairment:
	  Moderate impairment: Start with 20 mg/d, max of 80 mg/d
	  Severe impairment: Start with 20 mg/d, max of 40 mg/d
		CPY450 metabolism: 3a4
		Half-life: 18–31 hours
		Affected by food: Yes

Olanzapine (Zyprexa) Tablet: 2.5 mg, 5 mg, 7.5 mg, 10 mg, 15 mg, 20 mg ODT: 5 mg, 10 mg, 15 mg, 20 mg	Pediatrics (13–17): 10 mg/d Adults (more than 18 years): 10–20 mg/d Renal impairment: No adjustment Hepatic impairment: May need lower doses	CPY450 metabolism: 1a2 and 2d6 Half-life: 21–54 hours for IM solution Affected by food: No

(continued)

TABLE 17.2 U.S. FOOD AND DRUG ADMINISTRATION-APPROVED ATYPICAL ANTIPSYCHOTICS FOR TREATMENT OF PSYCHOTIC DISORDERS (CONTINUED)

Generic (Trade) Formulations	Maintenance Dose Range by Age/Renal/Hepatic Impairment Dosing	Pharmacokinetics

Olanzapine injection (Zyprexa Relprevv)
Short-acting injection: 10 mg/2mL
Zyprexa Relprevv: 210 mg, 300 mg, 405 mg
	Pediatrics: Not approved
	Adults (more than 18 years): Olanzapine short-acting injection: 2.5–10 mg/d
	Zyprexa Relprevv:
	  150–300 mg every 2 weeks
	  300–405 mg every 4 weeks
	Renal impairment: No adjustment
	Hepatic impairment: May need lower doses
		CPY450 metabolism: 1a2 and 2d6
		Half-life:
		  Olanzapine short-acting injection: 21–54 hours
		  Zyprexa Relprevv: 30 days
		Affected by food: No

Olanzapine-samidorphan (Lybalvi)
Capsule: 5 mg/10 mg, 10 mg/10 mg, 15 mg/10 mg, 20 mg/10 mg
	Pediatrics: Not approved
	Adults (more than 18 years): 5 mg/10 mg–20 mg/10 mg
	Renal impairment: No adjustment
	Hepatic impairment: No adjustment
		CPY450 metabolism: 1a2 and 3a4
		Half-life:
		  Olanzapine: 35–52 hours
		  Samidorphan: 7–11 hours
		Affected by food: No

Paliperidone (Invega)
Tablet: 1.5 mg, 3 mg, 6 mg, 9 mg
	Pediatrics (12–17):
	  3–6 mg/d (weight less than 51 kg)
	  3–12 mg/d (weight more than 50 kg)
	Adults (more than 18 years): 6 mg
	Renal impairment:
	  Mild: Max 6 mg/d
	  Moderate and severe: 3 mg/d
	Hepatic impairment: No adjustment
		CPY450 metabolism: 2d6
		Half-life: 23 hours
		Affected by food: Yes

Paliperidone palmitate (Invega Sustenna, Invega Trinza, Invega Hafyera)
Invega Sustenna extended-release injectable solution: 39 mg, 78 mg, 117 mg, 156 mg
Invega Trinza extended-release injectable solution: 273 mg, 410 mg, 546 mg, 819 mg
Invega Hafyera extended-release injectable solution: 1,092 mg, 1,560 mg
	Pediatrics: Not approved
	Adults (more than 18 years):
	  Invega Sustenna: 117 mg/mo
	  Invega Trinza: 273–819 mg/3 mo
	  Invega Hafyera: 1,092–1,560 mg
	Renal impairment: Moderate to severe (GFR less than 50), not recommended
	Hepatic impairment: No adjustment
		CPY450 metabolism: 2d6 and 3a4
		Half-life
		  Invega Sustenna: 25–49 days
		  Invega Trinza: Deltoid 84–95 days; gluteal 118–139 days
		  Invega Hafyera: 148–159 days
		Affected by food: No

Quetiapine (Seroquel, Seroquel XR) Tablet: 25 mg, 50 mg, 100 mg, 150 mg, 200 mg, 300 mg, 400 mg Extended-release tablet: 50 mg, 150 mg, 200 mg, 300 mg, 400 mg	**Pediatrics (13–17):** 400–800 mg/d **Adults (more than 18 years):** 400–800 mg/d **Renal impairment:** No adjustment **Hepatic impairment:** May need lower doses	**CPY450 metabolism:** 3a4 **Half-life:** 6–7 hours **Affected by food:** May cause mild increase in absorption
Risperidone (Risperdal) Tablet: 0.25 mg, 0.5 mg, 1 mg, 2 mg, 3 mg, 4 mg, 6 mg ODT: 0.5 mg, 1 mg, 2 mg, 3 mg, 4 mg Liquid: 1 mg/mL	**Pediatrics (13–17):** 0.5–2 mg/d **Adults (18–64):** 2–8 mg/d **Geriatric (more than 65 years):** 0.5–2 mg/d **Renal impairment:** Dose should be reduced **Hepatic impairment:** Dose should be reduced	**CPY450 metabolism:** 2d6 **Half-life:** 20–24 hours **Affected by food:** No

Risperidone (Consta, Perseris)
Consta injection: 12.5 mg, 25 mg, 37.5 mg, 50 mg
Perseris injection: 90 mg, 120 mg
	Pediatrics: Not approved
	Adults (more than 65 years):
	  Consta: 12.5–50 mg every 2 weeks
	  Perseris: 90 or 120 once a month
	Renal impairment: First carefully titrate with oral risperidone
	Hepatic impairment: First carefully titrate with oral risperidone
		CPY450 metabolism: 2d6
		Half-life:
		  Consta: 3–6 days
		  Perseris: 4–6 hours and 10–14 days
		Affected by food: No

Ziprasidone (Geodon)
Capsule: 20 mg, 40 mg, 60 mg, 80 mg
Injection: 20 mg/mL
	Pediatrics: Not approved
	Adults:
	  Tablet: 40–200 mg/d
	  Injection: 10–20 mg/d
	Renal impairment: No adjustment
	Hepatic impairment: No adjustment
		CPY450 metabolism: 3a4
		Half-life
		  Tablet: 6–8 hours
		  Injection: 2–5 hours
		Affected by food: Yes

DDCAR, didesmethyl-cariprazine; GFR, glomerular filtration rate; IM, intramuscularly; ODT, orally disintegrating tablet.

Source: Data from Stahl, S. M. (2020). *Prescriber's guide: Stahl's essential psychopharmacology* (7th ed.). Cambridge University Press.

INDIVIDUAL CONSIDERATIONS

Pediatrics
A. Educate parents, teachers, and siblings on the signs and symptoms of brief psychotic disorders, and report concerns to the school nurse, pediatrician, or APRN for further evaluation.
B. Although the prevalence of brief psychotic disorders is low in the pediatric population, it is essential to be vigilant of any acute changes in behavior, speech, and ability to complete independent activities of daily living (ADLs).

Pregnancy
A. Pregnancy is considered a high-risk time for women. In the 4 months postpartum, women have a high risk of brief psychotic episodes and should be carefully monitored for signs of psychosis. During the peripartum period, some women may have hallucinations telling them to hurt or kill the baby, or have visual hallucinations about the baby having a deformed body part.
B. Educate the family, the spouse, and the patient on the signs and symptoms of psychosis and what to report to the APRN.

Geriatrics
A. Older adults may have multiple medical comorbidities and take several medications that can induce brief psychotic episodes.
B. The APRN should educate healthcare givers and spouses on the signs and symptoms of psychosis and what to report to the healthcare providers.

Partners/Family
A. Psychoeducation of partners and family is pivotal to positive outcomes in treating brief psychotic episodes. The APRN should discuss during office visits the treatment plan options, medications, and nonpharmacologic options, as well as the importance of reporting acute changes in behavior, speech, or inability to carry out independent activities of daily life.
B. Partners and family should be encouraged to participate in activities with the patients and maintain fluid communication with the APRN to assist the patient in recovery.

RESOURCES
A. Early Assessment and Support Alliance (EASA): www.easacommunity.org
B. National Alliance on Mental Illness (NAMI): www.nami.org
C. Prodrome and Early Psychosis Program Network (PEPPNET): https://med.stanford.edu/peppnet.html

REFERENCES AND BIBLIOGRAPHY
American Psychiatric Association. (2013). *Diagnostic and statistical manual of mental disorders* (5th ed.). https://doi.org/10.1176/appi.books.9780890425596

Catalan, A., Salazar de Pablo, G., Vaquerizo Serrano, J., Mosillo, P., Baldwin, H., Fernández-Rivas, A., Moreno, C., Arango, C., Correll, C. U., Bonoldi, I., & Fusar-Poli, P. (2020). Annual research review: Prevention of psychosis in adolescents—systematic review and meta-analysis of advances in detection, prognosis and intervention. *Journal of Child Psychology and Psychiatry*, 62(5), 657–673. https://doi.org/10.1111/jcpp.13322

Fusar-Poli, P., Salazar de Pablo, G., Rajkumar, R. P., López-Díaz, L., Malhotra, S., Heckers, S., Lawrie, S. M., & Pillmann, F. (2022). Diagnosis, prognosis, and treatment of brief psychotic episodes: A review and research agenda. *The Lancet Psychiatry*, 9(1), 72–83. https://doi.org/10.1016/s2215-0366(21)00121-8

Griswold, K. S. (2015, June 15). Recognition and differential diagnosis of psychosis in primary care. *American Family Physician*, 91(12), 856–863. https://www.aafp.org/pubs/afp/issues/2015/0615/p856.html

Hull, M. (2023, June 11). *Psychosis & psychotic disorder statistics*. The Recovery Village. https://www.therecoveryvillage.com/mental-health/psychosis/psychosis-statistics

National Institute of Mental Health. (n.d.). *Understanding psychosis*. https://www.nimh.nih.gov/health/publications/understanding-psychosis

Provenzani, U., Salazar de Pablo, G., Arribas, M., Pillmann, F., & Fusar-Poli, P. (2021). Clinical outcomes in brief psychotic episodes: A systematic review and meta-analysis. *Epidemiology and Psychiatric Sciences*, 30, Article e71. https://doi.org/10.1017/s2045796021000548

Riches, S., Pisani, S., Bird, L., Rus-Calafell, M., Garety, P., & Valmaggia, L. (2021). Virtual reality-based assessment and treatment of social functioning impairments in psychosis: A systematic review. *International Review of Psychiatry*, 33(3), 337–362. https://doi.org/10.1080/09540261.2021.1918648

Smith, C. M., Komisar, J. R., Mourad, A., & Kincaid, B. R. (2020). COVID-19-associated brief psychotic disorder. *BMJ Case Reports*, 13(8), e236940. https://doi.org/10.1136/bcr-2020-236940

Stephen, A., & Lui, F. (2023, June 25). *Brief psychotic disorder*. StatPearls Publishing. https://www.ncbi.nlm.nih.gov/books/NBK539912

Sullivan, S. A., Kounali, D., Cannon, M., David, A. S., Fletcher, P. C., Holmans, P., Jones, H., Jones, P. B., Linden, D. E., Lewis, G., Owen, M. J., O'Donovan, M., Rammos, A., Thompson, A., Wolke, D., Heron, J., & Zammit, S. (2020). A population-based cohort study examining the incidence and impact of psychotic experiences from childhood to adulthood, and prediction of psychotic disorder. *American Journal of Psychiatry*, 177(4), 308–317. https://doi.org/10.1176/appi.ajp.2019.19060654

World Health Organization. (2023). *ICD-10-CM diagnosis code F23: Brief psychotic disorder*. ICD10Data. https://www.icd10data.com/ICD10CM/Codes/F01-F99/F20-F29/F23-/F23

Zakhari, R. (2020). *The psychiatric-mental health nurse practitioner certification review manual*. Springer Publishing Company.

DELUSIONAL DISORDER

DEFINITION
A. Delusions are false beliefs despite evidence to the contrary. These beliefs are fixed based on erroneous interpretations of what reality presents.
B. The individual must have at least 1 month of reporting and/or experiencing delusion(s), but no other psychotic symptom should be present.
C. People diagnosed with delusional disorder can function and lead productive lives compared with those diagnosed with psychotic disorders such as schizophrenia.
D. In some cases, the delusion may interfere to a greater degree in their occupational and social functioning.
  1. The functional impairment is closely related to the delusion and manifested in overt psychotic symptoms.
E. The delusional disorder can occur in younger individuals; however, this disorder is more prevalent in older individuals.
F. Different types of delusions can be used as the basis for diagnosis. A delusional disorder diagnosis is made when a person reports at least one of the types of delusions. Most delusions are perceived misconceptions of reality; however, some can be a minimal deviation from reality. Some cultural practices and beliefs may accentuate the delusion content; however, delusions do not significantly affect the level of functioning of a person. The person can express delusions for a month or more. There are no other culprits after ruling out substance-induced, physiologic, medical, or mental conditions.
G. Other criteria used for diagnosis include ruling out schizophrenia and if there are reported hallucinations related to the delusion.
H. Some psychotic disorders might be caused by a medical condition or the use of substances or medications. In these

cases, the APRN should review the history in detail and complete an exhaustive assessment of the current presentation.
  1. In cases where a substance or medication causes suspicion, the agent should be discontinued or removed from the patient's medication regimen, and the patient should be closely monitored.
  2. In cases of psychosis due to a medical condition, an interprofessional collaboration with the primary care provider should be established, and the physiologic consequences of such a medical condition should be treated.
I. Some people suffering from psychotic disorders might have cognitive impairments leading to declining independent functioning.
J. The most commonly reported delusions include the following:
  1. Delusions of jealousy: belief that one's partner, spouse, or lover is unfaithful
  2. Erotomanic delusion: belief that another person is in love with the person; most commonly reported that famous people artist is in love with the person
  3. Grandiose delusions: belief that the person is famous, intelligent, rich, and has incredible talent
  4. Persecutory delusions: belief that someone is out to get them, that they are being surveilled, and that someone is conspiring against them
  5. Somatic delusions: belief that something in their body is sick or not functioning
  6. Thought broadcasting: belief that others hear their thoughts
  7. Bizarre delusions: belief that the impossible has occurred ("Someone took my internal organs and replaced them with computer chips to monitor me."); no evidence, no bruises, surgical incisions, or scars
  8. Thought insertion: belief that an external force is inserting their thoughts

INCIDENCE
A. According to *DSM-5* (American Psychiatric Association, 2013a), the prevalence of delusional disorder is about 0.2% and is much rarer compared with other thought disorders such as schizophrenia.
B. It is believed that people suffering from delusional disorder can generally function despite delusions and do not seek mental healthcare unless they exhibit other symptoms.
C. The most commonly reported delusion is persecutory.
D. There are no significant gender differences in the overall frequency of the delusional disorder.
  1. Women commonly report erotomanic delusions, while men report delusions of jealousy and persecutory types.
  2. Premenopausal women have more erotomanic delusions than postmenopausal women who suffer from jealousy and somatic delusions.
E. Cultural backgrounds should be considered as those that might influence the content of the delusions.

PATHOGENESIS
A. Delusional disorders have a later onset, with a mean age of onset at 40 years; however, diagnosis may range from 18 to 90 years of age. The delusional disorder directly affects the limbic system and basal ganglia; however, some delusions can be caused by medical and neurologic conditions and substances.
B. Delusional disorders are also related to the dysregulation of dopamine in the midbrain. People with delusional disorders can function well, presenting with some preoccupation and normal psychological functioning unless talking about their specific delusion.

PREDISPOSING FACTORS
A. Family history of psychosis
B. Personality disorder
C. Substance use
D. Immigrants who have language barriers
E. Older adults diagnosed with dementia
F. Individuals who are deaf or visually impaired
G. No access to healthcare services
H. People residing in rural areas
I. Member of a minority group
J. Low level of education
K. Gender (women may depend on their spouse for financial support and transportation)
L. Cultural beliefs

COMMON COMPLAINTS
A. "I am a member of royalty and do not deserve to be here."
B. "The FBI planted chips inside my head to experiment with me."
C. "I cannot trust my husband/boyfriend because he cheats on me."
D. A postmenopausal woman is reporting a pregnancy.

OTHER SIGNS AND SYMPTOMS
A. Labile behavior if confronted about the delusion
B. Consistently holding grudges based on delusion
C. Preoccupation with being contaminated and having an incurable disease
D. Persistent refusal of treatment changes due to a lack of insight into the illness
E. Treatment and medication nonadherence

SUBJECTIVE DATA
A. See "Subjective Data" in the "Schizophrenia" section.

PHYSICAL EXAMINATION
A. See "Physical Examination" in the "Schizophrenia" section.
B. See "Psychometric Tools" in the "Schizoaffective Disorder" section.
C. Ask if the delusion has been present for over 1 month.
D. Rule out other causes of the delusional disorder.

DIAGNOSTIC TESTS AND SCREENING
A. See "Diagnostic Tests and Screening" in the "Schizophrenia" section.
B. See "Psychometric Tools" in the "Schizoaffective Disorder" section.
C. Consider CT, and MRI, if applicable, to rule out an organic cause of the delusion.

DIFFERENTIAL DIAGNOSES
A. Obsessive-compulsive disorder
B. Delirium—major neurocognitive disorder
C. Psychotic disorder due to another medical condition
D. Substance/medication-induced psychotic disorder
E. Schizophrenia and schizophreniform disorder
F. Depression with psychotic features
G. Bipolar disorder
H. Schizoaffective disorder

PLAN

General Treatments and Interventions

A. See "General Treatments and Interventions" in the "Brief Psychotic Disorder" section.

B. The APRN should prepare a comprehensive treatment plan to address the delusional disorder and problems with the patient's lack of insight and possible resistance to treatment. Other considerations for biological, physical, and psychological differences in response to treatment modalities are related to sex and gender. General treatment and interventions should include the following:

1. Initiate a therapeutic conversation with the patient by using clinical skills such as discussing issues (delusions), addressing the purpose of the discussion, and finalizing the list of recommendations. Establishing rapport with the patient, providing empathic listening, and emphasizing the importance of working together in the treatment plan are essential.
2. Psychotherapy using the CBT modality has been demonstrated to be effective in reducing the frequency of delusions. CBT is more effective than supportive counseling.
3. The APRN should review all the laboratory results and other tests, including the mental status examination (MSE), and complete the physical.
4. Educate the patient on the signs and symptoms and how the clinician came to a diagnosis. Discuss the treatment modalities, including pharmacotherapies and psychotherapy.
5. Discuss the importance of safety and create a safety plan. If there are safety concerns, it is recommended that the patient be admitted for stabilization.
6. Discuss the prognosis, emphasizing the importance of treatment adherence. The prognosis is approximately 50% of patients responding positively to pharmacotherapy and at least 20% of those patients reporting a decrease in symptoms. The overall prognosis is favorable when the patient has a higher level of education and occupational functioning.
7. Use the Clinician-Rated Dimensions of Psychosis Symptom Severity. This scale assists clinicians in assessing patients with primary symptoms of psychosis.

COMMON MEDICATIONS

A. Pharmacologic treatment with antipsychotic medications (see Tables 17.1 and 17.2)

PATIENT TEACHING

A. Educate patient about the signs and symptoms of delusional disorders.
B. Discuss the consequences of untreated delusions, such as legal issues for people with an erotomanic delusion or a persecutory delusion.
C. Discuss potential barriers to treatment due to the delusion and mistrust of others.
D. Discuss the importance of family involvement and social support to assist the patient with the recovery process.
E. Discuss treatment modalities and their risks versus benefits.
F. Educate on medication side effects.

FOLLOW-UP

A. If the patient is treated in the community, the APRN should schedule an initial follow-up visit 2 weeks after the initiation of treatment. This visit is to review/update the treatment plan and monitor the patient's clinical progress.
B. If the patient was discharged from the hospital, the patient should be seen as soon as possible to discuss the treatment plan, review medication and nonpharmacologic treatment, and discuss continued care with the APRN.
C. After the initial follow-up visit, the patient should be seen every 4 to 6 weeks for continued monitoring of symptoms and possible changes or adjustments to the treatment regimen.

CONSULTATION AND REFERRALS

A. It is recommended that the proposed treatment has input from an interdisciplinary team. The APRN can consult with a psychologist, a neurologist, primary care providers, and social workers to ensure that a solid treatment plan is prepared for the patient. Any referrals to services not provided by the APRN or other specialties should be initiated as needed.

INDIVIDUAL CONSIDERATIONS

Pediatrics

A. Although delusional disorders are not common in this population, educating the parents, teachers, and others in the patient's support system on the signs and symptoms of delusion and what to report to the psychiatric nurse practitioner is essential.
B. Educate on the importance of maintaining safe environments.
C. Educate on the importance of monitoring activities and maintaining a healthy lifestyle where all physiologic and psychological needs are met.

Pregnancy

A. Pregnancy can be a risk factor for some patients as they can suffer from postpartum psychosis, putting at risk the safety of the mother or the baby or the safety of both.
B. Some patients, after having a miscarriage, might develop a delusion of pregnancy, although they are no longer pregnant. Educating the patient, their partner, and other treatment providers on the binding effect of providing support to the patient is essential.

Geriatrics/Older Adults

A. The APRN should educate the patient and all caregivers on the signs and symptoms of delusions and what to report to the APRN.
B. Educate on the importance of monitoring ADLs, including that all physiologic and psychological needs are met. The older adult should be eating, sleeping, maintaining hygiene, and adhering to any treatment regimen they may have.
C. Older adults are at high risk of delusional disorders that can be confused with delirium due to medications or a medical condition.
D. Discuss safety planning.

Partners/Family

A. The support system, such as partners and family, is pivotal to patient monitoring, treatment planning, and recovery. It is essential to educate them on the signs and symptoms of the delusional disorder, the treatment modalities, the objectives of treatment, and what to report to the APRN.
B. Discuss cultural beliefs and how those can affect the patient or can be misinterpreted by other cultures.

RESOURCE

A. *Mental health.* (2019, December 19). www.who.int/health-topics/mental-health

REFERENCES AND BIBLIOGRAPHY

American Psychiatric Association. (2013a). Diagnostic and statistical manual of mental disorders (5th ed.). https://doi.org/10.1176/appi.books.9780890425596

American Psychiatric Association. (2013b). *Desk reference to the diagnostic criteria from DSM-5*. American Psychiatric Association Publishing.

Delusional disorder: Causes, symptoms, types & treatment. (n.d.). Cleveland Clinic. https://my.clevelandclinic.org/health/diseases/9599-delusional-disorder

González-Rodríguez, A., Esteve, M., Álvarez, A., Guàrdia, A., Monreal, J. A., Palao, D., & Labad, J. (2019). What we know and still need to know about gender aspects of delusional disorder: A narrative review of recent work. *Journal of Psychiatry and Brain Science, 17*(12), 4583. https://doi.org/10.20900/jpbs.20190009

González-Rodríguez, A., & Seeman, M. V. (2020). Addressing delusions in women and men with delusional disorder: Key points for clinical management. *International Journal of Environmental Research and Public Health, 17*(12), 4583. https://doi.org/10.3390/ijerph17124583

Joseph, S. M., & Siddiqui, W. (2023, March 27). *Delusional disorder*. StatPearls Publishing. https://pubmed.ncbi.nlm.nih.gov/30969677

Joyce, E. M. (2018). Organic psychosis: The pathobiology and treatment of delusions. *CNS Neuroscience & Therapeutics, 24*(7), 598–603. https://doi.org/10.1111/cns.12973

PSYCHOTIC DISORDER DUE TO ANOTHER MEDICAL CONDITION

DEFINITION

A. Psychotic disorders due to another medical condition have specific criteria for diagnosis.
  1. Evident psychotic symptoms include hallucinations or delusions.
  2. There is evidence that psychotic symptoms are a consequence of another medical condition.
  3. Another mental disorder does not better explain the psychotic disorder.
  4. The psychotic symptoms are not occurring concurrently with delirium.
  5. The psychotic symptoms cause impairment in functioning and occupational, social, and significant distress to the patient.

INCIDENCE

A. The prevalence of psychotic disorders due to another medical condition is estimated from 0.21% to 0.54%. Adults older than 65 years of age have a higher prevalence of 0.74% due to medical comorbidities and taking several prescribed medications.
B. For people with specific medical comorbidities, such as metabolic, autoimmune disorders, and temporal lobe epilepsy, there is evidence of a higher prevalence of psychosis.
C. Individuals suffering from traumatic brain injuries, brain tumors, thyroid disease, central nervous system conditions, autoimmune disorders, and epilepsy are at higher risk of developing psychotic symptoms. People with epilepsy have approximately 7% risk of experiencing psychotic disorders.

PATHOGENESIS

A. The psychotic disorder due to another medical condition is due to changes in brain function and neurotransmitter pathways connectivity that are associated with the primary medical condition.
B. Various medical conditions can interfere with normal functioning, leading to behavioral changes and psychotic symptoms such as hallucinations and delusions.
C. Neurotransmitters such as dopamine, glutamate, N-methyl-d-aspartate (NMDA), gamma-aminobutyric acid (GABA), and acetylcholine play roles in psychotic disorders.
D. Chronic medical conditions may predispose an individual to have psychotic episodes, with recurrence depending on the course of the medical condition.

PREDISPOSING FACTORS

A. Dementia
B. Epilepsy
C. Huntington disease
D. Multiple sclerosis
E. Stroke
F. HIV/AIDS
G. Lupus
H. Advanced age
I. Endocrine disorders
J. Lyme disease
K. Alcohol and other substance use

COMMON COMPLAINTS

A. Depressed mood
B. Increased anxiety
C. Mood lability with periods of anger and agitation
D. Insomnia
E. Increased suspiciousness

OTHER SIGNS AND SYMPTOMS

A. Reported hallucinations
B. Verbalized delusions
C. Forgetfulness
D. Acute change in behavior or cognition
E. Acute change in vital signs, including blood pressure and temperature

SUBJECTIVE DATA

A. See "Subjective Data" in the "Schizophrenia" section.
B. Patient also exhibits inability to care for self and loss of independence.

PHYSICAL EXAMINATION

A. See "Physical Examination" in the "Schizophrenia" section.
B. Review the complete list of medications, including OTC agents.

DIAGNOSTIC TESTS AND SCREENING

A. Similar to schizophrenia (see "Diagnostic Tests and Screening" in the "Schizophrenia" section)
B. HIV
C. CT, MRI, EEG
D. Lumbar puncture
E. Rheumatology or immunologic workup

DIFFERENTIAL DIAGNOSES

A. Delirium
B. Psychotic disorder
C. Substance/medication-induced psychotic disorder

PLAN

General Treatment and Interventions

A. Identifying the underlying medical condition causing the psychotic symptoms is critical before initiating any treatment.
B. Antipsychotic medications are the gold standard for treatment of psychosis; however, the clinician must review for potential drug–drug interactions.
C. CBT and group therapy are also crucial in treating psychosis due to a medical condition.

D. The APRN should complete an exhaustive review of the patient's medical records and consult and collaborate with the patient's primary care provider.
E. The APRN should order tests and laboratory work to rule out the causes of psychotic symptoms.
F. Educate the patient, family, and other caretakers on the signs and symptoms of psychotic disorders due to a medical condition.
G. Discuss the treatment modalities, including close monitoring of symptoms, safety, and any other acute changes in behavior or symptomatology.
H. Prepare a safety plan that might include inpatient admission for initiation of treatment, order tests, and taper medications if applicable.

COMMON MEDICATIONS
A. The pharmacologic modality used to treat psychosis due to another medical condition is selected based on the treatment of the underlying medical condition before attempting to control the psychosis. Upon resolution of the underlying medical condition that caused the psychotic symptoms and treatment necessary for continued psychosis, the use of psychotropic medications can be considered (see Tables 17.1 and 17.2). The use of benzodiazepines, antidepressants, and antipsychotic medications is available to treat psychosis.

PATIENT TEACHING
A. The patient should be educated on the signs and symptoms of psychosis due to medical conditions and what to report to the psychiatric nurse practitioner.
B. The patient should be educated on the treatment modalities, the risks versus the benefits of such modalities, the importance of medication, and adherence.

FOLLOW-UP
A. The patient should be seen soon after discharge from the hospital. If seen in the community, an initial visit is to complete a comprehensive intake and start planning the treatment.
B. After the intake visit, the patient should be seen weekly if medications were started to review clinical progress and titrate medications.
C. The subsequent visit should be every 3 to 4 weeks, as applicable.
D. The safety plan should be reviewed on every visit with the clinician.

CONSULTATION AND REFERRALS
A. The psychiatric-mental health nurse practitioner (PMHNP) should actively involve the patient's primary care provider and other providers of healthcare services and initiate referrals as appropriate.

INDIVIDUAL CONSIDERATIONS
Pediatrics
A. It may be pertinent to educate the patient and their family on the signs and symptoms of psychosis due to another medical condition and when to report them to the healthcare provider, although this is not prevalent in this population.

Pregnancy
A. Pregnancy can be a risk factor for developing psychosis. The patient and their family should be educated on the signs and symptoms and when to report them to the APRN.

Geriatrics/Older Adults
A. Older adults are at high risk of suffering from psychotic episodes due to medical conditions and should be closely monitored.

Partners/Family
A. Partners and family are essential elements to consider during treatment planning and serve as allies while treating patients suffering from psychosis due to medical conditions. They should be educated on the signs and symptoms and what to report to the psychiatric nurse practitioner.

REFERENCES AND BIBLIOGRAPHY
Calabrese, J., Al Khalili, Y. (2023, May 1). *Psychosis*. StatPearls Publishing. https://www.ncbi.nlm.nih.gov/books/NBK546579
Freudenreich, O. (2012, December 3). *Differential diagnosis of psychotic symptoms: Medical "Mimics."* Psychiatric Times. https://www.psychiatrictimes.com/view/differential-diagnosis-psychotic-symptoms-medical-mimics
National Institute of Mental Health. (n.d.). *Understanding psychosis*. https://www.nimh.nih.gov/health/publications/understanding-psychosis
Psychology Today. (2021, October 5). Psychotic disorder due to another medical condition. https://www.psychologytoday.com/us/conditions/psychotic-disorder-due-another-medical-condition
Psychosis. (n.d.). Cleveland Clinic. https://my.clevelandclinic.org/health/symptoms/23012-psychosis

SCHIZOAFFECTIVE DISORDER
DEFINITION
A. Schizoaffective disorder is a chronic, serious mental health illness with features of schizophrenia and a mood disorder.
B. The individual may experience symptoms of schizophrenia concurrently with symptoms of a major depressive or manic episode.
C. There are two subtypes of schizoaffective disorder: schizoaffective bipolar type and schizoaffective depressive type.
D. Treatment usually involves medications and therapy.
E. Refer to the *DSM-5* (American Psychiatric Association, 2013) for diagnostic criteria.

INCIDENCE
A. The lifetime prevalence of schizoaffective disorder is approximately 0.3%.
B. The age of onset for schizoaffective disorder is usually during early adulthood, with males developing the disorder at an earlier age than female individuals.
C. Males and females seem to be affected equally by this disorder.
D. It has been suggested that schizoaffective disorder bipolar type is more common in younger adults than the depressive type. Conversely, the depressive type may be more common in older adults when compared with younger adults.
E. Diagnosis is often delayed due to first being diagnosed with schizophrenia or a mood disorder.

PATHOGENESIS
A. As in schizophrenia, the etiology of schizoaffective disorder is not well-understood and is thought to be multifactorial.
B. Genetics, environmental factors, neurobiology, and brain structure also seem to play a role in the etiology of schizoaffective disorder (see "Pathogenesis" in the "Schizophrenia" section).

C. Progressive functional consequences in schizoaffective disorder are variable, as with schizophrenia.
D. When compared with schizophrenia, the schizoaffective disorder has a better prognosis, but not when compared with mood disorders.

PREDISPOSING FACTORS
A. Family history of schizophrenia, schizoaffective, and mood disorder in first-degree relatives
B. Prenatal and perinatal adverse events
  1. Prematurity
  2. Low birth weight/fetal malnutrition
  3. Perinatal hypoxic events
  4. Infections during pregnancy
C. Social adversities
  1. History of trauma: emotional abuse, physical abuse, sexual abuse, neglect, bullying
  2. Low socioeconomic status
  3. Living in overcrowded urban areas
  4. Belonging to a migrant group
  5. Drug use: cannabis use in adolescence

COMMON COMPLAINTS
A. Auditory hallucinations
B. Delusions
C. Disorganized thinking
D. Memory problems
E. Impaired attention
F. Anhedonia
G. Low mood
H. Sleep problems

OTHER SIGNS AND SYMPTOMS
A. Positive symptoms such as delusions, hallucinations, disorganized speech, and/or disorganized behavior, including catatonia
B. Negative symptoms (typically begin before positive symptoms)
  1. Blunted affect: diminished range of emotions
  2. Alogia: poverty of speech
  3. Anhedonia: decreased ability to experience pleasure
  4. Apathy/social withdrawal
  5. Avolition: decreased ability to perform goal-oriented tasks
C. Cognitive symptoms (typically present before positive symptoms)
  1. Prioritizing tasks/planning
  2. Working memory
  3. Focusing and sustaining attention
  4. Working memory
  5. Self-regulation
  6. Problem-solving
D. Depressive symptoms (may be present before positive symptoms)
  1. Depressed mood
  2. Feelings of guilt or worthlessness
  3. Changes in weight or appetite
  4. Fatigue
E. Psychomotor retardation
F. Suicidal ideation
G. Manic symptoms (may be present before positive symptoms)
  1. Grandiosity
  2. Talkative/pressured speech
  3. Distractibility
  4. Racing thoughts
  5. Psychomotor agitation/goal-directed activity
  6. Risky behavior (e.g., sexual activity, gambling, buying sprees, substance use)

SUBJECTIVE DATA
A. Review past psychiatric history, including hospitalizations and outpatient treatment, especially if there is any history of a mood disorder.
B. See "Subjective Data" in the "Schizophrenia" section.

PHYSICAL EXAMINATION
A. See "Physical Examination" in the "Schizophrenia" section.

DIAGNOSTIC TESTS AND SCREENING
A. Complete blood cell (CBC) count with differential
B. Comprehensive metabolic panel (CMP)
C. Thyroid function
D. Urine drug screen
E. Blood alcohol
F. Vitamin B_{12} and vitamin D levels
G. Pregnancy test for patients of childbearing age
H. EKG (baseline EKG recommended before starting some psychotropic medications)

Psychometric Tools
A. Clinical Global Impression for Schizoaffective Disorder Scale (CGI-SCA): The CGI-SCA is used to assess the severity of illness and the degree of change in schizoaffective disorder.
B. Positive and Negative Syndrome Scale (PANSS): The PANSS is used for rating positive and negative symptoms in schizophrenia.
C. Brief Psychiatric Rating Scale (BPRS): The BPRS is used to measure symptoms of psychosis, depression, and anxiety.
D. Calgary Depression Scale for Schizophrenia (CDSS): The CDSS is used to assess depression in individuals with schizophrenia.
E. Patient Health Questionnaire-9 (PHQ-9): The PHQ-9 is used to screen and track symptoms of depression.
F. Young Mania Rating Scale (YMRS): The YMRS is used to rate the severity of mania symptoms.
G. Rapid Mood Screener (RMS): The RMS is used to screen for bipolar I disorder.

DIFFERENTIAL DIAGNOSES
A. Delusional disorder
B. Schizophreniform disorder/brief psychotic disorder
C. Schizophrenia
D. Bipolar disorder
E. Major depressive disorder
F. Schizotypal personality disorder
G. Substance-induced psychotic disorder
H. Psychotic disorder due to another medical condition
I. Obsessive-compulsive disorder
J. Posttraumatic stress disorder (PTSD)/complex PTSD
K. Autism spectrum disorder

PLAN

General Treatment and Interventions
A. The management of schizoaffective disorder includes pharmacologic and nonpharmacologic treatment modalities. These treatments should be person-centered, based on the individual's clinical presentation and severity of symptoms,

disorder type (depressive, bipolar), biological markers, and personal preferences.
   1. See "General Treatment and Interventions" in the "Schizophrenia" section.
   2. Nonpharmacologic treatments: See nonpharmacologic treatments in the "Schizophrenia" section.
   3. Pharmacologic treatments: Schizoaffective disorder is a chronic illness that may require the lifelong use of medications to control symptoms. Pharmacologic treatment of the schizoaffective disorder is primarily composed of three types of medications: antipsychotics, mood stabilizers, and antidepressants (Tables 17.1 and 17.2).

COMMON MEDICATIONS
A. Currently, the only medication approved by the U.S. Food and Drug Administration (FDA) for treatment of schizoaffective disorder is paliperidone. Nevertheless, a combination of antipsychotics, mood stabilizers, and antidepressants is frequently prescribed off-label to treat symptoms of schizoaffective disorder (see Tables 17.1 and 17.2, or refer to *Prescriber's Digital Reference* [PDR]).

PATIENT TEACHING
A. Provide patient and family psychoeducation. Provide written patient education material on topics that were covered, including the following:
   1. Definition of schizoaffective disorder
   2. Symptoms of schizoaffective disorder
   3. Pathogenesis
   4. Treatment modalities
   5. Addressing adherence issues
   6. Lifestyle modifications, including nutrition and exercise
   7. When to seek help, along with important numbers to call when help is needed

FOLLOW-UP
A. Follow-up care for individuals with schizoaffective disorder should include a patient-centered approach. It is recommended that the psychiatric nurse practitioner incorporate comprehensive assessments, medication management, and supportive therapy during follow-up visits.
B. Assess treatment efficacy using psychometric tools (see "Psychometric Tools").
C. Monitor for medication side effects, including metabolic syndrome and abnormal movements.
D. Conduct metabolic syndrome screening and monitoring at baseline, at 4 months, and then yearly after starting treatment.
E. Order and review the results of a fasting blood glucose or hemoglobin A1c, comprehensive lipid panel, blood pressure, and waist circumference.
F. Assess for abnormal movements every visit, including akathisia, drug-induced parkinsonism, and dystonia. Use the Abnormal Involuntary Movement Scale (AIMS) to assess for tardive dyskinesia at baseline and then at least every 6 to 12 months depending on risk level.
G. Assess for treatment adherence at every visit. Review and update treatment plan as needed.
H. Schedule clinical visits monthly once the individual is stabilized.

CONSULTATION AND REFERRALS
A. Coordinate care and consult with an interprofessional team including primary care, specialty, social work, and case management services.
B. Consult or refer the individual to psychiatry subspecialists (e.g., addiction, neuropsychiatry, perinatal, liaison, forensic psychiatry) if warranted.
C. Refer the individual to a higher level of care during periods of decompensation that cannot be managed in the outpatient behavioral health setting. The services can include the Comprehensive Psychiatric Emergency Program (CPEP) and Mobile Crisis Outreach.
D. Refer the individual to case management and community-based services that support recovery and address problems with social determinants of health (e.g., ACT program).

INDIVIDUAL CONSIDERATIONS
Pediatrics
A. Schizoaffective disorder is mostly diagnosed in early adulthood, but it can also occur in adolescence.
B. Negative and cognitive symptoms of schizoaffective disorder can be observed in late adolescence during the premorbid and prodromal period of schizoaffective disorder, much the same as in schizophrenia disorder.
C. Individuals may also present with mood disorder symptoms in adolescence before they exhibit positive symptoms.
D. There are no FDA-approved medications to manage symptoms of schizoaffective disorder in the pediatric population. Antipsychotics, mood stabilizers, and antidepressants are used off-label much in the same way as with the adult population.

Pregnancy
A. Pregnancy can make schizoaffective symptoms worse. This is particularly true if the individual has stopped taking their medication.
B. Controlled human studies have not been conducted to assess the effect of most antipsychotics during pregnancy.
C. Withdrawal symptoms have been observed in infants whose mothers were taking antipsychotics.
D. Use of anticonvulsant medications is contraindicated during pregnancy due to their potential for congenital anomalies.

Geriatrics/Older Adult
A. Schizoaffective disorder depressive type is more common in older adults, whereas the bipolar type is more common in younger adults.
B. Compounding age-related complications such as comorbidities, cognitive decline, mobility problems, and social isolation can exacerbate schizoaffective symptoms.
C. Polypharmacy can pose a significant challenge in this population. Medication interactions need to be carefully considered.
D. There is an increased risk of mortality in older adults with dementia who are prescribed antipsychotics.

Partners/Family
A. A comprehensive treatment plan should include the individual's partner and other caregivers.
B. Family and partners can benefit from joining community organizations such as the National Alliance on Mental Illness (NAMI).

REFERENCE AND BIBLIOGRAPHY
American Psychiatric Association. (2013). *Diagnostic and statistical manual of mental disorders* (5th ed.). https://doi.org/10.1176/appi.books.9780890425596

National Alliance on Mental Illness. (n.d.). *Schizoaffective disorder*. https://www.nami.org/About-Mental-Illness/Mental-Health-Conditions/Schizoaffective-Disorder

SCHIZOPHRENIA

DEFINITION

A. Schizophrenia disorder is a chronic, serious mental illness that can include thought process, behavioral, and emotional dysfunction.
B. Symptoms include delusions, hallucinations, disorganized speech and behavior, and negative symptoms (see "Other Signs and Symptoms"). No single one of these symptoms is exclusively characteristic of schizophrenia.
C. Many of the symptoms of schizophrenia can also be exhibited by individuals with other schizophrenia spectrum and psychotic disorders.
D. Schizophrenia can lead to impaired social/interpersonal, occupational, and personal care levels of functioning compared with before the onset of the disease process.
E. Schizophrenia disease process is variable. Most individuals with schizophrenia experience a recurrent exacerbation of symptoms, although some also experience sustained remission.
F. Refer to the *DSM-5* (American Psychiatric Association, 2013) for diagnostic criteria.

INCIDENCE

A. Schizophrenia affects nearly 1% of the population in the United States.
B. Approximately 25% to 50% of individuals with schizophrenia attempt suicide. There is a 5% suicide completion rate for individuals with schizophrenia.
C. Individuals with schizophrenia have a life expectancy of 20 to 30 years lower than the general population.
D. the age of onset is usually in the late teens to early 30s.
E. On average, males have an earlier age of onset of schizophrenia compared with females.
F. Ethnic and racial differences also vary depending on the geographic areas of origin.

PATHOGENESIS

A. The etiology of schizophrenia is not well-understood, but it is thought to be multifactorial.
B. Genetics, environmental factors, neurobiology, and brain structure may play an essential role in the etiology of schizophrenia.
  1. Genetics: Twin studies indicate that schizophrenia has a strong genetic component. These findings do not account for the other subset of twins that do not go on to develop schizophrenia, but seem to suggest that epigenetics or environmental factors that can create changes in gene expression may also play a significant role in the schizophrenia phenotype.
  2. Environmental factors: Pregnancy and adverse birth events have been implicated with schizophrenia. Other environmental events, such as social adversities and substance use, have been associated with schizophrenia.
  3. Neurobiology: Schizophrenia and other psychotic disorders have been associated with neurotransmitter dysfunction. The three leading hypotheses involve the neurotransmitters dopamine, glutamate, and serotonin. The dopamine hypothesis is the oldest, and suggests a link between psychosis and dopamine hyperactivity in the mesolimbic pathway in D2 receptors. The glutamate hypothesis suggests that there is an NMDA receptor hypoactivity. The serotonin hypothesis suggests that there is hyperactivity of the 5-hydroxytryptamine receptor 2A (5HT2A) receptors in the cortex.
  4. Brain structure: Brain imaging of individuals with schizophrenia has demonstrated potentially decreased brain matter volume and enlarged ventricles compared with individuals without the disorder.
C. Schizophrenia disease progression is thought to start with a prodromal period heralding the start of a decreased level of functioning followed by episodes of disease exacerbation with periods of treatment response and failures. These recurrent disease exacerbations have been associated with treatment resistance and loss of brain tissue.

PREDISPOSING FACTORS

A. Family history of schizophrenia
B. Prenatal and perinatal adverse events, including prematurity, low birth weight/fetal malnutrition, perinatal hypoxic events, and infections during pregnancy
C. Social adversities
  1. History of trauma: emotional abuse, physical abuse, sexual abuse, neglect, bullying
  2. Low socioeconomic status
  3. Living in overcrowded urban areas
  4. Belonging to a migrant group
  5. Drug use: cannabis use in adolescence

COMMON COMPLAINTS

A. Auditory hallucinations
B. Delusions
C. Disorganized thinking
D. Memory problems
E. Impaired attention
F. Anhedonia

OTHER SIGNS AND SYMPTOMS

A. Positive symptoms include delusions, hallucinations, disorganized speech, and/or disorganized behavior, including catatonia.
B. Negative symptoms include the following:
  1. Blunted affect: diminished range of emotions
  2. Alogia: poverty of speech
  3. Anhedonia: decreased ability to experience pleasure
  4. Apathy/social withdrawal
  5. Avolition: decreased ability to perform goal-oriented tasks
C. Cognitive and negative symptoms typically begin before the onset of the first psychotic episode and may worsen as it progresses. Cognitive dysfunction symptoms include the following:
  1. Prioritizing tasks/planning
  2. Working memory
  3. Focusing and sustaining attention
  4. Working memory
  5. Self-regulation
  6. Problem-solving

SUBJECTIVE DATA

A. Assess onset, course, and duration of symptoms.
B. Review factors that precipitate or exacerbate symptoms.
C. Assess if cognitive deficits or negative symptoms were present before positive symptoms.
D. Assess for the previous level of social functioning.
E. Review past psychiatric history, including hospitalizations and outpatient treatment.

F. Assess history of suicidal ideation and attempt.
G. Assess for current and past substance use, including history of substance use treatment and participation in peer-based support group programs such as Alcoholic Anonymous (AA) or Narcotics Anonymous (NA).
H. Assess for a history of substance use withdrawal symptoms.
I. Review legal history.
J. Assess for any history of aggression or impulsivity.
K. Review psychiatric family history.
L. Review past medical history in the context of presenting symptoms.
M. Assess if there was a history of head trauma or seizure disorder.
N. Review social history. Include any perinatal complications, history of trauma (including neglect), socioeconomic status, education, occupational history, and relationships.
O. Review cultural, religious beliefs, and migration history.
P. Assess for coping mechanisms and support system.

PHYSICAL EXAMINATION
A. A full review of systems and physical exams should be conducted to rule out other illnesses.
   1. Vital signs: temperature, blood pressure, heart, and respiration rate
   2. Weight, height, and body mass index (BMI) for baseline data
   3. Constitutional
   4. Examination of general appearance (Does the individual look unkempt and/or disorganized?)

Head, Eyes, Ears, Nose, and Throat
A. Check for abnormal eye movement, including rapid blinking and saccadic eye movement.
B. Assess for poor oral hygiene.
C. Examine the thyroid.

Musculoskeletal
A. Assess for abnormal gait.
B. Assess for muscle strength and tone and abnormal movements.

Neurologic
A. Assess cranial nerves.
B. Examine deep tendon reflexes.
C. Assess the sensation.

Psychiatric
A. Conduct a mental status exam.

DIAGNOSTIC TESTS AND SCREENING
A. CBC count with differential
B. CMP
C. Hemoglobin A1c
D. Thyroid function
E. Urine drug screen
F. Blood alcohol
G. Pregnancy test for women of childbearing age
H. EKG (baseline EKG recommended before starting some psychotropic medications)

Psychometric Tools
A. PANSS: The PANSS is a scale for rating positive and negative symptoms in schizophrenia.
B. BPRS: The BPRS is a schizophrenia severity scale.
C. CDSS: The CDSS assesses for depression in individuals with schizophrenia.

DIFFERENTIAL DIAGNOSES
A. Delusional disorder
B. Schizophreniform disorder/brief psychotic disorder
C. Schizoaffective disorder
D. Bipolar disorder
E. Major depressive disorder
F. Schizotypal personality disorder
G. Substance-induced psychotic disorder
H. Psychotic disorder due to another medical condition
I. Obsessive-compulsive disorder
J. PTSD/complex PTSD
K. Autism spectrum disorder

PLAN
General Treatment and Interventions
A. Assess the severity of symptoms.
   1. Ensure safety.
   2. Stabilize the patient.
   3. Assess for other comorbid conditions.
   4. Monitor progress.
B. Ensure maintenance of stability.
   1. Assess the individual's treatment goals.
   2. Use shared decision-making to create a plan.
   3. Consider developmental and cultural issues.
   4. Consider the treatment setting.
   5. Assess for adherence issues.
   6. Ensure the treatment plan is multidisciplinary.
C. Schizophrenia treatment modalities can be divided into pharmacologic and nonpharmacologic treatments. These treatments should be individualized based on the individual's clinical presentation and severity of symptoms, biological markers, and personal preferences.
   1. Nonpharmacologic treatments
      a. Psychoeducation (see "Patient Teaching")
      b. Cognitive behavioral therapy for psychosis (CBTp): designed to decrease symptoms of psychosis and improve function
      c. Cognitive remediation: therapy used to improve cognitive functioning
      d. Family therapy: focuses on family interactions; usually solution-oriented
      e. Group therapy: provides a supportive, safe environment; focuses on the management of psychotic symptoms and interpersonal relationships
      f. Social skills therapy: uses behavioral techniques to improve function
      g. Vocational therapy: program to assist individuals with schizophrenia to integrate into a work environment appropriate to their functional level
      h. Intensive case management
      i. ACT: program that helps individuals with a serious mental illness live in the community through assistance with housing, case, stress, medication management, and crisis intervention, among other programs
   2. Pharmacologic treatments
      a. Schizophrenia is a chronic illness that may require lifelong use of medications to control symptoms. Schizophrenia is primarily treated with antipsychotics. Unfortunately, most antipsychotics that are currently ▶

approved by the FDA for schizophrenia mainly treat positive symptoms. Negative and cognitive symptoms generally persist even with antipsychotic treatment (Tables 17.1 and 17.2).

COMMON MEDICATIONS

A. Tables 17.1 and 17.2 list the most common FDA-approved conventional and atypical antipsychotics used to manage schizophrenia disorder and include a description of available formulations, dose range, and pharmacokinetics for both antipsychotics.
B. Please refer to the *PDR* for a complete medication profile. Table 17.3 lists the most common medications used to manage antipsychotic-induced movement disorders.

PATIENT TEACHING

A. Provide patient and family psychoeducation. Provide written patient education material to the patient and their family on the following topics:
  1. Definition of schizophrenia
  2. Symptoms of schizophrenia
  3. Pathogenesis
  4. Treatment modalities
B. Address adherence issues.
  1. Discuss lifestyle modifications, including nutrition and exercise.
  2. Discuss when to seek help. Provide important numbers to call when help is needed.

FOLLOW-UP

A. Follow-up for patients with schizophrenia should include a person-centered approach.
B. Assess treatment efficacy using psychometric tools (see "Psychometric Tools").
C. Monitor for medication side effects, including metabolic syndrome and abnormal movements.
D. Conduct metabolic syndrome screening and monitoring at baseline, at 4 months, and then yearly after starting treatment. Monitoring should include ordering and reviewing fasting blood glucose or hemoglobin A1c, comprehensive lipid panel, blood pressure, and waist circumference.
E. Assess for abnormal movements at every visit, including akathisia, drug-induced parkinsonism, and dystonia.
F. Use the AIMS to assess for tardive dyskinesia at baseline and at least every 6 to 12 months, depending on risk level.
G. Assess for treatment adherence at every visit.
H. Schedule clinical visits monthly once the individual is stabilized.

CONSULTATION AND REFERRALS

A. Coordinate care and consult with an interprofessional team, including primary care, specialty, social work, and case management services.
B. Consult or refer the individual to psychiatry subspecialists (e.g., addiction, neuropsychiatry, perinatal, liaison, forensic psychiatry) if warranted.
C. Refer the individual to a higher level of care during periods of decompensation that cannot be managed in the outpatient behavioral health setting. Services can include the CPEP and Mobile Crisis Outreach.
D. Refer the individual to case management and community-based services that support recovery and address problems with social determinants of health (e.g., ACT program).

TABLE 17.3 ANTIPSYCHOTIC-INDUCED MOVEMENT DISORDERS

Condition	Presentation	Typical Onset	Treatment Modalities
Acute dystonia	• Muscle spasm of the neck (torticollis), face, tongue • Laryngeal spams, difficulty swallowing • Oculogyric crisis	Less than 1 week	• Stop offending agent • Anticholinergic (benztropine, diphenhydramine)
Akathisia	• Restlessness • Pacing • Fidgeting	More than 2 weeks	• Lower dose or change offending agent • Anticholinergic • Beta-blocker (propranolol) • Benzodiazepine
Drug-induced parkinsonism	• Muscle rigidity (cogwheel type) • Resting tremor • Masked facies • Shuffling gait	Less than 3 months	• Lower or change offending agent • Amantadine (preferred agent) • Anticholinergic
Neuroleptic malignant syndrome	• Fever • Muscle rigidity • Mental status changes • Autonomic instability	Less than 1 month	• Stop offending agent immediately • Provide supportive care • May benefit from benzodiazepines; use is controversial
Tardive dyskinesia (condition often irreversible)	Repetitive involuntary movement involving: • Grimacing • Rapid blinking • Chewing movements • Sticking tongue out • Arms and legs may also be affected with jerking movements (chorea)	More than 3 months	• VMAT2 inhibitor (deutetrabenazine, valbenazine)

VMAT2, vesicular monoamine transporter 2.

Sources: Data from Stahl, S. M. (2020). *Prescriber's guide: Stahl's essential psychopharmacology* (7th ed.). Cambridge University Press; Zakhari, R. (2020). *The psychiatric-mental health nurse practitioner certification review manual.* Springer Publishing Company.

INDIVIDUAL CONSIDERATIONS

Pediatrics
A. It is rare for individuals under 13 years of age to develop schizophrenia.
B. When schizophrenia is diagnosed before the age of 18, it is called *early-onset schizophrenia*.
C. Negative and cognitive symptoms of schizophrenia can be observed in late adolescence during the premorbid and prodromal period of schizophrenia.
D. Pediatric FDA-approved antipsychotic medications for schizophrenia are listed in Table 17.2.

Pregnancy
A. Pregnancy can make schizophrenia symptoms worse. This is particularly true if the individual has stopped taking their medication.
B. Controlled human studies have not been conducted to assess the effect of most antipsychotics during pregnancy.
C. Withdrawal symptoms have been observed in infants whose mothers were taking antipsychotics.
D. Use of anticonvulsant medications is contraindicated during pregnancy.

Geriatrics/Older Adult
A. There are more women than men with late-onset (more than 45 years of age) schizophrenia.
B. Compounding age-related complications such as comorbidities, cognitive decline, mobility problems, and social isolation can exacerbate schizophrenia symptoms.
C. Polypharmacy can pose a significant challenge in this population. Medication interactions need to be carefully considered.
D. There is an increased risk of mortality in older adults with dementia who are prescribed antipsychotics.

Partners/Family
A. A comprehensive treatment plan should include the individual's partner and other caregivers.
B. Family and partners can benefit from joining community organizations such as NAMI. See the "Resources" section.

RESOURCES
General patient information about schizophrenia from the National Alliance on Mental Illness (NAMI): www.nami.org/About-Mental-Illness/Mental-Health-Conditions/Schizophrenia

Patient information on drug safety during pregnancy and lactation: https://mothertobaby.org

REFERENCES AND BIBLIOGRAPHY
American Psychiatric Association. (2013). *Diagnostic and statistical manual of mental disorders* (5th ed.). https://doi.org/10.1176/appi.books.9780890425596

Fraser, S., Hides, L., Philips, L., Proctor, D., & Lubman, D. I. (2012). Differentiating first episode substance induced and primary psychotic disorders with concurrent substance use in young people. *Schizophrenia Research, 136*(1–3), 110–115. https://doi.org/10.1016/j.schres.2012.01.022

National Alliance on Mental Illness. (n.d.). *Schizophrenia*. https://www.nami.org/About-Mental-Illness/Mental-Health-Conditions/Schizophrenia/Support

SCHIZOPHRENIFORM DISORDER

DEFINITION
A. Schizophreniform disorder is an acute-onset psychotic disorder similar to schizophrenia.
B. Symptoms must include at least two of the psychotic symptom clusters of schizophrenia (delusions, hallucinations, disorganized speech, disorganized behavior, and negative symptoms).
C. Symptoms last over 1 month but less than 6 months.
D. There is usually no prolonged prodromal period.
E. Baseline functioning goes back to normal after symptoms resolve.
F. Refer to the *DSM-5* (American Psychiatric Association, 2013a) for diagnostic criteria.

INCIDENCE
A. Schizophreniform disorder affects approximately 0.1% of the population in their lifetime.
B. There is a higher risk of schizophreniform in men than in women.
C. The disorder occurs more often in adolescents and younger adults.

PATHOGENESIS
A. The etiology of schizophreniform disorder is not well-understood.
B. The cause of the schizophreniform disorder is thought to be multifactorial, as seen in schizophrenia.
C. Etiologic factors include genetic, environmental, neurobiological, and brain structural factors, as described in the "Schizophrenia" section in this chapter.
D. There is some evidence supporting schizophreniform disorder association with two disorders: mood disorders and schizophrenia. Individuals with a schizophreniform disorder associated with mood disorder symptoms have a better outcome than those with symptoms that align more closely with schizophrenia.
E. About 60% to 80% of patients with schizophreniform disorder go on to develop schizophrenia.

PREDISPOSING FACTORS
A. Individuals with schizophreniform disorders tend to have a family history more associated with mood disorders than psychotic disorders when compared with schizophrenia disorder.
B. Other predisposing factors include environmental, neurobiological, and brain structural factors, as described for schizophrenia.

COMMON COMPLAINTS
A. Auditory hallucinations
B. Delusions
C. Disorganized thinking
D. Memory problems
E. Impaired attention
F. Anhedonia

OTHER SIGNS AND SYMPTOMS
A. Positive symptoms such as delusions, hallucinations, disorganized speech, and/or disorganized behavior, including catatonia
B. Negative symptoms
  1. Blunted affect: diminished range of emotions
  2. Alogia: poverty of speech
  3. Anhedonia: decreased ability to experience pleasure
  4. Apathy/social withdrawal
  5. Avolition: decreased ability to perform goal-oriented tasks

SUBJECTIVE DATA
A. See "Subjective Data" in the "Schizophrenia" section.

PHYSICAL EXAMINATION
A. See "Physical Examination" in the "Schizophrenia" section.

DIAGNOSTIC TESTS AND SCREENING
A. Routine initial tests to establish a baseline include the following:
1. CBC count with differential
2. CMP
3. Hemoglobin A1c
4. Thyroid function
5. Urine drug screen
6. Blood alcohol
7. Pregnancy test for women of childbearing age
8. EKG (baseline EKG recommended before starting some psychotropic medications)

Psychometric Tools
A. See "Psychometric Tools" in the "Schizophrenia" section.

DIFFERENTIAL DIAGNOSES
A. Delusional disorder
B. Brief psychotic disorder
C. Schizoaffective disorder
D. Schizophrenia
E. Bipolar disorder
F. Major depressive disorder
G. Schizotypal personality disorder
H. Substance-induced psychotic disorder
I. Psychotic disorder due to another medical condition
J. Obsessive-compulsive disorder
K. PTSD/complex PTSD
L. Autism spectrum disorder

PLAN

General Treatment and Interventions
A. Schizophreniform management involves pharmacologic and nonpharmacologic treatments.
B. See "General Treatment and Interventions" in the "Schizophrenia" section.
C. Nonpharmacologic treatments: See nonpharmacologic treatments in the "Schizophrenia" section.
D. Pharmacologic treatments: As in schizophrenia, the mainstay of pharmacologic treatment for schizophreniform disorder is antipsychotics.

COMMON MEDICATIONS
A. See Tables 17.1 and 17.2.

PATIENT TEACHING
A. Provide patient and family psychoeducation. Provide written patient education material to the patient and their family on the following topics:
1. Definition of schizophreniform disorder
2. Symptoms of schizophreniform disorder
3. Pathogenesis
4. Treatment modalities

B. Address adherence issues.
C. Discuss lifestyle modifications, including nutrition and exercise.
D. Discuss when to seek help. Provide important numbers to call when help is needed.

CONSULTATION AND REFERRAL
A. See "Consultation and Referrals" in the "Schizophrenia" section.

INDIVIDUAL CONSIDERATIONS

Pediatrics
A. It is rare for individuals under 13 years of age to develop schizophreniform disorder.
B. There are no FDA-approved medications to manage symptoms of schizophreniform disorder in the pediatric population, but antipsychotics are commonly used off-label to treat psychotic symptoms in the pediatric population.

Pregnancy
A. Pregnancy can worsen schizophreniform disorder symptoms. This is particularly true if the individual has stopped taking their medication.
B. Controlled human studies have not been conducted to assess the effect of most antipsychotics during pregnancy.
C. Withdrawal symptoms have been observed in infants whose mothers were taking antipsychotics.

Geriatrics/Older Adult
A. There are more women than men with late-onset (more than 45 years of age) psychotic spectrum disorders like schizophrenia.
B. Compounding age-related complications such as comorbidities, cognitive decline, mobility problems, and social isolation can exacerbate psychotic spectrum disorder symptoms.
C. Polypharmacy can pose a significant challenge in this population. Medication interactions need to be carefully considered.
D. There is an increase in mortality rates in older adults with dementia who are prescribed antipsychotics.

Partners/Family
A. A comprehensive treatment plan should include the individual's partner and other involved caregivers.
B. Family and partners can benefit from joining community organizations (e.g., NAMI).

RESOURCES
A. National Alliance on Mental Illness: www.nami.org

SUBSTANCE/MEDICATION-INDUCED PSYCHOTIC DISORDER

DEFINITION
A. The substance/medication-induced psychotic disorder is caused by using substances or prescribed medications that induce psychotic symptoms. According to the *DSM-5* (American Psychiatric Association, 2013a), the diagnostic criteria include the following:
1. At least one symptom is a hallucination or delusion.
2. The reported symptom started after the use of a substance or if withdrawing from the substance and after ingestion of a medication.
3. The substance or medication can induce a hallucination or a delusion.
4. The psychotic episode does not meet the criteria for another psychotic disorder that is not substance/medication-induced.

5. The psychotic episode is not related to delirium or occurring concomitantly.
6. The psychotic episode causes significant impairment in occupational, functional, and general distress.

B. For coding and charging purposes, the clinician should use the guidelines from the *International Classification of Diseases*, 11th Revision (*ICD-11*; World Health Organization, 2019).
C. Some psychotic disorders can occur after the use of alcohol, cannabis, hallucinogens, anxiolytics, sedatives, hypnotics, and other unknown substances.
D. Psychotic disorders can also occur during periods of withdrawal from substances. Other medications that induce psychotic symptoms include anticonvulsants, anesthetics, analgesics, antimicrobials, chemotherapeutic agents, and others.
E. Results from a systematic review by Wilson et al. (2018) provided information on a weaker relationship between substance-induced psychotic disorders and a family history of psychotic disorder.
F. Individuals presented with better insight into their illness and a balance between the negative and positive psychotic symptoms, however with increased symptoms of depression and anxiety.
G. Another risk associated with delayed treatment of substance/medication-induced psychosis is the potential conversion of the disorder from a transient to a chronic condition, such as schizophrenia or bipolar disorder, frequently seen in cannabis users.

INCIDENCE

A. The prevalence of substance/medication-induced psychotic disorder in the general population is between 7% and 25% of people with the first episode of psychosis. In younger adults, there is no exact percentage; however, it is estimated to be higher due to the increased number of youth using substances such as cannabis.
B. It is important to emphasize that the use of substances, either prescribed or for recreational purposes, causes, exacerbates, and leads to poor prognosis of psychosis.
C. Beckmann et al. (2020) provided statistical information on the use of cannabinoids in adolescents aged 12 to 17, with 12.4% at least using it once per year. This percentage increased to 35% in individuals ages 18 to 25. Many researchers provide supportive evidence of the direct link between cannabis and other tetrahydrocannabinol (THC) substances causing psychosis.
D. Amphetamines can also contribute to psychotic symptoms; cocaine causes paranoia approximately 90% of the time.
E. Other substances readily available to people over 21 years old, such as nicotine, can also be a precursor of psychosis and potential substance use disorder.
F. Laboratory-prepared substances, commonly known as *club drugs*, can also be lethal or cause psychosis. Some commonly prescribed medications, including steroids and antibiotics, may have undesirable side effects that include psychosis.

PATHOGENESIS

A. The presentation of symptoms can vary depending on the substance/medication used. Most substances have pathogenetic mechanisms containing higher levels of dopamine (in hallucinogens, stimulants); cannabinoid receptor agonists (in cannabis-related substances); 5HT2A-receptor agonists for hallucinogenic plants, which can affect mood; and antagonists of NMDA receptors (in ketamine and k-opioid receptor activation). Several theories indicate that some substances create a dysregulation of dopamine levels in the mesolimbic pathway. Other researchers provide evidence of the important role of neurotransmitters like dopamine and glutamate and how disrupting normal levels can alter the neurotransmission in the pathways located in the hippocampus, midbrain, corpus striatum, and prefrontal cortex, leading to the emergence of psychotic symptoms. The dysregulation of neurotransmitter receptors, agonists, and antagonists directly affects psychotic symptoms.

PREDISPOSING FACTORS

A. History or current use of alcohol, cocaine, amphetamines, hallucinogens, and cannabis
B. Family history of psychotic disorders
C. Use of novel psychoactive substances
D. Severe mental illness
E. History of impulsivity, aggression, and violence
F. History of medication and treatment nonadherence
G. History of hospitalizations for mental health reasons
H. History of detox programs
I. Traumatic brain injury
J. Dementia
K. Side effects of prescribed medications including steroids, antiepileptics, antimalarials, and antiretrovirals

COMMON COMPLAINTS

A. Labile vital signs such as tachycardia, tachypnea, elevated blood pressure, diaphoresis, and fever
B. Feeling that something is crawling under their skin
C. Persecutory delusions
D. Anxiety
E. Mood lability
F. Visual hallucinations
G. Increased or decreased appetite
H. Insomnia
I. Inability to perform independent ADLs
J. Hypersensitivity to noise, temperature, and light
K. Tremors

OTHER SIGNS AND SYMPTOMS

A. Psychomotor agitation
B. Aggression (verbal and physical)
C. Hallucinations or delusions
D. Odd behavior that is not congruent with reported mood or affect

SUBJECTIVE DATA

A. See "Subjective Data" in the "Schizophrenia" section.

PHYSICAL EXAMINATION

A. See "Physical Examination" in the "Schizophrenia" section.
B. Assess for substance use disorder.
C. Conduct an exhaustive review of medications, including OTC.

DIAGNOSTIC TESTS AND SCREENING

A. See "Diagnostic Tests and Screening" in the "Schizophrenia" section.
B. See "Psychometric Tools" in the "Schizoaffective Disorder" section.

DIFFERENTIAL DIAGNOSES

A. Substance intoxication or substance withdrawal
B. Psychotic disorder due to another medical condition
C. Primary psychotic disorder

PLAN

General Treatments and Interventions

A. For adolescent patients and after screening for substance use disorder, the APRN should use a parallel or integrated treatment approach, which is the gold standard in this population.
B. Comprehensive treatment approaches are recommended to treat substance/medication-induced psychosis. A comprehensive assessment and review of the laboratory and other test results should include psychosocial individual or group therapy, pharmacotherapy, and the patient's social support involvement, including family and other healthcare providers.
C. Ensure close observation for signs of withdrawal, agitation, and confusion, or for safety, as some patients may attempt to hurt themselves or others during periods of withdrawal.
D. Ensure low stimulus environment with decreased noise, appropriate temperature, and access to basic needs of food and water.
E. Preparation of a safety plan: Many patients may express suicidality or homicidal in response to hallucinations or as a side effect of the substance.
F. The offending agent/substance should be tapered down; sometimes, the patient must complete a detox program.
G. Initiation of psychotherapy: CBT is an evidence-based treatment option, as well as motivational interviewing.

COMMON MEDICATIONS

A. The initial recommendation to treat substance/medication-induced psychosis is to remove the offending agent and wait until symptoms resolve.
B. The second recommendation is to initiate antipsychotic medications (see Tables 17.1 and 17.2). Other pharmacologic treatment recommendations include the use of benzodiazepines to treat withdrawal symptoms.

PATIENT TEACHING

A. Educate the patient/family/caretakers on the signs and symptoms of substance/medication-induced psychosis and what to report to the APRN.
B. Discuss the risks associated with substance use that cause or worsen psychotic symptoms and can interfere with treatment, leading to a grimmer prognosis.
C. Educate on treatment options and the importance of patient adherence to recommendations and treatment.

FOLLOW-UP

A. Patients diagnosed with substance/medication-induced psychosis must be closely monitored in inpatient settings.
B. After the intake, the APRN must prepare a safety and treatment plan to include pharmacotherapy and psychotherapy.
C. Patients discharged from the hospital or a detox program should be seen as soon as possible to continue treatment. After the initial meeting, a second visit should be scheduled in 2 weeks to review clinical progress, review the safety plan, and make medication and treatment adjustments. The objective of close monitoring and frequent initial visits is to prevent symptom relapse.
D. It is recommended that the patient have concomitant treatment (pharmacologic and psychotherapy).

CONSULTATION AND REFERRALS

A. The APRN should know various treatment modalities and interventions to help individuals with substance/medication-induced psychosis. The clinician should consult substance use specialists, geriatricians, pediatricians, psychologists, and social workers, and initiate appropriate referrals for services outside the scope of practice. Interdisciplinary collaboration is essential as it helps make a robust treatment plan.

INDIVIDUAL CONSIDERATIONS

Pediatrics

A. Screen for substance use disorder using the CRAFFT (**C**ar, **R**elax, **A**lone, **F**orget, **F**riends, **T**rouble).
B. Discuss the high risk of psychosis associated with substance use such as cannabis.

Pregnancy

A. Educate on the risk factors associated with substance use inducing psychotic symptoms and affecting the fetus.
B. Educate on the risk of maternal infections and drug toxicity that can affect the fetus.

Geriatrics/Older Adults

A. Educate the patient and caretakers on the signs and symptoms of psychosis.
B. Discuss potential side effects of prescribed medications that might induce psychosis.
C. Discuss safety planning and nonpharmacologic interventions, such as psychotherapy.

Partners/Family

A. Educate the caretakers on the signs and symptoms of psychosis and the risks associated with the use of substances.

RESOURCES

A. CRAFFT: https://crafft.org

REFERENCES AND BIBLIOGRAPHY

American Psychiatric Association. (2013a). *Diagnostic and statistical manual of mental disorders* (5th ed.). https://doi.org/10.1176/appi.books.9780890425596

American Psychiatric Association. (2013b). *Desk reference to the diagnostic criteria from DSM-5.* American Psychiatric Association Publishing.

Beckmann, D., Lowman, K. L., Nargiso, J., McKowen, J., Watt, L., & Yule, A. M. (2020). Substance-induced psychosis in youth. *Child and Adolescent Psychiatric Clinics of North America, 29*(1), 131–143. https://doi.org/10.1016/j.chc.2019.08.006

Dryden-Edwards, R. (2023, April 12). *How is substance-induced psychosis treated? Drug abuse symptoms.* MedicineNet. https://www.medicinenet.com/how_is_substance-induced_psychosis_treated/article.htm

Fiorentini, A., Cantù, F., Crisanti, C., Cereda, G., Oldani, L., & Brambilla, P. (2021). Substance-induced psychoses: An updated literature review. *Frontiers in Psychiatry, 12*(12). https://doi.org/10.3389/fpsyt.2021.694863

Hjorthøj, C., Starzer, M. S. K., Benros, M. E., & Nordentoft, M. (2020). Infections as a risk factor for and prognostic factor after substance-induced psychoses. *American Journal of Psychiatry, 177*(4), 335–341. https://doi.org/10.1176/appi.ajp.2019.19101047

Niebrzydowska, A., & Grabowski, J. (2022). Medication-induced psychotic disorder. A review of selected drugs side effects. *Psychiatria Danubina, 34*(1), 11–18. https://doi.org/10.24869/psyd.2022.11

Wilson, L., Szigeti, A., Kearney, A., & Clarke, M. (2018). Clinical characteristics of primary psychotic disorders with concurrent substance abuse and substance-induced psychotic disorders: A systematic review. *Schizophrenia Research, 197*, 78–86. https://doi.org/10.1016/j.schres.2017.11.001

World Health Organization. (2019). *International statistical classification of diseases* (11th rev.). https://icd.who.int

World Health Organization. (2023). *ICD-10-CM diagnosis code F19.959: Other psychoactive substance use, unspecified with psychoactive substance-induced psychotic disorder, unspecified.* ICD10Data. https://www.icd10data.com/ICD10CM/Codes/F01-F99/F10-F19/F19-/F19.959

III SPECIAL POPULATIONS AND CARE SETTINGS

18 CULTURAL CONSIDERATIONS

Marie Smith-East

INTRODUCTION

Understanding cultural backgrounds and beliefs can considerably impact the effectiveness of psychiatric-mental health treatment. It is vital for APRNs to be aware of cultural differences and to approach treatment with cultural sensitivity. This includes understanding the impact of cultural stigma on mental health and the importance of involving family and community in the treatment process. Additionally, language barriers and access to healthcare resources must be addressed to ensure equitable care for all. This chapter provides an overview of the challenges to cultural considerations in providing psychiatric-mental healthcare and solutions for providing that care across the life span.

CULTURAL COMPETENCE DEFINED

A. Cultural competence is a necessary component in providing patient-centered, high-quality care to an ever-changing population of diversity in culture, race, ethnicity, gender, and sexuality.
B. Many schools of nursing (in addition to various healthcare disciplines) often integrate the teaching of cultural competency as it translates into practice and the development of clinician skills.
C. Cultural competency is often a mandated training for staff members in healthcare settings.
D. Cultural competence can be learned. The American Nurses Association (ANA) includes culturally congruent care in the *Nursing: Scope and Standards of Practice*.
  1. *Cultural competency* in nursing refers to the ability to understand and effectively interact with people from diverse cultures, including being aware of one's own cultural biases and assumptions, as well as developing skills to communicate and collaborate with individuals from different backgrounds.
  2. Providing culturally congruent care in evidence-based nursing care involves respecting the patient's cultural values, beliefs, worldview, and practices to ensure that they receive equitable and effective services regardless of their cultural background.

CULTURAL HUMILITY DEFINED

A. *Cultural humility*, a term introduced in 1998 in clinical training within multicultural education in the United States, describes a dynamic and ongoing process of self-reflection and self-critique of personal biases (Tervalon & Murray-Garcia, 1998).
  1. Cultural humility essentially acknowledges the understanding of "the complexity of identities—that even in the sameness there is a difference" (Khan, 2021, para. 4).
  2. In following a framework of cultural humility, the healthcare provider "will never be fully competent about the evolving and dynamic nature of a patient's experience" (Khan, 2021, para. 4), particularly within an ever-changing healthcare system and society, yet is willing to commit to a lifelong self-evaluation in providing culturally effective care.

FOUR MODELS OF CULTURAL COMPETENCE TO DELIVER CULTURALLY CONGRUENT CARE

Definition: Cultural competence is reflected in a nurse's capacity to not only understand differences but also appreciate the individual's background and life experience. This applies to a person's cultural, racial, ethnic, gender, and sexual identities. Being open and understanding to the values, practices, and beliefs of persons whose lived experiences are different from the nurse's allows the APRN to fit the treatment plan to the patient's needs, increasing the probability of adherence to prescribed behavioral and environmental changes. Other phrases used when discussing cultural competence are *cultural humility, cultural proficiency*, and *cultural responsiveness*.

A. Cultural competence model (CCM; Deering, 2024)
  1. Increases awareness, attitude, knowledge, and skills to improve and expand culturally responsive daily interactions
  2. Uses language that is understood by patients, increasing mutual respect and trust between provider and patient, and promotes patient and family inclusion in healthcare
B. Transcultural nursing model (Leyva-Moral & Bernabeu-Tamayo, 2021)
  1. Provides holistic care that respects the differences, beliefs, and values of people from diverse backgrounds
  2. Brings a relationship between cultural competence and Watson's Human Caring
  3. Promotes providing care with kindness and honesty, presenting your authentic self in delivering care, and taking into account the perspectives of others
C. Leininger's sunrise model (Farokhzadian et al., 2022)
  1. Takes into consideration patient's physical, spiritual, and cultural needs through an anthropological lens
  2. Utilizes three different concepts of care: cultural care maintenance and preservation, cultural care negotiation and accommodation, and cultural care restructuring and repatterning
D. Purnell model for cultural competence (Purnell, 2019)
  1. 12 domains of nursing ranging from heritage and communication to death rituals and healthcare professionals
  2. Examines culture from the global society and the community with the individual at the center
  3. Domains help the APRN evaluate diverse characteristics of different groups of individuals

CHALLENGES AND SOLUTIONS: APPLYING CULTURAL CONSIDERATIONS APPROACHES IN CLINICAL PRACTICE

A. Cultural factors can influence the manner in which patients perceive and utilize mental healthcare services.

B. Incorporating cultural considerations into the patient's treatment plan can improve patient satisfaction and help build trust and rapport with patients, leading to better mental health outcomes.
  1. According to a national study on racial and ethnic disparities among children/adolescents who were Black, Indigenous, and people of color (BIPOC), psychiatric and behavioral problems in school often led to punishment or incarceration and rarely ever to mental healthcare, despite about 50% to 75% of youth in the juvenile justice system meeting the criteria for a mental health disorder (Leblanc, n.d.).
  2. According to the National Institute of Mental Health (2023), the prevalence of any mental illness was highest among adults reporting two or more races (34.9%), followed by American Indian/Alaskan Native (AI/AN) adults (26.6%).

C. Challenges to providing culturally considerate psychiatric-mental healthcare include systemic social inequities, language barriers, differing beliefs about mental illness, stigma, the clinician's awareness of one's own biases, and the clinician's ability to navigate the complexities of cultural differences in order to provide effective treatment.
  1. According to McKnight-Eily et al. (2021), persistent systemic social inequities and discrimination can worsen stress and associated mental health concerns for people of color; this was true especially during the COVID-19 pandemic.

D. Solutions for overcoming challenges to providing culturally considerate care include the following, which can be adapted both in clinical practice and in training:
  1. Mindfulness of self-reflection through self-assessment
  2. Simulations and immersion experiences demonstrating cultural competemility
  3. Classroom assignments or peer-to-peer assessments in courses and in clinical practice
  4. Preceptorships in diverse communities and/or healthcare providers
  5. Assessment tools for patients (e.g., Iowa Cultural Understanding Assessment-Client Form) and tools for assessing cultural competence (e.g., Self-Assessment Checklist for Personnel Providing Services and Supports to Children and Youth With Special Health Needs and Their Families)

E. Assessment tools may be integrated within the electronic health record to take into account social determinants of health such as housing, food, and employment. These factors could contribute to poorer mental health.

MEDICATIONS, PSYCHOTHERAPY, AND TREATMENT PLANS

A. When prescribing psychiatric medications, it is essential to consider cultural factors that may impact treatment.
  1. Medication metabolism may vary greatly by individuals of various cultural backgrounds due to genetic and environmental factors.
  2. Cultural beliefs and practices may affect a patient's willingness to take medication(s), their understanding of mental illness, and their expectations for treatment outcomes.

B. Clinicians must demonstrate cultural competence while working with a patient to develop a treatment plan that is culturally sensitive and effective. Considerations may include the following:
  1. Education regarding traditional healing practices
  2. Involving family members in treatment
  3. Utilizing interpreters for language barriers
  4. Adjusting medication dosages to account for differences in metabolism
      a. For example, African populations have been found to metabolize some psychiatric medications differently from other populations (Rajman et al., 2017). This can lead to variations in drug efficacy and potential side effects, which can affect treatment adherence.
      b. Indigenous North American populations may have a higher risk of adverse reactions to psychiatric medications due to genetic differences in drug metabolism (Henderson et al., 2018).
      c. Factors such as diet, weight, and environment are also areas that contribute to the variation in the pharmacogenetics of medications, highlighting once more the importance of individualized patient-centered treatment.

C. Treatment plans should consider addressing and processing traumatic experiences (e.g., through psychotherapy) that may have been influenced by cultural or systemic factors, and the clinician should demonstrate cultural humility and sensitivity when developing a treatment plan with the patient (and possibly their family).

SUMMARY

Developing a deeper understanding of the unique challenges faced by various cultural groups and how care could be tailored to meet their specific needs is imperative in providing psychiatric-mental healthcare. Applying cultural competence in clinical practice is essential for providing quality healthcare to diverse patient populations. Solutions for incorporating cultural considerations in clinical practice include using cultural competence frameworks for assessment and care, utilization of interpreters, awareness of culturally relative norms surrounding illness, and providing treatment that respects religious and dietary restrictions. Incorporating beliefs regarding treatment—as they relate to psychiatric medications and psychotherapy—as part of providing culturally competent care can enhance patient adherence and ultimately improve mental health outcomes.

REFERENCES AND BIBLIOGRAPHY

American Nurses Association. (2021). *Nursing: Scope and standards of practice*. (4th ed.). https://www.nursingworld.org/nurses-books/nursing-scope-and-standards-of-practice-4th-edit

Deering, M. (2024, May 3). Cultural competence in nursing. *NurseJournal*. https://nursejournal.org/resources/cultural-competence-in-nursing

Farokhzadian, J., Nematollahi, M., Dehghan Nayeri, N., & Faramarzpour, M. (2022). Using a model to design, implement, and evaluate a training program for improving cultural competence among undergraduate nursing students: A mixed methods study. *BMC Nursing*, 21(1), Article 85. https://doi.org/10.1186/s12912-022-00849-7

Henderson, L. M., Claw, K. G., Woodahl, E. L., Robinson, R. F., Boyer, B. B., Burke, W., & Thummel, K. E. (2018). P450 pharmacogenetics in Indigenous North American populations. *Journal of Personalized Medicine*, 8(1), 9. https://doi.org/10.3390/jpm8010009

Khan, S. (2021, January 13). *Cultural humility vs. cultural competence—and why providers need both*. HealthCity (Boston Medical Center). https://healthcity.bmc.org/policy-and-industry/cultural-humility-vs-cultural-competence-providers-need-both

Leblanc, D. (n.d.). *Black, Indigenous, and People of Color (BIPOC) mental health fact sheet*. Resources to Recover, Laurel House. https://www.rtor.org/bipoc-mental-health-equity-fact-sheet

Leyva-Moral, J. M., & Bernabeu-Tamayo, M. D. (2021). Chapter II: The theoretical background and history of transcultural nursing. In A. Yava & B. Tosun (Eds.), *Transcultural nursing: Better & effective nursing education for improving transcultural nursing skills (BENEFITS)* (pp. 32–52). Ankara Nobel Tıp Kitabevleri Ltd. https://www.researchgate.net/profile/Mirko-Prosen/publication/358891245_Migration_Globalisation_and_Nursing/links/622473759f7b32463413593b/Migration-Globalisation-and-Nursing.pdf#page=32

McKnight-Eily, L. R., Okoro, C. A., Strine, T. W., Verlenden, J., Hollis, N. D., Njai, R., Mitchell, E. W., Board, A., Puddy, R., & Thomas, C. (2021). Racial and ethnic disparities in the prevalence of stress and worry, mental health conditions, and increased substance use among adults during the COVID-19 pandemic—United States, April and May 2020. *Morbidity and Mortality Weekly Report*, *70*(5), 162. https://doi.org/10.15585/mmwr.mm7005a3

National Institute of Mental Health. (2023, March). *Mental illness*. https://www.nimh.nih.gov/health/statistics/mental-illness

Olafuyi, O., Parekh, N., Wright, J., & Koenig, J. (2021). Inter-ethnic differences in pharmacokinetics—is there more that unites than divides? *Pharmacology Research & Perspectives*, *9*(6), e00890. https://doi.org/10.1002/prp2.890

Purnell, L. (2019). Update: The Purnell theory and model for culturally competent health care. *Journal of Transcultural Nursing*, *30*(2), 98–105. https://doi.org/10.1177/1043659618817587

Rajman, I., Knapp, L., Morgan, T., & Masimirembwa, C. (2017, March). African genetic diversity: Implications for cytochrome P450-mediated drug metabolism and drug development. *EBioMedicine*, *17*, 67–74. https://doi.org/10.1016/j.ebiom.2017.02.017

Tervalon, M., & Murray-Garcia, J. (1998). Cultural humility versus cultural competence: A critical distinction in defining physician training outcomes in multicultural education. *Journal of Health Care for the Poor and Underserved*, *9*(2), 117–125. https://doi.org/10.1353/hpu.2010.0233

19 SPECIAL CONSIDERATIONS FOR THE LGBTQ+ POPULATION

Dallas Ducar, Hyun-Hee Kim, and Kai Camara

THE IMPORTANCE OF IDENTITY

Every patient in any clinical setting will have some relationship to their identity. Whether identity is related to one's religion, job, community, or family, everyone draws their sense of self from their relationships with others. Philosophers Hegel and Heidegger, as well as Gestalt psychologists, all recognized alignment with the philosophy of *ubuntu* (humanity), which posits, "I am because of you." Mugubate and Chereni (2020) highlighted the application of *ubuntu* in social work, but it is relevant in all of healthcare, including advanced practice nursing. People exist in intersecting communities, and because of this their identities cannot be separated from their sense of community.

The skill of effectively discussing identity is crucial to APRNs because a person's identity is crucial to the development of a sense of self. Developing the therapeutic relationship is fundamental to assisting patients who are on a journey to understand their own sense of self and their relationship to others. Whether engaging in psychotherapy or psychopharmacology, the APRN, like other healthcare and psychiatric providers, actively seeks to understand, via dialogue, how the individual's identity relates to the choices they make. Whether it is a choice of medication, a choice of a therapeutic modality, or a choice to fundamentally engage in treatment—it is all up to the patient. Recognizing the importance of autonomy and the patient's right to choice is crucial. Respecting the principle of autonomy centers the patient's right to self-determined care. Recognizing patients as the agents of change is critical to the therapeutic alliance and supporting their identity development.

REFERENCE AND BIBLIOGRAPHY
Mugubate, J., & Chereni, A. (2020). Now, the theory of Ubuntu has its space in social work. *African Journal of Social Work, 10*(1). https://www.ajol.info/index.php/ajsw/article/view/195112

HISTORICAL PERSPECTIVE

The modern healthcare system is built on patriarchy. The medical system, similar to most social and cultural systems, is rooted in the centering and prioritization of the voices of affluent, cisgender, straight, White men. Medicine not only reflects this social construct of gender bias, it has successfully absorbed and silently enforced it since ancient Greece (Cleghorn, 2021). Modern healthcare still embraces, to a large extent, institutionally privileged systems, which elevate and respond to the voices of those who have privilege. The population consisting of LGBTQ+ individuals is diverse in culture, socioeconomics, geographic backgrounds, religion, ethnicity, and race, but singular in their experience of stigma and fear of biases (Cabaj, n.d.). Therefore, one of the first steps in caring *with* LGBTQ+ (queer) individuals is to engage in serious self-examination of motive: "You have chosen to work with LGBTQ+ individuals. Can you explain why?"

Self-reflection on sexuality and gender allows the APRN to examine long-held, as well as recently learned, belief systems. Self-understanding and honesty open the APRN to consider biases, implicit or explicit, and answer why the choice has been made to work *with* queer people as a professional goal. APRNs are guides on a path of respectful caring in relationship to the patient. This is not to say that it is not crucial to center interventions in evidence-based treatment; however, it is essential to pay attention to those who center the voices that have been pushed to the margins. APRNs, although well-intentioned, should be cautious of falling into the savior complex (Berrett-Koehler, 2020). The phrase *caring with*, rather than *caring for*, is used intentionally in this chapter to demonstrate the deeply held belief that no one person has all the answers.

Queer patients experience disproportionate polydiscrimination and are unlikely to receive care from persons with the same lived experience. Trans women—specifically, Black trans women—are locked out of labor markets (Reisner et al., 2020; Sherman et al., 2022). In many states, it can be nearly impossible for a Black trans woman to become a physician due to the systemic racial barriers implicit in this system. Trans voices are often silenced in our healthcare systems, forced into a paradigm of being recognized only as patients. This "others" the patient and magnifies a divide between those who are in positions of power and those who are not. This divide only worsens at the intersection between race and gender. Psychiatric APRNs have the moral responsibility to provide care to assist both physical and emotional healing, as well as to be the voice of advocacy for all patients, especially those who have been silenced. Advocacy entails not only supporting patients on an individual level, but also promoting the development of a just healthcare system. It requires each healthcare provider to critically reflect on their own biases and have the courage to respond ethically and responsibly.

A system that persists since ancient Greece is not unintentional, and it can also be identified in the history of nursing. As recent as 1952, homosexuality was considered a sociopathic personality disturbance in the first edition of the *Diagnostic and Statistical Manual of Mental Disorders* (*DSM-1*; American Psychiatric Association, 1952), which was not changed until the *DSM-II* (American Psychiatric Association, 1968), when it was recategorized as a sexual orientation disturbance diagnosis (Cabaj, n.d.).

Entire books can be written (and have been written) on the history of psychiatry and queer folks. Human beings have been pathologized for their sexual attraction since the dawn of modern psychiatry. The fact that trans and gender-diverse (trans) patients went largely unrecognized in many parts of the world does not mean that they did not exist. Western cisgender, White male-dominated medical academia omitted the spectrum of gender diversity from historical accounts. There is evidence that trans individuals have existed since the neolithic era (Robb & Harris, 2018). There is also historical evidence that trans youth transitioned in the early 1900s and later without experiencing any pushback (Gill-Peterson, 2021).

To declare anyone an "LGBTQ+ specialist" or a "specialist in affirming care" risks medicalizing an identity even further. No person's identity should rely on the existence of any healthcare system. Identity is something people discover for themselves and with their community, but it should never rely on prior authorizations or insurance executives. Throughout the 20th century, the queer community depended on itself to care for itself. To say that one speaks for another is to further deprive queer individuals of their right to self-determination. Instead, it is essential to lift up the voices of those at the margins. To emphasize one central authority on one's individual identity is to act in direct opposition to what it means to be queer: to be self-determined and to decide for themselves what healthcare choices are best for them.

Understanding this historical perspective is crucial to caring with the LGBTQ+ population. An APRN who desires to practice with this population and provide affirming care must do so with a deeply rooted awareness of context and self-awareness. Many queer individuals are in desperate need of care that recognizes their own identity, resists discrimination, and forwards affirmation. Understanding this history improves the APRN's ability to provide just and engaged care and emphasizes that the APRN's awareness of the context of queer communities mandates a recognition of their own relationship to this context.

Every APRN, regardless of gender identity, is able to provide affirming care, not just those who identify as LGBTQ+. While the literature on identity concordance versus discordance is somewhat mixed, cultural competence might be a factor in communication deficit (Shen et al., 2018). Modern healthcare should not rely on those at the margins leveraging their own personal identities, but instead on all healthcare providers focusing on patient-centeredness, information-giving, partnership building, and patient engagement in communication (Shen et al., 2018).

When the APRN understands the historical context upon which healthcare is situated, a cognitive self-examination of biases can lead to developing compassion for others, thereby reducing the APRN's implicit bias and the effect it has on providing care. This includes recognizing the role that *disinformation* can play, as seen especially in 2023, when there was a global proliferation of hate speech and disinformation against this community (Strand & Svensson, 2021). Therefore, ensuring access to reliable and truthful information to combat disinformation and myths is essential to caring with LGBTQ+ individuals. The combination of this knowledge and self-examination will help the APRN examine their own myths and preconceived biases and make the needed corrections.

REFERENCES AND BIBLIOGRAPHY

American Psychiatric Association. (1952). *Diagnostic and statistical manual of mental disorders* (1st ed.). Author.
American Psychiatric Association. (1968). *Diagnostic and statistical manual of mental disorders* (2nd ed.). Author.
Cabaj, R. (n.d.) *Working with LGBTQ patients*. American Psychiatric Association. https://www.psychiatry.org/psychiatrists/diversity/education/best-practice-highlights/working-with-lgbtq-patients
Cleghorn, E. (2021, June 17). *Medical myths about gender roles go back to ancient Greece. Women are still paying the price today.* Time Magazine. https://time.com/6074224/gender-medicine-history/
Gill-Peterson, J. (2021, April 5). *Transgender childhood is not a 'trend.'* The New York Times. https://www.nytimes.com/2021/04/05/opinion/transgender-children.html
Love, A. (2020, September 9). Allies, accomplices and Saviors: Knowing the difference to maximize impact. bkconnection. https://ideas.bkconnection.com/allies-accomplices-saviors-knowing-the-difference-to-maximize-impact
Reisner, S. L., Chaudhry, A., Cooney, E., Garrison-Desany, H., Juarez-Chavez, E., & Wirtz, A. L. (2020). 'It all dials back to safety': A qualitative study of social and economic vulnerabilities among transgender women participating in HIV research in the USA. *BMJ Open*, 10(1), e029852. https://doi.org/10.1136/bmjopen-2019-029852
Robb, J., & Harris, O. (2018). Becoming gendered in European prehistory: Was neolithic gender fundamentally different? *American Antiquity*, 83(1), 128–147. https://doi.org/10.1017/aaq.2017.54
Shen, M. J., Peterson, E. B., Costas-Muñiz, R., Hernandez, M. H., Jewell, S. T., Matsoukas, K., & Bylund, C. L. (2018). The effects of race and racial concordance on patient-physician communication: A systematic review of the literature. *Journal of Racial and Ethnic Health Disparities*, 5(1), 117–140. https://doi.org/10.1007/s40615-017-0350-4
Sherman, A. D. F., Balthazar, M. S., Daniel, G., Bonds Johnson, K., Klepper, M., Clark, K. D., Baguso, G. N., Cicero, E., Allure, K., Wharton, W., & Poteat, T. (2022). Barriers to accessing and engaging in healthcare as potential modifiers in the association between polyvictimization and mental health among Black transgender women. *PLoS One*, 17(6), e0269776. https://doi.org/10.1371/journal.pone.0269776
Strand, C., & Svensson, J. (2021, July). *Disinformation campaigns about LGBTI+ people in the EU and foreign influence*. European Parliament. https://dspace.ceid.org.tr/xmlui/bitstream/handle/1/1805/QA0921283ENN.en.pdf?sequence=1&isAllowed=y

THE DANGERS OF DISINFORMATION AND BIAS

A. Many myths exist when it comes to caring for LGBTQ+ communities.
    1. These myths are founded on the notion that queer individuals are increasing over time, as reflected in recent media reports that more LGBTQ+ people are coming out.
        a. There is a belief in the United States that the increase in queer individuals is related to media presence to teaching more neoliberal ideas, which is completely unfounded.
        b. Instead, there is direct evidence that society has become more accepting over the past generation, and this has led to increasing acceptance of queer individuals (Andersen & Fetner, 2008; Charlesworth & Banaji, 2019; Twenge et al., 2015).
            i. In the mid-1900s, there was increasing activism to destigmatize left-handed individuals, and as a corollary the amount of reported left-handed individuals increased (Barnes, 2013).
            ii. The same phenomenon is likely occurring with queer individuals: With an increase in acceptance comes an increase in people who feel safe enough to come out.

B. Despite increasing acceptance, the United States is seeing increasing political attacks against LGBTQ+ individuals.
    1. Recent studies have shown that these attacks have a direct effect on patient stress levels (Hughto et al., 2021).
        a. The messages that queer individuals, specifically queer youth, receive from the media have the added effect of perpetuating minority stress (Hughto et al., 2021).
    2. Therefore, dispelling disinformation is a critical and important step in reducing the possibility of unconscious biases in healthcare workers across the country.

C. Political health policy across the United States has only contributed to myths and disinformation.
    1. Legislation banning medical treatment of trans children was introduced as recently as 2021 (Krishnakumar, 2021). These bills claimed that gender-affirming care was experimental.

a. For example, in 2021, Alabama's *Vulnerable Child Compassion and Protection Act* (SB10) exemplified a growing trend of state-level legislation targeting access to gender-affirming care for transgender youth. By proposing to criminalize the provision of puberty blockers and hormone therapy, the bill disregarded established medical consensus from organizations such as the American Academy of Pediatrics (AAP) and the American Medical Association (AMA), which recognize these treatments as medically necessary and evidence-based interventions (AAP, 2018; AMA, 2021). SB10 not only threatened healthcare providers with severe penalties but also posed significant risks to the mental health and well-being of transgender youth by removing access to care that has been shown to reduce rates of depression, anxiety, and suicidality (Turban et al., 2020).
2. Such legislation disregards the growing body of research that demonstrates the positive mental health benefits for trans youth who have access to gender-affirming care (Tordoff et al., 2022).

D. These same bills claim that gender-affirming care is too widely available.
1. Despite claims to the contrary, gender-related medications are not prescribed simply by request. Instead, medical therapies for trans youth are pursued only after much consideration and input from both medical and mental health providers.
   a. Care is begun by establishing a relationship with the patient and their family.
   b. Medications are provided only after it has been determined that the child has a consistent gender identity that does not align with sex assigned at birth, and only after a thorough discussion with youth and their families about all potential associated risks and benefits.
   c. Healthcare for transgender youth is highly individualized. In fact, up to a quarter of patients at some gender clinics do not end up receiving medications related to gender. In rural areas, a quarter of individuals surveyed reported no access to gender-affirming care (Almazan et al., 2023).
2. APRNs want their patients to thrive, and lawmakers who forward this harmful legislation openly reject this fundamental fact.

E. Gender-affirming care is evidence-based. Healthcare for transgender youth is grounded in longitudinal data and research spanning decades at multiple centers internationally.
1. Gender clinics in the United States have more than a decade of experience consistently supporting the benefits of gender-affirming care.
2. Pubertal suppression, a treatment also deemed safe for cisgender children, leads to decreased suicidal ideation in trans youth.
3. Research demonstrates improved quality of life and health after receiving gender-affirming gonadotropin-releasing hormone (GnRH) agonists and hormones.
4. When trans youth are allowed to access gender-affirming care, lives are saved (Green et al., 2022; Tordoff et al., 2022; Turban et al., 2020).

F. Even if gender-affirming care is banned, it is likely that many patients will seek treatment in unsafe ways, such as obtaining hormones illegally and using online platforms to seek advice on medication dosing. The "War on Drugs" has had this effect.

1. Providers of gender-affirming healthcare have a unified perspective that these laws will be devastating to youth (Hughes et al., 2021).
   a. Gender-affirming care is already difficult to access due to the limited availability of local clinics and insurance restrictions.
   b. Bills banning access to care for trans youth would effectively make standard medical care inaccessible to many vulnerable adolescents.
   c. It is therefore paramount for APRNs to stand up and advocate against such political movements to prevent the possibility of further unconscious bias; this includes psychoeducation and advocacy not only for patients, but for the public.

G. Trans children, like all children, thrive when they feel supported and affirmed.
1. For trans youth with supportive parents, rates of mental illness fall to levels equal to those of their cisgender peers (Fuller & Riggs, 2018).
2. Lack of this affirmation can perpetuate into adulthood and leave many patients with the experience of being disconnected from the self, their own needs, or others.
3. Even if one has not been abjectly harmed, myths and disinformation have systemic effects. When these myths and disinformation are perpetuated, rates of discrimination—whether intentional or unintentional—may increase.

H. Discrimination in healthcare is a very real issue. Whether it is unconsciously or intentionally reinforced, discrimination is extremely harmful (Cicero et al., 2019).
1. Common experiences of discrimination in healthcare for transgender youth begin with ambivalence and uncertainty on the part of the healthcare provider. This reinforces established power and stigmatizing attitudes, resulting in a reduced access to care for queer individuals (Hughto et al., 2015; Poteat et al., 2013).
   a. Discrimination sends a message that queer individuals in general should not be believed. When one's very existence goes unacknowledged, it is unsurprising that a patient would also feel that their needs are not being seen or responded to appropriately.
   b. It is through examination of one's own biases, appropriate education, and action, therefore, that one can resist and fight back against the systemic effects of discrimination within healthcare for transgender patients.

I. Unconscious biases, or beliefs for or against a group that the individual is unaware of, are most pernicious at the intersection of race and gender.
1. According to the literature, Black trans patients experience higher rates of discrimination and insurance refusal, resulting in avoidance of healthcare.
   a. This avoidance does not make the issue go away, but rather increases the cost to the individual and to the system.
   b. If empathic communication, shared decision-making, investment in trauma-informed care, and patient centeredness are fostered, it will undoubtedly lead to an increase in patients who feel safe seeking care.
   c. Increased engagement, in turn, will likely lead to increased utilization of "high value" interventions in primary care, leading to better health outcomes for those who have been pushed to the margins.
2. In short, examining biases and investing in more equitable care can lead to better outcomes for individuals, populations, and the healthcare system.

J. Patients who have been previously discriminated against, but who are able to receive affirming healthcare, are more likely to consider those affirming healthcare providers and clinics to be their medical "home" (Cicero, 2019; Howell & Maguire, 2023).

1. They find a place where they want to show up, thereby improving adherence and engagement in primary prevention.
2. Over time, this results in decreased underuse of value-based care, promotes improvements in overall population-based health outcomes, and decreases waste, overutilization, and underuse.
3. Affirming healthcare, not just preventive healthcare, can be one of many keys to reducing waste and increasing value.

REFERENCES AND BIBLIOGRAPHY

Almazan, A. N., Benyishay, M., Stott, B., Vedilago, V., Reisner, S. L., & Keuroghlian, A. S. (2023). Gender-affirming primary care access among rural transgender and gender diverse adults in five northeastern U.S. states. *LGBT Health*, 10(1), 86–92. https://doi.org/10.1089/lgbt.2021.0391

American Academy of Pediatrics. (2018, October). Ensuring comprehensive care and support for transgender and gender-diverse children and adolescents. *Pediatrics*, 142(4), Article e20182162. https://doi.org/10.1542/peds.2018-2162

American Medical Association. (2021, April 26). AMA to states: Stop interfering in health care of transgender children [Press release]. https://www.ama-assn.org/press-center/press-releases/ama-states-stop-interfering-health-care-transgender-children

Andersen, R., & Fetner, T. (2008). Cohort differences in tolerance of homosexuality: Attitudinal change in Canada and the United States, 1981–2000. *Public Opinion Quarterly*, 72(2), 311–330. https://www.jstor.org/stable/25167627

Barnes, H. (2013, September 7). *Do left-handed people really die young?* BBC News. https://www.bbc.com/news/magazine-23988352

Charlesworth, T. E. S., & Banaji, M. R. (2019). Patterns of implicit and explicit attitudes: I. long-term change and stability from 2007 to 2016. *Psychological Science*, 30(2), 174–192. https://doi.org/10.1177/0956797618813087 https://journals.sagepub.com/doi/full/10.1177/0956797618813087?casa_token=lW1_2jQ1pewAAAAA:7tk_IfvySjeJY3PMWFP7uB_yMhkCMFtaS0-RlP4LaeuSxRA0MP9rkNzEKnrYtHzOr0gKCQ3gc0s

Cicero, E. C., Reisner, S. L., Silva, S. G., Merwin, E. I., & Humphreys, J. C. (2019). Healthcare experiences of transgender adults: An integrated mixed research literature review. *Advances in Nursing Science*, 42(2), 123–138. https://doi.org/10.1097/ANS.0000000000000256

Fuller, K. A., & Riggs, D. W. (2018). Family support and discrimination and their relationship to psychological distress and resilience amongst transgender people. *International Journal of Transgenderism*, 19(4), 379–388. https://doi.org/10.1080/15532739.2018.1500966

Green, A. E., DeChants, J. P., Price, M. N., & Davis, C. K. (2022). Association of gender-affirming hormone therapy with depression, thoughts of suicide, and attempted suicide among transgender and nonbinary youth. *Journal of Adolescent Health*, 70(4), 643–649. https://www.sciencedirect.com/science/article/pii/S1054139X21005680

Howell, J. D., & Maguire, R. (2023). Factors associated with experiences of gender-affirming health care: A systematic review. *Transgender Health*, 8(1), 22–44. https://doi.org/10.1089/trgh.2021.0033

Hughes, L. D., Kidd, K. M., Gamarel, K. E., Operario, D., & Dowshen, N. (2021). "These laws will be devastating": Provider perspectives on legislation banning gender-affirming care for transgender adolescents. *Journal of Adolescent Health*, 69(6), 976–982. https://doi.org/10.1016/j.jadohealth.2021.08.020

Hughto, J. M. W., Pletta, D., Gordon, L., Cahill, S., Mimiaga, M. J., & Reisner, S. L. (2021). Negative transgender-related media messages are associated with adverse mental health outcomes in a multistate study of transgender adults. *LGBT Health*, 8(1), 32–41. https://doi.org/10.1089/lgbt.2020.0279

Hughto, J. M. W., Reisner, S. L., & Pachankis, J. E. (2015). Transgender stigma and health: A critical review of stigma determinants, mechanisms, and interventions. *Social Science & Medicine*, 147, 222–231. https://doi.org/10.1016/j.socscimed.2015.11.010

Krishnakumar, P. (2021, April 15). *Anti-transgender legislation in 2021: A record-breaking year*. https://www.cnn.com/2021/04/15/politics/anti-transgender-legislation-2021

Poteat, T., German, D., & Kerrigan, D. (2013). Managing uncertainty: A grounded theory of stigma in transgender health care encounters. *Social Science & Medicine*, 84, 22–29. https://doi.org/10.1016/j.socscimed.2013.02.019

Tordoff, D. M., Wanta, J. W., Collin, A., Stepney, C., Inwards-Breland, D. J., & Ahrens, K. (2022). Mental health outcomes in transgender and nonbinary youths receiving gender-affirming care. *JAMA Network Open*, 5(2), e220978. https://doi.org/10.1001/jamanetworkopen.2022.0978

Turban, J. L., King, D., Carswell, J. M., & Keuroghlian, A. S. (2020, February 1). Pubertal suppression for transgender youth and risk of suicidal ideation. *Pediatrics*, 145(2), Article e20191725. https://doi.org/10.1542/peds.2019-1725

Twenge, J. M., Carter, N. T., & Campbell, W. K. (2015). Time period, generational, and age differences in tolerance for controversial beliefs and lifestyles in the United States, 1972–2012. *Social Forces*, 94(1), 379–399. https://www.jstor.org/stable/24754257

RESEARCH TIPS: APPROACHING RESEARCH WITH CARE, CONSIDERATION, AND RESPECT

A. Researchers should be aware, when soliciting populations for participation in any kind of study, that obtaining institutional review board (IRB) approval prior to even recruiting subjects is mandatory. The rights of the participant are guaranteed and federally protected by the common rule (HHS, 1991). After obtaining IRB approval and participant consent, the researcher must understand that asking someone to engage in dialogue about their experiences can be taxing for the individual. Establishing trust and beginning each encounter with care and consideration are necessary.

B. Due to current legal protections for LGBTQ+ populations, which are identified as inadequate, the research must proceed with extreme caution when collecting information and asking for participants' sexual and minority status. Disclosure can negatively impact the participants' lives and/or livelihoods. Secure processes for protecting confidentiality or anonymity should be put in place (Smith 2020).

C. Researchers should approach research with this population with a beginner's mind, understanding that those who are marginalized face disproportionate risk in healthcare. Researchers who study LGBTQ+ populations are tasked with determining how to adequately contextualize the complex nature and unique lived experience of trans and queer people while remembering that research itself can have the potential to exacerbate risk.

SAMPLING IN HARD-TO-FIND POPULATIONS

A. Identifying and gathering a sample from the intended population may be difficult, particularly if that population has been marginalized by society and prefers to stay hidden, in a sense, for safety reasons.

1. LGBTQ+ patients may be hesitant to participate in research due to fear of inadvertent outing or having their personal information revealed online, also known as *doxxing*.

   a. *Outing* is the process by which a person's gender identity or sexual orientation is disclosed to others without their consent. *Doxxing* is a by-product of the information age, providing the online means for potentially dangerous individuals to access sensitive data about a person's identity. This information could include their physical location, making the threat of physical violence a credible concern.

B. Key practices that may help when seeking participants are to look close to home, to network, and to tap the resources one already has access to.
  1. Nonprobability methods of sampling can be incredibly helpful when sampling hard-to-find populations.
  2. Snowball sampling allows researchers to use current participants—even if there are only a few—to identify others who may be appropriate for the study, who then identify others, and so on. This method of networking recognizes that queer people know other queer people. Often, their communities are vast and resilient, and they know and can recommend the study to others.
  3. Convenience sampling can also be an effective method of pulling together a sample. However, when using convenience sampling, it is important to be mindful of and control for bias where possible. In clinical or qualitative research designs, this approach can be particularly useful, especially if accessibility is a concern, because it can be less time-consuming and less expensive overall.
  4. Probability-based approaches such as time-location sampling and respondent-driven sampling are also worth considering.

C. Knowing what question the research seeks to answer, or the clinical problem it would like to solve, will help determine whether a quantitative or qualitative study would be more beneficial, and this will determine the level of accessibility to the target population. The researcher should also consider using the nursing theory framework to help structure ideas in planning.

D. Part of the reason transgender or gender-diverse patients in particular may be difficult to sample is not only safety concerns, but also the idea of "passing," or the invisibility offered by the "stealth effect."
  1. If a trans patient has reached the point in their gender affirmation where they are visually assumed to be aligned with their expressed gender identity, they lose some of their "otherness" and become part of the heteronormative mainstream. Successfully "passing" based on outward gender expression offers a sense of safety for the individual who is less likely to be singled out as transgender because of societal assumptions.
  2. This level of invisibility seeks social acceptance and avoids marginalization, stigma, or social exclusion. It may cause the individual to be hesitant to participate in research that focuses on that well-masked otherness.

UNDERSTANDING CULTURAL CONTEXT AND PRACTICING PURPOSEFUL ENGAGEMENT IN RESEARCH

Political Context

A. Politics and religion in the United States often attempt to label trans people and those in same-sex relationships as sexual deviants despite evidence to the contrary. These types of accusations create a hostile social climate and play a role in the health risk profile disparities seen in this patient population.
  1. Although LGBTQ+ people face disparate levels of risk, these risks are not inherent but rather are a by-product of society's stigmatization. Fear for personal safety can be a large driving factor for participation in studies, so creating an affirming and safe space in which participants can engage will be paramount.
  2. There are national and local organizations, as well as local groups and even student-led organizations, that researchers can tap as resources in order to offer mindful and purposeful engagement that remains culturally competent. Reaching out to local chapters of LGBTQ+-led organizations can provide access to information and resources that will strengthen the researcher team's ability to approach their project with care, compassion, and safety.

B. Researchers should strive to remain flexible to changing situations and keep an open mind to the views of the participants, actively listening to their stories. The idea of "nothing about us without us," a 1990 slogan from the South African disability rights movement, is of utmost importance when doing the work to study a particular group of people facing systemic oppression.
  1. Work to center the voices of those with whom the researcher is working. When the sample consists of non-White, LGBTQI+ women, for example, care should be taken to make sure the subject's perspectives are used. Each person is the expert of their own unique experience.
  2. There may be times when differences between the interviewer and the interviewee exist. The researcher should strive to get comfortable in the uncomfortable.
  3. Questions the researcher can pose to themselves before engaging with the interviewee include the following:
     a. Is the researcher able to sit in silence until the interviewee gathers their thoughts?
     b. Does the researcher's own anxiety cause a need to fill quiet spaces?
     c. Can the researcher provide consideration that gives the participant time to finish what they want to say, in the moment of the conversation, even if it requires sitting in absolute silence for a period of time?

SMARTIE GOALS

A. George Doran, Arthur Miller, and James Cunningham (1981) developed the SMART goals. This format is often used in nursing education to assess whether one's stated objective is **s**pecific, **m**easurable, **a**ttainable, **r**elevant, and **t**imely.

B. Recently, many healthcare providers are making a move toward SMARTIE goals as a more comprehensive approach. The traditional framework remains, but "I" and "E" add two questions: Is it **i**nclusive, and is it **e**quitable? This extra step moves practice toward a more inclusive care model by recognizing that disparities exist and that researchers can actively choose to address them in planning.

REFERENCES AND BIBLIOGRAPHY

Doran, G. T. (1981). There's a S.M.A.R.T. way to write management's goals and objectives. *Management Review, 70*(11), 35–36. https://community.mis.temple.edu/mis0855002fall2015/files/2015/10/S.M.A.R.T-Way-Management-Review.pdf

Smith, T. (2020). *Why IRBs must scrutinize collection of LGBTQ information.* American Medical Association. https://www.ama-assn.org/delivering-care/population-care/why-irbs-must-scrutinize-collection-lgbtq-information

U.S. Department of Health and Human Services. (1991). *What regulations protect research participants?* Office for Human Research Protections. https://www.hhs.gov/ohrp/education-and-outreach/about-research-participation/protecting-research-volunteers/principal-regulations/index.html

RISK FACTORS AND PROTECTIVE FACTORS IN THE SPECIFIC CARE SETTING

BACKGROUND

A. Numerous health disparities and inequities have been well-documented in the literature for LGBTQ+ populations.

These health disparities should be understood in a culturally and politically specific context that normalizes and upholds cisgender and heterosexual identities and oppressive gender norms, as within the minority stress model (Testa et al., 2015), rather than as an inevitable outcome that is etiologically bound to gender or sexual diversity.

B. Under the minority stress model, LGBTQ+ individuals experience stressors specific to their minoritized identity, which leads to health disparities and negative outcomes compared with nonminoritized populations. Health can be negatively impacted by distal processes, such as being assaulted for perceived gender identity or sexual orientation; or proximal processes, such as psychological distress from long-standing internalized negative beliefs.

C. Although the minority stress model may be criticized for its emphasis on the *individual* response to *socially* generated stressors and may often fail to examine why such stressors exist, the positive aspects of minority identities, or coping and resilience, it is a helpful starting point for understanding health disparities as a social outcome rather than as a result of individual pathology.

  1. LGBTQ+ people of color (POC) may experience distal and proximal stressors along multiple axes of identity (e.g., racism as well as homophobia or transphobia).
  2. It is helpful to apply an intersectional approach to understand these experiences. These factors are not simply additive but interact in complex ways to produce a myriad of differences in health and socioeconomic outcomes.

D. Minority stress has a significant impact throughout the course of an individual's life, leading to disparities at all developmental stages.

  1. LGBTQ+ youth are much more likely than heterosexual youth to report suicidal thoughts, depression, anxiety, and substance use.
  2. Trans youth are far more likely to have been hospitalized psychiatrically, been diagnosed with depression or anxiety, engaged in substance use, or disproportionately endorsed suicidal thoughts or self-injurious behavior (Reisner et al., 2015).
  3. LGBTQ+ adults and adolescents are both at a higher risk of eating disorders and subclinical disordered eating behaviors.
  4. Given the neurotoxic effect of stress on the hippocampus and the prefrontal cortex, LGBTQ+ older adults may be at a greater risk of cognitive decline.
  5. Trans older adults are at a significantly higher risk of overall poor physical health, disability, depression symptoms, and perceived stress compared with cisgender older adults.
     a. Gender and sexual minority adults were less likely to endorse protective factors for their health, such as having insurance, having a doctor, or receiving preventive care (flu shots, Pap tests, etc.).
     b. Although some within-group differences exist (e.g., bisexual youth are noted to be generally at higher risk of poor mental health outcomes than lesbian, gay, or heterosexual youth), the general trend of negative health outcomes holds true broadly for the LGBTQ+ populations that have been studied.

UNIVERSAL AND LGBTQ+-SPECIFIC RISK FACTORS

A. There are universal risk factors for negative mental health outcomes, such as adverse childhood events (ACEs). These may be experienced by any individual, regardless of gender identity or sexual orientation, and are not necessarily specific to the experience of being LGBTQ+.

  1. Studies of LGBTQ+ adults have shown consistently that they were more likely to have experienced ACEs as children, such as abuse and neglect, living in a household with a family member experiencing mental illness, familial substance use, or parental incarceration.
  2. LGBTQ+ youth (particularly LGBTQ+ youth of color, those living in alternative residential settings such as foster care, those living in rural settings, or those of low socioeconomic status) are much more likely to endorse the highest number of ACEs (4+) compared with their non-LGBTQ+ counterparts.
  3. ACEs lead to tremendous difference in downstream effects: LGBTQ+ students who had experienced two or more ACEs had 13 times the odds of suicidal ideation and attempts than heterosexual students who had not experienced any ACEs.
  4. Even within the same family, LGBTQ+ youth may be at a higher risk of abuse than their heterosexual siblings.
     a. LGBTQ+ adults were also more likely to report lifetime psychological maltreatment and intimate partner violence.
     b. Such elevated incidences of ACEs are likely to compound and increase the likelihood of additional risk factors for negative mental health outcomes, such as substance use and sexual risk-taking behaviors.

B. In the United States, policing and hyperincarceration have been noted to be key perpetuating factors for racial inequality and poverty.

  1. LGBTQ+ communities have been historically subject to, and continue to face, similar police surveillance and brutalization.
  2. As adolescents, LGBTQ+ youth are disproportionately represented among homeless youth (Morton et al., 2018), directly as a result of familial rejection, which puts them at greater risk of police surveillance and violence due to criminalization of poverty.
  3. LGBTQ+ youth are overrepresented in juvenile detention settings, and LGBTQ+ adults are much more likely to have been incarcerated than their cisgender and heterosexual counterparts (Robinson, 2020). Similar to racial profiling, trans and gender-expansive youth often experience trans-profiling ("walking while trans"), harassment, and criminalization by law enforcement officers, who often assume that such youths are engaging in sex work (Robinson, 2020).
     a. Such police profiling also reflects the reality of many LGBTQ+ people who face marginalization in the labor market. In the United States, as access to healthcare is tied to health insurance, most commonly provided by an employer, poverty and unemployment have an enormous influence on health.

C. Beyond law enforcement, trans youth are also subject to disciplinary actions by institutions for perceived transgression of gender norms (e.g., being unable to wear uniforms consistent with gender identity, having no alternative uniform options at gender-segregated schools) and provided LGBTQ+ exclusionary education in biology or health classes (Jones et al., 2016), which may contribute to external victimization by peers or internalization of negative beliefs.

D. In the context of a therapeutic relationship, APRNs can provide a source of counterbalance to societal stigma and victimization by taking an affirmative stance, challenging internalized negative beliefs, and naming one of the causes of distress as systems of oppression.

E. As seen in the examples discussed previously, identity-specific factors (experiences of stigma and discrimination related to being LGBTQ+) can interact with universal risk factors.

BULLYING

A. Bullying is a common experience in schools, with 10% to 30% of all youth reporting victimization by peers (Hymel & Swearer, 2015); however, LGBTQ+ youth may specifically be targets of bias-based bullying (bullying based on some perceived or actual aspect of one's gender, sexual orientation, race, ethnic, or other identity), which seems to worsen negative outcomes related to being bullied.

    1. LGBTQ+ youth who have experienced bullying specifically around their sexual orientation report higher rates of depression, suicidal ideation, suicide attempts, and substance use.

        a. Although LGBTQ+ status is consistently and strongly correlated with increased suicide risk, there can be mitigating sociopolitical factors.

        b. LGBTQ+ youth in school settings with gay–straight alliance groups or antidiscrimination and antibullying policies were 20% less likely to attempt suicide than those in settings without protective policies or gay–straight alliance groups (Hatzenbeuler, 2011).

B. APRNs may aid in advocating for the patient, helping educate family members, working collaboratively with other APRNs, liaising with school officials, and attending school meetings.

COMMUNITY RISK FACTORS

A. Broader community-level risk factors have been noted for adults.

    1. In a study of LGBTQ+ adults in the United States, those living in states without state-level legal protections for sexual orientation were more likely to report depression and anxiety compared with those living in states with specific legal protection (Hatzenbeuler et al., 2009).

    2. At least one study indicates that general LGBTQ+ acceptance does not appear to be sufficient. LGBTQ+ climate index correlated positively with markers of good health (routine healthcare use, self-rating measures, health insurance) in LGBTQ+ adults, but only in states with antidiscrimination laws (Solazzo et al., 2018).

    3. To measurably improve the health of LGBTQ+ patients, changing hearts and minds may not be enough. Meaningful legal protections; public health and economic policies that promote the well-being of *all* citizens, including the most marginalized members of our community; and institutional changes are necessary. APRNs should understand advocacy as both part of their professional obligation and their civic duty.

PROTECTIVE AND RESILIENCE FACTORS

A. Resilience factors

    1. For LGBTQ+ patients can be thought of broadly in terms of individual-level, family-level, and community-level factors (Testa et al., 2015) that are associated with positive outcomes or those factors that buffer relationships with negative outcomes. It may be difficult to cleanly separate these categories as factors likely influence each other in complex ways.

        a. Resilience is not an immutable characterological trait but rather a quality that is developed over the life span through a combination of protective factors and adversities.

        b. Resilience helps people cope with negative events and allows them to take calculated risks, knowing that they have the internal or external resources to recover from potential failures.

B. Individual-level factors

    1. On the individual level, factors for resilience, positive self-regard (self-esteem, acceptance), health-promoting behavioral/cognitive styles (proactive coping, self-care, self-efficacy, cognitive ability to mediate stress), and spirituality have been identified as intrapersonal factors for resilience.

    2. Higher self-esteem has been associated with higher self-forgiveness, being less prone to shame, early recognition of LGBTQ+ identity, active coping, outness, and lower anxiety on the individual level.

        a. Higher self-esteem is also associated with family acceptance, social connectedness, and support, all of which likely help foster healthy self-esteem and positive identity pride.

        b. Rather than adopting a neutral therapeutic stance, APRNs can help counter ubiquitous cis- and heteronormativity by taking an actively LGBTQ+-affirming stance in care settings.

        c. Affirming APRNs can help foster self-esteem and identity pride and provide education countering negative and inaccurate stereotypes and assumptions about LGBTQ+ people.

C. Family-level factors

    1. Family acceptance has been shown to be a consistent protective factor for LGBTQ+ people and has been well-studied for LGBTQ+ youth.

        a. Youth who were out to their parents about their LGBTQ+ identity reported less internalized homophobia/transphobia.

        b. Parental rejection has been associated with numerous negative outcomes and risk-taking behaviors, particularly for youth, such as higher rates of depression, suicide, and problem substance use.

        c. Given the incredible impact families can have on LGBTQ+ youth, APRNs should educate families on the power of their acceptance and support. Parents may have a range of reactions to initial disclosure, oftentimes experiencing stages of grief. While the most common trajectory over time is that of acceptance, APRNs should help minimize the potential harm of a less-than-welcoming reaction.

        d. APRNs may consider holding separate parent-only sessions to help them process difficult, complex emotions. Parents may need assistance connecting to support systems of their own, whether existing relationships or community-based supports such as a local chapter of PFLAG (Parents, Families, and Friends of Lesbians and Gays), because parents of LGBTQ+ youths can also experience stigma and marginalization.

D. Community-level factors

    1. It should be noted that social- or community-level resilience factors may not be universally or equally applicable and must be considered in their specific context.

2. Although social connectedness is generally shown to be a protective factor, this may not fully hold true for all LGBTQ+ people in all circumstances, particularly for POC.
  a. Vance et al. (2021), in an observational study of teens and mental health, identified that Black and Latinx transgender youth were found to have similar rates of mental health symptoms as White transgender youth, but school connectedness and supportive adult relationships were protective for White transgender youth and not for Black and Latinx transgender youth.
  b. Similarly, Aguilera and Barrita (2021), in a study of LGBTQ+ men, identified that connectedness to the LGBTQ+ community played a stronger role in mediating the relationship with stress for White men than it did for non-White men.
    i. Experience of ethnic/racial stigma in LGBTQ+ spaces was indirectly associated with stress and disconnection from the LGBTQ+ community for White men but not for men of color, who may experience such stigma in all contexts of their lives.
    ii. Trans women of color (TWOC) who experienced significant trauma and high levels of transphobia and racism also reported pride in their identities as TWOC despite adversities, or perhaps because of the resilience necessary in overcoming them.

Risk and Resilience

A. Risk and resilience factors and different facets of an individual's identity are not additive in a simplistic way.
  1. While a common assumption may be that LGBTQ+ POC are more likely to experience negative mental health outcomes than their White peers given the additional stress due to their racial or ethnic identity, this disparity has not been consistently demonstrated.
  2. This suggests that LGBTQ+ POC may gain resilience from early life experiences related to their experience of being a racial or ethnic minority, which later helps them navigate later life stresses related to their gender or sexual orientation identity.
B. Social connectedness to peers and family is obviously helpful on an intimate and immediate level (e.g., being able to rely on a support network for money, housing, or transportation).
  1. On a community level, institutions can also provide affirming spaces for LGBTQ+ people.
    a. Drop-in centers may be particularly beneficial for youth in positive identity and relationship development.
    b. Additionally, larger group affiliations may help marginalized individuals contextualize their own struggle in a historical sense, as contiguous and inextricably linked with the struggle of many others.
    c. This sort of understanding and affiliation may help counter internalization of shame and stigma and promote social and political involvement, which helps mitigate a sense of powerlessness, and increase engagement in meaningful activities.
C. Impact of the American healthcare model
  1. The American model of healthcare, with its focus on the patient as an atomized consumer, makes individualization of resilience and risk a tempting focus, particularly for the compassionate APRN wishing to alleviate psychological distress.
  2. However, such a single-minded focus on cultivating resilience in the individual patient to mitigate negative health outcomes implies that it is the marginalized individual's responsibility to effectively adapt to existing oppression that is the source of their suffering.
  3. APRNs should be wary of solely quantifying resilience by metrics of success as defined by capitalism or thinking of resilience as the ability to maximally adapt oneself to an oppressive society. In a more nuanced understanding of resilience, it may be seen as a necessary human quality for overcoming challenges, not for simply surviving in an oppressive society but for being able to change society itself by engaging in the collective work of dismantling systems of oppression.

REFERENCE AND BIBLIOGRAPHY

Aguilera, B., & Barrita, A. (2021). Resilience in LGBTQ PoC. In J. J. Garcia (Ed.), *Heart, brain and mental health disparities for LGBTQ people of color* (pp. 137–148). Springer International Publishing.

Hatzenbuehler, M. L. (2011). The social environment and suicide attempts in lesbian, gay, and bisexual youth. *Pediatrics, 127*(5), 896–903. https://doi.org/10.1542/peds.2010-3020

Hatzenbuehler, M. L., Keyes, K. M., & Hasin, D. S. (2009, December). State-level policies and psychiatric morbidity in lesbian, gay, and bisexual populations. *American Journal of Public Health, 99*(12), 2275–2281. https://doi.org/10.2105/AJPH.2008.153510

Hymel, S., & Swearer, S. M. (2015). Four decades of research on school bullying: An introduction. *American Psychologist, 70*(4), 293–299. https://doi.org/10.1037/a0038928

Jones, T., Smith, E., Ward, R., Dixon, J., Hillier, L., & Mitchell, A. (2016). School experiences of transgender and gender diverse students in Australia. *Sex Education, 16*(2), 156–171. https://doi.org/10.1080/14681811.2015.1080678

Reisner, S. L., Chaudhry, A., Cooney, E., Garrison-Desany, H., Juarez-Chavez, E., & Wirtz, A. L. (2020). 'It all dials back to safety': A qualitative study of social and economic vulnerabilities among transgender women participating in HIV research in the USA. *BMJ Open, 10*(1), e029852. https://doi.org/10.1136/bmjopen-2019-029852

Robinson, B. A. (2020). The lavender scare in homonormative times: Policing, hyper-incarceration, and LGBTQ youth homelessness. *Gender & Society, 34*(2), 210–232. https://doi.org/10.1177/0891243220906172

Solazzo, A., Brown, T. N., & Gorman, B. K. (2018, January). State-level climate, anti-discrimination law, and sexual minority health status: An ecological study. *Social Science and Medicine, 196*, 158–165. https://doi.org/10.1016/j.socscimed.2017.11.033

Testa, R. J., Habarth, J., Peta, J., Balsam, K., & Bockting, W. (2015). Development of the Gender Minority Stress and Resilience Measure. *Psychology of Sexual Orientation and Gender Diversity, 2*(1), 65–77. https://doi.org/10.1037/sgd0000081

Vance, S. R., Boyer, C. B., Glidden, D. V., & Sevelius, J. (2021, March 26). Mental health and psychosocial risk and protective factors among Black and Latinx transgender youth compared with peers. *JAMA Network Open, 4*(3), Article e213256. https://doi.org/10.1001/jamanetworkopen.2021.3256

ASSESSMENT NEEDS

A. The key to successful interaction and assessment in all patient populations lies in the healthcare provider's willingness to learn about those who differ from them.
  1. Resonating with those who share a similar background is less challenging than trying to understand people from different backgrounds.
  2. This practice may be referred to as *cultural competence* or as *inclusivity*, but the primary objective is the same: recognizing that each person is inherently worthy of individual consideration, respect, and dignity.
B. Fear is a barrier to care.
  1. One of the most prominent reasons given by trans patients for why they avoid seeking care is fear.
    a. This includes fear of discrimination or denial of care, or fear of having to take on the role of a teacher with their own clinical provider (Von-Vogelsang et al., 2016).

b. One of the unique aspects of nursing practice is its focus on the whole person approach.
    i. Nursing, as a discipline, recognizes the holarchy that is the patient. It maintains space for how each piece, or holon, from a person's environment relates to their specific physiology.
    ii. Nursing requires the APRN to interact both individually and together with the patient to form a complete picture of health and well-being, including emotional, psychological, and physical dimensions.

2. LGBTQ+ patients have health risk profile disparities, such as increased risk of anxiety and depression, suicidal ideation and attempt, eating disorders, and substance use.
  a. To ensure that culturally competent care is being practiced, healthcare models must periodically update best-practice framework.
  b. This involves working with members of the community to understand the impact of action, or inaction, and working to dismantle systems that force the patient into a reductionist model.
  c. This also requires APRNs to reflect on their own assessment styles and work to approach each patient with a holistic, nonpathologic stance.

MOVING BEYOND THE BINARY

A. In Western society, binary methods of thinking, which involve limiting thought to two choices (right/wrong, good/bad, black/white, male/female) are entrenched in society, and healthcare has largely followed this same model.

B. In general, APRNs may consider, as a default, that certain disease processes and anatomic structures are inherently male or female based on sex assigned at birth.

C. To provide culturally consistent and just care, APRNs must move away from this binary framework and toward a more inclusive and complete way of assessing patients.
  1. Health is a human condition. All patients, including cisgender patients, LGBTQ+ patients, and those presenting with intersex traits, whose needs have largely been discarded by a normative healthcare assessment, require health support. (Patients with intersex traits include persons for whom chromosomes, hormones, reproductive anatomy, and external presentation of genitalia vary greatly on a spectrum from person to person.)
  2. By recognizing that humans are diverse, APRNs can begin to diversify their own assessment capabilities and competencies.

Physical Assessment

A. Typically, when learning advanced assessment skills, one of the first things an APRN does is take a visual inventory of the patient before them.

B. Outward visual cues can help determine a rapid list of considerations and help inform questioning as the APRN moves through the assessment.
  1. Some things the APRN might objectively observe include overall body composition, visible malformations, rashes, lesions, and whether the patient presents as well-fed or malnourished or shows any signs of abuse or neglect.
  2. Objectively, a lot of data exist within a cursory glance, and APRNs use this information to begin a list of differential diagnoses to include or rule out.

C. Binary systems have the potential to become harmful when they cloud professional judgment due to assumptions.
  1. An example is a patient walking into an exam room who presents as outwardly masculine.
    a. Upon initial objective examination of their presentation, the APRN notes they have a full beard and no visible breast tissue and checks the "male" box on their intake forms. One may default to assuming, based on presentation, that the patient was assigned male at birth and has specific organs.
    b. If this patient had come in for right lower quadrant abdominal pain of unknown etiology that seems to be getting worse, a differential that might jump out is a possible appendicitis. The differential diagnoses will change if this patient is trans and their specific anatomy still includes ovaries, fallopian tubes, and a uterus.
    c. This will open up many new possible routes of treatment that could have been missed based on the assumption that this person was assigned male at birth and had specific organs.

PERSON-CENTERED INTAKES AND ORGAN INVENTORY

A. Using an organ inventory form during patient intake is one way to ensure accurate and up-to-date information that is both inclusive and patient-specific.
  1. Organ inventories go beyond the idea that a patient fits neatly into predetermined boxes by allowing for any and all possible combinations of anatomic structures and hormonal and chromosomal profiles.
  2. Beyond LGBTQ+ health, this method of data collection makes it possible to account for all patient types.
    a. Some patients are born with conditions that place them outside of binary health models even if they are not LBGTQ+ (e.g., vaginal agenesis; Mayer–Rokitansky–Küster–Hauser syndrome, in which a patient is born with a congenitally absent vagina or uterus; ovotesticular disorder, in which a person is born with both ovarian and testicular tissue; Menon et al., 2009).
    b. An inability to adapt and encompass all patient presentations renders binary health models out of date. Best practice should strive to be considerate of diversity, and patients should be able to expect a high level of care across specialties regardless of their intersectionality.

LANGUAGE AND TERMINOLOGY

A. To paraphrase Maya Angelou, when we are better learners, we are better providers. Words, and the intent behind words, matter.
  1. In the development of language, the imperative is to understand one another and to be able to communicate the unique experience had by the individual in a way that makes it accessible to others.
  2. Each community of people tends to create a language and identifiers of their shared experience, and LGBTQ+ patients are no different.
  3. As understanding within the community grows and changes, so too must healthcare's usage of language grow and change.

B. Previously, the words *transitioning* and *changing* were used to describe the journey made by a trans individual as they claimed their identity. In listening to and centering the voices of trans people, the APRN should know that these terms may not be accurate or reflective of patient experience.

TABLE 19.1 LGBTQ+ INCLUSIVE TERMINOLOGY

LGBTQ+	An individual who identifies as lesbian, gay, bisexual, transgender, queer, nonbinary, intersex, asexual, or another nonheterosexual and noncisgender identity; an individual with intersex traits
Sex assigned at birth	A gender assignment made at birth, using male/female identifiers based on visible external genital anatomy, chromosomes, and hormones
Gender identity	An individual's internal sense of being male or female, both, neither, or some combination of the two
Intersex	An individual who identifies as a member of the intersex community
Individual with intersex traits	An individual born with external genitalia, internal reproductive anatomy, and hormone/chromosomal combinations that fall outside the XX/XY presentation; may or may not identify as a member of the intersex community
Gender expression	External means of presenting one's gender identity; may use things such as clothing, mannerisms, social roles, or hairstyles to outwardly portray their chosen gender
Transgender	A person who identifies/asserts as a gender incongruent with their sex assigned at birth, with this assertion not matching the sex assigned at birth and remaining consistent/persistent
Nonbinary	An individual whose gender identity exists outside of a binary framework
Cisgender	A person who identifies and expresses as their sex assigned at birth
Social affirmation	The act of changing one's gender identity/expression socially, such as using a new chosen name or specific pronouns, cutting hair, or styling hair or clothing differently, in order to align with one's affirmed gender instead of one's sex assigned at birth
Gender dysphoria	A clinical symptom related to *DSM-5* criteria; includes a sense of alienation from some or even all of the social expectations and physical characteristics of one's sex assigned at birth, which causes distress
Gender-affirming/affirming	Previously called "transition/ing" or "change/ing"; the process by which a trans person identifies and claims their identity and gender

DSM-5, Diagnostic and Statistical Manual of Mental Disorders, Fifth Edition.

1. While *transitioning* or *changing* may be used by some, others may opt for *affirming* or just *being*.
2. *Gender-affirming care* has become the more predominant term used for this journey by many in the Western world. Other words and phrases have been better defined or replaced by more inclusive and accurate language, which is necessary as healthcare strives to be both accurate and precise (Table 19.1).

C. Language can be inclusive in any setting and is not exclusive to this patient population, but, like anything else, it takes practice.

1. When treating pediatric patients, for example, the APRN cannot assume that their family unit consists of one mother and one father, and so instead of saying "Your parents," APRNs may say "Your grownups."
   a. This way of speaking still conveys the correct information, but leaves room for all caregivers in the child's life, such as grandparents, aunts or uncles, same-sex parents, and foster parents.
   b. Small changes in the ways information is delivered can have a significant impact on patient well-being and satisfaction. Instead of using the term *wife* or *husband*, APRNs can ask about a patient's partner or significant other. When navigating the topic of pregnancy, which can be difficult or even painful for some patients, APRNs can ask if the patient is sexually active and, if so, with egg- or sperm-producing partners.
   c. This leaves room for all gender identities and expressions and remains sensitive around a topic that can bring unnecessary harm to the patient otherwise.

REFERENCES AND BIBLIOGRAPHY
Menon, A., Biswas, M., Kochar, S., Bal, H., Abhichandani, R., & Singh, S. (2009). Vaginal agenesis in Mayer Rokitansky Kuster Houser syndrome. *Medical Journal Armed Forces India*, 65(3), 287–288. https://doi.org/10.1016/S0377-1237(09)80033-6

Von Vogelsang, A.-C., Milton, C., Ericsson, I., & Strömberg, L. (2016). 'Wouldn't it be easier if you continued to be a guy?'—A qualitative interview study of transsexual persons' experiences of encounters with healthcare professionals. *Journal of Clinical Nursing*, 25(23–24), 3577–3588. https://doi.org/10.1111/jocn.13271

UNDERSTANDING THE STEPS OF GENDER-AFFIRMING CARE

A. A person's gender identity is valid regardless of their level of affirmation.

B. Some patients will go on to receive any and all medical affirmation procedures, up to and including gender-affirming surgery. Others, whether by choice or by limitation, may stop at any point along the affirmation pathway.

1. For some patients, social affirmation is enough to feel fully affirmed in their gender identity, while for others surgical intervention may be necessary.
2. Gender-affirming care can be costly and difficult for many to access, and while some patients may choose not to pursue more invasive procedures, others desperately want them and cannot afford or access them.
   a. It is this reality that makes it so important to recognize that even in marginalized communities, privilege exists.
   b. Sensitivity to an individual's situation and presentation is paramount.

C. Disinformation and bias have an impact on APRN care.
1. Due to disinformation or bias, many patients and APRNs may not understand the nature of the possible steps of gender-affirming care.
2. Social media, and the spread of misleading claims, can often leave patients feeling anxious or confused. It is the APRN's duty to educate themselves and be ready to dispel disinformation.
3. It is the APRN's responsibility to identify resources to ensure that patients and family members or friends can begin to educate themselves.

D. There is generally a large gap between when one becomes first aware of their own gender identity (in childhood) and when one proceeds with clinical intervention.
1. Most youth who come to understand their own identity are too young for any clinical intervention, and the recommendation is social transition.
2. Psychological analyses in children and adolescents have found that adult patients who identified as transgender or gender-diverse were aware of their own gender difference during childhood at an average of 8½ years old, with some as young as 2 years (Olson et al., 2015).
3. When considering the time gap between the age of identity realization and the time of clinical intervention, the APRN should support the child as much as possible and lead with social affirmation.

SOCIAL AFFIRMATION

A. Social affirmation is the first line of treatment in patients of prepubescent age who are exploring their gender identity.
B. Social affirmations are nonclinical in nature and are completely reversible but offer an immediate actionable response that serves as a signal of support to a child exploring their gender identity and expression.
1. The process of social affirmation includes changing clothing or hairstyling and using a new name or pronouns.
   a. For many families, these changes often start out at home and gradually branch out to include their child's school, friends, and extended family members.
   b. Children as young as toddlerhood may benefit from being allowed to identify and express themselves in this safe and exploratory way.
   c. Social affirmation is a safe and effective way to offer a child the chance to explore their own identity without an expectation of maintaining that identity and without any long-term or irreversible effects.

ROLE OF GONADOTROPIN-RELEASING HORMONE AGONISTS

A. Initiating gender-affirming treatment modalities beyond social affirmation requires analysis not only for physical readiness but also for psychological and emotional readiness.
B. Taking a step-based approach can be viewed as a development-dictated schedule that can be followed to provide age-considerate and incremental intervention toward affirmation over time.
C. The AAP, among others, has published research that points to a decreasing average age of puberty onset for youth in the United States; consensus for pubertal onset was age 8 to 13 years for youth assigned female at birth (AFAB) and age 9 to 14 years for those assigned male at birth (AMAB; Wolf et al., 2016).
1. Although it is unclear where the decrease originates from, further research of early pubertal onset is known to be associated with negative health outcomes regardless of sex assigned at birth.
2. Early thelarche, or breast development, is associated with an increased lifetime risk of developing breast cancer (CCG, 2010), and there is evidence to suggest that early-onset puberty in AMAB youth is correlated to increased risk of developing diabetes (Ohlsson et al., 2020). Ohlsson et al. (2020) studied 30,000 baby-boomer era males and found that those who had entered puberty earlier or had their pubertal growth spurt earlier were approximately twice as likely to develop early type 2 diabetes and that the disease was more serious, often requiring insulin to control; in contrast, males who had experienced later puberty and an adolescent growth spurt beyond 15 years of age saw their risk reduced by nearly 30%.

D. GnRH agonists
1. Consideration of this decrease in pubertal onset age leads to the second step of intervention and the first medically facilitated intervention: use of GnRH agonists, also called *puberty blockers*.
2. Originally approved by the U.S. Food and Drug Administration (FDA) to treat conditions such as precocious puberty and congenital adrenal hyperplasia, GnRH agonists halt the production of estrogen and testosterone in the body, effectively pausing the emergence into puberty for the duration of use. The effects of GnRH agonists are reversible upon discontinuation.
3. The use of GnRH agonists allows for increased assessment and diagnostic time by temporarily delaying the onset of puberty.
4. Once GnRH agonists are withdrawn, unless they are replaced with cross-sex hormone therapy, the adolescent will enter puberty congruent with their sex assigned at birth. If, however, during the assessment and diagnostic time the healthcare team and family agree that hormone replacement therapy is a viable option for them, suppressants will be withdrawn and replaced with cross-sex hormone therapy to initiate puberty congruent with their identified gender.
5. Current guidelines suggest that gender-diverse youth should have reached, at a minimum, Sexual Maturity Rating stage 2 regardless of sex assigned at birth before initiating pubertal suppression.

E. Onset of puberty brings with it a host of physical characteristics that may not be desirable to someone who identifies as gender-diverse.
1. These physical characteristics may be modifiable later with surgical or pharmaceutical intervention, but changes may be limited due to the nature of trying to change what already exists.
2. Once AMAB trans youth experience a pubertal phase congruent with their sex assigned at birth, they can be left with a larger/taller frame than is typical in their cisgender counterparts. They may also have a lower/deeper voice than they desire, and thus may pursue voice coaching to address.
3. In the same regard, AFAB trans youth who experience puberty congruent with their sex assigned at birth may feel they are shorter in stature than they desire and may have less muscle mass or a more curvaceous body fat distribution.
   a. In both cases, gender dysphoria and perseverance over things like facial or jaw structure, body hair growth, and breast development—either "too much"

or "not enough"—can cause emotional and psychological distress that manifests as the previously mentioned mental health concerns.

   b. Of course, many nonbinary patients may feel dysphoria regarding different experiences of their body or may not desire any intervention.

ROLE OF GENDER-AFFIRMING HORMONE THERAPY

A. Gender-affirming hormone therapy (GAHT) is the subject of much scrutiny in society today. In part, this is due to the spread of disinformation and the idea that healthcare providers are approving and administering hormones to children. GAHT does not become an option for any gender-diverse youth until they are ready to enter puberty, and it requires agreement among the patient, their caregivers, and their clinical providers.

B. A well-documented and consistent diagnosis of gender dysphoria will have been evaluated for and confirmed, and the patient will have been deemed an appropriate candidate for this level of medical affirmation. This confirmation of appropriateness is based on both psychological and physiologic readiness for puberty.

C. GAHT is an intervention that carries with it some irreversible effects.

   1. APRNs typically have multiple conversations around fertility and family planning as well as gender identity for months to years before initiating the withdrawal of GnRH agonists and the administration of GAHT.

   2. Hormones may include testosterone injections, creams, implants, or patches, as well as a combination of estrogen/progesterone with androgen blockers.

   3. Labs will be closely monitored throughout treatment to ensure the patient reaches safe levels of hormone sufficient to initiate the desired pubertal onset.

D. APRNs should consider the following:

   1. It is important to remember that hormone administration carries with it some risk.

      a. For example, estrogen has been studied in birth control and is shown to increase the risk of blood clots.

      b. For this reason, many patients who opt for GAHT can be safely prescribed only a certain amount of estrogen, and often this amount is not enough to completely suppress male puberty.

      c. Androgen blockers are often used in conjunction with GAHT in order to safely achieve the desired result without prescribing a dangerous level of estrogen.

   2. When assessing this population, it is important to keep in mind how hormones affect the body as the differential diagnoses are compiled to ensure safe and accurate diagnosis; the body inventory can be incredibly helpful in obtaining appropriate insight into a patient's whole health picture so the APRN does not inadvertently miss something important or possibly life-threatening.

ROLE OF SURGICAL AFFIRMATION

A. If a patient chooses to pursue surgical intervention, stringent criteria must be met, including a documented diagnosis of gender dysphoria over time, a letter from a trained mental health clinician, and general administration of GAHT by a licensed clinician.

B. Preoperative requirements for surgery are generally decided by insurance companies' requirements for medical necessity in combination with generally accepted clinical guidelines.

   1. Some states may have fewer requirements than others.

   2. Surgical intervention levels vary and include procedures such as chest reconstruction (via either breast removal or augmentation), phalloplasty, orchiectomy, vaginoplasty, and tracheal shave.

   3. Referrals for these types of surgical interventions require letters of clearance from healthcare providers and often entail lengthy wait times to book consultations.

REFERENCES AND BIBLIOGRAPHY

Cancer Collaborative Group. (2010). Insulin-like growth factor 1 (IGF1), IGF binding protein 3 (IGFBP3), and breast cancer risk: pooled individual data analysis of 17 prospective studies. *The Lancet Oncology, 11*(6), 530–542. https://doi.org/10.1016/S1470-2045(10)70095-4

Ohlsson, C., Bygdell, M., Nethander, M., & Kindblom, J. M. (2020). Early puberty and risk for type 2 diabetes in men. *Diabetologia, 63*(6), 1141–1150. https://doi.org/10.1007/s00125-020-05121-8

Olson, K. R., Key, A. C., & Eaton, N. R. (2015). Gender cognition in transgender children. *Psychological Science, 26*(4), 467–474. https://doi.org/10.1177/0956797614568156

Wolf, R. M., & Long, D. (2016). Pubertal development. *Pediatrics in Review, 37*(7), 292–300. https://doi.org/10.1542/pir.2015-0065

INCLUSION OF FAMILIES IN PROVISION OF CARE

A. APRNs working with LGBTQ+ youth will likely be working with their families and guardians, given legal limitations on minors' rights to consent to medical care.

B. Parents, spouses/partners, children, and guardians (biological relatives such as grandparents, aunts, or uncles, or court appointed nonbiologically related adults) may be an important part of care.

C. This care could persist throughout the patient's life span.

   1. Compared with decades past, many more young adults live with their parents, participate in higher education, delay marriage, and live in periods of familial interdependence for extended years into their adulthood.

   2. Even for those patients whose families are no longer legally obligated to participate in treatment, family involvement may be practically necessary for the APRN or requested by the patient, family, or both.

   3. Family and other caregivers may also be an integral part of care for geriatric patients, medically complex patients, and those with intellectual or developmental disabilities who may have limitations in their decision-making capacity.

D. Since legalization of same-sex marriage in the United States in 2015 in *Obergefell v. Hodges*, same-sex couples and parents now enjoy marriage equality with the tax and legal benefits this entails; prior to this, same-sex partners were often denied hospital visitation rights when visitations were restricted to "immediate family members."

   1. Unmarried same-sex partners were denied right to make medical decisions for an incapacitated partner, and nonbiological parents (in same-sex partnerships) were not granted the same degree of parental legal rights as stepparents in heterosexual partnerships.

   2. Now, much more formal legal protections exist for same-sex married couples. Nevertheless, LGBTQ+ patients may still have negative experiences in clinical settings related to their partner (legally recognized or not), such as their partner being prohibited from joining appointments or clinicians making assumptions about their sexuality or their partner.

3. APRNs should be aware that such protection, unfortunately, does not extend to nonmarried partners or chosen families.
   a. APRNs should not necessarily elevate married partnerships above other types of relationships.
   b. For patients with disabilities receiving state assistance (such as Supplemental Security Income), the question of marriage is even more complex because marriage can lead to significant reduction or loss of necessary benefits.
   c. Involvement of a patient's loved ones in care need not be limited to biologically or legally recognized relationships but should be considered for the individual patient's situation.

E. Although working with families (whether kin or chosen families) and partners can often present a complex dynamic to navigate, their involvement in a patient's psychiatric treatment can be invaluable.
   1. Family members or partners residing in the same house can be a helpful source of collateral information.
   2. They can advocate for patients in clinical settings when patients may have difficulty communicating, assist patients in adhering to a consistent medication regimen, provide transportation to and from appointments, and encourage patients to participate in home practices between therapy sessions.
   3. In moments of crisis, they can be part of a safety plan, whether in keeping the patient safe at home or in helping access emergency services.
      a. Such partner or family support may be of particular importance for LGBTQ+ patients who have experienced medical trauma.
      b. The main caregivers for youth will often be the most reliable sources of developmental history, early medical history, and treatment history, which the patient themselves may be too young to recall.
      c. Developing a therapeutic rapport with both the patient and their family may be difficult, but once established it may help to continue to engage the patient in treatment.

F. Family involvement programs have been noted to reduce relapse rates in psychosis programs, particularly early on in treatment.
   1. Parents and families often highly motivate youths with substance use disorders to enter and stay in treatment, and their involvement can have positive impacts on overall therapeutic gains.
   2. There are varying degrees of evidence supporting efficacy of family involvement programs for adult mental health patients in treatment for substance use disorder (improving engagement), bipolar disorder (improved symptoms), posttraumatic stress disorder (PTSD; improving engagement), and unipolar depression (improved symptoms, relationship satisfaction).

PRACTICAL GUIDANCE

A. Families of choice and support networks
   1. Most of the studies in current literature focus on kin relationships and significant others; however, of particular importance for LGBTQ+ patients are chosen families, friends, and other informal support networks.
   2. Given the dearth of literature on the specific impact of such types of support (data are mixed regarding the relative importance of influence of chosen family vs. family of origin) and whether programs designed for kin relationships may also apply to chosen families, this section focuses primarily on involvement of kin and significant others in treatment, although this clinical approach may be applied to all close relationships of relevance to the patient.

B. Guiding principles
   1. Although close relationships are generally positive, protective factors for a patient, APRNs should not make assumptions.
      a. Kin relationships for some LGBTQ+ patients may be fraught and a source of trauma.
      b. LGBTQ+ people are also at higher risk of experiencing intimate partner violence, yet face additional barriers to receiving assistance due to their identity.
   2. The APRN's duty is to the patient.
      a. While the patient may be impossible to "divorce" entirely from their greater familial or interpersonal context, APRNs should act with the *patient*'s best interest in mind.
      b. This may require first establishing the patient's safety and balancing the patient's autonomy (respecting their decision to involve other parties or not) against the APRN's duties of beneficence and nonmaleficence (helping patients discern whether such involvement is in their best interest and minimizing any potential harm).

C. Institutional and state regulations
   1. In the United States, the age of majority is 18 years, at which point the patient is legally deemed to be competent to make medical decisions on their own behalf.
      a. Legally emancipated minors (those who are married, have children, are in the military, or are otherwise substantially independent from their caregivers) are also deemed competent to make their own medical decisions.
      b. Most states have some decision-making provision for adolescents to consent to their own care regarding medical treatments, usually for medical care related to pregnancy, abortion, contraception, or sexually transmitted infection (STI); in emergencies when parental consent cannot be reasonably obtained; or in cases of potential harm in delaying care. Recent state rulings on abortions vary and should be known to the APRN.
      c. There may be additional institutional recommendations and practices regarding medical decision-making when parents share joint decision-making custody.
      d. In contentious relationships or when significant medical risks or complex medical procedures are involved, APRNs should seek counsel from their institutional legal team (typically a hospital or clinic risk management department).
      e. Advice and supervision from more senior colleagues are sometimes warranted.
   2. It may be necessary to clarify and request documentation regarding custody arrangements for caregivers (e.g., to ascertain that one parent has sole legal custody to consent to treatment) or regarding specific court-determined roles (e.g., a conservatorship does not typically grant powers over medical decision-making, while a guardianship does).
      a. Family members themselves may need education on what legal roles may entail and when they become relevant.

b. For example, durable power of attorney for healthcare is not activated until a person is deemed incapable of making their own medical decisions by clinicians.

3. Importantly, the patient's consent to involve other parties in their care is not a one-time decision. It is an ongoing decision open for revision as circumstances change.

4. APRNs may find it helpful to check in regularly on the patient's level of comfort with family or partner involvement, especially around major transition points, such as reaching the age of 13 years (many health systems have different medical record privacy rules for teens vs. younger children) or the age of 18 years (privacy settings again often change for healthcare proxies of adult patients vs. proxies of minor patients).

D. Disclosures

1. The Health Insurance Portability and Accountability Act (HIPAA) regulations must be adhered to.

2. Even for patients whose family or guardian involvement may be legally mandatory (minors, patients with legally appointed guardians), APRNs must respect the patient's right to privacy.

    a. It is helpful to establish with all parties involved what can be reasonably disclosed and what patients may expect to remain confidential.

    b. Explicit communication with the patient about *how* the APRN will disclose certain issues may help them feel at ease. The APRN and the patient may even come up with what they will say together. This helps avoid situations in which patients may be unpleasantly caught by surprise when they learn that an unexpected detail had been divulged.

3. For both patients and families, the APRN's professional obligations as a mandated reporter should be clearly outlined at the beginning of treatment.

    a. Many POC are subject to heightened police and institutional surveillance, leading to greater rates of incarceration and police violence, which perpetuate inequalities.

    b. Immigrants with undocumented family members may be under unique stress in interacting not just with police, but with *any* state agency.

    c. Poverty, regardless of race, is also significantly correlated with higher rates of reported and actual maltreatment, and families below the poverty line are disproportionately represented in reports of abuse and neglect. Even when well-intended, police presence for *any* reason may bring greater scrutiny and potential harm to marginalized communities.

4. When emergency services are necessary, APRNs should be aware of the historical impact of policing on marginalized communities and empower families and patients to choose the least potentially traumatic option while ensuring the safety of the patient in crisis.

    a. Patients may opt to go to a psychiatric crisis center or to have a family member bring them to the ED, rather than have 911 called.

    b. Peer supervision can be a useful tool in gaining perspective on difficult family situations and questions around neglect or abuse.

    c. When there is a necessary mandated report, APRNs may find transparency to be a helpful tool. APRNs and parents may opt to call child protective services together or discuss voluntary services.

E. Supporting patients and their loved ones

1. Inclusion of significant others should be beneficial to patient outcomes. If and when involvement becomes detrimental to the patient's treatment (if the presence or involvement of significant others becomes disruptive or therapy-interfering for the patient), APRNs may need to find alternative arrangements.

    a. This may mean scheduling individual and couples sessions separately or requesting phone updates from the parents prior to or after the individual session.

    b. Caregiver burden is well-known, and caregivers can experience significant negative physical and mental health issues related to their caregiving duties. When such disruptive behaviors may be related to the family member's or partner's own mental health concerns, the APRN may need to connect them to care of their own.

F. Special considerations for working with families of trans youth

1. Given the current politicization of gender-affirming care for trans youth, APRNs may increasingly find themselves in challenging situations with trans youth and their families.

2. APRNs should educate themselves on what gender-affirming treatment entails to be able to help families differentiate actual clinical practice from provocative and inaccurate media coverage.

    a. Prepubertal children do not receive hormones; they explore their gender in therapy or in supportive settings and may begin social affirmation or transition (e.g., changing haircuts, buying new clothes, choosing a new name).

    b. As puberty begins (Tanner stage 2), children and families may opt for pubertal suppression with GnRH agonists to stop the distressing physical changes associated with puberty.

        i. This allows children more time to explore gender expression and gender identity and to mature psychologically and cognitively.

        ii. Puberty blockers may be stopped at any point to allow endogenous puberty to resume. Adolescents (typically 14 years and older) are offered GAHT.

    c. Not all trans youth will opt to begin GAHT. Some youth desire only social or nonmedical forms of affirmation (e.g., wearing a binder, shaper, or makeup) or menstrual suppression with oral contraceptives. They may later seek gender-affirming surgeries without GAHT.

    d. While the World Professional Association for Transgender Health (WPATH) Standards of Care Version 8 now allows for 15-year-olds to be considered for chest reconstruction surgery ("top surgery"), most surgical affirmation procedures are reserved for adults. In the authors' experience, any surgical affirmation for minors, even older teens, is quite rare.

3. APRNs should be familiar with and understand the well-established benefits and safety of gender-affirming treatment. Severe side effects are very rare.

    a. GAHT has been consistently shown to lead to many positive outcomes, such as improvements in overall psychological functioning and quality of life (Murad et al., 2010).

    b. Gender-affirming surgeries have also been shown to be associated with significant improvements

in overall mental health outcomes (Almazan & Keuroghlian, 2021).
4. Beyond safety, APRNs help families appreciate that delaying or denying gender-affirming care is *not* neutral.
   a. Patients who desired and were able to initiate GAHT in a timely manner as an adolescent were significantly less likely to experience negative health outcomes, such as suicidal ideation, problematic substance use, and psychological distress, compared with patients who desired GAHT but had to delay care until adulthood (Turban et al., 2022).
   b. Experiences of dysphoria or being denied access to care necessary for gender embodiment goals are distressing for many patients.
5. Family reactions to initial disclosure are often variable, but the overall trajectory of families over time is generally positive.
   a. Family members may undergo their own processes of grief or loss, which are often expected and anticipated by the youth; however, care must be taken to minimize the harmful impact of perceived rejection on the patient.
   b. Families may benefit from psychoeducation on the impact of family rejection. In the authors' experience, caregivers benefit enormously from having their own space to process with the APRN.
   c. Cultivating a positive relationship with families can help them progress in the journey to becoming more confident and nurturing advocates for their child.
6. The traditional assessment-first model of gender-affirming healthcare is problematic and is generally associated with medical gatekeeping.
7. Assessment of a patient's diagnosis of gender dysphoria or gender incongruence does not lead to a road map of future affirmation treatment and may instead lead to falsification of narratives in order to fit a mold.
   a. The informed consent model approach is much less pathologizing of gender variance, better respects the patient's autonomy, and is more practically helpful in ascertaining the patient's gender embodiment goals and tailoring specific treatment. This approach, contrary to traditional gatekeeping, allows room for more honest and frank discussion of ambivalence, worries, hopes, and expectations, as patients are free to present as their complex, authentic selves rather than as idealized, fictitious candidates. Informed consent is not merely signing a document; it is an ongoing discussion between the APRN, the patient, and the caregivers, a process that unfolds along with treatment and is subject to change as the patient's needs, goals, and risk calculus change.

CHALLENGES AND TOOLS

A. Identify barriers to care in order to address any existing systemic inequity among patient populations.
   1. For the LBGTQ+ population, health risk profile disparities exist in a myriad of forms, from social and political factors to economic constraints, and each poses its own set of challenges.
   2. By and large, the biggest barrier to care is the lack of access to care.
      a. Many APRNs are not trained in affirming LGBTQ+ healthcare, and this can lead to discrimination and lack of access to care.
      b. The lack of an affirming care environment can directly lead to a patient delaying care and thereby increasing harm to the body and cost to society.
      c. Access to care is decreasing in today's environment due to disinformation campaigns that seek to directly attack healthcare institutions and threaten healthcare providers with harassment and, in some cases, violence.

SOCIOPOLITICAL CLIMATE AND REGULATORY RESTRICTIONS

A. In the United States, societal beliefs and political positioning heavily influence one another. This symbiotic relationship, coupled with disinformation campaigns, represents one of the largest challenges to providing equitable, safe, and efficacious healthcare to patients.
B. With the rise of social media and the removal of the fairness doctrine in mass media, it has become increasingly difficult to correct misleading, false, and harmful narratives that can have a significant impact on patient care.
   1. Often, the policies and laws governing how to practice as a clinician are dictated by politicians who write and pass those laws.
      a. The politicians that write laws based on disinformation are generally not clinicians.
      b. Recent political events demonstrate the growing influence by a radical and often violent politically motivated group seeking to define LGBTQ+ people in a negative light.

Influence of Politics on Gender Care

A. Anti-trans, anti–gender-affirming care
   1. The political climate in the United States in 2024 reflects a negative attitude toward equal rights for the LGBTQ+ community.
      a. Recent legislation in states like Florida and Texas, as well as other highly conservative states, demonstrates a coordinated effort to prescribe to political platforms founded on legal challenges to LBGTQ+ rights, women's rights, immigrant rights, and other minority-specific rights (ACLU, 2023).
      b. This political philosophy is often framed as a misleading argument about returning to "American values."
         i. Nationally, more than 120 bills restricting LGBTQ rights were introduced in 2023 alone (ACLU, 2023).
         ii. These bills target LGBTQ freedom of expression, access to healthcare for transgender persons, and safety for transgender youth.
B. Some legislation used specifically to define rights for all Americans except LGBTQ+ people
   1. House Bill 2 (HB2) in North Carolina, also known as the *Public Facilities Privacy and Security Act*, defines "biological sex" and has been used as the basis for further legislation to remove legal protections for trans people.
   2. Florida's *Don't Say Gay* bill is another attempt to limit recent social acceptance through education and discourse surrounding sexual orientation and gender identity (Florida Education Association, American Federation of Teachers, & National Education Association, 2022).
   3. The Governor of Texas, Greg Abbott, faced backlash in 2022 over a directive that classified gender-affirming care for minors as child abuse, mandating the Texas Department of Family and Protective Services to investigate families

providing such care. This order was halted by the courts. However, in 2023, Abbott signed Senate Bill 14 into law, which fully bans gender-affirming treatments like puberty blockers and hormone therapy for minors. This new law, effective since September 2023, is facing ongoing legal challenges and has sparked national controversy (Goodwyn, 2022; Nguyen & Melhado, 2023).

4. The political environment is becoming increasingly hostile toward clinicians who provide LGBTQ+ competent care. This, combined with reduced economic access to care, creates an increasingly difficult landscape for LGBTQ+ patients and families.

ECONOMIC CONSTRAINTS TO ACCESS

A. LGBTQ+ people are more likely to be locked out of access to economic resources and experience more economic instability in general (Jarrett et al., 2020).

B. Some of the most common concerns are finances and insurance issues, lack of service availability, and fears or worries (Puckett et. al, 2018).

   1. In general, lack of employment protections can lead to LGBTQ+ individuals being discriminated against in the workplace and not being able to work.

   2. This landscape has recently changed as the Supreme Court of the United States issued *Bostock v. Clayton County*, which held that the prohibition against sex discrimination in Title VII of the Civil Rights Act of 1964 (Title VII) includes employment discrimination against an individual on the basis of sexual orientation or gender identity.

   3. Despite this, the economic landscape has not significantly improved, resulting in many LGBTQ+ individuals earning less than non-LGBTQ+ individuals and at times resorting to sex work, which can increase the likelihood of contracting infectious diseases.

C. One way to improve the lives of LGBTQ+ individuals is to ensure access to affordable healthcare.

   1. APRNs should work to analyze social determinants of health and reduce the effect of these whenever possible.

      a. This can include ensuring information is presented in a way that is accessible and understandable to the patient.

      b. Additionally, clinics and institutions can provide reduced-cost care to those who meet need-based guidelines. Importantly, organizations should consider working to increase diversity at their institution and hire more individuals from communities at the margins.

      c. Direct employment can be one of the best methods of increasing an individual's economic stability in life and improving diversity and cultural competency at an institution. While APRNs should not rely on marginalized colleagues to teach them, employing these colleagues will result in a more diverse and thoughtful care environment.

OUTING, DOXXING, AND SAFETY CONCERNS

A. Some APRNs who provide affirming care may be LGBTQ+ themselves. This poses a significant challenge to those who are already at risk of violence.

B. Healthcare providers who are not publicly LGBTQ+ can be at an increased risk of being outed.

   1. Outing is the involuntary revealing of someone's sexual orientation or gender identity without their consent to others.

   2. If the APRN is publicly known as LGBTQ+, they can also experience doxxing. This is when one's address is posted publicly online for the purpose of harming the individual.

   3. More recently, some violent groups have taken to *swatting*, which is a criminal harassment technique wherein an emergency service is deceived to send law enforcement to an individual's address. These are direct attempts to cause harm to healthcare providers and to instill fear to prevent further care by the APRN.

C. Violence is not new to healthcare. There is a history of violence at places like reproductive health clinics where moral and religious objectors have resorted to threats and physical harm in an effort to elevate their argument against reproductive choice.

   1. These threats became so egregious that the Clinton Administration signed into law the Freedom of Access to Clinic Entrances Act (FACE Act) of 1994, which imposed heavy fines and prison sentences for violent offenders of the law.

      a. Despite this, threats against healthcare providers have persisted since the COVID-19 pandemic, coupled with the rise in disinformation (Larkin, 2021).

      b. Trans POC are under specific threat, with more than 30 trans individuals of color murdered in 2022 (HRC, 2022).

      c. Additionally, 2022 saw a strong increase in threats against hospitals and healthcare providers, namely those who provide affirming healthcare (O'Reilly, 2022).

         i. This is combined with a general rise in threats to healthcare providers and clinicians in general (Boyle, 2022).

         ii. The threats of violence are real, and affirming-care clinicians, healthcare providers, clinic administrators, hospital executives, law enforcement, politicians, and more must take a stand against such violence.

D. Core to nursing is advocacy. Healthcare providers, dedicated to promoting health and doing no harm, must stand together against violence in all forms.

   1. In a world with increasing disinformation, more and more patients are responding with physical threats and violence when faced with information they do not agree with.

   2. Nurses in 2023 maintained their 22-year role as the most trusted professional in the workforce in the United States and have the unique ability to band together as one of the nation's most populous portions of the labor force. Voices are stronger together, and all clinicians, everywhere, must not stand for violence.

REFERENCES AND BIBLIOGRAPHY

Almazan, A. N., & Keuroghlian, A. S. (2021). Association between gender-affirming surgeries and mental health outcomes. *JAMA Surgery, 156*(7), 611–618. https://doi.org/10.1001/jamasurg.2021.0952

American Civil Liberties Union. (2023). *Over 120 bills restricting LGBTQ rights introduced nationwide in 2023 so far*. https://www.aclu.org/press-releases/over-120-bills-restricting-lgbtq-rights-introduced-nationwide-2023-so-far

Boyle, P. (2022, August 18). *Threats against health care workers are rising. here's how hospitals are protecting their staffs*. Association of American Medical Colleges. https://www.aamc.org/news-insights/threats-against-health-care-workers-are-rising-heres-how-hospitals-are-protecting-their-staffs

Florida Education Association, American Federation of Teachers, & National Education Association. (2022). *What you need to know about Florida's "Don't Say Gay" and "Don't Say They" laws, book bans, and other curricula restrictions*. https://www.nea.org/sites/default/files/2023-06/30424-know-your-rights_web_v4.pdf

Goodwyn, W. (2022, March 22). *Families in Texas with transgender children say they're under attack*. NPR. https://www.npr.org/2022/03/22/1087991657/families-in-texas-with-transgender-children-say-theyre-under-attack

Human Rights Campaign. (2022). *Fatal violence against the transgender and gender non-conforming community in 2022*. https://www.hrc.org/resources/fatal-violence-against-the-transgender-and-gender-non-conforming-community-in-2022

Jarrett, B. A., Peitzmeier, S. M., Restar, A., Adamson, T., Howell, S., Baral, S., & Beckham, S. W. (2020). Gender-affirming care, mental health, and economic stability in the time of COVID-19: A global cross-sectional study of transgender and non-binary people. *MedRxiv: The Preprint Server for Health Sciences*. https://doi.org/10.1101/2020.11.02.20224709

Larkin, H. (2021). Navigating attacks against health care workers in the COVID-19 era. *JAMA*, 325(18), 1822–1824. https://doi.org/10.1001/jama.2021.2701

Murad, M. H., Elamin, M. B., Garcia, M. Z., Mullan, R. J., Murad, A., Erwin, P. J., & Montori, V. M. (2010, February). Hormonal therapy and sex reassignment: A systematic review and meta-analysis of quality of life and psychosocial outcomes. *Clinical Endocrinology*, 72(2), 214–231. https://doi.org/10.1111/j.1365-2265.2009.03625.x

Nguyen, A., & Melhado, W. (2023, June 2). Gov. Greg Abbott signs legislation barring trans youth from accessing transition-related care. *The Texas Tribune*. https://www.texastribune.org/2023/06/02/texas-gender-affirming-care-ban

O'Reilly, K. B. (2022, October 6). *Terrifying bomb threats against children's hospitals must stop*. American Medical Association. https://www.ama-assn.org/practice-management/physician-health/terrifying-bomb-threats-against-childrens-hospitals-must-stop

Puckett, J. A., Cleary, P., Rossman, K., Mustanski, B., & Newcomb, M. E. (2018). Barriers to gender-affirming care for transgender and gender nonconforming individuals. *Sexuality Research and Social Policy*, 15(1), 48–59. https://doi.org/10.1007/s13178-017-0295-8

Turban, J. L., King, D., Kobe, J., Reisner, S. L., & Keuroghlian, A. S. (2022, January 12). Access to gender-affirming hormones during adolescence and mental health outcomes among transgender adults. *PLoS One*, 17(1), Article e0261039. https://doi.org/10.1371/journal.pone.0287283

REFERRALS, COMMUNITY PARTNERS, AND RESOURCES

CLINICAL REFERRALS

A. Ideally, every patient, regardless of any facet of their identity, would feel equally welcomed and appropriately treated at every medical facility; however, this is not yet reality for many patients.

B. LGBTQ+ patients may also have significant medical trauma or any number of negative experiences in clinical settings. APRNs working with LGBTQ+ patients should be aware of LGBTQ+-affirming clinics and services in their community to be able to provide appropriate referrals.

   1. In major cities, this may be a dedicated health center specifically for LGBTQ+ patients (e.g., The Fenway Institute in Boston, Callen-Lorde in New York City).

   2. Smaller health centers, mental health clinics, or primary care clinics dedicated to LGBTQ+ patients exist in smaller cities and towns.

   3. Most major academic medical centers have an LGBTQ+-focused health program, and many also have programs for gender-affirming healthcare for trans and gender-diverse patients.

C. With recent waves of anti-trans legislation, the future of trans health programs may be more uncertain, and threats toward clinics and healthcare workers may make it more difficult for those who are not yet patients there to get information about clinical services offered, making both a formal and an informal network of affirming clinicians all the more important for helping patients connect to care.

D. Professional organizations such as the Gay and Lesbian Medical Association: Health Professional Advancing LGBTQ Equality (GLMA) and the Association of Gay and Lesbian Psychiatrists (AGLP) maintain lists of affirming clinicians.

COMMUNITY RESOURCES

A. While connecting to medical specialists and formal mental health treatment is undoubtedly important, nonmedical resources are also crucial.

   1. Not every APRN may have access to dedicated social work or case management. APRNs should cultivate at least some understanding of the major LGBTQ+ community organizations in their county or state.

   2. There are likely already existing lists of LGBTQ+-friendly resources compiled by community organizations and mutual aid networks.

   3. It may be helpful to partner with such community organizations for referrals, shared patients, and larger collaborative projects.

Key Community Resources

The following are some key resources that APRNs should be able to refer to in their specific community:

A. LGBTQ+ community centers: The LGBTQ+ community center is often a significant resource of knowledge regarding existing community resources and various affirming services. Community centers commonly offer a number of health-related services such as STI testing, support or therapeutic groups, and referral resources. They are also a place for people to connect to peers, to socialize, and to gather with other LGBTQ+ people in a joyful context rather than a deficit-based context.

B. LBGTQ+ inclusive shelters: These are of particular importance for trans and gender-diverse persons experiencing housing insecurity, who often may not feel safe in gender-segregated settings that are not explicitly affirming.

C. LGBTQ+ inclusive domestic violence resources: Similar to housing shelters, many trans and gender-diverse persons may not be welcomed into domestic violence shelters or facilities, which tend to be typically designed for cisgender women and children.

D. Legal assistance: Patients may require assistance with a number of legal matters, including housing discrimination, labor violation, and changing legal documents. Many law schools partner with trans health programs to provide name-change clinics. Each state provides information about pro-bono or reduced cost legal services for those in financial need. The National Center for Transgender Equality (https://transequality.org) is also an excellent national resource.

E. Support groups: These may be around specific identities (e.g., trans and gender-diverse youth, parents of LGBTQ+ children), around specific concerns (e.g., trauma, bereavement, general mental health), or around specific stages of life (e.g., transitioning after age 30 years). Often, these are provided by LGBTQ+ community centers or community health clinics, but many smaller or private practice clinics may also run support groups or therapeutic groups. The *Psychology Today* directory (http://psychologytoday.com) is usually a helpful place to start.

F. The following are crisis resources that APRNs can refer to:

   1. Trans Lifeline (https://translifeline.org): Trans Lifeline is a peer support organization providing crisis support, run by and for trans people. Unlike many other crisis support lines, Trans Lifeline explicitly does not practice nonconsensual rescue. Given the historical and potential harm of police, and the possibility of past traumatic experiences with emergency personnel, this can often be a helpful thing to note for trans and gender-diverse patients hesitant to consider other crisis resources.

2. Trevor Line (www.thetrevorproject.org/get-help): The Trevor Project is a support line for LGBTQ+ youths. They also provide a dedicated, monitored, and safe social media space for LGBTQ+ youth.

3. Emergency mobile crisis/psychiatric crisis services: Each county or state generally has some type of crisis psychiatric service available. This may be a mobile crisis unit (team that goes into the community to provide assessments or connection to resources) or an urgent evaluation center. APRNs should be aware of the procedures for accessing services, and what can be expected, to be able to walk patients through such a process.

CONCLUSION

APRNs are tasked with being advocates for those patients who have been marginalized by society. Oftentimes, the LGBTQ+ community has been self-reliant out of necessity, when modern healthcare has attempted to reduce and atomize the presence of LGBTQ+ patients. The current trend to need to quantify and specialize is a disservice to healthcare delivery. Marginalized communities have witnessed a dearth of economic opportunities and have often been effectively disenfranchised by society. Recent trends in healthcare have led to the pathologization and reduction of LGBTQ+ individuals—specifically trans individuals—leading many APRNs to see LGBTQ+ as intrinsically suffering.

The affirming model of care is one in which each individual, regardless of who they are, can receive culturally competent, holistic, specific, compassionate, person-centered, trauma-informed care. This model requires the APRN to engage in active reflective and thoughtful practice while persistently considering their own beliefs as well as their positionality within the healthcare system. The APRN must meet the patient where they are and be an active advocate for them. This advocacy does not stop at the bedside or in the clinic. It means taking to the streets and actively fighting for a more just and liberatory future. In these troubling, uncertain times, when clinicians are under violent attack, it is up to healthcare providers, including APRNs, to stand up for science, freedom, and the right for all people to simply be.

20 SPECIAL CONSIDERATIONS FOR CHILDHOOD AND ADOLESCENT POPULATIONS

Michelle A. Peralta Westland, Hillary J. Chan, John Westland, Julia Farquharson, Carole Gionet, Maria Manalo, and VaLori R. Abad

INTRODUCTION

This chapter provides a guide for the APRN on special considerations when working with children and adolescents in healthcare settings. Children and adolescents are not small adults. Given the youth's developmental stage, clinicians are required to adapt their clinical approach, ensuring assessments and screening are well targeted to capture the young patient's specific medical and mental health needs. By focusing on the experience and relationship between the young patient and their clinician, important health topics can be accurately addressed with clarity, openness, and without prejudice or assumptions (Anderson & Lowen, 2010). Establishing a therapeutic relationship is a key component to receiving accurate health information when assessing any individual and supporting treatment adherence. Recognizing a young person's developmental stage supports how the clinician gathers pertinent information (e.g., family collateral), asks questions, and adapts their treatment approaches. Appreciating additional factors such as the impact of a young person's cultural and social environments, their understanding of family, typical and atypical developmental stressors impacting their lives, and/or past or current health concerns will help guide the clinician's approach (WHO, 2003).

Preventive care is a driving force when working with young people who may access care intermittently given their social or cultural constructs or accessibility to affordable healthcare (Neinstein, 2008). A supportive and open approach to care is essential for young people to accept or seek health services or advice; therefore, efforts to create an environment grounded in safety and trust will allow clinicians to raise sensitive topics about a young person's health and well-being (Anderson & Lowen, 2010). Since today's most common morbidities and mortalities are preventable, opening a dialogue on how a young person's behavior, environment, or social constructs impact their health can enhance a clinician's ability to promote preventive actions (Neinstein, 2008).

This chapter highlights key factors impacting a child and adolescent's therapeutic engagement with a clinician utilizing a trauma-informed perspective. It also addresses the possible misconceptions or biases that clinicians may internalize, which impact assessment, screening, and discussions around health information for sensitive health topics such as trauma, sexual health, suicide, or other mental health or socio-development needs. A review of parent/caregiver involvement in care is discussed, with specific considerations on how to incorporate them into the child and adolescent's care throughout the developmental process. Lastly, a brief discussion on the challenges and barriers that APRNs may encounter in pediatric mental health practice is presented.

The goal of this chapter is to guide advanced practice clinicians through a developmentally appropriate approach that supports the young patient, resulting in improved overall well-being that helps them reach their developmental milestones, thus enhancing their future health outcomes.

CARING FOR PATIENTS AND THEIR FAMILIES

CHILD AND ADOLESCENT DEVELOPMENT

A. According to the United Nations Convention on the Rights of the Child (UNCRC), a *child* is defined as an individual who is between the ages of 0 and 18 years old (United Nations, 1990; Sawyer et al., 2018). This definition is widely recognized and has been used as a framework for policies, laws, and programs related to children worldwide.

B. Erikson's theory of development breaks down childhood maturation into five stages of change (Table 20.1; Kozier et al., 2003).

1. Each stage describes an internal conflict within the child that must be resolved for them to move forward developmentally and psychosocially.
2. Each stage is categorized by the appropriate age range where certain behavioral milestones are observed and typically achieved.
3. Behavioral indicators (see Table 20.1) are examples of what a clinician may observe when interacting with a young patient. These behavioral indicators can help inform the clinician on how best to approach the young person and help them recognize if the patient is advanced or delayed in their development.

C. The United Nations (UN) and the World Health Organization (WHO) have defined *adolescence* as the period between 10 and 19 years of age, which is a critical developmental stage characterized by physical, emotional, cognitive, and social changes (UNICEF, n.d.; WHO, 2023). The adolescent period is further subdivided into the following substages of development:

1. Early adolescent: approximate ages 10 to 13, or middle school years
2. Middle adolescence: approximate ages 14 to 17, or high school years
3. Late adolescence: approximate ages 17 to 19
   a. Each period reflects developmental attributes specific to identity or social constructs that impact how a young person perceives or interacts with their surroundings (Table 20.2).
      i. It can help the clinician focus on what may be important to assess or screen for when an adolescent enters their care.

TABLE 20.1 ERIKSON'S PSYCHOSOCIAL DEVELOPMENTAL STAGES AND BEHAVIORAL INDICATORS

Stage/Age	Conflict/Crisis	Developmental Attribute/Outcome	Behavioral Indicators of Positive Resolution	Behavioral Indicators of Negative Resolution
Infancy (0–1 year)	Trust vs. mistrust	Hope	Seeking help or a response and anticipating to receive it Ability to share basic thoughts, ideas, and expressions	Inability to accept assistance or resistance to interact openly with others Engages in superficial conversation or cannot easily express thoughts or ideas
Toddler (1–3 years)	Autonomy vs. shame and doubt	Will	Increased socialization and acceptance of group rules with an ability to express disagreement when it is felt Ability to articulate an opinion Can accept delays with gratification or need fulfillment	Cannot easily express needs or share opinions Difficulty socializing and fitting into group norms Limited ability to tolerate needs being met
Preschool/primary grades (3–5 years)	Initiative vs. guilt	Purpose	Takes initiatives to start projects/tasks Asks a lot of questions and has a curiosity about understanding the world Starts to express original/individual thought	Apprehension about starting new projects/tasks Expresses guilt or embarrassment when making small mistakes Imitates or copies others' behaviors, ideas, and thoughts
School age (6–12 years)	Industry vs. inferiority	Competence	Completes tasks Collaborates with others Demonstrates good time management skills	Has difficulty completing tasks Difficulty collaborating or working with others Disorganized
Adolescence (12–18 years)	Identity vs. role confusion	Fidelity	Asserts their independence Future-oriented and planning realistically for place in the world Develops close social and/or intimate relationships	Adopts and internalizes the values or beliefs of others without question Failing to demonstrate any self-direction or to take responsibility and self-motivate Difficulty or failing to set life goals

Source: Adapted from Kozier, B., Erb, G., Bernman, A. J., Burke, K., Bouchal, S. R., & Hirst, S. P. (2003). *Fundamentals of nursing: The nature of nursing practice in Canada* (Canadian ed.). Pearson Education Canada.

    ii. It may also help the clinician appreciate the confounding factors that may interfere with or support the patient's abilities in decision-making, treatment adherence, or motivations to change.

D. A clinician's approach to assessment and screening should reflect the young person's developmental stage and their key priorities for accessing care. It is the clinician's responsibility to:
1. Have a robust awareness of developmental stages and needs of children and adolescents
2. Always look for ways to modify their approach to meet the needs of the child/adolescent
3. Look for ways to address all the needs of the young person

E. Applying a developmental approach to care will ensure that the clinician is able to capture the needs of their young patients and support them effectively to make informed health choices.

RECOGNIZING AND PREVENTING MENTAL HEALTH PROBLEMS IN CHILDREN

A. During all youth assessments (child and adolescent), even when the patient presents with a physical health concern, it is essential that the clinician uses a mental health lens, despite the tendency to separate physical from mental health conditions.
    1. Example: In a patient presenting with abdominal pain, the differentials should include anxiety in addition to the host of physical health concerns that may contribute to this presentation.
    2. The holistic APRN makes a conscious effort to understand the patient and the impact that illness or disease has on their life.

B. Clinicians may sometimes be reluctant to ask a patient about mental health symptoms because they are afraid of the "what if" (i.e., what if the patient says they are suicidal, what do I do) scenarios.
    1. The best approach is to ask questions and be familiar with resources. Early recognition of problems in the individual or the family during the adolescent stages of development can reduce the possibility of mental health problems in the next stages of development.

C. Signs of mental illness to recognize in children and adolescents include the following:
1. Decline in school performance
2. Poor grades despite strong efforts

TABLE 20.2 STAGES OF ADOLESCENCE

	Early Adolescence (10–13 years)	Middle Adolescence (14–16 years)	Late Adolescence (17–19 years)
Cognitive and moral	Concrete thought process Lack of ability to foresee long-term consequences of current decision-making	Development of abstract thought process Starting to question morals, principles, and beliefs	More future-oriented perspective Idealistic viewpoint of the world influencing a self-righteous stance Increased independent thinking
Self-concept/identity formation	Starting preoccupation with changing body Newly developed self-consciousness about appearance	Concern with attractiveness, "stereotypical adolescent"	More stable body image Attractiveness may still be a concern Firmer identify
Family	Beginning to seek more privacy	Conflicts over control and independence Wanting greater autonomy Struggle for acceptance	Emotional and physical separation from family Increase autonomy
Peers	Seeking of same-sex peer affiliation to counter instability	Intense peer group involvement and desire for acceptance and integration Preoccupation with peer culture and values Peers provide behavioral example	Peer group and values recede in importance Intimacy/possible commitment takes precedence
Sexuality	Increased interest in sexual anatomy/genital and body changes Limited desire to dating and intimacy relationships	Testing of ability to attract partner Initiation of relationships and sexual activity Exploration and questions of sexual orientation	Consolidation of sexual identity Focus on intimacy and formation of stable relationships

Source: Adapted from Bourns, A., Kucharski, E., Peterkin, A. D., & Risdon, C. (2022). *Caring for LGBTQ2S people: A clinical guide* (2nd ed.). University Toronto Press. pp. 77–78.

3. Constant worry or anxiety
4. School avoidance or refusal to take part in normal activities
5. Hyperactivity or fidgeting
6. Persistent nightmares
7. Persistent disobedience or aggression
8. Frequent temper tantrums
9. Depression, sadness, or irritability

RESILIENCE

A. Resilience is critical to maintaining positive mental health in children and adolescents. Khanlou and Wray (2014) describe *resilience* as a "life-long buffer to potential threats to wellbeing over time and transition" (p. 65).
B. A person is resilient when they can positively adapt to life circumstances. Resilient people are able to demonstrate flexibility in three domains of health—(a) emotional, (b) mental, and (c) behavioral—making them better able to adjust to internal and external forces that can impact well-being. This elasticity helps children and adolescents manage and learn from life's challenges.
C. Resilience is like the foundation that strengthens an individual's overall self. Tools that influence resilience include the following:
   1. Having a positive attitude toward self, fostering internal self-respect and self-compassion
   2. Developing prosocial skills that promote positive relationships
   3. Having flexible thinking habits, including skills that aid in task completion
   4. Developing positive thinking habits that can promote the skills necessary for task completion
D. Resilient children and adolescents are often self-aware, mindful of self, and have a positive attitude toward and foster positive relationships with others. Resilience is protective against risk factors that can erode an individual's mental health and well-being. It is important for clinicians to promote opportunities for children/adolescents to develop resilience.

ACADEMIC SUPPORT FOR CHILDREN AND ADOLESCENTS WITH MENTAL HEALTH ISSUES

A. When assessing children and adolescents, the clinician should inquire about any academic support they receive from a school. This will provide significant insight into the patient's development and functioning.
B. A fulsome set of questions related to school and school performance can be found in Chapter 5, "Conducting the Pediatric Psychiatric Assessment." This chapter provides a brief description of some of the school support strategies children can access both in Canada and in the United States.

INDIVIDUAL EDUCATION PLAN AND IDENTIFICATION, PLACEMENT AND REVIEW COMMITTEE: CANADIAN PERSPECTIVE

A. The Individual Education Program (or Plan; IEP) is a written document that outlines the special accommodations, education, or services a child/adolescent may require at school. They are created for children who have exceptionalities. These plans are based on assessment of the child's needs, abilities, and strengths.
B. Some children also receive an Identification, Placement and Review Committee (IPRC) in Canada. This committee will work collaboratively to identify areas of exceptionality and work together with the family on resource and placement planning with the goal of student success.

1. This is a committee comprising educational professionals, the school psychologist or social worker, the special education teacher or resource teacher, the principal, and any other members of the school community who can assist in planning for the child.

INDIVIDUAL EDUCATION PLAN AND THE CHILD STUDY TEAM: U.S. PERSPECTIVE

A. A child study team (CST) is a multidisciplinary educational team that is responsible for locating, identifying, evaluating, determining eligibility, and developing an IEP for students suspected of having educational disabilities.
B. The members of the CST include a school psychologist, a learning disabilities teacher-consultant, a school social worker, and in some cases a speech-language specialist.
1. Specialists provide consultative, evaluative, and prescriptive services to teachers and parents.
2. The team provides diagnostic services to children from 3 to 21 years of age who have been identified as having a potential disabling condition.

CAPACITY: ARE CHILDREN AND ADOLESCENTS CAPABLE OF HEALTHCARE DECISION-MAKING?

A. Our society places a strong emphasis on self-determination and individual patients' rights. Furthermore, various international laws and guidelines stress the importance of respecting the developing autonomy of children and involving minors in treatment decision-making (Coughlin, 2018; Grootens-Wiegers et al., 2017).
B. Many countries have laws specifying at what age children should be involved in decisions about medical treatment. Unfortunately, there is no universal agreement as to what age it is appropriate for children to be considered competent for medical decision-making (Grootens-Wiegers et al., 2017). Therefore, the clinician must be aware of the laws in their jurisdiction regarding age of consent.
1. How does the clinician navigate a situation where an adolescent is wanting a selective serotonin reuptake inhibitor (SSRIs) to treat their depression, but the parent/caregiver is refusing this treatment? According to Grootens-Wiegers et al. (2017), by the age of 12, children have the capacity to make medical decisions.
2. In some North American countries, age of consent has been eliminated and decision-making is decided based on the individual's capacity to make decisions. Therefore, irrespective of the individual age, a person is assumed capable of consenting or declining treatment unless found to be incapable.
3. It is essential that the clinician apply the legal test for capacity each time they are offering a treatment (Geist & Opler, 2010).
C. It may not be clear in a medical setting whether a child or adolescent of a certain age is sufficiently competent to make medical decisions.
1. Children and adolescents of the same age may have different maturity levels and development stages; this should be accounted for in deciding capacity in a child/adolescent.
2. Children who demonstrate sufficient competence for decision-making in certain situations can lack adequate competence in another. More specifically, adolescents may have the mental ability to make a reasonable decision, but certain situations (e.g., peer pressure) can impact the child/adolescent's competence (Grootens-Wiegers et al., 2017).
D. Decision-making capacity is defined by four standards: (a) communicating a choice, (b) understanding, (c) reasoning, and (d) appreciation.
1. For the child/adolescent to be considered competent to make a decision, all four capacity standards should be met.
2. Decision-making competence is dependent on the specific decision in the specific situation (Grooten-Wiegers et al., 2017).
    a. Competence can be affected temporarily or chronically by the state of an individual's mental health (e.g., psychosis).
    b. It is essential for clinicians to screen for mental health challenges before deciding if a child/adolescent is competent.
E. Determining medical decision-making capacity in a child/adolescent can be challenging. The brain in adolescence differs significantly from the brain of a child or adult.
1. Significant changes in the brain associated with processing rewards and risks, self-regulation, and the effect of peers on decision-making occur during adolescence. These neurologic changes can affect decision-making in general, as well as medical decision-making (Grootens-Wiegers et al., 2017).
2. The competence of adolescents to make a medical decision can vary per situation. Adolescents are prone toward increased risk-taking in emotional situations and when they are with their peers. This affects their decision-making competence mostly in emotional situations and when they are with their friends.
    a. For example, an adolescent diagnosed with attention deficit hyperactivity disorder (ADHD) can be aware of the benefits of regular physical activity and avoiding substance use (e.g., cannabis, alcohol, energy drinks, etc.). Yet participating in the treatment plan to avoid substance use can be much harder when the adolescent is with a peer group who decides to skip class to smoke cannabis and use other substances.
F. It is prudent for the clinician to fully inform the child/adolescent of their mental health or medical conditions and involve the individual in treatment planning. It is essential to consider the specific laws in your region while thinking critically about capacity and the rights of the child/adolescent and parents/caregivers.

MAINTAINING PATIENT CONFIDENTIALITY

A. A nursing code of ethics is developed by a governing body to help set the practice and professional conduct standards that nurses, of all classes, must follow in their day-to-day work.
1. A code of ethics provides guidelines that help nurses recognize their accountabilities to the public at large as well as to a single patient (Keatings & Smith, 2000).
2. They do not necessarily provide rules of morality, but similarly to laws they will be reflective of the values and beliefs that society holds.
3. In Canada, the *Code of Ethics for Registered Nurses* is held by the Canadian Nurses Association (CNA), and in the United States the primary *Code of Ethics for Nurses* was developed by the American Nurses Association (ANA).

B. Confidentiality is viewed as a core component of ethical nursing practice. The importance of maintaining confidentiality between the health practitioner and the patient cannot be emphasized enough, since without trust effective medicine cannot be delivered.

   1. Ethical dilemmas arise when the limits of confidentiality are tested.

      a. For example, if maintaining confidentiality of the information being shared between the patient and the clinician results in further harm to the patient or others (e.g., child abuse, suicidal ideation, or homicidal intent), then the clinician's accountability to disclose information and the need for informed consent to share personal information may shift.

   2. The perspective of the parents/caregivers can be valuable in formulating the full health picture of a young person; however, not all children or adolescents may want to reciprocate by disclosing their personal health concerns in return.

      a. Establishing trust will be a key component when assessing a child or adolescent and requires the clinician to support the limits of confidentiality and the practice of gaining consent when gathering or sharing health information (Dulcan, 2010).

      b. Clinicians will have an obligation to familiarize themselves with the regulatory and governing laws around confidentiality and disclosure of personal health information as directed by their licensing province, state, or country before proceeding with information sharing.

C. From an ethical standpoint, confidentiality needs to be maintained regardless of age and should only be broken with careful thought, consideration, and legal/ethical examination.

   1. Clinicians should not assume that just because a patient is a minor that their personal health information is not protected. This means that personal health information should not be automatically disclosed to a parent or guardian.

   2. Obtaining explicit consent from the child or adolescent is an excellent exercise in professional relationship and trust building and can be attained simply by asking "Are you okay if I share this with your parents?" Or "It may be important to share this with your parents with you present, how can we do this together?" It also demonstrates a sophisticated style of practice that aims to maintain the autonomy of the child or adolescent.

   3. The clinician must be mindful of how the child or adolescent's age and developmental stage impacts their capacity to understand and appreciate their current situation.

      a. Involvement of a child or adolescent's parents in care may not only be dependent on their developmental stage but also the presenting concern.

      b. Working with a young person to understand the social implications of information sharing in their life may provide insights as to why someone may be reluctant to share information with a parent.

         i. For example, a young person who engages in self-harm may not want to disclose to their parents that they are cutting daily. However, appropriate questioning such as "Why are you afraid to let your family know? What will it mean if they find out?" may help identify a fear of being put on medication or simply a fear of disappointing a parent. In either case, the clinician must decide whether the findings require further investigation to support disclosure.

D. Children and adolescents have a right to refuse information sharing and it is up to the clinician to ask themselves if a breach in confidentiality will have a greater benefit to the young person's health outcomes (Keatings & Smith, 2000).

   1. If a young person's safety is compromised or cannot be maintained due to a lack of information, then the clinician has the duty to work with that individual to support sharing the information.

   2. If the young person refuses to be an active participant in sharing, then the clinician should respectfully inform them about the plan to disclose the information and with whom it will be shared.

   3. The clinician should proceed with caution if a breach of confidentiality is determined to be in the young person's best interest.

   4. Careful documentation of the proceedings and any consultation with professional colleagues or legal experts should be captured.

      a. For example, a young person discloses they have a vague plan to kill themselves someday but insists this information not be shared with their parents/caregivers. This young person lives in the same home as their parents/caregivers and upon further investigation would have the means and access to carry out their plan. Although the plan is not imminent, the risk of self-harm remains high, and a lack of action may have dire consequences. In this case, the clinician is obligated to inform the parents/caregivers about the situation despite the young person's persistent refusal. In some instances, helping a young person understand why it could be important to share with a parent/caregiver or trusted adult may help them process what is happening.

E. In all cases, the clinician must carefully review the risks of breaching confidentiality by taking the time to understand the implications of their decisions and determining how to best include the patient in that process.

COLLABORATION: THE INCLUSION OF THE PATIENT AND THE PARENTS/CAREGIVER IN CARE

A. A child or adolescent's functioning and psychological well-being are highly dependent on the family and school setting. Although the adolescent is the primary patient, parents/caregivers cannot be overlooked, and the adolescent cannot be assessed in isolation (Neinstein, 2008).

B. Definitions of family include single-parent families, stepfamilies, blended families, foster families, adoptive families, extended families, and families of choice.

C. Dynamics and relationships of the subsystems (spouse, parent/child, or sibling) must be understood, as does the family cultural and ethnic background. A clinician who wishes to provide comprehensive care to adolescents must feel comfortable working with families (Neinstein, 2008).

D. The adolescent patient may be very conscious of stigma associated with mental health issues. Fear of judgment, being seen as "crazy," and fearing that the professional will share information with their parents or caregivers can all act to prevent the adolescent from speaking openly with their mental healthcare provider.

1. Parents and other caregivers can be an important source of information about what may be happening for the young person in their life. They can provide history that the adolescent may not be aware of (e.g., developmental history) or unwilling to share (e.g., academic challenges).
2. Fully understanding the adolescent and effecting change require gathering information from diverse sources, including the family, school, and other agencies involved, in addition to the patient themselves.
3. Speaking with the adolescent and the parents/caregivers together is also an opportunity to observe the relationship between them. When speaking with the adolescent and the parent/caregiver together, it is important not to appear to take one person's side against the other. Focusing on how people are feeling about an issue rather than the accuracy or details of conflicting facts can ensure that both parties feel supported.
4. If an adolescent is accompanied to their appointment by their parent/caregiver, many clinicians may opt to see the adolescent first, alone. This is a strong signal that the clinician respects the patient's autonomy, privacy, and confidentiality.
    a. The parent may join the session following the individual meeting with the patient to further explore any joint issues and gather information from the parents'/caregivers' perspective.
    b. Some clinicians ask the teen if they would like their parent to join them for the first few minutes, and then ask the parent to leave so that the clinician and the patient can meet independently of the parent.
E. It is extremely important to explain the limits of confidentiality so that both the parent and the adolescent hear what is and is not confidential.
1. This helps establish realistic expectations about boundaries for conversations, especially the boundary surrounding the communication between the clinician and the adolescent.
2. If situations arise where it is in the best interest of the adolescent for their parents to be made aware of what is happening, or recommendations being made, the clinician can communicate this to the adolescent and cocreate a plan to enlist the parents' support.

UNCONSCIOUS BIASES AND MYTHS

A. Many children and young adults who struggle with mental issues hide their suffering. Oftentimes, risky or maladaptive behaviors are used to express emotions. This results in lack of or no therapeutic care, mostly due to the stigma of fear, shame, and misunderstandings regarding mental health disorders. Dispelling misconceptions about youth mental health is essential to ensure that children and young adults receive the support and education they need.
B. The following are common myths and misconceptions:
1. A child with a psychiatric disorder is damaged for life.
2. Psychiatric problems result from personal weakness.
3. Psychiatric disorders result from *bad parenting*.
4. A child can manage a psychiatric disorder through willpower.
5. Therapy for children is a waste of time.
6. Children with mental health challenges are overmedicated.
7. Children grow out of mental health problems.

TRAUMA: SCREENING FOR ADVERSITY IN CHILDREN AND ADOLESCENTS

A. Adverse childhood experiences (ACEs) are stressful, traumatic events that occur in childhood, prior to the age of 18, with the potential to destabilize the child's sense of safety and stability (Matjasko et al., 2022). ACEs are grouped into three categories: abuse, neglect, and household dysfunction.
B. When children experience multiple adverse experiences, the result can lead to toxic stress that is disruptive to child development. Toxic stress can result in damaged, weakened physical systems and brain architecture with permanent effects if the stress response is long-lasting, prolonged, and the child lacks access to supportive relationships (Franke, 2014).
C. Signs and symptoms exhibited in children who experience traumatic experiences can mimic ADHD, anxiety, oppositional defiant disorder, and depression. If unaddressed or unrecognized, ACEs can have profound, cumulative, lifelong effects. Early detection and timely intervention can reduce the likelihood of adverse health problems and enhance quality of life.
D. The aim of health screening tools is to improve health outcomes through early interventions of disease recognition. ACEs screening questionnaires are accessible screening tools that can be utilized for early identification of typical childhood traumas. By identifying ACEs and providing the needed interventions, the sequelae that increase a person's risk of premature death can be mitigated or reduced. The development of a trusting relationship between patients and healthcare providers through routine interactions with children and their families may enable patients to disclose ACEs. Regular screening allows for at-risk children to be identified so anticipatory guidance can be offered before symptoms are exhibited.
E. Explain the screening process for ACEs.
1. Depending on the tool selected, the process should take less than 10 minutes to complete.
2. Explain that questions are based on experiences and exposures about emotional stressors known to impact current and future health.
3. Inform the patient and their caregiver that the tool is being offered to all patients to identify stresses early to aid in lessening them.
4. Inform the patient and their caregiver that the identification of specific symptoms will determine whether referral for additional services is clinically indicated.
5. Clarify that answers are confidential, except in situations when the patient is at considerable risk of abuse or neglect.
F. Screen for ACEs.
1. Choose a screening tool that includes modifications from the original adult questionnaire, is focused on childhood experiences, and is based on the needs of your patient population.
2. Explain the rationale and screening process, as noted above, to the patient/caregiver. Patients over the age of 12 may complete the screening with the clinician or answer verbally during the appointment. Patients under the age of 12 can verbally answer questions asked by the clinician.
3. Review and score the screening. Explain the ACE score by discussing the next steps. Remember: Early identification and appropriate intervention are paramount to physical and mental health.

4. Offer nonjudgmental support and incorporate trauma-informed care into the treatment plan. Collaborate with community partners, as needed, to provide the patient/family with evidence-based interventions that can address ACEs, including individual/family psychotherapies and/or treatment of substance use disorders or co-occurring conditions. Protect patient privacy but share results with other healthcare providers to avoid duplicate screening and the potential for retraumatization.
5. Plan to rescreen periodically in the pediatric population, per facility policy, as exposure to ACEs may occur after initial screening and throughout childhood and adolescence.
6. Provide the young adult/caregiver with behavioral health resources to support health and well-being.

G. Clinicians should notify child protective services immediately with concerns of suspected abuse or neglect.

H. Know when to screen for ACEs.
1. The clinician should determine the best time to screen.
2. Some clinicians chose to screen upon intake, while others wait until a trusting relationship is established.
3. Screening may be administered face-to-face between the patient and the clinician, or may be completed independently.
4. Choosing whether to ask patients about their exposure to situations (e.g., physical abuse) is a crucial decision when screening for exposure to trauma and adversity. Others require patients to report the total number of categories of adversity experienced in order to triage patients appropriately.
5. Some healthcare experts believe that treatment can be better targeted to the needs of the individual when specific adversities or traumas are disclosed.

AVAILABLE TOOLS FOR SCREENING ADVERSE CHILDHOOD EXPERIENCES AND TRAUMA

A. The following tools originated from the Center for Youth Wellness (CYW) to support screening for ACEs and trauma in practice. These tools are available in English and Spanish and take approximately 2 to 5 minutes to complete.

1. There are three age-specific CYW Adverse Childhood Experiences Questionnaires (ACE-Qs) available (Bucci et al., 2015). The CYW ACE-Q is a clinical screening tool that determines cumulative exposure to ACEs in patients aged 0 to 19. It is based on the instrument designed by Vincent Felitti and Robert Anda for use with adults.
2. The CYW ACE-Q is designed for use in pediatric and family practice settings to identify children who are more likely to experience long-term health issues, learning challenges, behavioral and mental health issues, and developmental issues due to changes in brain architecture and developing organ systems brought on by exposure to extreme and prolonged stress (Bucci et al., 2015). These screenings differ from the original ACEs screening tool in that the patient or the caregiver is asked to tally the total number of statements that apply to their experiences, as opposed to answering "yes" or "no" to specific experiences. The patient or the caregiver is asked NOT to mark or identify which statements apply.

THE HEADSS ASSESSMENT

A. The HEADSS assessment (Table 20.3) is a valuable screening tool that a clinician can utilize when looking for a brief way of assessing children and adolescents for mental health issues (Goldenring & Rosen, 2004). It allows the clinician to assess risks that can be impacting on the patient's mental health.
B. By using this screening tool, the clinician can gather pertinent psychosocial information that will help with the formulation and diagnosis of the patient.
C. This model structures questions in a manner that facilitates communication between the clinician and the adolescent. It is meant to be used when interviewing the patient alone unless the patient requests that their family be present.
D. The clinician should communicate to the adolescent that their response to the HEADSS assessment will be kept confidential unless the adolescent discloses information where the clinician has concern there is imminent harm to the patient or others (Goldenring & Rosen, 2004).

TABLE 20.3 THE HEADSS ASSESSMENT

Assessment Category	Sample Questions
Home and environment Need to establish if the adolescent is living in a safe and supportive environment	• Who lives at home with you? Where are you living? • How many brothers and sisters do you have? Are they healthy? • Are you happy with your living arrangements? Do you feel safe? • Are your parents healthy? What do your parents do for a living? • Are your parents together? If not, where are they? • How do you get along with your siblings, parents? What kinds of things do you and your family argue about the most? What happens in the house when there is disagreement? • What are the rules like at home? • Is there anything you would like to change about your family?
Education/**E**mployment Need to establish if the adolescent is in school and/or working	• Which school do you go to? What grade are you in? Any recent changes in schools? • What do you like best and least about school? Favorite subjects? Worst subjects? • What were your most recent grades? Are these the same or different from the past? Have you ever failed or repeated any years? • How many hours of homework do you do daily? • How much school did you miss last/this year? Do you skip classes? Have you ever been suspended? • What do you want to do when you finish school? Any future plans/goals? • Do you work now? How much? Have you worked in the past? • How do you get along with teachers, employers?

(continued)

TABLE 20.3 THE HEADSS ASSESSMENT (CONTINUED)

Assessment Category	Sample Questions
Activities *Need to ask about activities as they are critical to building rapport and it gives an understanding of the day-to-day life of the adolescent*	• Are most of your friends from school or somewhere else? Are they the same age as you? • Do you hang out with mainly people of your same sex or a mixed crowd? • Do you have one best friend or a few friends? Do you have a lot of friends? • Do you spend time with your family? What do you do with your family? • Do you see your friends at school and on weekends, too? Are there a lot of parties? • Do you do any regular sport or exercise? Hobbies or interests? • Do you have a religious affiliation, belong to a church, or practice some kind of spiritual belief? • How much television do you watch? What are your favorite shows? • Do you read for fun? What do you read? • What is your favorite music? • Do you have a car? Do you use a seat belt? • Have you ever been involved with the police? Have you ever been charged? Do you belong to a group/gang?
Drugs *Need to assess whether their drug use impacts their lives*	• Many young people experiment with drugs, alcohol, or cigarettes. Have you or your friends ever tried them? What have you tried? • When you go out with your friends or to party, do most of the people that you hang out with drink or smoke? Do you? How much and how often? • Do any of your family members drink, smoke, or use other drugs? If so, how do you feel about this? Is it a problem for you? • Have you or your friends ever tried any other drugs? Specifically, what? Have you ever used a needle? • Do you regularly use other drugs? How much and how often? • Do you or your friends drive when you have been drinking? • Have you ever been in a car accident or in trouble with the law, and were any of these related to drinking or drugs? • How do you pay for your cigarettes, alcohol, or drugs?
Sexuality *Need to assess whether their sexual feelings and activity are impacting negatively on their well-being*	• Have you ever been in a relationship? When? How was it? How long did it last? • Have you had sex? Was it a good experience? Are you comfortable with sexual activity? Number of partners? Using contraception? Type and how often (e.g., 10%, 50%, or 70% of the time). • Have you ever been pregnant or had an abortion? • Have you ever had a discharge or sore that you are concerned about? Have you ever been checked for a sexually transmitted disease? Knowledge about sexually transmitted infections and prevention? • Have you ever had a Pap smear? • Do you have any concerns about hepatitis or AIDS? • Have you had an experience in the past where someone did something to you that you did not feel comfortable with or that made you feel disrespected? • If someone abused you, who would you talk to about this? How do you think you would react to this?
Suicide, depression, and homicide *Need to identify symptoms of anxiety or depression since suicidal ideation can exist with depression/anxiety.*	• Have you been depressed lately? What does being depressed mean to you? • What do you do when you get depressed? Have you been hospitalized? • Has anyone in your family ever been depressed? Died by suicide? • Have you ever tried to hurt yourself? How? • Have you ever felt like killing yourself? What happened? • Do you feel suicidal now? Do you have a plan? • Have you ever felt like hurting someone else?
Safety *Important to ask questions regarding an adolescent's safety at school and home and during their free time*	• Have you ever been seriously injured? How? • Do you always wear a seat belt in your car? • Have you ever ridden in a car with someone who was drunk or high? • Is there any violence in your home? • Have you ever been picked on or bullied? • Have you ever felt the need to carry a weapon to protect yourself?

Source: Adapted from Goldenring, J. M., & Rosen, D. S. (2004). Getting into adolescent heads: An essential update. *Contemporary Pediatrics, 21,* 21–64.

TREATMENT ADHERENCE

A. A collaborative approach to care will positively affect how well the patient follows the recommendations of the clinician. *Treatment adherence* is then defined as the willingness and ability of the patient to follow through with the agreed-upon treatment plan. Patients and their parents/caregivers can struggle to remain on track with the agreed-upon care plan for many reasons. Medication adherence can be a significant struggle for children/adolescents. This type of nonadherence is defined as "missing 20% or more of prescribed medications" (McVoy & Levin, 2023, p. 366).

B. There are several barriers to adherence for patients with mental health issues, including being a child/adolescent, having mood lability, having risky behavioral events, the cognitive and developmental level of the individual, the efficacy of the patient's working memory, and the patient's and the parents'/caregivers' feelings toward the treatment (McVoy & Levin, 2023).

C. Risks associated with general medical treatment non adherence include the following:
  1. Biomedical factors: medication side effects, scheduling, comorbid conditions, severity of symptoms, perceived susceptibility to the illness, consequences of the illness, perception of treatment disadvantages, and treatment cessation upon symptom resolution
  2. Psychological factors: lack of insight, specific cultural beliefs, poor memory, poor self-esteem, high levels of stress, being in denial, personal beliefs about treatment, and developmental milestones
  3. Social factors: attitudes of friends and family, lack of support (perceived or actual), poor therapeutic alliance with treatment team, cost of treatment, feelings of rejection, and history of poor adherence

CONSEQUENCES OF NONADHERENCE

A. Nonadherence to treatment can have significant consequences for the patient and the family. Challenges with adherence can place a strain on the patient–clinician relationship, the patient–parents/caregiver relationship, and the patient–family system relationship. There is a direct relationship between nonadherence and morbidity and mortality from several chronic conditions.
B. Consequences of nonadherence include the following:
  1. Patient has poorer health outcomes.
  2. Nonadherence interferes with treatment decision-making. When a patient does not adhere to treatment, this can lead to treatment failure, adversely affecting the clinician's choices of treatment. The clinician may consider the treatment to be noneffective when, in this case, the effectiveness is related to adherence.
  3. Patient incurs higher healthcare costs due to the morbidity correlated with treatment nonadherence.
  4. Nonadherence can be burdensome to the family/caregivers (e.g., parents/caregivers having to take more time off from work, increased cost for transportation).
  5. Patient has poorer quality of life (e.g., the child/adolescent misses out of favorite activities, school, sports).

IMPACT ON THE FAMILY RELATIONSHIP

A. Impact on adolescent development, particularly the separation–individualization process between the patient and the parent/caregiver, which may be hindered or delayed
B. Feelings of guilt for both the patient and the parent/caregiver
C. Parents/caregivers feeling uncertain or questioning their ability to set appropriate limits
D. Increased family stress and strain on the family dynamic as the family unit tries to constantly balance the health needs of the patient with those of "normal life."
E. Negative impact on siblings and sibling relationships

ENHANCING TREATMENT ADHERENCE

A. One of the best ways to positively influence patient adherence is to develop a positive relationship with patients and their parents/caregivers. Having a reflective practice can also positively enhance treatment adherence.
B. Strategies to help with preserving a sense of normalcy include the following:
  1. Understand the context in which the adolescent is living.
     a. How do they view themselves in the world?
     b. Who are their friends?
     c. What are their social activities?
     d. How do they cope (at school, with friends, etc.) with chronic illness?
  2. Promote healthy relationships.
     a. Foster strong open relationships with the clinical team and the parent/caregiver with the collaboration of the patient.
     b. Parents/caregivers should serve as practical support.
  3. Encourage patients/caregiver and patients to seek support (e.g., connecting with community mental health agencies, community health team resources).
  4. Encourage healthy, positive, and motivating friendships as emotional support for the patient and the parents/caregivers.
C. Adherence-promoting strategies include the following:
  1. Address all comorbid issues that can affect adherence (e.g., mental health issues, developmental challenges, learning disabilities, medical conditions).
  2. Foster collaborative relationship between the clinician and the patient/parents/caregivers.
  3. Frequently check in with the patient and parents/caregivers about treatment efficacy. Is the treatment working the ways that they understood it might?
  4. Use motivational enhancement strategies (e.g., motivational interviewing [MI] strategies or play therapy for younger children).
  5. Offer concrete strategies.
  6. Set out a plan together that encourages achievable gains.
  7. Use peer support (Santer et al., 2014):
     a. Peer groups
     b. Friends
  8. Consider the needs of the patient with adhering to the plan while at school or in social/recreational activities (Santer et al., 2014).
  9. Use technology (e.g., electronic reminders for appointments or medication refills) especially with adolescent population.
D. Strategies to optimize the adolescent–clinician relationship include the following:
  1. Adolescents' perception of their healthcare provider's behavior contributes to their willingness to adhere to treatment and follow through with returning for visits (Neinstein, 2008). Neinstein (2008) provided general considerations for optimizing the adolescent–clinician relationship:
     a. Encourage open communication.
        i. Use an empathic, nonjudgmental approach (warmth and respectful with a tone of curiosity). Use sensitive, nonstigmatizing language.
        ii. Listen to the adolescent.
        iii. Treat their comments seriously.
     b. Avoid power struggles.
     c. Be flexible.
     d. Strive for cleanliness, honesty, respect, and carefulness.
     e. Maintain the limits of confidentiality.
     f. Provide experience and equal treatment of all patients.
     g. Use direct encouragement.
E. Become an influencer for change.
  1. People have internal and external drivers of change. Sources of influence include personal motivation, a supportive environment to promote change, and having positive social support. The goal of MI is to enhance a person's internal motivation to change. MI has been used in a range of clinical settings to promote adherence to treatment or to influence positive health behaviors (Schaefer & Kavookjian, 2017).

THE CLINICIAN ROLE

APPLYING TRAUMA-INFORMED CARE TO PRACTICE

A. A patient's knowledge of health needs, how the patient makes decisions, and how they collaborate and adhere to treatment are affected by the relationship built between them and the clinician (Fleishman et al., 2019).
B. This relationship needs to be mutually trusting, emotionally supportive, and collaborative in nature (Fleishman et al., 2019). Recognizing that children/adolescents can have trauma experiences and that this experience can affect their interactions with clinicians and the healthcare system is vital to the development of a safe space that promotes collaboration through trust and transparency (Fleishman et al., 2019).
C. A method for implementing trauma-informed practice is to follow the OPTIMAL approach to care:
    1. Open/nonthreatening body language: Be empathic in your approach.
    2. Privacy is essential. Safeguard your patient's private and confidential information. Ensure your patients are aware of the limitations of confidentiality.
    3. Touch: Clinicians sometimes need to touch their patients to provide care. Assure patients that their permission will always be sought prior to touching them or anything that belongs to them (e.g., mobility or communication device). Consider personal equipment that is attached to the patient, used to aid in their activities of daily living, as an extension of their body and ask permission first before touching these items as well.
    4. Introduce oneself and state one's role.
    5. Messaging should be clear and consistent between clinicians caring for the same patient.
    6. Anticipatory guidance is a key element of care that can help reinforce what a patient can do to prevent unsafe situations or healthcare challenges from occurring.
    7. Language: The language used to communicate with the patient should be simple and easy to understand. Be mindful of nonverbal communication and its impact on patients. Both the clinician employing paraphrasing after listening to the patient and the patient using a teach-back approach when being provided health education can improve the communication between patients and clinicians.

THE ROLE OF THE ADVANCED PRACTICE REGISTERED NURSE IN PEDIATRIC MENTAL HEALTHCARE

A. APRNs can help increase access to mental healthcare in primary care settings, especially for children and adolescents who have limited access. Collaboration and partnership are key elements of the work of increasing access to services.
B. Many pediatric patients present with a combined picture, straddling both the physical and mental health realms of care. APRNs practice holistically, a well-suited approach to care for these young individuals.
    1. The APRN can provide a combination of services that include both physical and mental health direct patient care, health promotion activities, and service navigation for patients needing to access further mental health resources.
    2. APRNs have the expertise to identify and address system gaps.
    3. Research shows that the services provided by APRNs result in excellent patient outcomes and more patient satisfaction as compared with other healthcare professional groups providing similar services.

CHALLENGES FOR THE ADVANCED PRACTICE REGISTERED NURSE

A. In recent years, there has been national recognition that there is a lack of access to mental healthcare. The issue of access has been identified as being primarily due to a lack of qualified healthcare providers, especially in the community and rural settings (AAP, 2021; Moroz et al., 2020).
B. To address this gap in care, it has been proposed that increasing funding for mental health providers, especially pediatric provider, will be the main solution.
    1. In the United States, psychiatric-mental health nurse practitioners (PMHNPs) have an essential role in access to mental healthcare. PMHNPs face various barriers to practice, such as state-to-state variations on scope of practice and autonomy, reimbursement restrictions, and education.
    2. State-specific variations have led to a lack of clarity on nurse practitioner (NP) scope and have also likely elicited declining numbers of qualified PMHNPs (Hudspeth & Klein, 2019).
    3. A core concern for PMHNPs identified in the literature is psychopharmacologic education and treatment challenges. NPs practicing in the field of pediatric mental health have reported significant concerns around decision-making on treatment plans, treatment adherence, and monitoring drug-related symptoms (Mangano et al., 2020).
    4. Treatment planning for the pediatric patient can be complicated by patient and/or parental disagreement, particularly because age of consent for medical testing and treatment varies state to state from 12 to 18 years of age.
    5. Because there is a lack of pediatric mental health research, many psychopharmacologic treatments are used off-label in this population, and therefore comfort with prescribing certain treatments is a challenge for NP clinicians (Mangano et al., 2020).
C. Treatment adherence is a common challenge across many health-related specialties and is encountered frequently in mental health.
    1. The main factors for nonadherence have been noted to be related to stigma associated with psychotropic medications, concern regarding dependence on medications, patient knowledge regarding illness and treatment choices, as well as the therapeutic alliance between the patient and the healthcare provider (Laranjeira et al., 2023).
D. Burnout is a common theme in healthcare workers across all disciplines. Rates of burnout in mental health specialties tend to be higher, and according to the American Psychological Association mental health worker burnout is between 21% and 61% (2018). Major factors contributing to burnout are many and can be mitigated by smaller caseloads, workplace flexibility, and a focus on healthcare provider self-care (APA, 2018).

OPPORTUNITIES FOR PARTNERSHIP

A. Collaboration between various other mental healthcare providers and primary care providers is essential to the integration of mental health in pediatric primary care. According to the American Academy of Child and Adolescent Psychiatry, successful partnerships are characterized by effective ▶

collaboration, communication, and coordination between psychiatrists, other mental health providers, and primary care providers, in consultation with the children and their families.
B. A working relationship between the APRNs, psychiatrists, and other allied mental health practitioners can enhance the mental health services for children and adolescents. These partnerships can reduce gaps in services by reaching larger numbers of children and their families through promotion of prevention, early intervention, and treatment of childhood psychiatric illness (AACAP, 2010).
   1. APRNs with the skill and knowledge to treat children and adolescents with mental illness can help address the gaps and services that exist today. However, collaboration with other mental health professionals and agencies can result in more positive outcomes.
   2. Engage with social workers/psychotherapists/psychologists for ongoing therapy, consult with psychiatrists if symptoms are worsening and diagnostic clarification and additional treatment options are needed, collaborate with psychologists for psychoeducational assessment, and/or include child protective services for resource and community support.
C. APRNs are uniquely positioned to partner with primary care providers and specialized mental health providers to advocate for collaborative and integrated care at the provincial, state, or federal levels. Wissow et al. (2021) outlined four key areas of advocacy initiatives:
   1. Transforming pediatric practice to address family psychosocial needs
   2. Financially feasible pediatric integrated care
   3. Development of a more diverse and larger integrated care workforce
   4. Efforts in developing more research programs to study the process and interventions that will bring integrated care to full practice

PURSUING EVIDENCE-BASED PRACTICE WITHIN THE PEDIATRIC POPULATION

A. Most mental illnesses have their origins in early childhood and can possibly be related to prenatal events (Dalsgaard et al., 2020; Weir, 2012). Improving pediatric psychiatric research and mental healthcare for the pediatric population will serve to prevent mental illness and improve the population's quality of life into adulthood.
B. Trends in pediatric mental health have changed dramatically over the past decade, with significantly increasing rates of anxiety, depression, and other mental health diagnoses (Lebrun-Harris et al., 2022).
   1. Research in pediatric psychiatry must consider the ethical care of these populations and how this may inform clinical and health policy decisions.
   2. Using the biopsychosocial model, understanding determinants of health, health literacy, and working in unison with patients and their families, clinicians must build a trusting and therapeutic relationship in order to provide unbiased and thorough support and care.
   3. Research that includes and focuses on cultural competency and humility addresses the disparity in health equity that exists in healthcare systems in North America as populations become more diverse (Kibakaya et al., 2022).
C. A core competency of nursing is to advocate for patients' optimal health, and in doing so to uphold social justice and continually improve the healthcare environment (American Association of Colleges of Nursing, 2021; College of Nurses of Ontario, 2019). APRNs are prepared with the knowledge, skill, and judgment to provide family-centered, culturally humble care and are well-positioned as leaders in furthering pediatric research.

A GUIDE TO MOTIVATIONAL INTERVIEWING IN ADOLESCENT AND PEDIATRIC POPULATIONS

A. Motivational interviewing (MI) can be described as a method to improve a person's intrinsic motivation for change. It is a person-centered collaborative process during which an individual is guided by the clinician to elicit and reinforce their motivation for change.
   1. MI involves a gentle and respectful form of communication that encourages the growth of motivation in order to pursue a healthier and more meaningful life.
   2. It is often associated with treatment of substance use disorders. However, this effective approach to behavior change has been applied in a wide array of clinical settings, including obesity management, eating disorders, diabetes management, and adherence to treatment.
B. MI is not simply a way to get people to do what you want them to do, or to do as you ask. It is not even a way to encourage others to follow your advice. There are specific principles, techniques, and mnemonics to help you understand and implement this approach in your practice. However, the main elements or the spirit behind MI is much more important than any of the specific techniques or tools.

WHY PEOPLE CHANGE

A. It is natural for people to feel ambivalent or to have mixed feelings about changing something in their life. There are always pros and cons behind the decision to make a change. This applies whether one is talking about the possibility of abstaining from alcohol use, starting an exercise program, or leaving an unhealthy relationship. The use of logic or the weight of an argument shared with the patient may not affect their decision-making process in the way you would expect or hope.
B. Think for a moment of a scenario where you do not like the person whom a close friend is dating. The person they are dating is disrespectful of your friend. Since you care about them, you want the best for them. Can you picture having a conversation during which you try to convince them to end the relationship or at least share with them your concerns? Now, can you imagine how they might respond to what you are sharing? When this question was put to participants in dozens of MI training sessions, most participants reported that their friend became defensive or angry. Triggering this response in people does not motivate them to change. In fact, this can encourage people to push back, defending their decision not to change or actively moving in a direction opposite to that which one is hoping to influence the person. The more one confronts someone about change, the more they may resist. If you take a more reflective and supportive stance, the patient's resistance decreases (Miller & Rollnick, 2013).
C. The more people talk about the possibility of change with their healthcare provider, the more likely it will occur. This is supported by research that shows that people tend to believe what they hear themselves say.
D. Clinicians may believe that a person's main motivation to change behavior is the relief or avoidance of the distressing stimuli (e.g., pain). However, there are many other things that

influence a person's motivation to change, including beliefs, knowledge, confidence in their own abilities, or importance of the change happening.

E. Many healthcare professionals seek to encourage change in their patient's behavior and help make things right. This is referred to as the *righting reflex*. MI encourages clinicians to resist this righting reflex because when you try to persuade the patient to change their behavior it can inadvertently encourage the patient to resist change. We recognize that in the primary care setting you will mostly be applying MI in a brief interaction with your patient. The following guide can help you apply the core concepts of MI in your daily practice:

MOTIVATIONAL INTERVIEWING IS PERSON-CENTERED

A. Focusing on the concerns and perspectives of the patient
  1. "I'm not worried about my drug use, my mother is."
B. Encouraging the patient to share their thoughts and feelings
  1. "She gets so upset over nothing. I hate it."
C. Allowing the patient to determine the direction and destination of the conversation
  1. "I just want her off my back."

MOTIVATIONAL INTERVIEWING GUIDES THE PERSON

A. The clinician intentionally addresses ambivalence.
B. Effort is made to elicit and reinforce things the patient says about healthy changes to their behavior. This is referred to as *change talk* (Skinner, 2017).
C. The clinician listens for things the patient says that relate to change (change talk) and then reflects this back to the patient.
  1. "You really hate how upset your mom gets over your drug use."

RECOGNIZING CHANGE TALK

A. *Change talk* refers to anything the patient says that relates to the possibility of change happening. Typically, the clinician is focused on a target behavior, such as drug use, exercise, self-harm, diabetes management, and so on. Using MI involves listening for and selectively reinforcing this change talk. However, if one takes a systemic approach, one can listen for and reinforce any talk that relates to change happening. Clinicians can reflect on and reinforce change talk using reflective listening, which will be discussed in more detail.

B. Change talk can be remembered by the mnemonic DARN-CAT (Miller & Rollnick, 2013):
  1. **Desire to change**
     a. "I want to feel less burnt out from smoking" or "I wish she wouldn't bother me so much about smoking."
  2. **Ability to change**
     a. "I've gone a couple of days without smoking" or "I can stop whenever I want."
  3. **Reasons to change**
     a. "I've spent all my savings on weed" or "I'd like to be able to save money for a car."
  4. **Need to change**
     a. "I can't stand all the arguing about weed; it isn't worth it" or "If I keep getting suspended, I'm not going pass this year."
  5. **Commitment to change**
     a. "I'm going to stop smoking during lunch so I can get to my classes in the afternoon."
  6. **Actions identified**
     a. "I can ask my friend if they will play basketball with me over lunch."
  7. **Taking steps**
     a. "I smoked at lunch yesterday, but not as much" or "I ate with my best friend yesterday then played on my phone for a while."

GUIDING THE PATIENT IN A SPECIFIC DIRECTION

A. Even though MI is person-centered and is focused on the concerns and perspectives of the patient, the clinician has a direction in mind for the conversation. The metaphor used in MI is one of dancing rather than wrestling. Dancing is a cooperative activity where both parties are moving for a common purpose! They are on the same side, and no one wins or loses. Even though one person may be leading and the other is following, the result can appear seamless. This is in stark contrast to wrestling, where the two parties are adversaries and they are acting at opposite purposes. There is a clear winner and loser and winning comes at the expense of the other party.

B. Applying this metaphor to MI, one does not try to force, persuade, or convince the patient of anything. There is no attempt to win over the patient to see your way of seeing things. Instead, there is a respectful conversation where the patient feels accepted and heard and does not feel the need to defend their choices.

C. Engaging in self-reflection during a session with a patient is quite useful, even for a moment. If it feels like you are wrestling rather than dancing with your patient, it is time to change your approach. If you have ever said to yourself "This feels like pulling teeth," that is a sign that a change of approach is called for. There is a famous line from the play Hamilton where Aaron Burr tells Alexander Hamilton to "…Talk less…smile more…" (Miranda & McCarter, 2016, p. 24). One could apply that to clinical work, and perhaps replace "…smile more…" (Miranda & McCarter, 2016, p. 24) with *listen more*.

ENHANCING INTRINSIC MOTIVATION

A. People often deal with extrinsic motivators or pressures, such as suspensions, having phones confiscated, or allowances cut off. MI encourages the exploration of intrinsic motivators, even if they are associated with extrinsic sources.
B. Do ask:
  1. "How is it for you when your mom gets so upset?"
  2. "How did you feel about being suspended?"
  3. "How important is it for you, to have your phone back?"
  4. Unless the patient feels that the change is in their best interest, at least to some extent, it is not going to happen. Asking them about things that matter to them can encourage motivation to change. If the patient feels coerced, it will be difficult for them to pursue change in a committed way.
C. Do not say:
  1. "Well, if you want to get your phone back, I guess you'll have to stop smoking!"
D. Do not ask:
  1. "Why don't you quit smoking since you know it upsets your mom?"
  2. This statement can encourage defensiveness in the patient. It can even inadvertently encourage them to state why they want to continue to use drugs, or as a bigger risk it could even discourage them to further pursue any type of healthcare.

THE FOUR ELEMENTS OF MOTIVATIONAL INTERVIEWING

A. The spirit of MI can be described using the following elements: partnership, acceptance, compassion, and evocation (Skinner, 2017):
  1. Partnership
     a. People are seen as being their own experts. Although people may be coming to you to benefit from your expertise, the person who is seeking you out still knows themselves better than anyone else. This applies whether it is knowledge of their symptoms, what their health goals are, or how they experience pain or what level of risk they are willing to take in their treatment. For example, if asked for ideas about how to address an issue, you can invite the patient to brainstorm with you or ask what has been even partially helpful in the past.
  2. Acceptance
     a. Acceptance is different from approval. You do not have to agree with your patient's choices, but when you communicate that you accept them for who they are and respect their autonomy, people are more likely to contemplate engaging in change. If the patient is unhappy about the consequences of their actions and not yet ready to pursue change that would address those consequences, offer support rather than judgment or instruction. For example, "That's such a challenging place to be: wanting your mom off your back about drug use, and also wanting marijuana to try to manage your anxiety."
  3. Compassion
     a. Compassion might be described as putting empathy into action. The clinician demonstrates that they are listening and seeking to understand the patient's experience. The clinician may also engage with the patient to support them to access tangible and intangible things that support their personal goals and values. For example, "You really don't like it when your mom gets so upset. It really bothers you."
  4. Evocation
     a. The clinician attempts to draw out of the patient their goals and values and parts of them that are in favor of change.
        i. "You really care about your relationship with your mom."
        ii. "How would it be for you if your mom had more trust in you?"
        iii. "What do you think you can do to help build that trust?"
        iv. "What's the worst thing that could happen if your situation doesn't change?"
        v. This last example asks the patient to think about what negative outcome they would rather avoid. It does not identify what the situation is, so that the patient can identify whatever matters to them. The answer to this question can provide a concrete reason for them to change their behavior (change talk).
        vi. If the patient says, "The worst thing would be if my mom told me I had to go to inpatient rehab, if I don't stop smoking," the clinician can respond with "You really don't want to go to rehab," said in a compassionate tone, rather than an instructive tone. This reinforces the patient's expressed goal of not attending rehab. You can follow up with "What do you think you can do to try to make sure this doesn't happen?"

THE MAIN PRINCIPLES OF MOTIVATIONAL INTERVIEWING

A. The mnemonic DARES can help you recall the principles of MI (Peterson, 2019).
  1. **D**evelop discrepancy.
  2. **A**void arguing.
  3. **R**oll with resistance.
  4. **E**xpress empathy.
  5. **S**upport self-efficacy.

B. Develop discrepancy.
  1. Develop discrepancy between the patient's present state and where they want to be. Help the person identify their own goals and values and allow them to present their own arguments for change.
     a. "You really want to have a better relationship with your mom."
     b. "What has to happen in order for you to get your cell phone back?"

C. Avoid arguing.
  1. Try to refrain from being the sole source of change. If you are the instigator of change, this leaves your patient in a passive position. The more active your patient is, the more invested they will be in any attempt at change. When you have information to share, advice to give, or perspectives that are different from your patient's, use the "elicit, provide, elicit" method to provide information to your patient that is gentle and therefore more easily accepted (Skinner, 2017):
  2. Elicit, provide, elicit.
     a. Elicit.
        i. Ask permission to raise an issue or look at a specific topic.
           (1) If your patient is using marijuana to help them manage their anxiety, you can state: "Would it be OK if we spent a few moments looking at how marijuana and anxiety relate to each other?"
           (2) If they answer "yes," then ask: "What has your experience been?" or "What have you heard?"
     b. Provide.
        i. After listening carefully to what your patient shares and not interrupting or displaying any judgmentalism about what they have said, state "Thank you for all you shared with me. Would it be OK if I shared with you what I have heard from my other patients?" (or "…what I have seen/read about/my understanding of how they relate to each other?").
           (1) Then, go ahead and share whatever information you feel would be useful for your patient to know.
     c. Elicit.
        i. After you have shared what you would like your patient to know, ask them: "How does that sound to you?" or "What do you make of what I have shared?"
        ii. Do not merely ask "Do you understand?" They may understand or think they understand, yet totally disagree with what you have spoken about. You need to know how they feel about what you have shared so that you can reply with a compassionate response and offer clarification if needed.
        iii. If your patient answers "no" to your request to spend a few moments talking about a topic, ask them to help you understand why. For example, ▶

"Can you help me understand how come you would rather not talk about this?" or "What is it about (this topic) that makes it something you would rather not talk about?"

   iv. Your patients may share with you that they have already had lectures from their parents or other adults about the topic and do not want to hear any more. You can express compassion for this experience and let them know that you were seeking to have a conversation about the topic and were interested in hearing their experiences and opinions. They will not be expecting this statement from the clinician, which demonstrates respect for their feelings, experiences, and wishes, even if they do not engage in any further conversation about the topic.

D. Roll with resistance.
   1. If your patient asks, "When are we done," or starts checking their cell phone in the middle of an interview, respond with compassion: "I have until 10 a.m., is that still OK for you?" or "Do you have somewhere you need to be?" asked compassionately, not sarcastically. A patient may tell you that they need to use the washroom. If your patient is repeatedly doing something on their phone, you can state: "Wow, someone is really trying to get hold of you." This acknowledges that they are on their phone without being judgmental or instructive. Your patient may then acknowledge what this activity means to them: an activity to focus on that makes it easier to talk, an app that has prompted them to feel compelled to respond to, or a text that they just remembered they needed to send.

E. Express empathy.
   1. When people feel that they are understood and accepted, they tend to be more open with those around them. Accepting people appears to have the effect of giving them space to change. When people feel that they are not accepted, it can engender a feeling of resistance to change.
      a. "You really hate it when your mom gets so upset."
      b. "Things sound really stressful for you right now."

F. Support self-efficacy.
   1. Your patient is ultimately the one responsible for pursuing any changes in their life. A person's belief in the possibility of them creating change is an important motivator. The clinician's own expressed belief in the patient's abilities can also be a reinforcer of the person's motivation. For example, "You went for an entire weekend without smoking! How did you do that?" expressed with a tone of admiration and curiosity.

PUTTING THE PRINCIPLES INTO PRACTICE: THE OARS+ APPROACH

A. Open questions
   1. The patient should be doing most of the talking. Open-ended questions cannot be answered with a simple yes or no and encourages the patient to explore what their experience is.
      a. "What kinds of things create stress for you in your life?"
      b. "What made you decide to come to speak with me today?"
      c. "How do you manage your stress when you don't have any marijuana?"

B. Affirmation
   1. Communicating affirmation to your patient can help them feel that change is possible and builds rapport and self-efficacy. You can point out strengths, abilities, and efforts they make.
      a. "You really care about yourself."
      b. "You're really determined."
      c. "You really know what you want."
      d. "You put so much effort into…"

C. Reflective listening
   1. Reflective listening, or reflections, are statements rather than questions. The clinician paraphrases or reflects back to the patient what they have heard, or what they sense the patient may be thinking or feeling.
   2. In MI, the clinician is listening particularly for change talk. When the clinician hears it, or senses that the patient is feeling or thinking something that is aligned with change, they reflect it, as a statement.
      a. "You really want to get your mom's trust back."
      b. "It would feel horrible if you had to go to inpatient rehab."
      c. "It seems like things feel pretty uncomfortable between you and your mom right now."
   3. If you hear the patient talking about reasons to not change their behavior, it is important to refrain from reflecting these statements. You don't want to reinforce their thoughts about maintaining a behavior that is unhealthy.
      a. For example, your patient might say: "I love weed. It calms me down. I just wish my mom would calm down about it." You can reply: "You really wish your mom would be less stressed about your smoking weed."
      b. You are selectively reinforcing the change talk.

D. Summarizing
   1. By summarizing what the patient has said, particularly about change, you provide an opportunity for the patient to hear their own words about change a third time: once when they said it; a second time when you reflected it; and a third time when you provide a summary of what has been talked about. This can happen at the conclusion of a topic you have discussed, partway through an appointment, or at the end of the appointment with the patient. This reinforces what has been said about change.
      a. "You're really serious about making changes that will increase trust with your mom. It even includes changing how much you smoke."

E. Eliciting change talk
   1. There are several things a clinician can do to elicit talk that is about change.
      a. Ask evocative questions.
         i. "How could you tell if your use of marijuana was causing issues in your life?"
         ii. "If you had to stop using weed for a while, how long do you think you could stop?"
         iii. "What would you do to make that possible?"
      b. Ask for the patient to elaborate.
         i. "What else have you done to try to stay healthy?"
         ii. "How did you make that happen?"
      c. Ask about extremes.
         i. "What's the worst thing that could happen if things don't change with your mom?"
         ii. Use a scaling question: "On a scale of 0 to 10 how confident are you that you would be able to stop or decrease using weed?"
         iii. When the patient provides a number, perhaps 5, then ask the patient about why they did not report a lower number: "Why isn't it just a 3 or a 4?" This question helps the patient focus on what they are

able to do, their strengths, and their confidence. It highlights what they can do and why they can do it, so they can build on it, rather than focusing on what they cannot do or what they have not attained.

KEY POINTS TO REMEMBER

A. The four elements of MI are more important than any of the skills or techniques.
B. Focus on helping your patient pursue the healthy things that they value.
C. See things through your patient's eyes.
D. Listen for and reinforce their desire for change.
E. Compassion and acceptance facilitate trust and change.

SUMMARY

This chapter emphasizes the importance of adapting the APRN's clinical approaches when working with children and adolescents. It highlights the barriers that can hinder effective support to young patients with mental health issues, including population-specific research and a lack of understanding on the impact of development on the therapeutic alliance. Clinicians must tailor their approaches to suit the developmental stage of their patients and focus on developmentally appropriate preventive care strategies, screenings, and assessments. By practicing mindfully and addressing the unique needs of this patient demographic, clinicians can break down assumptions and biases and optimize young people's health outcomes.

REFERENCES AND BIBLIOGRAPHY

Academy of Eating Disorders. (2016). *Eating disorders: A guide to medical care* (3rd ed.). AED Report. https://www.massgeneral.org/assets/mgh/pdf/psychiatry/eating-disorders-medical-guide-aed-report.pdf

American Academy of Child and Adolescent Psychiatry. (2015). Practice parameter for the assessment and treatment of children and adolescents with eating disorders. *Journal of the American Academy of Child & Adolescent Psychiatry, 54*(5), 412–425. https://www.jaacap.org/article/S0890-8567(15)00070-2/pdf

American Academy of Pediatrics. (2021). *AAP-AACAP-CHA declaration of a national emergency in child and adolescent mental health*. https://www.aap.org/en/advocacy/child-and-adolescent-healthy-mental-development/aap-aacap-cha-declaration-of-a-national-emergency-in-child-and-adolescent-mental-health

American Association of Colleges of Nursing. (2021). *The essentials: Competencies for professional nursing education*. https://www.aacnnursing.org/Portals/0/PDFs/Publications/Essentials-2021.pdf

American Nurses Association. (2015). *Code of ethics for nurses with interpretive statements*. https://www.nursingworld.org/practice-policy/nursing-excellence/ethics/code-of-ethics-for-nurses

American Psychiatric Association. (2013). *Diagnostic and statistical manual of mental disorders* (5th ed.). https://doi.org/10.1176/appi.books.9780890425596

American Psychological Association. (2018). Research roundup: Burnout in mental health providers. *Practice Update*. https://www.apaservices.org/practice/update/2018/01-25/mental-health-providers

Anderson, J., & Lowen, C. (2010). Connecting youth with health services: Systematic review. *Canadian Family Physician, 56*, 778–784. PMID: 20705886.

Bourns, A., Kucharski, E., Peterkin, A. D., & Risdon, C. (2022). *Caring for LGBTQ2S people: A clinical guide* (2nd ed., pp. 77–78). University of Toronto Press.

Bucci, M., Gutiérrez Wang, L., Koita, K., Purewal, S., Silvério Marques, S., & Burke Harris, N. (2015). *Center for Youth Wellness ACE-Q: User guide for health professionals*. Center for Youth Wellness. https://www.nursing.umaryland.edu/media/son/academics/professional-education/religion-and-ethics/CYW-ACE-Q-USer-Guide-copy.pdf

Canadian Nurses Association. (2017). *Code of ethics for registered nurses*. https://www.cna-aiic.ca/en/nursing/regulated-nursing-in-canada/nursing-ethics

College of Nurses of Ontario. (2019, April). *Entry to practice competencies for registered nurses*. https://www.cno.org/globalassets/docs/reg/41037-entry-to-practice-competencies-2020.pdf

Coughlin, K. W. (2018). Medical decision-making in pediatrics: Infancy to adolescence. *Pediatric Child Health, 23*(2), 138–146. https://doi.org/10.1093/pch/pxx127

Dalsgaard, S., Thorsteinsson, E., Trabjerg, B. B., Schullehner, J., Plana-Ripoll, O., Brikell, I., Wimberley, T., Thygesen, M., Madsen, K. B., Timmerman, A., Schendel, D., McGrath, J. J., Mortensen, P. B., & Pedersen, C. B. (2020). Incidence rates and cumulative incidences of the full spectrum of diagnosed mental disorders in childhood and adolescence. *JAMA Psychiatry, 77*(2), 155–164. https://doi.org/10.1001/jamapsychiatry.2019.3523

Diemer, E. W., Grant, J. D., Munn-Chernoff, M. A., Patterson, D. A., & Duncan, A. E. (2015). Gender identity, sexual orientation, and eating-related pathology in a national sample of college students. *Journal of Adolescent Health, 57*(2), 144–149. https://doi.org/10.1016/j.jadohealth.2015.03.003

Dulcan, M. (2010). *Dulcan's textbook of child and adolescent psychiatry*. American Psychiatric Association Publishing.

Emmons, K. M., & Rollnick, S. (2001). Motivational interviewing in health care settings: Opportunities and limitations. *American Journal of Preventive Medicine, 20*(1), 68–74. https://doi.org/10.1016/S0749-3797(00)00254-3

Felitti, V. J., Anda, R. F., Nordenberg, D., Williamson, D. F., Spitz, A. M., Edwards, V., Koss, M. P., & Marks, J. S. (1998). Relationship of childhood abuse and household dysfunction to many of the leading causes of death in adults: The Adverse Childhood Experiences (ACE) study. *American Journal of Preventive Medicine, 14*(4), 245–258. https://doi.org/10.1016/s0749-3797(98)00017-8

Fleishman, J., Kamsky, H., & Sundborg, S. (2019) Trauma-informed nursing practice. *Online Journal of Issues in Nursing, 24*(2), 1–12. https://doi.org/10.3912/OJIN.Vol24No02Man03

Franke, H. A. (2014). Toxic stress: Effects, prevention and treatment. *Children, 1*(3), 390–402. https://doi.org/10.3390/children1030390

Gaudiani. J. L. (2019). *Sick enough: A guide to the medical complications of eating disorders*. Routledge.

Geist, R., & Opler, S. E. (2010). A guide for health care practitioners in the assessment of young people's capacity to consent to treatment. *Clinical Pediatrics, 49*(9), 834–839. https://doi.org/10.1177/0009922810363610

Ghane, A., Huynh, H. P., Andrews, S. E., Legg, A. M., Tabuenca, A., & Sweeny, K. (2014). The relative importance of patients' decisional control preferences and experiences. *Psychology & Health, 29*(10), 1105–1118. https://doi.org/10.1080/08870446.2014.911873

Goldenring, J. M., & Rosen, D. S. (2004). Getting into adolescent heads: An essential update. *Contemporary Pediatrics, 21*, 21–64.

Golden, N. H., Katzman, D. K., Sawyer, S. M., Ornstein, R. M., Rome, E. S., Garber, A. K., Kohn, M., & Kreipe, R. E. (2015). Update on the medical management of eating disorders in adolescents. *Journal of Adolescent Health, 56*(4), 370–375. https://doi.org/10.1016/j.jadohealth.2014.11.020

Grootens-Wiegers, P., Hein, I. M., van den Broek, J. M., & de Vries, M. C. (2017). Medical decision-making in children and adolescents: Developmental and neuroscientific aspects. *BMC Pediatrics, 17*(1), 1–10. https://doi.org/10.1186/s12887-017-0869-x

Hornberger, L. L. (2021). Identification and management of eating disorders in children and adolescents. *American Academy of Pediatrics, 147*(1), e1–e23. https://doi.org/10.1542/peds.2020-040279

Hudspeth, R. S., & Klein, T. A. (2019). Understanding nurse practitioner scope of practice: Regulatory, practice, and employment perspectives now and for the future. *Journal of the American Association of Nurse Practitioners, 31*(8), 468–473. https://doi.org/10.1097/JXX.0000000000000268

Ito, H. (2013). What should we do to improve patients' adherence? *Journal of Experimental & Clinical Medicine, 5*(4), 127–130. https://doi.org/10.1016/j.jecm.2013.05.001

Katz, A. L., & Webb, S. A. (2016). Informed consent in decision-making in pediatric practice. *Pediatrics, 138*(2), 1–7. https://doi.org/10.1542/peds.2016-1485

Katzman, D. K., & Findlay, S. M. (2011). Medical issues unique to children and adolescents. In D. Le Grange & J. Lock (Eds.), *Eating disorders in children and adolescents: A clinical handbook* (pp. 137–147). Guilford Press.

Kaye, L., Warner, L. A., Lewandowski, C. A., Greene, R., Acker, J. K., & Chiarella, N. (2009). The role of nurse practitioners in meeting the need for child and adolescent psychiatric services: A statewide survey. *Journal of Psychosocial Nursing and Mental Health Services, 47*(3), 34–40. https://doi.org/10.3928/02793695-20090301-07

Keatings, M., & Smith, O. B. (2000). *Ethical & legal issues in Canadian nursing* (2nd ed.). C.V. Mosby Canada.

Khanlou, N., & Wray, R. (2014). A whole community approach toward child and youth resilience promotion: A review of resilience literature. *International Journal of Mental Health and Addiction, 12*(1), 64–79. https://doi.org/10.1007/s11469-013-9470-1

Kibakaya, E. C., & Oyeku, S. O. (2022). Cultural humility: A critical step in achieving health equity. *Pediatrics, 149*(2), e2021052883. https://doi.org/10.1542/peds.2021-052883

Klein, D. A., Goldenring, J. M., & Adelman, W. P. (2014). HEEADSSS 3.0: The psychosocial interview for adolescents updated for a new century fuelled by media. *Contemporary Pediatrics, 1*, 1–16.

Kozier, B., Erb, G., Bernman, A. J., Burke, K., Bouchal, S. R., & Hirst, S. P. (2003). *Fundamentals of nursing: The nature of nursing practice in Canada* (Canadian ed.). Pearson Education Canada.

Kumar, A., Kearney, A., Hoskins, K., & Iyengar, A. (2020). The role of psychiatric mental health nurse practitioners in improving mental and behavioral health care delivery for children and adolescents in multiple settings. *Archives of Psychiatric Nursing, 34*(5), 275–280. https://doi.org/10.1016/j.apnu.2020.07.022

Laranjeira, C., Carvalho, D., Valentim, O., Moutinho, L., Morgado, T., Tomás, C., Gomes, J., & Querido, A. (2023). Therapeutic adherence of people with mental disorders: An evolutionary concept analysis. *International Journal of Environmental Research and Public Health, 20*(5), 3869. http://doi.org/10.3390/ijerph20053869

Lebrun-Harris, L. A., Ghandour, R. M., Kogan, M. D., & Warren, M. D. (2022). Five-year trends in US children's health and well-being, 2016–2020. *JAMA Pediatrics, 176*(7), e220056. https://doi.org/10.1001/jamapediatrics.2022.0056

Loeb, K. L., Brown, M., & Goldstein, M. M. (2011). Assessment of eating disorders in children and adolescents. In D. Le Grange & J. Lock (Eds.), *Eating disorders in children and adolescents: A clinical handbook* (pp. 156–185). Guilford Press.

Maddick, A. F., & Laurent, S. (2012). Consent, competence and confidentiality for children and young people: Case problems from osteopathic practice. *International Journal of Osteopathic Medicine, 15*(3), 111–119. https://doi.org/10.1016/j.ijosm.2012.04.002

Mangano, E., Gonzalez, Y., & Kverno, K. S. (2020). Challenges faced by new psychiatric-mental health nurse practitioner prescribers. *Journal of Psychosocial Nursing and Mental Health Services, 58*(10), 7–11. https://doi.org/10.3928/02793695-20200915-01

Martyn, K. K., Martin, J., Gutknecht, S. M., & Faleer, H. E. (2013). The pediatric nurse practitioner workforce: Meeting the health care needs of children. *Journal of Pediatric Health Care, 27*(5), 400–405. https://doi.org/10.1016/j.pedhc.2013.03.005

Maser, C., & Vandermorris, A. (2022). 2SLGBTQ children and youth. In A. Bourns & E. Kucharski (Eds.), *Caring for LGBTQ2S people* (pp. 75–107). University of Toronto Press.

Matjasko, J. L., Herbst, J. H., & Estefan, L. F. (2022). Preventing adverse childhood experiences: The role of etiological, evaluation, and implementation research. *American Journal of Preventive Medicine, 62* (6 Suppl 1), S6–S15. https://doi.org/10.1016/j.amepre.2021.10.024

McVoy, M., & Levin, J. B. (2023). Updated strategies for the management of poor medication adherence in patients with bipolar disorder. *Expert Review of Neurotherapeutics, 23*(4), 365–376. https://doi.org/10.1080/14737175.2023.2198704

Miller, W. R., & Rollnick, S. (2013). *Motivational interviewing: Helping people change* (3rd ed.). Guilford Press.

Miranda, L., & McCarter, J. (2016). *Hamilton: The revolution: Being the complete libretto of the Broadway musical, with a true account of its creation, and concise remarks on hip-hop, the power of stories, and the new America*. Grand Central Publishing.

Moroz, N., Moroz, I., & D'Angelo, M. S. (2020) Mental health services in Canada: Barriers and cost-effective solutions to increase access. *Healthcare Management Forum, 33*(6), 282–287. https://doi.org/10.1177/0840470420933911

Motivational Interviewing Network of Trainers. (2021). *Learning motivational interviewing. MINT excellence in motivational interviewing.* Accessed May 2, 2023. https://motivationalinterviewing.org

Neinstein, L. S. (2008). *Adolescent health care: A practical guide* (5th ed.). Wolters Kluwer Lippincott Williams & Wilkins.

Peterson, A. L. (2019, January 25). *What is… motivational interviewing.* Mental Health @ Home. https://mentalhealthathome.org/2019/01/25/what-is-motivational-interviewing

Psychology Today. (2022, June 7). *Do you talk yourself into the wrong choices? New research shows how easy it is to convince yourself a bad idea is a good one.* https://www.psychologytoday.com/us/blog/fulfillment-any-age/202206/do-you-talk-yourself-the-wrong-choices

Rome, E. S., & Strandjord, S. E. (2016). Eating disorders. *Pediatric Review, 37*(8), 323–336. https://doi.org/10.1542/pir.2015-0180

Rosen, D. S., & the Committee on Adolescence. (2010). Identification and management of eating disorders in children and adolescents. *Pediatrics, 126*(6), 1240–1253. https://doi.org/10.1542/peds.2010-2821

Santer, M., Ring, N., Yardley, L., Geraghty, A. W. A., & Wyke, S. (2014). Treatment non-adherence in pediatric long-term medical conditions: Systematic review and synthesis of qualitative studies of caregivers' views. *BMC Pediatrics, 14*(1), 63–63. https://doi.org/10.1186/1471-2431-14-63

Sawyer, S. M., Azzopardi, P. S., Wickremarathne, D., & Patton, G. C. (2018). The age of adolescence. *The Lancet Child & Adolescent Health, 2*(3), 223–228. https://doi.org/10.1016/S2352-4642(18)30022-1

Schaefer, M. R., & Kavookjian, J. (2017). The impact of motivational interviewing on adherence and symptom severity in adolescents and young adults with chronic illness: A systematic review. *Patient Education and Counseling, 100*(12), 2190–2199. https://doi.org/10.1016/j.pec.2017.05.037

Schwalbe, C., & Gearing R. (2012). The moderating effect of adherence-promoting interventions with clients on evidence-based practices for children and adolescents with mental health problems. *American Journal of Orthopsychiatry, 82*(1), 146–155. https://doi.org/10.1111/j.1939-0025.2011.01133.x

Skinner, W. (2017). *The essentials of … series: Motivational interviewing.* Canadian Centre on Substance Use and Addiction. https://www.ccsa.ca/sites/default/files/2019-04/CCSA-Motivational-Interviewing-Summary-2017-en.pdf

Sokol, J. T. (2009). Identity development throughout the lifetime: An examination of Eriksonian theory. *Graduate Journal of Counseling Psychology, 1*(2), Article 14. https://epublications.marquette.edu/gjcp/vol1/iss2/14

UNICEF. (n.d.). *Adolescent development and participation.* https://www.unicef.org/adolescence

United Nations. (1990, September 2). *Convention on the rights of the child.* https://www.unicef.org/child-rights-convention/convention-text

Weir, K. (2012). The roots of mental illness: How much of mental illness can the biology of the brain explain? *Monitor on Psychology, 43*(6). https://www.apa.org/monitor/2012/06/roots

Wissow, L. S., Platt, R., & Sarvet, B. (2021, April). Policy recommendations to promote integrated mental health care for children and youth. *Academic Pediatrics, 21*(3), 401–407. https://doi.org/10.1016/j.acap.2020.08.014

World Health Organization. (2003). *Caring for children and adolescents with mental disorders: Setting WHO directions.* https://apps.who.int/iris/handle/10665/42679

World Health Organization. (2021). *Child health.* https://www.who.int/health-topics/child-health#tab=tab_1

World Health Organization. (2023). *Adolescent health.* https://www.who.int/health-topics/adolescent-health#tab=tab_1

21 AGING AND OLDER ADULT POPULATIONS

Suzanne Drake and Helen Jones

INTRODUCTION

As advances in healthcare in the United States have extended the lives of older adults, it is estimated that by 2030 older adults will comprise 20% of the people living in the United States. Since 2019, the Gerontological Society of America's Reframing Aging Initiative has trained facilitators nationwide to use research-backed strategies to change the narrative around getting older. People are living longer, and they are living longer successfully. The Reframing Aging Initiative stresses the need to reframe aging as a dynamic process where older people "gather momentum through the build-up of unique experiences and insights" (Busso et al., 2019, p. 562).

DEFINITION AND DESCRIPTION

Older adults, defined as people who are 65 years of age and older, are the largest growing segment of the population in the United States. Even if a practitioner is not dealing directly with this population, it is vital to understand the needs of this population as older adults may be living with their children, caring for their grandchildren, and/or may be a source of concern for their younger adult children. This population will have an impact on their younger family members and on the communities in which they live. Some may be living alone without friends, whom they have outlived, and/or without family, who may be living in other parts of the country or from whom they are estranged. They may be living independently, living with their adult children or grandchildren, or living in retirement villages, assisted living arrangements, or long-term care (LTC) settings. They may be unhoused.

The more APRNs understand the unique needs of older adults, the better equipped they will be to manage the related needs of their younger patients, who may be providing care/support for their aging relatives. APRNs play an important role in educating those who provide direct care or supportive services to older adults.

UNIQUE CHALLENGES OF AGING AND OLDER ADULT POPULATIONS

A professional understanding of community care settings for this population is essential to providing comprehensive, accessible, and culturally sensitive psychiatric-mental healthcare to the aging and older adult population. Deep knowledge of the immediate needs of older adults is necessary for planning and providing care for their psychiatric-mental healthcare and thus contributing to their overall quality of life and well-being. Some factors to consider include the following:

A. Older adults may experience a range of mental health issues, including depression, anxiety, dementia (including Alzheimer disease), and late-onset schizophrenia. The prevalence of these conditions necessitates specialized care and support.
B. Older adults often have comorbid physical health conditions (e.g., heart disease, diabetes, arthritis), which can complicate the diagnosis and treatment of psychiatric conditions. A professional understanding of community care settings allows for integrated care approaches that address both mental and physical health needs.
C. Cognitive, emotional, and social changes are part of the normal aging process. APRNs need to distinguish between these normal changes and signs of mental health disorders. This understanding is critical in community settings where aging individuals interact daily.
D. Older adults may face barriers in access to mental health services (e.g., mobility issues, stigma, lack of awareness). APRNs who understand community care settings can work toward improving accessibility, outreach, and tailoring services to meet the unique needs of older adults.
E. Community care settings often involve not just the individual but also their support networks, including family, friends, and community services. A professional understanding helps in mobilizing these networks effectively to provide support and care.
F. Ethical considerations such as autonomy, consent, and capacity are paramount to caring for older adults, especially those with cognitive impairments. Moreover, sensitivity to cultural backgrounds and values is essential in a community setting. Professionals need to navigate these considerations with care and respect.
G. In community settings, professionals can engage in preventive measures and early interventions that can significantly impact the quality of life of older adults. Understanding the community context allows for targeted strategies that address risk factors and leverage protective factors inherent in the community.
H. Effective psychiatric-mental healthcare for older adults often requires collaboration across various disciplines, including psychiatry, psychology, nursing, social work, and occupational therapy. A comprehensive understanding of the community care setting facilitates this interdisciplinary approach, ensuring a holistic care model.
I. Understanding the specific needs and challenges of the aging population in community settings aids in effective resource allocation. It ensures that resources are directed toward the most impactful interventions and support services.
J. Professionals with a deep understanding of community care settings are better equipped to advocate for policies and programs that support the mental health of older adults. This advocacy is crucial to developing age-friendly communities and enhancing the overall well-being of this population.

THE DANGERS OF MYTHS AND PRECONCEIVED BIAS

A. Unconscious biases and myths associated with the older adult population can significantly impact the quality of care and interaction older adults receive from healthcare providers, caregivers, and society at large. Recognizing and addressing these biases is crucial to improving the overall well-being and treatment of older individuals.

B. Some common unconscious biases and myths include the following:

1. There is a prevailing myth that cognitive and physical decline is an inevitable and natural part of aging. While aging is associated with changes, many older adults maintain high levels of cognitive and physical function. This bias can lead to underestimating an older adult's capabilities and contributions.

2. A common stereotype is that older adults are unable or unwilling to use technology. This can lead to their exclusion from digital services and innovations designed to improve quality of life, despite evidence that many are capable of learning and using new technologies effectively.

3. Older adults are often perceived as being set in their ways and resistant to change. This stereotype can lead to their preferences and needs being overlooked, especially in care planning and decision-making processes.

4. There is a misconception that the aging population primarily represents an economic burden due to healthcare costs and pensions. This view overlooks the significant contributions older adults make to society, including volunteering, mentoring, and the transmission of knowledge and cultural values.

5. Treating the older adult population as a homogenous group ignores the vast diversity in experiences, preferences, health status, and capabilities among individuals. This can lead to a one-size-fits-all approach in services and policies, which may not effectively meet the needs of all older adults.

6. The myth that aging automatically leads to a decline or cessation of sexual desire and activity can contribute to the neglect of sexual health and intimacy needs among older adults in healthcare and residential settings.

7. There is a bias that mental health issues like depression and anxiety are just part of aging, which can lead to underdiagnosis and undertreatment. Recognizing mental health conditions as treatable is essential in improving the quality of life of older adults.

8. The belief that older adults have a diminished capacity for enjoyment, particularly in terms of leisure activities, learning, and social engagement, can lead to their exclusion from various programs and initiatives aimed at enhancing well-being.

9. There can be a fatalistic attitude toward health in older age, with the assumption that health promotion and preventive measures are less effective or important. This can result in missed opportunities for enhancing health and longevity.

C. While some older adults may require assistance, the assumption that all are dependent can lead to paternalistic attitudes and practices, undermining the autonomy and self-determination of older individuals. Combating these unconscious biases and myths requires ongoing education, self-reflection, and systemic changes in how society views and interacts with the older population. Promoting an accurate, respectful, and nuanced understanding of aging is essential in fostering a more inclusive and supportive environment for older adults.

THE AGING AND OLDER ADULT POPULATION, COMMUNITY CARE SETTING, AND UNIQUE CIRCUMSTANCES

A professional understanding of the aging and older adult population and community care settings is essential in providing comprehensive, accessible, and culturally sensitive psychiatric-mental healthcare to the aging and older adult population. This understanding can potentially address the immediate needs of older adults, as well as contribute to their overall quality of life and well-being.

A. In attempting a deeper understanding of this population, one must recognize that there is a significant gap in evidence-based research specifically targeting mental disorders in the older adult, as well as a pressing need to enhance the structure of psychiatric care for this demographic, as noted by Petrova and Khvostikova (2021).

B. Self-neglect among older adults is a particularly underresearched area. *Self-neglect* is defined by an individual's refusal or inability to attend to their basic personal needs, such as hygiene, nutrition, and financial management.

C. One such research initiative in Texas enrolled over 300 older adult individuals to study the impact of self-neglect, highlighting the importance of this focus area. However, the challenge posed by the lack of psychometrically validated tools to measure self-neglect forced researchers to depend on nonstandardized methods or subjective judgment, complicating data collection and analysis.

D. Until such tools are developed, the role of collaboration between research teams and social service agencies will continue to be paramount to identifying older adults who are at risk of self-neglect.

E. Barriers to evidence-based learning about this population create unparalleled challenges for researchers in studying vulnerable populations like these, including but not limited to navigating environments with poor lighting, gas leaks, structural dangers, and infestations, which can impact the research process.

RISK AND PROTECTIVE FACTORS IN AGING

A. In the context of the aging and older adult population, deep understanding is important in promoting health, preventing disease, and ensuring a high quality of life. These factors can influence physical, mental, and social well-being. Here is an overview:

B. Risk factors:

1. Older people, especially those in LTC, are at greater risk of harm due to physical frailty, presence of multiple comorbidities, complex drug regimens, and the need for care coordination. Conditions like heart disease, diabetes, hypertension, and osteoarthritis increase vulnerability to further health complications.

2. Conditions such as Alzheimer disease and other forms of dementia pose significant risks to older adults' autonomy and quality of life. How decisions are made in the setting of cognitive impairment needs to be more carefully considered as the process of decision-making is important (Ibrahim et al., 2019).

3. Reduced mobility due to muscle weakness, joint problems, chronic pain, or neurologic conditions increases the risk of falls and associated injuries. *Patient safety*, as per the World Health Organization (WHO), means preventing errors and harm in healthcare. This definition has led to the belief that harm from professional mistakes should never happen. This hinders the promotion of "dignity of risk," where personal dignity includes autonomy and taking risks for personal growth and a better life (Ibrahim & Davis, 2013).

4. Vision and hearing loss and other sensory impairments can lead to difficulties in communication, increased risk of accidents, and social isolation. One in three older adults fall each year, and falls are a leading cause of injury in this age group.
5. Loneliness and social isolation are key risk factors for mental health conditions in later life. Lack of regular social contact can lead to depression and worsened physical health. Older people are more likely to experience many of the risk factors that can cause or exacerbate social isolation or loneliness, such as the death of loved ones, worsening health and chronic illness, new sensory impairment, retirement, or changes in income.
6. Mental health in older adults is influenced by physical and social environments, cumulative effects of earlier life experiences, and aging-related stressors such as adversity, loss of capacity, declining function, bereavement, and ageism.
7. Reduced income and purpose in retirement are financial difficulties that can limit access to healthcare, nutritious food, and other resources essential for well-being.
8. Use of multiple medications increases the risk of adverse drug reactions and interactions.
9. Geriatric syndromes such as incontinence, dental issues, hearing loss, and mobility issues can cause isolation from embarrassment. Conditions such as depression, anxiety, and substance abuse are significant sequelae of social isolation, and decreased quality of life adds to the cycle.
10. Poor nutrition from difficulty getting out to shop, depression, solitary eating, and financial or dental problems can exacerbate chronic conditions and weaken the immune system.
11. Inadequate housing, exposure to pollution, and lack of access to green spaces can negatively impact health.

C. Protective factors:
1. Exercise can help maintain mobility, muscle strength, cardiovascular health, and cognitive function. Chair yoga may help older adults with certain health conditions, such as arthritis, exercise without putting pressure on joints. It may improve balance, strength, and range of motion. It also reduces the fear of falling and helps people who are not used to exercise begin improving their strength and balance.
2. A balanced diet of fruits, vegetables, whole grains, and lean proteins can protect against chronic diseases. Studies have shown that many older people, in general, need guidance regarding their unique nutrient requirements.
3. Active and regular participation in social activities and maintaining close relationships can support mental health and cognitive function.
4. Engaging in mentally stimulating activities (like reading, solving puzzles, and lifelong learning) can help preserve cognitive health.
5. Regular health screenings and access to medical care are crucial to early detection and management of health issues.
6. Effective stress management and resilience training can protect against mental health disorders.
7. A safe home free from fall hazards and with adequate support (like grab bars in bathrooms) can prevent injuries.
8. Access to services such as transportation, home healthcare, and senior centers can help older adults maintain independence and quality of life.
9. Feeling useful and having a sense of purpose through volunteering or caregiving roles can enhance well-being.
10. Sufficient income to cover basic needs and healthcare is a significant protective factor.

D. Addressing risk factors and bolstering protective factors require a multimodal approach, including individual lifestyle changes, community and societal support, and policy initiatives aimed at creating age-friendly environments. This can help ensure that older adults not only live longer but also enjoy a higher quality of life in their later years.

ASSESSING THE NEEDS OF THE AGING AND OLDER ADULT POPULATION

A. Assessing the needs of the aging and older adult population within a community or specific setting involves a comprehensive approach that considers the physical, psychological, social, and environmental aspects of their lives. A thorough needs assessment can inform the development of targeted interventions, services, and policies to support the well-being of older adults in a variety of settings.

B. Developing a comprehensive assessment will serve toward a greater goal of advancing a community that is age-friendly. This assessment will include a review of municipal programs, services, and amenities currently offered to older adults. Gathering information about what is already offered will help plan for future programs and services that either expand upon successful measures or identify gaps in service programs.

ASSESSMENT

A. It is essential to select what specific aspects of needs are being assessed. It may include, but is not limited to, healthcare needs, social support services, housing, specialized needs of minority groups, as well as transportation services. As the assessment evolves, identify service gaps, discrimination practices, and barriers to access.

B. By including a wide range of stakeholders, there will be a stronger probability that diverse perspectives and needs will emerge. The list of stakeholders will include older adults, caregivers, healthcare providers and professionals, community leaders, and legislative policy makers.

C. Focus groups are useful in gathering a broad range of stakeholders. When health and social care groups work together, share information, and trust each other's judgment, this reduces duplication and ensures that the range and the complexity of an older person's needs are accurately identified and addressed in a way that addresses their wishes and preferences.

ASSESSMENT TOOLS

A. Investigate the wide variety of standardized assessment tools and frameworks that will be appropriate to the determined goals of the targeted group(s). Common tools for assessing older population demographics include the comprehensive geriatric assessment (CGA) for healthcare needs. Select technological and data analytics that will enhance data collection and analysis while ensuring privacy.

B. In the context of a community assessment, surveys can be an effective way to assess a community's perceived strengths, weaknesses, needs, and existing structures. Surveys can be general or targeted to specific segments of the community. Surveys can be delivered by email, phone, or in person, and each method has advantages and disadvantages in terms of collecting useful information.

C. The data collection process includes surveys, scales, checklists, interviews, and questionnaires to gather essential information on health status, social connections, economic stability, living conditions, and access to services. These tools must be culturally sensitive, reliable, and valid if they are to inform professional judgment.

D. The interviews can be structured or semistructured, including focus groups, with a wide range of stakeholders to gather qualitative and quantitative insights into their experiences, challenges, and identified needs.

    1. Site visits to homes, community centers, healthcare facilities, and other relevant environments will provide current information about living situations, accessibility issues, available resources, and gaps in service needs. This will include data from medical records, service usage reports, and demographic studies.

E. Are primary care providers accessible and specialist services, mental health support networks, and rehabilitative services already in place? It is also important to determine the level of social engagement, available social activities currently in place, and ways to access community center or social groups.

F. Ask about healthy affordable food options and existing meal programs like Meals on Wheels or food pantries.

G. Determine whether transportation services are available for older adults to access healthcare services, shopping needs, and social events. Identify whether the services that exist are financially viable for the population in need. Assess for barriers, including physical, financial, awareness, or cultural/language features.

ANALYSIS AND RECOMMENDATIONS

A. *Data analysis* can be grouped into *four* main categories: descriptive analysis, diagnostic analysis, predictive analysis, and prescriptive analysis. Simply put, descriptive and diagnostic analytics ask "What?" and "Why?" and predictive analytics asks "What next?" The point of prescriptive analytics is to answer the question "What should we do about it" and stresses the need to formulate a plan. Rather than simply projecting future outcomes as predictive analytics does, prescriptive analytics evaluates the various aspects of multiple data sources and then delivers recommendations as to how to reach the most optimal outcome.

B. Based on the analysis of the assessment findings, the next step is to develop targeted recommendations for ongoing support of current strengths, as well as listing identified needs and gaps in service delivery. These should be specific, actionable, and feasible, acknowledging the resources and constraints of the specific community or setting.

COMMUNICATING AND SHARING RESULTS

A. The final step is to prepare a comprehensive report detailing the assessment process, findings, and recommendations. This report will be openly shared with stakeholders, policy makers, and legislators.

B. As this process evolves, collaborate with relevant organizations and agencies that will be needed to endorse and implement changes. The more they are involved in the process, the higher likelihood they will "own" it and be eager to operationalize the anticipated changes.

C. Ethical considerations: Throughout the assessment process, the dignity, privacy, and autonomy of older adults must be meticulously guarded. Informed consent is imperative for participation in surveys, interviews, and other data collection activities.

D. Reassessment: A well-conducted needs assessment is a dynamic process that should be revisited periodically to adapt to the changing needs of the aging population and the evolution of community resources and services. This will complete the process of gathering feedback to complete the loop moving forward. Changes fuel the never ending process of transforming care in the future.

INCLUDING PATIENT FAMILIES IN PROVIDING CARE

A. Including the patient's family in providing care, often referred to as *family-centered care*, recognizes the pivotal role family members play in the patient's health and well-being. However, while there are significant benefits to this approach, it also presents various challenges.

    1. Importance of including family in care:

       a. Families provide emotional, social, and sometimes physical and financial support, contributing to the patient's overall well-being. This is not a new role for families. People have always provided emotional, physical, and financial support to family members and other people they feel close to (Schulz et al., 2020).

       b. Family members often assist in daily care routines, maintain and oversee safety, manage medications, manage transportation to appointments, and ensure continuity of care outside the clinical setting.

       c. Family caregivers often report positive experiences from caregiving, including a sense of giving back to someone who has cared for them, satisfaction of knowing that their loved one is receiving good care, personal growth, and increased meaning and purpose in one's life. This sense of meaning can have important benefits to caregivers well after their role has ended (APA, 2021).

       d. Family members can advocate for the patient's needs and preferences, especially in cases where the patient may be unable to communicate effectively due to age or health conditions. Their most important role is to advocate, as they strive to ensure the best life possible for their loved ones when they are vulnerable and unable to advocate for themselves.

          i. Involving the family can improve communication between healthcare providers and patients, working together to ensure that care plans are understood and followed correctly.

          ii. Families can provide essential insights into the patient's cultural background and preferences, aiding in culturally sensitive care delivery.

          iii. In cases of severe illness or cognitive impairment, family members often play a critical role in decision-making processes, including advance care planning and end-of-life decisions.

    2. Challenges in including family in care:

       a. The number of people taking on this role, the duration and intensity, and the complexity of the care provided have changed over the past three decades.

       b. Complex family relationships and dynamics can complicate care, especially if there are disagreements about care decisions or family roles (Riffin, 2021).

       c. Including families in patient care can be difficult due to patient autonomy, potential for disagreements, and intrusiveness.

       d. Balancing the patient's right to privacy with family involvement can be challenging, especially in sensitive situations or when the patient's wishes conflict with the family's views.

e. The emotional burden on families, particularly in chronic or terminal illnesses, can be significant, potentially leading to caregiver burnout and strained family relationships (Schulz et al., 2020).

f. Time and resource constraints can make it challenging to involve family members in care discussions and education, especially when family members disagree on care options.

g. Differences in cultural backgrounds, values, and individual preferences can lead to misunderstandings or conflicts between healthcare providers, patients, and their families.

h. Healthcare providers can become overly reliant on families for providing care, potentially relegating too much responsibility to families who may need the reprieve and neglecting to provide adequate support services and resources.

i. Navigating legal and ethical considerations, such as consent and autonomy, can be complex, particularly when family members' views do not align with the patient's expressed wishes.

STRATEGIES TO ADDRESS CHALLENGES

A. Strategies for managing these challenges include collaborating, dividing, and focusing, depending on the patient's cognitive status and health. Collaborating and patient-directed focusing are generally well-received by patients and caregivers (Riffin, 2021).

B. Establish open, honest, and regular communication channels between healthcare providers, patients, and families.

C. Provide education and resources to families to equip them with the knowledge and skills needed for caregiving.

D. Implement strategies for mediation when conflicts arise, ensuring that the patient's best interests remain the focus.

E. Offer access to support services for families, such as counseling and caregiver support groups, to mitigate emotional stress and burnout.

F. Ensure that the patient's wishes and autonomy are respected in all care decisions involving them as much as possible.

G. Foster cultural competence among team members. Appreciate and incorporate diverse cultural perspectives in planning care.

H. Adopting family-centered care practices and strategies can enhance patient outcomes, support families in their caregiving roles, and ensure ethical and compassionate care delivery.

I. While including the patient's family in care delivery is essential for holistic and effective healthcare, it requires careful navigation of potential challenges. Adopting family-centered care practices and strategies can enhance patient outcomes, support families in their caregiving roles, and ensure ethical and compassionate care delivery.

CHALLENGES AND TOOLS FOR THE APRN

A. Healthcare providers face many challenges in delivering care, particularly in environments with diverse patient populations, such as the increasing number of older people with multimorbid and chronic mental illness. The issues can span clinical, administrative, ethical, and interpersonal domains. Addressing these requires a combination of skills, resources, and tools. Common issues encountered as well as tools and strategies to deal with them are as follows:

1. Aging leads to a range of organic changes in health, affecting different bodily systems and mechanisms and resulting in unpredictable clinical outcomes. Older adults and patients with chronic conditions often present with complex, multifaceted health needs, requiring comprehensive management.

2. Due to the complexity of aging and geriatrics, it is imperative to consider older adults' diverse clinical conditions, mortality risk, and functional abilities within a comprehensive, personalized care approach to provide effective care (Roller-Wirsberger, 2019).

3. Use integrated care models, adopt multidisciplinary team approaches, and continuously engage in professional education to stay abreast of best practices in managing complex health conditions.

4. The fast pace of medical advancements challenges staying updated with the latest treatments and technologies. The amount of medical knowledge is said to double every 73 days. Yet not keeping up with the latest information can put APRNs at risk.

5. To stay current, one must engage in ongoing professional development. Besides subscribing to relevant journals, APRNs should participate in workshops, conferences, and online learning platforms.

6. To save time and stay current, APRNs can get daily briefs from newsletters such as the American Association of Nurse Practitioners (AANP) SmartBrief, medical podcasts, or subscription services like Medscape, UpToDate, and Epocrates, providing quick access to medical updates and clinical guidelines, which can enhance the quality of patient care and improve decision-making.

B. Diagnostic uncertainties:

1. Older populations may be more vulnerable to diagnostic error for reasons that relate to both the patient and the clinician (Skinner et al., 2016). Atypical presentations of diseases in older adults can lead to diagnostic challenges.

2. Common diagnostic criteria for specific diseases derived and validated in younger populations may not apply to older individuals (Skinner et al., 2016). Older adults may attribute their symptoms as normal signs of aging.

3. Tools and strategies: The diagnostic process for older adult patients often requires patience, persistence, and a multidimensional assessment to accurately diagnose and provide appropriate care. APRNs must be well-versed in clinical characteristics and tests that differentiate between the presence and absence of diseases in this unique population (Skinner et al., 2016).

4. Geriatric-specific diagnostic criteria, decision support tools, and algorithms are utilized, along with CGAs to aid in accurate diagnoses. In challenging cases, it is wise to seek second opinions or consult with geriatricians or specialists with expertise in the care of older adults.

C. Resource limitations such as administrative and systemic challenges:

1. Our healthcare system is unprepared for the complexity of caring for a burgeoning population of older adults. Limited access to care, constraints on time, staffing, and financial resources all impact the quality of care.

2. Tools and strategies: Use efficient practice management software and telehealth services to extend care reach, and learn management techniques to optimize resource use.

3. On a micro and macro level, APRNs can work with policy makers, stakeholders, and educators to create an

adequately prepared workforce; strengthen the role of public health; remediate disparities and inequities; develop, evaluate, and implement new approaches to care delivery; allocate resources to achieve patient-centered care and outcomes, including palliative and end-of-life care; and redesign the structure and financing of long-term services and support (Fulmer et al., 2021).

4. APRNs can apply these goals to the extent possible within their own setting. If these priorities are addressed proactively, an infrastructure can be created that promotes better health and equitable, goal-directed care that recognizes the preferences and needs of older adults (Fulmer et al., 2021).

D. Healthcare system navigation:
1. Patients and families often find healthcare systems complex and difficult to navigate, leading to challenges in accessing needed services. Patients suffer due to poor care coordination, miscommunication, unnecessary procedures, and high costs. Often, care seems uncoordinated as caregivers are unaware of each other's actions, leading patients to consult numerous unconnected health professionals who lack knowledge of the patient's medical history, resulting in fragmented care and conflicting treatments.
2. Tools and strategies: Patient navigators or care coordinators can guide patients through the system, and clear informational resources can be provided to help patients understand their care pathways.
3. APRNs can lead by example by:
   a. Initiating, promoting, and participating in interdisciplinary collaboration
   b. Bridging the communication gaps, ensuring that each team player's perspective is valued and considered in the patient's care
   c. Leveraging technology to facilitate communication and collaboration among team members, thus overcoming barriers of distance and time, allowing for more integrated and coordinated care planning and delivery
   d. Mentoring and educating peers and students about effective interdisciplinary collaborative teamwork
   e. Participating in policy making to advocate for structural changes that support this, including reforming payment systems to encourage APRN role recognition

E. Documentation burden:
1. The increasing demands of documentation and electronic health records (EHRs) can be time-consuming. Studies show EHR benefits are often evaluated from a user's viewpoint, focusing on single tasks rather than overall care delivery impacts.
2. While EHR may not significantly reduce documentation time, it can save time in other areas, such as accessing patient charts or managing reports.
3. Tools and strategies: Consider EHR optimization, voice recognition software for note-taking, and training on efficient documentation practices.
4. APRNs can champion change by collaborating with administration, clinicians, and information technology (IT) professionals to identify inefficiencies and suggest EHR utilization strategies that enhance workflow rather than disrupt it.
5. APRNs can leverage EHR systems to enhance patient education, engagement, and self-management, utilizing patient portals and other EHR functionalities to improve communication and care outcomes.

F. Ethical and legal challenges:
1. There are a variety of areas in which ethical issues can emerge, including complex family dynamics, end-of-life wishes, preserving dignity and respect, promoting independence, and keeping the individual safe. There are various factors that can make older adults vulnerable to abuse, neglect, and ill intent (American Society on Aging [ASOA], 2021).
2. Ensuring patient privacy and confidentiality, especially in digital communication and records, is crucial. Secure communication platforms, regular training on confidentiality practices, and strict adherence to data protection regulations.
3. Informed consent and autonomy become a major element in decisions about leaving a healthcare facility against medical advice. If the APRN believes that the older adult lacks the cognitive ability to leave the hospital against medical advice and believes it is unsafe to discharge the patient, the APRN must select a policy by which to prevent release.
4. Determine if the person meets the criteria for an involuntary psychiatric hold or meets the criteria for a "medical capacity hold," which is generally based on hospital protocol. A medical capacity hold indicates that the person does not have a mental illness and does not meet the criteria for an involuntary hold.

G. Factors affecting an older adult's wish to leave against medical advice
1. These factors include concerns about financial costs of treatment, fear of infection from the hospital, family concerns, pain management, and miscommunication.
2. Tools and strategies: The next step is to involve social services, assure pain management, and communicate clearly and openly with the patient, the family members, and the primary care physician. These strategies optimize adherence to recommendations about hospitalization and treatment plans.
3. Determine if the older adult lacks the decision-making ability to refuse treatment and lacks the ability to provide rational explanations about their desire to leave the hospital.
4. Provide ethical consultation services, clear informational materials for patients and families, and connection to legal advice when necessary.

H. End-of-life care decisions:
1. Discussions and decisions around end-of-life care can be challenging and emotionally charged. Situations that create ethical difficulties for healthcare professionals regarding end-of-life decisions are resuscitation, mechanical ventilation, artificial nutrition and hydration, terminal sedation, withholding and withdrawing treatments, euthanasia, and physician-assisted suicide.
2. Tools and strategies: Consider use of advanced care planning tools, palliative care consultations, and training in communication skills around end-of-life care.
3. Withholding or withdrawing treatment requires fully understanding the ethical and legal implications.
4. APRNs must guide the team in identifying a firm ethical approach regarding end-of-life care.
5. Consider the law, guidance from legal bodies, clear evidence base, and resources available.
6. Formulate a clear ethical approach understanding that their own perspective is not influencing the process. Establish moral justification and realistic solutions.

I. Interpersonal challenges:
  1. Communication barriers: Effective communication with patients who have hearing, cognitive, or language barriers can be difficult.
     a. Tools and strategies: Interpreters, communication aids (visual tools or hearing devices), and training in culturally sensitive communication practices are used.
  2. Managing expectations: Patients and families may have expectations that are not aligned with clinical realities or best practices.
     a. Often the therapeutic confidential dyad must include the family or guardian, as well as the older adult.
     b. In addition to verbal information, it may be helpful to provide written information that can be processed at a time more conducive to making an informed and rational decision and that is compatible with the clinical realities of the situation.
     c. Tools and strategies: Ensure clear, empathetic communication of treatment options and outcomes, setting realistic goals, and involving patients in decision-making. Transparency and honesty with the older adult and family members, if they are involved, are essential to preserve the therapeutic alliance.
J. Emotional and psychological stress:
  1. APRNs deal with patient suffering and often need to make high-stakes decisions.
  2. Listen empathetically to the guardian, especially if a family member is appointed. The person will offer their own thoughts, wishes, and fears about the older adult's care. When ethically appropriate, share the patient's wishes with the guardian, who will have a stronger platform on which to make critical treatment-related decisions.
  3. Provide as much information as possible to help the guardian make a decision that is in keeping with their loved ones' wishes and belief systems.

OPPORTUNITIES TO REFER AND PARTNER WITH OTHERS

A. There are significant opportunities for healthcare providers to partner with others and provide referrals, which can enhance patient care, extend the scope of services offered, and ensure a holistic approach to health and well-being. Such collaborations and referrals can be within the healthcare sector or involve community-based organizations, social services, and other sectors. Here are where partnerships and referrals are particularly valuable:
  1. Interdisciplinary healthcare teams and specialist providers: Collaborating with specialists in areas like cardiology, neurology, or geriatrics can provide patients with comprehensive care tailored to their specific needs.
  2. Allied health professionals: Working with physiotherapists, occupational therapists, dietitians, and speech therapists can address the wide range of health issues patients may face.
  3. Mental health services: Referring patients to psychologists, psychiatrists, or mental health counselors can address the mental and emotional aspects of health, which are crucial to overall well-being.
  4. Social services: Partnerships with social workers or community health workers can help address social determinants of health, such as housing, food security, and access to care.
  5. Community and support groups: Connecting patients with community resources and support groups, such as those for chronic diseases, caregiver support, or aging populations, can provide them with additional emotional and social support.
  6. Home healthcare and palliative care services: Collaborating with home health agencies and palliative care services can ensure that patients receive the care they need in the comfort of their homes, especially for those with chronic conditions or terminal illnesses.
  7. Rehabilitation services: Referrals to rehabilitation services, including physical, occupational, and speech therapy, can be crucial to recovery from injuries, surgeries, or managing chronic conditions.
  8. Legal and financial services referrals to legal and financial advisory services can be important, especially for older adults, for issues related to healthcare directives, guardianship, and financial planning.
  9. Educational and vocational services: For patients recovering from injuries or dealing with chronic illnesses, referrals to educational and vocational rehabilitation services can support their return to work or adaptation to new life circumstances.
  10. Technology and innovation partners: Collaborating with technology providers can bring innovative solutions like telehealth, remote monitoring, and health apps into the care plan, enhancing accessibility and patient engagement.
  11. Public health and preventive services: Partnering with public health initiatives for vaccination, screening, and health promotion campaigns can play a key role in disease prevention and health education.
  12. Fitness and wellness programs: Referrals to fitness programs, yoga classes, or wellness centers can support patients' physical and mental health beyond the clinical setting.
  13. Nutritional services: Dietitians and nutritional counseling services can provide patients with personalized dietary plans to manage or prevent health conditions such as diabetes, obesity, and heart disease.
B. When establishing partnerships and making referrals, it is important to ensure that the services are reputable, accessible to the patient, and aligned with the patient's health goals and needs. Effective communication and follow-up can help in coordinating care and evaluating the outcomes of such partnerships and referrals.

RESOURCES

Numerous resources are available for helping older adults, ranging from governmental and nonprofit organizations to online platforms and community services:

A. AARP (American Association of Retired Persons): The AARP offers resources on health, travel, retirement planning, and discounts for members over the age of 50. The goal of AARP Foundation's Connect2Affect is to reduce social isolation among older adults. This service offers a way to connect with others and find local resources and services.
B. National Council on Aging (NCOA): The NCOA provides a wide range of services including benefits checkup, falls prevention, and healthy aging tips.
C. Administration on Aging (AoA): Part of the U.S. Department of Health and Human Services, the AoA advocates for older individuals and their concerns at the federal level.

D. Alzheimer's Association: The Alzheimer's Association offers resources and support to individuals and families affected by Alzheimer's and other dementias.
E. Meals on Wheels America: Meals on Wheels delivers meals to individuals at home who are unable to purchase or prepare their own meals. Beyond providing nutritious meals, many Meals on Wheels programs also offer friendly visitation services, providing companionship along with meal delivery.
F. Eldercare Locator: The Eldercare Locator is a public service of the U.S. AoA that connects you to services for older adults and their families. Local services include social and community groups aimed at reducing isolation.
G. Senior centers: Senior centers are local community centers providing a range of services, activities, and support for older adults. Many senior centers offer a variety of activities, classes, and events that provide opportunities for socializing and making new friends.
H. Legal aid for seniors: Organizations like the National Elder Law Foundation (NELF) offer legal assistance and advice on issues like estate planning and rights protection.
I. Medicare: Medicare is the federal health insurance program for people who are 65 or older, certain younger people with disabilities, and people with end-stage renal disease.
J. National Institute on Aging: The National Institute on Aging offers health information and research updates related to aging.
K. Veterans Affairs (VA) services for seniors: VA provides healthcare, financial, and support services for older veterans.
L. Area Agencies on Aging (AAA): The AAA are local agencies that provide a range of services designed to support older adults and caregivers.
M. Long-Term Care Ombudsman Program: This program advocates for residents of nursing homes, board and care homes, assisted living facilities, and other adult care facilities.
N. Family Caregiver Alliance: Family Caregiver Alliance offers information and support to families and friends providing LTC at home.
O. Senior Companions Program: Part of the Corporation for National and Community Service, Senior Companions connects older volunteers with their peers to provide companionship and support to those who are homebound or isolated.
P. The Friendship Line at Institute on Aging: This is a 24-hour toll-free crisis line for people 60 years of age and older as well as adults living with disabilities. It is also a warm line providing emotional support and offering a caring ear for people who might be lonely or isolated.
Q. Faith-based organizations: Many churches, synagogues, mosques, and other religious centers have groups specifically for older members, offering both spiritual support and social interaction.
R. Volunteering: Engaging in volunteer work can be a great way for older adults to stay active, meet people, and make new friends while giving back to the community.
S. Online communities and forums: These include websites and online platforms specifically designed for older adults that can provide opportunities to connect with peers from around the world, share experiences, and find friendship.
T. Local libraries and community centers: These often host events, workshops, and clubs tailored to older adults, providing opportunities to meet others with similar interests.

REFERENCES AND BIBLIOGRAPHY

American Psychological Association. (2021). *Positive aspects of caregiving*. https://www.apa.org/pi/about/publications/caregivers/faq/positive-aspects

American Society on Aging. (2021). *Ethical considerations for working with older adults*. https://www.asaging.org/web-seminars/ethical-considerations-working-older-adults

Busso, D. S., Volmert, A., & Kendall-Taylor, N. (2019). Reframing aging: Effect of a short-term framing intervention on implicit measures of age bias. *The Journals of Gerontology: Series B, 74*(4), 559–564. https://doi.org/10.1093/geronb/gby080

Densen, P. (2011). Challenges and opportunities facing medical education. *Transactions of the American Clinical and Climatological Association, 122*, 48–58. https://www.ncbi.nlm.nih.gov/pmc/articles/PMC3116346

Fulmer, T., Reuben, D. B., Auerbach, J., Fick, D. M., Galambos, C., & Johnson, K. S. (2021). Actualizing better health and health care for older adults. *Health Affairs, 40*(2), 219–225. https://doi.org/10.1377/hlthaff.2020.01470

Ibrahim, J. E., & Davis, M.-C. (2013). Impediments to applying the 'dignity of risk' principle in residential aged care services. *Australasian Journal on Ageing, 32*(3), 188–193. https://doi.org/10.1111/ajag.12014

Ibrahim, J. E., Holmes, A., Young, C., & Bugeja, L. (2019). Managing risk for aging patients in long-term care: A narrative review of practices to support communication, documentation, and safe patient care practices. *Risk Management and Healthcare Policy, 12*, 31–39. https://doi.org/10.2147/RMHP.S159073

Petrova, N. N., & Khvostikova, D. A. (2021). Prevalence, structure, and risk factors for mental disorders in older people. *Advances in Gerontology, 11*(4), 409–415. https://doi.org/10.1134/s2079057021040093

Pickens, S., Burnett, J., Trail Ross, M. E., Jones, E., & Jefferson, F. (2023). Meeting the challenges in conducting research in vulnerable older adults with self-neglect-notes from a field team. *Frontiers in Medicine, 10*, Article 1114895. https://doi.org/10.3389/fmed.2023.1114895

Pless Kaiser, A., Cook, J. M., Glick, D. M., & Moye, J. (2018). Posttraumatic stress disorder in older adults: A conceptual review. *Clinical Gerontologist, 42*(4), 359–376. https://doi.org/10.1080/07317115.2018.1539801

Richeson, J. A., & J. Nicole Shelton. (2013). *A social psychological perspective on the stigmatization of older adults*. National Academies Press (US). https://www.ncbi.nlm.nih.gov/books/NBK83758

Riffin, C., Wolff, J. L., Butterworth, J., Adelman, R. D., & Pillemer, K. A. (2021). Challenges and approaches to involving family caregivers in primary care. *Patient Education and Counseling, 104*(7), 1644–1651. https://doi.org/10.1016/j.pec.2020.11.031

Roller-Wirnsberger, R., Thurner, B., Pucher, C., Lindner, S., & Wirnsberger, G. H. (2019). The clinical and therapeutic challenge of treating older patients in clinical practice. *British Journal of Clinical Pharmacology, 86*(10), 1904–1911. https://doi.org/10.1111/bcp.14074

Schulz, R., Beach, S. R., Czaja, S. J., Martire, L. M., & Monin, J. K. (2020). Family caregiving for older adults. *Annual Review of Psychology, 71*(1), 635–659. https://doi.org/10.1146/annurev-psych-010419-050754

Skinner, T., Scott, I., & Martin, J. (2016). Diagnostic errors in older patients: A systematic review of incidence and potential causes in seven prevalent diseases. *International Journal of General Medicine, 9*, 137–146. https://doi.org/10.2147/ijgm.s96741

World Health Organization. (2024, October 1). *Ageing and health*. https://www.who.int/news-room/fact-sheets/detail/ageing-and-health

22 PHYSICAL AND MENTAL DISABILITIES IN THE PEDIATRIC POPULATION

Steven E. Curtis

INTRODUCTION

Physical and mental disabilities refer to physical and neurodevelopmental disorders that start before birth or in the early developmental period of childhood. The term *physical and mental disabilities* includes the disorders described by the term *developmental delay* or *developmental disability*.

The *International Classification of Diseases*, 11th Edition (*ICD-11*; World Health Organization [WHO], 2019), identifies developmental disability in the category of neurodevelopmental disorders, which includes disorders related to intellectual development, speech or language disorders that are developmental in nature, autism spectrum disorders (ASDs), learning disorders that are developmental in nature, developmental coordination disorders, attention deficit hyperactivity, and stereotyped movement disorder. In both the *Diagnostic and Statistical Manual of Mental Disorders*, Fifth Edition, Text Revision (*DSM-5-TR*; American Psychiatric Association, 2022), and the *ICD-11* (WHO, 2019), specifiers are included to focus the diagnosis as intellectual, language, medical or genetic, and mental health. There are discussions related to the fact that all disorders that begin in childhood or adolescence should be viewed as neurodevelopmental disorders; however, this is not how the diagnosis is currently framed (Stein et al., 2020).

In this chapter, the author will use person-first language (e.g., child with autism spectrum disorder vs. an "autistic child"). In addition, the terms *disability* and *disorder* will be utilized, instead of *differences*. The writer is sensitive to these issues surrounding person-first language, and differences versus disorders, and has chosen to choose terminology frequently used in the medical community. One exception is that the term *neurodiversity* will be utilized to indicate that people overall have a diversity in behavior, learning, and so on. For more information, readers are encouraged to read *NeuroTribes* by Steve Silberman (2016).

PHYSICAL AND MENTAL DISABILITIES: DEFINITION

PHYSICAL DISABILITIES OF CHILDHOOD

A. Definition: This includes children who experience paralysis of one or more limbs, muscular tone difficulties, impaired balance, impact on larger or gross motor movements reducing the child's ability for mobility or coordination, and reduced ability for fine motor movements.
B. Etiology: Etiology may include a traumatic brain injury (TBI), acquired brain injury (stroke), spinal cord injury, cerebral palsy (CP), muscular dystrophy, spina bifida, and loss of limbs.
C. Prevalence: One in six children in the United States have at least one developmental disability or delay.
D. The Centers for Disease Control and Prevention (CDC) identifies eight specific, selected conditions in developmental disabilities, including attention deficit hyperactivity disorder (ADHD), ASD, CP, fragile X syndrome, intellectual disabilities, language disorders, learning disorders, and Tourette syndrome.
E. Common physical disabilities include the following:
  1. CP: CP is caused by nonprogressive disturbances in fetal or infant brain, manifested by challenges with muscle tone, movement, posture, cognition, communication, and/or behavior. Diagnosis is based on history, physical examination, neuropsychological evaluation, and imaging depending on the age of the child. Most children with CP are diagnosed during the first 2 years of life. Examples of professionals who specialize in the diagnosis of CP include pediatric neurologists and developmental pediatricians. Two to three children out of 1,000 have CP.
  2. Spina bifida: This is a neural tube defect that can cause damage to the spinal cord and nerves. It can be the etiology for both physical and intellectual disabilities. It is usually diagnosed during pregnancy or shortly after birth. Spina bifida, which does not cause any physical or intellectual disability, is often undiagnosed or diagnosed later in life.
  3. Childhood/juvenile arthritis: This idiopathic diagnosis affects over 220,000 children and adolescents each year. It can result in permanent physical damage to joints, affecting a child's activities of daily living. Rheumatologists should be consulted with these patients.
  4. Spinal cord injury: This refers to any injury that causes damage to the nerves and nerve fibers receiving signals from the brain (NIH, 2023). About 5% of all spinal cord injuries occur in the pediatric population, and 60% to 75% occur in the neck area, with 20% occurring in the chest and/or upper back. The remainder occur in the lower back.
  5. Epilepsy: Pediatric epilepsy is diagnosed when the patient has two or more seizures of unknown etiology. It is one of the most common pediatric disorders of the nervous system. It is estimated that about 0.6% (470,000) of U.S. children up to the age of 17 have epilepsy.
  6. Muscular dystrophy: This is an inherited condition that presents as progressive weakness and muscle wasting due to skeletal muscle degeneration. It is an inherited X-linked recessive disorder affecting boys more than girls (1 in 3,500 live boy births). Onset is usually between 3 and 5 years of age. This congenital myopathy is one of the most common congenital myopathies to affect U.S. children.

NEURODEVELOPMENTAL DISORDERS

A. Neurodevelopmental disorders, as defined by the *DSM-5-TR* (American Psychiatric Association, 2022), are a

group of disorders that typically begin in childhood and that can be chronic conditions persisting throughout the life span.
1. Neurodevelopmental disorders include disorders that manifest in all developmental domains, including the following:
   a. Intellectual disability (ID), which includes intellectual and adaptive behavior deficits in the areas of conceptual, social, and practical domains
   b. Communication disorders (CD), which includes deficits in language, speech, and communication
   c. ASD, which is manifested by deficits in communication and social interaction, and restricted, repetitive patterns of behavior, interests, or activities
   d. ADHD, a persistent pattern of inattention and/or hyperactivity that interferes with functioning or development
   e. Specific learning disorder (SLD), difficulties learning and using academic skills in the basic skills areas of reading, writing, and math
   f. Motor disorders (MD), which include delays in gross motor and fine motor skills
      i. MDs also include repetitive and purposeless motor behavior and tic disorders (e.g., Tourette).
B. It is rare for a single neurodevelopmental disorder to occur in isolation, and there is a large overlap with other similar disorders (homotypic comorbidity) and other psychiatric issues (heterotypic comorbidity).
C. Examples of disorders commonly comorbid with physical and mental disabilities are major depressive disorder (MDD; a type of depressive disorder), generalized anxiety disorder (GAD; a type of anxiety disorder), and obsessive-compulsive disorder (OCD).
D. Many of these children have experienced trauma and/or attachment issues due to abuse, neglect, bullying, and/or accidents. Elimination disorders (e.g., enuresis and encopresis) are also common.
E. Some are initially masked and become more clinically apparent with age.
   1. ASD in females is frequently recognized in later adolescence, or early adulthood, when there is demand for more effective and complex socialization.
   2. Females with ASD are able to blend in until the social demand becomes too great.
F. Sensory processing disorder (SPD) is an additional disorder not currently recognized by the psychiatric community. SPD is a disorder in which the child is overly sensitive to certain stimuli (e.g., loud noises) in the environment. These sensitivities may result in the child with SPD avoiding certain situations or becoming overly excited or active in others. SPD is diagnosed by occupational therapists. Even though SPD is not officially recognized, the concept makes sense intuitively. Children with ASD frequently have sensory sensitivities that impact their behavior and performance.

Causal Factors
A. For most physical and mental disabilities, causal factors involve a complex interaction of genetic, prenatal, postnatal, and environmental events.
   1. For example, in one child, CP is caused by a lack of oxygen in the brain, due to exceptionally low blood pressure in the mother. However, in many cases, the exact cause of CP is not known.
   2. Another example is ADHD. It is often said that ADHD is related to an imbalance of neurotransmitters (e.g., dopamine) in the brain; however, this does not point to the cause of this imbalance. The exact cause of ADHD is not fully understood, and it is mostly due to a combination of factors.
B. Giftedness is a common characteristic that is overlooked by clinicians and parents. We all come into this world with a certain potential to learn. Some people are very challenged with learning activities of all kinds. Others find most learning easy. Then there are those individuals who have an extremely high level of cognitive talent, and these individuals may be found to be "gifted."
   1. Gifted children are often misdiagnosed as having attention problems or even ASD. However, upon closer examination, these children may demonstrate behaviors that are typical of gifted children.
   2. Gifted children with physical and mental disabilities are frequently conceptualized as "twice-exceptional," meaning that they have significant cognitive strengths, and at the same time struggle with a disorder such as ASD, ADHD, or even an SLD.

WHY ADDRESS PEDIATRIC PHYSICAL AND MENTAL DISABILITIES?

A. Children account for 22% of our nation's population. Two to three out of 1,000 children have CP.
B. The prevalence of at least one neurodevelopmental disorder is 15% to 20%, which often goes undetected.
C. The prevalence of the most studied neurodevelopmental disorders, such as ADHD (9.04%), ASD (1.74%), and SLD (7.74%), has increased over time.
D. There is higher prevalence of any neurodevelopmental disorders with boys, older children, children of birth weight lower than 2,500g, non-Hispanic White children, children with public insurance, children with mothers with less than a college education, and children living in a household less than 200% of the federal property line.
E. The increased prevalence and the higher prevalence with non-Hispanic White children may be related to improvements in awareness and access to care. The COVID-19 pandemic has placed an extreme amount of stress on children, and their families, which has made the struggles for those with neurodevelopmental disorders even more difficult.
F. One out of five children encountered in a pediatric or family practice setting will have at least one neurodevelopmental disorder. In a clinic specializing in psychiatry, the encounters will be even more frequent.
G. The presence of a possible physical or mental disability, and the need for treatment, constitutes a common reason for consultation in pediatric settings.
H. Recognizing disability and associated comorbidities, as well as understanding overall care, specific strategies for treatment, and where to refer when more care or information is needed, are the APRN's professional responsibilities.

CONSIDERATIONS WHEN WORKING WITH PARENTS

INTERPROFESSIONAL COLLABORATION
A. When confronted with challenging behavior or other issues, the difficult task for the parents is in trying to understand their child's needs. The needs of their child are not always clear, and this is the main reason professional help is sought.

B. Initially the child will be brought to the general practitioner with questions from the parents.
1. "Our child has been identified by the teacher and school as possibly having ADHD."
2. "Should we go to a neurologist or neuropsychologist?"
3. "Are there any tests we can do to try and find a diagnosis to help our child?"
C. The child is referred to an expert in the field.
1. The child is ultimately brought to an expert in the field because the child is a puzzle for all those concerned.
2. The parents and the teachers are not sure if the child has an attention disorder, some type of ASD, SPD, or some other type of undiagnosed disorder. This is when they come to the APRN for help.
D. Common pathway for seeking professional help includes the following:
1. Teachers
a. A teacher of a particular child with seemingly puzzling behavior becomes concerned that something is critically wrong with the child. Symptoms can include the following:
i. The child seems not to listen to the teacher's directions or discussions.
ii. The child acts immature for chronological age and does not make friends like the other children.
iii. The child is very physically active in class and impulsively blurts out answers without raising a hand.
b. To address any type of concern, the teacher will follow educationally prescribed interventions:
i. Speak with the student about the behaviors.
ii. Set up a rewards system to reinforce good behaviors.
iii. Take disciplinary actions, such as detention, loss of play time, or being sent to the principal.
iv. Seek school recommendation for professional help/diagnosis. Refer to the school psychologist, social worker, or nurse.
2. If treatment by the first professional is seen by the parents and teachers as effective, then all is well. However, often, one treatment is not entirely successful, and the parents continue their quest for help by turning to another healthcare provider.
a. Many times, parents visit with four or five professionals before settling on a solution that is acceptable. Some parents may visit with as many as 15 professionals.
b. Parents may also use parent coaches, who may or may not be successful.
c. When no solution is found, parents may just give up and hope for the best.
E. Parents often embark on a journey that can be a long, intensive, and expensive search to arrive at an adequate understanding of their child's needs. This search hopefully results in the discovery of comprehensive understanding and effective solutions. However, many times, this journey leaves parents frustrated, financially drained, and without any answers to the challenges they face.

BARRIERS TO DIAGNOSIS AND TREATMENT
Implicit Bias
A. Parents are often labeled as "overinvolved" or enmeshed in their child's life.
1. Parenting can be quite challenging. Some children are fussy, cry frequently, are delayed with several developmental milestones (e.g., in speech and language), and are overly hyperactive and emotionally reactive from birth.
2. Parents of children with neurodevelopmental disorders are frequently criticized and shunned socially as well as by some professionals.
a. The divorce rate of parents with children with special needs has been noted to be higher than with parents without children with special needs, although this is not always supported in research.
b. When parents bring their child with a physical and mental disability to healthcare professionals, they often feel that they are not taken seriously.
B. Disabilities that are "visible" are more accepted as legitimate versus those that are "hidden."
1. For example, a child with a broken arm is clearly accepted as temporarily disabled.
2. However, a child with an expressive language delay may not be seen by a healthcare provider as having a disability because this "hidden" disability is not easily seen.
C. When children present to healthcare providers with hyperactivity, learning challenges, or social skills deficits, parents may feel that the healthcare provider lacks empathy for what the family is experiencing.
1. Implicit bias toward highly involved parents can interfere with the healthcare provider's ability to see the difficulties of the family unit and the challenges faced by the youth.
2. It is rare that a pediatric patient is brought in for evaluation or treatment for a physical and mental disability only because they have parents who are overly concerned or who are making it up.
D. Examine the school system model.
1. Historically, without a major battle of litigation and protests, schools have been reluctant to open their doors to women, students of color, students with disabilities, or LGBTQ+ students.
2. In order to overcome these barriers, parents learn the skill of assertiveness and fight for their student's rights. This might increase the perception that they are overly involved, overly concerned, and enmeshed in their student's life.
3. Increased involvement results when parents of children with disabilities hear things like:
a. "Special education is taking all the school's money."
b. "We cannot have your child in this classroom because of disruption to the other students."
c. "We cannot offer that service here (even if it is the law to provide this)."
E. The APRN whose patients include the family unit, especially that of a parent of a child with a physical and mental disability, should do the following:
1. Check for implicit beliefs that might interfere with proper diagnosis.
2. Reserve time to listen to the frustrating journey the parents have taken.
3. Establish a therapeutic relationship with the parents as well as the child. This listening will go a long way in developing wonderful rapport and will help the parents be active participants in their child's care.

THE IMPACT OF HOPEFULNESS AND HOPELESSNESS
A. Children with neurodevelopmental disorders can be especially challenging, and intervention strategies frequently fail to produce any immediate noticeable effects.

B. Parents may go through a cycle of hopefulness and hopelessness.
  1. Parents of these children seem to go through ups and downs. Some days they feel like they are on top of things. Other days they feel depressed, as if nothing is getting any better, and they do not feel that they can cope.
  2. Teachers of children with these disorders also experience this emotional lability.
  3. The children themselves can also move through this cycle.
     a. Focus on the progress that has been made, on the little changes that have occurred over time.
     b. Direct the parents, teachers, and students to review the information that has been gathered and how it can be applied toward progress.
C. Provide intervention.
  1. The APRN, along with the treatment team, provides realistic encouragement to the parents, allowing them to sit back, take a deep breath, and let the team work with them toward positive outcomes.
  2. Encourage parents to think small and appreciate the progress that has been made thus far.
  3. Support the parents, reminding them to take care of themselves, avoiding caregiver burnout.
  4. Provide the parents with information and encouragement to engage in self-care (yoga, walking, reading) and to seek support from self-help groups, such as the following:
     a. Self-help groups for parents with children with developmental disorders: https://blog.bayada.com/be-healthy/eight-support-groups-for-parents-raising-children-with-special-needs
     b. Self-care for parents of children with mental health needs: www.nationwidechildrens.org
     c. Training skills from the World Health Organization: www.who.int/teams/mental-health-and-substance-use/treatment-care/who-caregivers-skills-training-for-families-of-children-with-developmental-delays-and-disorders
  5. If the parents/guardians demonstrate signs of depression, anxiety, or burnout, provide information on and referrals to mental health professionals.
     a. Psychiatric NP
     b. Therapists with expertise in caregiver burnout
     c. Psychiatrist

FRAMEWORK FOR UNDERSTANDING AND HELPING

THE PROBLEM-SOLVING APPROACH TO UNDERSTANDING

A. Taking time to understand a human being takes much effort. When we are dealing with children with physical and mental disabilities, the causes of challenges and solutions for interventions are not always obvious.
B. In most cases, it is best to develop a comprehensive understanding of the child by investigating potential causal factors in an orderly way.
  1. Healthcare providers approach the investigation of any type of illness or challenge in a nonjudgmental, holistic, and systematic fashion. This assists in avoiding implicit bias or underlying beliefs about a person or a diagnosis.
C. The healthcare provider follows a diagnostic algorithm, a sequence of steps, and decision trees to best understand the situation and decide what to do.
  1. This process may not be obvious to the untrained observer.
  2. Most healthcare professionals, however, follow a thoughtful assessment system that is well-documented in professional literature.
D. Using a problem-solving approach to understanding assists the healthcare provider in understanding the pediatric patient with a physical or mental disability.
  1. A step-by-step procedure helps clarify concerns and systematically investigate possible causes of the behavioral, social, or learning challenges in the pediatric patient.
  2. Information is gathered and "working theories" are developed along the way that attempt to explain the current concerns. These theories are modified as new information is obtained.
  3. Healthcare providers continue to problem-solve and investigate until they are satisfied with the information they have obtained and the resulting level of understanding of the child.
     a. Scenario:
        i. A child is referred due to little motivation to complete schoolwork and who has been identified as lazy and oppositional.
           (a) Parents and teachers may prematurely conclude that the child needs some type of punishment when the schoolwork is not completed.
           (b) More careful investigation may reveal that the child has some type of learning difficulty that makes it incredibly hard for them to keep up with the other children.
           (c) In-depth investigation and problem-solving strategies can aid parents and teachers in finding the true source of the child's difficulties.

PROFILE-BASED APPROACH TO INTERVENTION

A. Neurodiverse and neurotypical: Everyone's brains are different. Those who are neurotypical fall into the mean or average brain development. Neurodivergent brains are those identified as outside the average. This approach identifies that brains are different, not better or worse.
B. *Neurodiversity* is not a medical term nor is it a diagnosis.
  1. The neurodiverse child includes those with ASD, ADHD, or dyslexia.
  2. There is no strict definition for which conditions fall under the neurodiverse category, which can include tics and anxiety, as well as ID, depression, and schizophrenia.
C. Support the success of neurodivergent children.
  1. Explain the "neurodevelopmental profile."
     a. This profile consists of many systems, including social thinking, attention-control, memory, higher thinking, motor, sequential ordering, spatial ordering, and language systems.
     b. These work together to form our mind.
  2. Identify the child's strengths and weaknesses in each of these areas to begin to "cultivate their minds" (i.e., addressing the weaknesses and building up the strengths). This concept and strategy are more fully described in *All Kinds of Minds* (https://allkindsofminds.org).
     a. Strengths can include such talents as being able to build, having a high level of vocabulary, being able to draw, and having unique musical ability.
        i. Oftentimes in schools, children with challenges are only reinforced when they demonstrate certain skills (e.g., reading, writing, sharing in groups).
        ii. Other skills do not get reinforced as often (e.g., being able to design a building).

iii. Since we are all "wired" differently, the child with the natural proclivity to do well in reading and writing excels in school. The child with the natural proclivity to be nonverbal and build may be deemed as "odd" and not do as well on language-based tasks.
3. Develop a profile for the child once sufficient data are obtained about the areas of strength as well as those needing more growth.
   a. For example, a child may be very good at social conversation but has great difficulty conducting math calculations. This profile is just a description of the child's natural proclivities and learning thus far. This may be an activity that is foreign to health professionals since we typically focus on pathology. However, this activity can be extremely helpful.
   b. Utilize and share the profile.
      i. This information can be used for intervention planning.
      ii. This profile is combined with the theory generated through the problem-solving mentioned earlier to obtain a holistic view of the child. Interventions can then be designed based on this information.
4. Interventions for the weak areas can be conducted using traditional intervention methods from such fields as special education, clinical psychology, speech/language pathology, or occupational therapy.
5. Interventions for areas of strength can be implemented using information from such fields as the booming area of "positive psychology" and other methods that are shown to improve that skill.
   a. Positive psychology, as described by Martin Seligman in his book *Authentic Happiness* (2002), is an approach to behavioral difficulties that focuses on what we can do to make ourselves happier and function better. This is considerably different from the more traditional approach of targeting interventions only to reduce the problem behavior or other challenges.

ASSESSMENT STEPS

Step 1: View Challenges Holistically, Versus Categorically, at First

A. Conduct a full physical and mental health evaluation.
   1. Pediatric physical and developmental assessment
      a. The developmental assessment systematically assesses the child's growth and development in the areas of motor, language, cognitive, and social emotional development.
         i. It assists in the early identification of any possible delays and disorders, as well as emotional and adaptive skills.
         ii. It can guide intervention/treatment plan.
   2. Pediatric psychological assessment
      a. The pediatric assessment evaluates the whole child. This comprehensive assessment reviews family, community, and school supports.
         i. Consider the source of referral (e.g., school, parents, social group).
         ii. This assessment includes an examination of memory and attention, as well as intelligence, behavioral, social, and emotional developmental milestones and achievements.
B. Avoid narrow thinking.
   1. One risks misdiagnosing an issue when thinking things like "I am going to do an evaluation of ADHD, or ASD."
      a. This is too narrow of thinking when a child with a possible physical and mental disability is initially assessed.
      b. Thinking only of ADHD, the clinician may use the common questionnaire for ADHD (e.g., Vanderbilt Scales) and will thus be more than likely to prematurely find that the child meets the criteria for ADHD.
   2. A physical and mental disability frequently has comorbidities. Evaluating ADHD seems simple on the surface, but misdiagnoses are common since the child may have another neurodevelopmental disorder that is the primary reason for the challenge.
      a. A child with an SLD in reading (e.g., dyslexia) may demonstrate attention issues in the classroom that look like ADHD. These learning issues may not even be recognized by the teacher or parent and reported on the Vanderbilt Scales. Evaluating for ADHD is not like diagnosing diabetes by measuring the patient's blood glucose level. The state of our diagnostic process in this area is not that easy or specific yet.
C. Instead of thinking initially in categorical terms, the NP holistically views the challenge as "puzzling behavior."
   1. The term *puzzling behavior* is used by the author to initially describe children with undiagnosed challenges related to a possible physical and mental disability.
   2. When a child is said to have "puzzling behavior," the implication is that there is something different about the child in comparison with peers. However, the term *puzzling* does not mean that something is necessarily wrong.
   3. The child may or may not have some type of behavioral, social, or learning challenge. The child may or may not have some type of sensory processing issue. The child may have a disorder or be found to be completely normal. Puzzling only means that the child demonstrates behavior that is of concern in some manner and is perplexing to understand. The word *puzzling* helps postpone judgment about the presence of, or lack of, a disorder until more investigation is conducted.
D. There are many examples of puzzling behavior, but common concerns presented to healthcare professionals are as follows:
   1. Noncompliance with requests
   2. Overly excited behavior
   3. Attention or learning difficulties at school
   4. Delayed socialization with others
   5. Angry and disruptive behavior
   6. Can also pertain to concerns of low self-esteem, anxiety, depression, or some type of sensory issue
   7. Other common scenarios
      a. "My child is extremely bright and loves to learn. However, he has difficulty behaving appropriately in groups and frequently gets overexcited. When he is overly excited, he becomes disruptive and is asked to leave. His teacher wants to kick him out of her classroom."
      b. "Joseph is in second grade, and he is so behind others in his reading. However, he loves to listen to stories and has wonderful conversations with others. He is beginning to hate school because he feels stupid all the time. Joseph is very happy at home, but when he is at school, he is beginning to act out."

c. "Renee sits and stares at school. She seems like she is just not engaged. At home, she demonstrates the same behavior. She often does not seem to hear what is said and has great trouble following my directions. She is happiest when she engages in make-believe play."

E. A parent questionnaire may be utilized, initial background interview with the parents (if under 12) may be conducted, and initial background interview with the parents and patient may be conducted (if over 12).
1. This questionnaire and interview consists of the standard questions asked in most psychiatric assessments of children. In addition, a "broad-band" questionnaire (the Behavior Assessment System for Children-Third Edition [BASC-3]) is used and is sent to the parents, and pediatric patients if appropriate, to complete.
2. A "broad-band" questionnaire is a norm-referenced measure that helps assess a variety of mental health challenges, strengths, and adaptive behavior levels.

F. A mental status/observation session (we call it a neurobehavioral status evaluation) is then conducted. In this session, the standard procedures for a pediatric mental status examination are performed, and additional questions are asked given the results of the questionnaire.
1. During this initial stage of assessment, it is helpful to put the concerns brought forth by the parents in behavioral terms.
   a. For example, if a parent brings their child in and states the child is "emotionally reactive" and "aggressive," what do these three words about behavior really mean? The key is to ask questions about what the behavior looks like, what comes before the behavior, what comes after the behavior, when does it occur, how often does it occur, and so on. The goal is to ask enough questions that you can visualize the child performing these behaviors in real life.
   b. This process is very therapeutic because it forces the clinician to listen very closely. In the fields of applied behavioral analysis, school psychology, and special education, we call this process a "functional behavioral assessment" or FBA.
   c. In special education, conducting an FBA is a legal requirement before a child with behavior challenges can be placed in a more restrictive setting. However, the FBA is primarily a strategy to fully understand the behavior presented.

Step 2: Use "Narrow-Band" Questionnaires to Pinpoint Diagnoses
Classification and Assessment Methods
A. When NPs begin the quest for understanding their pediatric patient's puzzling behavior, they can take two paths. Down the first path, the NP asks, "What behaviors can I impact?" On the second path, the NP asks, "What is wrong with the child?" These are two fundamentally different approaches.
B. Professional psychologists who have a good understanding of developmental psychopathology will use both approaches when they attempt to understand and intervene with a particular child.
1. In the first approach, the behavior of concern is clarified, and specific behaviors are analyzed systematically. In the second approach, the healthcare provider looks for specific causes of the puzzling behavior.
2. In this step, the NP uses a classification system (e.g., DSM-5-TR; American Psychiatric Association, 2022) that pinpoints patterns of challenges that are consistent with certain types of disorders.

C. In Step 1, The broad-band questionnaires and clinical interviews may have revealed no evidence of a physical and mental disability, evidence of one disability, or evidence of multiple disabilities with several comorbidities.
1. This is now the time to use more "narrow-band" questionnaires, or procedures, such as the Vanderbilt Scales for ADHD, Screen for Child Anxiety Related Disorders (SCARED) for anxiety disorders, or Gilliam Autism Rating Scale (GARS) for possible ASD.

D. Utilize neurodiversity questionnaires.
1. Camouflaging Autistic Traits Questionnaire (CAT-Q)
   a. A 25-item self-report for patients 16 and older who may be camouflaging autistic traits
   b. Considers gender differences
   c. Test–retest of .77 and Cronbach's alpha of .94
   d. Free download, scoring, interpretation, and psychometric properties, and can be found online at https://novopsych.com.au/assessments/formulation/camouflaging-autistic-traits-questionnaire-cat-q/?swcfpc=1
2. Ritvo Autism Asperger Diagnostic Scale-Revised (RAADS-R)
   a. Assesses "higher functioning" ASD in adults
   b. Examines the patient's social relatedness problems, circumscribed interests, language, and areas of sensory motor functioning
   c. Free download, scoring, interpretation, and psychometric properties, and can be found online at https://novopsych.com.au/assessments/diagnosis/ritvo-autism-asperger-diagnostic-scale-revised-raads-r/?swcfpc=1
3. Multidimensional Assessment of Interoceptive Awareness-Version 2 (MAIA-2)
   a. Has 37 items and is for patients 18 and older
   b. MAIA-Y for patients between 7 and 17 years of age for assessing interoceptive awareness
   c. Includes eight scales assessing five dimensions of body awareness
   d. Free download, scoring, interpretation, and psychometric properties, and can be found online at https://novopsych.com.au/assessments/formulation/multidimensional-assessment-of-interoceptive-awareness-version-2-maia-2/?swcfpc=1
4. Autism Spectrum Quotient (AQ)
   a. Utilized for screening for ASD in adults and adolescents aged 16 years and over
   b. Free download, scoring, interpretation, and psychometric properties, and can be found online at https://novopsych.com.au/assessments/diagnosis/autism-spectrum-quotient/?swcfpc=1
5. Autism Spectrum Screening Questionnaire (ASSQ)
   a. Used for screening for "high-functioning" ASD in children or adolescents (6–17 years of age)
   b. Free download, scoring, interpretation, and psychometric properties, and can be found online at https://novopsych.com.au/assessments/diagnosis/autism-spectrum-screening-questionnaire-assq/?swcfpc=1
6. Vanderbilt ADHD Diagnostic Parent Rating Scale (VADPRS)
   a. Used for screening for ADHD in children (6–12 years of age)

b. Free download, scoring, interpretation, and psychometric properties, and can be found online at https://novopsych.com.au/assessments/diagnosis/vanderbilt-adhd-diagnostic-parent-rating-scale-vadprs/?swcfpc=1

E. Psychiatric disorders such as MDD, GAD, and conduct disorder may be diagnosed based on history taking, mental status examination, broad-band questionnaires, and age-appropriate, narrow-band questionnaires.
 1. A thorough physical examination, with common lab tests, should have recently been conducted to rule out medical, vision, and hearing issues related to the concerns.
 2. ADHD can also be diagnosed with this step, but many prefer to gather additional psychological testing before a firm diagnosis of ADHD is made.

F. Diagnoses of ID, CD, SLD, and MD are typically made after additional cognitive, academic, speech, language, fine motor, gross motor, and/or adaptive behavior assessment has been conducted. This information is combined with the information from Steps 1 and 2 and compared with the criteria for each of these diagnoses.
 1. Diagnosis of SLD using the *DSM-5-TR* (American Psychiatric Association, 2022) is based on the presence of a discrepancy of expected achievement (often estimated by using overall IQ) and actual achievement. Public schools also use this method.
 2. Increasingly, public schools are using a "Response to Intervention (RTI)" approach to the classification of a student having a "specific learning disability." RTI involves screening children who are at risk of learning challenges, providing them with intensive research-based intervention and then assessing their progress. If a student does not demonstrate any improvement after this evidence-based intervention, then a determination of qualification for special education services as a student with a specific learning disability is made. Sometimes psychologists using different methods of diagnosing learning challenges confuse parents as to which method of assessment is best. Both methods are accepted in the field.

G. A diagnosis of ASD is frequently made with additional assessment using the Autism Diagnostic Observation Schedule, Second Edition (ADOS-2). ADOS-2 is a standardized assessment tool that uses semistructured play and interviews to obtain information about symptoms or behaviors consistent with ASD. Information from ADOS-2 is combined with information obtained from the previous assessment steps. This information is then compared with the criteria for a diagnosis of ASD presented in the *DSM-5-TR* (American Psychiatric Association, 2022). Additional cognitive, academic, adaptive behavior, speech, language, and other neuropsychological testing is often used to obtain the current level of performance.

Team Evaluations

A. Because of the common comorbidities and multiple causal factors, the assessment and treatment of children with physical and mental disabilities can be very complex and not always straightforward.

B. Team assessment is the state of the art and may include multiple professionals, including NPs, pediatricians, family practice physicians, psychiatrists, neurologists, psychologists, occupational therapists, speech/language pathologists, and special education teachers.

C. Assessment frequently includes not only assessment for diagnostic purposes and determination of comorbidities, but also for current levels of functioning to help with intervention.

D. Clinicians in nonpublic school settings typically use the *DSM-5-TR* (American Psychiatric Association, 2022) and/or *ICD-10* (WHO, 1990) for diagnostic purposes. School professionals recognize these diagnostic systems, but typically use classification guidelines for special education eligibility as defined by the Individuals with Disabilities Education Act (IDEA).

E. Treatment, or intervention, may involve one type of intervention (e.g., psychotropic medication for ADHD), or multiple interventions involving a school-based team of professionals (e.g., to address the needs of a child with an intellectual delay).
 1. The school-based team often includes a school counselor, school psychologist, speech/language pathologist, occupational therapist, special education teacher, and general education teacher.
 2. Many children with physical and mental disabilities are provided with special education services as part of an Individualized Education Program (or Plan; IEP).

STRENGTH-BASED APPROACH TO INTERVENTION

A. A comprehensive assessment can help clarify specific concerns, obtain an accurate diagnosis, identify comorbidities, and identify causal factors to help create a theory as to what is happening with the child. In addition, a comprehensive assessment can help collect data on the strengths of a child to formulate a neurodevelopmental profile. There are two approaches to interventions:
 1. Implement research formulated to treatment strategies based on the diagnosis obtained.
 2. Make a developmental profile and design strength-based interventions.

B. There are many ways through which interventions can be designed, depending on the type of problem presented.
 1. Sometimes the intervention may be purely behavioral in focus, whereby the strategy is modifying some aspect of the patient's puzzling behavior.
 2. At other times, the intervention may require the use of medication or some type of therapy.

C. Form and participate in a team of care providers focused on the needs of the pediatric patient.
 1. Schools
  a. In schools, teams consisting of teachers, administrators, and specialists frequently develop intervention strategies for children.
   i. If the patient has a difficulty related to school, it may be helpful to set up a meeting to discuss the patient with these individuals.
   ii. Schools develop IEPs for students with special learning needs.
   iii. If the difficulty is not related to school, it may still be possible to get a team meeting together, but this is not always so easy since the involved professionals may be in different parts of the community, making it difficult for everyone to come together. With the increased use of telehealth, meetings with the team have become much more doable. This coordination of care can be very helpful.

Traditional Treatment Approaches

A. Utilize clinical decision-making apps.

1. "UpToDate" database: UpToDate is a fee-for-service app. Medscape (www.medscape.com/public/medscapeapp) is a free alternative to UpToDate. Epocrates (www.epocrates.com) has a free version for use as a clinical resource toolkit.
   a. For each of the physical and mental disabilities discussed in this chapter, there are research-based interventions that are articulated in scientific journals and databases. This author uses the UpToDate database to research strategies, especially those involving medication.
   b. For example, if a 10-year-old pediatric patient is diagnosed with ADHD, the UpToDate database presents treatment considerations and strategies. This information combined with a prescribing app such as Epocrates can provide expert guidance on how to provide best practices. In addition, other resources such as Stahl's *Prescriber's Guide: Children and Adolescents* (2019) and so forth can be extremely helpful.

Strength-Based Approach

A. During the assessment activities, the healthcare provider is encouraged to take note of the child's strengths and interests. It is often easier to build upon what a child is already interested in.
B. Many patient care plans include a section for strengths. Even plans, such as the IEP in schools, are primarily a deficit-oriented approach.
C. In locating areas of strength, it is helpful to think about the positive aspects of the pediatric patient.
   1. Questions to ask: What does this patient excel at? What is this patient interested in?
      a. Pay attention to the subtle aspects of the child's behavior and social skills.
         i. If the child is argumentative, perhaps one area of strength is the child's verbal reasoning ability.
         ii. It is challenging to argue effectively without good verbal skills. An example of a profile created for a particular child is as follows:
            (a) LM is a 10-year-old boy in the fourth grade who has a long history of difficulties with hyperactivity, impulsivity, and inattentiveness. He clearly meets the criteria for ADHD. Areas of strength and weakness were identified by his mother to include the following: (a) areas of strength include being able to build, imitating cartoon characters, learning different languages, and singing; (b) areas of weakness include having difficulties with thinking before acting, being aggressive toward his younger brother, and not listening in class.
D. By identifying the child's strengths and weaknesses, the NP is developing a "profile" for the pediatric patient.
   1. Areas of strength, as well as areas of need, are carefully articulated.
   2. Interventions can then be designed to address both areas.
      a. For example, for the above patient, the child can be enrolled in an art class with a focus on drawing cartoons.
      b. At the same time, the patient can be prescribed a stimulant to help decrease impulsivity.

CHALLENGES FOR THE APRN

A. Time factor: One of the many challenges facing the APRN when working with children demonstrating physical and mental disabilities is that the assessment and intervention process can be extremely time-consuming.
   1. In a medical setting, it can be almost impossible to put aside adequate time to fully implement the strategies discussed earlier. This is when it is helpful to decide what part of the assessment and treatment activities the NP can do and cannot do.
   2. In a psychiatric outpatient setting, it is possible to space out assessment and treatment sessions to have adequate time to do what needs to be done. In this situation, it works well to inform the parents that in order to be comprehensive several sessions are needed and that it will take time to conceptualize the concerns and how to best address them.
B. Parents of children with physical and mental disabilities may express urgency in figuring how to help their child and may even put pressure on you "to do something."
   1. Best to get it right, then to get it done!
   2. It is recommended that the APRN refrains from being forced to rush.
C. When patience supports quality work, an effective treatment plan can be formulated, meeting the needs of the patient and the parents.

OPPORTUNITIES TO PARTNER WITH OTHERS AND PROVIDE REFERRALS

A. A benefit of working with pediatric patients with physical and mental disabilities is the number of specialty professionals involved.
   1. If the APRN is new to this area, it is recommended to attend team meetings held either at the school or other agency. This is an opportunity to learn, network, collaborate, and problem-solve with other members of the team.
   2. When the APRN is unsure about the diagnoses or treatment strategy, meeting with the team can provide the NP with additional information. Reaching out to other specialists assists in proper diagnosis and treatment planning.
      a. Multidisciplinary meetings can be extremely helpful and rewarding. Much of the time, healthcare professionals are working independently and this is a chance to be part of a team.
   3. After attending a number of these team meetings, the APRN can become part of the consulting network, serving as a referral for and to future patients.

RESOURCES

A. American Academy of Child and Adolescent Psychiatry: www.aacap.org
B. American Psychological Association Society of Clinical Child and Adolescent Psychology (Division 53): https://sccap53.org
C. Association for Play Therapy: www.a4pt.org
D. Council for Exceptional Children: www.cec.sped.org
E. International Dyslexia Association (Washington State Branch): www.wabida.org
F. National Association of School Psychologists: www.nasponline.org
G. Society for Developmental and Behavioral Pediatrics: www.sdbp.org
H. Society of Pediatric Psychology: www.societyofpediatricpsychology.org

REFERENCES AND BIBLIOGRAPHY

American Psychiatric Association. (2022). *Diagnostic and statistical manual of mental disorders* (5th ed., text rev.). https://doi.org/10.1176/appi.books.9780890425787

Centers for Disease Control and Prevention. (2023). *Developmental disabilities*. U.S. Department of Health and Human Services. https://www.cdc.gov/ncbddd/developmentaldisabilities/index.html

Delahooke, M. (2019). *Beyond behaviors: Using brain science and compassion to understand and solve children's behavioral challenges*. PESI.

Dulcan, M. K., Ballard, R. R., Jha, P., & Sadhu, J. M. (2018). *Concise guide to child and adolescent psychiatry* (5th ed.). American Psychiatric Association.

Harrison, P., & Thomas, A. (2014). *Best practices in school psychology: Student level services*. National Association of School Psychologists.

National Institutes of Health. (2023). *Spinal cord injury*. https://www.ninds.nih.gov/health-information/disorders/spinal-cord-injury

Seligman, M. E. (2002). *Authentic happiness*. HarperCollins.

Silberman, S. (2016). *NeuroTribes: The legacy of autism and the future of neurodiversity*. Avery.

Stahl, S. M. (2019). *Prescriber's guide: Children and adolescents* (1st ed.). Cambridge University Press

Stein, D. J., Szatmari, P., Gaebel, W., Berk, M., Vieta, E., Maj, M., de Vries, Y. A., Roest, A. M., de Jonge, P., Maercker, A., Brewin, C. R., Pike, K. M., Grilo, C. M., Fineberg, N. A., Briken, P., Cohen-Kettenis, P. T., & Reed, G. F. (2020). Mental, behavioral and neurodevelopmental disorders in the *ICD-11*: An international perspective on key changes and controversies. *BMC Medicine, 18*(21). https://doi.org/10.1186/s12916-020-1495-2

World Health Organization. (1990). *International statistical classification of diseases and related health problems* (10th rev). https://icd.who.int/browse10/2019/en

World Health Organization. (2019). *International statistical classification of diseases* (11th rev.). https://icd.who.int

23. MENTAL AND PHYSICAL DISABILITIES IN ADULTS

Colin Hemmings

INTRODUCTION

INTELLECTUAL DISABILITY

Almost all psychiatric APRNs and other mental health clinicians will see people with disabilities, no matter the service in which they work. Disabilities take many forms, but an important type is intellectual disability (ID), formerly known by various other terms, such as *mental retardation*.

People with ID are more likely than people with typical intelligence quotient (IQ) to be further disabled by other disorders, mental and physical, including neurodevelopmental disorders. It is not uncommon to see complex presentations of mental illness, neurodevelopmental disorders, physical health problems, and challenging behaviors concomitantly in patients with ID. This chapter focuses on the mental healthcare of people with ID and includes some practical guidance to help the APRN assess and manage these patients.

MENTAL HEALTH OF INTELLECTUAL DISABILITY

The mental healthcare of people with ID has developed into a well-recognized area of clinical practice and research. It is widely agreed that this field includes the assessment and management of challenging behaviors, accompanied by major risk to the patient or to others, as well as diagnosable mental disorders. It differs in focus from the general medical healthcare of people with ID and the practice and delivery of their social care and education.

DEFINITIONS

INTELLECTUAL DISABILITY

A. The *Diagnostic and Statistical Manual of Mental Disorders*, Fifth Edition (*DSM-5*; American Psychiatric Association, 2013), defines *ID* as a neurodevelopmental disorder that begins in childhood and is characterized by intellectual difficulties as well as impairments in conceptual, social, and practical areas of living. The *DSM-5* (American Psychiatric Association, 2013) requires the meeting of all three of the following criteria for a diagnosis of ID:
   1. Deficits in intellectual functioning, such as reasoning, problem-solving, planning, abstract thinking, judgment, academic learning, and learning from experience, confirmed by clinical examination and standard IQ testing
   2. Deficits in adaptive functioning that significantly impair the ability to conform to developmental and sociocultural standards for the individual's independence and ability to meet their social responsibility
   3. The onset of the preceding two deficits occurring during childhood

B. The *DSM-5* (American Psychiatric Association, 2013) has moved away from using IQ scores to diagnose ID and has placed emphasis on a person's deficits in adaptive functioning. However, there is still the broad notion that people with ID have an IQ that is at least 2 SD less than the average IQ (i.e., IQ of 70 or less). Using this IQ level, the prevalence of ID would be around 2.5%, but the need for adaptive deficits to confirm the diagnosis means that the prevalence of ID may be somewhat less (1%–2%).

AUTISTIC SPECTRUM DISORDER

A. Autistic spectrum disorder (ASD) is a lifelong neurodevelopmental disorder affecting social interaction, communication, and behavior. Many people with ID also have ASD, but a significant proportion of people with ASD do not have ID.

B. Although the exact etiology of ASD is unknown, it is thought that a wide range of genetic and environmental factors can play a role.

C. The core features of autism include abnormalities in communication and social interaction, and restricted, repetitive, and stereotyped patterns of behavior, interests, and activities.

D. Associated features vary across the spectrum but may include a delay in or lack of development of language, deficits in nonverbal communication (e.g., abnormalities in eye contact and body language), deficits in understanding and using gestures, difficulties adjusting behaviors to different situations, limited range of facial expressions, stereotyped and repetitive use of language, lack of responses to people's emotions, poor integration of verbal and nonverbal communication, reduced sharing of emotions and interests, repetitive movements, lining up of objects, preoccupation with specific objects, insistence on sameness, extreme distress at changes in daily routines, and difficulties with transitions.

E. People with ASD tend to have cognitive processing difficulties, which means that they can easily become overwhelmed when presented with too much information or stimuli. They often have sensory hypersensitivities and so they can have unpredictable negative reactions to noise, smells, and lights. They struggle with lack of structure in their daily lives, they frequently find their environment unpredictable and changes confusing, and they may experience common daily activities as meaningless.

F. It is difficult to be precise about the prevalence of ASD, especially since the idea of a spectrum disorder rather than core autism has been accepted by *DSM-5* (American Psychiatric Association, 2013); however, it is in the region of 1% to 2% of the population.

ATTENTION DEFICIT HYPERACTIVITY DISORDER

A. Another important neurodevelopmental disorder that can be present in people with ID is attention deficit hyperactivity disorder (ADHD), with core features of impulsivity, inattention, and hyperactivity.

B. Evidence is increasing to support the diagnosis of ADHD in adults with ID.

C. Diagnosing ADHD/hyperkinetic disorder in a person with ID can be difficult because ID, to some extent, can often be associated with poor attention and hyperactivity; therefore, the APRN who conducts the diagnostic assessment must be satisfied that the level of distractibility or restlessness is significantly more severe than would be expected in a person with ▶

ID and that it is not caused by a mental health or physical health problem, both of which are common in this population group.
D. The diagnosis of ADHD is even more difficult when ID and ASD are both present.
E. Prevalence estimates of ADHD vary widely but are usually around 4% to 8% of the population.

GENETIC SYNDROMES

A. Most people with ID do not have recognized genetic syndromes. In around half of cases, there is no clear cause.

Down Syndrome

A. Down syndrome is associated with a wide range of causes; in the majority of cases, the cause is thought to be multifactorial and thus influenced by multiple genes and environmental factors.
B. Down syndrome is the most common genetic cause of ID, with an estimated incidence of around 1 in 1,000 live births worldwide. This condition is well-known to the general public. In Down syndrome, there is extra genetic material in chromosome 21 (or trisomy 21).
C. People with Down syndrome have characteristic physical features, such as flattened facial appearance; low-set, small ears; small nose; and small mouth.
D. People with Down syndrome have an increased risk of specific physical health conditions such as hypothyroidism, leukemia, and cataracts, as well as early-onset dementia and Alzheimer disease.

Behavioral Phenotypes

A. Some genetic syndromes have been found to be associated with certain temperaments or patterns of behavior. For example:
   1. People with Down syndrome are often cheerful and sociable, albeit stubborn.
   2. People with Prader–Willi syndrome are often compulsive overeaters.
   3. Many people with Lesch–Nyhan syndrome are prone to self-injurious behaviors.
B. In many cases, the presence of genetic syndromes does not add anything in itself to the assessment and management of mental health problems in people with ID.

PHYSICAL DISABILITIES

A. People with ID often have more physical health problems, including an increased prevalence of neurologic conditions.
B. Epilepsy can lead to problems with diagnosis (e.g., differentiating temporal lobe epilepsy from mental illness) because symptoms such as hallucinations can occur in some types of epileptic seizures. Epilepsy can also cause difficulties in treatment as psychiatric medications can make seizures more likely.
C. The phenomenon of "forced normalization" in epilepsy can occur, whereby a reduction in seizures following the introduction of antiepileptic medication can be associated with an exacerbation of a psychosis.
D. In ID, the prevalence of epilepsy increases in parallel with the degree of ID (i.e., up to 50% of people with the most severe level of ID have epilepsy).
E. People with ID also have much higher rates of sensory problems, such as hearing and visual impairments, making them more susceptible to misinterpreting things they see and hear.

PROFESSIONAL UNDERSTANDING OF THIS POPULATION

A. Virtually all health professionals will see patients with ID in their clinical practice.
B. People with ID account for 1% to 2% of the population depending on how strictly criteria are applied. However, they are disproportionally likely to have a range of other comorbidities and to need healthcare.
C. People with ID who also have mental health problems are dually disadvantaged.
   1. They have higher morbidity and mortality rates when compared with people without ID.
   2. They are vulnerable to exploitation, abuse, and neglect and find it harder to access care.
   3. They are more likely to be socially excluded.
   4. Not only are people with a disability more likely to also have mental and physical health problems, they are also harder to assess and treat.

UNDERSTANDING THIS POPULATION

CLASSIFICATION SYSTEMS

A. Mental disorders are diagnosed using standardized language-based criteria, such as in the *DSM-5* (American Psychiatric Association, 2013) and the World Health Organization's (WHO's) *International Classification of Diseases*, 11th Revision (*ICD-11*; WHO, 2019). These standardized, largely language-based diagnostic criteria become less and less useful in people with increasingly severe ID as people are less and less able to express their internal mental states verbally.
B. Due to the limitations of *DSM-5* and *ICD-11* in diagnosing mental disorders in people with ID, the *Diagnostic Manual-Intellectual Disability* (DM-ID) was developed in the United States and the *Diagnostic Criteria for Psychiatric Disorders for Use With Autistic Spectrum Disorders/Mental Retardation* (DC-LD) was developed in the United Kingdom.
   1. These also take into account atypical symptoms, which can be a change in frequency or intensity of challenging behaviors, a decline in a person's functioning or a deterioration of their skills, or increased social withdrawal, rather than the more obvious symptoms such as hallucinations.
   2. The reduction in functioning may be temporary, but long-standing mental health problems may lead to a prolonged or even permanent reduction in a person's functioning.

PREVALENCE

A. There are two fundamental facts about the mental health of people with ID that are still not known widely outside the field, despite several decades of evidence:
   1. People with ID experience the range of mental health problems like the rest of the population, although sometimes with atypical presentations.
   2. People with ID experience higher rates of mental health problems than the rest of the population.
B. Some mental disorders are significantly more prevalent in people with ID (e.g., schizophrenia), while the prevalence of others is often similar to, or at least not substantially greater than, that in people without ID.
C. When challenging behaviors are not included, the prevalence of mental disorders overall in people with ID is still higher than that of the general population, but not so marked. ▶

D. People with ID have higher rates of mental health problems compared with the general population for a variety of reasons. These are thought to include:
  1. Increased genetic predisposition
  2. Increased psychosocial stressors
  3. Physical comorbidities and more limited coping strategies
E. Rates may be underestimated because mental health problems are generally more difficult to detect and diagnose in people with ID.

CHALLENGING BEHAVIORS

A. Many people with ID can display challenging behaviors, such as aggressive, self-injurious, and destructive behaviors.
B. The behavior can have a range of possible underlying causes, including mental illness, physical health problems, communication difficulties, long-standing impaired learned behavior, environmental changes, or a combination of any of these.
C. There is no universal definition of challenging behavior, but it is commonly cited as "culturally abnormal behavior of such an intensity, frequency or duration that the physical safety of the person or others is likely to be placed in serious jeopardy, or behavior which is likely to seriously limit use of, or result in the person being denied access to, ordinary community facilities" (Emerson, 1995, p. 233).
D. Challenging behaviors can often fluctuate over years and thus be chronic in duration. The mainstay of interventions for challenging behaviors should always include psychological (including behavioral) interventions, possibly coupled with changes to the person's social and physical environment.
E. It is important that a person with ID and challenging behaviors is screened to check for all other factors that may be causing or exacerbating the challenging behaviors. However, it is important to remember that some challenging behaviors may also be developmentally appropriate behaviors in a person with ID.
F. Some factors associated with challenging behaviors include the following:
  1. Learned behaviors
  2. Response to life events (e.g., change of key worker, bereavement)
  3. Attachment problems
  4. Relationship problems
  5. Physical environment
  6. Communication difficulties
  7. Sensory difficulties
  8. Genetic syndromes/behavioral phenotypes
  9. Physical health problems (e.g., pain, infections, constipation)
  10. Dementia
  11. Epilepsy
  12. Drug and alcohol use and withdrawal states
  13. Mental illness
  14. Personality disorder
  15. Autism
  16. ADHD

Relationships Between Mental and Physical Health Problems and Challenging Behaviors

A. It is widely accepted that mental health problems can sometimes be associated with challenging behaviors in people with ID. The relationship between psychiatric symptoms and challenging behaviors could work in different ways.
  1. Some challenging behaviors might actually be atypical symptoms of a mental illness.
  2. Mental illnesses may also produce conditions for the expression of challenging behaviors that are maintained by behavioral processes.
  3. Events or demands on a person with ID might become aversive only if the person experiences psychiatric symptoms.
  4. Physical problems such as constipation and infection may be an important or even primary contributory factor to some challenging behaviors.
B. The majority of challenging behaviors are not likely to be associated with physical or mental health problems.
C. It is important to neither overplay nor underplay the importance of mental health problems when considering challenging behaviors in people with ID. In complex cases, single answers or diagnoses are unlikely to explain all of the presentation or lead to a simple solution. Multifactorial causation in complex cases of challenging behaviors may be more the norm than the exception.

DANGERS OF MYTHS AND PRECONCEIVED BIASES

Diagnostic Overshadowing

A. Diagnostic overshadowing is an important factor in the underdiagnosis of mental health problems in people with ID. Diagnostic overshadowing was originally (and usually still is) described as a health professional's ascribing a person's mental health symptoms to their ID, rather than looking further for the cause. It can also happen because symptoms are ascribed to other diagnoses present, such as autism or epilepsy.

RISK FACTORS

A. It is not easy to draw clear conclusions about offending behaviors in people with ID because challenging behaviors, such as aggression to others and destructiveness, are usually not processed through the criminal justice system.
B. For people with ID, the risk factors for offending behaviors are often similar to those for people without ID. However, people with ID may have increased difficulties with retaining information and internalizing coping strategies from treatment due to cognitive limitations.
  1. Impulsivity and deficits in consequential thinking are common in people with ID.
  2. There may be more pronounced difficulties with problem-solving, empathy, and perspective taking; impulsivity; and poor consequential thinking in this population.
  3. Some more severe adverse life events, such as exposure to violence, are known to be more common among people with ID.
  4. People with ID experience much higher rates of abuse than the general population. They are vulnerable adults and can be exploited in all ways, including sexually and financially. In some situations in which the law is broken, they may be perpetrators and victims simultaneously.

ASSESSMENT NEEDS

PSYCHIATRIC ASSESSMENT IN INTELLECTUAL DISABILITY

A. The psychiatric assessment of a person with ID makes use of different methods. Of most importance is usually the history, including the person's early life and development and their usual mood, speech, behaviors, and baseline levels of functioning. The timing of the onset of symptoms is crucial.

B. If the person with ID is able to speak, a direct interview will usually be conducted, along with a history of the presenting problems from key people such as carers and relatives, the use of rating instruments, a consideration of previous medical records and reports from sources such as education and social care, a physical examination, and medical investigations.

C. Holistic mental health assessments may be conducted by differing practitioners, who may include nurses, psychiatrists, psychologists, and other healthcare and social work professionals.

D. For the most complex presentations, a joint assessment may be helpful, including practitioners from two or more professional disciplines. This should provide complementary perspectives.

HISTORY

A. While adapting the assessment to the individual is vital, a number of key questions and topics should be asked. All patients can be assessed, even if they have no verbal communication skills.

B. A detailed history of someone's early life and development is crucial to help establish the right diagnosis. This developmental history needs to be complemented by a detailed knowledge of the person, including their mood, speech, and behaviors. It is important to get as many reliable accounts as possible about how the person usually is.

C. For the history, informants are often important sources of information. However, different individuals (carers, family members, professionals) may have competing agendas.

D. Some particular issues that should be considered are the interaction of medication with mental health, epilepsy (which can cause many associated mental health issues), and pain or discomfort (which can lead to mood problems or challenging behaviors).

E. It is often difficult to establish whether difficulties are primarily mental, physical, psychological, or psychosocial in nature, or whether they are multifactorial. It is important to take a careful history that covers all aspects of the person's life, including their vulnerability.

INFORMANT HISTORY

A. It is usually necessary to obtain information from a range of sources. The referred person may find it difficult to explain their difficulties or may even have no verbal communication at all.

B. Speaking to the staff who support the person will give a valuable insight into their concerns.

C. Different staff working with the same person may have widely differing views. When possible and appropriate, it will be helpful to speak to family members also. They are usually the only people who can give a full developmental history.

D. It is important to bear in mind that narratives from care staff and relatives may be competing and be influenced by differing agendas.

INTERVIEW

A. Questions to consider in an assessment of mental health in a person with ID include the following:
  1. Is this experience or behavior new or very different for this person?
  2. Is this experience or behavior unusual for this person?
  3. Does this experience or behavior seem to trouble this person?
  4. What is the usual mood or temperament of the person with ID? Have there been any changes in their usual routines?
  5. Is this person in good physical health? Has their physical health been checked recently?
  6. Are there any dangers in these experiences or behaviors, for the person or for others?
  7. What can the person tell you about their thoughts, feelings, and behaviors?
  8. Does this experience or behavior appear to trouble or distress the person?
  9. Is there a detailed, pregnancy/birth to adulthood, developmental history?
  10. Is there a family history of any mental illness?
  11. What is the usual temperament or mood of the person?
  12. Have there been any changes in their usual routines?
  13. Is the person in good physical health and have they had relevant investigations?
  14. Are there any changes in the person's sleep, appetite, weight, or energy/activity level?
  15. Can any recent upsets or negative events explain any changes in the person?
  16. Have any changes in the person been reported by more than one informant?
  17. Have any changes in the person been reported in more than one environment?
  18. What are the possible functions or meanings for the person's experiences or behaviors?
  19. Is the behavior motivated by gaining something pleasant or avoiding something unpleasant?

OBSERVATIONS

A. It may be appropriate to observe the person in their home or in another place, such as a day center, to better understand the influence of their environment.

B. A tentative diagnosis may be made more on the basis of observations than on a person's account.
  1. An example of behavior that suggests auditory hallucinations is a person with ID shouting at people who are not present when this has not been their previous behavior.
  2. Suspiciousness and social withdrawal not previously part of the person's personality and behavior could also be suggestive of mental health problems.
  3. Nonverbal evidence for possible mental health problems by necessity becomes of greater importance in assessment in people with ID who have limited verbal abilities.

BIOLOGICAL INVESTIGATIONS

A. Results of biological investigations are usually important to obtain.
  1. Blood tests, EKGs, EEGs, and brain scans might be helpful when considering underlying medical conditions as well as safety of treatment.
  2. A physical examination may sometimes be useful, including targeted examinations (e.g., hearing, vision).
  3. Sensory impairments such as cataracts and partial hearing loss may make people with ID more susceptible to misinterpreting things they see and hear.

RATING INSTRUMENTS

A. Rating instruments used in the general population to assist diagnosis have debatable validity when used in people with ID.

B. Several dedicated instruments for people with ID have been developed.
  1. The Glasgow Anxiety Scale and the Glasgow Depression Scale were designed for people with ID to complete.

2. Such questionnaires require the person to have a level of verbal ability.
C. Other questionnaires are designed for family or staff to complete (e.g., Autism Diagnostic Interview-Revised, or ADI-R) to assess for possible ASD.
D. If it is helpful to understand more about the person's cognitive functioning, an IQ test, such as the Wechsler Adult Intelligence Scale-Fourth Edition (WAIS-IV), may be administered. This can help in developing a picture of the person's strengths and difficulties.
E. Staff may also be asked to record the details for all challenging behaviors for a few weeks, using the Antecedent-Behavior-Consequence (ABC) chart, which would then be analyzed by the mental health professional. The patient may be asked to complete mood charts for a few weeks to give information about the person's mood alongside details of activities.
F. Screening tools for mental health problems in people with ID include the Mini Psychiatric Assessment Schedule for Adult with Developmental Disability (PAS-ADD), which is a short, structured questionnaire that can be completed by nonspecialist healthcare professionals. This screening tool can be used to suggest when referral for more specialist assessment is needed.
G. The Developmental Behavior Checklist (DBC-A) can be used to assess the behavioral and emotional problems of adults with ID.

DIAGNOSIS

A. One of the aims of assessment is accurate diagnosis, followed by appropriate treatment.
B. APRNs combine information from various sources to build up an overall guide to the possible diagnosis of mental illness in a person with ID. Some of this evidence can be contradictory, and thus it can often be impossible to give a conclusive diagnostic opinion.
C. When trying to assess the mental health of a person with ID, one must remember these guiding principles:
   1. Symptoms of mental illness tend to come in clusters. Therefore, one odd or unusual experience on its own may be of less significance for a psychiatric diagnosis than if the person with ID has a pattern of symptoms.
   2. Mental illness is more likely if the person has had a previous psychiatric episode.
   3. People with ID who have a family history of mental health problems are also more likely to develop mental health problems than those with no family history.
   4. The basis of healthcare is an accurate diagnosis followed by appropriate treatment. However, there are circumstances in which, even though the diagnosis of mental health problems is not clear-cut, it may still be justifiable, ethical, and in the best interests of the person with ID to prescribe a trial of a medication. The response, or lack of response, to the medication can then be used to help determine (but not prove) whether the tentative diagnosis of mental health problems was correct.

INTERVENTIONS

Medications

A. The principles of treatment in people with ID are similar to those in the general population. Medication treatments for mental health problems in ID appear broadly similar in efficacy.
B. Many clinicians have reported that effective dosage levels of medications for mental health problems often appear to be lower in people with ID, although there is minimal published evidence to support this widely accepted view.
C. Some medications can make thinking, remembering, and word-finding more difficult, and also make people more at risk of having epileptic seizures than usual.
D. People with ID are more likely to have general physical health problems, and a view that they tend to be more sensitive to medication is widely held. However, there is no clear published evidence that they experience more side effects than people without ID. It is sometimes the case that any preexisting problems in people with ID may make some side effects appear worse.
E. Medication can have side effects that patients with ID might struggle to identify and report. It is preferable, therefore, to start medications at low doses and increase the dose gradually ("start low, go slow").
F. There is a consensus that medication prescribing often needs to be instigated and increased more cautiously in patients with ID.
G. Deb et al. (2006) recommend that antipsychotic drugs be considered to manage challenging behavior only if psychological or other interventions alone do not produce change within an agreed time, if treatment for any coexisting mental or physical health problem has not led to a reduction in the behavior, or if the risk to the person or others is very severe. The current published evidence for the use of antipsychotic medications such as risperidone and aripiprazole to reduce associated features of ASD, such as anxiety, aggression, stereotyped behaviors, and hyperactivity, is limited, but the practice is commonplace. For some people with ID and ASD, these medications can sometimes produce evident benefits.

Psychosocial Interventions

A. Most psychological interventions can be used for adults with an ID, with adaptations to account for the person's intellectual level.
B. Many people with ID are able to engage with regular therapy sessions.
C. Assessment of challenging behavior seeks first to accurately describe what is happening and understand the person's reasons for engaging in the behavior of concern, and then to work with the system of caregivers for the person.
D. Positive behavior support seeks to prevent or reduce the behavior of concern by meeting the person's needs in alternative, beneficial ways.
E. It is common that the person's social circumstances have a significant effect on their mental health and that changing or improving the person's environment, social care, or daily activities may be the most effective way of reducing the person's distress.

DIFFICULTIES IN THE PSYCHIATRIC ASSESSMENT OF PEOPLE WITH INTELLECTUAL DISABILITY

A. A person with ID may have the following difficulties with mental health assessment:
   1. Understanding the purpose of the assessment
   2. Understanding questions about their mental state
   3. Understanding concepts or ideas beyond the concrete or literal
   4. Expressing emotions verbally and nonverbally
   5. Communicating internal experiences or motivations
   6. Interpreting the behaviors or speech of others
   7. Finding the mental health assessment process itself difficult and stressful

CHALLENGES FOR THE ASSESSOR

A. Eliciting psychiatric symptoms depends to a great extent on the person with ID being able to articulate their experiences, thoughts, and beliefs.
B. It is impossible to diagnose mental health problems with certainty in people with limited verbal communication—in practice, this means people with ID who have an IQ below approximately 45.
C. Second, the difficulty of differentiating psychiatric symptoms and features related to a person's ID (and comorbid conditions such as ASD and ADHD, if present) may also lead to mental health problems being underdiagnosed or wrongly diagnosed.
D. The focus on psychotic illness in this chapter illustrates this balance between under- and overdiagnosing in people with ID.

Psychotic Illness

A. Psychotic illnesses are more common in people with ID than in the general population. They can include brief, stress-related illnesses as well as schizophrenias.
B. Psychoses are more difficult to detect, and often the symptoms are subtler or less typical than those in the general population.
C. People with ID can be susceptible to developing short-lived psychotic episodes that are brought on by stressful life events because they often have more limited coping abilities.

Assessment of Delusions

A. It is often difficult to determine whether a person with ID has true delusional beliefs. For example, they may have fantasies that they are famous (e.g., that they are a successful singer). They then may be wrongly thought to have grandiose delusions.
B. Because of their reduced opportunity to take part in normal life experiences, the delusions of people with ID disorders, when they occur, may not be complicated. This makes it harder to judge whether beliefs are delusional. In schizophrenias, people sometimes have delusions that they are being controlled (delusions of passivity).
C. People with ID may have a real lack of autonomy, or at least a perceived lack of control over their lives, and they may complain. This can sometimes be misunderstood as a delusion.
D. People with ID are also often sensitive to how they are perceived by others. This can often be based on real-life experiences of being mocked.

Egosyntonic or Egodystonic?

A. A guide to whether or not an odd or unusual belief may be delusional is whether or not the experiences or beliefs are distressing for the person with ID. A person does not generally tend to fantasize or voluntarily imagine hearing or seeing things that are frightening or upsetting or to believe things that cause them distress.
  1. Egosyntonic beliefs are in harmony with or acceptable to the needs and goals of the person or consistent with their ideal self-image.
  2. Egodystonic beliefs are in conflict or dissonant with the needs and goals of the person or in conflict with their ideal self-image.
B. This egosyntonic/egodystonic distinction for odd beliefs can only be a rough aid to diagnosis because psychotic symptoms are not necessarily always upsetting for the person with ID.
  1. The presence or absence of distress may still be important to help decide whether treatment should be offered.
  2. It has also been suggested that people with ID are more likely to be able to be temporarily persuaded that delusional beliefs are false because of their increased suggestibility.
C. There are additional difficulties in assessing delusional beliefs when people with ID also have ASD:
  1. People with both ID and ASD have additional problems to varying degrees with theory of mind. So the beliefs of a person with ID and ASD may sometimes appear persecutory because they lack the ability to understand another person's motivations. They also may have problems understanding nonverbal communication, leading to misinterpretations.
  2. Unusual preoccupations or odd ideas held rigidly by people with ID and ASD may be particularly difficult to differentiate from delusions. For example, they may have grotesque or violent fantasies that they even seem to enjoy to some extent, particularly if these seem to arouse strong (and thus for them more easily understood) emotions in others. They also have problems understanding nonverbal communication and social cues, which can lead to misinterpretations.
  3. As people with both ID and ASD find their environment confusing and are unable to understand everything that happens around them, they can sometimes become paranoid about others (e.g., they might think that other people are talking about them), and this can be misinterpreted as evidence of persecutory delusions.
  4. People with ID and ASD may more commonly have "magical thinking" or have a lifelong blurring of the boundaries between reality and fantasy, which again may be complicating factors in psychiatric assessment. Sometimes psychosis may be indicated by a change in the intensity of the magical thinking or in the degree of conviction to which the fantastical beliefs are held. These more subtle shifts in thinking can be hard to discern with certainty.

Assessment of Hallucinations

A. Hallucinations can be hard to diagnose with certainty. It is often thought, for example, that "hearing voices" is an indicator of psychosis. There could, however, be other explanations for someone with ID hearing voices.
  1. Talking to themselves may be a coping mechanism for managing anxiety and thus be more prominent at times of stress.
  2. People with ID may often recall previous conversations and rehearse them or think out loud. They often do not recognize that this is considered socially odd.
  3. People with ID may also experience their own thoughts as voices. It may be harder for a person with ID to distinguish between their inner thoughts or speech ("self-talk") and external "voices," compared with those without ID.
  4. Conversations with imaginary friends or fantasy figures are also more common in people with ID. They will not recognize that this is often considered socially odd.
  5. Behaviors that may be appropriate for someone with ID at a certain developmental stage may be wrongly interpreted as psychotic behaviors. These can all be appropriate for a person's developmental stage if they also have ID.
B. The internal experiences of a person with ID must be assessed with very careful questioning, avoiding, for example,

asking leading questions or using words that may be taken too literally.
C. The delusional interpretation of a person regarding their own experiences would signify that the voices are true hallucinations.
D. Complex hallucinations, such as hearing voices giving them a running commentary of what they are doing, are also less commonly reported by people with ID.

Assessment of Thought
A. Some people with ID have information-processing impairments that affect their thinking and language. They can speak in idiosyncratic ways. Incoherent speech may also be hard to judge in people with ID as it can sometimes be difficult to follow the thread of their speech, especially if they have unusual preoccupations or when they are excited or anxious.
B. Therefore, language difficulties can appear that are similar to the thought disorder or disordered speech sometimes found in psychosis because they are often odd, irrelevant, and socially inappropriate.
C. Incoherent speech may also be hard to judge in people with ID as it can be difficult to follow the thread of their conversation, especially if they have unusual preoccupations and they are excited or anxious.

Assessment of Behavior
A. People with ID can show gross disorganization of behavior when under stress. Their mannerisms and stereotyped behaviors may become marked or extreme.
B. People with ID who experience increased levels of anxiety (e.g., due to changes in their routine) can potentially engage in new, bizarre behaviors as a coping mechanism.
C. People with ID have higher rates of cognitive processing problems and often have limited coping strategies when they experience by sensory overload, and this can result in distress and odd and challenging behaviors.

Assessment of "Negative" Psychotic Symptoms
A. Some symptoms of long-standing mental health problems are described as "negative" symptoms; these can include social withdrawal, reduced speech, and reduced motivation.
B. Flattened and odd moods, reduced motivation, social withdrawal, poor nonverbal communication, and low amounts of speech can be seen in ID as well as in schizophrenia, particularly if ASD is also present.
C. Negative symptoms of psychosis may be mimicked by lack of spontaneity and movement when people with ID are asked to perform tasks that have no meaning for them. These apparent "symptoms" can be misattributed to mental health problems when they may be being influenced by a great many other factors, such as institutionalization, oversedation, lack of stimulation, and problems with processing information.

RELATIONSHIP BETWEEN AUTISTIC SPECTRUM DISORDER AND SCHIZOPHRENIA
A. Differentiating schizophrenia from ASD in people with ID can be difficult.
B. Social withdrawal and lack of empathy can often occur in schizophrenia as well as in ASD.
C. Unusual preoccupations held rigidly by people with ID and ASD may be particularly difficult to differentiate from delusions.
D. People with ASD can be concrete and often preoccupied with their special interests and their view of themselves, and this world can appear so odd to others as to appear delusional.
E. A very detailed history of the person's early life and development is necessary to help establish the right diagnosis.
F. A very detailed developmental history, ideally from more than one source, may be the only method to determine if psychosis has occurred comorbidly on a background of ID and ASD. Unfortunately, this history is not always possible to obtain, especially if people with ID have moved around as children or been in care.
G. The term *autism* was first used to describe social impairment in schizophrenia. However, it is recognized that ASD and schizophrenia are separate conditions. People can have one or other of the conditions, or less commonly they may have both.
H. Often, people who develop schizophrenia in adolescence or early adulthood have been found to have had problems with communication and reciprocal social interaction and to have had obsessions, rituals, and bizarre thinking dating from childhood, well before any psychotic symptoms such as delusions or hallucinations developed.
I. People with ID and ASD may be more susceptible to developing short-lived psychotic episodes that can be triggered by life events because they have more limited ability to cope with stress. However, a pragmatic approach is needed that is less concerned with definitive diagnostic labeling and more focused on the actual symptoms or impairments. For example, many people with schizophrenia may benefit from psychosocial strategies such as social skills training aimed at their autistic-type features, whether they are formally diagnosed with comorbid ASD or not.
J. ASD and the schizophrenias are spectrum disorders that share a lot of similarities. They are recognized as neurodevelopmental disorders of atypical brain developments with overlapping symptoms and features and overlapping genetic and environmental risks.
K. Emotional expression and nonverbal communication are often diminished in both ASD and schizophrenia. Neuropsychological deficits in theory of mind and executive function and lack of empathy can often occur in schizophrenia as well as autism. Both people with ASD and those with schizophrenia can show other similarities, such as concrete thinking and stereotyped behaviors.

Catatonia
A. Catatonia is more common in ASD as well as in schizophrenia.
B. Catatonia can include gross disturbances of movement, such as adopting a motionless posture for long periods.
C. Alternatively, in a catatonic state, the person may become overactive and be in a state of constant excitement.
D. Catatonia may be part of the presentation of schizophrenia, may be part of ASD, or may be manifested in some people with ASD who also have comorbid schizophrenia, or be found in individuals who have neither diagnosis.

INTELLECTUAL DISABILITY, AUTISM SPECTRUM DISORDER, AND MOOD
A. Diagnosing a mood disorder in a person with ID and ASD can be quite difficult because they may not be able to understand how they are feeling or communicate how they are feeling.

B. Excessive excitement about special interests, overactivity, and pressurized and loud speech can be mistaken for symptoms of mania.
C. ASD is associated with a generally unstable mood that can change rapidly, depending on the person's environment. People with both ASD and ID have difficulty recognizing and describing their emotional states or moods. People with ID and ASD can present with flattened, restrictive, or odd affect, in addition to difficulties with eye contact, limited emotional expression, and poor social interactions, which can be misinterpreted as low mood.
D. The restrictive pattern of interests of people with ID and ASD may appear as a lack of or a reduced interest in general activities. It is crucial to establish a functional baseline for the person. Sometimes people with ID and ASD can have difficulties acknowledging emotional distress, which is instead expressed through somatic complaints such as headaches and abdominal pains.

CHALLENGES FOR NURSE PRACTITIONER AND TOOLS TO DEAL WITH CHALLENGES

CAPACITY AND CONSENT
A. Patients need to have the capacity (or ability) to consent to their healthcare assessment and treatment. Practitioners are therefore required to make a capacity assessment before carrying out any care or treatment of people with ID. The practitioner needs to assess the patient's ability to understand information given to them about a given healthcare decision, for example, to take medication. The patient needs to be able to retain that information and then to weigh it up to make a decision. The patient then needs to have the ability to communicate that decision, verbally or nonverbally. It is vital for the practitioner to consult others who know the person, such as family members.
  1. If the person is deemed to have capacity about a decision, they can make whatever decision they choose even if others think it is unwise.
  2. If the person is deemed to lack capacity, the decision should be made for them, following a best interests process.
  3. If the person with ID lacks capacity to decide about their own mental health and treatment, an approach of ethical pragmatism is often taken. For example, if they lack capacity to decide about medication, it can still be considered using a best interests process involving family wherever possible.

GUIDELINES TO AID PRACTICE: CHALLENGING BEHAVIORS
A. Reiss (1994, p. 70) offers useful guidance for practitioners when considering challenging behaviors:
  1. They must assess whether or not there has been a clear change in behavior from baseline levels of fluctuation.
  2. They must then consider whether any behavioral disturbance may be part of a symptom pattern that corresponds to a mental disorder.
  3. They should remember that there is always the possibility that challenging behaviors may be exacerbating a coexisting mental disorder, and also that mental disorders can manifest as new or increased challenging behaviors.
  4. Allowances should be made for the impact that differing levels of intellectual functioning have on the expression of the symptoms.
  5. Accept that the cause of the behaviors may ultimately be ambiguous. In more severe ID, diagnoses of mental disorders can often only be tentative.

INCLUSION OF THE PATIENT AND FAMILY IN CARE

REASONABLE ADJUSTMENTS
A. Owing to the difficulties people with ID present to assessment, the APRN must provide them with "reasonable adjustments" to help them access best care.
  1. Assessment in people with ID normally requires increased time due to both communication difficulties and complexity of problems.
  2. The APRN must adapt the words used for each person assessed to elicit the quality of information required to complete a good quality assessment. The APRN needs to be creative about which words work best for each patient.
  3. Understanding must be constantly checked. Sometimes the best advice an APRN can give themselves in the assessment of a person with ID is just to "slow down" in general.
B. People with ID might not have the experience of being listened to. They may have had repeated experiences of losses due to high care staff turnover or being in care. For these reasons, they may have attachment difficulties and need more time to develop a trusting therapeutic relationship.
C. People with ID should be supported to express their rights and choices, which will also help with rapport and trust. Adapted communication methods (e.g., easy-to-read leaflets, pictures) may be necessary in assessments and also in discussing the role of treatments such as medication.
D. Adaptations might include keeping verbal and written language as simple as possible. Sometimes nonverbal creative techniques, such as drawing, can help. Allowances may also be required for difficulties understanding time and numbers—for example, having a visual diary of sessions and not trying to establish in minute detail exactly how or when something happened if this is beyond the person's ability.
E. It might also be helpful to adapt assessment times to account for the person's ability to concentrate. Assessment may need to take place over a number of sessions rather than just one, and in different places. A person's support network (e.g., family, support staff, care management, other professionals) may need to be involved in supporting an intervention. However, this would always need to be considered with the person's views, ability to consent, and best interests in mind.

ACQUIESCENCE AND SUGGESTIBILITY
A. The APRN must be aware of the potential influence of acquiescence and suggestibility. People with ID are more likely than the general population to agree with whatever they are asked, especially if they do not fully understand.
B. Asking questions using different wording and experimenting with complexity of vocabulary and opposite meanings can help clarify whether suggestibility is having an impact on the assessment. For example, an answer of "Yes" to both "Do you feel happy?" and "Do you feel sad?" may point to suggestibility.
C. People with ID may have learned to agree with, or acquiesce to, professionals even if they do not actually agree or understand, perhaps in deference to perceived authority, as a way of masking their ID, or out of a need to be accepted ("social desirability"). APRNs will need to be creative to ask ▶

questions in different ways or state that it is all right for the person to disagree.

D. Psychiatric and behavioral disorders can be a major concern for families and carers of people with ID. Such difficulties are a common source of stress and negative emotions in carers. Challenging behaviors, which can often be the outward manifestation of mental health problems, often present major difficulties for families and carers. Behavioral or psychiatric problems are important sources of stress experienced by caregivers, and that stress intensifies with the increasing severity of the carer's experience. Psychiatric and behavioral disorders are related to carer burden and coping and are perceived to have a negative impact on families. However, high levels of satisfaction, uplift, and quality of life as a result of caring have also been reported by family carers.

E. In residential care settings, the presence of challenging behaviors and interpersonal difficulties is related to lower job satisfaction, increased anxiety, emotional exhaustion, depersonalization or cynicism, and staff burnout.

OPPORTUNITIES TO PARTNER WITH OTHERS AND TO PROVIDE REFERRALS

BIOPSYCHOSOCIAL APPROACHES

A. The assessment and management of challenging behaviors is a perfect illustration of how approaches to the mental health of people with ID need to be multidisciplinary. People with ID are more likely to have complex needs than people without it. It is not uncommon to find people with ID who also have mental illness, multiple physical health problems, sensory needs, and communication difficulties, as well as a range of unmet social needs. This makes assessment much more complicated.

B. Because causes of challenging behaviors are invariably multifactorial, it is important not to reduce them to simply biological or psychiatric in nature or simply "behavioral" and thereby dismiss any possible mental disorder. The term *behavioral overshadowing* refers to a clinician ascribing a psychopathology to learned behavior, rather than considering whether it is perhaps a symptom of a mental illness.

C. If behavior is thought to be "behavioral," then it is often considered to serve a function, but if it is considered to be psychiatric then any possible functional component is disregarded. Even if some behaviors are biologically driven, the environment can still reinforce them, or the behaviors can provide some function for the individual that may make them amenable to behavioral approaches.

NEED FOR A MULTIDISCIPLINARY TEAM

A. There is perhaps no other field in health and social care that has greater need of a holistic (biopsychosocial) and integrated approach than the mental healthcare of people with ID, with partnerships between agencies and with relatives and paid care staff. Various ways of understanding, such as "medical" or "biological," "behavioral," or other models, are ultimately only different aids that should be considered simultaneously.

B. A multidisciplinary approach is advised; for example, in one complex patient, these could include the following:
1. Occupational therapy input regarding sensory issues
2. Speech and language therapy input regarding communication difficulties
3. Behavioral support specialist input regarding specific challenging behaviors
4. Dietitian input
5. Educational and vocational interventions because people with autism really struggle with unstructured time and need to be engaged in meaningful activities during the day
6. Family interventions (e.g., educating and supporting families), including family therapy, which might be appropriate when the main problem appears to be the relationship or interaction between the person with autism and ID and a member(s) of their family
7. Medication (e.g., for mental illness, ADHD, or some of the associated features of ASD)
8. Other interventions as needed

RESEARCH

A. Many of the concepts described in this chapter are still not widely known or universally understood by mental health clinicians, especially by those not trained in the mental health aspects of ID.

B. There are many well-documented difficulties in conducting research in people with ID, including funding and recruitment. Mental health research has therefore frequently excluded this group.

C. The increasingly stringent ethical clearance for research in people with ID may unfortunately lead to less research in people with ID being carried out in the future. This unintended outcome is not in the best interests of these patients, and it is therefore important that practitioners, as well as paid care staff and relatives, support and participate in research into the mental health of people with ID to further develop the evidence base.

SUMMARY OF KEY POINTS

A. Most mental health problems found in the wider population can also occur in people with ID.

B. The prevalence of mental health problems, including challenging behaviors where a mental illness is not diagnosable, is higher in people with ID.

C. The prevalence of some mental illnesses (e.g., schizophrenia) is significantly increased in people with ID. The prevalence of others, such as depression, is also increased, but less so.

D. Comorbid neurodevelopmental conditions, such as autism and ADHD, are much more common in people with ID than in the general population.

E. Comorbid physical health problems, including epilepsy and sensory problems, are more common in people with ID.

F. Abuse and exploitation are extremely common among those with ID and should be considered whenever a person with ID presents with mental health problems.

G. Bereavement can have a disproportionately large effect on adults with ID, likely due to limited understanding of the concept of death.

H. Mental health problems in people with ID can be both under- and overdiagnosed.

I. Mental health problems are more difficult to detect in people with ID, and often the symptoms are more subtle or less typical than those in the general population.

J. People with ID are more likely to have "atypical" symptom presentations, through behavior disturbance, self-harming behavior, or disruption in daily functioning.

K. People with ID often have a combination of symptoms based on the complex interaction of mental illness, physical illness, and environmental factors.

L. The increased prevalence of mental health problems in ID is due to a complex relationship among genetic, biological, and environmental factors.

M. Wrongly describing problems as being due to a person's ID and not their mental illness is known as *diagnostic overshadowing*.

N. Mental health problems, including challenging behaviors, are usually multifactorial phenomena that require an integrated, multimodal approach to assessment and treatment.

O. Assessment of mental health of adults with ID should always consider and inquire about adverse life events.

P. Observational, nonverbal evidence for possible psychosis becomes of greater importance by necessity in assessment, especially when a person with ID has more limited verbal abilities.

Q. Comorbid neurodevelopmental conditions, such as autism, and physical health problems, such as epilepsy, make assessment more complex.

R. The treatment of mental health problems in ID broadly follows that for people without ID.

S. People with ID are often unable to report the side effects of medications.

T. A multidisciplinary approach to treating mental illness in people with ID is necessary.

U. If someone lacks the capacity to consent, a decision to use medication must be in the person's best interests.

V. In the absence of a diagnosable mental illness, medication for challenging behaviors should not be first-line and should be part of a management plan that includes psychosocial interventions.

RESOURCES

A. Hemmings, C. (2018). *Mental Health of Intellectual Disabilities: A complete introduction to assessment, intervention, care and support* (5th ed.). Hove: Pavilion Press.

B. Hemmings, C., Bouras, N. (Eds.). (1999). *Psychiatric and behavioural disorders in developmental disabilities and developmental disabilities* (4th Ed.). Cambridge University Press.

REFERENCES AND BIBLIOGRAPHY

American Psychiatric Association. (2013). *Diagnostic and statistical manual of mental disorders* (5th ed.). https://doi.org/10.1176/appi.books.9780890425596

Buckles, J. (2016). The epidemiology of psychiatric disorder in adults with intellectual disabilities. In C. Hemmings & N. Bouras (Eds.), *Psychiatric and behavioural disorders in intellectual and developmental disabilities* (4th ed., pp. 34–44). Cambridge University Press.

Deb, S., Clarke, D., & Unwin, G. (2006). *Using medication to manage behaviour problems among adults with a learning disability: Quick reference guide*. University of Birmingham, MENCAP, The Royal College of Psychiatrists.

Einfeld, S. L., & Tonge, B. J. (2002). *Manual for the developmental behaviour checklist: Primary carer version (DBC-P) & teacher version (DBC-T)* (2nd ed.). Monash University Centre for Developmental Psychiatry and Psychology.

Emerson, E. (1995). *Challenging behaviour: Analysis and intervention in people with learning disabilities*. Cambridge University Press.

Fletcher, R., Loschen, E., Stavrakaki, C., & First, M. (Eds.). (2007). *Diagnostic manual—intellectual disability: A textbook of diagnosis of mental disorders in persons with intellectual disability*. NADD Press.

Hemmings, C. (2007). The relationship between challenging behaviours and psychiatric disorders in people with severe intellectual disabilities. In N. Bouras & G. Holt (Eds.), *Psychiatric and behavioural disorders in developmental disabilities and mental retardation* (3rd ed., pp. 62–75). Cambridge University Press.

Hemmings, C. (2016). Reflections. In C. Hemmings & N. Bouras (Eds.), *Psychiatric and behavioural disorders in developmental disabilities and developmental disabilities* (4th ed., pp. 279–288). Cambridge University Press.

Lord, C., Rutter, M., & Le Couteur, A. (1994). Autism diagnostic interview-revised: A revised version of a diagnostic interview for caregivers of individuals with possible pervasive developmental disorders. *Journal of Autism and Developmental Disorders, 24*, 659–685. https://doi.org/10.1007/BF02172145

Prosser, H., Moss, S., Costello, H., Simpson, N., Patel, P., & Rowe, S. (1998). Reliability and validity of the mini PAS-ADD for assessing psychiatric disorders in adults with intellectual disability. *Journal of Intellectual Disability Research, 42*(4), 264–272. https://doi.org/10.1046/j.1365-2788.1998.00146.x

Reiss, S. (1994). Psychopathology in mental retardation. In N. Bouras (Ed.), *Mental health in mental retardation: Recent advances in practice* (pp. 67–78). Cambridge University Press.

Reiss, S., Levitan, G.W., & Zyszko, J. (1982). Emotional disturbance and mental retardation: Diagnostic overshadowing. *American Journal of Mental Deficiency, 86*, 567–74. PMID: 7102729

Royal College of Psychiatrists. (2001). *DC-LD: Diagnostic criteria for psychiatric disorders for use with autistic spectrum disorders/mental retardation*. Gaskell Press.

Unwin, G. L., & Deb, S. (2011). Family caregiver uplift and burden: Associations with aggressive behaviour in adults with intellectual disability. *Journal of Mental Health Research in Intellectual Disability, 4*(3), 186–205. https://doi.org/10.1080/19315864.2011.600511

World Health Organization. (2019). *International statistical classification of diseases and related health problems* (11th rev.). https://icd.who.int

Xenitidis, K., Paliokosta, E., & Maltzos, S. (2007). Assessment of mental health problems in people with autism. *Advances in Mental Health and Learning Disabilities, 1*(4), 15–22. https://doi.org/10.1108/17530180200700038

24 HOMELESS AND INDIGENT POPULATIONS

Rosa Landinez and Sandra Ojurongbe

INTRODUCTION

The term *homeless* was first used in the 1870s to describe people traveling around the country searching for a job. These individuals were seen as immoral and threatening to the fixed values of "home life." Most homeless individuals were men, described as "vagrants" who were escaping family obligations and wandering without purpose. In the early 20th century, the creation of affordable and available housing was envisioned as an initial solution to the homelessness crisis. However, with the industrial revolution, the need for workers increased and opened opportunities for homeless men to find steady jobs in different trades. An increase in migration from farms to urban areas was then seen.

In the history of homelessness in the United States, several important periods marked substantial changes to legislation and the creation of programs to address homelessness. After the Civil War, homelessness declined due to increased opportunities to work in the national railroad system, urbanization, and the vast movement of young White men returning from the war who began working. World War II also served as an initial economic booster to the nation, intending to put the nation to work. However, this boom was primarily seen in White males. Homelessness also disproportionately affected older people who either have disabilities or are dependent on social security or welfare benefits.

Today, *homelessness* is a modern term that refers to the state of having inadequate or unstable living places. The definition has changed due to legislation and a need for more consensus between governmental agencies. Some agencies might advocate for using a common vocabulary and preestablished criteria, including standard demographic data shared by all agencies working to help homeless people.

The deinstitutionalization of individuals with mental health disorders in the early 1980s, accompanied by the gentrification of the inner city, the emergence of HIV/AIDS, high unemployment rates, inadequate or nonexistent affordable housing opportunities, and lack of funding for projects aimed at helping homeless people, caused detrimental consequences to those in need of a place to stay or to live. Deep cuts in the supplemental security income and increased barriers to accessing disability benefits for most applicants further increased the number of homeless Americans. The homeless population was younger (i.e., younger than 40 years) and had co-occurring medical, mental health, and substance use disorders (SUDs). This period also marked an increase in women and families experiencing homelessness. Some researchers also provide evidence to support the causality or co-occurrence of AIDS and homelessness during this time; those experiencing homelessness who were residing in a shelter had a 9% risk of having AIDS.

REFERENCES AND BIBLIOGRAPHY

National Academies of Sciences, Engineering, and Medicine. (2018a). Addressing homelessness in the United States. In *Permanent supportive housing: Evaluating the evidence for improving health outcomes among people experiencing chronic homelessness* (pp. 19–37). The National Academies Press. https://doi.org/10.17226/25133

National Academies of Sciences, Engineering, and Medicine. (2018b). The history of homelessness in the United States. In *Permanent supportive housing: Evaluating the evidence for improving health outcomes among people experiencing chronic homelessness* (pp. 175–184). The National Academies Press. https://doi.org/10.17226/25133

HOMELESSNESS

DEFINITION

A. The U.S. Department of Housing and Urban Development (HUD) defines *homeless* as an "individual or family who lacks a fixed, regular, and adequate nighttime residence," such as those living in emergency shelters, transitional housing, or places not meant for habitation; *or* an "individual or family who will imminently lose their primary nighttime residence, provided that (i) residence will be lost within 14 days of the date of application for homeless assistance; (ii) no subsequent residence has been identified; and (iii) the individual or family lacks the resources or support networks needed to obtain other permanent housing"; *or* "unaccompanied youth under 25 years of age, or families with children and youth, who do not otherwise qualify as homeless under this definition, but who: (i) are defined as homeless under the other listed federal statutes; (ii) have not had a lease, ownership interest, or occupancy agreement in permanent housing during the 60 days prior to the homeless assistance application; (iii) have experienced persistent instability as measured by two moves or more during in the preceding 60 days; and (iv) can be expected to continue in such status for an extended period of time due to special needs or barriers"; *or* "any individual or family who: (i) is fleeing, or is attempting to flee, domestic violence; (ii) has no other residence; and (iii) lacks the resources or support networks to obtain other permanent housing" (HUD, 2012, p. 1).

B. Natural or human-caused disasters, war, family dissolution, involuntary migration, lack of affordable and adequate housing, health problems or untreated mental health problems, loss of employment, poverty, or a combination of these factors are legitimate circumstances that plummet individuals or families into homelessness. Depending on the factor or factors, the resultant state of homelessness can be transitional, episodic, or chronic.

C. Homelessness is further categorized into sheltered, unsheltered, and chronic.

  1. Sheltered homelessness: This includes people who are staying in emergency shelters, transitional housing programs, or safe havens.

  2. Unsheltered homelessness: This includes people whose principal nighttime locale is a public or private place not assigned for, or ordinarily used as, a regular sleeping accommodation for people (e.g., streets, vehicles, parks).

  3. Chronic homelessness: This includes individuals with disabilities who have been uninterruptedly homeless for at least a year or have experienced at least four episodes of homelessness in the last 3 years. The combined length of time they were homeless on those occasions is at least 12 months.

INCIDENCE AND PREVALENCE

A. In 2017, a report from the National Institutes of Health indicated that approximately 550,000 people in the United States were experiencing homelessness (meaning they were staying in shelters or places such as the street). This number showed a 30% decrease from 2016, but remained a concerning statistic.

B. In 2019, the estimated homeless population in the United States was approximately 568,000, with approximately 1.4 million people requesting access to a shelter or transitional housing yearly. At least 14% of homeless people are veterans, with approximately 90% being male; a small percentage are transgender or gender nonconforming veterans.

C. Gender and ethnicity are essential demographics when discussing homelessness.
  1. Men experience more homelessness than women.
  2. Of those experiencing homelessness in the United States, 48% are White, 41% are African American, and 22% are Hispanic/Latinx American. These numbers are conservative and might not present the actual state of homelessness in the United States.

D. The National Institutes of Health report also provides information on other variables affecting subsets of populations in the United States and stratifies those experiencing homelessness into three main categories:
  1. Transient (approximately 80%): those who spent at least a night at a shelter
  2. Episodic (approximately 10%): those who used a shelter multiple times, but stays remained brief; most likely to have mental health issues and involvement with social services
  3. Chronic (approximately 10%): those who spent long periods in a shelter and had been homeless for at least 1 year (may include those who have a nuclear family member with a disability) or had been homeless at least four times in the past 3 years

E. Approximately 30% of people who are chronically homeless have a severe mental illness.

F. The 2022 HUD report indicated the consistent overrepresentation of people of color, specifically Black, African American, or African people, as well as Indigenous people (including Native Americans and Pacific Islanders), experiencing homelessness relative to the U.S. population.
  1. A slight increase was noted in 2022, when it was reported that roughly 582,500 people experienced homelessness. This increase indicates a 3% increase in unsheltered homelessness, offset by a 2% decline in sheltered homelessness.
  2. Between 2021 and 2022, sheltered homelessness increased by 7%, or 22,504, as COVID-19 restrictions lifted and sheltered locations increased capacity. The most updated count on the homeless population with collected information from outreach field teams from a program called the Point-In-Time (PIT) count, a tally completed every year during the last 10 days of January since 2010, is an estimate of 550,000 to 650,000 people experiencing homelessness in the United States.
  3. In 2022, 50% of all people experiencing homelessness identified as White and 24% of people identified as Hispanic or Latinx. Hispanic or Latinx people make up about 16% of the total U.S. population.
  4. Between 2020 and 2022, the number of families with children experiencing homelessness declined by 6%, indicating a total decline of 36% since 2010. The number of people under 25 years old who experienced homelessness alone as "unaccompanied youth" also declined by 12% (Table 24.1).

G. During the school year 2019 to 2020, public schools identified 1,280,886 students who experienced homelessness, representing 2.5% of all students enrolled in public schools.
  1. Students of color continued to dominate the majority of students who were homeless.
     a. Hispanic and Latinx students accounted for 28% of the general student population but 38% of homeless students.
     b. Black and African American students accounted for 15% of the overall student body but 27% of homeless students.
     c. Students identified as Asian and White were underrepresented; White students accounted for 46% of public school enrollment, representing 26% of students experiencing homelessness.

REFERENCES AND BIBLIOGRAPHY

"582,462 and counting." (2023, February 3). *The New York Times*. https://www.nytimes.com/2023/02/03/business/economy/us-homeless-population-count.html

Frazer, K., & Kroll, T. (2022). *Understanding and tackling the complex challenges of homelessness and health*. MDPI. https://www.mdpi.com/1660-4601/19/6/3439

Iwundu, C. N., Santa Maria, D., & Hernandez, D. C. (2020). Commentary: The invisible and forgotten. *Family Community Health*, 44(2), 108–109. https://doi.org/10.1097/fch.0000000000000287

Keller, M. J., Conard, P. L., & Armstrong, M. L. (2022, July/August). Homelessness: Women veterans without billets. *Medsurg Nursing*, 31(4), 233–238. https://www.proquest.com/scholarly-journals/homelessness-women-veterans-without-billets/docview/2709977599/se-2

Lopez, G. (2022, July 15). America's homelessness crisis is getting worse. *The New York Times*. https://www.nytimes.com/2022/07/15/briefing/homelessness-america-housing-crisis.html

National Academies of Sciences, Engineering, and Medicine. (2018a). Addressing homelessness in the United States. In *Permanent supportive housing: Evaluating the evidence for improving health outcomes among people experiencing chronic homelessness* (pp. 19–37). The National Academies Press. https://doi.org/10.17226/25133

National Academies of Sciences, Engineering, and Medicine. (2018b). The history of homelessness in the United States. In *Permanent supportive housing: Evaluating the evidence for improving health outcomes among people experiencing chronic homelessness* (pp. 175–184). The National Academies Press. https://doi.org/10.17226/25133

Substance Abuse and Mental Health Services Administration. (2021, March). *Advisory: Behavioral health services for people who are homeless* (Publication No. PEP20-06-04-003). U.S. Department of Health and Human Services. https://store.samhsa.gov/product/advisory-behavioral-health-services-people-who-are-homeless/pep20-06-04-003

Substance Abuse and Mental Health Services Administration. (2024, January). *Definitions of homelessness used by SOAR and SSA*. U.S. Department of Health and Human Services. https://soarworks.samhsa.gov/sites/default/files/media/documents/2023-10/Definitions%20of%20Homelessness.pdf

Union of International Associations. (2021). *The Encyclopedia of World Problems and Human Potential*. https://uia.org/encyclopedia

U.S. Department of Housing and Urban Development. (2012, January). *Criteria and recordkeeping requirements for definition of homelessness*. HUD Exchange. https://www.hudexchange.info/resource/1974/criteria-and-recordkeeping-requirements-for-definition-of-homeless

U.S. Department of Housing and Urban Development. (2022, September 27). *HUD Releases 2021 Annual Homeless Assessment Report Part 1*. https://www.hud.gov/press/press_releases_media_advisories/hud_no_22_022

TABLE 24.1 DEMOGRAPHIC CHARACTERISTICS OF PEOPLE EXPERIENCING HOMELESSNESS

	All People		Sheltered People		Unsheltered People	
	n	%	n	%	n	%
All people	582,462	100	348,630	100	233,832	100
Age						
Under 18	98,244	16.8	87,960	25.2	10,284	4.2
18–24	40,177	6.9	26,981	7.7	13,196	5.6
Over 24	444,041	76.3	233,689	67.0	210,352	90.1
Gender						
Female	222,970	38.3	152,693	43.8	70,277	30.0
Male	352,836	60.6	193,366	55.5	159,470	68.3
Transgender	3,588	0.6	1,593	0.5	1,995	0.9
Gender that is not singularly female or male	2,481	0.4	846	0.2	1,635	0.7
Questioning	609	0.1	132	0.0	477	0.2
Ethnicity						
Non-Hispanic/non-Latinx	442,220	75.9	269,964	77.4	172,256	73.5
Hispanic/Latinx	140,230	24.1	78,666	22.6	61,564	26.5
Race						
American Indian, Alaska Native, or Indigenous	19,618	3.4	8,843	2.5	10,775	4.6
Asian or Asian American	8,261	1.4	3,909	1.1	4,352	1.9
Black, African American, or African	217,366	37.3	154,557	44.3	62,809	26.9
Native Hawaiian or Pacific Islander	10,461	1.8	4,692	1.3	5,769	2.5
White	291,395	50.0	157,637	45.2	133,758	57.2
Multiple races	35,383	6.1	18,992	5.4	16,391	7.0

Note: The demographic data for the unsheltered may not sum to the total because three community outreach centers (CoCs) did not report complete demographic information for the unsheltered data used in this report.

Source: de Sousa, T., Andrichik, A., Cuellar, M., Marson, J., Prestera, E., & Rush, K. (2022, December). *The 2022 Annual Homelessness Assessment Report (AHAR) to Congress.* Exhibit 1.5, p. 12. U.S. Department of Housing and Urban Development, Office of Community Planning and Development. https://www.huduser.gov/portal/sites/default/files/pdf/2022-AHAR-Part-1.pdf.

PATHWAYS TO HOMELESSNESS

Pathways to homelessness may involve several factors, including trauma, poverty, physical or mental illness, SUD, lack of affordable housing, and socioeconomic injustices. The COVID-19 pandemic also had a strong effect on homelessness.

A. The high prevalence of mental illness among homeless people is related to incessant privation in established models of care and secondary consideration of the design and implementation of community-based methods for housing and assistance.

  1. Lack of coordination between organizations responsible for healthcare and social services significantly exaggerates the obstacles faced by people with mental illness and experiencing homelessness.
  2. Untreated chronic mental illness can be pervasive and presents a significant obstacle for individuals seeking and needing healthcare services and housing. This problem can worsen for homeless people and members of minority groups.

B. Sustaining an injury or becoming ill can easily lead one to homelessness.

  1. It may result in excessive amounts of lost workdays, exhaustion of sick time, or the inability to efficiently manage or perform work functions, especially in the case of labor-intensive or physically demanding jobs.
  2. Loss of employment can restrict access to affordable healthcare treatment. Available funds and savings can quickly be depleted depending on the duration of the injury or illness. Without a stable income and the ability to make rent or mortgage payments, buy food, and afford medical expenses, poverty and homelessness may be inevitable.

C. The deinstitutionalization of individuals with mental illness in the 1960s and the lack of concrete plans to address the scarce housing available for individuals with mental illness discharged from hospitals contributed to a rise in homelessness.
D. The decrease in government funding for supplemental security income directly affected individuals with mental illness, members of vulnerable populations, and minorities. Efforts made by the government to enforce strict criteria to apply for disability benefits also presented as a barrier for homeless people with mental illness.
E. Changes in local policies to decriminalize offenses in public committed by individuals who were under the influence of alcohol or other substances are also seen as contributing factors to homelessness. Most individuals who were temporarily jailed due to minor offenses and discharged to the community seek shelter or simply stay on the street.

HOUSING INSTABILITY

A. According to Healthy People 2030, housing instability encompasses factors that challenge the ability to afford consistent, stable housing. Having difficulty paying rent, or spending 30% to 50% of household income on rent or mortgage, is a severe burden, leaving little left over for other essentials such as food, utilities, transportation, and healthcare needs. As a result, these individuals or families may live in overcrowded conditions, have to move frequently, or face evictions or foreclosures.
B. Housing instability affects specific populations disproportionately, including children whose parents move frequently, formerly incarcerated individuals, and individuals with severe mental illness.
C. Black and Hispanic households are nearly twice as likely to be cost-burdened compared with White households.
D. The economic impact of the pandemic has been especially salient on renters. The stringent restrictions enacted to curb the spread of COVID-19 resulted in job losses and a decline in household incomes. Low-income families were significantly affected, spiraling many into homelessness.

RACIAL INEQUITIES IN HOMELESSNESS

A. The HUD 2022 annual report revealed racial inequities among Americans experiencing homelessness. Among the racial groups experiencing sheltered homelessness, 37% were Black/African American, 50% were White, 6% identified as multiple races, 6% were Native American or Indigenous Peoples, 2% were Asian, and 1% were Pacific Islander.
B. A higher percentage of people in sheltered locations identified as Black (44% or 154,557 people) compared with people experiencing homelessness in unsheltered locations (27% or 62,809 people).
C. Black or African Americans make up 12% of the Census, yet they had an equivalent percent of the unsheltered population with Whites, who constitute 56% of the U.S. Census.
D. Colonization and the institution of slavery in the United States provide the historical context for the overrepresentation of people of color in the yearly PIT homeless count.
  1. Many enslaved Black people had no housing or less than habitable housing.
    a. After the abolition of slavery in the 19th century, vagrancy laws about people perceived as idle, disorderly, and jobless became the foundation of the Black Codes passed in most U.S. states, including those in the northern United States.
    b. The Black Codes were instituted to control the employment and movement of freed Black people after the end of the Civil War through the criminalization of Black unemployment.
    c. Therefore, without considerable government or charitable support, at the termination of the Civil War, millions of emancipated Black people were deemed homeless.
  2. Native Americans' fate followed a similar trajectory of enslavement and forceful appropriation of their land, resulting in the loss of cultural, ancestral, and spiritual value.
    a. Native American communities, including their homes, possessions, and livelihood, were destroyed.
    b. Native American lands became federally owned, and to incentivize the development of the American West and spur economic growth, Congress passed the Homestead Act of 1862. This legislation provided 160 acres of federal land to anyone who agreed to farm the land.
    c. The Homestead Act essentially legalized the embezzlement of copious amounts of Native American land, leaving many Native Americans homeless in the process.
E. The 19th century was also an inflection point for homelessness in the Latinx population. After the end of the Mexican-American War in 1848, the Treaty of Guadalupe Hidalgo was signed, which resulted in the Mexican government signing over 500,000 square miles of territory to the United States.
  1. Ultimately, this acquisition resulted in thousands of residents being dispossessed of their ancestral land by White settlers and U.S. courts.
  2. Vagrancy laws such as California's Anti-Vagrancy Act of 1855 spotlighted Mexican Americans and Native Americans for perceived unemployment, similar to the Black Codes for emancipated Black people.
F. Federal housing policies fortified the racial inequities in homelessness.
  1. Federal housing programs in the 1930s and 1940s subsidized the construction of exclusively White suburbs, enforcing the racial boundaries of urban neighborhoods and concentrating racial minorities in inner-city ghettos.
  2. Millions of White Americans were provided mortgage loans while simultaneously establishing redlining and preserving racial segregation in the metropolitan real estate market.
G. The ability to afford a house is intrinsically linked to poverty. The disparate inequities in educational attainment, employment, and wages due to systemic racism hinder the socioeconomic advancement of people of color and their ability to afford and maintain stable housing.
  1. Systemic racism also inhibits the ability to accumulate and transfer wealth across generations.
    a. Enslaved Black people were considered property and were not given land to farm after the abolition of slavery. Native Americans' lands were forcefully taken and resettled on reservations, and the California Land Act of 1851 dispossessed Mexican Americans of their land to attract White settlers to the region.
    b. In contrast, White Europeans who came to North America involuntarily as vagrants, prisoners, political offenders, or servants between the 15th and 19th centuries eventually found opportunities to acquire land and in so doing could evade homelessness and establish intergenerational wealth.

H. Empirical evidence unanimously supports racial inequities among homeless people. In a recent study, Olivet et al. (2021) concurred with the disparate inequities among people of color.

1. Despite the resounding evidence, they reported that limited research explains the inequities or examines whether disparities in receiving homeless services such as shelters, housing programs, and other aspects of communities' homelessness response are forthcoming or surreptitious. It was posited that more research is needed to comprehend the correlation between structural racism and homelessness and assist in developing efficacious policy and practice interventions.
2. The study used data from the Supporting Partnerships for Anti-Racist Communities (SPARC) Initiative. This mixed-methods study included eight cities from 2016 to 2019 to examine structural racism and homelessness.
3. The aims of the primary study were to (a) document racial/ethnic disproportionality among people experiencing homelessness across multiple communities to determine patterns of overrepresentation; (b) explore the experiences of people of color across pathways into homelessness, experiences with the homelessness response system, and barriers to exiting homelessness; and (c) examine racial disparities in housing outcomes.
4. To determine pathways to homelessness and identify factors of outcomes, 195 participants were interviewed. Findings indicated that Black/African Americans and Native Americans were the most overrepresented among those experiencing homelessness in each community. Also elucidated from the findings were suggestions that factors linked to homelessness for people of color included impediments to housing and economic mobility, racism and discrimination within homeless services, and criminal justice involvement.

GLOBAL HOMELESSNESS

A. Worldwide, marginalized communities inordinately encounter homelessness. Homelessness is increasingly frequent among people living in poverty and among minorities in terms of race/ethnicity, sexual orientation and identity, the institutionalized, and those with physical and mental disabilities when compared with the general population.

B. The United Nations estimates that worldwide there are 1.6 billion people living in inadequate housing, with 15 million forcefully evicted annually. This estimate includes individuals living in shelters, in inadequate housing, or on the street, and reports that as many countries are at war, refugee migration continues to increase this grave social problem. Homelessness is closely related to and a result of global poverty affecting approximately 9.2% of the world's population, with poverty linked to systemic problems such as lack of access to housing and healthcare services, decreased life expectancy, and overall poor quality of life.

C. Indigenous pathways to homelessness likely include poverty, physical and mental illness, SUD, lack of affordable housing, and socioeconomic inequities. In addition, current injustices in the health of Indigenous peoples are linked to past and present colonial policies that created and sustained systemic racism, cultural oppression, disempowerment, and dispossession of Indigenous people's lands.

1. In Australia, the Aboriginal communities represent 3% of the population, yet they constitute a quarter of the people receiving homeless services.
2. The Indigenous community in Canada is 10 times more likely to use homeless shelters than non-Indigenous people. Moreover, Indigenous people experiencing homelessness are eight times more prevalent in Canada than are other groups. Indigenous people comprise about 6% of British Columbia's population, yet in 2018 they accounted for 40% of Vancouver's homeless, of whom 46% are unsheltered.
3. In New Zealand, Maori homelessness has been reported to be five times that of non-Maori.

D. Within the past 10 years, there has been a 70% increase in homelessness among the nations that make up the European Union (EU), with 24 of the 28 member nations reporting an increase in homelessness over the past two to three decades, with only Finland reporting a decrease over the same time frame. According to the European Federation of National Organisations Working with the Homeless (FEANTSA), on any given night in the EU, approximately 700,000 people experience homelessness.

COVID-19

A. The COVID-19 pandemic accelerated an existing crisis affecting the homeless and indigent populations. Significant increases were noted in unsheltered, chronically homeless individuals. Racial inequities were glaring as African Americans, Native Americans, and Pacific Islanders persisted as groups overrepresented among the homeless population.

1. Homeless people had an increased risk of infection due to exposure to COVID-19 and inability to access soap and water, face masks, or hygienic facilities.
2. Homeless people faced housing and economic instability, or inability to pay for stable housing due to lack of financial means.
3. Homeless people lacked access or had limited access to healthcare services, including medical and mental healthcare, leading to an extreme disparity in managing chronic medical conditions, decreased life expectancy, adverse health outcomes, untreated and worsening mental health issues, and revictimization of this vulnerable population.
4. Homeless people were also affected by lack of access to vital social services (e.g., food banks, community clinics), a decreased number of beds in shelters and other facilities, and mandates to stay off the streets due to the pandemic.

B. The COVID-19 pandemic gravely worsened the homelessness crisis by plunging many Americans into economic hardship through job loss or job insecurity, medical debt, reduced homeless shelter capacity or availability, and reduced social services. Most individuals or families disproportionately affected were low-income families, people of color, and Indigenous people. Although federal, state, and local authorities instituted an assortment of interventions to mitigate homelessness during the pandemic, including the American Rescue Plan Act (ARP) for rental support, direct financial support, and eviction moratoriums, these temporary efforts may not be enough to lift the individuals or families from their economic pitfalls into affordable housing.

C. Undocumented migrant communities (e.g., refugees, asylum seekers, those with ambiguous immigration status) encountered restrictive immigration statutes. In the EU member states, these restrictions resulted in inadequate access to housing, limited employment prospects, discrimination, and exclusion from public funding. Many became homeless and as a result sought homeless service providers for basic support and consultation concerning eligibility for assistance.

D. Individuals experiencing homelessness faced many challenges daily, and the COVID-19 pandemic brought other issues.
   1. People experiencing homelessness were mostly unable to comply with all the restrictions placed by the government and local communities. The recommendations to stay home, perform frequent handwashing (with soap and water), use hand sanitizer, use face masks, and keep social distance were measures with which individuals experiencing homelessness could not comply.
   2. The allocation of shelter spaces for homeless people was reduced, and many had to stay on the street, with no access to hygienic spaces in which to wash their hands or maintain daily hygiene and no funds to purchase appropriate face masks or to buy nutritious food. Homeless people had minimal options, and some resorted to going to EDs, risking exposure to COVID-19.
   3. Recommendations and mandates to maintain physical distance were impossible to enforce in shelters or for people living in their cars due to reduced spaces. Most homeless people faced challenges in maintaining their health during the pandemic, and veteran women had higher rates of unemployment due to COVID-19 with limited or no access to vital healthcare and financial services.
   4. Access to hot meals was limited as meal distribution facilities closed.
   5. Access to COVID-19 testing was limited as testing was initially offered in drive-through or open-lot settings, and most homeless individuals do not have a car.
E. The pervasive health inequities that individuals experiencing homelessness endured during the COVID-19 pandemic increased social isolation and hindered efforts to prevent the spread of disease and access to treatment.
   1. Researchers believe that health literacy became another barrier for homeless people during the COVID-19 pandemic, with misleading information creating confusion about the prevention and treatment of COVID-19 illness.
   2. Local governments focused on the general population and not on vulnerable groups such as the homeless population.
F. Homeless shelters started implementing strict measures to contain the spread of the virus by often closing beds, mandating frequent testing, and setting a stricter curfew. Some of these measures were initially helpful; however, due to the high turnover rate of people seeking shelter and the lack of structured measures and surveillance, some shelters had outbreaks of COVID-19.
   1. Researchers made recommendations to include preventive measures, including frequent screening and appropriate treatment.
   2. According to Baggett and Gaeta (2021), there was a high prevalence of asymptomatic individuals tested at a shelter. Thirty-six percent of the shelter population was infected, but 88% of them had no symptoms at the time of diagnosis.
      a. The issue of asymptomatic people living in crowded quarters such as shelters and unknowingly infecting others was seen as a dramatic problem causing public health risks.
      b. The results of this study supported the U.S. implementation of polymerase chain reaction (PCR) testing as a prevention measure.
   3. Other issues arose because some individuals were underreporting symptoms and/or changing shelters, visiting the ED, or staying on the street. There is a contrast with results from other research indicating that unsheltered individuals are at a lower risk of contracting COVID-19. The consensus is that homeless individuals have adverse health effects and poor health outcomes.
G. Homeless veterans in the United States were also affected by the COVID-19 pandemic.
   1. A research study conducted in six states (California, Florida, Iowa, Kentucky, Massachusetts, and New Jersey) indicated that the vaccination rates for those receiving care from primary care providers were approximately 40% to 60%, and among those who resided in transitional housing programs were 20% to 90%.
   2. Homeless veterans and the healthcare staff attempting to reach them faced multiple barriers to vaccination.
      a. Systemic barriers included difficulty scheduling, not meeting the eligibility criteria, and insufficient availability to transport the veterans to a vaccination location.
      b. Other barriers included distrust of the government, vaccine mandates, and strict protocols for vaccination when eligible.
   3. The results of this study proposed less restrictive guidelines to attract and increase the number of homeless veterans who got vaccinated, including improving access to vaccination and education campaigns from healthcare professionals whom the veterans trust.
   4. Homeless veteran women were also significantly affected during COVID-19 due to being unable to find appropriate care in community centers for mental healthcare, trauma-related, and because some refused to apply for supportive services. These women veterans might have neglected to obtain treatment for chronic medical and mental healthcare conditions, leading to crises.
H. The COVID-19 pandemic created an economic crisis in the United States.
   1. Many industries were forced to close, national unemployment rates rose, and people were forced to stay home due to government restrictions.
   2. Lockdowns were mandated, schools were closed, travel was restricted, and only specific businesses were allowed to remain open to have the minimal workforce to sustain cities.
I. In early 2020, approximately 43 states plus Washington D.C. implemented moratoriums on evictions due to the COVID-19 pandemic.
   1. These moratoriums positively impacted the mental health of renters at risk of eviction or eviction processes that had been initiated before the pandemic's beginning.
   2. The results of the study by Ali and Wehby (2022) provided evidence of the potential short-term effects on the mental health of renters. They proposed that this be considered in future policies related to housing stability.
   3. Stable housing promotes decreased levels of stress and improved overall health (Ali & Wehby, 2022).
J. During the COVID-19 pandemic interval, FEANTSA members faced new housing challenges, compounding the already overtaxed prepandemic housing predicament.
   1. The war in Ukraine overwhelmed the already stressed homeless regions as countries struggled to house refugees arriving from Ukraine.
   2. The COVID-19 pandemic exacerbated barriers to services available to migrants. Initially, services for homeless

people were limited; homeless shelters had reduced capacity due to isolation guidelines.

3. As the public health threat posed by the pandemic intensified, EU governments provided access to safe accommodations in hotels and hostels, irrespective of immigration status. Accommodation was short-lived, however, as circumstances returned to prepandemic conditions when restrictions were lifted.

MENTAL AND PHYSICAL ILLNESS

A. Between 20% and 25% of individuals experiencing homelessness suffer from mood disorders, and 30% of individuals experiencing chronic homelessness have a severe mental illness.
B. There is a high prevalence of men experiencing homelessness and residing in shelters who have tested positive for tuberculosis and hepatitis C and are also infected with HIV.
  1. Hepatitis C has a prevalence ranging from 19% to 69% in people who are homeless.
  2. Other concerning statistics include hospital readmission rates, higher use of EDs, and a more significant number of substance use-related disorders.
C. Individuals experiencing homelessness have a higher prevalence of chronic medical conditions (e.g., asthma, diabetes, hypertension, chronic obstructive pulmonary disease [COPD], and cancer).
D. Homeless individuals have a lower life expectancy of approximately 20 years less of life and are at a higher risk of premature death due to poor health. Other issues include exposure to infectious diseases due to overcrowding and lack of appropriate areas for sanitation leading to poor hygiene.
E. People experiencing homelessness often carry a diagnosis of chronic mental illness due to lack of treatment, revictimization, exposure to environmental hazards, and difficulty with accessing social services.
  1. Homeless individuals have a higher prevalence of chronic mental health conditions such as anxiety, SUDs, depression, and posttraumatic stress disorder (PTSD).
  2. Homeless individuals have comorbid chronic medical conditions affecting their daily activities. Untreated comorbid conditions lead to decreased life expectancy, poor quality of life, prolonged hospitalizations, and increased frequency of ED visits.
  3. Homeless individuals have an increased risk of suicide due to untreated mental health conditions and barriers to accessing healthcare services. The multiple barriers include lack of healthcare insurance, inability to afford transportation, and lack of limited facilities with multidisciplinary social and mental health services in areas where they stay.

SOCIAL DETERMINANTS OF HEALTH

A. According to the World Health Organization (WHO), social determinants of health (SDH) are the nonmedical factors that influence health outcomes (Figure 24.1).
  1. These are conditions in which people are born, grow, work, live, and age, and the broader set of forces and systems shaping the conditions of daily life.
  2. These include economic policies and systems, development agendas, social norms, social policies, and political systems.
B. SDH exert a significant influence on health inequities. SDH can influence health equity in positive or negative ways.
  1. Income and social protection
  2. Education

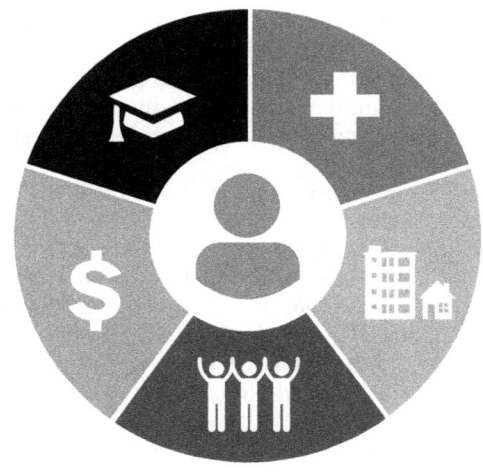

FIGURE 24.1 Social determinants of health.

Source: U.S. Department of Health and Human Services, Office of Disease Prevention and Health Promotion. (n.d.). *Healthy People 2030: Social determinants of health.* https://health.gov/healthypeople/priority-areas/social-determinants-health.

  3. Unemployment and job insecurity
  4. Working life conditions
  5. Food insecurity
  6. Housing, basic amenities the environment
  7. Early childhood development
  8. Social inclusion and nondiscrimination
  9. Structural conflict
  10. Access to affordable health services of decent quality.

C. The causes of homelessness are complex and multifaceted and must be investigated at the macro, meso, and micro levels of determinants.
  1. Macro-level determinants: pertain to economic situations concerning discrimination, income, employment, and housing availability
  2. Meso-level determinants: interpersonal conflicts that result in violence, child neglect or abuse, breakdown of relationships, or weakened social support systems
  3. Micro-level determinants: characteristics at the individual level, such as medical or mental health problems, SUD, and resilience

D. The various levels of determinants are interconnected with risk factors that can ultimately lead to homelessness.
  1. An individual may be affected by the SDH of exorbitant neighborhood housing costs and insufficient living wage employment opportunities, which lead to the risk of housing instability or homelessness.
  2. Housing stability is progressively jeopardized by factors such as elevated eviction rates, foreclosure, gentrification, and natural disasters.
  3. Losses in employment and earnings at the onset of the pandemic posed significant challenges in rent affordability, especially for individuals or households already experiencing a financial crisis. Households of color were more vulnerable socioeconomically and were far more likely to suffer losses in income. According to Household Pulse Survey data for early 2022, 25% of Hispanic households reported lost employment income early in the pandemic. The percentage for Black households and households identifying as mixed race was 20%. Asian

households were reported as 12% and White households at only 11%.

4. Income inequalities are partially a consequence of deep-rooted discrimination in employment, economic, and housing markets that propagate considerable disparities in wealth.
   a. The median net wealth reported in 2023 is $121,700 for all U.S. households.
   b. The median for White households was roughly $190,000, which was eight times that of Black households ($24,000), more than five times that of Hispanic households ($36,000), and about two-and-a-half times that of all other households, including Asian households, mixed racial households, and those of another race ($75,000).

5. Undocumented immigrants, many of whom are people of color, are susceptible to housing insecurity and homelessness.
   a. Poverty rates are usually high due to low-wage employment and limited job opportunities, making it difficult to afford rising housing costs.
   b. These are more pronounced in big cities such as Los Angeles and New York City, with high concentrations of immigrants and homeless populations.
   c. Those who do not speak English find this another barrier to accessing services. It is pivotal to address the specific factors affecting the homeless and indigent population.
   d. SDH are crucial to improving overall quality of life.

MENTAL HEALTH AND SUBSTANCE USE DISORDER

A. Mental health and homelessness appear to be closely associated, with experimental findings supporting a positive correlation between them.

1. Empirical evidence has not definitively determined a causal relationship between one and the other because of the juxtaposition of determinants.
2. Moschion and van Ours (2021) studied the inception of the relationship between homelessness and mental illness, how the use of mental health and housing support services relates to experiences of homelessness, and whether episodes of mental illness increase the likelihood of future homelessness.
   a. The study focused on five mental health diagnoses: depression, anxiety, bipolar affective disorder, schizophrenia, and PTSD.
   b. Results indicated that episodes of depression increased the probability of becoming homeless. However, this was not the case for other mental health conditions.
   c. Associations between mental health episodes and homelessness are complex and are most unlikely to be causal.

B. Although causality might be an elusive determinant, mental illness may hinder one's ability to sustain stable housing. Symptoms of mental illness, particularly serious mental illness (SMI) such as a psychotic disorder, bipolar disorder, major depressive disorder, or PTSD, may trigger behavioral problems and/or cognitive decline, challenging one's ability to earn a stable income.

1. Individuals with SMI usually have difficulty managing or resolving conflicts with landlords, increasing the probability of evictions.

2. Psychiatric symptoms such as psychosis and cognitive deficits can hinder managing and maintaining household functions and social relationships.

C. Various reports from the government, private organizations, advocate agencies, and academic researchers present evidence of the high prevalence of specific psychiatric diagnoses in people experiencing homelessness compared with the general population in the United States. Also discussed are the adverse effects of untreated mental illness and homelessness on health outcomes, including retraumatization, skin disorders, exposure to infectious diseases, HIV, hepatitis C, and COVID-19.

D. People with mental illness are also more likely to experience SUD than those without a mental illness. According to the Substance Abuse and Mental Health Services Administration (SAMHSA) 2018 National Survey on Drug Use and Health, approximately 9.2 million adults in the United States have a co-occurring SUD (SAMHSA, 2019).

1. SUD can negatively affect relationships with friends and family, resulting in loss of employment. For individuals previously struggling financially, employment loss can lead to eviction and/or homelessness.
2. Sustaining an SUD is expensive, leaving little money to maintain secure housing and stable employment.

INTIMATE PARTNER VIOLENCE

A. According to the Centers for Disease Control and Prevention (CDC), about one in three women and one in four men self-reported severe physical violence from an intimate partner in their lifetime, and 14% of women and 5% of men report being stalked by an intimate partner.

1. Intimate partner violence (IPV) can result in homelessness and housing insecurity along direct and indirect avenues.
   a. Some perpetrators of violence may deliberately ruin their victim's credit, prohibit them from working, or intimidate or stalk them at work, resulting in loss of employment.
   b. Victims of violence may be forced to leave their homes and stay in shelters or with family to escape victimization and violence.
   c. Trauma experienced as a result of IPV often precipitates depression or PTSD, and the cascade of events leads to housing instability or homelessness for victims and possibly children.
   d. Domestic violence is a central risk factor for adolescents' homelessness.

REFERENCES AND BIBLIOGRAPHY

Allen, J., & Vottero, B. (2020). Experiences of homeless women in accessing health care in community-based settings: A qualitative systematic review. *JBI Evidence Synthesis*, 18(9), 1970–2010. https://doi.org/10.11124/jbisrir-d-19-00214

Ali, A. K., & Wehby, G. L. (2022). State eviction moratoriums during the COVID-19 pandemic were associated with improved mental health among people who rent. *Health Affairs*, 41(11), 1583–1589. https://doi.org/10.1377/hlthaff.2022.00750

Baggett, T. P., & Gaeta, J. M. (2021). COVID-19 and homelessness: when crises intersect. *The Lancet Public Health*, 6(4), e193–e194. https://doi.org/10.1016/s2468-2667(21)00022-0

Balut, M. D., Gin, J. L., Alenkin, N. R., & Dobalian, A. (2022). Vaccinating veterans experiencing homelessness for COVID-19: Healthcare and housing service providers' perspectives. *Journal of Community Health*, 47(5), 727–736. https://doi.org/10.1007/s10900-022-01097-1

Baptista, I., & Marlier, E. (2019, September 13). *Fighting homelessness and housing exclusion in Europe: A study of national policies*.

https://op.europa.eu/en/publication-detail/-/publication/2dd1bd61-d834-11e9-9c4e-01aa75ed71a1/language-en

Barbu, S., Barranco, S. P., & Silk, R. (2020). The impact of COVID-19 on homeless service providers and homeless people: The migrant perspective. *Cityscape, 23*(2), 361–379. https://www.huduser.gov/PORTAL/periodicals/cityscpe/vol23num2/ch19.pdf

Bingham, B., Moniruzzaman, A., Patterson, M., Distasio, J., Sareen, J., O'Neil, J., & Somers, J. M. (2019). Indigenous and non-Indigenous people experiencing homelessness and mental illness in two Canadian cities: A retrospective analysis and implications for culturally informed action. *BMJ Open, 9*(4), e024748. https://doi.org/10.1136/bmjopen-2018-024748

Cash, J. C. (Ed.). (2020). *Family practice guidelines* (5th ed.). Springer Publishing Company.

Centers for Disease Control and Prevention. (2017, March 2). *Homelessness as a public health law issue: Selected resources*. U.S. Department of Health and Human Services. https://www.cdc.gov/phlp/php/publications/homelessness.html

Chang, C. D. (2019). Social determinants of health and health disparities among immigrants and their children. *Current Problems in Pediatric and Adolescent Health Care, 49*(1), 23–30. https://doi.org/10.1016/j.cppeds.2018.11.009

Đoàn, L. N., Chong, S. K., Misra, S., Kwon, S. C., & Yi, S. S. (2021). Immigrant communities and COVID-19: Strengthening the public health response. *American Journal of Public Health, 111*(S3), S224–S231. https://doi.org/10.2105/ajph.2021.306433

FEANTSA. (2021, February 12). *Report: Investment in affordable & social housing solutions: Reaching the "Locked Out" in Europe*. https://www.feantsa.org/en/report/2021/02/12/feantsa-report-investment-in-affordable-social-housing-solutions-reaching-the-locked-out-in-europe

Fowle, M. Z. (2022). Racialized homelessness: A review of historical and contemporary causes of racial disparities in homelessness. *Housing Policy Debate, 32*(6), 940–967. https://doi.org/10.1080/10511482.2022.2026995

Fowler, P. J., Hovmand, P. S., Marcal, K. E., & Das, S. (2019). Solving homelessness from a complex systems perspective: Insights for prevention responses. *Annual Review of Public Health, 40*(1), 465–486. https://doi.org/10.1146/annurev-publhealth-040617-013553

Gabrielian, S., Hamilton, A. B., Gelberg, L., Koosis, E. R., Johnson, A., & Young, A. S. (2019). Identifying social skills that support housing attainment and retention among homeless persons with serious mental illness. *Psychiatric Services, 70*(5), 374–380. https://doi.org/10.1176/appi.ps.201800508

Joint Center for Housing Studies of Harvard University. (2022a). *America's rental housing: 2022*. https://www.jchs.harvard.edu/americas-rental-housing-2022

Joint Center for Housing Studies of Harvard University. (2022b). *The state of the nation's housing: 2022*. https://www.jchs.harvard.edu/state-nations-housing-2022

Kapadia, F. (2022). Ending homelessness and advancing health equity: A public health of consequence, March 2022. *American Journal of Public Health, 112*(3), 372–373. https://doi.org/10.2105/ajph.2021.306704

Marçal, K. E. (2021). Intimate partner violence exposure and adolescent mental health outcomes: The mediating role of housing insecurity. *Journal of Interpersonal Violence, 37*(21–22), NP19310–NP19330. https://doi.org/10.1177/08862605211043588

Moschion, J., & Van Ours, J. C. (2021). Do transitions in and out of homelessness relate to mental health episodes? A longitudinal analysis in an extremely disadvantaged population. *Social Science & Medicine, 279*, 113667. https://doi.org/10.1016/j.socscimed.2020.113667

National Academies of Sciences, Engineering, and Medicine. (2018a). Addressing homelessness in the United States. In *Permanent supportive housing: Evaluating the evidence for improving health outcomes among people experiencing chronic homelessness* (pp. 19–37). The National Academies Press. https://doi.org/10.17226/25133

National Academies of Sciences, Engineering, and Medicine. (2018b). The history of homelessness in the United States. In *Permanent supportive housing: Evaluating the evidence for improving health outcomes among people experiencing chronic homelessness* (pp. 175–184). The National Academies Press. https://doi.org/10.17226/25133

National Health Care for the Homeless Council. (2022, November 16). *Our work*. https://nhchc.org/our-work

National Park Service. (2022). *What are civil rights?* U.S. Department of the Interior. https://www.nps.gov/subjects/civilrights/civil-rights-overview.htm

Olivet, J., Wilkey, C., Richard, M., Dones, M., Tripp, J., Beit-Arie, M., Yampolskaya, S., & Cannon, R. (2021). Racial inequity and homelessness: Findings from the SPARC study. *The ANNALS of the American Academy of Political and Social Science, 693*(1), 82–100. https://doi.org/10.1177/00027162219910140

Ralli, M., Arcangeli, A., De-Giorgio, F., Morrone, A., & Ercoli, L. (2021). COVID-19 and homelessness: Prevalence differences between sheltered and unsheltered Individuals. *American Journal of Public Health, 111*(8), e13–e15. https://doi.org/10.2105/ajph.2021.306382

Rubin, R. (2021). Helping people who are homeless stay healthy during the pandemic. *JAMA, 325*(6), 517. https://doi.org/10.1001/jama.2020.23436

Substance Abuse and Mental Health Services Administration. (2019, August). *2018 National Survey on Drug Use and Health*. https://www.samhsa.gov/data/release/2018-national-survey-drug-use-and-health-nsduh-releases

Substance Abuse and Mental Health Services Administration. (2023, December 5). *Homelessness programs resources*. U.S. Department of Health and Human Services. https://www.samhsa.gov/homelessness-programs-resources

Swope, C. B., & Hernández, D. (2019). Housing as a determinant of health equity: A conceptual model. *Social Science Medicine, 243*, 112571. https://doi.org/10.1016/j.socscimed.2019.112571

Trivedi, C., Adnan, M., Shah, K., Manikkara, G., Mansuri, Z., & Jain, S. (2022). Psychiatric disorders in hospitalized homeless individuals. *The Primary Care Companion for CNS Disorders, 24*(6). https://doi.org/10.4088/pcc.21m03209

U.S. Census Bureau. (2022, June 10). *The chance that two people chosen at random are of different race or ethnicity groups has increased since 2010*. https://www.census.gov/library/stories/2021/08/2020-united-states-population-more-racially-ethnically-diverse-than-2010.html

Zhao, E. (2022). The key factors contributing to the persistence of homelessness. *International Journal of Sustainable Development World Ecology, 30*(1), 1–5. https://doi.org/10.1080/13504509.2022.2120109

HEALTH ADVOCACY FOR THE HOMELESS AND INDIGENT POPULATIONS

A. Health advocacy is an essential step in helping homeless and indigent populations. There are various ways to initiate and be involved in health advocacy. These include the following:

1. Involvement in community organizations that support and provide services to homeless and indigent populations
2. Lobbying through local, regional, and national organizations that work in programs to help homeless people
3. Pro-bono work in community clinics, mobile healthcare services, and telehealth
4. Active involvement in legal organizations and volunteering in organizations that work in pro-homeless and indigent populations

B. The report from the National Institutes of Health 2018 indicates that people experiencing homelessness have adverse health outcomes due to lack of resources, programs, and access to healthcare for homeless people.

1. Evidence suggests that homelessness may cause deterioration of health, especially for individuals who have chronic medical conditions such as diabetes or hypertension or those suffering from a mental disorder.
2. Individuals experiencing homelessness are exposed to skin disorders and trauma (physical and psychological).
3. They are at risk of exposure to communicable diseases in the street or shelters due to poor living conditions and crowded spaces.
4. A research study in 1990 provided insight into the gravity of this issue related to tuberculosis, with 43% of positive tuberculosis skin tests (Mantoux tuberculin skin test [TST]) or active tuberculosis in men residing in homeless shelters.

C. The psychiatric-mental health nursing scope and standards of practice provide explicit guidelines for clinical practice.

1. These guidelines are also followed by APRNs and include competence in recovery models such as person-centered care, recovery-oriented public care models, prevention, screening, and early intervention.
2. An essential element that must be considered by APRNs is disparities in mental health treatment for vulnerable members of racial minority groups. The causes of these disparities include lack of access to healthcare services, language barriers, social barriers, financial reasons, severe mental illness, and homelessness.
3. Efforts should be made to improve access to services and provide opportunities for efficient care that is coordinated and interdisciplinary. APRNs should ally with patients to promote recovery and wellness.
4. Establishing evidence-based care models to include an interdisciplinary approach and care coordination is important to prevent duplication of services. A unified front to help the homeless and indigent populations is pivotal to engaging the patients and using funding effectively.
5. APRNs should strive to obtain and apply knowledge of available services for homeless people, especially women and families.
6. APRNs must advocate for the homeless population, including women and their families, who are especially at risk, to ensure equitable provision of care. Homeless women will seek healthcare services as long as healthcare providers are accessible and empathic and provide a positive experience for them, leading to improved health outcomes.

REFERENCES AND BIBLIOGRAPHY

Allen, J., & Vottero, B. (2020). Experiences of homeless women in accessing health care in community-based settings: A qualitative systematic review. *JBI Evidence Synthesis, 18*(9), 1970–2010. https://doi.org/10.11124/jbisrir-d-19-00214

Guido, G. W. (2019). *Legal and ethical issues in nursing*. Pearson Education.

Keller, M. J., Conard, P. L., & Armstrong, M. L. (2022, July/August). Homelessness: Women veterans without billets. *Medsurg Nursing, 31*(4), 233–238. https://www.proquest.com/scholarly-journals/homelessness-women-veterans-without-billets/docview/2709977599/se-2

National Academies of Sciences, Engineering, and Medicine. (2018). Addressing homelessness in the United States. In *Permanent supportive housing: Evaluating the evidence for improving health outcomes among people experiencing chronic homelessness* (pp. 19–37). The National Academies Press. https://doi.org/10.17226/25133

HOMELESSNESS AS HEALTH HAZARD

A. Individuals experiencing homelessness and individuals who are indigent face barriers to appropriate nutrition and may reside in minimally hygienic conditions, in small spaces, or on the street.
1. Individuals experiencing homelessness are exposed to harsh environmental conditions daily and lack access to adequate healthcare services or preventive care, all leading to adverse health outcomes.
2. Many individuals experiencing homelessness have medical and chronic mental health problems that cannot be addressed or cared for due to systemic barriers to care, exacerbating adverse health outcomes.
3. Individuals experiencing homelessness and individuals who are indigent have an increased risk of exposure to infectious diseases due to poor sanitation and close quarters.

B. Individuals experiencing homelessness or families without stable or permanent housing face massive health inequities across a plethora of health conditions and may experience poor health outcomes.
1. Individuals experiencing homelessness are three times more likely to report chronic diseases such as asthma, COPD, diabetes, and heart disease, which increase their risk of complications, or SUDs and drug-related infectious diseases.
2. SUD is three times as prevalent, and depression and hepatitis C are more than six times as prevalent, among the homeless population.

C. People experiencing homelessness access primary care infrequently due to uninsured status and marginalization and stigma by healthcare organizations.
1. Care is limited to ED visits presenting with untreated co-occurring health conditions that are more critical.
2. Individuals experiencing homelessness are hospitalized at a rate of approximately four times the general population and with longer and costlier inpatient stays.
3. A study by Subedi et al. (2022) substantiated the disparate health outcomes of homeless people. The study sought to compare hospital readmission rates among patients experiencing homelessness and patients who were not homeless and assess the impact of different clinical and demographic characteristics on acute care utilization among patients experiencing homelessness.
    a. Two salient measures of acute care utilization were examined: time to acute care (ED and inpatient) readmission and 30-day readmission rates.
    b. The results revealed that the 30-day readmission rate was 42.8% among patients experiencing homelessness compared with 19.9% among matched patients not experiencing homelessness.
    c. The hazard of 30-day readmission among patients experiencing homelessness was 2.6 (95% CI = 1.93, 3.53) times higher than the matched nonhomeless group.
    d. For homeless patients, conditions such as SUD, major depressive disorder, chronic kidney disease, obesity, arthritis, HIV/AIDS, and epilepsy were associated with shorter readmission times.
    e. Being Black or African American was associated with shortened readmission times.
4. D'Sa et al. (2020) appraised the current knowledge on the psychological impact of homelessness in children from a global perspective.
    a. The study posited that children experiencing homelessness might undergo development delays compared with children of their chronological age.
    b. Academic performance was also impaired due to high rates of absenteeism and attention problems interfering with cognition, resulting in poor academic performance.
    c. Behavioral problems, including aggression, were more common in children experiencing homelessness.
    d. High levels of anxiety, depression, and PTSD were also noted, especially among girls, increasing the risk of hopelessness and suicide.
5. Homeless children are also in jeopardy of poor physical health. A scoping review by Gultekin et al. (2019) provided striking evidence supporting the detrimental effects of homelessness on children.
    a. Homeless children suffered higher rates of asthma, respiratory infections, severe allergies, and ear infections than stably housed children.

b. Children and adolescents were at greater risk of food insecurity; adolescents were at risk of pregnancy, miscarriage, and unprotected and unsafe sex.
c. Adolescents were also at risk of trafficking and exploitation in exchange for safety, shelter, food, and clothing.
d. These risky behaviors also expose adolescents to sexually transmitted infections and substance use.

THE CHRONICITY OF MEDICAL, MENTAL HEALTH, AND SUBSTANCE USE DISORDERS AMONG THE HOMELESS POPULATION

A. A lack of coordinated services promotes fragmentation of care and lead to poor health outcomes for homeless people seeking healthcare services.

1. Hospitals, community clinics, medical offices, and outreach services are not prepared to care for the influx of homeless individuals with special needs, especially after they come from the street and potentially are exposed to diseases or have a history of untreated chronic illness.
2. Individuals experiencing homelessness can be considered a burden to healthcare systems due to a lack of adherence, untreated mental illness, and SUDs.
3. Individuals experiencing homelessness have a high rate of ED visits, sometimes leading to inpatient admissions and longer lengths of stay.

B. Women experiencing homelessness who seek healthcare services in the community face several roadblocks due to the inadequacy of the healthcare system.

1. Current healthcare is driven by economics and stops people who are uninsured or do not have the financial means to pay for services.
2. Practitioners can perceive women experiencing homelessness as being dependent on the healthcare system. These women are also subjected to discriminatory practices, disrespected by the practitioners and staff, and refused service.

C. Homeless and indigent individuals strain the current healthcare systems due to increased use of ED for routine care or accessing care when their chronic conditions are advanced to the point of requiring often lengthy inpatient hospitalizations.

1. Cost associated with frequent encounters with healthcare systems increases service costs and puts a strain on limited budgets for healthcare services.
2. Chronic medical and mental health issues and a lack of supportive social services and preventive care create a challenging situation for homeless people.
   a. In most encounters, homeless and indigent people require access to patient-centered care models and continued healthcare management by healthcare systems and clinicians.
   b. Individuals experiencing homelessness require special consideration with healthcare and social support services and rely on public programs such as Medicaid and Medicare.

DECREASED LIFE EXPECTANCY

A. Empirical studies have supported the association between homelessness, increased mortality, and reduced life expectancy.

1. Reports indicate the average life expectancy of people who experience homelessness is about 50 years, approximately 25 years shorter than the general life expectancy of females and males in the United States.

2. Poor physical or mental health can be a precursor to homelessness. Once homeless, the risk of exacerbating existing health problems and developing additional ones, including poor oral health, skin and foot problems, tuberculosis, hepatitis C, and HIV, significantly increases.
3. During homelessness, many health problems go untreated or are only sporadically addressed due to lack of access to medical care.
4. Individuals younger than 65 years who experience homelessness have a mortality risk five to nine times higher than the general population in the United States.

B. Morbidity and mortality are linked to numerous disease processes such as infectious diseases, cardiovascular disease, cancer, unforeseen injury, suicide, homicide, and substance use. Unsheltered homeless people carry a significant burden, with higher mortality than sheltered homeless people.

C. Compared with the general population, the prevalence of suicidal ideation and suicide attempts is immensely high in homeless individuals with mental illness. In a large sample of homeless adults with SMI, around 8% reported a suicide attempt within the previous month.

REFERENCES AND BIBLIOGRAPHY

Ahuja, N. J., Nguyen, A., Winter, S. J., Freeman, M., Shi, R., Rodriguez Espinosa, P., & Heaney, C. A. (2020). Well-being without a roof: Examining well-being among unhoused individuals using mixed methods and propensity score matching. *International Journal of Environmental Research and Public Health*, 17(19), 7228. https://doi.org/10.3390/ijerph17197228

Allen, J., & Vottero, B. (2020). Experiences of homeless women in accessing health care in community-based settings: A qualitative systematic review. *JBI Evidence Synthesis*, 18(9), 1970–2010. https://doi.org/10.11124/jbisrir-d-19-00214

Balasuriya, L., Buelt, E., & Tsai, J. (2020, November 16). *The never-ending loop: Homelessness, psychiatric disorder, and mortality*. Psychiatric Times. https://www.psychiatrictimes.com/view/never-ending-loop-homelessness-psychiatric-disorder-and-mortality

Centers for Disease Control and Prevention. (2017, March 2). *Homelessness as a public health issue: Selected resources*. U.S. Department of Health and Human Services. https://www.cdc.gov/phlp/php/publications/homelessness.html

D'Sa, V., Foley, D., Hannon, J., Strashun, S., Murphy, A. M., & O'Gorman, C. (2020). The psychological impact of childhood homelessness—a literature review. *Irish Journal of Medical Science*, 190(1), 411–417. https://doi.org/10.1007/s11845-020-02256-w

Gultekin, L. E., Brush, B. L., Ginier, E., Cordom, A., & Dowdell, E. B. (2019). Health risks and outcomes of homelessness in school-age children and youth: A scoping review of the literature. *The Journal of School Nursing*, 36(1), 10–18. https://doi.org/10.1177/1059840519875182

Katz, M. H. (2017). Homelessness—challenges and progress. *JAMA*, 318(23), 2293. https://doi.org/10.1001/jama.2017.15875

Keller, M. J., Conard, P. L., & Armstrong, M. L. (2022, July/August). Homelessness: Women veterans without billets. *Medsurg Nursing*, 31(4), 233–238. https://www.proquest.com/scholarly-journals/homelessness-women-veterans-without-billets/docview/2709977599/se-2

National Academies of Sciences, Engineering, and Medicine. (2018). Addressing homelessness in the United States. In *Permanent supportive housing: Evaluating the evidence for improving health outcomes among people experiencing chronic homelessness* (pp. 19–37). The National Academies Press. https://doi.org/10.17226/25133

National Center for Education Statistics. (2017, July 12). *Student homelessness in urban, suburban, town, and rural districts*. NCES Blog. https://nces.ed.gov/blogs/nces/post/student-homelessness-in-urban-suburban-town-and-rural-districts

Subedi, K., Acharya, B., & Ghimire, S. (2022). Factors associated with hospital readmission among patients experiencing homelessness. *American Journal of Preventive Medicine*, 63(3), 362–370. https://doi.org/10.1016/j.amepre.2022.02.004

MYTHS

A. The causes of homelessness are multifaceted and consist of systemic failures, structural factors, and individual circumstances. Unfortunately, homeless individuals are often stereotyped and stigmatized with myths that focus only on the individual level. Myths about homelessness can be barriers to positive solutions and interventions to end homelessness.

B. Myth 1: Homelessness is a moral failing.
  1. Homelessness is not a moral failure nor is it deserved. Adverse childhood experiences (ACEs), which include physical, emotional, or sexual abuse; subjection to violence or victimization; neglect; and dysfunctional family relations, generate toxic stress.
     a. Toxic stress is a prerequisite to physical and mental ailments, and occasionally premature death, poor health, and social outcomes in adulthood.
     b. Ostensibly, the scores on the ACE scale are predictive of risk for homelessness across the life span; the higher the score, the greater the likelihood of a homeless trajectory.

C. Myth 2: People experiencing homelessness just do not want to work.
  1. A 2021 study conducted by the University of Chicago, between 2011 and 2018, disclosed that roughly 53% of people living in homeless shelters and 40% of unsheltered people were employed, either full-time or part-time. Earnings were not substantial enough to afford rent.
  2. Earnings sufficient to afford rent does not equate to stable housing for some. Impediments such as landlord's bigotry against past or current homeless people, eviction history, a criminal record, and even income source can hinder one from achieving housing security.

D. Myth 3: People experiencing homelessness are dangerous, violent, or criminals.
  1. A person who is experiencing homelessness is no more likely to be a criminal than a person who is housed.
     a. In many cities, people who are homeless break the law merely by being unhoused.
        i. Many of the major cities within the United States (e.g., Philadelphia, San Francisco, Seattle, Hillsborough, Miami) have enacted legislation that criminalizes behaviors associated with homelessness such as sleeping, sitting, lying, panhandling, and loitering in public spaces.
        ii. The criminalization of homelessness is principally focused on making individuals experiencing homelessness less conspicuous by forcing them out of public spaces with the threat of arrest if necessary.
        iii. Other techniques may be employed to criminalize homelessness informally by demolishing homeless encampments or using police officers to reduce the visibility of homelessness on subways.
     b. Most spend their time and resources trying to survive and improve their situation.
     c. People who are homeless are more likely to be victims of a crime than to commit a crime, especially if they are a homeless woman, teen, or child.

E. Other myths include the following:
  1. Homeless and indigent people lack motivation to engage in care and to get better.
  2. Homeless and indigent people lack trust in healthcare systems and providers.
  3. Homeless individuals have communicable diseases.
  4. Homeless individuals are afraid of revictimization and do not want to seek care.
  5. Healthcare professionals' intrinsic bias toward specific populations is a barrier to providing fair and qualified care.

REFERENCES AND BIBLIOGRAPHY

Davidson, S. (2021, December 3). Homelessness in Fredericton, New Brunswick: Debunking myths and working toward solutions. *Journal of New Brunswick Studies [Revue d'études sur le Nouveau-Brunswick]*, 13(2), 3–7. https://journals.lib.unb.ca/index.php/JNBS/article/view/32607

Pagaduan, J. (2022, December 15). *Employed and experiencing homelessness: What the numbers show*. National Alliance to End Homelessness. https://endhomelessness.org/blog/employed-and-experiencing-homelessness-what-the-numbers-show

United Nations. (2021). *United Nations Resolution on Homelessness*. https://www.wgehomelessness.org/unresolutions

BARRIERS TO CARE

A. Stigma
  1. Homeless residents encounter ubiquitous stigma and stereotypes in the form of fallacious hypotheses, myths, and misconceptions ignorant of the factors that spawned the loss of residence.
     a. Homeless individuals are normally regarded as societal rejects, insignificant, and burdensome, lacking the fortitude to lead a "normal" life.
     b. The media perpetuates negative stereotypes by portraying the homeless population unpropitiously, often associating them with numerous social problems that jeopardize the welfare state of the community.
  2. Stigma on homeless and indigent individuals is a systemic issue that fails to address solutions to prevent homelessness.
     a. This stigma is exhibited in various ways, including discrimination, ethnocentric beliefs, and negative stereotypes.
     b. Healthcare providers need to learn about the barriers that the stigma of homelessness creates to servicing that population, potentially leading to a lack of engagement and fear of rejection if they come to receive care.
     c. Stigma and negative stereotypes can lead to enacting rules and regulations that directly affect the homeless population.
     d. Stigma has negative consequences on homeless individuals perpetuating trauma, worsening psychological problems, anxiety, mistrust, and poor health outcomes.
  3. Homeless individuals with mental illness and SUD are especially vulnerable to stigma and discrimination, in addition to the criticism they receive for being poor, homeless, unemployed, and dependent on social support benefits.
     a. Experiences of stigma and discrimination emanate from a variety of settings, including healthcare, law enforcement, and social service environments.
     b. The experiences of stigma and discrimination in these settings are birelational: homeless status and co-occurring health status such as being HIV-positive or having mental health disorders.
  4. Stigma and discrimination can have catastrophic effects on the general well-being, health, and recovery of persons experiencing homelessness, with and without mental disorders.

      a. Researchers have determined that the aforementioned negative stereotypes entrenched within communities can become internalized by people living with SMI.
      b. Research indicates that discrimination is directly associated with elevated emotional distress and impaired interpersonal relationships, while higher levels of internalized stigma are associated with worse mental health symptoms, such as depressive and psychotic symptoms and suicidal ideation.

B. Other barriers affecting the homeless and indigent population
   1. Long wait periods and increased healthcare provider caseloads
   2. Decreased number or lack of healthcare providers in the community
   3. Accurate statistics on homeless and indigent people not readily available, leading to inequality in the allocation of funding for services for homeless people
   4. Fewer clinicians in remote suburban areas, with a concentration of healthcare providers in large cities, leading to a need for more services in needed places
   5. Individuals experiencing homelessness not having the financial means to make copayments and most lacking healthcare insurance
   6. Language barriers
   7. Undocumented individuals experiencing homelessness lacking identification and might be afraid to seek care, risking being reported to authorities
   8. Individuals experiencing homelessness not having the financial means to pay for public transportation
   9. Women experiencing homelessness possibly being the only caretaker for their children and they cannot leave them alone for medical appointments

C. Lack of therapeutic communication and approaches to working with those experiencing homelessness as a significant barrier to care
   1. Clinicians who are unable or unwilling to empathize with the patients during initial interactions and who lack knowledge about cultural competence lead to patients having a bad initial experience and most likely provide ammunition to a subsequent refusal to follow-up care services.
   2. A calm and respectful demeanor provides a sense of closeness with the healthcare provider.
   3. APRNs who are professional and willing to assist the patient with information on services and educate them are valued by homeless women who come seeking care.
   4. APRNs who take the time to listen to the patient and to explain using simple terminology give a positive impression to patients, in contrast to APRNs who use technical terms, are judgmental with the patients, and lack cultural sensitivity, leading to patients having a bad experience during the clinical encounter.

REFERENCES AND BIBLIOGRAPHY

Allen, J., & Vottero, B. (2020). Experiences of homeless women in accessing health care in community-based settings: A qualitative systematic review. *JBI Evidence Synthesis, 18*(9), 1970–2010. https://doi.org/10.11124/jbisrir-d-19-00214

Mejia-Lancheros, C., Lachaud, J., O'Campo, P., Wiens, K., Nisenbaum, R., Wang, R., Hwang, S. W., & Stergiopoulos, V. (2020). Trajectories and mental health-related predictors of perceived discrimination and stigma among homeless adults with mental illness. *PLoS ONE, 15*(2), e0229385. https://doi.org/10.1371/journal.pone.0229385

Paat, Y. F., Morales, J., Escajeda, A. I., & Tullius, R. (2021). Insights from the shelter: Homeless shelter workers' perceptions of homelessness and working with the homeless. *Journal of Progressive Human Services, 32*(3), 263–283. https://doi.org/10.1080/10428232.2021.1969719

Waynor, W. R., Eissenstat, S. J., Yanos, P. T., Reinhardt-Wood, D., Taylor, E., Karyczak, S., & Lu, W. (2019). The role of illness identity in assertive community treatment. *Rehabilitation Counseling Bulletin, 63*(4), 216–223. https://doi.org/10.1177/0034355219886916

IMPORTANCE OF CULTURAL COMPETENCY

A. Cultural competency and cultural humility are essential to healthcare providers working with indigent and homeless populations.
   1. Cultural competency equips healthcare professionals with the necessary tools to address the specific healthcare needs of these populations. These needs are related to their various backgrounds and demographics, such as race, ethnicity, cultural customs, language, religion, and sexual orientation.
   2. Cultural competency assists APRNs in establishing better rapport with patients and creating an inclusive and welcoming environment to improve confidence and trust in healthcare services.

B. The transcultural nursing theory by Madeleine Leininger proposes the following:
   1. Each APRN should have a basic understanding and knowledge of cultural competence.
      a. This entails having the ability to respect cultural values, beliefs, and attitudes toward healthcare systems and healthcare providers.
   2. Everyone should be treated fairly regardless of race, ethnicity, gender, culture, language, or religion.

C. Lack of empathy, cultural competency, cultural humility, and patience can harm the clinical relationship with patients.
   1. APRNs who are vague and evasive with their responses denote disrespect for the patients and may create a more significant gap in valuable healthcare services for those experiencing homelessness.
   2. Individualized care that attends to the specific needs of the population served is also essential.
   3. Providing healthcare services should include respect for all individuals, education about the goals and how to attain them, mutual agreement, an understanding of how and what the healthcare provider's and the patient's roles are, active listening, and treatment expectations.
   4. The APRN should include patient-centered care treatment models to improve communication with the patient, target treatment plans to address the specific problems of each patient, and establish a continuous relationship (patient–APRN) to last for the duration of care.

D. APRNs and other healthcare professionals should be aware of their personal bias, transference, and countertransference issues.
   1. APRNs should:
      a. Have awareness of body and verbal language to convey respect and importance of trust and understanding of norms, common expectations of treatment, and maintaining fluid communication with individuals experiencing homelessness and those who are indigent.
      b. Be aware of specific healthcare needs for the homeless and indigent population, focusing on preventive care and tailoring treatment to support patient-centered care.

c. Assist in closing the gaps and fragmentation of care by actively engaging homeless and indigent individuals in treatment.

d. Use the cultural competency model to improve healthcare outcomes by using practices that motivate homeless and indigent people to seek, engage, and continue treatment.

2. Countertransference has been one of the most commonly reported barriers to the care of homeless individuals.

a. Homeless individuals with a mental illness are subjected to countertransference from staff taking care of them as they are seen as problematic, complicated, and demanding.

b. There is a stigma attached to homeless individuals who seek care as being unable to pay for services and nonadherent with treatment. It is important to also include that most homeless individuals encounter hospital and healthcare systems in times of crises or during emergencies.

c. Walker et al. surveyed 23 nursing staff using the Health Professionals' Attitudes Toward the Homeless Inventory (HPATHI). The results indicated a more positive attitude toward caring for homeless people postintervention. The important element was to include education about vulnerable populations and the positive aspect in the overall level of care given to the patient.

SYSTEMIC RACISM

A. Systemic racism was initially mentioned in the 1900s by a social scientist to describe racial discrimination in the labor market, schools, and other places.

B. Individuals experiencing homelessness and individuals who are indigent have been subjected for decades to various forms of systemic racism, including racial inequality and discriminatory practices, when seeking healthcare services. Current healthcare systems are insurance-based, preventing those who lack insurance or financial means from obtaining services.

C. Systemic racism in homeless and indigent populations perpetuates structural and systemic inequalities, leading to poor health outcomes, lack of access to healthcare services, and suboptimal quality of services. Systemic racism can also be seen in the following:

1. Treatment inequality: longer wait times to be seen by a healthcare provider, limited or no access to preventive care
2. Increased exposure to disease due to environmental hazards: options for temporary residence, which might expose them to infectious diseases, unsanitary conditions, and enclosed spaces with minimal privacy
3. Limited or lack of access to care: discriminatory practices due to lack of insurance, immigration status, valid identification, and modes of transportation to obtain services
4. Healthcare provider bias: lack of cultural competency and use of discriminatory practices among APRNs when serving underserved populations
5. Limited or lack of financial resources and personnel in community clinics: understaffed community clinics that provide care for large underserved populations, resulting in long wait periods and limited schedules, which prevents access to appropriate care

D. APRNs can address issues of systemic racism in clinical practice by acknowledging current limitations of the healthcare system, learning about the care needs of homeless and indigent populations, serving as advocates of vulnerable people, and providing care that meets standards, with empathy, respect, and professionalism.

HEALTHCARE LITERACY

A. Healthcare literacy is vital as it allows individuals to understand healthcare, illness, the importance of making informed decisions, and navigating healthcare and social services systems.

B. Those experiencing homelessness and those who are indigent may lack knowledge about their health, the importance of preventive services, how to access available services, or the importance of adherence to treatment plans and regimens.

C. Healthcare literacy empowers individuals to gain control over healthcare decisions. It also helps improve health outcomes.

REFERENCES AND BIBLIOGRAPHY

Allen, J., & Vottero, B. (2020). Experiences of homeless women in accessing health care in community-based settings: A qualitative systematic review. *JBI Evidence Synthesis, 18*(9), 1970–2010. https://doi.org/10.11124/jbisrir-d-19-00214

American Academy of Family Physicians. (2024, April). *Institutional racism in the health care system.* https://www.aafp.org/about/policies/all/institutional-racism.html

Braveman, P. A., Arkin, E., Proctor, D., Kauh, T., & Holm, N. (2022). Systemic and structural racism: Definitions, examples, health damages, and approaches to dismantling. *Health Affairs, 41*(2), 171–178. https://doi.org/10.1377/hlthaff.2021.01394

James-Conterelli, S., Dunkley, D., McIntosh, J. T., Julien, T., Nelson, M. D., & Richard-Eaglin, A. (2023). The impact of systemic racism on health outcomes among Black women. *The Nurse Practitioner, 48*(2), 23–32. https://doi.org/10.1097/01.npr.0000000000000001

Nurse Theorists & Nursing Theories: Madeleine Leininger. (2023, October 18). Hoffman Family Library. https://goodwin.libguides.com/nursingtheory/madeleineleininger

Office of Disease Prevention and Health Promotion. (n.d.). *Health literacy in Healthy People 2030.* U.S. Department of Health and Human Services. https://health.gov/healthypeople/priority-areas/health-literacy-healthy-people-2030

Walker, J. N., Vanderhoef, D., Adams, S. M., & Fleisch, S. B. (2021). The impact of an educational intervention on nursing staff attitudes toward patients experiencing homelessness and mental illness. *Journal of the American Psychiatric Nurses Association, 28*(6), 474–479. https://doi.org/10.1177/10783903211011669

HOW ARE DATA COLLECTED TO DETERMINE HOMELESSNESS AND INDIGENT POPULATIONS?

A. Data on homeless and indigent populations are challenging to obtain due to difficulty in accessing areas where these individuals stay and correctly identifying them in the community.

B. Although current data collection methods may produce discrepancies in the exact numbers of homeless, they provide a better understanding of trends, demographics, and specific needs of this population.

C. Data are collected by a combination of self-reporting and official counts.

1. The most common methods are homeless counts, mostly done by groups of volunteers doing outreach in the community.
2. A second method is by review of medical records on healthcare facilities that serve homeless and indigent populations.
3. A third method is by conducting surveys in areas where homeless and indigent people stay, such as in shelters or single-room occupancy (SRO) facilities.

4. The last way is by conducting qualitative research.
D. Each year, the HUD requires continuum of care (CoC) organizations to count the number of people experiencing homelessness (individuals or families) in the geographic area that they serve through the PIT count. The PIT count is conducted by most CoC organizations during the last 10 days of January. The count includes people served in shelter programs every year.
   1. Additionally, every odd-numbered year, CoC organizations are responsible for counting the unsheltered. Some communities count the unsheltered yearly, including Boston, Denver, Miami, New Orleans, Orlando, Philadelphia, and San Diego.
   2. Staff and volunteers are enlisted to survey the streets and other locations to identify and count people experiencing homelessness.
   3. Data collected during the PIT count are essential to effective planning and performance management toward the goal of ending homelessness for each community and nationwide.
   4. Counting those who are unsheltered ensures that many of the people with the highest needs are included in community planning.
   5. The PIT count is also the main data source for measuring progress on the goals of Opening Doors, the federal strategic plan to prevent and end homelessness. Through the PIT count, communities identify important data on the general homeless population and subpopulations, including veterans, families, chronically homeless individuals, and youth. These counts also help identify areas of progress and areas where efforts need intensifying.
E. The U.S. Department of Education provides homeless counts for school-age children and defines children experiencing homelessness as those who lack a fixed, regular, and adequate nighttime residence, including those:
   1. Sharing the housing of other people
   2. Living in motels, hotels, trailer parks, or campgrounds
   3. Living in emergency or transitional shelters
   4. Abandoned in hospitals
   5. Residing in places not designed for or generally used as regular sleeping accommodations for human beings (e.g., cars, parks, public spaces, abandoned buildings, substandard housing, bus or train stations, or similar settings)
F. According to the U.S. Government Accountability Office (GAO), data collected through the PIT count have limitations for measuring homelessness.
   1. While the HUD has taken steps to improve data quality, the data probably miscalculate the size of the homeless population because identifying people experiencing homelessness is innately difficult.
   2. Some CoCs' total and unsheltered PIT counts have large year-over-year fluctuations, which cast doubts about data accuracy.
   3. The GAO found that the methodologies used by CoCs for data collection are not meticulously scrutinized to guarantee HUD's standards are upheld.
   4. HUD's instructions to CoCs on probability sampling techniques to estimate homelessness were incomplete.
   5. Some CoC representatives reported that the assistance rendered by the HUD on data collection inconsistently meets their needs.
G. CoCs use the Homeless Management Information System (HMIS) software, applications designed to record and confidentially store data collected on individuals and families who access any homeless services throughout the year.
   1. Services used include but are not restricted to emergency shelters, transitional housing, permanent supportive housing (PSH), or rapid rehousing.
   2. People who are unsheltered are only included in HMIS if they use organizations that participate in the HMIS, such as day shelters, or if a local CoC selects to include their own customized domains on unsheltered people to their database.
   3. Some organizations that provide services for specific homeless groups are also excluded from the HMIS, such as those entering Violence Against Women Act-funded programs for survivors of domestic violence, and homeless Native Americans or those seeking homeless services on tribal lands.

RESEARCH TIPS AND UPDATES ON CURRENT RESEARCH ON HOMELESSNESS

A. Families who experienced homelessness in the past 12 months are at risk of being investigated for child mistreatment, and children whose families were in the shelter system were more likely to be placed in foster care and had a decreased chance of returning to their families, leading to staying more extended periods in the foster care.
   1. This systematic review provided insight into the limitations of current programs working with children and families who are homeless.
   2. There is a need to conduct more research on the topic. Future research should look for the mechanisms of the relationship between housing insecurity and foster care involvement with samples that reflect the general population.
B. Women experiencing homelessness confront multiple intrinsic and extrinsic barriers when accessing healthcare services. Allen and Vottero (2020) provided insight into the importance of further research on this topic to include studies in settings around the world to have a more comprehensive global perspective on the issue. These researchers also recommended that research on the attitudes of healthcare providers toward caring for homeless women is an opportunity to identify research gaps and improve access to healthcare services for homeless women.
C. ACEs are considered a major risk factor for homelessness in adults. These early adverse experiences are predictors and contributors to poor health outcomes and decreased social functioning. These also contribute to other barriers individuals experiencing homelessness meet when seeking help. They are also considered risks for higher morbidity and mortality individuals experiencing homelessness. In a systematic review, Liu et al. (2021) reported that approximately 9 of 10 adults who are experiencing homelessness have a history of at least one ACE of trauma and that this is a high predictor of suicidality, mental illness, and substance use. There is also a correlation between ACEs and involvement with the legal system. A focus on further research on ACEs with prevention strategies and education on trauma-informed care is needed to provide competent care to this population.
D. The dearth of diversity among research participants is a major deterrent in reducing health disparities.
   1. Inadequate data from minority populations can result in disparate skews in cost for healthcare needs and resources, leading to poor health or even premature death.
   2. Researchers in the United States traditionally have difficulty recruiting participants from minority populations due to past history of unethical practices involving

minority populations (e.g., Tuskegee syphilis study, Henrietta Lacks, Havasupai Tribe genetic studies, the infection of Guatemalans with sexually transmitted infections), resulting in mistrust.

3. Mistrust may also stem from the feeling that they or their interests are not adequately represented.

E. A combination of inflexible work schedules, childcare difficulties, or transportation issues are also barriers to research involvement.

F. Another major barrier to research involvement is the dearth of minority researchers and study staff. Having researchers who are members of the minority group being investigated may increase trust. Minority researchers may build the confidence of community leaders and stakeholders who are instrumental in engaging the interest of the community. Mentoring minority researchers to work with underserved communities is also important in enhancing the recruitment of ideal participants. It is also imperative that the researchers can communicate effectively with participants to ensure that contextualization is not compromised due to cultural misinterpretations.

G. Advancing the nation's capacity to protect and improve health equitably is unobtainable if large cross sections of the U.S. population, often those with the greatest health challenges, are less able to benefit from the findings due to underrepresentation in research studies, although according to the 2020 U.S. Census people identifying as White have decreased in number and racial/ethnic diversity has increased the nation's health disparities. Lack of representation perpetuates inequities and health disparities by shifting the direction of research toward majority groups, feeds mistrust, and compromises generalizability of research findings.

REFERENCES AND BIBLIOGRAPHY

Allen, J., & Vottero, B. (2020). Experiences of homeless women in accessing health care in community-based settings: A qualitative systematic review. *JBI Evidence Synthesis*, *18*(9), 1970–2010. https://doi.org/10.11124/jbisrir-d-19-00214

Bai, R., Collins, C., Fischer, R., Groza, V., & Yang, L. (2020). Exploring the association between housing insecurity and child welfare involvement: A systematic review. *Child and Adolescent Social Work Journal*, *39*(2), 247–260. https://doi.org/10.1007/s10560-020-00722-z

Bibbins-Domingo, K., & Helman, A. (2022). *Improving representation in clinical trials and research: building research equity for women and underrepresented groups (Consensus Study Report)*. National Academy Press.

Liu, M., Luong, L., Lachaud, J., Edalati, H., Reeves, A., & Hwang, S. W. (2021). Adverse childhood experiences and related outcomes among adults experiencing homelessness: A systematic review and meta-analysis. *The Lancet Public Health*, *6*(11), e836–e847. https://doi.org/10.1016/s2468-2667(21)00189-4

Mosites, E., Morris, S. B., Self, J., & Butler, J. C. (2021). Data sources that enumerate people experiencing homelessness in the United States: Opportunities and challenges for epidemiologic research. *American Journal of Epidemiology*, *190*(11), 2432–2436. https://doi.org/10.1093/aje/kwab051

Rubin, E. J. (2021). Striving for diversity in research studies. *The New England Journal of Medicine*, *385*(15), 1429–1430. https://doi.org/10.1056/nejme2114651

Sierra-Mercado, D., & Lázaro-Muñoz, G. (2018). Enhance diversity among researchers to promote participant trust in precision medicine research. *The American Journal of Bioethics*, *18*(4), 44–46. https://doi.org/10.1080/15265161.2018.1431323

Substance Abuse and Mental Health Services Administration. (2023, December 5). *Homelessness programs resources*. U.S. Department of Health and Human Services. https://www.samhsa.gov/homelessness-programs-resources

U.S. Government Accountability Office. (2020, August 13). *Homelessness: Better HUD oversight of data collection could improve estimates of homeless population*. https://www.gao.gov/products/gao-20-433

SOCIOECONOMIC PROGRAMS: FEDERAL, STATE, AND LOCAL

The government national and local levels have created several programs to assist individuals who are homeless.

A. Temporary housing models (THM): THM is an interim option for individuals who became homeless due to job loss, domestic violence, or economic hardship.

B. Emergency shelters (ES): ES is a temporary option for women and children who need a safe place to stay due to domestic violence.

C. Transitional housing (TH): TH offers shelter to individuals and families for up to 24 months in a supervised setting. These programs may offer care management services and assistance with finding a permanent housing option.

D. Medical respite programs (MRP): MRP offers a transitional venue where homeless individuals who need primary medical care during recovery receive the needed care until they can be well enough to go to other, more independent programs.

E. Mental health respite programs (MHRP): MHRP offers temporary shelter opportunities to individuals transitioning from inpatient care to the community or who have no place to stay due to their mental illness. These programs only assist between 7 and 12 days.

F. Permanent housing programs: These are community-based programs run by federal and local agencies. These include PSH exclusively for homeless individuals who have a disability, including mental illness, and those individuals who need rapid rehousing. Some of these housing programs include SROs.

G. Housing assistance programs: These are commonly known as *Section 8 Housing Choice Voucher* for individuals who meet specific criteria (low-income housing) and are a longer term option for qualified individuals.

H. Healthcare for the Homeless: This is a federally sponsored program run by community-based organizations to deliver care to homeless people with mental health issues and SUDs.

RISK FACTORS AND PROTECTIVE FACTORS FOR HOMELESS AND INDIGENT POPULATIONS

A. When engaging individuals experiencing homelessness in treatment, or helping them to navigate social and healthcare services, APRNs must consider that homeless and indigent people are vulnerable populations who frequently face challenges when obtaining necessities due to poverty, history of trauma, SUDs, and mental illness. APRNs should establish interdisciplinary collaborations to prepare patient-centered care models for the individuals under their care.

B. Competent healthcare providers are considered an important protective factor for vulnerable populations by assisting with healthcare access opportunities and addressing the special medical and psychiatric needs of homeless and indigent people. Other protective factors that help these individuals include education, access to affordable housing, and access to social support services. Each of these protective factors can help reduce the challenges faced by homeless and indigent people and empower them to maintain well-being.

ASSESSMENT AND OUTREACH INTERVENTIONS FOR THE HOMELESS POPULATION

A. Assessment should focus on this population's particular needs, including addressing their specific challenges when seeking healthcare services.

B. The advanced practice nurse should include in each assessment a comprehensive medical history, SUDs, mental health evaluation, treatment history, safety, social history, and issues with accessing services (food, work, housing).

ESTABLISH THERAPEUTIC RAPPORT DURING THE INITIAL ENCOUNTER

A. Patients value an empathic, respectful, and culturally competent APRN.
B. An initial encounter with an APRN who introduces themselves to the patient, who uses active listening and uses time appropriately to gather information, complete evaluations, provide psychoeducation, and answer questions in a nonjudgmental manner helps establish an alliance with the patient.
C. Research indicates that patients who felt disrespected during initial encounters with an APRN are less likely to return for follow-up care.
D. Using simple language to educate the patients, respecting personal space, and using reflection during interactions with the patients lead to positive impressions and increase the likelihood of the patients returning to care and adhering to treatment.
E. The initial encounter impression of the APRN can last a long time. Encounters with patients allow the APRN to learn about the patient and establish a professional relationship.
F. The APRN must know about cultural competency tenets. All healthcare providers must abide by the regulations of Title VI of the Civil Rights, which indicates that care should meet the standards of care regardless of the patient's race, ethnicity, religion, and beliefs.

PROVIDE TRAUMA-INFORMED CARE PRACTICES DURING ASSESSMENT

A. Nine out of 10 homeless adults have a history of a traumatic experience.
B. The prevalence of traumatic experiences leads to poor physical and mental health outcomes and increased healthcare service costs.
C. The principles of trauma-informed care include safety, collaboration, trustworthiness, choice, and empowerment, and should be included in the treatment approaches offered to homeless people. Exposure to traumatic events such as physical, verbal, and emotional abuse may have long-lasting consequences. The introduction of programs oriented to assist homeless people, with trained APRNs providing competent and appropriate trauma-informed care, might assist in motivating homeless individuals to start and continue treatment.
D. Healthcare providers must rescind the focus on causes at the individual level and focus rather on the systemic matters that precipitated the individual's current predicament. Consequently, trauma-informed care dictates that healthcare providers have a systems-level analysis of the lived experience of the homeless population and recognize the factors that accelerate people toward a trajectory of poverty, homelessness, incarceration, substance use, and other associated interrelated phenomena.
E. APRNs have learned the tenets of trauma-informed care as an evidence-based approach to treating and helping vulnerable populations, including homeless and indigent populations. The emphasis on adopting universal trauma precautions into practice should be a standard element during all patient interactions. Using screening tools to assess trauma and applying universal trauma precautions should contribute to the standard of care, allowing the APRN to engage the patient in treatment and provide clear and specific information on the treatment's value, leading to positive outcomes and less resistance from the patient to accept care.

Adopting a Trauma-Informed Approach: Key Principles

A. The U.S. Interagency Council on Homelessness (2020) adopted SAMHSA's six key principles of a trauma-informed approach for professionals interfacing with and providing services for the homeless population:
  1. Safety: People experiencing homelessness and program staff feel physically and psychologically safe. Physical settings and interpersonal interactions should promote a sense of safety for every child, young person, family, veteran, person living with a disability, or individual adult experiencing homelessness.
  2. Trustworthiness and transparency: Homelessness service systems and programs should operate and make decisions in ways that are transparent to everyone, building and maintaining trust with people experiencing homelessness, staff, and other stakeholders.
  3. Peer support: Peers are integral to establishing and maintaining safety and hope, building trust, enhancing collaboration, and using their lived expertise to help others with housing stability and other goals, like recovery and healing.
  4. Collaboration and mutuality: Value is placed on relationship, partnership, and leveling power differences between staff and patients to promote shared power and decision-making across the program. There is recognition that everyone has a role to play in advancing trauma-informed approaches.
  5. Empowerment, voice, and choice: The homelessness service system and organizations within it foster a belief in people's resilience and the ability of individuals and communities to heal from trauma. People's strengths and experiences are recognized, honored, and built upon. Consumers are supported in shared decision-making, choice, and goal setting to determine their own housing and service needs.
  6. Cultural, historical, and gender issues: Homelessness services systems and programs actively identify and address inequities and biases caused or perpetuated by their service delivery models. They promote access to culturally and gender-responsive services; leverage the healing values of traditional cultural connections; adapt programs, policies, and procedures to the racial, ethnic, and cultural needs of consumers; and recognize and address the impacts of historical trauma.

SAFETY ASSESSMENTS

A. Safety assessments are completed for all patients regardless of the diagnosis (medical or psychiatric).
B. In the case of vulnerable populations, safety assessments are vital to ensure that both risk factors and protective factors are discussed with each patient. It is the best opportunity for the APRN to provide psychoeducation and support and to engage the individual in strategies to prevent harm to themselves or others.
C. Safety assessments must consider that homeless individuals are at risk of violence perpetrated by others, and also that they are constantly exposed to environmental hazards (extreme weather conditions while in the street), untreated chronic mental illness, SUDs, and chronic medical comorbidities, leading to adverse outcomes and poor health quality. Including safety assessments during clinical encounters with

homeless and indigent individuals helps motivate recovery processes, helps prevent harm, and assists them with tools to manage crises. In a basic format, it should include:
   1. Triggers and stressors that may put the patient at emotional risk
   2. What warning signs may put the patient at risk of having a crisis
   3. What are the internal coping strategies that help the patient de-escalate
   4. Social settings or people who the patient feels provide distraction
   5. Names of people/contacts who the patient can call to ask for support
   6. Names of healthcare professionals or support agencies that the patient can call during a crisis
   7. What the APRN needs to do to make the environment safe
   8. One thing that is important for the patient and worth living for
D. Each APRN who is completing the safety assessment might include other items that are deemed appropriate for each patient, including if the individual has a pet as their only family support and who may provide a safety net.

COMMUNITY HEALTH ADVANCED PRACTICE NURSING
A. Community health APRNs provide healthcare outreach services in the community.
B. The APRN should identify available resources in the community, identify the needs of homeless people, and prioritize services according to the need. Awareness of current barriers, gaps, and roadblocks is imperative in providing healthcare services to this population.
   1. Prepare education materials and advertisement paraphernalia in different languages.
   2. Identify and train staff to provide bilingual services.
   3. Educate staff on cultural sensitivity and cultural competency.
   4. Develop programs focusing on identification and prevention.
C. Interdisciplinary collaboration and involvement with care coordination are essential, as is appropriate discharge planning, including follow-up care services.

Types of Outreach
A. Accessing healthcare can be challenging for individuals and families experiencing homelessness. Keeping appointments without means of transportation, affording medications, and having resources for communication devices such as phones and computers, as well as the physical space to safely store them, are arduous challenges for homeless people.
B. Complicating these challenges can be the existence of physical, mental health, and SUDs hindering one's ability to navigate the homeless service system.
C. Unsheltered homeless people who sleep on the streets may experience emotional and physical trauma and have difficulty trusting healthcare organizations or providers due to the stigmatization or criminalization of homeless people.
D. In providing care for homeless people, the onus is on the healthcare providers to build trusting relationships. One strategy for building trusting relationships with people who need medical services is for agencies to deliver healthcare, including medical treatment and behavioral healthcare, directly to the places where individuals reside. This may mean delivering services on the street, in shelters or soup kitchens, in encampments, or—in more rural areas—in the woods. This approach to care provision is broadly referred to as *outreach work*, and in practice encompasses a variety of approaches, including street medicine.
E. Essentially, outreach is an integral connection between the unstably housed and the available housing services and resources. Outreach programs are unconventional interventions that involve professionals networking to meet the needs of an individual experiencing homelessness, through patient engagement. Outreach programs may be in urban or rural settings, incorporated into other programs at a clinic, or a hybrid or traditional clinic. The professionals in the network meet the patients on their turf, assessing their needs and connecting them with the relevant services and providers.
F. APRNs must "think outside the box," for example, by visiting local food banks weekly to provide healthcare services and connecting individuals to local resources while they are there for a meal. The APRN should know cultural competency tenets, including culture, language, and customs, and have a basic understanding of trauma care and boundaries related to personal space; physical touch, especially when performing a physical exam; and the importance of empathy, respect, and giving undivided attention to the person. The APRN should explain to the patient the purpose of the examination and educate on the risks versus the benefits of having a complete physical exam done during the encounter. It is also important to explain each examination step, including its reason. There are basically four types of outreach. The first three types are primarily preoccupied with building relationships and breaking down barriers to care:
   1. The first is connecting individuals with clinical settings. Housing and other community resources are also involved.
   2. Assisting patients with a specific transactional task. This includes tasks such as assistance with Medicaid enrollment or phone distribution.
   3. Registering patients in a coordinated entry system (CES) within their jurisdiction. The CES is a process in which the most vulnerable homeless patients are matched with available and appropriate housing resources.
      a. This kind of work is more goal-specific than generalized outreach, but it builds a long-term relationship in the interest of facilitating active engagement with the region's CES as an entry point into services.
   4. The fourth type of outreach type involves asking the patient what they need and connecting them with peer specialists, community health workers (CHWs), and outreach workers.
      a. This work is oriented around patients' or communities' goals and encompasses regular contact in an attempt to build relationships, understand the specific needs of a specified community, and help patients identify and achieve goals that may eventually result in the pursuit of a linkage to care.
      b. Outreach care may be delivered from backpacks or vans, through ongoing programs or one-time campaigns, with the assistance of case managers, CHWs, emergency services workers, doctors, nurse practitioners, nurses, or behavioral health specialists.

Community Engagement
A. Community outreach programs are critical to providing needed services to the homeless and indigent populations in the United States.

1. Providers include government agencies, faith-based organizations, local and state programs, healthcare systems, advocacy groups, and volunteers.
2. Some outreach programs are staffed by interdisciplinary members, including healthcare professionals, social workers, peer specialists, and volunteers.

B. The services provided can include street outreach programs, food banks, soup kitchens, mobile outreach teams, community centers run by faith-based organizations, community outreach programs, public facilities with showers, and respite centers.
1. These programs facilitate access to services that otherwise would not be available to homeless or indigent people.
2. Community outreach programs have demonstrated several benefits, including providing screening, prevention, treatment, access to food, clothing, referrals, and linkages to social and specialized healthcare services.

C. Street outreach programs can be designed as a community-based initiative through a community outreach center (COC) led by faculty and university students to engage vulnerable people in comprehensive healthcare services.
1. Using an interdisciplinary team of students and faculty is an exemplary interprofessional education (IPE) approach to experiential learning, facilitating clinical practice while providing much-needed healthcare services to homeless and underserved populations.
2. An example of an interdisciplinary program was implemented by Doran and Doede (2020), nursing professors at the University of Maryland, Baltimore, Maryland.
   a. They developed a street outreach program subsidized through a partnership between the university and a COC located in Baltimore's central city.
   b. The COC provided a variety of preventive and crisis services.
   c. Although a considerable number of the people who used the services at the COC either were homeless or had recent experience with homelessness, only a small percentage of the people used the preventive services specifically.
   d. The program was instituted to connect with the neighbors, build trust and rapport, and encourage them to engage the full gamut of services provided at the center.
   e. Such collaborative programs are invaluable to underserved communities. Local clinics and centers usually lack the ability to conduct street outreach programs due to limited funding.
   f. The team consisted of social work, nursing, and medical students who provided medical, psychiatric, SUD, and social services in the form of assessments, wound care, monitoring vital signs, hygiene kits, condoms, documentation forms, referral materials, and lists of community resources.
   g. Students and faculty traversed the community on foot and performed outreach in places that homeless individuals frequented or resided in, such as encampments. Recruitment also included people waiting at bus stops, panhandling, or socializing in public areas. Students performed services based on their program specialty; nursing students performed physical assessments and/or wound care, social work students provided referrals and coordinated case management with the COC, and medical students provided health and behavior modification education. Although this specific project had medical students, APRN students can perform similar services.

Street Medicine

A. Street medicine is health and social services developed specifically to address the unique needs and circumstances of unsheltered homeless people, delivered directly to them in their environment.
B. The principal method of street medicine is to involve homeless people precisely where they are and on their own terms to significantly reduce or eradicate barriers to care, access, and follow-through. Visiting people where they live—in alleys, under bridges, or within urban encampments—is a necessary strategy to build trust with this socially marginalized and highly vulnerable population.
C. Street medicine is an effective medium to provide much-needed medical, mental health, and social care through assertive, coordinated, and collaborative care management.
D. Street medicine teams are made up of approximately four to five individuals and should include committed full-time outreach workers, some of whom have lived experience of homelessness; healthcare providers, either physicians or nurse practitioners; and a peer navigator or support person to assist with navigating social issues.
1. Teams may also include learners: medical students, nurse practitioner students, occupational therapists, nursing students, or medical residents.
2. Practitioners of street medicine transport their supplies with them and principally walk to patients' locations to provide care.
3. In addition to medical supplies, the team might provide other items that are necessary to people living on the streets, such as socks.
4. Essential components of a street medicine bag include the following:
   a. Pain management supplies
   b. Medical supplies for dealing with skin infections and wounds
   c. Blood pressure measurement tools
   d. Gloves and masks
   e. Flashlights
   f. Harm reduction supplies, such as Narcan, fentanyl test strips, and clean needles
   g. Feminine hygiene products
   h. Referral information downloaded to a phone

E. Having a consistent, reliable schedule is a central approach to street medicine because consistency helps people know where to obtain services when needed. At encampment sites, the team attends to wound care needs or mental health medications, as well as harm reduction strategies for SUD, such as syringe service programs, naloxone distribution, and medications for opioid use.
F. The Keck School of Medicine (KSOM) of the University of Southern California (USC) developed an innovative street medicine program consisting of a clinical provider (APRN or physician), a nurse, and a CHW.
1. The CHW, someone with a lived experience of homelessness, was the patient navigator, connecting with the patients and building relationships as the patients were guided through the available resources, benefits, and community-based services.

2. The street medicine program provided comprehensive primary care where the patients resided, under bridges, on the sidewalk, or where the patient preferred to receive care.
3. The patients were accessed on foot, with the medical supplies in backpacks. The team was mindful of building trust at every patient encounter as they collected medical and psychosocial histories. Trauma-informed care principles formed the basis of the interactions. The team understood that homeless patients may have childhood traumatic experiences as well as traumatic experiences as a result of the homeless experience. Trauma-informed care and empathetic listening helped build resilience as the healthcare providers listened to the patients' stories and authentically attended to their needs.
4. High-quality care provided included a wide range of clinical services such as chronic disease management, wound care, routine vaccinations, antiretroviral therapy, and monitoring for people living with HIV. In addition to treating acute health issues, preventive health screenings such as cancer screening were also provided.

Mobile Clinics

A. A mobile clinic is a motor vehicle tailored specifically to travel to communities to provide healthcare services. Services are provided by a team of healthcare professionals such as physicians or nurse practitioners, nurses, CHWs, and other health professionals. Mobile health units help underserved communities overcome barriers that frequently hinder access to healthcare.
B. Mobile clinics operate in all 50 states, the District of Columbia, and Puerto Rico. Many are stationed in densely populated cities around the country, such as Atlanta, Boston, Chicago, Dallas, Denver, Houston, Los Angeles, New York, Orlando, Phoenix, San Francisco, San Jose, Seattle, and St. Louis. Mobile health clinics commonly deliver care to some of the country's most vulnerable populations, including people of color, people experiencing poverty and/or homelessness, uninsured people, people in rural communities, veterans, and immigrants.
C. The medium of mobile health service can be combined to meet the unique needs of the target population.
1. One such service was developed in Orange County, California, to address the gap in services for people who were homeless with serious mental health needs. The goal of the combined mobile services was to make behavioral and mental health services and housing more accessible for homeless people with SMI. The team aimed to accomplish this goal by interacting with and listening to the people to assess their needs, develop individualized service plans, provide mobile treatment, and address barriers to treatment and housing. To offer these services effectively, two staffed vans were used, one for outreach and one for treatment services.
2. The outreach team went to several sites in the communities where homeless people were located to assess whether they needed outreach services, housing, employment assistance, or transportation.
3. The treatment team provided mobile short-term behavioral and mental health treatment services and linkage to long-term mental health services to patients examined by the outreach team. The outreach team included two case managers and two peer support specialists, one of whom was the driver. The treatment team consisted of a nurse practitioner, two case managers, a peer support specialist, and a peer recovery specialist who was also the driver. Each team had a team leader.

REFERENCES AND BIBLIOGRAPHY

Centers for Disease Control and Prevention. (2022, June 2). *Infographic: 6 Guiding principles to a trauma-informed approach.* U.S. Department of Health and Human Services. https://stacks.cdc.gov/view/cdc/138924

Doran, K., & Doede, M. (2020). An interdisciplinary street outreach program to engage vulnerable neighbors in care. *Public Health Nursing, 38*(2), 141–144. https://doi.org/10.1111/phn.12829

Cash, J. C. (Ed.). (2020). *Family practice guidelines* (5th ed.). Springer Publishing Company.

Liu, M., Luong, L., Lachaud, J., Edalati, H., Reeves, A., & Hwang, S. W. (2021). Adverse childhood experiences and related outcomes among adults experiencing homelessness: A systematic review and meta-analysis. *The Lancet Public Health, 6*(11), e836–e847. https://doi.org/10.1016/s2468-2667(21)00189-4

Malone, N. C., Williams, M. M., Smith Fawzi, M. C., Bennet, J., Hill, C., Katz, J. N., & Oriol, N. E. (2020). Mobile health clinics in the United States. *International Journal for Equity in Health, 19*(1). https://doi.org/10.1186/s12939-020-1135-7

National Health Care for the Homeless Council. (2022, November 16). *Our work.* https://nhchc.org/our-work

Rubin, R. (2021). Helping people who are homeless stay healthy during the pandemic. *JAMA, 325*(6), 517. https://doi.org/10.1001/jama.2020.23436

Stefanowicz, M., Feldman, B., & Robinson, J. (2021). House calls without walls: Street medicine delivers primary care to unsheltered persons experiencing homelessness. *The Annals of Family Medicine, 19*(1), 84–84. https://doi.org/10.1370/afm.2639

Total Care for the Homeless Coalition. (n.d.). *Home.* https://tchcsc.org

Varghese, L., & Emerson, A. (2021). Trauma-informed care in the primary care setting: An evolutionary analysis. *Journal of the American Association of Nurse Practitioners, 34*(3), 465–473. https://doi.org/10.1097/jxx.0000000000000663

Zarnello, L. (2023). Implementing trauma-informed care across the lifespan to acknowledge childhood adverse event prevalence. *The Nurse Practitioner, 48*(2), 14–21. https://doi.org/10.1097/01.npr.0000000000000002

TREATMENT PLANS

A. Typical treatment plan modalities for homeless and indigent individuals include case management, mental health and medical treatment, medication management, SUD treatment, peer support, the inclusion of social support, and information/guidance on employment and housing assistance programs.
B. The treatment plans should include available interventions and interdisciplinary and patient-centered approaches. The APRN should initiate the treatment by addressing the most pressing issues first, including ensuring the safety of the patient, completing an assessment, and educating the patient on the risks versus the benefits of getting appropriate treatment and care. The APRN should be knowledgeable of cultural competency tenets, cultural humility, local agencies that help homeless people, community services, and the ability to initiate referrals within the community for services. The expectation is not for the APRN to address every issue the patient presents but to initiate and make recommended treatment. The APRN should check for immunization and educate on lifestyle modifications and treatment options for common medical comorbidities.
C. Supportive systems are vital to the successful recovery of patients. APRNs should always consider including family and members of supportive systems during treatment planning. Having different perspectives and learning more about the patients are essential, and those who know them best can

help. Family and loved ones are great allies during the recovery process as they can relay information to the APRN and report any issues with nonadherence, side effects, or acute changes in condition or behavior.

D. It is the ethical and clinical obligation of the APRN to provide empathic and competent care to everyone under their care. Research indicates that patients who feel respected and heard are motivated to engage and continue in treatment. Empathic approaches, such as putting oneself in the patient's shoes, can go a long way and assist in recovery. Patients motivated to seek treatment and continue in treatment have better health outcomes.

REFERENCES AND BIBLIOGRAPHY

Allen, J., & Vottero, B. (2020). Experiences of homeless women in accessing health care in community-based settings: A qualitative systematic review. *JBI Evidence Synthesis, 18*(9), 1970–2010. https://doi.org/10.11124/jbisrir-d-19-00214

American Psychiatric Nurses Association. (2014). *Psychiatric-mental health nursing: Scope and standards of practice* (2nd ed.). American Nurses Association.

Cash, J. C. (Ed.). (2020). *Family practice guidelines* (5th ed.). Springer Publishing Company.

Guido, G. W. (2019). *Legal and ethical issues in nursing.* Pearson Education.

Walker, J. N., Vanderhoef, D., Adams, S. M., & Fleisch, S. B. (2021). The impact of an educational intervention on nursing staff attitudes toward patients experiencing homelessness and mental illness. *Journal of the American Psychiatric Nurses Association, 28*(6), 474–479. https://doi.org/10.1177/10783903211011669

SPECIAL CONSIDERATIONS RELATED TO AGE, GENDER, AND BEING A MEMBER OF A GROUP/COMMUNITY

A. Multiple agencies (local, state, and federal) offer programs to assist homeless and indigent people. These programs include the HUD Exchange Homeless Assistance, National Runaway Safeline, National Alliance to End Homelessness, National Coalition for the Homeless, and National Health Care for the Homeless Council. Each agency services specific groups (e.g., adolescents, veterans, children, women, LGBTQ+). Other community agencies, such as the Young Men's Christian Association (YMCA) or Young Women's Christian Association (YWCA), religious-based pantries, and community day programs are also available.

B. The APRN working with homeless and indigent patients should consider the specific needs of homeless individuals when attempting to obtain services. Essential factors include demographics such as age, gender, sexual orientation, and ethnic group. Each element demands a clear understanding of healthcare and social services' different needs and views. In the case of gender, there is evidence supporting the prevalence of physical and sexual assault and pervasive discriminatory practices exerted on people of specific gender or expressed sexual orientation. The APRN must incorporate cultural competency, cultural humility, patient-centered care, and trauma-informed care services in clinical practice.

REFERENCES AND BIBLIOGRAPHY

Cash, J. C. (Ed.). (2020). *Family practice guidelines* (5th ed.). Springer Publishing Company.

James-Conterelli, S., Dunkley, D., McIntosh, J. T., Julien, T., Nelson, M. D., & Richard-Eaglin, A. (2023). The impact of systemic racism on health outcomes among Black women. *The Nurse Practitioner, 48*(2), 23–32. https://doi.org/10.1097/01.npr.0000000000000001

Zarnello, L. (2023). Implementing trauma-informed care across the lifespan to acknowledge childhood adverse event prevalence. *The Nurse Practitioner, 48*(2), 14–21. https://doi.org/10.1097/01.npr.0000000000000002

CHALLENGES FOR THE APRN TO PROVIDE SERVICES TO THIS POPULATION AND TOOLS TO ADDRESS THOSE CHALLENGES

A. COVID-19 brought detrimental disruptions to accessibility, availability, and mode of providing care. These challenges also included a fast change from in-person to telehealth modalities, leading to loss of continuity of care, especially for those with no access to a computer or another electronic device with visual capabilities. The sudden closure of community clinics, outpatient programs, and medical offices affected most people, especially those who were homeless or indigent. Mental healthcare providers were also forced to change clinical practices and adjust to follow mandates. The new norm was to continue providing care using a different delivery system, such as telehealth, and at the same time begin to learn how to protect the privacy of the patient, how to bill for services and complete assessments, and how to conduct therapy sessions remotely. Going forward, the option of telehealth services is still essential for those in rural areas and for those who, due to physical or mental disability, are unable to go to clinics or EDs.

   1. The positive impacts of the switch to telehealth were increased and frequent communication between the patient and the healthcare provider, decreased cancellation of appointments rates and no-show rates, and improved communication between healthcare providers and opportunities for interprofessional collaboration.

B. There is no database registry to know the number of homeless individuals in a given community.

C. There is implicit bias in the healthcare system, with statistics not reflecting the actual number or percentage of homeless individuals or of urban versus suburban homeless individuals.

D. There is a limited number of identified community care teams for the homeless population.

E. There is a need for a hospital/agency alternative resource program for providing healthcare services such as screening for infectious diseases with vaccinations and psychiatric evaluations.

F. There is a lack of programs/care coordination and protocols to identify homeless people on admission to the ED. Many homeless individuals resort to using hospital EDs out of necessity for healthcare services. Most hospital EDs lack alternative services to help homeless people with comprehensive services, including prevention, screening for infectious diseases, vaccination, and specialized care such as psychiatric-mental health services. There also is a lack of a hospital/agency program that can meet the immediate needs of homeless people before discharge from an ED or hospital. Individuals who walk to an ED might be turned away, discharged prematurely, or subjected to unnecessary and costly tests and exams and then discharged without follow-up care. This creates the pervasive situation of fragmentation of care.

   1. A more downstream, patient-centered care approach to patients visiting the ED should include triage with an assessment and subsequent transfer of care to the appropriate specialty, possibly outside of the ED in an urgent care area. The initial triage can be done in person or via telehealth to decrease wait times in the ED waiting areas. Staff should be educated on appropriate etiquette, including using cultural competency tenets. A program to meet the needs of homeless people upon discharge should

supply food, prescription medications, transport to a shelter or wherever they are staying, and appropriate clothing for the weather.

REFERENCE AND BIBLIOGRAPHY

Marcus, R., Meehan, A. A., Jeffers, A., Cassell, C. H., Barker, J., Montgomery, M. P., Dupervil, B., Henry, A., Cha, S., Venkatappa, T., DiPietro, B., Boyer, A., Radhakrishnan, L., Laws, R. L., Fields, V. L., Cary, M., Yang, M., Davis, M., Bautista, G. J., … Mosites, E. (2022). Behavioral health providers' experience with changes in services for people experiencing homelessness during COVID-19, USA, August–October 2020. *The Journal of Behavioral Health Services Research, 49*(4), 470–486. https://doi.org/10.1007/s11414-022-09800-9

POTENTIAL SOLUTIONS THE APRN CAN USE TO MITIGATE BARRIERS TO PROVIDING ADEQUATE CARE TO HOMELESS AND INDIGENT INDIVIDUALS

A. The APRN should be proactive and involved with clinics/healthcare providers in the community that serve these individuals.

  1. Develop a network of healthcare professionals, street nurses, medical students, interested and caring people, local clinics, hospitals, EDs, needle exchanges, local churches, volunteers, food cupboards, and mental health providers to sustain the momentum.

  2. Organize mobile health clinics to meet with homeless people where they live and where they frequent.

  3. Organize local/community health fairs as part of community programs or street fairs.

  4. Develop relationships and collaborate with local agencies, community leaders, community healthcare providers, mental health advocacy/support groups and agencies, and local clergy by meeting with the people to find what healthcare providers can teach them and how to help them.

  5. Educate local community leaders on the importance of opening programs to provide healthcare/mental healthcare services to homeless and indigent people in their community.

INTERPROFESSIONAL COLLABORATION

A. APRNs and other healthcare providers are equipped with valuable tools to help homeless and indigent people. Interprofessional collaboration is an efficient model to ensure comprehensive healthcare and social delivery of services.

B. Collaboration among clinicians with different areas of specialty and expertise provides an opportunity to address various issues and needs of homeless and indigent people.

C. Models such as care coordination—the collaboration between agencies and clinicians by sharing information—and active involvement in advocacy and peer support help improve opportunities for better health outcomes for vulnerable populations.

D. Interprofessional collaboration allows the APRN to expand the resources used for healthcare linkages, networking, and referrals to other services not provided in their clinical practice. It is also important to prepare patient-centered treatment care plans that lead to improved patient outcomes, comprehensive treatment, improved access to care, and reduced overall cost.

CRISIS INTERVENTION

A. In New York City (NYC), there is a program that provides intervention for people in crisis.

  1. A multidisciplinary team of behavioral health professionals provides outreach services in the community to individuals experiencing a behavioral health crisis.

  2. Approximately 24 mobile crisis teams cover the city and can be activated by contacting NYC Well via text, phone, or email. Each team assists with short-term care, linkages to services, assessment, counseling, and crisis intervention services.

B. Other states in the United States have similar teams providing outreach in the community; some include police as part of their staff.

TELEHEALTH

A. Telehealth is the use of telecommunication technologies and electronic information to provide care and promote patient–healthcare provider interactions remotely. It consists of two forms:

  1. Two-way, synchronous, interactive patient–healthcare provider communication through audio and video equipment (also referred to as *telemedicine*)

  2. Asynchronous telemedicine, which involves acquiring medical data, then transmitting these data to a healthcare provider or medical specialist at a convenient time for assessment offline

B. Telehealth, as a medium for providing service, has been used in clinical settings for over 60 years and empirically studied for just over 20 years.

C. Telehealth has the advantage of increasing access to screening, assessment, treatment, recovery support, crisis support, and medication management covering various behavioral health and primary care settings.

D. Telehealth affords healthcare providers the opportunity to connect patients in numerous locations such as at a home, in private spaces, in a clinical setting, or in another location in the community. Telehealth methods can be applied by a myriad of healthcare providers (e.g., psychiatrists, primary care providers, mental health counselors, social workers, psychologists, addiction counselors, case managers, opioid treatment providers, peer workers). Additionally, practitioners can use telehealth with a hybrid approach for increased flexibility. It is an invaluable medium especially between healthcare providers and rural or underserved areas.

E. Improved access is necessary to provide medical care to homeless and indigent populations in a cost-effective manner.

F. People experiencing homelessness often encounter barriers to healthcare, such as means of transportation, cost, and lack of insurance.

  1. Telehealth mitigates transportation barriers and has become an essential care delivery method during the pandemic especially for people living on the streets and in encampments.

  2. Telehealth is recommended by the CDC for provision of primary care, nonemergency acute care, and chronic disease management.

  3. In March 2020, the Centers for Medicare & Medicaid Services expanded access to Medicare telehealth services. The types of services Medicaid covered via telehealth were also expanded. Prior to this, neither Medicaid or Medicare would cover the cost of most audio-only telehealth services.

  4. Medicare also expanded the list of healthcare providers who could provide telehealth services to Medicare patients. Formerly, only specific groups of healthcare providers were eligible to receive payment for telehealth services. However, as a result of changes during the pandemic, all healthcare providers eligible to bill Medicare received payment for professional telehealth services. Similarly, at the state level, legislation was enacted to allow private insurance companies licensed within the state to cover the cost for telehealth services.

G. A recent study evaluated the efficacy of telehealth in improving access to healthcare for homeless people using needs assessment surveys completed by patients at an urban drop-in center for people experiencing homelessness.

   1. The project site was an urban drop-in center in a mid-sized North Carolina city that provided legal, mental health, social work, and medical services for homeless people.

   2. Medical services include a telehealth clinic and an in-person walk-in clinic.

   3. At the telehealth clinic, healthcare providers interfaced with patients via an internet-based, two-way audio/visual system.

   4. Telehealth equipment allowed for the remote use of assessment tools such a stethoscope, ophthalmoscope, and dermatoscope.

   5. A total of 63 people completed the survey. The results showed common health challenges encountered were mental (58.7%) and physical (52.4%) as was ED use (75.9%, $n = 54$). Surveys were also completed by patients from both clinics.

      a. Results of the surveys after in-person and telehealth clinical visits showed patient satisfaction was greater than 90% for both visit types ($n = 125$, 44.0% telehealth and 56.0% in person).

      b. A profound finding was that without telehealth visits, 29.1% of patients would have gone to the ED and 38.2% would not have gotten care.

H. Homeless and indigent individuals are a population that, unfortunately, continues to grow. The systemic inequalities and challenges that they meet daily are many. Psychiatric-mental health nurse practitioners (PMHNPs) must assist in addressing the critical issues affecting this vulnerable portion of the population—active involvement in healthcare programs that promote the prevention and treatment of medical and medical illnesses.

I. Considering the unique and specific needs of homeless people to prepare patient-centered care treatment plans is necessary to improve the overall health quality of homeless and indigent people.

REFERENCES AND BIBLIOGRAPHY

Adams, C. S., Player, M. S., Berini, C. R., Perkins, S., Fay, J., Walker, L., Buffalo, E., Roach, C., & Diaz, V. A. (2021). A telehealth initiative to overcome health care barriers for people experiencing homelessness. *Telemedicine and E-Health, 27*(8), 851–858. https://doi.org/10.1089/tmj.2021.0127

Alvarado, H. A. (2021, December 29). *Telemedicine services in substance use and mental health treatment facilities.* Substance Abuse and Mental Health Services Administration. https://www.samhsa.gov/data/report/telemedicine-services

Legislative Analysis and Public Policy Association. (2021). *Telehealth and substance use disorder services in the era of COVID-19: Review and recommendations.* https://legislativeanalysis.org/?s=telehealth+services

25 VETERANS AND SURVIVORS OF WAR

Pamela Herbig Wall, Connie Braybrook, and Katie St. Pierre

INTRODUCTION

This chapter provides an overview of military and veteran culture and brings attention to the opportunities and challenges unique to caring for these individuals and their families. It provides information on the military healthcare system and how service members transition from active duty to the Veterans Health Administration (VHA) to receive benefits. There is information on the elements of culturally informed assessment techniques and how to ask questions to maintain a therapeutic alliance with the veteran. Information on military-specific mental health challenges and barriers to care, assessment, and treatment opportunities is provided.

DEFINITION

A. The U.S. Title 38 of the Code of Federal Regulations defines *veteran* as "a person who served in the active military, naval, air, or space service and who was discharged or released under conditions other than dishonorable" (38 C.F.R. § 3.1 d, 2023).
  1. Since the organization of the Continental Army in 1775, veterans have served in all five branches of the Armed Services in war and peacetime. Approximately 16.5 million veterans of our Armed Forces live throughout the United States.
  2. Today's veterans have served on military installations within the continental United States, overseas, and in the following conflicts: World War II, Korean War, Vietnam War, Gulf War, and Iraq and Afghanistan wars.
  3. The most significant number of veterans served during the years between 1964 and 1975, or the Vietnam era. The second largest served during peacetime.
B. The number of veterans is declining as the population is aging.
  1. In nearly two decades, the number of veterans has decreased from 26.4 million to 18 million in 2018.
  2. By the year 2045, the veteran population is projected to decline to less than 12 million.
C. Today's veterans are primarily male (14.84 million). A significant minority of veterans identify as female (1.66 million), most of whom have served since the 9/11 event.
  1. 9.8 million veterans access healthcare within the veterans healthcare system.
  2. The MISSION (Maintaining Internal Systems and Strengthening Integrated Outside Networks) Act of 2018 supports 10.2 million to seek healthcare outside of the traditional governmental conduits.
  3. It is imperative to increase military and veteran awareness among APRNs.
D. Many veterans do not believe that the public understands the unique perspective of their service experience. A survey found that only 13% of healthcare providers met the criteria for military cultural readiness, including the threshold for evidence-based care.
  1. Despite the inevitable transition to civilian life, only clinicians who worked in the Veterans Administration (VA) and military healthcare settings were more likely to be successful in delivering culturally competent care.
  2. It is our responsibility as civilian and veteran healthcare practitioners to address this gap in practice to provide accessibility to healthcare that is inclusive of the U.S. veteran population.
E. In response to this cultural competency disparity in 2011, Michelle Obama and Dr. Jill Biden launched Joining Forces to support military service members and their families.
  1. Part of the program was an initiative to generate interdisciplinary education in medicine and nursing focused on cultural competencies and wellness trajectories for military service members, veterans, and their family members. Of the 104 responding medical schools, fewer than a quarter rallied by including military cultural competencies within their curriculum.
F. Lack of military and veteran competencies and absence from formal medical education and training have consequences. Failure to understand the veteran or earn their trust can potentially decrease the therapeutic alliance and negatively affect adherence and outcomes.
G. As healthcare professionals take steps to dismantle stigmatization and increase accessibility for marginalized groups, it is imperative to consider both visible and invisible aspects of veteran culture to provide comprehensive and equitable healthcare.

MILITARY CULTURAL COMPETENCIES

A. Cultural competency as it relates to the military is an understanding of the customs, knowledge, experiences, and belief systems that are taught to and learned by service members and their families as they move through their service obligations.
B. Familiarization with military culture is critical to understanding the connections among values, health beliefs, needs, health-seeking behaviors, and mental health outcomes for service members and veterans, ensuring that the healthcare provider conveys respect and understanding of the veteran's experience.
C. Military culture encompasses three basic overlapping features: an organization governed by rules and regulations; a culture defined by norms, language, values, and symbols; and a social group characterized by norms, roles, and collectives.

The views expressed in this article are those of the author(s) and do not necessarily reflect the official policy or position of the Department of the Navy, Department of Defense, Uniformed Services University of the Health Sciences, or the United States Government.

MILITARY ORGANIZATION

A. The military organization or structure is ruled by Congressional mandate, Department of Defense (DOD) policies and regulations, service policies and regulations, and other internal rules and morals.

1. It is a hierarchal chain of command with officers in control, with subordinate roles for junior officers and enlisted members.
2. Immersion into military culture started when veterans crossed the boundary into their first officer candidate school, boot camp training, or Reserve Officers' Training Corps (ROTC) training in college.
3. Service members absorb the history and traditions of their respective service, expected behaviors (saluting, marching), and beliefs and norms that are universal to most of those who have served in the Armed Forces.

MILITARY NORMS, LANGUAGE, VALUES, AND SYMBOLS

A. The military or warrior ethos is the idea that the group or the collective earns supremacy over the self.

B. Conformity to military rules, regulations, norms, and beliefs is behaviorally and psychologically modified. The group, the team, and the collective reinforce this compliance.

1. Service members eat the same food, dress in the same uniforms, and wear the same headgear, outerwear, gloves, coats, and shoes.
2. Service members are all trained to the same physical readiness standards and must be "ready" 24/7 to respond to any global crisis.
3. Service members have rules of conduct (Uniform Code of Military Justice) that apply during work and off-duty hours.

C. This warrior ethos rhetoric can become so embedded that they become part of the service members' self-identity.

1. Ideas such as mission first, leaving no person behind, honesty, integrity, loyalty, selflessness, never quitting, never accepting defeat, pride, love, and "family" become the service member's worldview and lens.
2. This warrior/military ethos is regarded as a zero-failure mentality. Universally applied to every day, every situation, and every decision, these beliefs and standards may be viewed as unattainable, leading to either a strength or an opportunity for vulnerability (Table 25.1).

MILITARY AS A SOCIAL GROUP

A. The military as a social unit is a combined perspective of the interwoven military, family, and social connections with the military experience at the center.

1. Military service members live on and around military bases and treatment facilities.
2. Educational, faith-based, recreational, and other social experiences are shared on and off base.
3. Military-related and volunteer organizations serve the social culture of the military service member and meet the military family's needs (e.g., Veterans Service Organizations [VSO]; community services; Morale, Welfare, and Recreation [MWR]; United Service Organizations [USO]).

B. The interconnectedness between the "occupational role" of the military service member and the "social" group often carries with it the same set of values, beliefs, and norms from their military experiences, which sometimes manifest within the structure and morals of the veteran.

MILITARY 101

A. Civilians control the military's Armed Forces via the President of the United States in the role of Commander in Chief. Only Congress has the power to declare war. The Commander in Chief then delegates power through the Secretary of Defense to the DOD through the combatant commanders (10 serving in geographic areas around the globe) and then the Joint Chiefs of Staff and Service Chiefs of Staff, who manage the six branches of service: Army, Navy, Air Force, Marines, Space Force, and Coast Guard.

B. There are three military departments: the Department of the Army, the Department of the Navy (including the U.S. Marine Corps), and the Department of the Air Force (including the Space Force). The U.S. Coast Guard is under the Department of Homeland Security during peacetime missions.

C. There are two ways to serve in the military active component or reserve component.

1. Active components or "active duty" are those who are serving full-time.
2. The reserve component has two groups: the Reserves and the National Guard or Air National Guard Units.

D. There are three types of military ranks: officer, enlisted, and warrant officer.

TABLE 25.1 MILITARY ETHOS STRENGTHS AND VULNERABILITIES

Strength	Trait	Vulnerability
Placing the welfare of others above one's own welfare	Selflessness	Not seeking help for a health problem because personal health is not a priority
Commitment to accomplishing missions and protecting comrades in arms	Loyalty	Survivor guilt and complicated bereavement after losing friends
Toughness and ability to endure hardships without complaint	Stoicism	Not acknowledging significant symptoms and suffering after returning home
Following an internal moral compass to choose "right" over "wrong"	Moral code	Feeling frustrated and betrayed when others fail to follow a moral code
Meaning and purpose when defending societal values	Social order	Loss of meaning or betrayal when rejected by society
Becoming the best and most effective professional possible	Excellence	Feeling ashamed of (or not acknowledging) imperfections

Source: Data from DVA (2014), Module 4. Center for Deployment Psychology. (2014). Faces of military culture: Core competencies for healthcare professionals. https://deploymentpsych.org/test-face

1. Officers ranks can include lieutenant, captain, commander, colonel, general, and admiral. Warrant officer ranks are from W-1 to W-5.
2. Enlisted ranks can include private, corporal, sergeant, seaman, petty officer, and airman.

E. The U.S. Army is the largest uniformed service, with the Air Force, the Navy, and the Marine Corps trailing. The Space Force is the newest and has the fewest numbers.
1. Two-thirds of its active force are 30 years of age or younger, male (17% female), and ethnically diverse. Almost 50% of those serving in the U.S. military are married; 5% are dual military marriages (i.e., both spouses serving in the Armed Forces).

F. Each service member is assigned a military occupational specialty (MOS) code equivalent to a job designation.
1. These can range from administrative assignments to pilots, infantry, healthcare providers, or logisticians.
2. Identification of the veteran's MOS is critical to understanding service members' identity in the military and any military-related exposures.

LIFE CYCLE OF SERVICE

A. Recruitment: The recruitment process is different for each veteran depending on the time that they served. The military is primarily an all-volunteer force. However, many of those who served in the Vietnam War were drafted via the selective service. Their experiences may have been vastly different due to their recruitment process.

B. History: Upon being drafted or volunteering for service, individuals undergo a criminal history check and a mental and physical screening for any issue or condition that might prohibit service entry.

C. Training: Once the service member is cleared for service, they then proceed through their requisite training programs and enter their operational units. There they continue with constant on-the-job training, field exercises, deployments, and further education during their tenure in service.

D. Promotion and reenlistment: Service members must be selectively promoted to the next higher ranks and reenlist or face discharge from service after their initial service obligation.

E. Separation: If the service member faces conduct or behavioral problems while in service, they may face involuntary separation at any time during service. If the service member develops a health condition deemed incompatible with continued military service, they may be separated or retired via the Medical Evaluation Board. Here they may be assigned a disability status with the Department of Veterans Affairs (VA), resulting in additional benefits and compensation.

F. Retirement: The service member is typically eligible for retirement starting at 20 years of service and is required to retire after 30 years. Pension is determined based on salary and length of service.

MILITARY EXPOSURES

A. Life in the military is stressful and full of occupational exposures, requiring an expanded healthcare lens to think beyond typical occupational exposures that civilian counterparts do not experience.
1. Exposures occur in the workplace, in the training environment, where they live, and on deployment.
2. Exposures may include diesel fuel, inhalants, radiation, asbestos, industrial solvents, coolants, and lead paint.

B. Cause and effect relationships related to exposures are integral in determining the risk of adverse health outcomes.

1. Hearing loss is a primary source of occupationally derived injury in the military. Those at greater risk for hearing loss include men, those who have deployed, and those who have suffered acoustic trauma from improvised explosive devices (IEDs).
2. Those who suffer from blast trauma are also at risk for ocular trauma; 78% of all eye injuries from the wars post-9/11 resulted from blast.
3. Musculoskeletal injuries, diseases, and injuries continue to account for many medical encounters in the military medical health system. These injuries can be explained by the expectation of constant physical and field training and worsened by working in austere and deployed environments.

C. Toxic exposures can occur during deployments, some unique to the service member who served in wartime activities.
1. Potential exposure to Agent Orange for those who served in Vietnam. Nineteen million gallons of Agent Orange, an herbicidal defoliant, used by the U.S. Air Force, were sprayed over 9,000 miles of Vietnam to rid the North Vietnamese Army of the protective cover of vegetation and food.
   a. Agent Orange contains 2,3,7,8-tetrachlorodibenzop-dioxin, responsible for the adverse health outcomes of these exposed veterans.
   b. Health outcomes include bladder cancer, chronic B-cell leukemia, Hodgkin disease, multiple myeloma, non-Hodgkin lymphoma, prostate cancer, respiratory cancers, some soft tissue sarcomas, Parkinson, high blood pressure, and diabetes.
2. In the 1990 to 1991 Gulf War, 250,000 U.S. service members became ill from many unexplained and chronic symptoms. These included rashes, fatigue, gastrointestinal (GI) issues, muscle and joint pain, and neurologic problems.
   a. In May 2022, genetic research confirmed that Gulf War syndrome was caused by exposure to the fallout and plume from bombing a chemical weapons storage and production facility (sarin gas).
3. During the wars after 9/11, two unique exposures created the opportunity for adverse health outcomes: exposure to depleted uranium (DU) and burn pits.
   a. DU: DU is a by-product of uranium enrichment products and is used in military munitions.
      i. Exposure occurs when drinking contaminated water, inhaling fumes, or being wounded with DU munitions.
   b. Burn pits: Open-air burning of trash and solid waste occurred in Southwest Asia, Afghanistan, and other forward-deployed areas.
      i. Health outcomes include neurologic deficits, insomnia, allergies, hypertension, and cancers.
      ii. Information on the assessment and registries for military exposures can be found on the VA website (www.publichealth.va.gov/exposures/index.asp). Registration for these exposures may afford veteran healthcare eligibility, disability compensation, and other VA benefits.

MILITARY FAMILY

A. The military family consists of immediate and extended families of active-duty service members, members of the National Guard and Reserve, veterans, and those who have lost their lives in service.

B. Acknowledgment of the exposures and stress placed on the service member led to the institution of the federally funded Family Readiness Groups in 1950 to provide support and information to families.
C. Military family members outnumber those who have served. As of 2020, there are 15,669,841. The military family endures a great deal of uncertainty, change, and stress.
  a. Risks to children include neglect and abuse, secondary trauma related to exposure to their family member's injuries or posttraumatic stress disorder (PTSD), bullying, and the potential for deteriorating academic achievement.
  b. Risks to partners and spouses include limited access to support systems, potential economic disruption, lack of cultural engagement, and feeling of being unrecognized in a community.
  c. Spouses may face higher rates of mental health disorders such as depression, anxiety, and insomnia.

MILITARY AND VETERAN HEALTHCARE

MILITARY HEALTHCARE
A. The Defense Health Agency (DHA) is the headquarter for all military treatment facilities. The goal/requirement is to provide:
  1. A *ready medical force* ensuring medical personnel are ready to deploy and provide the medical skill necessary for the operational setting
  2. Improve performance through the quadruple aim strategy: (a) improved readiness, (b) improved population health, (c) the experience of care for both the patient and the healthcare provider, and (d) reduced cost.
B. Military treatment facilities meet all national standards and certifications to provide quality care compared with civilian institutions.

VETERANS' HEALTH AFFAIRS
A. When transitioning from active-duty to civilian status, understanding the healthcare system can be overwhelming for a veteran. When service members separate or retire from the military, they are *not* automatically qualified or entitled to medical care with the VA healthcare system. The requirements can be found at www.va.gov/health-care/eligibility.
B. The VA is the most extensive healthcare system in the United States. The VA has medical centers and outpatient clinics. Once eligible for VA healthcare, a veteran can receive care from primary care managers and specialists. The VA MISSION Act of 2018 created reform in the VA to improve access to care for veterans.
  1. A veteran can receive care through community healthcare providers if they meet specific eligibility requirements (VA does not provide service, does not meet accessibility standards, or is not within driving distance).

CHALLENGES
A. Challenges associated with caring for the active-duty and veteran population include clinicians' lack of cultural competency, focus on readiness, access to care, and encouraging veterans to seek treatment.
B. Caring for this large population who have served during different decades and different wars can make it difficult for clinicians to understand their service's intricacies. In addition, this population lives worldwide, requiring clinicians from all specialties to have a breadth of cultural competency for this population.
C. While the MISSION Act enables veterans to access specialty care as needed, specialty care outside the VA may have longer wait times, may lead to duplicative tests and procedures, and is associated with difficulty in accessing health information from other electronic health records.
D. Service members and veterans are less likely to seek care due to long wait times for appointments, difficulty with paperwork, and difficulty navigating the healthcare system.

CLINICAL APPLICATION OF MILITARY CULTURAL COMPETENCE

A. The warrior ethos and military culture is one that values collectivism amid an American individualistic society, thus making it crucial for healthcare providers to be aware of potential implicit bias. The unit, the mission, and the team come first.
  1. The service member knows that if they take time out to care for themselves, their absence might impact their unit.
  2. They might be perceived as "weak," which adds to the stigma of seeking care. This stigma is amplified when the veteran may have been troubled with mental health symptoms.
  3. The military operational readiness model is founded on "resilience" modeling algorithms.
  4. Personal readiness for training and deployment as well as suitability are framed by preserving and maintaining health behaviors within and across physical, emotional, social, spiritual, and family dimensions essential to personal readiness.
B. While it can be uplifting to be "resilient," it can also be exhausting to maintain this status. Some view the military resiliency model as a zero-failure or black-or-white mentality in which one is either resilient or not resilient, which furthers unwillingness to seek healthcare within the military health system.
C. Reluctance to seek care has secondary and tertiary effects. If the service member fails to seek care, there is no record of the illness or injury. If there is no record, the VHA remains unaware and unable to assess the veteran for service-connected disability. Additionally, as service members fail to engage in the immediacy of care, their physical and mental health erodes, impacting family and unit capabilities.

CULTURAL ASSESSMENT
A. Performing a culturally sensitive assessment for veterans encompasses the same principles as assessing a patient from any other cultural background.
  1. The first task of the healthcare provider is to verify that the patient self-identifies as a veteran. If they do not, ask if they have served. Then ascertain which branch they served with. Next, ensure that they wish to identify with that culture or group.
  2. Ask if they feel safe speaking about their experiences.
  3. Engage in trauma-informed care. Use assumption and judgment-free assessment strategies and questions.
  4. Ensure that personal biases and beliefs are set aside from the assessment. Sharing personal beliefs can potentially erode the therapeutic relationship and create opportunities for adverse outcomes in clinical care.
B. Additional competencies are available when assessing military family members. The *I SERVE 2: A Pocketcard for Healthcare Providers Caring for Military* and *Serving on the Homefront* was developed by nurse practitioners and researchers

invested in military family care (https://dbhds.virginia.gov/assets/doc/bh/msmvf/i-serve2card_virginia-edition.pdf). Questions on each pocket card guide the clinician in ascertaining risks and exposures to the military family member and their children to prompt appropriate referrals.

MENTAL HEALTH DISORDERS SPECIFIC TO THE VETERAN POPULATION

Veterans and survivors of war face a higher risk for various mental health conditions compared with the civilian population. The prevalence of suicide, PTSD, and substance abuse disorder (SUD) among veterans is especially high, with significant numbers who seek mental healthcare due to distressing experiences such as deployment and combat. Witnessing traumatic events and separation from family and other support systems add to the stress of military life. Diagnosis of depression cases has increased significantly among military personnel.

VETERAN SUICIDE
A. Veterans are at particular risk of mental health struggles, with a suicide rate that is 1.5 times higher than that of the overall U.S. population. According to the 2021 National Veteran Suicide Prevention Annual Report, fewer than 50 percent of returning veterans who need mental health treatment receive it (Office of Mental Health and Suicide Prevention, 2021). The U.S. DOD and VA have prioritized suicide prevention.

Assessment
A. Assessing the risk factors and protective factors and stratifying the risk are critical to developing an evidence-based plan of care for the veteran to ensure safety and optimal outcomes.
B. Screening for suicide is complex. In those who died by suicide, only 24% had a mental health diagnosis in the weeks before their death; only one-third had healthcare visits in the 7 days prior to suicide; primary care and outpatient visits were the most common.
C. The use of a well-validated screening tool is recommended to identify those who are at risk for suicide and suicide-related behavior. The Columbia-Suicide Severity Rating Scale (C-SSRS) is a validated, evidence-based screening tool that is recommended for use in the veteran population. It is available for use in 114 languages.
D. Asking about suicide does *not* increase the risk of suicide. If the patient screens positive for suicidal thoughts, evaluate the patient for intent, plan, means, and past suicidal experiences. If the patient has a positive overall screen for suicidal ideation, intent, or means, a more comprehensive evaluation of those risk and protective factors is recommended.
E. Risk stratification is part of a comprehensive assessment package and can help think about and communicate suicide risk (see www.mirecc.va.gov/visn19/trm).

Treatment and Prevention
A. Interventions for suicide vary depending on the stratification of risk. There are nonpharmacologic and pharmacologic options for care.
   1. Suicide safety plan: A collaborative management strategy for developing coping strategies and support systems during times of high risk for suicide is called a *suicide safety plan*. There is a mobile app titled SAMHSA Suicide Safe available on Google Play and the App Store or at www.ptsd.va.gov/appvid/mobile/safety_plan_app.asp. In any patient who has suicidal ideation or who is in crisis, a comprehensive risk assessment should be completed first. Then collaborate with the patient to develop a plan, acknowledging any potential barriers to enacting the plan.
      a. Include warning signs for suicide, coping strategies, social support contacts, family member contacts, professional contacts, and ideas to make the environment safe.
      b. When collaborating with the patient, ensure patient-centered care principles: open-ended questions, collaboration, and respect for the patient's values and beliefs.
      c. Use the patient's own words and ideas when developing the plan, problem-solve to address any roadblocks to the utilization of the plan, identify the likelihood of how and when the patient will use the plan, role-play, and attend to the patient's environment of care.
      d. Limit access to lethal means such as weapons, guns, and medications that the patient has considered in their suicide planning.
   2. Cognitive behavioral therapy (CBT): CBT is an evidence-based therapeutic intervention for reducing suicidal ideation and focuses on how the patient thinks about their stressors and environment. It teaches them to challenge their negative cognitions. It is framed by the stress diathesis model for reducing suicidal behaviors. The diathesis for suicide is based on a combination of genetic and environmental influences and exposures, including current support systems.
      a. CBT programs for suicide are delivered in person or via the internet; both are efficacious in mitigating suicidal ideation and behaviors.
   3. Pharmacologic management: In patients with mixed psychiatric conditions, the addition of lithium resulted in a reduction of the odds of suicide when compared with no intervention or placebo. Clozapine also reduces the odds of suicide in those diagnosed with a mental health disorder.

Barriers to Seeking Care
A. Barriers to care include but are not limited to perceptual, attitudinal, and structural barriers.
   1. Perceptual barriers are the top reasons veterans and nonveterans face barriers to care due to individuals lacking a perceived need for mental healthcare.
   2. Attitudinal barriers include a desire to handle one's problems independently of outside care. Individuals may additionally source their perceived lack of severity of illness as an attitudinal barrier believing that one's mental health will improve without intervention or treatment. The stigma around receiving mental healthcare is another barrier to care for all mental illnesses.
   3. Logistical and structural barriers can include a lack of available mental health and primary care providers, long wait times to access care, long drive times to reach VA facilities in rural communities, inability to access care due to illness or lack of broadband internet capabilities, and lack of hospital bed space or insurance.

B. Barriers to care should be addressed and mitigated by utilizing a patient-centered approach.
1. Management strategies include performing universal stratified suicide risk assessments at every visit, even in primary care.
2. A comprehensive evaluation for stressors and protective factors and culturally sensitive collaborative treatment plans are essential in mitigating suicidal behaviors.
3. Allowing the veteran to involve their military and veteran family and friends for a support system in a trajectory of well-being and optimal outcomes helps facilitate connectedness and reduce the likelihood of veteran suicide.

MILITARY SEXUAL TRAUMA

A. *Military sexual trauma* (*MST*) is a term established by the U.S. VA based on federal law and encompasses sexual harassment or sexual assault that occurs during military service. MST includes occurrence on and off duty and on or off military installations. MST perpetrators can be anyone, including individuals of any gender, military personnel, civilians, strangers, friends, or intimate partners.
B. In fiscal year 2021, 8.4% of active-duty women and 1.5% of activity-duty men surveyed reported experiencing unwanted sexual contact in the previous 12 months. Universal screening data from the VA estimate that 1 in 3 women and 1 in 50 men have reported military sexual assault during their service.
C. MST is not a diagnosis; however, the experience of MST is associated with problematic mental and physical health outcomes.
1. Reactions may vary depending on several factors: the type of abuse, if it were an isolated event or repeated event, if there was violence, if the event was reported, individual and institutional responses to the victim, and the victim's history of previous trauma.
2. Diagnoses associated with MST include PTSD, depression, substance use disorder, eating disorders, and physical health problems (e.g., headaches, pelvic pain, GI distress, chronic fatigue).
3. Other problems include relationship distress, employment problems, and a crisis of faith.
D. An individualized, trauma-focused approach to the mental health and medical treatment and care of individuals who have experienced MST strengthens the patient–healthcare provider relationship and the well-being of the service member or veteran.

Barriers to Seeking Care

A. MST is underreported, with an increased impact in the military community due to the increased risk of sexual victimization compared with civilian individuals.
B. Stigma-related barriers are more contributory to psychopathology than logistical barriers. The focus of military culture on values that promote strength and masculinity can create unique barriers based on fear of victimhood/weakness, resulting in an impact on career or image as a service member/veteran, which should be considered in the treatment and access to care for MST.
C. Traditional logistical barriers are seen in reporting and seeking care for MST, such as transportation, affordability, and access; however, the intersection of anticipated public stigma and military culture results in barriers more specific to MST.

BOX 25.1 SCREENING FOR MILITARY SEXUAL TRAUMA

"While you were in the military..."
Did you receive uninvited and unwanted sexual attention, such as touching, cornering, pressure for sexual favors, or verbal remarks?
Did someone ever use force or threat of force to have sexual contact with you against your will?
An affirmative response to either item is a positive screen for military sexual trauma.
A positive screen does not indicate the veteran's current subjective distress, diagnosis, interest in, or need for treatment.

Source: Street, A., & Stafford, J. (2013, July). Military sexual trauma information for behavioral health providers: Information from the National Center for PTSD—Military sexual trauma: Issues in caring for veterans. National Center for Posttraumatic Stress Disorders. https://www.mirecc.va.gov/cih-visn2/Documents/Provider_Education_Handouts/Military_Sexual_Trauma_Information_Sheet_for_BHPs_Version_3.pdf

Screening and Assessment

A. The VHA's approach consists of universal screening for MST and is considered to be best practice in the care of service members and veterans (Box 25.1).
B. Screening should be performed in a comfortable, private environment and include a clear understanding of MST. Including a rationale for universal screening normalizes the process, and MST screening is best received when delivered concisely and nonjudgmentally. As MST is not a diagnosis, assessment should include a functional assessment, including basic information about the MST experience and the individual's priorities for treatment and diagnostic assessment.

Treatment and Resources

A. MST is associated with many adverse mental health outcomes (e.g., PTSD, depression, anxiety, substance use disorders, eating disorders, dissociative disorders, and personality disorders).
B. Treatment should be individualized and focused on the mental and physical outcomes of experiencing MST.
C. Treatment should align with the best practices for the diagnostic criteria met by the individual as not all individuals who experience MST will develop psychopathology.
D. Consider the adverse impacts on physical and sexual health and the subsequent effect on the individual's mental well-being. Due to high prevalence, prioritize PTSD and suicidal ideation in the diagnostic assessment of the individual who has experienced MST.
E. Treatment of MST begins with establishing safety and rapport with the healthcare provider and treatment team, addressing the patient's basic needs for stabilization, and managing interpersonal relationships.
1. Initiate trauma-informed care using PTSD or diagnostic-specific psychotherapy approaches, such as CBT, prolonged exposure, and eye movement desensitization and reprocessing (EMDR) therapies.
2. A final component of care focuses on reintegration into the community, including integrating loved ones and the individual's support system into their care.
3. The process of coping, processing, and reconnecting highlights the need to ensure adequate boundaries and skills for the individual to utilize before initiating trauma processing, if indicated.

F. The VA provides robust MST resources for healthcare providers and veterans, including accessibility to free care and an MST coordinator at each facility to guide care or local resources.

G. It is normal for healthcare providers to have strong reactions when working with trauma survivors, making clinician self-care an essential priority. Clinicians should utilize formal support (e.g., a team approach) and informal support (e.g., consultation with colleagues) to support themselves when treating individuals with MST.

POSTTRAUMATIC STRESS DISORDER

A. PTSD was not codified by the American Psychiatric Association until 1980, but it is believed that the veteran descriptions of shell shock from World War I, war neurosis from World War II, and combat fatigue from the Vietnam War exemplify the qualifying *Diagnostic and Statistical Manual of Mental Disorders*, Fifth Edition (*DSM-5*; American Psychiatric Association, 2013), symptoms. Exposures to a traumatic event followed by psychological distresses are qualifying criteria.

B. Patient presentations are unique and varying. Some might present with more reoccurring symptoms, some with more behavioral/reactive symptoms, and some with more thought distortions.

C. See Chapter 9, "Anxiety Disorders," for information on treatment of PTSD.

TRAUMATIC BRAIN INJURY

A. Traumatic brain injury (TBI) is an injury that occurs because of an external force, typically caused by falls, accidents, sports injuries, and military conflicts. TBI is a significant cause of mortality and disability among service members and veterans. Military members are not only vulnerable to TBI due to motor vehicle accidents, falls, or assaults, exposure to combat-related exposures such as blasts or explosive devices is also a risk to service members while deployed or during training.

B. Explosive or blast devices, a significant source of military casualties in Iraq and Afghanistan, were responsible for approximately two-thirds of all U.S. service members killed and wounded. They are a varied group of brain injuries; the causality, severity, pathogenesis, and resulting outcomes are clinically different for every person affected.

C. Direct and indirect traumatic forces can cause brain damage. Direct forces such as a bullet, shrapnel, or blunt trauma to the head can cause focal injury to brain tissue. Indirect forces, such as acceleration/deceleration and rotational head movement, result in the brain being "shaken" within its casing.
   1. Acceleration/deceleration is responsible for damage to the gray matter on the brain's surface, causing cortical contusions and bleeding, while rotational forces are more likely to cause deep cerebral white matter injury, called *diffuse axonal injury*, via physical stretch or shearing.
   2. Both direct and indirect forces constitute the primary injury or the immediate effects of these forces on brain tissue.

D. Secondary injuries result from the consequent inflammatory cascade of physiologic responses to the primary injury. This secondary reaction, designed to be neuroprotective and promote healing, can become maladaptive, resulting in vascular damage, edema, hypoxia, tissue destruction, and permanent neurologic dysfunction, and interferes with neurogenesis.

E. TBI has three categories (Table 25.2): (a) mild, (b) moderate, and (c) severe.

F. Acute symptom resolution in patients with TBI usually occurs within several days to weeks after the initial injury. If symptoms persist, the cluster of unresolved symptoms is called *persistent postconcussive syndrome*. The clinical symptoms associated with persistent postconcussive syndrome are grouped into three categories:
   1. Somatic symptoms: These include headache, fatigue, sensitivity to light or noise, sleep disturbances, drowsiness, dizziness, and visual disturbances.
   2. Cognitive disturbances: These include memory difficulties and problems concentrating.
   3. Psychological symptoms: These include emotional liability, irritability, anxiety, and depression.

G. TBI is a significant cause of mortality and disability in the U.S. military. The incidence of TBI in the military population is disputed.
   1. 20% of those who have served since 9/11 have sustained a TBI.
   2. There have been 450,000 service members diagnosed with TBI since 2000; most cases were categorized as "mild" (82.2%) and disproportionately concentrated within the U.S. Army population.
   3. The highest incidence of TBI in the military for those who have never deployed and those who have previously deployed are in service members who work in combat-specific or armor/motor transport occupations.

H. TBI is associated with PTSD, with adverse mental health and physical outcomes, neurodegenerative disorders, damaging quality of life, and overall poor health ratings. Additionally, those with TBI are more likely to be medically retired than those with other combat-related disabilities, decreasing the overall readiness of the U.S. military.

I. Blast-related TBI: Proximity to blasts and explosions is an occupational hazard for veterans and military service members.
   1. Blast-related TBI results from exposure to a detonated explosive device that has produced pressure waves and acoustic, electromagnetic, light, and thermal energies. Blast-related TBI can result in four types of injuries:

TABLE 25.2 TRAUMATIC BRAIN INJURY SEVERITY

Category	Loss of Consciousness	Glasgow Coma Scale	Posttraumatic Amnesia	Structural Imaging
Mild	Less than 30 minutes	13–15	Less than 24 hours	Normal
Moderate	30 minutes–24 hours	9–12	1–7 days	Abnormal, transient changes
Severe	More than 24 hours	3–8	More than 7 days	Abnormal, lasting changes

a. Primary: the transmission of the blast pressure wave to the brain
b. Secondary: consists of penetration of projectiles through the skull and into the brain
c. Tertiary: related to acceleration/deceleration effects (getting thrown into a fixed surface)
d. Quaternary: through thermal, chemical, and other injuries to the head, face, and respiratory tract

2. The mechanism of injury for the primary blast injury occurs due to shock waves that travel across the tissue, causing acceleration deformation of the tissue or by the indirect transmission of kinetic energy.
3. The level of injury sustained from an event is multifactorial: distance from the explosion, the amount of blast energy released, the level of personal protection worn, the number of exposures, and environmental factors (open vs. closed spaces).
4. Management depends on the severity and type of symptom that has manifested, with a focus on early identification and return to work/activity after resolution of symptoms.
5. Clinical signs and symptoms of blast-related TBI are difficult to predict. However, vestibular ocular motor screening (VOMS) with sports and military patients with brain injury successfully detects signs and symptoms of concussion.
a. Those who have been exposed to mild blast TBI exhibit abnormalities of white brain matter structural integrity, more frequent and severe postconcussive symptoms (headache, confusion, amnesia, difficulty concentrating, and short-term memory loss), reduced cerebral glucose metabolism, eye trauma, tinnitus and hearing impairment, and vestibular symptoms.
b. There is evidence that those exposed to blast injuries experience changes in noradrenaline and serotonin. This disruption leads to many neurocognitive symptoms, including processing speed, learning and memory, and executive function.

J. Repetitive mild TBI: The risk of repetitive mild TBI is significant for military service members. They run the risk of exposure to blast and focal TBI from training exercises, deployment-related activities, and sports-related activities (e.g., football, hockey, rugby).
1. Those exposed to repetitive mild TBI are at increased risk for the following: neurodegenerative diseases, chronic traumatic encephalopathy, functional impairment, more persistent cognitive deficits, slower rates of learning, more progressive behavioral impairments, depression, and longer recovery time.
2. Additionally, they have a triple incidence of subsequent concussions after experiencing three or more prior concussions. Repeated exposures are associated with significantly longer reaction times, lower neurocognitive performance scores, and increased symptom reporting.

Barriers to Seeking Care

A. Most who seek care for their injuries do so within days to weeks following the injury. However, some do not seek care within that window of time.
B. During the high operational tempo in deployed and combat settings, a medical illness and failure to return to duty may significantly impact the service member's intent to seek treatment. This stigma and the warrior ethos create continued barriers to seeking care for those who suffer from head injuries in the military and veteran populations.
C. Of those who suffered concussions, only 52% sought care. Of those who did not seek care, 62% had a health belief that the injury was not severe enough to warrant care, and 18% believed that if they sought help it might impact their military career—28% of those with mild TBI reported stigma in seeking care (Escolas et al., 2020).

Screening and Assessment

A. The Boston Assessment of Traumatic Brain Injury-Lifetime (BAT-L; https://heartbrain.hms.harvard.edu/bat-l-boston-assessment-traumatic-brain-injury-lifetime) is available to evaluate and diagnose TBIs in the veteran population. It includes a comprehensive assessment of blast and non–blast-related TBIs over the veteran's lifetime and any postconcussive sequelae.
B. All individuals presenting with postconcussive symptoms should be assessed for cognitive, physical, and behavioral changes (Table 25.3). Once finished with the screening, educate the veteran and family members (if relevant) of the status of their evaluation and available resources in the area, and then work toward a consensus decision on the veteran's desired treatment goals.

Treatment and Resources

A. The Defense and Veterans Brain Injury Center's (DVBIC) mission is to provide research, clinical acumen, and education on military-related TBI. The DVBIC is a network of 18 clinical sites established in 1992 by Congressional mandate.
B. The Centers for Disease Control and Prevention has information on TBI and concussion, including patient and healthcare provider education and statistical data on incidence, prevalence, and risks.
C. The VA and the DOD have a joint clinical practice guideline for the management of concussion and mild TBI published in 2016 and updated in 2021. A pocket card is part of the clinical practice guideline (www.healthquality.va.gov/guidelines/Rehab/mtbi/mTBICPGClinicianPocketCard50821816.pdf) that guides the healthcare provider through assessment and management algorithms unique to the military veteran's care. Management strategy guidelines are available for each significant symptom cluster common to concussions/mild TBI, including headache, dizziness, tinnitus, visual symptoms, sleep disturbance, behavioral disturbances, cognitive symptoms, fatigue, and hearing and hearing olfactory deficits.

TABLE 25.3 COMMON SYMPTOMS PRESENT AFTER TRAUMATIC BRAIN INJURY/POSTCONCUSSIVE SYMPTOMS

Cognitive Deficits	Behavioral	Physical
Attention Concentration Executive function Judgment Language Memory Perception Speech Visual spatial function	Agitation or aggression Anxiety Depression Disinhibition Irritability	Ataxia Blurry vision Dizziness Fatigue Headaches Noise/light sensitivity Sleep disturbance Tinnitus

REFERRAL SOURCES

A. During the transition from active-duty to civilian life, there is an opportunity to provide additional services to assist the service member. Any service member is eligible to receive benefits through the program.

B. The *In Transition* is a program designed to assist service members who need mental health resources, coaching, and other help associated with permanent change of station (PCS) moves, coming home from or going to a deployment, transitioning from active-duty to reserve component service, and those who are preparing to leave the military.

C. The *In Transition* program can be accessed via many military websites, including health.mil, militaryonesource.mil, woundedwarrior.mil, and others. Communication with the *In Transition* program provides free resources including a licensed psychological health clinician/coach and is confidential. Any psychiatric-mental health nurse practitioner (PMHNP) can refer a service member to the program. Skilled counselors and coaches are assigned to all service members referred to the *In Transition* program.

D. For veterans navigating the VHA for benefits, refer them to the nearest VSO. Over 100 officially VA-recognized VSOs work closely with the VA in support of the military veteran. No two VSOs are alike; they all have different missions and visions. However, they are alike in that they assist veterans in understanding their VA benefits and the claims process and readjusting to civilian life. The federal government does not operate VSOs, and the VA does not recognize all of them. It is recommended that veterans receive assistance from an accredited organization. Accredited VSOs have received training, obtained continuing education, and have been reviewed by the VA Office of General Counsel. An accredited VSO may provide legal representation for their disability claim or any other service. A list of the recognized VSOs is found here: www.va.gov/ve/docs/traditionalVeteranOrganizations.pdf.

E. The VA also has a program for homeless veterans or those experiencing housing instability. The program consists of coordinated outreach efforts seeking out homeless veterans, and connecting veterans with housing solutions, healthcare, community employment solutions, or any other necessary support. It allows collaboration with other federal, state, and local agencies to expand veterans' employment opportunities and housing options. The program has a $2 billion budget that supports 6,000 field positions, 100 homeless program office staff, and $700 million for contracts and grants. A list of all community resources and referral centers (CRRCs) for the VA homeless program can be found here: www.va.gov/HOMELESS/Crrc.asp. The VA homeless program's most recent results indicate an 11% decline in veteran homelessness since early 2020. One of the programs that assist in increasing housing options for veterans is the Shallow Subsidy Initiative, a group of 238 nonprofit organizations that provide rental assistance to low-income veterans. The VA uses a "Housing First" approach, which prioritizes housing so they can tend to necessities (food) before getting a job or addressing their substance/mental health issues (Liu, 2023). The "Housing First" approach has undergone domestic and international studies and multiple literature reviews, resulting in clear evidence demonstrating the practical solution to homelessness.

RESOURCES

MILITARY CULTURAL COMPETENCIES

A. Center for Deployment Psychology: https://deploymentpsych.org/military-culture-course-modules
B. Veterans Administration Community Provider Toolkit: www.mentalhealth.va.gov/communityproviders
C. PsychArmor: https://psycharmor.org
D. D'Aoust, R. F., & Rossiter, A. G. (2021). *Caring for veterans and their families: A guide for nurses and healthcare professionals.* Jones & Bartlett Learning. The Military Family.
E. Cozza, S. J., Goldenberg, M. N., & Ursano, R. J. (Eds.). (2014). *Care of military service members, veterans, and their families.* American Psychiatric Pub.
F. Sheehy, S. and Schwartz, L. S. (2021). *Ask the question: "have you ever served?" Caring for military members and veterans in civilian healthcare.* https://doi.org/10.1097/01.NURSE.0000795268.34720.a9

CLINICAL PRACTICE GUIDELINES FOR VETERAN RELATED ILLNESSES

A. VA website: www.healthquality.va.gov

MILITARY-RELATED EXPOSURES

A. VA website: www.publichealth.va.gov/exposures

POSTTRAUMATIC STRESS DISORDER

A. National Center for PTSD and Veterans: www.ptsd.va.gov/understand/common/common_Veterans.asp
B. Wounded Warrior Project: www.woundedwarriorproject.org/programs/mental-wellness/Veteran-ptsd-treatment-support-resources
C. Cohen Veterans Network: www.cohenVeteransnetwork.org

TRAUMATIC BRAIN INJURY

A. Traumatic Brain Injury Center of Excellence: https://health.mil/Military-Health-Topics/Centers-of-Excellence/Traumatic-Brain-Injury-Center-of-Excellence
B. BrainLine: www.brainline.org/resource/defense-and-Veterans-brain-injury-center-0
C. Defense and Veterans Brain Injury Center: www.militaryonesource.mil/resources/gov/defense-center-of-excellence-for-traumatic-brain-injury
D. Brain Injury Family Caregiver Guide: www.health.mil/Reference-Center/Publications/2021/07/07/Traumatic-Brain-Injury-A-Guide-for-Caregivers-of-Service-Members-and-Veterans

IN TRANSITION/TRANSITION ASSISTANCE

A. Military OneSource: www.militaryonesource.mil/transition-retirement/separation/transition-assistance-programs-and-resources
B. USO Pathfinder Transition Program: www.uso.org/programs/uso-pathfinder-transition-program

DEPARTMENT OF VETERANS AFFAIRS DISABILITY INFORMATION

A. VA Disability Information: www.va.gov/disability
B. VA Website Information on how to file a claim: www.va.gov/disability/how-to-file-claim

VETERAN SERVICE ORGANIZATIONS

A. VA Accredited VSO Representative List by State: www.benefits.va.gov/vso/varo.asp

VETERAN HOMELESS ORGANIZATIONS
A. VA Homeless Programs: www.va.gov/homeless

VETERAN CRISIS INFORMATION
A. Veterans Crisis Line (Dial 988 then Press 1): www.Veteranscrisisline.net
B. VA Suicide Prevention: www.va.gov/health-care/health-needs-conditions/mental-health/suicide-prevention

VETERAN SUICIDE
A. VA/DoD Clinical Practice Guideline: www.healthquality.va.gov/guidelines/MH/srb/index.asp
B. Columbia-Suicide Severity Rating Scale (C-SSRS): www.samhsa.gov/resource/dbhis/columbia-suicide-severity-rating-scale-c-ssrs
C. VA Health Systems Research: Suicide Prevention: www.hsrd.research.va.gov/research_topics/suicide.cfm

REFERENCES AND BIBLIOGRAPHY

Agoston, D., Arun, P., Bellgowan, P., Broglio, S., Cantu, R., Cook, D., da Silva, U. O., Dickstein, D., Elder, G., & Fudge, E. (2017). Military blast injury and chronic neurodegeneration: Research presentations from the 2015 International State-of-the-Science Meeting. *Journal of Neurotrauma*, 34(S1), S-6–S-17. https://doi.org/10.1089/neu.2017.5220

American Psychiatric Association. (2013). *Diagnostic and statistical manual of mental disorders* (5th ed.). https://doi.org/10.1176/appi.books.9780890425596

Anderson-Barnes, V. C., Weeks, S. R., & Tsao, J. W. (2010). Mild traumatic brain injury update. *Continuum: Lifelong Learning in Neurology*, 16(6), 17–26. https://doi.org/10.1212/01.CON.0000391450.48225.73

Averill, L. A., Fleming, C. E., Holens, P. L., & Larsen, S. E. (2015). Research on PTSD prevalence in OEF/OIF veterans: Expanding investigation of demographic variables. *European Journal of Psychotraumatology*, 6(1), 27322. https://doi.org/10.3402/ejpt.v6.27322

Belanger, H. G., Kretzmer, T., Yoash-Gantz, R., Pickett, T., & Tupler, L. A. (2009). Cognitive sequelae of blast-related versus other mechanisms of brain trauma. *Journal of the International Neuropsychological Society*, 15(1), 1–8. https://doi.org/10.1017/S1355617708090036

Clever, M., & Segal, D. R. (2013). The demographics of military children and families. *The Future of Children*, 13–39. https://doi.org/10.1353/foc.2013.0018

D'Anci, K. E., Uhl, S., Giradi, G., & Martin, C. (2019). Treatments for the prevention and management of suicide: A systematic review. *Annals of Internal Medicine*, 171(5), 334–342. https://doi.org/10.7326/M19-0869

Escolas, S. M., Luton, M., Ferdosi, H., Chavez, B. D., & Engel, S. D. (2020). Traumatic brain injuries: Unreported and untreated in an army population. *Military Medicine*, 185(Suppl. 1), 154–160. https://doi.org/10.1093/milmed/usz259

Finley, E. P., Noël, P. H., Mader, M., Haro, E., Bernardy, N., Rosen, C. S., Bollinger, M., Garcia, H., Sherrieb, K., & Pugh, M. J. V. (2017). Community clinicians and the veterans choice program for PTSD care: Understanding provider interest during early implementation. *Medical Care*, 55, S61–S70. https://doi.org/10.1097/MLR.0000000000000668

Fulton, J. J., Calhoun, P. S., Wagner, H. R., Schry, A. R., Hair, L. P., Feeling, N., Elbogen, E., & Beckham, J. C. (2015). The prevalence of posttraumatic stress disorder in operation enduring freedom/operation Iraqi freedom (OEF/OIF) Veterans: A meta-analysis. *Journal of Anxiety Disorders*, 31, 98–107. https://doi.org/10.1016/j.janxdis.2015.02.003

Greer, N., Sayer, N., Kramer, M., Koeller, E., & Velasquez, T. (2017). *Prevalence and epidemiology of combat blast injuries from the military cohort 2001–2014*. Department of Veterans Affairs (US)

Haley, R. W., Kramer, G., Xiao, J., Dever, J. A., & Teiber, J. F. (2022). Evaluation of a gene–environment interaction of PON1 and low-level nerve agent exposure with Gulf War illness: A prevalence case–control study drawn from the US military health survey's national population sample. *Environmental Health Perspectives*, 130(5), 057001. https://doi.org/10.1289/EHP9009

Hanrahan, N. P., Judge, K., Olamijulo, G., Seng, L., Lee, M., Wall, P. H., Leake, S. C., Czekanski, E., Thorne-Odem, S., & DeMartinis, E. E. (2017). The PTSD toolkit for nurses: Assessment, intervention, and referral of veterans. *The Nurse Practitioner*, 42(3), 46–55. https://doi.org/10.1097/01.NPR.0000488717.90314.62

Hoge, C. W., & Warner, C. H. (2014). Estimating PTSD prevalence in US veterans: Considering combat exposure, PTSD checklist cutpoints, and DSM-5. *The Journal of Clinical Psychiatry*, 75(12), 6657. https://doi.org/10.4088/JCP.14com09616

Liu, S. (2023, December 18). *VA's implementation of Housnig First over the years*. VA Homeless Programs: U.S. Department of Veterans Affairs. https://www.va.gov/HOMELESS/featuredarticles/VAs-Implementation-of-Housing-First.asp

McDiarmid, M. A., Gaitens, J. M., Hines, S., Condon, M., Roth, T., Oliver, M., Gucer, P., Brown, L., Centeno, J. A., & Dux, M. (2017). The US Department of veterans' affairs depleted uranium exposed cohort at 25 Years: Longitudinal surveillance results. *Environmental Research*, 152, 175–184. https://doi.org/10.1016/j.envres.2016.10.016

National Academies of Sciences Engineering Medicine. (2019). *Strengthening the military family readiness system for a changing American society*. National Academies Press.

Office of Mental Health and Suicide Prevention. (2021, September). 2021 national veteran suicide prevention annual report. U.S. Department of Veterans Affairs. https://www.mentalhealth.va.gov/docs/data-sheets/2021/2021-National-Veteran-Suicide-Prevention-Annual-Report-FINAL-9-8-21.pdf

Ouimette, P., Vogt, D., Wade, M., Tirone, V., Greenbaum, M. A., Kimerling, R., Laffaye, C., Fitt, J. E., & Rosen, C. S. (2011). Perceived barriers to care among veterans health administration patients with posttraumatic stress disorder. *Psychological Services*, 8(3), 212. https://doi.org/10.1037/a0024360

Peterson, A. L., Luethcke, C. A., Borah, E. V., Borah, A. M., & Young-McCaughan, S. (2011). Assessment and treatment of combat-related PTSD in returning war veterans. *Journal of Clinical Psychology in Medical Settings*, 18(2), 164–175. https://doi.org/10.1007/s10880-011-9238-3

Risdall, J. E., & Menon, D. K. (2011). Traumatic brain injury. *Philosophical Transactions of the Royal Society B: Biological Sciences*, 366(1562), 241–250. https://doi.org/10.1098/rstb.2010.0230. http://rstb.royalsocietypublishing.org/content/366/1562/241.full.pdf+html

Robinson-Freeman, K. E., Collins, K. L., Garber, B., Terblanche, R., Risling, M., Vermetten, E., Besemann, M., Mistlin, A., & Tsao, J. W. (2020). A decade of mTBI experience: What have we learned? A summary of proceedings from a NATO lecture series on military mTBI. *Frontiers in Neurology*, 11, 836. https://www.ncbi.nlm.nih.gov/pmc/articles/PMC7477387/pdf/fneur-11-00836.pdf

Rossiter, A. G., Dumas, M. A., Wilmoth, M. C., & Patrician, P. A. (2016). "I Serve 2": Meeting the needs of military children in civilian practice. *Nursing Outlook*, 64(5), 485–490. https://doi.org/10.1016/j.outlook.2016.05.011

Ruff, R., Ruff, S., & Wang, X. F. (2010). Veterans with mild TBI from combat explosions had persisting neurological deficits compared with veterans who had civilian TBI. *Brain Injury*, 24(3), 408–409.

Simmons, A. N., & Matthews, S. C. (2011). Neural circuitry of PTSD with or without mild traumatic brain injury: A meta-analysis. *Neuropharmacology*. https://doi.org/10.1016/j.neuropharm.2011.03.016

Sue, D. W., Sue, D., Neville, H. A., & Smith, L. (2022). *Counseling the culturally diverse: Theory and practice*. John Wiley & Sons.

Tanielian, T., Farris, C., Batka, C., Farmer, C. M., Robinson, E., Engel, C. C., Robbins, M., & Jaycox, L. H. (2014). *Ready to serve: Community-based provider capacity to deliver culturally competent, quality mental health care to veterans and their families*. RAND Corporation. https://www.rand.org/content/dam/rand/pubs/research_reports/RR800/RR806/RAND_RR806.pdf

Trockel, M., Karlin, B. E., Taylor, C. B., Brown, G. K., & Manber, R. (2015). Effects of cognitive behavioral therapy for insomnia on suicidal ideation in veterans. *Sleep*, 38(2), 259–265. https://doi.org/10.5665/sleep.4410

U.S. Department of Defense. (2022). *Annual report on sexual assault in the military (Fiscal Year, 2021)*. https://www.sapr.mil/reports

U.S. Department of Veterans Affairs. (2022a). *Help veterans overcome barriers to mental health treatment*. U.S. Department of Defense. https://www.mentalhealth.va.gov/suicide_prevention/docs/FSTP-Barriers.pdf

U.S. Department of Veterans Affairs. (2022b). *National veteran suicide prevention annual report*. U.S. Department of Defense. https://www.mentalhealth.va.gov/docs/data-sheets/2022/2022-National-Veteran-Suicide-Prevention-Annual-Report-FINAL-508.pdf

U.S. Department of Veterans Affairs. (2023). *Title 38: Pensions, bonuses, and veterans' relief (38 C.F.R. § 3.1)*. U.S. Government Publishing Office. https://www.ecfr.gov/current/title-38/part-3/section-3.1

U.S. Department of Veterans Affairs & Department of Defense. (2019). *VA/DOD clinical practice guidelines for the assessment and management of patients at risk for suicide*. U.S. Department of Defense. https://www.healthquality.va.gov/guidelines/MH/srb/VADoDSuicideRiskFullCPGFinal5088212019.pdf

Weiser, M., McCabe, P., Lomax, R., & Aubut, J. A. (2010). Blast injuries and traumatic brain injury. *Brain Injury*, 24(3), 349–350. https://doi.org/10.1007/s10439-011-0424-0

Wilkinson, S. T., Ballard, E. D., Bloch, M. H., Mathew, S. J., Murrough, J. W., Feder, A., Sos, P., Wang G., Zarate, Jr, C. A., & Sanacora, G. (2018). The effect of a single dose of intravenous ketamine on suicidal ideation: A systematic review and individual participant data meta-analysis. *American Journal of Psychiatry*, 175(2), 150–158. https://doi.org/10.1176/appi.ajp.2017.17040472

Wilson, L. C. (2018). The prevalence of military sexual trauma: A meta-analysis. *Trauma, Violence, & Abuse*, 19(5), 584–597. https://doi.org/10.1177/1524838016683459

26 PROVISION OF PSYCHIATRIC CARE IN ACUTE SETTINGS

Se Min Um

INTRODUCTION

Clinicians in the acute care setting face many challenges meeting the needs of the patients in both inpatient and outpatient environments. Interdisciplinary and interdepartmental collaboration in the inpatient setting, as well as engaging in meaningful collaborative care in the outpatient setting, helps establish guidelines for best practices in either setting while also supporting seamless transition in care. Patient-centered care guides the practice of including the patient and family into the provision of care and is associated with better patient outcomes. Identifying and understanding the inherent risk and protective factors within the specific population are crucial to delivering the necessary and appropriate care.

INPATIENT PSYCHIATRIC UNITS

A. Inpatient psychiatric units are acute care settings. These units are often stand-alone facilities or departments within a hospital.
B. Licensure for these units depends on the types of services provided to the population.
  1. Services can range according to age: from child and adolescent care to adult care
  2. Diagnosis and treatment: substance treatment and dual diagnosis treatment
  3. Level of care: intermediate adult care, long-term adult care, and forensic psychiatric care
  4. Type of admission: voluntary or involuntary
C. Treatment modalities and guidelines vary depending on the population served; patient/family-centered care is best practice.

UNDERSTANDING THE POPULATION

A. Understanding the makeup and needs of the patient population served is vital to planning and provision of psychiatric-mental healthcare.
B. Treatment modalities should be appropriate to the age and to physical and developmental levels of the patient.
  1. Evidence shows that group and individual therapies have an important role in the treatment and recovery than was previously believed.
  2. Interaction with peers, families, and clinicians in the milieu is more beneficial among members of like ages and cognitive development.
C. Treatment needs should be informed by the patient's symptoms.
  1. Treatment can include pharmacotherapy, group/individual therapy, and psychoeducation.
  2. Other treatment strategies should be based on short- and long-term symptom management.
D. Helping the patient return to or achieve a certain level of functioning should be the realistic goal.
  1. Goals are established with the patient.
  2. Families and caregivers should be informed of realistic goals so as to be able to understand limitations and possibilities and support the patient's recovery.
E. Symptoms help formulate a diagnosis, but each patient with the same diagnosis may not have the same needs.
  1. Treating the patient as a unique individual with unique needs and goals will help personalize the care given.
  2. Pharmacotherapy can be random in its results. Prescriber knowledge and experience often determines how quickly a patient can reach a good prognosis.
F. Treatment compliance can be a major barrier to recovery.
  1. Clinicians' soft skills, establishing a therapeutic environment and relationship with the patient, can be a key factor in improving compliance.
  2. Engaging the patient in the recovery process early and supporting an ongoing sense of self-efficacy improve compliance.
G. Disposition and aftercare collaboration are also barriers that social workers and case planners often contend with. By getting to know the patient and their capabilities, support, and needs, a realistic but feasible plan can be attained.
H. Age and physical and mental/cognitive developmental level of the patient are essential factors in determining the type of treatment modalities.
  1. Age and body weight of the individual are key factors in pharmacotherapy.
  2. Medication dosages are not only based on these factors but also on patient presentation and any other underlying conditions.
I. Psychoeducation must be based on the educational level of the patient and their family.
  1. A patient's inability to comprehend communication from the clinician puts treatment compliance at risk.
  2. Clinicians must assess and determine the patient and their family's level of understanding and their ability to follow instructions.
J. Tailor activities and therapies to the patient's physical abilities.
  1. Identify the patient's strengths and weaknesses.
     a. Underlying medical conditions can limit the patient's ability with certain modalities such as exercise, walking, and other physical activities such as singing, dancing, or painting.
     b. Knowing the patient's interest in an activity or modality of care can improve patient engagement.
  2. Participation in activities should be within the patient's level; certain conditions and medications may contribute to further physical limitations.
  3. Individual therapy and group therapy are proven components of psychiatric treatment.
     a. Individual and group therapy can help patients identify and understand their symptoms, medications, coping skills, and other strategies to help manage symptoms specific to their illness.

4. Patients diagnosed with mood disorders or other mental illnesses require psychoeducation to improve compliance with treatment and know when to seek help.
    a. Individual teaching can be beneficial to patients.
        i. Working with the individual is effective, especially patients with agoraphobia or anxiety. Individual teaching is also beneficial to review and evaluate.
        ii. Group teaching can guide and allow learning and feedback experiences while fostering a sense of community.
    b. Emphasize the person, not the diagnosis. Avoidance of stigmatizing words and phrases will increase the patient's sense of self-worth and community.
        i. Patients may feel ostracized and isolated due to their condition, but speaking with other people who are facing similar challenges can create a sense of unity and inclusion.
        ii. Using person-centered language can diminish the patient's sense of stigma.
            (a) This is quite common with substance users who carry a heavy stigma when referred to as criminals or "junkies" rather than an individual with a substance disorder.
        iii. Other words that have been identified as stigmatizing are "dirty urine" when talking about *positive urine drug tests*; "committing suicide" rather than stating *death by suicide*; "psychotic" rather than *someone with the lived experience of psychosis*; and "unsuccessful suicide attempt," which can be replaced by *survived a suicide*.
    c. Discussing emotional, personal, and traumatic life events that led to their worst moments within a nonjudgmental and accepting group can be cathartic and healing. This type of therapy has no objective measure and any sense of improvement in symptomology is subjective to the patient.
K. Understanding the community and setting is important in delivering appropriate care.
    1. The level of cultural diversity is likely to be greater within metropolitan city hospitals compared with hospitals in suburban areas.
    2. Culture and ethnicity may be specific to certain geographic areas. The socioeconomic status of patients may also differ depending on the hospital location.
    3. Violence, crime, homelessness, and substance use are factors to consider when treating patients, and the presentation can vary among communities.
L. Understanding the resources of the workforce as a community is also necessary in delivering appropriate care because the healthcare professional is also part of a community.
    1. Patients and staff members live and work in the same region and community.
    2. Things that are important to one community are often shared, acknowledged, or exposed to others.
        a. Awareness and understanding of cultural nuance can improve communication and establish therapeutic connections, thereby preventing negative experiences between the patient community and the healthcare community.

MYTHS AND UNCONSCIOUS BIASES

A. When discussing mental illness, a myth usually refers to a false belief or idea that is widely believed as true.

B. Implicit bias is a negative, prejudicial attitude that a person holds but is not consciously aware of. In the delivery of healthcare in a hospital setting, the presence of negative explicit and implicit bias toward patients who are marginalized due to race, ethnicity, or diagnosis can interfere with positive patient outcomes.
C. Treating patients with mental illnesses in hospital settings requires the clinician to actively combat the intrusion of implicit bias and myths.
D. The hospital or medical center can have trainings on implicit bias, but should also encourage the APRN to understand the local patient population cultures, actively avoid stereotyping, address bias when it appears, and be the unbiased voice of advocacy for the patient.
E. The Joint Commission emphasizes the following about implicit biases and myths:
    1. The Institute of Medicine (IOM) stresses equality and equity in treatment.
    2. Health inequity should be avoided as it leads to differential patient treatment.
    3. Bias and myths impact clinical decision-making and can put patients' safety and well-being at risk.
    4. The Joint Commission standards to reduce healthcare disparities in behavioral healthcare and human services must be followed to maintain accreditation (Standard RC.02.01.01, EP 26; The Joint Commission, 2023).
F. Myths and preconceived (unconscious) biases in psychiatry can lead to mental illness stigma impacting the patient's ability for recovery.
    1. Mental illness stigma includes discrimination, stereotypes, and prejudice.
    2. Such negative connotations result in harmful impacts on patients' recovery as well as on clinicians who engage in stigmatization.
    3. Implicit bias blinds the clinician to the patient's individual attributes and strengths. It can interfere with the partnership-building skills, which place the patient and the clinician on the same "team," working together to achieve the patient's recovery goals.
G. The impact of historical perspective on present day patient care:
    1. Myths regarding persons with mental illness were influenced by stories of patient mistreatment long before mental illness was understood.
    2. Throughout history, psychiatric patients underwent treatment that would today be considered inhumane (e.g., use of straitjacket, incarceration and isolation, frontal lobotomies, and long-term institutionalization).
    3. Today, an evidence-based approach to treatment instills a higher probability of repeated results that are deemed humane and safe.
    4. Therapeutic approaches to stigma reduction have not been widely addressed.
        a. Stigma continues to be a major barrier to treatment and recovery, resulting in a poor experience for the patient and a reduction in the quality of care and services.
H. Psychiatric emergencies occur when mental illness becomes so severe that immediate intervention is required.
    1. People experiencing psychiatric emergencies might not be able to function, may be experiencing extreme emotional distress, or may attempt to harm themselves or others.
    2. Patient behavior may stem from fear, anger, prejudice/stigma, and social isolation. Patients may believe self-harm

and even suicide are their only option to escape or stop these feelings and thoughts.
   3. The most prevalent psychiatric emergencies include suicidal/self-harming behaviors, mood disorders (depressive or manic), impaired judgment, self-neglect, and substance abuse.
      a. A nonjudgmental and understanding approach can better de-escalate the individual and prevent stigma.

CAUSES OF STIGMA FOR PSYCHIATRIC DISORDERS
A. Stigma stems from various sources, such as from one's thoughts, ideas, or beliefs. It can also stem from external factors such as society, media, family, and friends.
B. Knowledge deficits about the disease, the definition/meaning of the mental illness, or the physical symptoms related to the diagnoses are factors that can contribute to stigmatization.
C. Substance users are often referred to as "addicts," which can have a negative connotation, and people with this type of mental illness are often associated with criminals or the bottom rung of society.

VIOLENCE AS A POSSIBILITY
A. Agitation is a common symptom of patients with psychiatric disorders. Whether a patient becomes aggressive or violent is a result of their mental illness and the situation getting out of control.
   1. The stigma around patients with mental illness and their tendency to get aggressive or violent causes them to suffer unintended isolation and discrimination.
   2. Although evidence shows that mental illness does not predict violent behavior, studies have shown that a substantial portion of adults believe an individual with a mental disorder, such as schizophrenia, is likely to be violent toward others.
      a. Persons with mental illness are four times more likely to be the victim rather than the perpetrator of a violent act.
      b. Despite evidence to the contrary, even the criminal justice system treats persons with mental illness more like criminals than the general population.
   3. Mental illness with a co-occurring substance use problem can elevate the risk of violence. A small percentage of patients have substance use problems; it is unfair and biased to assume the risk of violence based on any specific diagnosis or situation.
B. Patients' physical behaviors are sometimes incorrectly interpreted as aggression.
   1. Psychomotor agitation is the unintentional movements caused by restlessness or anxiety, compromises a patient's autonomy, and can be distressing to the individual. Clinicians working with these patients should be mindful that the movements do not necessarily equate to aggression.
   2. Understanding that some illnesses can cause behavior that one may not be accustomed to and treating the individual like a person can help the patient feel more at ease and reduce violence.
   3. If a violence case were to be made, people with mental illness are more often victims than perpetrators of violence due to their vulnerable condition.

SHAME
A. Patients with mental illness and their families often experience a greater sense of shame and embarrassment related to stigma.
   1. Shame delays seeking treatment and causes stress and anxiety from trying to hide the problem.
   2. Parents of patients with mental illness may feel shame greater than that of families with other diseases.
   3. The history of psychiatric emergencies may be higher than what is revealed due to patients' unwillingness to seek treatment.
   4. Higher levels of education and female sex are positive indicators of the demand for treatment.
   5. Many patients with mental illness are unable to financially sustain themselves and do not seek treatment due to the cost.

LACK OF KNOWLEDGE
A. People often fear the unknown; many people are still unaware of the various diagnoses and etiologies in mental illness.
   1. Knowledge deficit and misunderstanding of persons with mental illness can result in stigma.
   2. Lack of insight or information on the disease process, in patients with mental illness, may interfere with their intention to seek treatment.
   3. Incorrect and sensationalized mass media depictions of mental illness often shape the public's understanding of mental illnesses.
      a. Negative and inaccurate portrayals perpetuate stigma.
      b. Distorted or even comedic portrayals of mental illness are harmful as they depict psychiatric emergencies as insignificant, when in fact a person's life may be in danger.
B. Individuals with appropriate understanding and knowledge about a psychiatric condition seek help early.
   1. Delays in the provision of therapeutic intervention can delay recovery.
   2. Recovery can occur more rapidly when the individual can access treatment. This can be due to the support of family who, when the patient lacks insight, can guide the patient to therapeutic interventions.
C. There is stigma surrounding suicidal ideations and actions.
   1. Patients who consider suicide as the action to relieve their emotional suffering often (but not always) provide those around them with "hints" of their plans.
      a. It is difficult for a family member to think that a loved one is considering death by suicide.
      b. The stigma surrounding suicide can increase the reluctance to seek help for individuals at risk for suicide.
   2. Clinicians can educate the family and other caregivers of the signs of suicidal ideation and teach them how to safely engage the patient in order to get assistance.
      a. Recognizing suicidal statements (e.g., "I wish I was dead," "the world would be better off without me") and behaviors (e.g., giving away personal items, a drastic improvement in behaviors and attitude) provides the family and the clinician opportunities to engage the patient considering suicide.
      b. Ask the patient directly: "Are you considering suicide?" or "Are you thinking about killing yourself?" Listen to the response.
         i. If the answer is no, stay with the person and contact the clinician, or if the patient is in the hospital alert the staff and review goals and plans with the patient.
         ii. If the answer is yes, ask: "Do you have a plan to do it?" If the person says yes, call 911 and stay with the person until help arrives. Assign one-to-one observation to assure patient safety.

NEGATIVE ATTITUDES

A. Negative attitudes, manifested by stigmatizing prejudice, can result in discriminatory practices as well as policies. Knowledge about mental illness influences the public's perceptions and social norms. The media often portrays those with mental and substance use disorders according to dangerous, negative stereotypes, and the public often relies upon these depictions in lieu of true understanding.

   1. APRNs understand that mental illness and substance use disorders are diseases. Part of their responsibility to the patient is to promote understanding through increasing the public's knowledge of the facts, especially when the patient is hospitalized on a nonpsychiatric unit.

   2. Patient treatment modalities for such individuals are complex and multifaceted and often involve help and support from various resources.

B. Structural stigma and mental illness

   1. When institutions adopt beliefs, behaviors, and attitudes that stigmatize the person with the lived experience, this increases the likelihood of discrimination and prejudicial treatment.

   2. Structural stigma impacts research funding, which affects the development of new treatments for people with lived experiences.

   3. There are parity laws in many states for providing behavioral health coverage for mental and substance use disorders.

      a. There is higher utilization of behavioral health services in states that have parity laws.

      b. Persons with mental and substance disorders have low insurance reimbursements, and this has contributed to less access to psychiatrists and other clinicians who accept insurance.

      c. It has been identified that increased access has not resulted in better evidence-based practice care.

C. Prevention initiatives and early interventions for mental illness include the following:

   1. A healthy lifestyle (e.g., nutrition, exercise, social factors) can decrease but not eliminate the possibility of disease, both mental and physical.

   2. Prevention of illness and treatment for mental health disorders should be taken just as seriously as other potentially harmful illnesses.

   3. Some ways in which APRNs can engage in prevention initiatives for patients with mental health concerns and diagnosis include the following:

      a. Psychoeducation for parents to nurture children and reduce traumatic experiences

      b. Education on mindfulness and other evidence-based methods to reduce stress

      c. Promotion of understanding of mental health and recovery through distribution of knowledge to the community

      d. Education of other nursing professionals to promote healthy sleeping, eating, and exercise habits in their patient populations

D. Celebrity disclosures of medical and mental disorders also impact stigma surrounding these disorders.

   1. Many celebrities have publicly disclosed their struggles with mental and physical illnesses. This increases the understanding of the illness and reduces stigma.

      a. Some patients find solace in hearing a famous person also struggles with health.

      b. Messages with a positive tone can help dispel myths, decrease the stigma, and reduce shame in seeking help.

E. Platforms to expose the public to accurate information (e.g., educational events, public safety messages) can help educate and prevent negative attitudes.

THE ATTITUDES AND BELIEFS OF HEALTH PROFESSIONALS

A. Clinician attitudes are key to a patient's perception of stigma and sense of being well cared for. This is especially true in settings of close contact and interaction with people with mental illness (e.g., ED, psychiatric unit).

B. Alleviating healthcare professionals' biases and fears is necessary to provide compassionate care.

   1. Ongoing education and training in de-escalation can improve staff confidence in handling difficult and escalating situations.

   2. Delivery of care in a nonjudgmental and objective manner is necessary.

C. Workplace culture may add to anxiety and stress of both patients and staff. Support and resources for the staff are necessary to provide timely and effective care. Staffing issues, security support, and an effective workplace violence plan all impact staff members' satisfaction and have a trickle-down effect on patient care. Traumatic patient-related events, such as suicide, can cause posttraumatic stress to the healthcare professionals who took care of the patient. A robust employee assistance program (EAP) that supports staff members to seek help can help them better understand and inform patients to do the same.

D. Patients experiencing psychiatric emergencies may not always be brought in voluntarily.

   1. Involuntary treatment is a result of the patient being considered a threat to themselves or others.

   2. They could be mandated into treatment by families, friends, clinicians, and even law enforcement.

      a. Patients held against their will, even when it is to keep them safe, can result in the person having feelings of fear, prompting behaviors of self-protection.

      b. Working with a person who is on nonvoluntary psychiatric admission requires high levels of patience and calm from the healthcare practitioner. This can reduce patient anxiety and foster a sense of a safe environment.

E. Health professionals' understanding of cultural and racial diversity increases trust, which promotes treatment seeking by persons with minority status.

   1. Patients from ethnic minorities often suffer the impact of being a double minority both from cultural/racial factors as well as being a person with mental illness.

   2. Nursing ethical principles include autonomy, beneficence, nonmaleficence, justice, fidelity, and veracity. This mandates the fair and equal treatment of all patients regardless of their race, creed, religion, ethnicity, gender, and diagnosis.

THE IMPACT OF THERAPEUTICS

A. Despite the evidence that therapeutic interventions benefit recovery outcomes, some patients may associate psychotherapeutic treatments with fear due to distorted beliefs, lack of knowledge, misinformation, and negative past experiences and memories.

   1. Medication compliance is beneficial to patients diagnosed with severe mental illness. This is especially true with patients diagnosed with schizophrenia and bipolar disorders.

2. Medication compliance is often a major factor in preventing relapse. Patients who are nonadherent to their medication are five times more likely to experience a relapse.
    a. Patients may feel that treatment is coercive when they have a limited ability to understand the benefits, providing them with a rationale to stop taking their medications after discharge.

B. Some patients may not have the necessary finances or the access to pharmacies to fill their prescriptions, which also leads to noncompliance. Psychotropic medications can be stigmatizing as they are often mislabeled by the layperson as "crazy pills."
1. The side effects can be unpleasant and take away the patient's autonomy and sense of self.
2. Some patients may feel they are dependent on these drugs and feel a loss of control, adding to their fear and anxiety.
3. These are all barriers to treatment that healthcare professionals must be aware of and navigate to improve treatment compliance.

C. Mechanical and pharmaceutical restraints
1. Problematic behaviors in the hospital setting may result in physical or pharmacologic restraints, which protect the patient and the clinician from harm.
2. Restraints limit the patient's freedom of movement.
    a. Either type of restraint might negatively impact the patient's memory of the hospitalization.
    b. Patients who experience restraints feel the stigma of shame and mistrust in the healthcare system.
    c. Training and continuing education for staff and healthcare teams and using any kind of restraint as a last resort are the responsibility of the medical institution and must be frequently reviewed to be compliant with laws and guidelines.

CONSEQUENCES OF STIGMA IN EMERGENCY CARE ACCESS

A. Not using person-first language (e.g., the "schizophrenic patient" instead of a patient diagnosed with schizophrenia) impacts patient treatment.
1. Patients report feeling a change in the way they are treated by hospital staff. This labeling affects their interaction with others.
2. Labeling by staff invites stigma. A diagnosis does not define the patient, but in many cases the patient feels as though diagnoses become their identity.
    a. This labeling impacts the patient's sense of self-worth, resulting in shame, guilt, and embarrassment.
    b. Patient labeling can exacerbate depression and increase thoughts of suicide. Stigma can impact the patient's social support, leading them to be more socially isolated. These factors can lead to a more severe state of illness and can prolong hospitalization.

EDUCATION AND TRAINING FOR CLINICIANS AND THE GENERAL PUBLIC

A. Education about mental illness has been shown to reduce stigma.
1. It provides an evidence-based, rational explanation of the disease and etiology, increasing an understanding about the signs and symptoms of mental illness.
2. APRNs can be instrumental in providing this information and becoming the educational arm to the general population.
3. As a spokesperson, the APRN can contribute to public service announcements, books, brochures, videos, and audio podcasts, which have been demonstrated to have the most significant impact on reducing stigma.

B. Educating healthcare workers who do not have frequent contact or interaction with persons with mental illness can increase awareness and dispel myths.
1. De-escalation training can help improve clinicians' confidence and create a sense of safety in the workplace.
2. Education related to responding to psychiatric emergencies can prepare the healthcare professional to treat patients with better quality care.

C. Evidence has shown that without knowledge healthcare workers can carry significant biases toward persons with mental illness, particularly those with substance use disorder.
1. Repeatedly taking care of patients who come back as if through a revolving door can be demoralizing and reduce motivation to treat the individual fairly.
2. Changing this attitude through self-awareness and positive thinking can be an effective strategy.
3. The healthcare professional can learn about the illness, understand that crises are temporary and will pass, be aware of one's attitudes and emotions when treating patients with mental illness, choose positive language when interacting with patients, always treat patients and family with respect and support, and be aware of and maintain patients' rights.
4. Healthcare professionals should also be supported in seeking help for their mental health without consequence and stigma.

CONTACT WITH PERSONS WITH MENTAL ILLNESS

A. Contact with persons with mental illness can dispel stigma and help people understand that an individual is a person and not a diagnosis.
1. Various forms of contact, such as one-to-one interaction, telephone, and audiovisual recordings, have all been shown to be effective, with personal contact being the most effective.
2. People with family or friends who suffer from mental illness have fewer biases as do healthcare professionals who work with patients with mental illness.
3. Familiarity and personal experience can be a powerful tool to reduce stigma.

LEGISLATIVE REFORM AND ADVOCACY

A. Advocating for people with mental illness can prevent discrimination and improve awareness of fair and equal treatment. This can also result in a trickle-down effect to help with education, employment, housing, and other social benefits.

B. Advocacy is multipronged and involves knowledge sharing, education, training, counseling, defending vulnerable populations, and upholding justice and ethics.

C. The Substance Abuse and Mental Health Services Administration (SAMHSA) has the Protection and Advocacy for Individuals with Mental Illness (PAIMI) Program, which protects and advocates for the rights of adults and children with serious/significant mental illness (www.samhsa.gov/paimi-program).
1. PAIMI ensures the enforcement of the constitutional rights of the individual.

2. PAIMI examines and provides support to review federal and state statutes for persons with mental illness.
D. The Joint Commission has standards on accreditation for behavioral health.
　1. *The R3 Report's* National Patient Safety Goal (NPSG) 15.01.01 is an NPSG for suicide prevention in healthcare settings approved by The Joint Commission (The Joint Commission, 2018).
　2. Accredited medical facilities can provide services to support multiple types of behavioral health interventions, from mental health services and addiction treatment to eating disorders and serving children and their families.
E. There are also state-based standards.
　1. Each state will have its services posted online in their Department of Human Services, Division of Mental Health and Addiction Services. Refer to your specific state for guidelines.
　2. In states like New Jersey, substance abuse treatment and reform offers hospitals and clinics the opportunity to participate in a pay-for-performance program to improve the quality of services.

RESEARCH TIPS

A. Communities are often defined by geography, race, ethnicity, culture, religion, or other characteristics specific to the group. By first learning the social structure (e.g., socioeconomic relationships, attitudes, values, and beliefs), researchers are able to obtain a deeper understanding of the makeup and needs of a community in order to better serve them.
B. A SWOT (**S**trengths, **W**eaknesses, **O**pportunities, and **T**hreats) analysis might be done to gather insight and feedback from within the community, identify problems, and discuss potential solutions.
C. Public forums such as town halls (including virtual on virtual platforms) allow for the expression of views regarding key issues of concern, along with potential solutions and expectations.
D. A plan should be developed for assessing local needs and resources.
　1. Needs are gaps between what is and what should be, and it can be something as simple as access to healthcare.
　2. Resources, or assets, can include individuals, organizations, equipment, or anything else that can be used to improve the quality of living.
　3. By understanding needs and resources, prioritization of which areas to focus on in the plan can be highlighted.
　4. Proper planning should also include community members to garner trust and collaboration.
E. A needs assessment survey can be conducted to help identify and prioritize areas of focus. A needs assessment survey may take the form of letters mailed out to the community, online survey, or door-to-door interviews.
F. Focus groups can also be conducted to gather information from small-group discussions guided by a trained leader. Focus groups provide responses that are opinions and typically spoken and open-ended. They can give a more accurate gauge of peoples' true thoughts and feelings on a topic.
　1. Gathers information and prioritizes needs
　2. Builds support, involvement, and sustainability because it is the idea of the group
G. Once a more meaningful understanding of the community and its needs has been established, the precise goal can be targeted. Mental health is difficult to measure, especially with subjective diseases such as mood disorders. We do not possess the technology to quantify a person's mood as we do with tangible measurements, such as blood pressure or electrolyte levels. These challenges result in a significant amount of underdiagnosis of persons with mental illness, and to obtain any sort of measurement mental health professionals assess psychological morbidity from face-to-face interviews and questionnaires.
　1. 12-Item General Health Questionnaire (GHQ-12): The GHQ-12 is one of the most widely used responses in quantitative social science and epidemiology for the analysis of mental health trends.
　　a. It contains 12 questions, each with four Likert response categories, which are conventionally summed to give a single score.
　　b. Ease of use, widespread distribution, and capacity to consistently produce accurate results make this tool the popular choice.
　　c. Initially used to focus on at-risk individuals, it has since been validated across multiple languages and countries as a population screening tool for depression.
　　d. Due to its repurposed nature, different disciplines treat the GHQ-12 differently, treating it either as an indicator of cases of ill health or as an indicator of population trends.
　2. Patient Health Questionnaire-9 (PHQ-9): PHQ-9 is a nine-item tool that corresponds to the *Diagnostic and Statistical Manual of Mental Disorders*, Fourth Edition (*DSM-IV*; American Psychiatric Association, 1994), criteria for major depression and provides a severity score ranging from 0 to 27 over 2 weeks. The tool is specific for screening of depression and has high reliability and sensitivity.
　3. Measurement-based care (MBC): MBC is an approach to clinical management involving the systematic collection of data using validated measures to monitor patient progress and directly inform clinical decisions.
　　a. MBC emerged in recent years as an effective strategy for improving outcomes in patients with mood disorders.
　　b. Using validated tools to collect data and monitor outcomes enables clinicians to respond timely to the changing course of illness and make appropriate adjustments to treatment plans when current treatments are not working.
　　c. MBC enhances the therapeutic relationship between the patient and the clinician, which can garner a more informed and proactively engaged patient.
　　d. The SAMHSA has added the MBC model to its registry of evidence-based practices.
　　e. The American Psychiatric Association guidelines recommend that MBC with standard and empirically validated measures be used when treating patients with mood disorders.
　　f. Research has shown that adding a clinician-rated assessment to an MBC program can add clinical value.
　4. Clinical Global Impression-Severity Scale (CGI-S): The CGI-S is a well-established standard measurement of patients with psychiatric illnesses. The National Institute of Mental Health (NIMH) sponsored collaborative studies of antipsychotic medications in schizophrenia, and the CGI-S was part of the various selection of assessments.
　　a. The CGI-S is a clinician-rated assessment of a patient's overall clinical condition before initiating a study medication and over the course of treatment.

b. The CGI-S is a reliable and valid measure that is sensitive to changes in the standard of care in psychiatric inpatient settings.

c. Adding the clinician-rated CGI-S with the patient-rated PHQ-9 in an MBC setting enhances the combined ability to predict risk of suicidal ideation and behavior in patients with mood disorders.

H. By understanding the mental health needs of a community through the various strategies, tools, and data discussed, an objective perspective can be gained. Through the efforts to get to know the people who make up the community, a "pulse" and "heartbeat" of the community can be sensed and a truly meaningful journey toward good mental health can be achieved.

RISK AND PROTECTIVE FACTORS

A. Mental illness is thought to be caused by a variety of multifactorial intrinsic and extrinsic factors, including genetics, epigenetics, environmental factors, and changes in brain chemistry and physiology.

1. The National Institutes of Health (NIH) identified some evidence of illness-associated genetics that can increase the likelihood of certain mental illnesses, including substance use disorders, schizophrenia, bipolar disease, and depression (NIH, 2013).

2. Prenatal exposure to environmental stressors (e.g., alcohol and drugs) can lead to mental illness, as can childhood abuse, trauma, or neglect.

3. Toxins and other environmental factors create a causal link between exposure and disease.

4. Neurotransmitters are what the body and brain use to communicate and regulate mood. When these neural networks are not functioning properly, mood disorders and reality disorders may occur.

B. Risk factors:

1. Risk factors are events and experiences that have adverse effects on a person's mental health. Some risk factors are:
   a. Genetic (e.g., a history of mental illness in a blood relative, such as a parent or a sibling)
   b. Homelessness, unemployment, and any prior history of mental illness
   c. Trauma; physical and psychological
   d. Substance use
   e. Psychosocial factors (e.g., discrimination, racial injustice, and other causes leading to social isolation)
   f. Stress (e.g., family conflict; family disorganization; emotional, social, physical, and financial stress; other stressful life events)
   g. Medical conditions (e.g., traumatic brain injury, stroke, epilepsy, and cancer)

2. Risk factors can increase a person's likelihood of developing a mental health challenge.
   a. Mental illness is common and occurs in approximately one in five adults in a given year. Mental illness can begin at any age, but most cases begin earlier in life.
   b. Effects of mental illness can be temporary with recovery and remission of symptoms, or long-lasting with chronic symptoms ongoing.
   c. Mental illness can also be co-occurring (e.g., depression and substance use disorder).
   d. Mental illness is a leading cause of disability, and untreated mental illness can cause severe emotional, behavioral, and physical health problems. A patient with severe depression may not be able to care for themselves and neglect their heart condition.

3. People with mental illness may not be able to express their needs or advocate for themselves, which can easily lead to complications of other conditions. Examples include:
   a. Decreased pleasure and enjoyment of life/activities
   b. Relationship conflicts/difficulties
   c. Work or school problems
   d. Social isolation
   e. Substance abuse
   f. Financial problems, poverty
   g. Legal issues
   h. Housing issues, homelessness
   i. Danger to self, others, environment, self-harm (including suicide, homicide)
   j. Health issues, exacerbation/deterioration of pre existing medical conditions

C. Protective factors:

1. Protective factors can support the strengthening of mental health and improve a person's ability to cope in difficult environments and events.

2. Protective factors are positive characteristics that can be individual- or community-based.

RISK AND PROTECTIVE FACTORS EXIST IN MULTIPLE CONTEXTS

A. People have their own unique set of biological and psychological characteristics that can make them vulnerable or resilient during stressful experiences.

1. Relationships, support systems, and personalities exist in multiple contexts.

2. A variety of risk and protective factors exist and operate within each of these contexts and influence each other.

B. Targeting these multiple contexts will assist in providing effective treatments. For example:

1. Relationship risk factors
   a. Parents/friends who use drugs and alcohol or who suffer from mental illness
   b. Child abuse, neglect, maltreatment, and inadequate supervision

2. Relationship protective factors
   a. Healthy relationships: a vital protective factor, for example, the presence and involvement of a loving, supportive adult
   b. Parental resilience and positive family and social connections
   c. Support that can be identified and counted on in times of need

3. Community risk factors
   a. Neighborhood poverty, crime, and violence
   b. Communities with easy access to substances (e.g., drugs, alcohol, tobacco)
   c. Areas of limited educational and economic opportunities and resources

4. Community protective factors
   a. Availability of resources and after-school activities
   b. Opportunities for economic and financial growth
   c. Access to medical and mental health resources
   d. Safe housing and neighborhoods

C. In society, risk factors can include norms and laws favorable to substance use, as well as racism and a lack of economic opportunity. Protective factors in this context would include hate crime/discrimination laws or policies limiting the availability of alcohol.

RISK AND PROTECTIVE FACTORS ARE CORRELATED AND CUMULATIVE

A. Risk factors tend to be positively correlated with other risk factors (the higher the risk factors in one area the higher in the other) and negatively correlated with protective factors (the more risk factors the fewer protective factors).
   1. Individual
   2. Risk and protective factors: tend to have a cumulative effect on the development or prevention of mental health issues
      a. Individuals with multiple risk factors have a higher chance of developing a condition that can impact their mental and physical health, while people with multiple protective factors are at a reduced risk.

B. Early identification of risk factors is key to providing early intervention, treatment, and support that target multiple risk factors whenever possible.

INDIVIDUAL FACTORS CAN BE ASSOCIATED WITH MULTIPLE OUTCOMES

A. A single negative life event can be associated with the development of mental illness, such as depression, substance abuse, anxiety, or suicide.
   1. Posttraumatic stress disorder (PTSD) may link a person's single trauma to various forms of mental illness like anxiety, depression, and substance abuse to cope with the aftereffects of the trauma.

B. Just as individual risk factors can have compounding effects, single positive factors can also be associated with multiple outcomes.
   1. Responsibility to one's own family/children can be associated with abstaining from self-harm, getting a job, and attending a program.

C. These factors can be influences over long periods of a person's life span.
   1. Risk factors such as poverty and family dysfunction often exist early in a young person's life and can contribute to the development of mental and/or substance use problems.

D. Factors can also influence or be influenced by factors in other contexts.
   1. Effective parenting has been shown to mitigate the effects of risk factors such as poverty, divorce, family mental illness, and substance use.

E. Medical institutions situated in high-risk areas are more likely to have patients whose health (physical and mental) has been affected.
   1. APRNs who have understanding of the risk and protective factors are better prepared to formulate more appropriate interventions for the patient.
   2. Access to mental healthcare in the neighborhood that a patient lives in is a protective factor.

UNIVERSAL, SELECTIVE, AND INDICATED PREVENTION INTERVENTIONS

A. With appropriate preventive interventions, personal and community risks to a person's mental health can be lessened. Prevention interventions are categorized into the following:
   1. Universal preventive interventions: These interventions are the broadest approach, designed to reach entire groups or populations. Universal prevention interventions might target schools, whole communities, or workplaces.
   2. Selective interventions: These interventions target biological, psychological, or social risk factors that are more prominent among high-risk groups than among the wider population (e.g., prevention education for immigrant families with young children, peer support groups for adults with a family history of substance use disorders).
   3. Indicated preventive interventions: These interventions target individuals who show signs of being at risk for a substance use disorder. These include referral to support services for young adults who violate drug policies or screening and consultation for families of older adults admitted to hospitals with potential alcohol-related injuries.

RISK AND PROTECTIVE FACTORS FOR SUICIDE

A. The correct nomenclature for suicidal thoughts or actions are suicidal ideation (thoughts of suicide) and death by suicide. Also, when a person dies by suicide, it is not correct to label it a success, or a successful suicide attempt. There is no success in death by suicide.

B. Suicide is a major health problem, reflected in the fact that it accounted for 1.3% of all deaths worldwide in 2019.
   1. Global suicide rates are over twice as high in men than in women. It is the fourth leading cause of death for persons aged 15 to 29.
   2. In 2023, more than 50,000 Americans died by suicide, the highest recorded number in a single year.

C. Suicide is a permanent action in response to a temporary or long-standing problem. Suicidal ideation and death by suicide are rarely caused by a single circumstance or event. Instead, a range of factors contribute to attempts at, or death by, suicide.

D. Factors that increase suicide risk include the risk factors discussed above, but can further be categorized as follows:
   1. Individual risk factors
      a. Previous suicide attempt
      b. History of depression and other mental illnesses
      c. Serious illnesses such as chronic pain
      d. Criminal/legal problems
      e. Job/financial problems or loss
      f. Impulsive or aggressive tendencies
      g. Substance use
      h. Current or prior history of adverse childhood experiences
      i. Sense of hopelessness
      j. Violence victimization and/or perpetration
   2. Relationship risk factors
      a. Bullying
      b. Family/loved one's history of suicide
      c. Loss of relationships
      d. High-conflict or violent relationships
      e. Social isolation
   3. Community risk factors
      a. Lack of access to healthcare
      b. Suicide cluster in the community
      c. Stress of acculturation
      d. Community violence
      e. Historical trauma
      f. Racial/ethnic/religious discrimination
   4. Societal risk factors
      a. Stigma associated with help-seeking and mental illness
      b. Easy access to lethal means of suicide among people at risk
      c. Unsafe media portrayals of suicide, glamorization, or glorification of death

E. Many factors can reduce the risk of suicide and can vary in range at the individual, relationship, community, and societal levels.
1. Individual protective factors
   a. Effective coping and problem-solving skills
   b. Reasons for living (e.g., family, friends, pets)
   c. Strong sense of cultural identity
2. Relationship protective factors
   a. Support from partners, friends, and family
   b. Feeling connected to others
3. Community protective factors
   a. Feeling connected to school, community, and other social institutions
   b. Availability of consistent and high-quality physical and behavioral healthcare
4. Societal protective factors
   a. Reduced access to lethal means of suicide among people at risk
   b. Cultural, religious, or moral objections to suicide

Suicide and the Hospitalized Patient With Mental Illness

A. The risk of suicide is 50 times higher in psychiatric institutions than in the general populations.
B. Suicidal risk and severity of depression are significantly associated.
1. Suicidal behaviors may occur after the initial acute psychiatric illness and hospitalization.
2. Some antidepressant black box warning messages in 2006 created an alarmist response, decreasing the use of medications by almost 50% in children and adolescents.
3. Psychoeducation by the APRN, related to the warning, can educate the patient and families on the benefits and avoidance of some of the risk.
C. Frequent assessments of risk for suicide should be implemented to monitor the patient and determine the need for constant observation.

ASSESSMENT NEEDS FOR THE HOSPITALIZED PATIENT WITH MENTAL ILLNESS

A. A census is a tool for compiling, analyzing, and disseminating demographic, economic, and social data about all persons in a country or a well-delineated part of a country at a specified time.
1. The information collected from a census can be evaluated in a demographic analysis, which is a method used to study the components of variation and change in demographic variables and the relationships between them.
2. Current or historical records can be analyzed with factors such as the following:
   a. Static aspects of a population are age, economic characteristics, marital status, race, and sex.
   b. Dynamic aspects of a population are fertility, nuptiality (marriage status), growth, migration, and mortality.
   c. The information obtained on a community/population should be incorporated when considering a needs assessment.
B. A needs assessment should focus on factors that include immediate, intermediate, and long-term individual needs.
1. These include access to care (e.g., COVID-19 immunization), ongoing mental health support, and access to pharmacies and exercise programs.
2. Community health needs assessment provides the organization with a comprehensive information about general population health status, needs, and issues that might exist within a specific community.
3. Information from the community can inform short- and long-term plans, leading to better allocation of resources that best fit the needs of the individual and the surrounding community.
4. The benefits of an assessment and improvement plan for the behavioral health unit include the following:
   a. Improved organizational and community coordination
   b. Increased community knowledge about public health and strengthened partnerships/collaboration with the community
   c. Identifying priority needs, strengths, and weaknesses, and obtaining data for a baseline on performance and benchmarks for improvement
C. The Public Health Accreditation Board defines *community health assessment* as a systematic examination of the health status indicators for a given population that is used to identify key problems and assets in a community.
1. The purpose and goal should be to formulate strategies to identify and address the community/population's health needs.
D. A community health needs assessment should be formed with the following foundations:
1. Multisector collaborations that support shared ownership of all phases of community health improvement, including assessment, planning, investment, implementation, and evaluation
2. Proactive, broad, and diverse community engagement to improve results
3. A definition of community that encompasses both a significant enough area to allow for population-wide interventions and measurable results and includes a targeted focus to address disparities among subpopulations
4. Maximum transparency to improve community engagement and accountability
5. Use of evidence-based interventions and encouragement of innovative practices with a thorough evaluation
6. Evaluation to inform a continuous improvement process
7. Use of the highest quality data pooled from, and shared among, diverse public and private sources
E. A long-term community health improvement plan can be implemented based on the results of a community health needs assessment.
1. The Public Health Accreditation Board defines a *community health improvement plan* as a long-term, systematic effort to address public health problems based on the results of community health assessment activities and the community health improvement process.
2. This long-term plan should exist in continued collaboration with community partners to set priorities and coordinate the allocation of resources.
3. Policy development and action plans should also help drive the sustainability of the plan and should address the strengths, weaknesses, opportunities, and threats (SWOT analysis) to improve the health status of the community.

4. The patient with behavioral health problems remains in the hospital for a short time before returning to the community. The hospital's ability to coordinate services with the community works to benefit the patient, community, and hospital. Better service can be a direct result of a comprehensive assessment of individual and population mental health needs.

PATIENT AND FAMILY ENGAGEMENT

A. Family engagement has been identified as a critical protective factor for patients with mental illness. Family assessment allows the APRN to identify what the patient needs in the way of monitoring and support resources, as well as gauging the family's understanding of mental illness.

B. Patient and family engagement creates an environment in which healthcare professionals, patients, and families work together as partners to improve the quality and safety of care, which is what all organizations should strive for. Strong leadership and a transparent environment are necessary to create and sustain a patient- and family-inclusive organization.

C. Engaged patients and families make better informed decisions and use resources aligned with the patient's priorities more wisely.
  1. With the many competing priorities that a healthcare professional must juggle, patients only have their safety and well-being as the primary factors.
  2. Healthcare professionals who are responsive, transparent, approachable, and inclusive promote mutual patient-to-staff accountability and understanding.

BARRIERS TO PATIENT AND FAMILY ENGAGEMENT

A. Certain factors deter patients' and families' willingness and participation in the plan of care. Researchers have identified five factors:
  1. Patients (demographic characteristics, health literacy)
  2. Health conditions (illness severity, acuity)
  3. Healthcare professionals (knowledge, attitudes, and beliefs)
  4. Tasks (whether a required patient safety behavior challenges the clinician's clinical abilities)
  5. Healthcare setting (primary or secondary care)

B. A key factor that may act as a barrier is the patient's perception of their role and status as being subordinate, or lower, to clinicians.
  1. The fear of being labeled as a "difficult" patient or taking on a passive role in their treatment can become a difficult hurdle in forming a good connection with their clinician.
  2. This can be addressed by improving communication and educating patients, families, and the healthcare professional.

STRATEGIES TO SUPPORT PATIENT AND FAMILY ENGAGEMENT

A. Hospital leaders can commit to patient and family engagement by being transparent and communicating their organization's mission and values to the patient, family, and community.
  1. Leaders should serve as role models for their organizations by partnering with patients and family members.
  2. Provide the necessary infrastructure and resources for the hospital staff to be able to engage with patients and families. Integrate the practices into the policy and culture of the organization.
  3. Leaders who openly communicate the mission and values of their organization help ensure the importance of patient and family engagement.
     a. Mission and vision statements create a pathway for change by fostering purpose and prioritizing critical elements.
     b. These statements should include a clear commitment to patient and family engagement, involve input from all involved parties, and should be easily replicable and sustainable.

B. An organization's strategic plan shapes processes and policies.
  1. Incorporation of patient and family engagement as part of a strategic plan guarantees that these values will be practiced and supported regularly in daily operations.
  2. For example, the "service excellence" strategic pillar would focus on patient- and family-centered care, including patient and family engagement.
  3. Best practices for improving engagement may include extended visiting hours, bedside shift reports, the inclusion of patients and families in various committees, and overall collaboration and communication between hospital staff, patients, and their families.
  4. By strengthening the strategic pillar of service excellence through patient and family engagement, leaders cultivate a culture that reinforces these values.

C. Leaders should remain transparent and consistent about the value and importance of engagement.
  1. Leaders lead by example and openly communicate to the staff through public forums, town halls, and emails, ensuring they are visible throughout the organization.
  2. Reminders and reporting of issues in daily huddles and encouraging frontline staff to bring issues to the forefront can help bring attention to solutions.
  3. Patient- and family-centered care values can also be incorporated into the annual appraisals listing and rating examples of how the employee applied these values annually.

D. Financial compensation in the form of bonuses or raises can be tied to measures of engagement.
  1. Informal and formal recognition of staff who go above and beyond to promote patient and family engagement can boost morale and create a healthy and competitive environment.
  2. Being clear with the expectations of the entire hospital staff without exception can help drive the message of the importance of engagement and inclusion.

E. Sharing stories or reading a patient letter highlighting the excellence in service and inclusion and what that did for the patient and their family reminds the staff of the positive outcomes that can result.
  1. Subjective and emotional effects can only be described through stories, letters, and word of mouth. Data and outcomes are objective information and sharing this information can help foster transparency and accountability.
  2. Sharing data with high marks helps validate the processes in place, while data with areas for improvement can identify processes that may need a closer look.

PROVIDING THE NECESSARY INFRASTRUCTURE AND RESOURCES

A. Major investments are not necessarily needed to implement and support patient and family engagement strategies.

1. From an actual department to a small committee for the patient- and family-centered care, the goal can be accomplished with a large or small team.
2. Staff will need time to plan, implement, integrate, and sustain various projects and processes.
3. If hiring new staff for these roles is not feasible, existing staff can be allocated judiciously to help support initiatives. Staff liaisons, patient advocates, and patient engagement champions are some roles and titles that can be created with existing resources.

B. Training, education, and support for the staff are critical to establishing and maintaining meaningful clinician–patient relationships.
1. Communication skills can be taught through different modes (e.g., seminars, training sessions, retreats).
2. Role-playing and simulation can provide real-time feedback on staff members' skill sets.
3. Temporary or permanent coaches can also be used to provide direct feedback on actual staff and patient interactions.
4. A train-the-trainer model is a good peer-to-peer learning method that can garner more following and support from within the staff.

C. Some long-term resources and infrastructure might be a patient portal or website that allows patients and families to access information regarding their care, communicate with their physicians, view personal health information, retrieve test results, and make appointments.
1. Engaging patients in monitoring and updating their medications or treatment plans allows them to stay active in their own care and assist the provider, and the community resources stay informed.
2. Upgrades to the environment that focus on patient comforts, such as quiet and spacious waiting areas, could also be considered.

CHALLENGES AND TOOLS

A. The U.S. population continues to have a high demand and need for APRNs and psychiatric-mental health nurse practitioners (PMHNPs).
1. The NIMH estimates that upwards of 20% of the U.S. population have a diagnosable mental health disorder. This statistic places great emphasis on getting more NPs into practice and into the hospitals and communities.

B. The expected PMHNP competencies required for psychopharmacologic practice include the following:
1. Developing an age-appropriate treatment plan based on evidence-based standards of care and practice guidelines
2. Planning care to minimize complications and promote optimal function and quality of life
3. Considering motivation and readiness to follow the plan
4. Explaining the risks and benefits of treatment to the patient and family/caregiver
5. Appropriately prescribing and managing pharmacologic interventions
6. Using individualized outcome measures to evaluate response to treatment
7. Seeking consultation when appropriate to enhance one's practice

C. With such a comprehensive list of expectations for the NP to provide for the patients and patients' families, the role of the NP is rife with challenges.

1. This also places immense pressure on NPs to take on larger caseloads and responsibilities.
2. With best-practice guidelines developed around patient-centered care, clinicians are expected to treat the patient as an individual and not just the disease.

D. Internal medicine produces objective results from labs, tests, and diagnostic studies that the clinician then analyzes to deduce a physical finding.
1. This finding is based on the pathophysiology and etiology of the disease, and treatment can be tailored to the findings.
2. In psychiatry, the signs and symptoms of psychiatric disorders can often overlap and comorbidities are quite common.
3. Although some symptoms are observable, such as restlessness, anxiety, and response to internal stimuli, it is often assessed subjectively using patient interviews.

E. The cluster of symptoms and diagnoses for each patient may not appear as they do in textbooks, and treatment modalities are certainly not one-size-fits-all.
1. Patients with schizophrenia may present with predominantly positive symptoms, negative symptoms, or a combination of both.
2. A patient with a depressive disorder might also have insomnia or hypersomnia, anxiety, psychomotor retardation, or anorexia.
3. Co-occurring disorders, such as substance use disorder, PTSD, and anxiety disorder, can all exist along with the primary presenting problem.
4. The symptoms of these various disorders can overlap or share the need for treatment.
5. Physical conditions such as hypertension, endocrine dysfunction, and metabolic disorders can make selecting the appropriate pharmacotherapy difficult and limit the clinician with choices due to the side effects and drug interactions of the medication plan.

F. The decisions are complex, which is why a flexible approach to treatment, such that patient and family concerns are addressed, education is provided, and risks for adverse effects are minimized, is required.

DECISION-MAKING AND TREATMENT NONCOMPLIANCE

A. Medication and treatment compliance can be the single most challenging barrier for patients. The reasons why patients do not adhere to treatment include:
1. Side effects (e.g., weight gain, fatigue, sexual dysfunction, and pharmacologic dependency)
2. Socioeconomic factors (e.g., homelessness, unemployment, access to care, access to pharmacies, transportation issues)
3. Clinician scarcity
4. Patient-centered barriers (e.g., fear of stigma and knowledge deficit regarding pharmacotherapy)

B. There are many different first-line medications to treat disorders, and choosing the right medication for the patient begins with shared decision-making. Barriers can include:
1. Access to pharmacies
2. Cost of the medications
3. Language barriers and knowledge deficits
4. Memory and cognitive disorders

C. To garner compliance with treatment while providing the most benefit to the patient, a shared decision-making practice is necessary.

1. Patients who want to dictate and be the sole decision-maker in their treatment would not have a professional understanding of symptoms, side effects, and etiology.
2. Clinicians who do not want the patient's input in their treatment would not get valuable feedback regarding response to treatment or adverse effects.
3. Clinicians can work with patients to consider tapering off of inappropriate drugs, such as benzodiazepines for treatment of chronic anxiety disorders, cross-titrating from one medication to another, and augmenting or switching formulations to reduce the number of medications they might require.

D. Titration of medications needs to be efficient, but also cannot be too fast. Failure to appropriately titrate medications can lead to adverse effects.
1. Habitual selections (e.g., giving citalopram to every patient with a major depressive disorder), first-line medication selection with greater risks for adverse effects when other choices are available, or prescribing multiple daily doses when a once-daily dose exists are practices that can lead to poor patient outcomes.
2. Different clinicians have their styles and preferences for prescribing and combining medications, and there can be significant variability in how closely best-practice guidelines or off-label prescribing strategies are followed.

E. Patients admitted into the inpatient setting are often coming into an unfamiliar environment. Safety measures in the inpatient psychiatric setting restrict many freedoms that patients normally have at home or in their residences.
1. Ligature risk is a major concern that requires shoelaces, belts, and other potentially hazardous items to be restricted.
2. Due to the sensitive nature of psychiatric admission, privacy concerns require limitations on such items as cell phones, cameras, and other electronic recording devices.
3. Visitations with family and friends need to be monitored and scheduled accordingly. These necessary safety limitations and requirements also contribute to inpatient noncompliance and patients and families requesting an early discharge.

ETHICAL AND LEGAL ISSUES

A. There may be legal and ethical issues to consider in the clinical decision-making process, which should be addressed by an interprofessional collaborative team.
1. Acting alone or without supervision can be a risky undertaking.
2. Members of the interprofessional team can provide insights and an alternative perspective on complicated cases.
3. More eyes are better than one, which is often the phrase that is often beneficial to the team members.

B. Transference and countertransference can occur with patients and their families.
1. Due to the stressful nature of appeasing patients and their families, positive or negative emotions may develop during treatment.
2. Remaining objective and keeping a clear head are necessary as a professional, and it can be difficult to assess interactions and situations when there is bias in either direction.

C. There is also the added risk of legal issues with the litigious aspects of current society.
1. Complaints or lawsuits cause undue stress to the clinician and the organization.
2. It is imperative that NPs "do no harm" to avoid being dragged into these unnecessary suits.
3. Sticking to evidence-based, best-practice guidelines will ensure that a consistent quality of care can be delivered without fear of unwarranted legal ramifications.

TOOLS TO DEAL WITH CHALLENGES

A. Encouraging patients and families to disclose their concerns about medications helps clinicians focus on providing information for decision-making and arrive at an acceptable plan. A teach-back method can be effective in evaluating patients' or family members' understanding of the treatment plan.

B. "Janicak et al. (2011) describe seven principles that are helpful to PMHNP practice:
1. The diagnosis, subject to revisions, is fundamental. More specifically, the diagnostic formulation that considers the symptoms, genetic risks, history and course of illness, temperament, behaviors, and significant life events to form a prioritized differential diagnosis and plan of treatment is fundamental. Failures to respond to treatment as delivered require practitioners to examine alternative etiologies for the signs and symptoms, reanalyze, and reformulate. ...
2. Pharmacotherapy alone is generally insufficient for complete recovery. Education and psychosocial interventions are almost always needed. Treatment responses are influenced by the meaning of the illness, expectations, and motivations for change.
3. The phase of the illness and the timing of the intervention are critically important in terms of the initial strategy and duration of treatment. Best-practice guidelines are useful in adjusting treatment from the acute to maintenance phases of illness.
4. The risk-to-benefit ratio must always be considered when developing a treatment strategy. History of drug dependence or other comorbid medical conditions, drug tolerability and efficacy, and major risks (e.g., U.S. Food and Drug Administration black box warnings) must be considered and discussed as part of the informed consent process.
5. Prior personal (and possibly family) history of a good or poor response to a specific agent usually dictates the first-line choice for a subsequent episode.
6. It is important to target specific symptoms and monitor their presence over an entire course of treatment.
7. It is necessary to observe for the development of adverse effects throughout the entire course of treatment. The goal of treatment is remission and improved quality of life whenever possible" (Mangano et al., 2020, pp. 10).

C. The *Diagnostic and Statistical Manual of Mental Disorders*, Fifth Edition (*DSM-5*; American Psychiatric Association, 2013), diagnoses are based on syndromes and not on pathophysiology or etiology. To assess improvement, symptoms and functional changes of the patient must be monitored and effectiveness of treatment evaluated. There are evidence-based tools to reliably assess symptom severity, such as the Columbia-Suicide Severity Rating Scale (C-SSRS) and the Abnormal Involuntary Movement Scale (AIMS).

COLLABORATIVE CARE AND REFERRALS

INPATIENT SETTING

A. In the general workflow, partnership and collaboration with other departments are necessary. The ED and neurology ▶

department are often the closest in line with the psychiatric department. Mental illness is heavily associated with a brain disorder and the neurology department also operates in this same realm.
  1. Neuropsychiatry is a field that is gaining ground, and the two specialties do have many similarities in common.
  2. The ED is the gateway to the hospital, and mental health issues such as suicide, substance abuse, and all other mental health needs are triaged and funneled through the ED.

B. Partnerships with other departments and specialties often occur on a case-by-case basis. Each patient comes with their own unique set of challenging issues. It is when the psychiatric component comes into play in their treatment that such partnerships can form.
  1. Patients presenting with medical issues may often be overlooked regarding their mental healthcare.
  2. Screening tools for depression and suicide are important in identifying at-risk patients and working with the patient's primary care team.
  3. The maternal child health and labor and delivery departments are also specialty areas where close partnerships can be formed. Postpartum depression screening can help identify patients with mental health needs and follow-up services.

C. Employee health services, the EAP, and the human resources department are also areas within the hospital setting where close partnerships can be formed. The most valuable resource to healthcare organizations is the workforce, and supportive services for their mental health needs require contributions from these key areas. Providing outlets for employees to seek mental health while maintaining privacy without stigma is important in making these supportive services meaningful.

OUTPATIENT SETTING

A. Collaboration and partnership with outpatient clinicians, clinics, and programs is necessary in maintaining mental health when patients are discharged from the inpatient setting. This process allows ample opportunities for important partnerships.
  1. Deciding on which clinician, clinic, or program to which the patient will be referred depends on the collaboration of the inpatient clinician and the patient and their family.
  2. As more and more referrals are sent, the caseload of certain reliable and respectable partners can begin to form. Clinical services should be the priority factor when selecting follow-up care, and secondary to this factor is the need for placement and residence.

B. Many patients with mental illness lack social and financial support. Basic needs such as stable housing are important in achieving and maintaining long-term health. Barriers to stable housing include financial issues, stigma from neighbors and landlords, and a lack of mental health support in the community.
  1. Supportive housing services have been shown to increase housing stability for people with mental illness and also contribute to improved patient outcomes, such as reduced hospitalization.
  2. Voluntary mental health support is a key component of supportive housing, and collaborative care as a team-based multidisciplinary approach is needed for mental illness management.

C. Structured care plans, scheduled follow-ups, and interprofessional communication form the basis of collaborative care. In shelters, a collaborative care model with a partnership between the clinician and shelter staff can be as effective as traditional models where psychiatric care is built into on-site primary care infrastructure. This equal sense of partnership can ease the burden of revolving door care by providing a more layered and sustainable plan for the patient to have the supportive services and assistance that they so desperately need.

CONCLUSION

Providing care to the hospitalized psychiatric patient requires a village effort, from the multiple resources, the families, the diverse clinical and supportive staff, and the patient. Organizational missions and values are infused into rules and regulations and guided by outside regulatory bodies and laws. Self-management support, clinical information system integration to facilitate information flow, clinician decision support, links to community resources, and organization support from the leadership level are key elements of collaborative care. Working alongside all the partners from inside and outside of the medical center, the patient with a psychiatric disorder can obtain the support needed to guide a successful recovery.

REFERENCES AND BIBLIOGRAPHY

Agency for Healthcare Research and Quality. (2022). *Supporting patient and family engagement: Best practices for hospital leaders*. U.S. Department of Health and Human Services. https://www.ahrq.gov/sites/default/fileswysiwyg/professionals/systems/hospital/engagingfamilies/howtogetstarted/Best_Practices_Hosp_Leaders_508.pdf

American Psychiatric Association. (1994). *Diagnostic and statistical manual of mental disorders* (4th ed.). Author.

American Psychiatric Association. (2013). *Diagnostic and statistical manual of mental disorders* (5th ed.). https://doi.org/10.1176/appi.books.9780890425596

Barker, L., Lee-Evoy, J., Butt, A., Wijayasinghe, S., Nakouz, D., Hutcheson, T., McCarney, K., Kaloy, R., & Vigod, S. (2022). Delivering collaborative mental health care within supportive housing: Implementation evaluation of a community-hospital partnership. *BMC Psychiatry, 22*(1), 36. https://doi.org/10.1186/s12888-021-03668-3

Centers for Disease Control and Prevention. (2022a). *Assessments & plans*. U.S. Department of Health and Human Services. https://www.cdc.gov/publichealthgateway/cha/plan.html

Centers for Disease Control and Prevention. (2022b). *Risk and protective factors*. U.S. Department of Health and Human Services. https://www.cdc.gov/suicide/factors/index.html

Chammas, F., Januel, D., & Bouaziz, N. (2022). Inpatient suicide in psychiatric settings: Evaluation of current prevention measures. *Front Psychiatry, 13*. https://doi.org/10.3389/fpsyt.2022.997974

da Silva, A. G., Baldacara, L., Cavalcante, D. A., Fasanella, N. A., & Palha, A. P. (2020). The impact of mental illness stigma on psychiatric emergencies. *Frontiers in Psychiatry, 11*, 573. https://doi.org/10.3389/fpsyt.2020.00573

Ghiasi, N., Azhar, Y., & Singh, J. (2023). *Psychiatric illness and criminality*. StatPearls Publishing. https://www.ncbi.nlm.nih.gov/books/NBK537064

Glazer, K., Rootes-Murdy, K., Van Wert, M., Mondimore, F., & Zandi, P. (2020). The utility of PHQ-9 and CGI-S in measurement-based care for predicting suicidal ideation and behaviors. *Journal of Affective Disorders, 266*, 766–771. https://doi.org/10.1016/j.jad.2018.05.054

Griffith, G. (2019). Understanding the population structure of the GHQ-12: Methodological considerations in dimensionally complex measurement outcomes. *Social Science & Medicine, 234*. https://doi.org/10.1016/j.socscimed.2019.112638

International Association of Suicide Prevention. (2023). *Creating hope through action*. https://www.iasp.info/wspd/references/#:~:text=An%20estimated%20703%20000%20people%20die%20by%20suicide%20worldwide%20each%20year.&text=Over%20one%20in%20every%20100,was%20the%20result%20of%20suicide.&text=The%20global%20suicide%20rate%20is,high%20among%20men%20than%20women.&text=Over%20half%20(58%25)%20of,age%20of%2050%20years%20old

Janicak, P. G., Marder, S. R., & Pavuluri, M. N. (2011). *Principles and practice of psychopharmacotherapy* (5th ed.). Lippincott, Williams, & Wilkins.

The Joint Commission. (2018, November 27). *National Patient Safety Goal for suicide prevention*. R³ Report, 18. https://www.jointcommission.org/-/media/tjc/documents/resources/patient-safety-topics/suicide-prevention/r3_18_suicide_prevention_hap_bhc_5_6_19_rev5.pdf

The Joint Commission. (2023). *New requirements to reduce health care disparities*. R³ Report, 36. https://www.jointcommission.org/standards/r3-report/r3-report-issue-36-new-requirements-to-reduce-health-care-disparities

Loots, E., Goossens, E., Vanwesemael, T., Morrens, M., Van Rompaey, B., & Dilles, T. (2021). Interventions to improve medication adherence in patients with schizophrenia or bipolar disorders: A systematic review and meta-analysis. *International Journal of Environmental Research and Public Health*, 18(19), 10213. https://doi.org/10.3390/ijerph181910213

Mangano, E., Gonzales, Y., & Kverno, K. S. (2020). Challenges faced by new psychiatric–mental health nurse practitioner prescribers. *Journal of Psychosocial Nursing*, 58(10), 7–11. https://doi.org/10.3928/02793695-20200915-01

Mayo Clinic Staff. (2022, December 13). *Mental illness*. Mayo Clinic. https://www.mayoclinic.org/diseases-conditions/mental-illness/symptoms-causes/syc-20374968

National Academies of Sciences, Engineering, and Medicine. (2016). Understanding stigma of mental and substance abuse disorders. In *Ending discrimination against people with mental and substance use disorders: The evidence for stigma change* (pp. 33–53). National Academies Press. https://www.ncbi.nlm.nih.gov/books/NBK384915

National Institute of Health. (2013). *Common genetic factors found in 5 mental disorders*. NIH Research Matters. https://www.nih.gov/news-events/nih-research-matters/common-genetic-factors-found-5-mental-disorders

National Institute of Health. (2022). *Demographic data*. https://www.nihlibrary.nih.gov/resources/subject-guides/health-data-resources/demographic-data

Ong, H. S., Fernandez, P. A., & Lim, H. K. (2021). Family engagement as part of managing patients with mental illness in primary care. *Singapore Medical Journal*, 62(5), 213–219. https://doi.org/10.11622/smedj.2021057

Substance Abuse and Mental Health Services Administration. (2019). *Risk and protective factors*. U.S. Department of Health and Human Services. https://www.samhsa.gov/sites/default/files/20190718-samhsa-risk-protective-factors.pdf

Volkow, N. D., Gordon, J. A., & Koob, G. F. (2021). Choosing appropriate language to reduce the stigma around mental illness and substance use disorders. *Neuropsychopharmacol*, 46(13), 2230–2232. https://doi.org/10.1038/s41386-021-01069-4 (2021).

World Health Organization. (2022). *Patient engagement*. https://apps.who.int/iris/bitstream/handle/10665/252269/9789241511629-eng.pdf

Xiao, J., Mi, W., Li, L., Shi, Y., & Zhang, H. (2015). High relapse rate and poor medication adherence in the Chinese population with schizophrenia: Results from an observational survey in the People's Republic of China. *Neuropsychiatric Disease and Treatment*, 11, 1161–1167. https://doi.org/10.2147/NDT.S72367

27 PROVISION OF CARE IN THE COMMUNITY

Christy Perry and Shirley Griffey

INTRODUCTION

This chapter focuses on the care of patients with mental illness in the community, including what is considered a community and how the APRN can provide appropriate care. There are many challenges to providing care to patients with mental illness, but resolutions have been identified that have improved health outcomes. Care in the community is a necessity for the overall well-being of patients with mental illness. The goals of community-based care are to increase accessibility to care, provide quality care, promote well-being, reduce mental health disorders, and enhance recovery. Community care can also reduce the stigma associated with seeking mental health treatment.

Mental health can be considered a public health issue. Good mental health among members of a community allows the community to thrive. Early intervention is needed to prevent the onset of some mental health diagnoses, especially substance use disorders. Early interventions can be health-promoting activities, and include education on the signs and symptoms of mental illness and the early treatment of mental illness. Health promotion and prevention can decrease the incidence of disability. Young people do not receive treatment as often as older people, which can delay treatment until much later in life. Delayed treatment can increase the risk of a patient dropping out of school, using substances more frequently, having a poor response to medication, having more hospitalizations, and possibly attempting suicide in the future.

DEFINITION OF COMMUNITY CARE

A. Community can describe a group of people in a geographic area, a specific culture, a race, or a group of people with similar healthcare needs.
B. For the purposes of this chapter, the community is a group of people with a mental health diagnosis. These diagnoses include bipolar disorder, major depressive disorder, generalized anxiety disorder, schizophrenia, schizoaffective, substance use disorders, neurodevelopmental disorders, and neurocognitive disorders. The recommended treatment is provided outside of an inpatient hospital setting.
C. According to the Centers for Disease Control and Prevention (CDC), the goal of treatment in the community is to promote healthy living, prevent chronic illness, and provide the greatest health benefit to the greatest amount of people.
D. Community mental health centers can provide medication management, case management, and outpatient psychotherapy.
E. Community mental healthcare should focus on the community's deficits as well as its strengths. Identifying a person's strengths to promote wellness will improve self-management of the illness.
F. Evidence-based treatment and patient involvement are critical to community care. Each community should be assessed to address specific needs and develop a plan to provide treatment that is accessible and appropriate.
G. Culture can affect the way a community reacts to mental illness. A person's culture may prevent them from seeking help or it may prevent others in their culture from helping.

WHY CARE IS NEEDED IN THE COMMUNITY

A. In 2019, there were one in five adults with a mental health diagnosis, or 51.5 million people. Of these, 13.1 million were diagnosed with a severe mental illness. Worldwide, one in every eight people (970 million) have a mental health diagnosis.
  1. Generalized anxiety disorder and major depressive disorder are the most common diagnoses. In 2020, people being diagnosed with these disorders rose to 26% and 28%. In 2019, 301 million people were diagnosed with an anxiety disorder, 280 million were diagnosed with depressive disorders, 40 million people were diagnosed with bipolar disorders, and 24 million people were diagnosed with schizophrenia.
B. In the United States, the annual prevalence of adults having a major depressive episode is 8.4%, adults with schizophrenia less than 1%, adults with bipolar 2.8%, adults with anxiety 19.1%, adults with posttraumatic stress syndrome 3.6%, adults with borderline personality disorder 1.4%, and adults with obsessive-compulsive disorder 1.2% (Figure 27.1; National Alliance on Mental Illness [NAMI], 2022a).
C. Care of patients with mental illness in the community is a necessity. In the 1950s and 1960s, the care of patients with mental illnesses began to shift from inpatient, long-term care to community-based outpatient care. The change was necessary due to the poor and sometimes inhumane living conditions of the hospitals, violations of human rights, and sometimes harmful treatments. Improvements in pharmacologic treatments also reduced symptoms and allowed patients to live in a less structured environment.

INPATIENT VERSUS OUTPATIENT CARE

A. There are differences worldwide in the number of patients receiving inpatient versus outpatient care. President John F. Kennedy signed the Community Mental Health Act (CMHA) of 1963, which proposed that comprehensive care should be provided in the community.
  1. The development of outpatient mental health centers supported this care with federal funding.
  2. Each state was encouraged to develop a system that best fits the people of their community.
  3. A provision was provided for more research on mental illness as well as prevention measures.

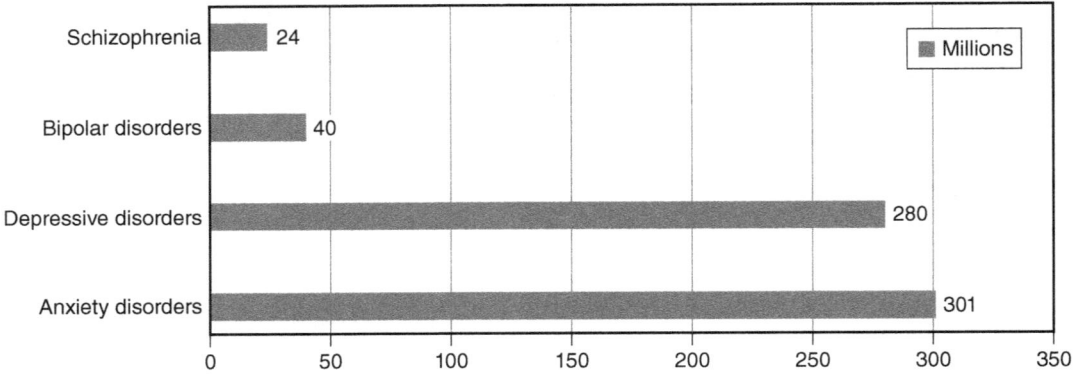

FIGURE 27.1 Worldwide diagnoses in 2019.

4. The main goal of the CMHA was to reduce the number of institutionalized patients. Government leaders were hopeful the newer pharmacologic therapies would reduce or eliminate mental illness. The medical profession agreed with the passing of the CMHA but had concerns that care in the communities was not equipped to provide the needed care. Medical professionals in the 1960s were concerned about some of the same stressors seen today, such as homelessness, housing, and other basic needs of patients with mental illness. The CMHA did fund some programs in the community, but they were not consistent programs and the National Institute of Mental Health (NIMH) could not regulate the programs. The expected number of community health centers was not developed and persons with serious mental illness did not receive the needed care due to the decrease in funding for inpatient care. In the early 2000s, state mental health hospitals had a 90% decrease in the census. European countries have had similar experiences, a decrease of inpatient care and inadequate community-based care.
5. To make a smooth transition, Fulone et al. (2021) identified six strategies to help communities continue with the implementation process of deinstitutionalization. These include psychoeducation, antistigma programs, case management, community mental health teams, assisted living, and interventions for acute psychosis.
   a. Psychoeducation includes teaching the patient, caregivers, and their families about their mental illness, possible symptoms they could experience, treatment options, and their prognosis and rehab potential by an individual or group that focuses on motivation, education, and behavioral techniques.
   b. Antistigma programs include interventions to reduce discrimination and negative impacts of mental illness. A study conducted by Brower found that ways to reduce stigma include having medical providers share their mental health stories, advocating governing entities to change inappropriate questioning about mental illness, expanding knowledge about mental illness, using evidence-based practice that decreases discrimination, and using language that does not stigmatize people.
   c. Case management includes an integrated healthcare system designed to provide flexible healthcare services.
   d. Community mental health team includes a multidisciplinary mental health team that follows the patient, such as an assertive community treatment (ACT) team.
   e. Assisted living should be designed to house deinstitutionalized people with mental illness.
   f. Interventions for acute psychosis include the use of a crisis intervention multidisciplinary team.

HOW TO DETERMINE WHAT CARE IS NEEDED IN A COMMUNITY

A. NAMI reports that one out of five people in the United States will experience a mental illness yearly.
B. In 2020, 52.9 million people or 21% of the U.S. population experienced mental illness. Only 46.2% of patients with mild to moderate mental illness received treatment, and the number increases to 64.5% with severe mental illness.
   1. Disparity in treatment warrants a community assessment (NAMI, 2022a).
      a. 53.8% of patients with mild to moderate mental illness are left untreated.
      b. 35.5% of people with severe mental illness are not adequately treated.
C. The CDC recognizes that communities need assistance with improving the health of their communities. To know what a community needs, a thorough assessment of the community should look at policy, targeted regulations, and community interventions. Communities should know current policies to effectively plan, identify, and create systems and environmental changes, and be able to monitor change over time.
   1. The CDC created the Community Health Assessment and Group Evaluation (CHANGE) Action Guide: Building a Foundation of Knowledge to Prioritize Community Health Needs in 2010. It is a data collection tool that can be utilized to help communities identify policy, systems, and environmental change to help communities organize data about their community, evaluate assets, and identify areas that need improvement.
   2. There are three main components of a community assessment: policy change, system change, and environmental change.
      a. Policy change consists of laws, rules, regulations, and protocol that guide community behavior and can either be organizational or legislative.
      b. System change is change in social norms, institutions, or systems for the entire community.
      c. Environmental change examines economic, physical, and social factors designed to influence behaviors of the entire community.

▶

3. The CDC uses a Framework for Program Evaluation to evaluate the information and make informed decisions. This measurement is completed using spreadsheets to collect data from schools, worksites, organizations, and healthcare systems.

D. Starting the process requires engagement of stakeholders, then focusing on design and collecting data. The process is finalized once data are analyzed and information is brought back to the stakeholders. Realizing that change can occur in many realms of the community, the socioecological model illustrates how multiple layers in a community influence one another. Community health is not only affected by individuals, relationships, economics, and culture, but also external factors like polices, environmental changes, and systems that give a better understanding of the impact on a community.

E. Although not all communities are the same, they exhibit many similarities that can affect change. Change can occur during a five-stage process of commitment, planning, assessment, implementation, and evaluation.

1. Commitment: This includes putting a community team together to address issues and to develop partnerships.
2. Assessment: This stage consists of gathering data and listening to community members' needs, as well as organizing strategies.
3. Planning: Once data are collected, the team can develop an action plan.
4. Implementation: This stage involves executing the developed plan with community members, stakeholders, and the newly developed partnerships.
5. Evaluation: Evaluation is the measurement used throughout the change process to see if key strategies are being implemented and if alternative interventions should be tried in the future.

F. The CHANGE tool and action guide had eight outlined steps in the original assessment but was narrowed to five steps in its 2013 revision. These are (a) planning a needs assessment, (b) conducting the assessment, (c) rating data, (d) recording and reviewing the consolidated data, and (e) developing a plan. These are summarized in the following:

1. Plan assessment: A multidisciplinary community team is assembled. The community to be assessed is defined, bylaws are created, operating procedures are discussed, and members of the community team are determined. The average size of a community team is 10 to 12 members. An example of who is on a community team is displayed in Figure 27.2.
2. Conduct assessment: The team develops a strategy, identifies the scope of the assessment, develops questions to ask, selects the sites, determines method of data collection, identifies the contact person in each sector, and documents findings. The CHANGE tool further breaks down this stage into five sectors including community-at-large, community institution/organizations, healthcare, schools, and worksites. The method of data collection should contain qualitative and quantitative data. The type of qualitative data includes individual interviews, focus groups, observations, postal surveys, telephone surveys, face-to-face surveys, and web-based survey.
3. Review and rate data: Prior to entering the data into the CHANGE tool, the team must develop a rating scale and know each site's environmental and policy change strategies (CDC, 2013).
4. Record and review consolidated data: One member of the team should enter the data into the spreadsheets using the CHANGE tool. An advantage to using the CHANGE tool is it calculates all data within each sector. After all data are entered, a summary of each sector can be obtained (CDC, 2013).
5. Develop a plan: The final step contains specific, measurable, attainable, realistic, and timely (SMART) objectives.

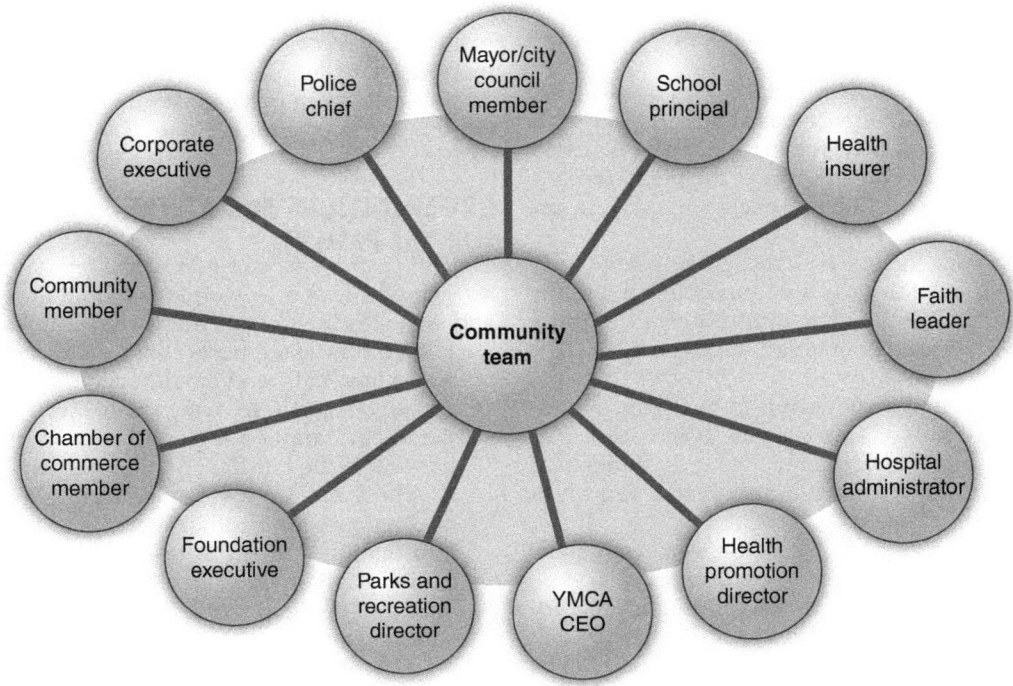

FIGURE 27.2 Example of community team.

CEO, chief executive officer; YMCA, Young Men's Christian Association.

MYTHS, STIGMA, AND BIASES REGARDING PEOPLE WITH MENTAL ILLNESS

A. Stigma and discrimination can impede mental healthcare. In some parts of the world, patients would rather suffer from a mental illness than be discriminated against when seeking treatment. Other people do not have the funds or insurance coverage to afford treatment (World Health Organization, 2022b). Stigma and discrimination may be a result of incorrect information by the public or myths held by communities or individuals. The following are some common myths:
   1. Children do not experience mental health symptoms.
   2. People with mental health problems are unpredictable and violent.
   3. People with mental health problems cannot be gainfully employed.
   4. Mental health problems are a result of character flaws or personal weakness.
   5. There is no hope for people with mental health problems.
   6. Therapy is not effective.
   7. Friends or family members cannot do anything to assist the person with mental health problems.
   8. There is no way to prevent mental health problems.

B. Half of all mental health symptoms present before the age of 14. Healthcare providers can screen for symptoms and educate families, patients, and other people who have ongoing contact with young people, such as teachers and other healthcare providers.

C. There is no evidence to support that people with mental illness are more likely to be violent compared with the person without mental illness. There is some evidence to support that the person with mental illness may be the victim of a violent act rather than the perpetrator of the violent act.

D. Mental illness is not the result of weakness or character flaws; it is like any other medical illness and should be treated in the same regard as any other medical illness.

E. Risk factors for mental illness include family history, genetics, physical illness, and environmental factors such as abuse or trauma.

F. There is hope for people with mental illness; recovery should be a treatment goal. Evidence-based research supports therapy as an effective treatment for many mental illnesses. Family and friends can be good support to the person receiving treatment. It is important to be respectful and not to use negative language.

G. Familiarity with risk factors and recognizing any early symptoms are important for early treatment and hopefully prevention of worsening of the symptoms (Substance Abuse and Mental Health Services Administration [SAMHSA], 2019, 2023).

H. Myths regarding mental health can lead to stigma against people with a mental illness. This can interfere with a person seeking mental health treatment. *Stigma* is defined as a negative belief or attitude toward a person due to trait or characteristic.

I. Stigma can be self-stigma or it can be perceived from others.
   1. Self-stigma is internalized negative thoughts regarding mental illness. Some examples of self-stigma are that the mental illness is a weakness, that treatment will not be effective, and/or feeling shame for asking for treatment.
      a. Stigma can lead to lower self-esteem, reduced hope, and possible resistance to seeking treatment.
      b. There is evidence that interactions with people with mental illnesses and education regarding common mental health diagnoses can reduce stigma.
   2. Public stigma is a negative view shared by people in the community against a specific population. Entire institutions (government or private organizations) can have stigma against a population who have mental illness, and this can limit services or opportunities based on the person's diagnosis.
   3. Stigma can create fear in the patient who is seeking treatment. The patient may be concerned that their complaint will not be taken seriously, or even worse that they may be harmed if they seek treatment. The NIMH recommends talking about mental health openly with other medical providers and people in the community to normalize it. Formal education to medical professionals is an effective way to reduce stigma.

J. A self-appraisal is helpful prior to caring for the patient with a mental illness. A self-appraisal can be part of a personal evaluation or a more formal evaluation in the workplace to address unrecognized biases. Healthcare providers can use inappropriate language when addressing patients with mental illness that can promote stigma, and education can reduce the use of this language (Table 27.1; Nyblade et al., 2019).

TABLE 27.1 APPROPRIATE LANGUAGE

Inappropriate Language	Appropriate Language
Addict Drug addict Alcoholic	Person with substance use disorder
Schizophrenic Crazy person Psychotic Nuts	Person with schizophrenia Person with mental illness
Committed suicide	Died by suicide Deceased
Clean drug screen or alcohol screen Dirty drug screen or alcohol screen	Negative screen Positive screen

ORGANIZATIONS FOR RESEARCH AND ASSISTANCE FOR THE PATIENT

A. The NIMH is a U.S. organization that is federally funded and is the leading organization on research on mental health.
   1. The NIMH supports clinicians and scientists at universities, hospitals, and small businesses via grants or other agreements. These researchers conduct basic, translational, and applied research to support and advance the mission of the NIMH.
   2. The NIMH provides education on various mental health topics for healthcare professionals as well as patient information. Patient education handouts can be downloaded digitally, and free-of-charge hard copies are also available. It also provides prevalence rates and other valuable statistics.
   3. The NIMH has an initiative titled "Brain Research Through Advancing Innovative Neurotechnologies" (BRAIN), which seeks to understand the individual cells and neural circuits of the brain with the hope of finding

new ways to treat and cure mental illness through medical, surgical, and behavior interventions.

B. NAMI is an organization that provides advocacy, education, support, and public awareness to individuals and families who are affected by mental illness. The vision of NAMI is to have a community who cares for the persons with mental illness. The focus is for the members of the community to help each other. NAMI has several important contributions to the community. It offers evidence-based educational programs and support for families and friends of someone who may be suffering from a mental illness. The organization is an advocate for the patient and is involved in shaping public policy to support people with mental illness. NAMI also provides peer-to-peer classes, many presentations, and a hotline.

RISK FACTORS OF CONCERN FOR PATIENTS IN THE COMMUNITY

A. Risk factors for developing mental illness can be vast. These factors can influence a person over the course of their life. One preventable risk, for example, is maternal substance use during pregnancy, which can produce mental health disorders later in life.
B. Biological risk factors cannot be changed, but some risks can be altered.
C. Factors that can be variable are life experiences, social contacts, financial situations, and health issues.
   1. Children and adolescents who have poor self-esteem and shyness may have anxiety later in life.
   2. Antisocial behavior, rebellious behavior, and early childhood emotional problems can lead to substance abuse.
   3. Head injuries and marijuana use can lead to psychiatric disorders.
   4. Early puberty, female, low self-esteem, insecure attachment, increased need for social approval, and poor social skills can lead to depressive symptoms.
   5. Risk factors related to young people that can increase the risk of all mental health disorders are poor parenting, abusive homes, and a parent with a history of mental illness and/or substance abuse.
D. Risk factors for suicide include access to lethal weapons, significant life events such as loss of a job or loss of relationship, social isolation, exposure to traumatic events, substance use disorders, mental health disorders, chronic health conditions, and social or familial connection with someone who has died by suicide. People living in poverty are at higher risk of suicide. Older adults and younger adults who are isolated are at higher risk.
E. There are many factors that can influence the development of a substance use disorder or mental illness. According to SAMHSA (2019), the risk factors for the development of a substance use disorder consist of genetic predisposition, community influences, and family and cultural influences.

PROTECTIVE FACTORS FOR PATIENTS IN THE COMMUNITY

A. A person may have risk factors but have or gain sufficient protective factors to avoid a mental health diagnosis.
B. Protective factors that decrease the incidence of children and adolescents developing mental health symptoms can be the exact oppositive of the risk factors. Protective factors include the following:
   1. High self-esteem
   2. Strong coping skills
   3. Strong emotional self-regulation
   4. Engagement with peers at school or community activities
   5. Successful academic development
C. Protective factors are provided by others to the young person and include a stable home, modeling of healthy relationships, and clear expectations of appropriate behavior.
D. Protective factors to prevent suicide are appropriate care for mental health and substance use disorders, supportive family and friends, and good coping skills.
E. Community risk factors can be cumulative, leading to poorer outcomes. Risk factors for a community can include the following:
   1. Poverty
   2. Lack of healthcare services
   3. High number of people using illicit substances
   4. High-crime areas
F. An increased number of protective factors improves outcomes for the people of the community. Strong community-based mental health clinics, access to this care, and care provided in a person's home are all considered protective factors. Education of mental health and appropriate treatments can be considered protective factors. Identification of problems early can help identify community-wide trends.
G. Protective factors are positive variables shown to lower negative outcomes. Protective factors for the community include the following:
   1. Access to quality healthcare
   2. Opportunities for employment
   3. Affordable housing
   4. Good educational programs
   5. Safe after-school activities for children
   6. Faith-based activities
   7. Low crime statistics
   8. Decreased substance use
H. Increasing community protective factors can improve individual protective factors. Improving childcare in a community can improve a child's risk factor of poor care. Improving public housing may eliminate an individual's risk of homelessness.

INDIVIDUAL PROVIDERS AND AGENCIES WHO CAN PROVIDE CARE IN THE COMMUNITY

A. Mental healthcare can be provided in a variety of settings, including traditional outpatient clinics (primary care offices as well as mental health offices), community mental health centers, intensive outpatient clinics, the school system, and in the home (Figure 27.3).
B. Some local governmental agencies operate community mental healthcare centers that care for patients with mild to severe mental health diagnoses.
C. Faith-based organizations also provide resources and care. Long-term relationships formed in faith-based organizations can be very supportive to a person with a mental illness and help build resilience.
D. The World Health Organization (WHO) has identified objectives for appropriate mental health treatment.
   1. One objective is to provide comprehensive, integrative, and responsive mental health in the community setting.

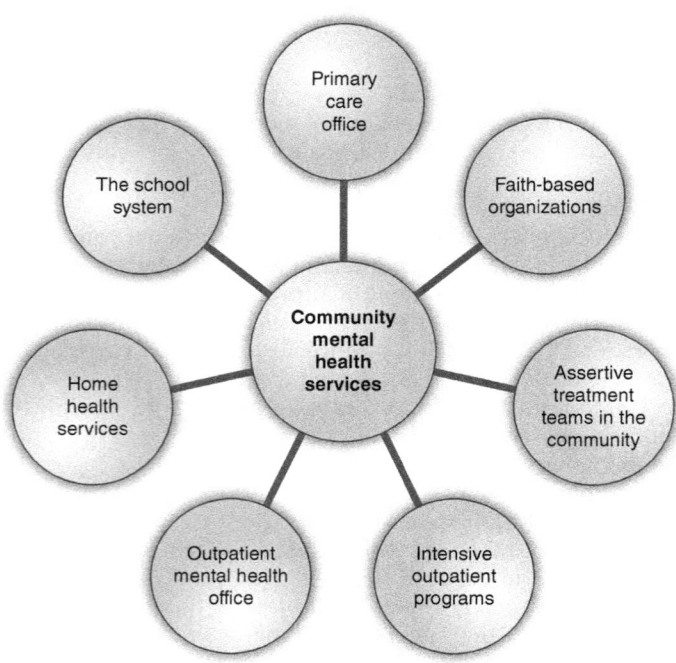

FIGURE 27.3 Providers in the community.

The care should include treatment of current illness, as well promoting wellness and recovery.

2. WHO identifies requirements of mental health providers, which are summarized in Box 27.1.

E. WHO recognizes that traumatic events may affect a community's mental health and require specific care at different times.

1. Natural disasters, civil unrest, or domestic violence may require a temporary increase in services. Mental health services should be incorporated into emergency responses and humanitarian responses.
2. The worldwide goals are to increase mental health services by half, to have 80% of the countries double their community mental health clinics, and to have mental health services integrated into primary care in 80% of countries by 2030.

F. Medical professionals and community members provide care to patients with mental illness as well as family members of the patients. Families of patients with mental illness are affected in many ways, such as having to provide additional time for needs not covered by insurance programs and mental health stigma. At least 8.4 million people in the United States assist with caring for an adult who has emotional or mental health issues. This averages 32 hours weekly that a family will provide unpaid services to their family members.

BOX 27.1 BASIC REQUIREMENTS OF COMPETENT MENTAL HEALTH PROVIDERS

- Listening and responding to patients
- Having a good understanding of their illness and their current health condition
- Knowing what helps the patient achieve wellness
- Being aware of community resources for housing, educational opportunities, and community activities for interaction with others to avoid isolation

G. Family caregivers do not have time to care for themselves, which leads to additional problems. A study conducted by Karimirad et al. (2022) found that caregivers feel exhausted (known as *caregiver burnout*), have trouble controlling or dealing with the patient's behavior, cannot be involved in leisure activities, and suffer from sleep issues and lack of physical exercise. Guilt can be another stressor if the family member does not provide the care. Addressing caregiver stress when providing treatment to the patient is essential.

H. ACT is a community-based program that has been beneficial to the patient and the family.

1. The concept behind the ACT team consists of a multidisciplinary team that creates a patient-centered relationship with consistent treatment among different members of the team. The principles of ACT are delivery of services in the community, outreach, holistic services, continuity of care, and integrated services. The team members include a psychiatrist, nurse, peer specialist, social worker, or case manager who has experience in various fields. ACT is an evidence-based approach to prevent hospitalization, improve quality of life, and assist with stabilization of people who are at risk of psychiatric crisis. The ACT team uses an assertive engagement protocol tool to ensure all avenues have been assessed prior to discharge.

I. The forensic assertive community team/treatment (FACT) is a model that emerged from ACT as a modified model and was established to prevent arrest and incarceration of adults with mental illness. The three essential elements that differentiate FACT from ACT are the inclusion of a forensic peer specialist, having one or two members as criminal justice liaisons, and having culturally diverse teams. Despite the need to assist patients who have both mental illness and criminal justice problems, barriers exist. These include training between FACT members and criminal justice employees, as well as problems existing with reimbursement and the additional policies that address financial, political, and sociolegal needs, which still need to be in place.

J. Socially integrating adults with mental illness can receive treatment in numerous ways, such as intensive case management and psychoeducation or mentoring, but these are costly and time-consuming. A more recent intervention is group-based programs, such as intensive outpatient programs (IOP). The IOP can design the program based on age of group members, setting, or diagnosis. Dalgaard et al. (2022) summarized that group-based interventions that focused on social reintegration and recovery had positive advantages over individual treatment options. A study by Pahwa et al. (2020) found that patients who integrated into community services had safety concerns related to their neighborhoods, stigma, loss of relationships, and homelessness, and concluded that many use group-related programs as a safe place from their environmental issues, a place to get support, and a place to learn appropriate coping skills and receive other necessary resources.

K. IOPs are not usually individually designed for psychosis. However, a study by Samplin and colleagues (2022) examined 92 patients with a diagnosis of psychosis by combining cognitive behavioral skills therapy (CBST) with medication management. The therapy consisted of 3 hours of CBST and 6 additional hours of therapy for approximately 8 weeks. Of the 92 patients, 77% completed the program, found improvement in five of the eight psychosis symptoms (hallucinations, disorganized speech, delusions, depression, and mania), and had high satisfaction.

CHALLENGES FOR PROVIDERS PROVIDING CARE IN THE COMMUNITY

A. Many of the minority populations and underserved populations lack insurance coverage, lack community-based programs, lack access to treatment, and experience stigma, and there may be a shortage of mental health workers in urban areas.
  1. Due to this disparity, approximately 60% of people with mental illness are treated by their primary care physician.
  2. Ways to overcome challenges for mental health providers include using more telepsychiatry and improvement in mental health training.
  3. The Housing Fast is a community-based program designed to assist with housing.
  4. The patient-centered medical home (PCMH) was created to treat the whole person with services such as primary care, behavioral health, and dental and social services regardless of their income or insurance.

B. WHO and the NIMH are creating programs for unserved communities. These programs include the Mental Health Gap Action Program (mh-GAP), which was started in 2008 to assist with mental health, substance use disorders, and neurology in a regular healthcare setting by a nonprofessional mental health specialist. A concept already in place is task sharing, which includes such programs as ACT or Mental Health First Aid (MHFA). The MHFA is a training program designed to raise mental health awareness, eliminate stigma, and promote treatment.

HEALTHCARE COST

A. Among the patients who received care for mental illness, 17.7 million had delayed or cancelled appointments, while 7.3 million experienced issues when picking up their medication and 4.9 million were unable to access mental health facilities. In the United States, severe mental illness causes $193.2 billion in lost wages every year. The economic impact of mental illness globally and regionally is significant. Arias and colleagues (2022) estimated that the economic value of disability related to mental illness could exceed $4.7 trillion. Regionally, this loss could account for 7.9% of the gross domestic product of North America.

SUBSTANCE ABUSE

A. One in fifteen adults in the United States have a dual diagnosis of a mental illness and a substance use disorder. The National Survey on Drug Use and Health conducted a survey in 2020 and found that 20.9% of adolescents ages 12 to 17 had a substance use disorder or diagnosed with major depression. Adults 18 years and older had a 29.3% risk of having a mental illness or substance use disorder.

HOMELESSNESS/SAFETY

A. According to NAMI, 20.8% of the homeless population have severe mental illness (2022). Mongelli et al. (2020) discussed that 2.5 to 3.5 million sleep in transitional housing, shelter, or in public places. Additionally, they report that the average life expectancy for a homeless person is 47 years old compared with the average age of 77 years old. Approximately one-third of the homeless population are children. Of homeless families, about 29% have a working adult, most of whom are women, and 63% of homeless women have been victims of domestic abuse.

POVERTY

A. The U.S. Department of Health and Human Services in 2020 estimated that 11.4% of the U.S. population are poor. The poverty guidelines for 2022 indicate that if a family of four has an income of less than $27,750 they are considered poor. Chin et al. (2022) examined the poverty–mental illness cycle and showed that children growing up in poverty are three times more likely to develop a mental illness. Additionally, poverty and mental illness occur through many disparities, such as malnutrition, trauma, violence, unemployment, and education. Snowden et al. (2022) found that different minority groups had higher odds of living in poverty, being arrested in the past, being unemployed, and were less likely to receive care.

SAFETY/SELF-HARMING BEHAVIORS

A. According to the CDC (2018), 46% of people who died by suicide had a known mental illness. The warning signs of suicide include increased consumption of alcohol or drug; aggressive behavior; socially withdrawing from family, friends, and community; change in mood; reckless behavior; or impulsivity (NAMI, 2019). Suicidal behaviors that are an emergency and need immediate attention include saving/collecting pills, buying a weapon, giving away treasured possessions, organizing personal matter, and saying goodbye to family and friends. There are many risk factors for suicide. These include a family history of suicide, substance use, intoxication, access to firearms, a chronic medical condition, being male, history of trauma or abuse, a recent loss, and prolonged stress.

CRIMINAL JUSTICE ISSUES

A. Nearly two out of five people incarcerated have a history of mental illness, approximately 37% in state and federal prisons and 44% in local jails. In this population, 66% of the women incarcerated has a mental illness.

RESOLUTIONS FOR THE CHALLENGES WHILE CARING FOR PATIENTS IN THE COMMUNITY

A. There are three categories of prevention interventions:
  1. Universal: a broad approach to reach an entire population, such as a school
  2. Selective: focuses on biological, social, and psychological, such as support groups
  3. Indicated: deals with individual interventions for high-risk individuals for substance use disorders, such as referral to outpatient services

RESOURCES

A. Community mental health alliance programs (National Alliance on Mental Illness [NAMI]): www.nami.org
B. National Institute of Mental Health: www.nimh.nih.gov
C. Substance Abuse and Mental Health Services Administration (SAMHSA): www.samhsa.gov
D. Mental Health.gov: www.mentalhealth.gov

REFERENCES AND BIBLIOGRAPHY

American Psychiatric Association. (n.d.). *Stigma, prejudice and discrimination against people with mental illness*. Psychiatry.org. https://www.psychiatry.org/patients-families/stigma-and-discrimination

Arias, D., Saxena, S., & Verguet, S. (2022, May 7). *Quantifying the global burden of mental illness and its economic value*. Papers.ssrn.com https://papers.ssrn.com/sol3/papers.cfm?abstract_id=4103145

Assertive Community Treatment. (2021, June 25). *Center for evidence-based practices*. Case Western Reserve University. https://case.edu/socialwork/centerforebp/practices/assertive-community-treatment

Assistant Secretary for Planning and Evaluation. (2024, January 17). *Poverty guidelines*. U.S. Department of Health and Human Services. https://aspe.hhs.gov/topics/poverty-economic-mobility/poverty-guidelines

Bond, G. R., & Drake, R. E. (2015). The critical ingredients of assertive community treatment. *World Psychiatry, 14*(2), 240–242. https://doi.org/10.1002/wps.20234

Brooks, A. (2019, March 4). *What is community health and why is it important?* Rasmussen University. https://www.rasmussen.edu/degrees/health-sciences/blog/what-is-community-health

Brower, K. J. (2021). The professional stigma of mental health issues: Physicians are both the cause and solution. *Academic Medicine, 96*(5), 635–640. https://doi.org/10.1097/acm.0000000000003998

Centers for Disease Control and Prevention. (2010). *Change health assessment and group evaluation (CHANGE) Action Guide: Building a foundation of knowledge to prioritize community needs*. U.S. Department of Health and Human Services. http://www.communitycommons.org/entities/4226783c-f5e8-4d3c-b20b-4c71d91c92f0

Centers for Disease Control and Prevention. (2013). *Community Health Assessment and Group Evaluation (CHANGE) tool*. U.S. Department of Health and Human Services. https://archive.cdc.gov/www_cdc_gov/nccdphp/dnpao/state-local-programs/change-tool/index.html

Centers for Disease Control and Prevention. (2018, June 7). *Suicide rising across the US*. CDC VitalSigns. U.S. Department of Health and Human Services. https://www.cdc.gov/vitalsigns/pdf/vs-0618-suicide-H.pdf

Chin, J. L., Garcia, Y. E., Blume, A. W. (2022). *The psychology of inequity: Motivation and beliefs*. Praeger.

Couser, G. P., Taylor-Desir, M., Lewis, S., & Griesbach, T. J. (2021). Further adaptations and reflections by an assertive community treatment team to serve clients with severe mental illness during COVID-19. *Community Mental Health Journal, 57*(7), 1227–1229. https://doi.org/10.1007/s10597-021-00860-3

Cuncic, A. (2019). *What to expect from assertive community treatment*. Verywell Mind. https://www.verywellmind.com/assertive-community-treatment-4587610

Dalgaard, N. T., Flensborg Jensen, M. C., Bengtsen, E., Krassel, K. F., & Vembye, M. H. (2022). PROTOCOL: Group-based community interventions to support the social reintegration of marginalised adults with mental illness. *Campbell Systematic Reviews, 18*(3), e1254. https://doi.org/10.1002/cl2.1254

Erickson, B. (2021). Deinstitutionalization through optimism: The community mental health act of 1963. *The American Journal of Psychiatry Residents' Journal, 16*(4), 6–7. https://doi.org/10.1176/appi.ajp-rj.2021.160404

Freeman, M. (2022). The world mental health report: Transforming mental health for all. *World Psychiatry, 21*(3), 391–392. https://doi.org/10.1002/wps.21018

Fulone, I., Barreto, J. O. M., Barberato-Filho, S., Bergamaschi, C. de C., Silva, M. T., & Lopes, L. C. (2021). Improving care for deinstitutionalized people with mental disorders: Experiences of the use of knowledge translation tools. *Frontiers in Psychiatry, 12*, 575108. https://doi.org/10.3389/fpsyt.2021.575108

Hoggett, P. (1993). What is community mental health? *Journal of Interprofessional Care, 7*(3), 201–209. https://doi.org/10.3109/13561829309014984

Ielmini, M., Lucca, G., Trabucchi, E., Aspesi, G. L., Bellini, A., Caselli, I., & Callegari, C. (2022). Assessing mental pain as a predictive factor of suicide risk in a clinical sample of patients with psychiatric disorders. *Behavioral Sciences, 12*(4), 111. https://doi.org/10.3390/bs12040111

Karimirad, M. R., Seyedfatemi, N., Mirsepassi, Z., Noughani, F., & Cheraghi, M. A. (2022). Barriers to self-care planning for family caregivers of patients with severe mental illness. *Journal of Patient Experience, 9*, 237437352210926. https://doi.org/10.1177/23743735221092630

Lamberti, J. S., & Weisman, R. L. (2021). Essential elements of forensic assertive community treatment. *Harvard Review of Psychiatry, 29*(4), 278–297. https://doi.org/10.1097/hrp.0000000000000299

Lamberti, J. S., Weisman, R., & Faden, D. I. (2004). Forensic assertive community treatment: Preventing incarceration of adults with severe mental illness. *Psychiatric Services, 55*(11), 1285–1293. https://doi.org/10.1176/appi.ps.55.11.1285

Mayo Clinic Staff. (2017, May 24). *Mental health: Overcoming the stigma of mental illness*. Mayo Clinic. http://www.mayoclinic.org/diseases-conditions/mental-illness/in-depth/mental-health/art-20046477

Misra, S., Jackson, V. W., Chong, J., Choe, K., Tay, C., Wong, J., & Yang, L. H. (2021). Systematic review of cultural aspects of stigma and mental illness among racial and ethnic minority groups in the United States: Implications for interventions. *American Journal of Community Psychology, 68*(3–4), 486–512. https://doi.org/10.1002/ajcp.12516

Nagy, J., & Fawcett, S. B. (n.d.). Chapter 19, Choosing and adapting community interventions: Section 2, Understanding risk and protective factors: Their use in selecting potential targets and promising strategies for intervention. In The University of Kansas Center for Community Health and Development, *Community toolbox*. https://ctb.ku.edu/en/table-of-contents/analyze/choose-and-adapt-community-interventions/risk-and-protective-factors/main

National Institute of Mental Health. (n.d.). *Technology and the future of mental health treatment*. https://www.nimh.nih.gov/health/topics/technology-and-the-future-of-mental-health-treatment

National Alliance on Mental Illness. (2019). *Risk of suicide*. https://www.nami.org/About-Mental-Illness/Common-with-Mental-Illness/Risk-of-Suicide

National Institute of Mental Health. (2020). *About the National Institute of Mental Health*. https://www.nimh.nih.gov/about

National Alliance on Mental Illness. (2022a). *Mental health by the numbers*. https://www.nami.org/mhstats

National Alliance of Mental Illness. (2022b). https://www.nami.org/home

Nyblade, L., Stockton, M. A., Giger, K., Bond, V., Ekstrand, M. L., Lean, R. M., Mitchell, E. M. H., Nelson, L. R. E., Sapag, J. C., Siraprapasiri, T., Turan, J., & Wouters, E. (2019). Stigma in health facilities: Why it matters and how we can change it. *BMC Medicine, 17*(1), 25. https://doi.org/10.1186/s12916-019-1256-2

Pahwa, R., Dougherty, R. J., Kelly, E., Davis, L., Smith, M. E., & Brekke, J. S. (2020). Is it safe? Community integration for individuals with serious mental illnesses. *Research on Social Work Practice, 32*(7), 826–838. https://doi.org/10.1177/1049731520951628

Samari, E., Teh, W. L., Roystonn, K., Devi, F., Cetty, L., Shahwan, S., & Subramaniam, M. (2022). Perceived mental illness stigma among family and friends of young people with depression and its role in help-seeking: A qualitative inquiry. *BMC Psychiatry, 22*(1), 107. https://doi.org/10.1186/s12888-022-03754-0

Samplin, E., Grzenda, A., & Burns, A. V. (2022). Feasibility and effectiveness of a psychosis-specific intensive outpatient program. *Psychiatric Research and Clinical Practice, 4*(3), 74–79. https://doi.org/10.1176/appi.prcp.20210030

Snowden, L. R., Cordell, K., & Bui, J. (2022). Racial and ethnic disparities in health status and community functioning among persons with untreated mental illness. *Journal of Racial and Ethnic Health Disparities, 10*(5), 2175–2184 https://doi.org/10.1007/s40615-022-01397-1

Stein, L. I., & Test, M. A. (1980). Alternative to mental hospital treatment. *Archives of General Psychiatry, 37*(4), 392–397. https://doi.org/10.1001/archpsyc.1980.01780170034003

Substance Abuse and Mental Health Services Administration. (2011). *Consumer-operated services: Getting started with evidence-based practices*. HHS Pub. No. SMA-11-4633. U.S. Department of Health and Human Services. https://store.samhsa.gov/sites/default/files/sma11-4633-getting-started.pdf

Substance Abuse and Mental Health Services Administration. (2013, July). *Community conversations about mental health: Information brief*. U.S. Department of Health and Human Services. https://store.samhsa.gov/sites/default/files/sma13-4763.pdf

Substance Abuse and Mental Health Services Administration. (2019). *Risk and protective factors*. U.S. Department of Health and Human Services. https://www.samhsa.gov/sites/default/files/20190718-samhsa-risk-protective-factors.pdf

Substance Abuse and Mental Health Services Administration. (2020, January 14). *Home page CBHSQ data*. U.S. Department of Health and Human Services. https://www.samhsa.gov/data

Substance Abuse and Mental Health Services Administration. (2023, April 24). *What is mental health?* U.S. Department of Health and Human Services. https://www.samhsa.gov/mental-health

Thornicroft, G., Deb, T., & Henderson, C. (2016). Community mental health care worldwide: Current status and further developments. *World Psychiatry, 15*(3), 276–286. https://doi.org/10.1002/wps.20349

Vermont.gov. (n.d.). *Risk and protective factors.* https://mentalhealth.vermont.gov/suicide-prevention/risk-and-protective-factors

Weimand, B. M., Israel, P., & Ewertzon, M. (2017). Families in Assertive CommunityTreatment (ACT) teams in Norway: A cross-sectional study on relatives' experiences of involvement and alienation. *Community Mental Health Journal, 54*(5), 686–697. https://doi.org/10.1007/s10597-017-0207

World Health Organization. (2021, September 21). *Comprehensive mental health action plan 2013–2030.* https://www.who.int/publications/i/item/9789240031029

World Health Organization. (2022a, May 18). *2022 progress report on the Global Action Plan for Healthy Lives and Well-Being for All: Executive summary.* https://www.who.int/publications/m/item/2022-progress-report-executive-summary

World Health Organization. (2022b, June 8). *Mental disorders.* https://www.who.int/news-room/fact-sheets/detail/mental-disorders

Youth.gov. (n.d.). *Risk and protective factors for youth.* https://youth.gov/youth-topics/youth-mental-health/risk-and-protective-factors-youth

IV CONCEPTION TO LAUNCH AND ESTABLISHING A PRACTICE

28 ESTABLISHING A PSYCHIATRIC APRN PRACTICE

Suzanne Drake

INTRODUCTION

The autonomy that APRNs achieve through practice ownership is viewed by many as an ideal toward which to strive. Starting a practice involves more than a wish; it requires careful thought and strategic planning. Transitioning from employee to a practice owner requires clinical experience and business skills. With various aspects to consider, such as understanding community needs and managing finances and legal responsibilities, the idea can feel overwhelming. Yet, for APRNs who have been trained to approach challenges, this task can be tackled with confidence. The nursing process acts as a guide that promotes thinking, problem-solving, and innovation—crucial skills for succeeding as an entrepreneur. By applying the steps of assessment, diagnosis, planning, implementation, and evaluation, APRNs can effectively navigate the intricacies of running a business while upholding quality care standards and ethical practices for development. This organized method not only improves results, but also opens doors for professional growth and fosters a culture of excellence in private practice environments.

This chapter examines the process of setting up a practice, highlighting benefits and obstacles from both the APRN and patient perspectives. Success factors include self-awareness, location selection, financial preparation, compliance with regulations, and marketing strategies. Insights from practice owners, literature review, and case studies demonstrate the practical application of these principles. Starting a practice offers independence and customization of patient care, but also entails challenges like costs, regulations, and effective marketing. Personal awareness, strategic location selection, and thorough planning are vital to predicting a practice's success.

IT STARTS WITH A THOUGHT

APRNs may start to consider establishing practice ownership through personal introspection, leading them to contemplate career goals and professional aspirations. When these self-reflective inquiries move beyond speculation, they promote deeper insights and thoughtful strategizing. Examining the initial inspiration for starting a private practice and the intended goals is necessary to move it beyond fantasy to actualization. Putting thoughts and musings to paper is a powerful tool in pressing forward.

BENEFITS TO THE APRN

Venturing into private practice presents many advantages for APRNs seeking career growth and enhanced care for their patients:

A. A sense of agency and authority emerges from the impotent subordination characteristic of employment relationships. Transitioning from employee to owner liberates one from the restrictive grip of bureaucratic systems, bringing a fresh sense of freedom, self-reliance, and power.
B. The APRN has autonomy and control over policies, workflow, and other business operations.
C. The APRN gains the freedom to make decisions about their work hours, patient care, what services are offered, and business operations.
D. The flexibility in scheduling contributes to job satisfaction and a better work–life balance.
E. Managing the practice fosters professional development and offers opportunities for creativity, innovation, and community engagement.
F. Cultivating lasting relationships with patients can engender loyalty and a positive reputation.
G. Specializing in market segments enables practitioners to provide services tailored to a particular demographic, their "ideal patient."
H. The APRN has creative freedom to design and implement the practice according to one's beliefs, values, aesthetics, preferences, and other personal benefits unique to one's circumstances.
I. While expenses may be involved, the financial benefits can outweigh those of positions, setting the APRN firmly in charge of their future.

BENEFITS TO PATIENTS

A. APRNs combine psychiatric expertise with medical knowledge, affording patients a broad range of care for the whole person.
B. APRNs often serve as a point of contact for patients, promoting continuity of care. This ongoing connection can deepen the understanding of a patient's history, enhance the management of long-term and chronic conditions, and boost the effectiveness of treatment.
C. APRNs can offer comprehensive and personalized care, resulting in less fragmented, more holistic care. Patients can benefit from better access to care in private practice.
D. APRNs may offer more flexible scheduling options and can effectively cater to urgent care needs.
E. APRNs typically spend more time with their patients in private practice, providing extensive patient education. Patient empowerment and engagement promotes greater participation in their healthcare.
F. When working autonomously, APRNs can readily focus on screening, prevention, health education, and other essential aspects of healthcare.
G. Private practice allows the APRN to promptly address patient concerns and modify treatments without the hurdles commonly seen in larger healthcare institutions. This personalized approach results in more responsive and adaptable care delivery.
H. APRNs can offer a wide array of psychiatric services, such as medication prescribing and medication management, as well as various modalities of psychotherapy, through independent practice.
I. Patients can benefit from faster access to high-quality psychiatric care at affordable cost.

J. Increased competition between healthcare providers can potentially lower healthcare costs for patients and the broader regional healthcare system.

POTENTIAL DOWNSIDES OF PRACTICE OWNERSHIP

A. Isolation can be a problem for the APRN, who might need more connection with the teamwork available in larger settings, potentially hindering professional development and peer assistance.
B. APRNs may need help to keep up-to-date with medical advancements due to limited access to inservice education and training compared with individuals in larger institutions.
C. Private practitioners must spend money and time on marketing efforts to attract and keep patients.
D. There is a considerable financial risk at play, which may include expensive initial investments and unpredictable earnings.
E. Having an unstable income can create challenges to financial planning. Operating a practice is also unpredictable as variables such as patient volume and regulations may fluctuate unexpectedly.
F. Owners must allocate significant time to managing operations, resulting in an imbalance between work and personal life.
G. Challenges may arise in ensuring sufficient coverage during emergencies or after-hours, which can impact the continuity of patient care.
H. Dealing with insurance contracts and navigating potential lower or delayed reimbursements can complicate financial stability.
I. Healthcare regulations increase the workload by demanding time-consuming and frustrating compliance.
J. The pressure and accountability of being the ultimate decision-maker can feel crushing.
K. Not everyone enjoys responsibilities such as managing payroll and ensuring compliance as they often distract from the joy of providing patient care.
L. APRNs encounter additional obstacles, such as obtaining admission privileges and understanding state regulations, which may restrict their potential for advancement.

DEVELOPING A PLAN

A. All nascent businesses begin with a plan. Using established strategies that have proven effective over time can significantly help when starting a new company. Employing a proven, effective method over seven decades as a foundational strategy can minimize the chance of making mistakes through guesswork and experimentation.
B. Modified from the scientific method, the nursing process is a decision-making approach that promotes critical thinking skills.
C. The nursing process will help craft a viable business plan. However, it will also be invaluable throughout the lifetime of the practice.
D. The nursing process is not linear but an organic, evolving, cyclic journey. This methodical approach promotes organized steps, from assessment to diagnosis, to planning, implementation, evaluation, and reassessment, cultivating a cycle of dynamic problem-solving and more effective solutions.
E. Think of the practice as your patient.

GOAL ASSESSMENT

Self-Assessment

A. As clinically skilled as a clinician may be, their practice will only survive if they understand that they will be operating a business. Opening a practice is a big undertaking; only some are cut out for it. While many may be qualified, not all should. Understanding oneself is vital to finding and following a fulfilling career path, which is a true advantage in business ownership. Having confidence in one's abilities is essential to pursuing goals with courage, and this confidence results from profound self-understanding.
B. Self-knowledge can be honed through therapy, journaling, mindfulness meditation, accepting feedback from others, and analyzing assessment tools. Self-inquiry is intended to inspire authentic self-awareness rather than pass judgment. Recognizing one's more negative characteristics or the "shadow side" is an essential aspect of truthful self-awareness.
C. By adding evidence-based assessments, one can comprehensively determine if one's personality aligns well with entrepreneurship. These assessment tools evaluate traits such as risk tolerance, leadership skills, adaptability, and resilience that are essential for business success.
   1. The Big Five Personality Traits evaluation (free open source available online) examines qualities such as openness and conscientiousness, both of which are linked to achievement.
   2. The DISC (**D**ominance, **I**nfluence, **S**teadiness, and **C**ompliance) profile (free version) focuses on traits like dominance and conscientiousness to provide insights into negotiation tactics and team leadership capabilities.
   3. The Grit Scale measures passion for reaching long-term goals in entrepreneurship.
   4. The Risk Taking Inventory and the Entrepreneurial Mindset Profile help gauge risk tolerance and overall suitability for entrepreneurship by examining traits such as independence and creativity.
D. If, after deriving insights into one's characteristics, the APRN does not entirely match the typical qualities of successful entrepreneurs and has average or below-average scores in these areas, there is still hope. With the assistance of a business coach, these characteristics can be cultivated.

Assessing Motivation and Goals

Starting a practice is often driven by many factors, including the desire for independence and a need for change or escape from current dissatisfaction.

A. APRNs contemplating this path typically begin by identifying what initially sparked their interest and reflecting on the positive aspects of owning a practice.
B. Setting goals involves defining the expected outcomes and considering how one's daily routine will be impacted. Together, these elements form an approach to motivation and goal setting that is essential to a successful establishment and growth of a private practice.
   1. Factors such as viability, potential earnings, and envisioning the environment are important considerations.
   2. Understanding the patient demographic and analyzing the competitive landscape help refine the practice's unique market position.
   3. Additionally, decisions regarding management structure, such as choosing between operating solo or involving partners in decision-making, need to be weighed.

4. Lastly, evaluating preparedness and securing funding before launching the practice are crucial.

Assessing Personal Financial Style

A. Effective and responsible financial management, whether personal or business, is critical to achieving success. Conversely, without it, the business will not survive. For APRNs struggling with financial management, helpful resources such as Dave Ramsey's *Complete Guide to Money* can provide crucial educational support.

B. Successful financial management involves essential habitual practices:
1. Successful financial management involves creating and adhering to budgets for personal and business expenses, spending responsibly, and ensuring bills are paid on time.
2. It is essential to save more money than one makes to prevent the buildup of debt. Being financially prudent means preparing for the future by saving money for retirement and other long-term objectives.
3. Monitoring and enhancing one's debt-to-income ratio and credit score are other crucial components of overall financial well-being.

C. Entrepreneurs can have a safety net while building their practice by having additional sources of income like savings, passive income, a financially stable partner, equity investments, or a side gig.

Assessing Executive Function

A business owner must have robust executive function skills.

A. Self-regulation entails maintaining composure and professionalism even during difficult situations. Emotional regulation is needed to make rational decisions and interact effectively with patients, employees, and colleagues.

B. Problem-solving skills are necessary as challenges are inevitable in business. The key is the ability to identify issues, analyze them critically, and devise solutions.

C. Starting and completing tasks on time is essential in maintaining the flow of business operations and building trust. Avoiding procrastination and promptly meeting obligations is also essential.

D. Making timely and well-informed decisions is derived from assessing data, weighing options, and considering the future impact of each choice on the company.

E. Effective prioritization and adept time management are needed to ensure seamless business operations and meeting deadlines. This includes delegating tasks as needed.

F. Business efficiency is critical to maintaining smooth operations within an organization. This involves organizing digital spaces to oversee financial records, patient information, and operational data to ensure easy accessibility and orderliness.

G. Strategic planning is vital to private practice. It is vital to establish long-term goals, create action plans, and adjust strategies as needed to achieve business objectives. This involves anticipating scenarios, preparing for contingencies, and managing risks.

Assessing Moral Compass

A. Markey et al. (2022) investigated the essence of integrity in leadership, reimagining personal and professional integrity as a gateway to leadership that prioritizes human connections. A commitment to ethical values in every aspect of life is imperative for a successful and effective leader.

B. APRNs who build their lives and practice around principles, stay true to core values, and consistently demonstrate honesty and transparency foster a sense of trustworthiness among colleagues and patients.
1. Embodying authenticity, they are consistent in words and actions, even through adversity. This demonstrates fortitude, tenacity, and credence.
2. Congruence and honesty engender reliability and promote trust.

C. Notable leaders are compassionate. They regularly express gratitude, kindness, and respect, actively seeking out and highlighting the strengths of their patients and colleagues.
1. They are fair and just. They take responsibility and hold themselves accountable.
2. They promptly acknowledge mistakes and take steps to resolve issues, reinforcing their integrity and commitment to ethical behavior.
3. They are assertive and demonstrate good boundaries for themselves and others.

Assessing Leadership Skills

A. Self-awareness includes being aware of how one is seen by others. Practice owners are in positions of leadership. Some people naturally garner the respect of others, becoming motivators who inspire those around them. How much weight others give to their opinions also plays a role in defining their leadership and influence.

B. Leadership styles vary greatly and can impact how a leader interacts with their team and the organization as a whole.
1. Autocratic leadership: The leader makes decisions independently, maintaining control over followers by setting rules and procedures. The group is expected to follow instructions without offering input, establishing a hierarchy, and enabling decision-making but potentially limiting creativity and involvement.
2. Democratic leadership: The democratic leader shares decision-making responsibilities with the group by supporting the interests of its members and promoting equality. This promotes collaboration and consensus building, improving group satisfaction and decision quality.
3. Laissez-faire leadership: Here, the leader provides tools, resources, and oversight but mostly steps back, allowing team members to take charge of how they achieve goals. While it can enhance initiative and creativity, it may lead to unclear role definitions and a lack of motivation.
4. Transformational leadership: Transformational leaders inspire and motivate followers by setting a vision that challenges and transforms the state. They focus on initiating change by aligning goals with objectives. This creates an enthusiastic work environment that fosters innovation.
5. Each style has its advantages and challenges.

Assessing Experience

A. It is imperative to evaluate whether the APRN has the skills and experience to operate autonomously before venturing into solo practice.

B. If reassurance is still needed or the APRN is relatively new in their field, it is premature to start practicing solo. Instead, the APRN is advised to focus on mastering their specialty's theoretical aspects and clinical skills.

1. During this phase, the APRN can improve their skills by taking a residency in their specialty and/or working in a private practice, with the added benefit of expanding their professional network.
2. Enrolling in business-related courses covering medical practice management, coding, and billing, as well as learning the nuances of insurance plans and contracts, will provide the APRN with essential administrative skills.
3. Continuing education and obtaining certifications within their specialty will also aid in establishing a niche for the APRN, setting them up to attract their ideal patients to their practice.

Assessing Family Circumstances

A. The influence of family opinions on business decisions and the level of commitment required should not be underestimated. It is essential to consider the needs and perspectives of one's family.
B. The duties and financial factors associated with managing a business can impact their support or resistance, especially in situations like parenthood or caring for older adults or relatives with disabilities. Economic conditions at home, such as student loan obligations and the need for two incomes, can also play a role.
C. Life events such as marriage, divorce, or having children may alter family dynamics and priorities. It is important to recognize and address family members' concerns as their apprehensions may be valid.
D. It is crucial to discuss and devise solutions to resolve them. If family concerns lack merit and differ from the goals of the APRN, having confidence can empower one to help allay family fears and show respect for their viewpoints while still moving forward.

Assessing Interprofessional Collaboration

A. In any new venture requiring more than a casual familiarity with small business ownership, procuring a mentor or coach can be invaluable.
B. Working in private practice can pose a risk of becoming siloed.
C. Highly complex health issues require more than one discipline to manage the patient's care.
D. Consider the following:
   1. Joining or creating a patient-centered team, for example, consulting regularly with patients' primary care providers and relevant specialists to coordinate care
   2. Establishing and/or leveraging a network of "go-to" people:
      a. Attorney: It is wise to obtain the help of an attorney from the start to advise on the right entity choice for your business and help with the business plan, specifically the pro forma. The American Association of Nurse Attorneys has a list of referrals for nurse attorneys in your state.
      b. Accountant: Hiring a certified public accountant (CPA) experienced in healthcare practice can help you get started and even grow the practice. An expert can handle payroll, quarterly taxes, deductions, exemptions, expenses, and receipts, leaving you with one less headache. Be sure to learn what and how everything is done, sign all checks, and review everything. Get recommendations from colleagues and interview a few until a good match is found.
      c. Bank manager: Get to know the bank's manager as they can be accommodating in many ways, including potential business loans and certified document signing.
      d. Help for the helper: This includes a therapist, business coach, peer supervision, and mentor.
      e. Operations support: This provides maintenance and technology support services.
      f. Outsource options: Determine what can or should be outsourced, such as billing, collections, and coding.
      g. A network of trusted competent practitioners/colleagues whose expertise enhances case collaboration and mutual referrals: Network growth via state and national professional organizations, digital forums, and listservs for APRNs, as well as local peer supervision groups, are invaluable.

PROFESSIONAL LIMITATIONS

A. Scope of practice laws mandate that APRNs practice in accordance with their education, national certification, and professional experience. These regulations ensure that APRNs deliver healthcare services that align with their training and qualifications.
B. APRNs are legally authorized to own practices. The APRN must consider the following:
   1. Understand their specialty role and the specific population foci.
   2. The APRN's practice must be fully aligned with their certification, training, and expertise.
   3. The APRN must be licensed and know the laws and regulations in the state where they are providing care. In most states:
      a. The degree and specifics of autonomy allowed to the APRN vary.
         i. Autonomous: It is legal to practice without physician oversight.
         ii. Supervisory or collaborative: In this state, a formal agreement for physician oversight is required. Learn the specifics of the agreement (e.g., chart review and frequency) and the cost for collaboration as a private practice owner.
         iii. Prescriptive authority: This includes Schedule II drugs and associated conditions.
      b. Laws for APRN medical staff membership vary, including admitting privileges and whether APRNs can sign end-of-life planning and treatment orders such as physician orders for life-sustaining treatment (POLST).

FEDERAL REGULATORY LAWS

The APRN in private practice must be familiar with specific federal laws that apply to their practice.

A. Health Insurance Portability and Accountability Act (HIPAA)
   1. The HIPAA mandates apply to all practices requiring practitioners to adhere to guidelines for safeguarding patient health information.
   2. These guidelines involve implementing measures, such as administrative and technical safeguards, to maintain the confidentiality and security of medical records and other protected health information (PHI).
   3. Private practitioners are also responsible for ensuring compliance through staff training, conducting risk assessments, and managing data access. Failure to comply can result in penalties, underscoring the importance of practices of all sizes to uphold an HIPAA compliance program.

B. Manual: Hospital Readmissions Reduction Program (HRRP)
  1. While its primary focus is on hospitals, it indirectly impacts practitioners by emphasizing the quality of discharges and postcare follow-up. Through HRRP, hospitals face reduced Medicare payments if they experience more than expected readmission rates for conditions. This encourages hospitals to collaborate with practitioners in improving discharge planning processes, promptly sharing comprehensive patient information, and ensuring effective follow-up care. By doing so, they aim to decrease readmissions and enhance overall patient outcomes.
C. Patient Safety and Quality Improvement Act of 2005 (PSQUIA)
  1. PSQUIA promotes practitioners' involvement in patient safety organizations (PSOs). By collaborating with PSOs, APRNs can securely exchange information regarding safety incidents without concerns about repercussions. This practice promotes a culture of safety and ongoing enhancement in healthcare procedures by enabling professionals to derive lessons from mistakes and adverse events, leading to the implementation of measures and enhancements in safety throughout their practices.
D. Centers for Medicare & Medicaid Services (CMS) and Children's Health Insurance Program (CHIP)
  1. The CMS and CHIP oversee significant health programs such as Medicare and CHIP, which hold vital importance to private practitioners. The CMS establishes reimbursement rates, policies, and compliance standards that practitioners must adhere to in order to secure funding and accreditation. CHIP offers health coverage to children from families that exceed the income threshold for Medicaid eligibility, impacting practitioners by broadening their patient pool and influencing the funding and delivery of pediatric care.
E. Medicare Access and CHIP Reauthorization Act (MACRA)
  1. MACRA changes the way that Medicare rewards clinicians for value over volume.
  2. MACRA revolutionizes how Medicare incentivizes clinicians based on value rather than volume.
  3. It consolidates quality initiatives into the Merit-Based Incentive Payment System (MIPS).
     a. For private practitioners, MACRA introduces the MIPS, which integrates various quality programs into a unified framework. It streamlines multiple quality programs under the new MIPS.
     b. This makes reporting easier by evaluating performance in four areas: quality, cost, improvement efforts, and enhancing care information.
     c. It gives bonus payments for participation in eligible alternative payment models (APMs).
     d. APRNs can enhance their payment adjustments by performing in these categories, encouraging standards of care and more effective practice management.
     e. Additionally, it offers payments for involvement in APMs. MACRA also promotes the participation of healthcare providers in APMs, such as accountable care organizations (ACOs) and patient-centered medical homes.
     f. These models prioritize quality and cost-effective care. Taking part in APMs can make practitioners eligible for payments and exempt them from MIPS requirements, providing significant financial incentives to embrace innovative care delivery practices with the goal of improved patient outcomes and enhanced practice sustainability.
F. No Surprises Act
  1. Started in January 2022, this Act includes clinicians providing outpatient and private practice care the requirement of providing a good faith estimate (GFE) to new and established patients who are uninsured, self-pay, or patients who are shopping for care, a GFE of costs for services that you provide.

NEEDS ASSESSMENT

MARKET ANALYSIS

A. Gathering as much information as possible about the potential area in which the practice will be located will assist in gaining insights into potential patient demographics, their needs, and current access to mental healthcare, as well as competitors. Start with location. The "where" may be the most important decision the APRN will make.
B. Explore the demographics of the area: the median age, occupations, education level, socioeconomic factors, family constellations, interests, or whatever other factors that may help predict how viable the practice can be. Sources of information include the U.S. Census Bureau and the U.S. Postal Service. Most importantly, determine if there is a need in this community.
  1. Identify the most common challenges and barriers residents face in seeking and receiving help.
     a. Economic stress
     b. Medical comorbidities
     c. Trauma, violence
     d. Stigma
     e. Under- or unemployment
     f. Logistical barriers such as transportation, language
     g. No insurance, unaffordable copays
  2. Identify the strengths of resources currently available (e.g., houses of worship, community health agencies, general hospital with behavioral health unit).
     a. Community's coping strategies, which may be adaptive (e.g., spirituality, social support) or maladaptive (e.g., alcohol and drugs)
     b. Existence of crisis services
     c. Federally qualified health centers (FQHCs)
     d. Medicaid
  3. Investigate:
     a. How mental health needs are currently being met and by whom (e.g., agencies, organizations, other private practice providers)
     b. Prevalence of self-help groups (e.g., National Alliance on Mental Illness [NAMI], 12-Step Programs, and self-management and recovery training)
     c. Availability and accessibility of recovery programs
     d. Wait time to see a mental health provider

Location Considerations Related to Population

Choose a location based on the population intended to be served: children, families, older adults, LGBTQ+ individuals, and marginalized populations, and those with serious mental illness (SMI) or substance use disorders (SUDs). Consider the "best" patient profile and what financial resources are available to them in order to access care. Consider going where the need is versus going where the money is.

A. Relocation: Consider personal preferences regarding relocation or remaining in the current community; ascertain that the preferred location is in alignment with the vision of the intended population to serve.

B. Family responsibilities: Consider commuting distance and proximity to childcare, school, and home.
C. Consider the demographics of the location, such as diversity and multiculturalism.
D. Consider the economic health of the community, such as income range, unemployment rate, and population growth.
E. Local businesses may provide insight into patients' ability to pay; new big-name businesses coming into the area are a good sign as they have most likely already done feasibility research in the area.
F. Cost of living may impact hiring and patients.
G. Identify the largest insurance payors and consider whether they align with revenue goals.
H. Estimate how far the business will reach; how far the "ideal" patient is willing to travel.
I. Explore incentives for small business startups.
J. Review regional salaries, minimum wage laws, property values, rental rates, business insurance rates, utilities, tax laws, and government licenses and fees.

THE IDEAL PATIENT

A. Private practitioners will be happier and more effective if they have an idea of who and where their ideal patient will be.
   1. For example, if one's ideal patient is health-conscious and motivated and the clinician's niche is working with women with perinatal anxiety and depression, would they establish a practice where the median age is 60? Or would they look for young families in their childbearing years?
B. Consider not only where the ideal patients live and what they do, but also whether they would be a good match for the clinician.
   1. Whether the ideal patient is in alignment with the clinician's values
   2. Motivations and behaviors of the ideal patient (e.g., needs, priorities, spending habits)
C. Be aware of others who will be competing to gain the favor of the ideal patient.

ECONOMIC ASSESSMENT

The *cost of living* refers to the overall expenses needed to sustain oneself in a specific location, including essential needs. Housing, food, and taxes are usually considered when calculating the cost of living, as well as other costs such as transportation, healthcare, entertainment, and education.

A. To determine how expensive it is to live there, compare the cost of living here: www.bankrate.com/real-estate/cost-of-living-calculator.
B. Explore the economic health of the area. Local civic organizations for business leaders can be very helpful. These groups focus on networking, community service, and advocacy for business interests. Consider the local Chambers of Commerce, Rotary Clubs, and Lions Clubs, as well as economic development corporations (EDCs), minority business associations, local nonprofit organizations, and foundations.
C. Talk to small business owners downtown to determine if the area is thriving and growing. Find out if there were large corporate employers that moved into or out of the community.
D. Research income range in the community.
E. Seek advice from a local residential real estate company and talk to commercial real estate specializing in medical practices regarding cost to buy or rent an office in the area.
F. Obtain specific details about the local housing market, the cost of the average home, and rental costs in various neighborhoods.
G. Explore industries in the target area. Seek to learn about the big players and the largest employers in the area. Find out about their employee benefits. (Make acquaintance with the Employee Assistance Program Department.)
H. Payment methods will dictate how patients will pay for services and thus how revenue is generated. Review regional payors:
   1. Public: Medicare/Medicaid
   2. Charity care
   3. Employee-based group private insurance plans
   4. State employee health plans
   5. Payment and reimbursement
      a. Requirements to get on their panels
      b. Credentialing barriers
      c. Discrimination in reimbursement for APRNs
      d. Reimbursement rates (e.g., in-network, out-of-network)
      e. Out-of-pocket (self-pay)
      f. Concierge

Behavioral Health Industry

A. The pandemic put behavioral health into the spotlight. The U.S. behavioral health market is projected to grow from $77.62 billion in 2021 to $99.40 billion in 2028 as favorable policies are implemented. Mental health services are growing at an explosive rate; this has bearing on competition.
B. Consider the growth potential and outlook in general for the behavioral health industry.
C. Evaluate the saturation of mental health professionals, supply and demand, and appointment wait times when choosing your target location.
D. The overall atmosphere in the community toward seeking treatment can differ by demographics. There may be stigma and embarrassment, or general acceptance of mental health treatment when necessary, or a more embracing attitude.
E. Consider the ideal patient's or payer's readiness, and value of and capacity to compensate for your services.

Competitive Analysis

A. Supply: Conduct a supply analysis.
   1. Recognize your competitors and gain insight from their strategies.
   2. Identify other healthcare providers offering comparable services in your region.
   3. Discover where the locals go for behavioral health services.
   4. Evaluate the market share owned by current healthcare providers.
   5. Assess the strengths and weaknesses of your rivals.
   6. Reflect on whether there are any indirect or secondary rivals that may influence your success.
   7. Conduct research on the typical fees locals pay for comparable services.
B. Demand: Determine if there is a need for your services in the local area.
   1. Market size: Approximate the size of the market for the services you provide.
   2. Review economic metrics like income level and unemployment percentage.

3. Evaluate the level of market saturation by determining the number of behavioral health practices, agencies, and programs that are accessible to the community.
4. Find out the cost of services like yours that are already available in the market.

C. Create a distinctive selling point or unique selling proposition (USP) to distinguish your company from competitors.

D. Utilize the gathered information to gain a competitive advantage by making strategic decisions that will impact the success of your business.

E. Determine a window of opportunity to enter the market.

Current Trends

A. New, revitalized, and upcoming payment models
   1. There is an increasing recognition by the public and policy makers of the need for access to behavioral healthcare.
   2. Shift from fee-for-service to value-based behavioral healthcare. This is not easy to do in behavioral care as outcomes are subjective and highly individual, relying on patient-reported outcomes. Observable improvements often take longer and are complex due to various treatment methods. Integration with physical health complicates care segmentation in value-based models. Patient engagement and lack of standardized benchmarks further complicate measuring care quality. Transitioning to value-based care (VBC) in behavioral health requires innovative approaches and collaboration to redefine success.
   3. Capitation is a payment model whereby healthcare providers are paid a fixed amount per patient annually for all needed services. It intersects with regulations and practices in various ways:
       a. MACRA/MIPS: Healthcare providers may impact their reimbursement adjustments based on cost efficiency and resource use measures.
       b. Mental Health Parity: Capitation must ensure equal funding for mental health and substance use treatments compared with other medical services.
       c. No Surprises Act: Healthcare providers under capitation must clarify network status and treatment coverage to avoid unexpected bills.
       d. GFE: Healthcare providers should still provide cost estimates for uninsured patients, even though capitation ideally covers all care costs.

B. New delivery models
   1. Expansion of telehealth after the public health emergency (PHE). Even before the pandemic, research has shown that clinical outcomes utilizing telepsychiatry are as good as or better than usual care.
   2. Biden/Harris initiatives to increase access to children's mental health services. Federal grants under the Expanding Access to Mental Health Services in Schools Act and the Bipartisan Safer Communities Act help schools hire more school-based mental health professionals and build a strong pipeline into the profession for the upcoming school year with the goal of doubling the number of mental health professionals.
   3. Trauma-informed services are provided in schools and elsewhere.
   4. Team-based integrative behavioral healthcare (IBH) aims to integrate the full spectrum of behavioral healthcare including SUD throughout primary care, social services, and early childhood, providing culturally informed person-centered care.
   5. Collaborative care model: The clinician is not necessarily present but actively collaborates with the primary care team. Integration requires collaboration as a precondition, but collaboration does not require integration.
   6. Disruptive technologies: Virtual medical office assistants; virtual and digital diagnostics; treatment and practice management support; digital phenotyping using smartphone apps to track behavior patterns, sleep, activity, and social interactions; and virtual reality to simulate challenging environments to the patient have shown promise in treating anxiety, phobias, depression, and post-traumatic stress disorder (PTSD).

C. Urgent and upward trending needs
   1. Impact of the pandemic, political unrest, and mass shootings on mental health still spiking; increase in anxiety, depression, and suicide ideation signals an increased need for identification and triage; greater recognition of the effect of long COVID and secondary trauma on mental health sequelae
   2. Trauma-informed care
   3. Alternative addiction treatments, increasing need for medication-assisted treatment (MAT) providers
   4. Emergent and urgent needs unique to specific communities such as mass shooting of specific populations or location

THE OFFICE

A. Secure an office that reflects the demographics and needs of the patients intended to serve and apply finishing touches that reflect the clinician's therapeutic style.

B. Many successful psychiatric practices start small and grow from there. The cost of office space is usually calculated by price per square foot. Common to all office selections is how much space is needed. Avoid costly wasted space especially in the initial phase of practice. In the growth phase, space can still be conserved while maintaining the ability to expand without having to move again. For example, once settled in the community, one might invest in purchasing a 500-square-feet office space. Take 100 square feet for consultation room, another 100 for common space such as a waiting room and a kitchen/business area, and rent out the rest. Expand into the rented space as the practice grows and leases are up.

C. Other considerations include the following:
   1. Consider accessibility and handicapped parking according to the Americans with Disabilities Act (ADA).
   2. Consider patients' method of transportation (e.g., accessible by public transit, adequate parking for those who drive).
   3. Real estate purchase: Purchasing an office can be risky and best planned for growth phase once consistent profits are secure.
   4. Buying an established practice can be complicated. Seek guidance from an attorney and CPA for due diligence to determine the value of the practice and whatever it is worth if the patients leave.
   5. Rent: When choosing offices to rent, think about size and workflow, and whether improvements or space reconfiguration will be necessary, and whether covered by property owner or by tenant.
   6. Virtual: The pandemic has legitimized virtual behavioral healthcare by increasing access to care for people who otherwise would not avail it. It is a great way to save on the cost of office space, and evidence has shown that it

is as effective or more than in-person visits. However, for some, there are downsides. Without person-to-person contact, it can be difficult to form a therapeutic alliance that relies on subtle cues perceived by all senses. HIPAA compliance is also more difficult.

7. Home office: Another cost-saving possibility is a home office. It may even be tax-deductible. However, to claim it as a tax deduction, the space must be 100% dedicated to your practice. Additionally, having a home office can cause boundary risks as patients enter the clinician's home space and minimize differentiation between work and home life for the clinician.

8. Other arrangements include the following:
   a. Cost sharing
      i. Sublet unused space to other therapists or sublet from them. Sublet an extra consultation room while sharing the waiting room and administrative staff or share a single room by the day or hour.
      ii. Group practice: Sharing the work with others usually results in less work but will likely reduce startup costs.
      iii. Coworking membership: Rent by specified days and times. These are fully furnished offices that even have conference rooms and all-inclusive administrative amenities.

D. Working with a commercial realtor can be helpful in finding a location within a desirable price range. One that specializes in medical or professional offices is advantageous. Typically, the seller/renter pays the commission, but sometimes it is split. These professionals can compare values by doing comparables (comps), assist in finding a suitable location for the ideal patient, and help negotiate the best deal.

E. Whether planning to buy, rent, sublet, build, or practice in a home office, be mindful to conform to the local zoning laws.

F. Whether renting, subletting, buying real estate, using a home office, or practicing virtually, finding a location with an address is an important first step before filing for basically everything, including loans. While the location may move in the near future, it is best to avoid using a home address and phone number from the beginning unless operating in a home office. Even then, consider a P.O. Box and a dedicated business phone.

G. Consider the configuration of the space.

1. The space has an entrance into a waiting room, with a nearby restroom.
2. Ideally, it will have a separate exit for patient privacy as well as yours.
3. There is space to be used for family or group therapy if needed.
4. Sharing the waiting area with another practitioner will determine the space needed.
5. If the practice will have staff, plan on a separate reception area off the waiting area that can be closed off and locked when not in use.
6. Consultation room(s) should have a window and enough room to feel (even if it is not) spacious.

COSTS

A. Profits: Businesses can only survive if they make money. Business owners must be able to control the difference between revenue and cost (i.e., profit), regardless of whether the practice is a taxable or tax-exempt entity.

B. Startup costs: Start by adding up all expenses for a full financial picture. This should be done long before launch. Being well-prepared is key. Bills will begin coming in before greeting the first patient. Understanding costs in advance will help ensure a successful launch.

C. Startup: Calculating startup costs helps estimate profits, conduct a breakeven analysis, secure loans, attract investors, and save money with tax deductions.

D. Furniture and fixtures: A psychiatric-mental health practice has a notoriously low overhead. However, some necessary considerations include the following:

1. Waiting room: Chairs, side tables, and magazine racks are useful, if not for magazine then for flyers and psychoeducational and other handouts. Consider beverages—coffee and water dispenser—and sound system for relaxing music or white noise.
2. Consultation room(s): Size will depend on the type of services offered. For psychopharmacology only, a desk and two or three chairs should be sufficient. If therapy is added, include a conversational arrangement with a sofa, stuffed chairs, coffee tables, and comfortable clinician chair.
3. Reception area: The area should have file cabinets, workstation with drawers and shelves, and ergonomic chairs.
4. Medical equipment: At minimum, this should include a scale, stethoscope, sphygmomanometer, or automatic blood pressure monitor.
5. Office supplies: These include paper shredder, printer, scanner, fax, computer, paper, pads, forms, writing implements, and other office supplies.
6. Technology: This includes cloud-based electronic medical records with e-Prescribing and billing software, as well as credit card processing accounting software.
7. Professional Costs: Determine the cost of licensure, Drug Enforcement Administration (DEA), certifications, insurances (general business and malpractice), continuing education, subscriptions, and professional memberships.

E. Fixed and variable costs: Plan not only to open but to have enough money to sustain until the business can break even. Consider fixed monthly costs and prepare for variable costs (Table 28.1).

TABLE 28.1 STARTUP, FIXED, AND VARIABLE COSTS IN A NURSE PRACTITIONER PRACTICE

Startup Costs	Fixed Costs	Variable Costs
First month's rent Security deposit Licenses and permits Legal fees Signage Furniture Fixtures Technology and software Capital improvement	Office rental or mortgage Salaries Collaborative agreement Taxes Insurance Licenses and certification renewals Loans Depreciation Website and electronic health records Online payment processing	Telephone Repairs Utilities Cable Office supplies Continuing education

Raising Startup Money

A. Credit matters. Establish and maintain good personal and business credit history to fund a practice. If the credit history is under the mark, the Federal Trade Commission has recommendations for credit improvement. Dun & Bradstreet is also a good source of recommendations for building business credit.
  1. Improve credit score, if necessary.
  2. Apply for business credit.
  3. Check and monitor credit score.
  4. Write a business plan to present to lenders.
  5. Prepare a pro forma using startup cost calculations.

B. Sources of capital may include personal savings, bank loans, small business loans, venture capital/crowdfunding, grants, or leveraging assets (e.g., first or second mortgage on property, selling of property).

Establishing a Business as a Legal Entity

A. While it is possible to file a business online using one of the online formation services, healthcare is one of the most regulated industries in the country, so seeking legal and financial counsel is advised.

B. Independent practice for APRNs is still considered innovative. Hire an attorney who is most familiar with the field.

C. The American Association of Nurse Attorneys offers a state-by-state directory. Talk to an attorney, a CPA, and colleagues with expertise in regulations and compliance early in the process. Discussing intentions before committing to establishing a practice allows the early formation to take shape while the stakes are low.

D. Be sure to incorporate! Some states mandate which entities one can and cannot change. There are many ways to structure a business. Based on one's professional goals and state laws, allow advisors to provide guidance on which entity is appropriate.

  1. Sole proprietorship: This is the simplest and least expensive entity. However, the individual clinician and their practice are one and the same in the eyes of the Internal Revenue Service (IRS). Losses are deducted from individual taxes, and gains are added and taxed accordingly. Liability rests entirely with the proprietor; there is no protection for the proprietor's assets, and the proprietor will be subject to self-employment tax. For tax filing, proprietors use Schedule C to submit only one return.

  2. Partnership: A partnership is an entity with two or more partners who form an agreement on their obligations to the partnership.
      a. Partners share the work burden, and individuals' work hours would most likely be reduced.
      b. A partnership offers some tax advantages; however, it carries the same liability as a sole proprietorship. The practice is taxed on profits and losses. Partnership owners file two tax returns, one using Form 1065, which is its own informational tax return, and each partner reports their portion on their personal tax returns using Schedule E.
      c. Partnerships may make obtaining funding for startup costs easier. The income generated by the entity is passed to the partners based on their respective ownership percentages.
      d. As with a sole proprietorship, check with the state and local government regarding requirements for business licenses or permits to do business. Partners may also need to file a DBA (Doing Business As...), but it is unnecessary to file anything with the state to form a partnership or sole proprietorship.

  3. Limited liability corporation (LLC), or similarly professional limited liability company (PLLC): Single-member LLCs allow the business owner to have corporate protection while being taxed as a sole proprietorship.
      a. If there is more than one member, the LLC can be taxed as a partnership or corporation. State laws differ, but in general LLCs are a hybrid offering the best of both worlds between a sole proprietorship and a corporation: the liability protection of an S-corp and the autonomy of a sole proprietorship.
      b. Under an LLC, there is no requirement for a board of directors. An LLC with more than one partner can elect in its first year to be taxed as a partnership and file those returns or taxed as a corporation, and the entity pays its own taxes.
      c. An LLC would have its own Employer Identification Number (EIN), and its assets and liabilities would be separate from those of the individual business owner (and partners, if applicable). Any profits and losses would be passed on to the business owner and taxed accordingly.
      d. The single-member LLC does not pay taxes. However, the business owner is taxed on profit and losses. Single-member LLCs are the most streamlined and flexible business entity that will protect the business owner's personal assets.

  4. S-corp: There must be a board of directors with strict rules, recordkeeping, regular meetings, and ongoing fees and filings to stay in compliance.
      a. This structure reduces managerial flexibility. Owners are stockholders who must be U.S. residents or citizens who can receive common stock but not preferred stock. The shareholders pay taxes on the profits, not the corporation, so the IRS only collects once.
      b. An S-corp can have up to 100 shareholders.
      c. An S-corp also protects the business owner from personal liability. The IRS wants to make sure there is a manager and payroll taxes are being paid. Income is passed to the owners through salary or profits or losses. Reasonable compensation rules apply to the S-corp.

DIAGNOSIS

A. A SWOT analysis is a diagnostic tool for strategic planning that involves identifying and evaluating Strengths, Weaknesses, Opportunities, and Threats (Figure 28.1; Humphrey, 1960s/1970s).

B. Once data have been collected, review the current state of facts and decide how to proceed.

C. Build a team of trusted colleagues, family, and/or friends who can provide honest feedback.

D. Brainstorm. Create a mind map or use a whiteboard or sticky notes. Consider all the factors in the assessment.
  1. List strengths. Be specific. Consider all the skills, resources, and advantages that can be built upon and offered to the community.
  2. List weaknesses. Address areas in need of improvement and known deficiencies.
  3. List opportunities. Identify factors that can be exploited to the advantage of the business.

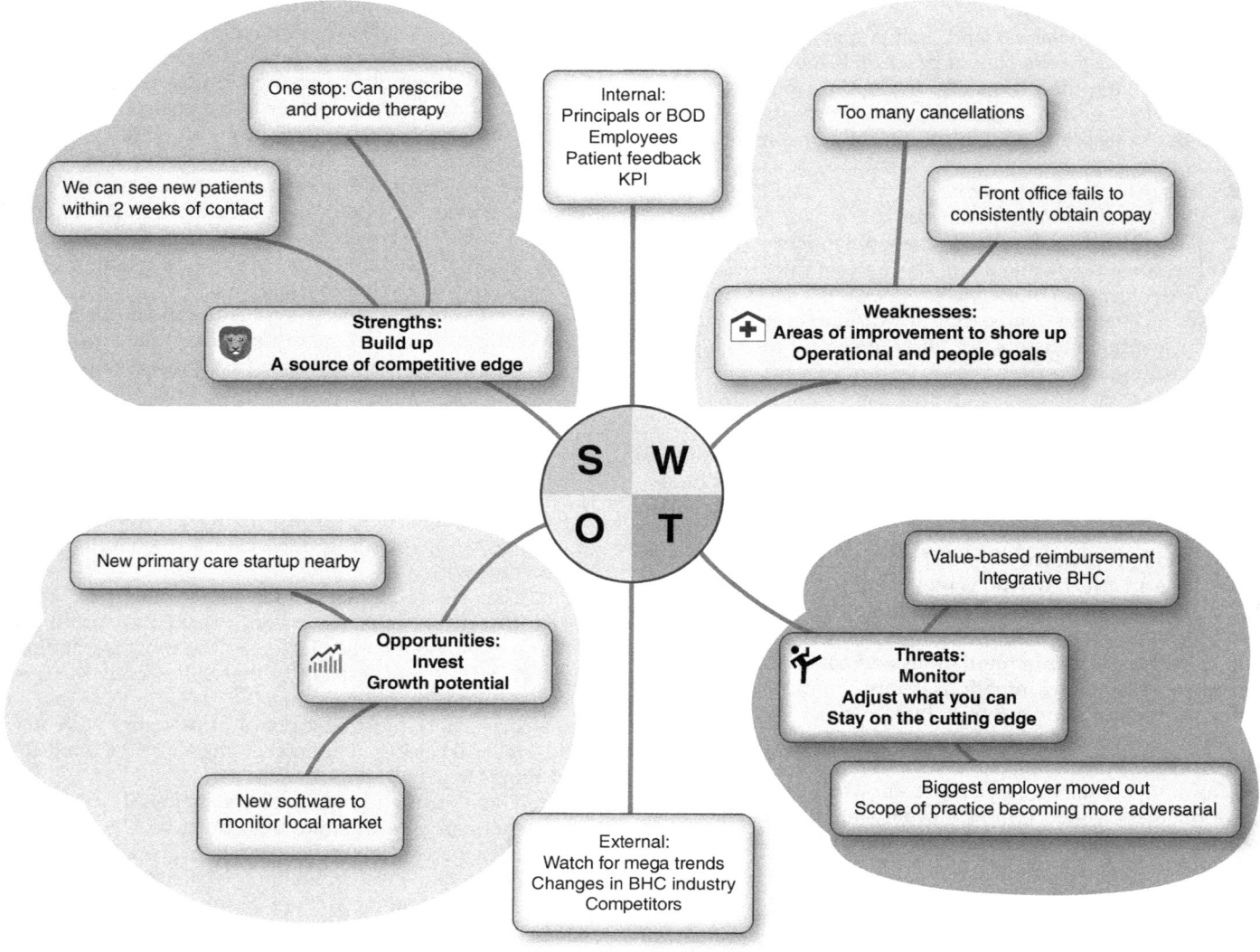

FIGURE 28.1 **S**trengths, **W**eaknesses, **O**pportunities, and **T**hreats (SWOT) analysis.

BHC, behavioral healthcare; BOD, board of directors; KPI, key performance indicator.

Source: Adapted from Humphrey, A. (1960s/1970s). SWOT analysis framework. Stanford Research Institute.

4. List potential and actual threats. Consider factors such as barriers, competitors, referral sources, regulations, insurance panels, hospital privileges, economic threats, and others.

E. Evaluate feasibility. A feasibility study will use all the data collected and calculate the potential for success by identifying the expected costs and projected benefits of going forward in detail.

1. Conduct a preliminary analysis.
   a. Define the goals, scope, and limitations of the project.
   b. Collect information about the market, competition, risks, and regulatory guidelines.
   c. Evaluate the feasibility of the project based on existing data.
2. Prepare a projected income statement using pro forma.
   a. Draft an income statement forecast detailing revenues, expenses, and profitability for a time frame (3–5 years).
   b. Make assumptions. Utilize market research to predict sales, costs, and financial outcomes.
   c. Assess project sustainability based on this forecasted income statement.
3. Prepare an opening-day balance sheet.
   a. Outline the project's assets, liabilities, and equity at launch by creating a balance sheet.
   b. Consider investments, loans, startup expenses, and other financial elements.
   c. Evaluate the status of the project at its inception.
4. Conduct a market survey.
   a. Develop and execute a market survey to gain insights into customer preferences, demand patterns, and competitor analysis.
   b. Utilize surveys, interviews, and secondary sources to gather information.
   c. Analyze survey results to grasp market trends and pinpoint opportunities or obstacles.
5. Develop a plan outlining the structure of the business staffing needs and operational procedures.
   a. Clearly define roles, workflow processes, and resource distribution.
   b. Consider regulatory factors relevant to the business.
   c. Summarize all data collected, including forecasts, market research results, and operational strategies.

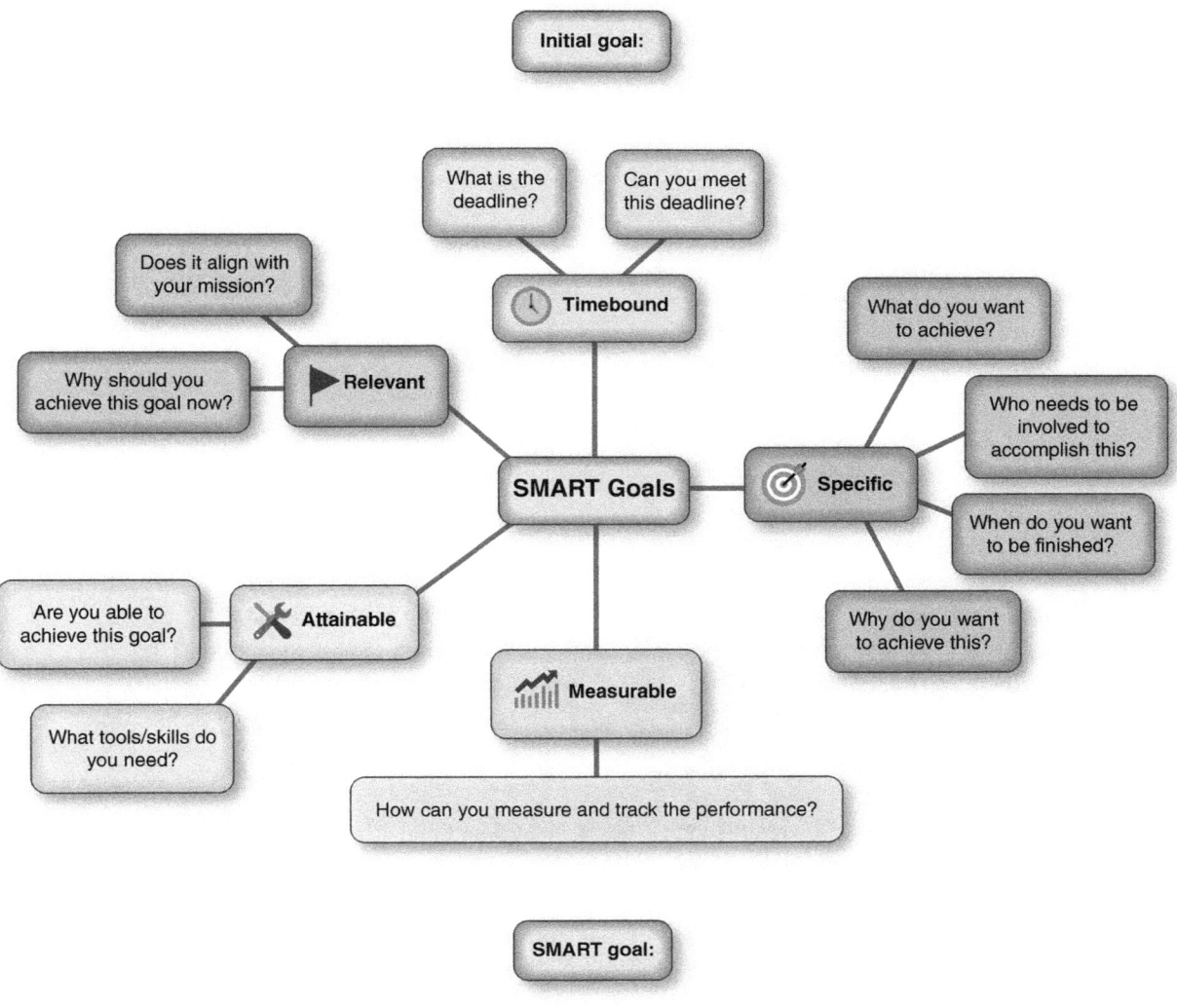

FIGURE 28.2 SMART (**S**pecific, **M**easurable, **A**chievable, **R**ealistic, and **T**imebound) goals.

Source: Adapted from Doran, G. T. (1981). There's a S.M.A.R.T. way to write management's goals and objectives. *Management Review, 70*(11), 35–36.

d. Look for insights, trends, and potential risks or uncertainties. Conduct sensitivity analysis to evaluate how different variables may impact the project's viability.
6. Make a go/no-go decision.
    a. Decide whether to proceed with the project after examining the feasibility study results about the project's goals and limitations.
    b. Evaluate if the project is financially feasible by reviewing income projections, balance sheets, and market surveys.
    c. Analyze risks and benefits before deciding to move forward or terminate the plan based on a thorough evaluation.
F. Once the entity's viability is determined, it is time to create a business plan. This is needed to obtain a small business loan, and/or it will serve as a living, renewable document to keep the business afloat and evolving.

BUSINESS PLAN/OUTCOMES

A. SMART (**S**pecific, **M**easurable, **A**chievable, **R**ealistic, **T**imebound) goals: The business plan is derived from the assessment and diagnosis. A SMART business plan helps focus on delivering results that will enable loans and funding to be secured. It is an organic, living document and an ever-changing plan that will keep the business operating (Figure 28.2; Doran, 1981).
B. Business plan: Informed by personal values, a business plan should be a statement of intent or mission that reflects the business's vision and purpose. Details should be specific, realistic, and have deadlines.
C. Base the business plan on data that have been gathered (Figure 28.3; McCarthy, 1960). Consider the following:
   1. Prove that there is a need for these services in this community.
   2. Prove that this community is interested in what will be offered.
   3. Identify the rationale for why this community will use the services.
   4. Confirm that patients or their third-party payors can reimburse services.
   5. Identify approaches to overcome any noted obstacles.
D. Including a pro forma in the business plan will show prospective investors how decisions are made based on hypothetical scenarios.

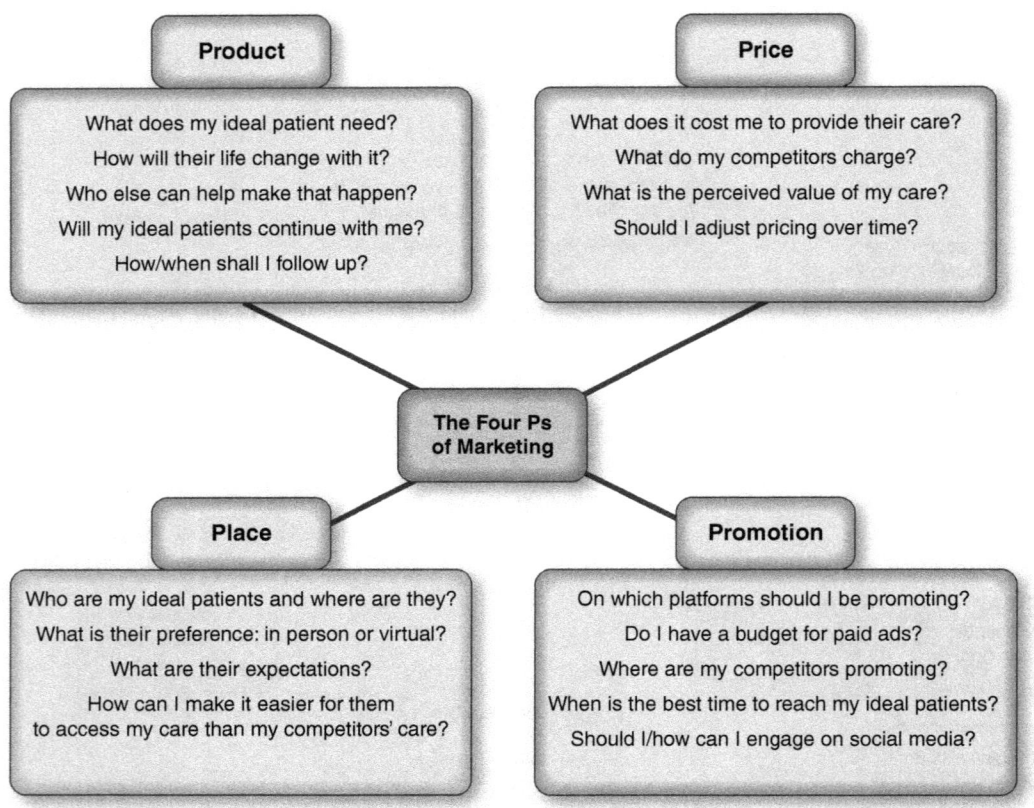

FIGURE 28.3 The 4 Ps of marketing.

Source: Adapted from McCarthy, E. J. (1960). *Basic marketing: A managerial approach.* Richard D. Irwin.

1. Project 1, 3, and 5 years out.
2. Startup costs are expenses incurred while creating a new business (e.g., research expenses, borrowing costs, technology), and postopening startup costs include advertising, promotion, and employee expenses.

E. Marketing plan: The plan should narrow the market to include specific targets based on the area's demographics (quantitative data) uncovered in a needs assessment.

F. Growth: Consider how profit is built into a business plan

LICENSURE AND CREDENTIALLING

A. Once the office address and business phone are established, proceed with obtaining important registrations. These may include:
 1. Malpractice insurance
 2. State professional license
 3. State registration or certification as an APRN
 4. State and federal narcotics authorization (controlled dangerous substances [CDS], DEA)

B. An EIN will be needed to register a business entity. A federal ID is primarily a social security number, employer identification number, or taxpayer identification number. When asked for an EIN, a tax identification number (TIN) can be provided; however, when asked for a TIN, the EIN cannot be used.

C. The national provider identification (NPI) is the standard unique health identifier for healthcare providers and suppliers and is assigned by the National Plan and Provider Enumeration System (NPPES). To obtain an NPI, register with the NPPES. Applying for the NPI is a process separate from Medicare enrollment. To obtain an NPI, apply online at https://nppes.cms.hhs.gov. For more information about NPI enumeration, apply for a business NPI here: https://npiregistry.cms.hhs.gov/search. The APRN may have their own, but it is advisable to use business entity NPI for billing to maintain clarity in recordkeeping processes.

D. One must obtain and furnish an NPI on the application to enroll in Medicare. Note: The name and Social Security number (SSN) provided and, if applicable, the legal business name (LBN) and TIN must be the same as those used to obtain the NPI.

E. Opting out of Medicare: Healthcare providers who do not wish to work with the Medicare program may "opt out" of Medicare. After that, Medicare does not pay for any covered items or services rendered by an opt-out healthcare provider except for an emergency or urgent need. If a patient still wishes to obtain services from an opt-out healthcare provider, the healthcare provider and the patient can set up payment terms through a private contract. Patients or opt-out healthcare providers must not submit any healthcare provider claims. Healthcare providers who opt out must do so for 2 years, which automatically renews every 2 years unless the healthcare provider requests not to renew their opt-out status.

F. Clinical Laboratory Improvement Amendments of 1988 (CLIA) application form should be completed and mailed to the address of the local state agency for the state in which the laboratory resides (Boss Health Care, n.d.).

G. Electronic data interchange (EDI) enrollment form must be completed before submitting any electronic media claims (EMCs) or other EDI transactions to Medicare. The agreement must be executed by each provider of healthcare services, either directly with Medicare or through a billing service or clearinghouse. For more information regarding the CMS Standard EDI Enrollment Form, contact the local Medicare administrative contractor (MAC) for processing Part A and Part B (A/B MAC), or the MAC for processing durable medical equipment (DME MAC).

H. CHIP provides low-cost health coverage to children in families that earn too much money to qualify for Medicaid but not enough to buy private insurance. CHIP applications are made through the individual states.

I. The Council for Affordable Quality Healthcare (CAQH) is a national third-party vendor that collects healthcare provider data for credentialing purposes. Any participating health plan with the CAQH may use the application, which streamlines the credentialing process for practitioners by reducing paperwork.

J. Private insurance plans credentialling: Identify which insurance companies are most active in the community served, then contact them with a letter of interest to ensure their panels are open. The insurance credentialing process must be followed to become a participating in-network healthcare provider with a particular insurance company. Being in-network prevents patients from having claims go toward their out-of-network deductible. Begin the process by requesting to join the insurance company's network and submitting information. Most large insurance companies utilize the CAQH to access the APRN's license, DEA, curriculum vitae (CV), and W9, and whatever else is required. A CAQH ID should be obtained to initiate the credentialing process. The process may take up to 6 months.

GOALS, PLANS, AND OBJECTIVES

A. A private practice is a business. Setting goals that align with the best interests of both patients and the practice is essential to keep the practice thriving.

B. Once a vision for the practice has been created, goals should be set to achieve the vision with clear accountability and performance benchmarks. Progressing in the right areas will result in satisfied patients and a thriving practice. Money is energy, and it must keep flowing. Cash flow problems signal the death knell of a practice.

C. A set of sample workflow goals follows. Each can be put into a SMART format.
1. Insurance plans and deductibles will be determined before the first visit.
2. The reimbursement rate per code will be planned ahead of time.
3. All copays will be collected before the start of the session.
4. Patients with high deductible plans will pay the out-of-pocket rate before each visit.
5. An agreement will be entered with each patient based on fee structure and reimbursement.
6. Credit card options will be available for patient-pay and incentives for prompt payment.
    a. Verify the credit card processing service meets the Payment Card Industry Data Security Standard (PCI DSS) standards and can securely manage transactions while protecting PHI. If you choose to use PayPal, make sure to use their services that are compliant with HIPAA regulations and sign a business associate agreement (BAA).
    b. Do not use Venmo, Zelle, or Cash App as they are not appropriate for processing HIPAA-compliant payments.
7. Financial projections pro forma will be reviewed and revised annually.
8. Practice will maximize profit by maintaining the lowest possible overhead and review yearly.
9. Practice will maximize claim reimbursement through regular contract negotiations.
    a. Timely, clean claims will be submitted through stringent documentation and coding management.
    b. New *International Classification of Diseases* (*ICD*) and *Diagnostic and Statistical Manual of Mental Disorders* (*DSM*) codes will be updated as they come out.
10. Payor contracts will be actively monitored and negotiated annually.
11. Practice will maintain scheduling productivity.
12. A no-show and short notice policy will be implemented, included in welcome documents, and discussed with and signed by each patient.
13. Patients will receive automatic appointment reminders X days prior to appointments.
14. Practice will earn extra revenue with the CMS's Chronic Care Management (CCM) and Transitional Care Management (programs for chronic care management and transitional care posthospitalization).

MARKETING AND ADVERTISING

A. Marketing is about change. It transforms culture, and the business owner is the change agent. The private practitioner is uniquely positioned to change culture for the good. The keys to success are the practitioner's intention, generosity, and authenticity.

B. Mission: Set the stage by stating the overall mission and purpose of the practice. The business brand should be built around fulfilling underlying human needs or desires. Market with people not at them.

C. Explain research: Research will be the foundation of a marketing plan and should include the following:
1. Competitive analysis
2. SWOT analysis
3. Ideal patient
4. Understanding how, when, where, and why the target market seeks or receives services, which is key to converting leads

D. Explain strategy: Describe business initiatives and strategies.
1. Define SMART goals.
2. Define the plan's contributors and their responsibilities.
3. Identify the USP. Competitive advantage relies upon specializing and differentiating the practice's niche. The USP should make these explicit.
4. Focus on the ideal patient and current competition.
5. Define a marketing budget.
6. Develop a brand. A great brand influences others' perceptions and attracts patients.
7. Define distribution channels.
    a. Advertisement: may include social media, television, or magazine advertisements
    b. Sales promotions: may include short-term promotions or deals for patients or prospective patients (e.g., free webinar on stress management)
    c. Direct marketing: directly reaching out to the target audience
    d. Public relations: presenting a favorable image of the brand
    e. Peer-to-peer (word of mouth)
    f. healthcare provider referrals

g. Networking
   h. Radio, YouTube, and podcasts
8. Consider digital marketing.
   a. Email marketing: Communicate or advertise through emails.
   b. Identify goals and the digital marketing tools needed. Precisely market through social media and record who shows interest and from which platform to target further.
   c. Create a great website with engaging content on the home page. Consider blogging regularly—search engines seek active sites.
   d. Search marketing: Search marketing generates leads from search engines to drive website traffic to a website or product.
   e. Implement a search engine optimization (SEO) strategy using precise keywords to improve search result ranking.

E. Define key performance indicators (KPIs) and measurement method: Begin measuring to establish a baseline and targets that reflect an improved return on investment (ROI).
   1. Measurement should be done before, during, and after—throughout the year, on a monthly or even weekly basis—to ensure that the plans indicate positive results and to shift them if they do not.

F. List principal strategy and strategic plans: Strategic plans, timelines, and calendars give life to ideas and strategies. Try focusing on four or five main strategies for the year and creating SMART plans for them. Throughout the year, and especially at the end, evaluate their effectiveness through KPIs and other benchmarks.

G. Financial budgeting: Capital expenses are a company's major purchases that depreciate over time. They are large investments, such as renovations, technology, equipment, or machinery. They are designed to be used over the long term. Operating expenses (OpEx) are a company's day-to-day expenses to keep its business operational.

IMPLEMENTATION

A. Implementing the plan is known as business operations and consists primarily of daily or recurring activities. The day-to-day activities can be optimized to generate sufficient value to more than cover expenses, making the business viable and profitable.

B. Employees participate in reaching measurable business goals by performing functions such as smooth workflow management, collecting copays, coding, billing, collections, accounting, and marketing.

C. The business operations of a professional practice are divided into front-end and back-end activities. Ensure that the two divisions are running efficiently to prevent laxity on one side, which can hinder the achievement of the objectives. On the front end, the business should focus on streamlining customer service delivery to increase customer satisfaction. It should also formulate a means of receiving customer feedback and complaints to understand their expectations and identify improvements in service delivery (business operations).

RISK MANAGEMENT

A. It is highly recommended that the APRN and all staff develop a risk management mind-set and incorporate it into everyday practice. The APRN must practice within the requirements of the state's Nurse Practice Act, in compliance with the practice or organization's procedures and policies, and within the national standard of care. "This is a 'plan or strategy, designed to limit the number of medical mistakes that occur' according to the ECRI Institute" (Servca, 2019, para. 1).

B. Maintain competencies by staying current with psychiatric professional journals and national and state specialty organization conferences and obtaining additional certification training in ancillary evidence-based techniques, such as dialectical behavioral therapy (DBT) and repetitive transcranial magnetic stimulation (rTMS).

C. Maintain clear and comprehensive documentation. All documentation must be accurate and honest, including assessment, and subjective and objective observations, and all communications and actions taken. Record each encounter accurately, objectively, and without delay.

D. Beware of false claims. This can include failing to report government overpayments, misrepresenting costs, billing for non-Food and Drug Administration-approved drugs or devices, performing unnecessary procedures, or records related to performance or quality, among others.

E. Contact an attorney promptly with concerns about patient care or practice issue. A decision to file a medical malpractice lawsuit is often driven by how the patient and the family feel the healthcare provider and staff treated them. Studies show that the quality of the relationship conveying a sense of caring can reduce the likelihood of a lawsuit (Relias Media, 2021).

F. Maintain files referencing one's character, such as patient recommendations, performance evaluations, and continuing education.

G. Follow appropriate communication standards.

H. Practice owner responsibilities include clear policies and procedures, hiring and credentialing, supervision, staff conduct, training, and outlining the duties and responsibilities of staff.

EVALUATION

A. A business evaluation is a direct assessment of the implemented business plan in which one considers whether the steps taken were adequate and whether the intended outcomes were achieved.

B. Some valid methods to measure outcomes include the following:
   1. Finances
      a. KPIs quantify the practice's SMART goals. KPIs measure performance against specific outcome goals, such as targeted quarterly revenue or targeted new patients per month. They are measurable indicators used to evaluate the performance and advancement of an entity (person or company) in reaching particular goals. These indicators offer concrete proof of achievement or areas requiring enhancement.
      b. Refer to the pro forma and determine if financial projections were met.
   2. Clinical outcomes
      a. The Partners for Change Outcome Management System and the Better Outcomes Now (www.betteroutcomesnow.com) offer easy-to-use software to measure outcomes. This is beneficial not only to patients and clinicians but also in measuring whether the services offered yield the expected results.

b. David Burns' Therapist's Toolkit is a highly recommended comprehensive collection of assessment and treatment forms including pre- and posttests and outcome measurements in analog and digital forms that allow clinicians and patients to measure progress and outcomes. Also included is a "Therapy Session Evaluation" for patients to fill out after each session. The toolkit is exceptionally user-friendly and has excellent psychometric properties. Most have reliability above 90%, with many above 95%, and are highly correlated with other well-established instruments (Burns, n.d.).

3. Staff evaluations
   a. Front- and back-office staff evaluations should be completed at least annually and more often for newer employees who need fast feedback.
4. Referral satisfaction
   a. The key to referral satisfaction is the quality of the work done with the referred patient. If the referral source is one of the patient's healthcare providers, getting the patient's consent to collaborate with them would be wise. A thank you note for the referral is more memorable than a phone call that may interrupt their workday.

CONCLUSION

When exploration of the concept of private practice ownership becomes more than a wish, the details may seem overwhelming. Evaluating factors such as the community's needs, financial viability, legal obligations, and one's own preparedness takes time and planning. Conducting research, crafting a business strategy, and consulting experts in the industry are crucial steps before committing to a choice.

APRNs are trained to approach challenges. The nursing process provides a framework that fosters thinking, problem-solving skills, and creativity, enhancing decision-making efficiency. By utilizing assessment, diagnosis, planning, implementation, and evaluation methods taught in this process, APRNs can effectively navigate the complexities of entrepreneurship while upholding quality care standards and ethical practices for long-term success in practice settings. This systematic approach not only enhances outcomes, but also promotes career growth and fosters a culture of excellence within private practice environments.

HIGHLY RECOMMENDED RESOURCES

A. Woodcock, E. (2016). *Operating Policies and Procedures Manual for Medical Practices* (5th ed.). MGMA.
B. Buppert, C. (2021). *Nurse Practitioner's Business Practice and Legal Guide* (7th ed.). Jones & Bartlett Learning.
C. Godin, S. (2018). *This Is Marketing: You Can't Be Seen Until You Learn To See*. Portfolio/Penguin.
D. Phillips, B. (2022). Business for healthcare providers: www.clinicianbusinessinstitute.com and https://npbusiness.org
E. No Surprises Act (effective January 1, 2022; ncpsychiatry.org): www.ncpsychiatry.org/no-surprises-act
F. Survey: Americans' financial behavior likely to be impacted by....: https://finance.yahoo.com/news/survey-americans-financial-behavior-likely-040100451.html
G. The U.S. behavioral health market is projected to grow from $77.62 billion in 2021 to $99.40 billion in 2028 at a CAGR of 3.6% in forecast period, 2021–2028: www.fortunebusinessinsights.com/u-s-behavioral-health-market-105298
H. Panorama Consultancy Services and Arbitration: https://panoconsultancy.com/our-services
I. How to pay for healthcare (*Harvard Business Review*): https://hbr.org/2016/07/how-to-pay-for-health-care
J. Fact sheet: Biden-Harris administration announces two new actions: www.ed.gov/news/press-releases/fact-sheet-biden-harris-administration-announces-two-new-actions-address-youth-mental-health-crisis
K. Healthcare IT governance: Why data governance is necessary: www.verizon.com/business/resources/articles/s/why-data-governance-in-healthcare-is-necessary
L. Starting a sole proprietorship FAQ (FindLaw): www.findlaw.com/smallbusiness/incorporation-and-legal-structures/starting-a-sole-proprietorship-faq.html
M. How to start an accounting business (wikiHow): www.wikihow.life/Start-an-Accounting-Business
N. Sole proprietorships, partnerships and LLCs (Wolters Kluwer): www.wolterskluwer.com/en/expert-insights/sole-proprietorships-partnerships-and-llcs-are-commonly-used-entities
O. What is the best business entity for a small business? (U.S. Chamber): www.uschamber.com/co/start/startup/best-business-entity-for-small-business
P. LLC vs. s-corp: What are they and how are they different? (*Forbes*): www.forbes.com/advisor/business/llc-vs-s-corp
Q. SWOT analysis (Skills for Leadership): www.skillsforleadership.co.uk/swot-analysis
R. Example marketing budget (Course Hero): www.coursehero.com/tutors-problems/Financial-Accounting/39220439--Your-company-is-selling-a-product-Product-A-at-a-price-of-90
S. Medicare enrollment application: Durable medical equipment, prosthetics, orthotics, and supplies (DMEPOS) suppliers (CMS-855S): www.hhs.gov/guidance/sites/default/files/hhs-guidance-documents/CMS-855S%20-%2011-2021.pdf
T. Medicare enrollment application: Physicians and non-physician practitioners (CMS-855I): www.cms.gov/Medicare/CMS-Forms/CMS-Forms/downloads/cms855i.pdf
U. Find providers who have opted out of Medicare (Centers for Medicare & Medicaid Services): https://data.cms.gov/tools/provider-opt-out-affidavits-look-up-tool
V. How to apply for a CLIA certificate (U.S. Department of Health and Human Services): www.hhs.gov/guidance/document/how-apply-clia-certificate-including-international-laboratories-0
W. How to enroll in Medicare Electronic Data Interchange (Centers for Medicare & Medicaid Services): www.cms.gov/Medicare/Billing/ElectronicBillingEDITrans/EnrollInEDI
X. Medicaid and CHIP (HealthCare.gov): www.healthcare.gov/medicaid-chip
Y. What is the insurance credentialing process? (Physician Practice): https://physicianpracticespecialists.com/credentialing/what-is-the-insurance-credentialing-process
Z. How to set goals for medical practices (Chron): https://smallbusiness.chron.com/set-goals-medical-practices-77920.html
AA. Where can I find demographic information about my community? (Candid Learning): https://learning.candid.org/resources/knowledge-base/demographic-information
AB. How to write a marketing plan (with sample templates; Vital Design): https://vtldesign.com/digital-marketing/digital-marketing-strategy/how-to-write-marketing-plan-template

AC. How to create a marketing plan for your business (domain): www.domain.com/blog/create-business-marketing-plan

AD. Nurse Spotlight: Defending your license (Free Online Library): www.thefreelibrary.com/Nurse+Spotlight%3a+Defending+Your+License.-a0669377101

AE. Risk management in private practice: How to reduce the likelihood of a claim (Servca): www.servca.com/blog/risk-management-reduce-negligence-claim

AF. Avoid the common mistakes that encourage patients to sue (Relias Media): www.reliasmedia.com/articles/147941-avoid-the-common-mistakes-that-encourage-patients-to-sue

AG. Business operations (CFI): https://corporatefinanceinstitute.com/resources/knowledge/strategy/business-operations

REFERENCES AND BIBLIOGRAPHY

Boss Health Care. (n.d.). *Medicare—Clinical Laboratory Improvement Amendments.* http://bosshealthcare.com/medicare-clinical-laboratory-improvement-amendments

Burns, D. (n.d.). Therapist's toolkit. *Feeling Good.* https://feelinggood.com/resources-for-therapists/therapists-toolkit

Davis, M., Hall, J., & Mayer, P. (2016). Developing a new measure of entrepreneurial mindset: Reliability, validity, and implications for practitioners. *Consulting Psychology Journal: Practice and Research, 68*(1), 21–48. https://psycnet.apa.org/record/2015-47632-001

Doran, G. T. (1981). There's a S.M.A.R.T. way to write management's goals and objectives. *Management Review, 70*(11), 35–36.

Duckworth, A. L., & Quinn, P. D. (2009). Development and validation of the short grit scale (Grit–S). *Journal of Personality Assessment, 91*(2), 166–174. https://doi.org/10.1080/00223890802634290

Harris, G., & Eikenberry, K. (2012). *Free DISC test - DISC personality testing.* The Kevin Eikenberry Group. https://discpersonalitytesting.com/free-disc-test

Humphrey, A. (1960s/1970s). *SWOT analysis framework.* Stanford Research Institute.

Karpen, S. (2018). The social psychology of biased self-assessment. *American Journal of Pharmaceutical Education, 82*(5), 441. https://doi.org/10.5688/ajpe6299

Markey, K., Moloney, M., Doody, O., & Robinson, S. (2022). Time to re-envisage integrity among nurse leaders. *Journal of Nursing Management, 30*(7). https://doi.org/10.1111/jonm.13557

McCarthy, E. J. (1960). *Basic marketing: A managerial approach.* Richard D. Irwin.

Relias Media. (2021, May 1). Avoid the common mistakes that encourage patients to sue. *Healthcare Risk Management.* https://www.reliasmedia.com/articles/147941-avoid-the-common-mistakes-that-encourage-patients-to-sue

Servca. (2019, September 17). *Risk management in private practice—How to reduce the likelihood of a claim.* https://www.servca.com/blog/risk-management-reduce-negligence-claim

Woodman, T., Barlow, M., & Bandura, C. (2013). *Risk taking inventory (RTI)* [Database record]. APA PsycTests. https://psycnet.apa.org/doiLanding?doi=10.1037%2Ft72214-000

29 ELECTRONIC HEALTH RECORDS AND TELEHEALTH

Suzanne Drake

ELECTRONIC HEALTH RECORDS

INTRODUCTION

Implementing an electronic health record (EHR) for a private practice requires thorough planning and some time-consuming implementation to guarantee a seamless transition and maximize the technology for improved patient care. Choosing an EHR is personal and unique to each specific practice.

Extensive research is well worth the time, as it is a crucial decision in the establishment of a practice. Thorough research is needed because it will affect the level of care, the effectiveness of the practice operations, and the platform's sustainability and importance. This chapter serves as a guide to efficient implementation of an EHR system in private practice to achieve improved clinical outcomes and increased patient satisfaction.

DEFINITIONS

Frequently, electronic medical record (EMR) and EHR are used interchangeably in many cases. However, the Office of the National Coordinator for Health Information Technology (ONC) states that they are essentially dissimilar (Garrett & Seidman, 2011; see Figure 29.1).

A. EMR: A patient's EMR is a digital representation of the paper charts in an office documenting their medical and treatment history. It enables healthcare providers to follow information over time, recognize patients in need of appointments, monitor health indicators, and enhance the quality of care at the facility. However, EMRs have limited capabilities for sharing information outside of the practice, which hinders their versatility and portability (Health Insurance Portability and Accountability Act [HIPAA]).

B. EHR: EHRs are more comprehensive than EMRs as they concentrate on the patient's overall well-being by combining regular clinical data and more extensive health information.

C. EHRs are designed for utilization across different healthcare settings, consolidating information from all healthcare professionals engaged in a patient's care to enhance teamwork and prioritize patient well-being. EHRs allow health information to travel with the patient, improving communication among care teams and enabling patients to take a more active role in their healthcare.

D. Types of EHR/EMRs include the following (Table 29.1):
  1. On-premise (local): All medical information is stored on-site on servers owned by individual healthcare providers, practices, or healthcare organizations. These systems require downloading and installation. The EMR may be hosted on a local server owned by the practice or by an outside company (remote) that sells and supports the software. These are often a more viable option for larger practices that employ information technology (IT) personnel to maintain the server and software.
  2. Remotely hosted: These systems store data on third-party servers owned by EHR/EMR vendors, often using cloud-based storage. These may include dedicated servers reserved for specific organizations and subsidized servers funded by the vendor.
  3. Cloud-based: Cloud-based systems are software applications that store and transmit data on dedicated off-site servers, known as "the cloud." These systems are increasing in popularity as solo and small group practices find this is easier to manage and more affordable, with less of a need to hire IT support staff.

E. This chapter primarily emphasizes EHRs instead of EMRs, as EHRs are more practical and widely used in small- to medium-sized private practices.

CONFIDENTIALITY IN ELECTRONIC COMMUNICATION

A. Maintaining privacy in digital communication is critical. The APRN must inform patients of restrictions and obtain consent when they begin communicating electronically, ensuring that patients are aware of potential breaches of confidentiality and associated risks. For instance, simply adding a disclaimer to an unsecured email is insufficient; instead, the APRN should use secure portals for private communication and avoid external communication.

B. Exercise extreme caution when using digital communication methods between two users via standard protocols like email, short message service (SMS), multimedia messaging service (MMS), and instant messaging. While it may be useful for certain purposes like simple yes-and-no information exchanges, it is especially important to be mindful when using these methods to protect privacy and confidentiality. Be aware that closed networks (e.g., social media direct messages) are dicey at best.

C. Adhere to professional standards for medical data and stay informed about regulations governing practitioner–patient interactions. Sending protected health information (PHI) through unencrypted emails, text messages, instant messaging apps, video conferencing, social media, or file-sharing platforms without safeguards is noncompliant.

D. Training employees in confidentiality and security measures is essential for safeguarding patient data.

E. Encryption use is mandatory for all PHI digital communication. Implement access controls, training, and policies. Control access to approved staff. Train employees on HIPAA regulations. Develop policies meeting HIPAA standards. Obtain business associate agreements (BAAs) from third-party service providers handling PHI.

PLANNING STAGE

It should be noted that this guidance mainly pertains to the United States. Different regulations and legal requirements regarding telehealth services and EHR systems may vary in

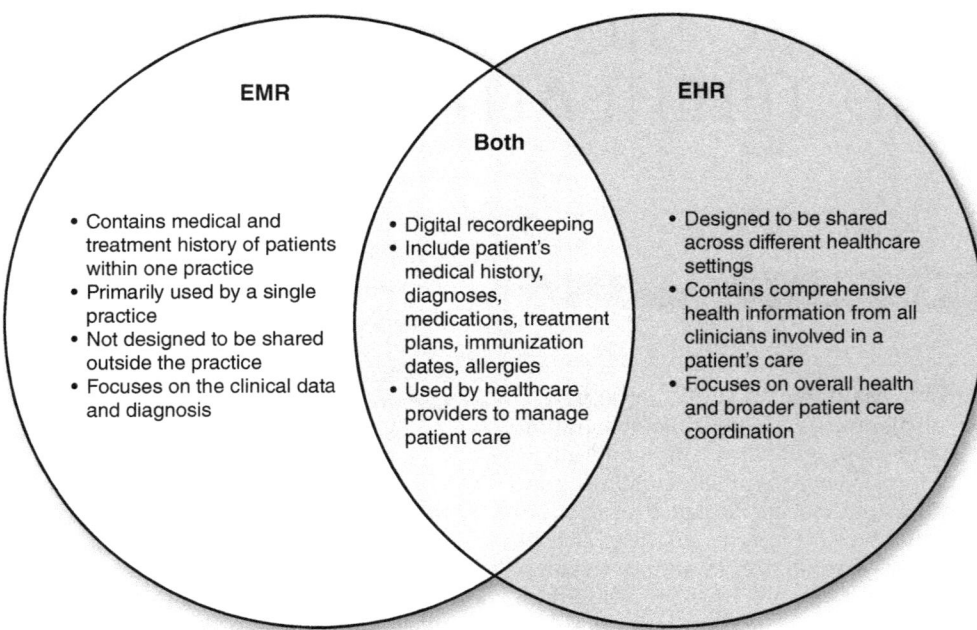

FIGURE 29.1 Comparison of electronic medical record (EMR) and electronic health record (EHR) features.

other countries. It is vital for the APRN to be aware of and comply with specific regulations and norms where they are providing services.

A. Evaluate needs.
  1. What are your practice goals now and in the future? What do you want an EHR to do for you?
  2. Consider your practice's size, patient volume, and growth potential.
  3. What types of services do you offer? Do you have specialty-specific requirements? What are your unique workflow needs? What do you need to enhance patient care, simplify operations, and help you comply with regulations?
  4. Who will be using the system? How many practitioners? How many employees? Who will be handling which data?
  5. How much data do you have now that will have to be moved into the EHR?
  6. Will you need to interface with other systems outside of yours?

TABLE 29.1 COMPARISON OF ON-PREMISE AND CLOUD-BASED ELECTRONIC HEALTH RECORDS PLATFORMS

Feature	Cloud-Based EHR Platforms	On-Premise EHR Platforms
Implementation cost	Lower initial costs, higher TCO over time	Higher upfront costs, lower annual costs
Time to implement	Can be set up quickly	Requires a more extended setup period
Data security	Often perceived as more vulnerable to breaches	Considered more secure, requires management of security protocols
Interoperability	High compatibility with other systems, easier integration with apps	Challenges in compatibility and integration
Scalability	Easily scalable	Requires additional resources for scaling
Customization	Limited options set by the vendor	Allows extensive customization
Data safety and backup	Vendor responsible for backups and security	Organization handles backups and disaster recovery
Support and maintenance	Often includes quick and efficient IT support	Requires in-house personnel and hardware maintenance
Accessibility	Needs stable internet, offers remote access	Does not require internet, not accessible remotely
Data management	Limited data management options	Allows centralized data control within the organization

EHR, electronic health record; IT, information technology; TCO, total cost of ownership.

Source: Data from O'Connor, K. (2024, February 23). *The 3 types of EHR systems to choose from.* Eldermark. https://www.eldermark.com/blog/the-3-types-of-ehr-systems-to-choose-from.

7. Will you need to access the system remotely? Home computer, smartphone?
8. What kind of hardware platforms will you need? PC or Mac? Mobile, tablets? Local and/or remote servers?
9. What is your budget? Some EHRs charge by the individual national provider identifier (NPI) numbers and others by the total employees who have access.
   a. The costs for cloud-based EHR range from $9 per month to over $650 per month, depending on many factors, such as features, number of users, infrastructure requirements, practice type and size, training availability, integrations, and storage.

B. List essential functionality and features.
   1. Consider the type of EHR and the pros and cons of each type (Table 29.2).
   2. Bare minimum requirements.
      a. Compliance and security: HIPAA compliance comes first and foremost. It guarantees patient health information privacy and security via encryption and control of who has access.
         i. Consider ONC-Authorized Testing and Certification Bodies (ONC-ATCB) certified platforms, ensuring that the EHR meets the standards of the Department of Health and Human Services (HHS). Healthcare providers participating in the Centers for Medicare & Medicaid Services (CMS) Medicare and Medicaid Meaningful Use (MU) program and Merit-Based Incentive Payment System (MIPS) are required to comply with this or face reduced payments. Other certifications exist ensuring compliance with data security standards. The HITRUST® certification is the gold standard of security in the healthcare industry.
         ii. Be sure that the EHR is covered by a BAA. This agreement is legally required when any third-party service providers handle PHI on behalf of the

TABLE 29.2 PROS AND CONS OF ELECTRONIC HEALTH RECORDS AND ELECTRONIC MEDICAL RECORD PLATFORMS

Pros of Cloud-Based EHR	Cons of Cloud-Based EHR
Accessibility: Care providers with authorization can retrieve resident information from any place and using any device that is approved.	Internet reliance: EHR is dependent on the internet. Users need an internet connection to access and make changes to EHR information.
Affordability: Many cloud-based EHR systems are priced affordably, enabling small practices and senior living communities with tight budgets to access them.	Ongoing expenses: Cloud-based services typically charge monthly usage fees.
Increased efficiency: Cloud storage allows for quick sharing of resident medical information with pharmacies, clinics, and other healthcare organizations.	Slow upload times: Large file uploads may occasionally experience delays.
SaaS: Benefits of using cloud-based EHR solutions often include extra software as a service enabling features such as integrated scheduling tools and payment gateways.	Limited customization: There may be fewer options to customize EHR software to suit unique organizational needs.
Secure storage: Data are securely stored off-site, providing peace of mind in case of a disaster.	Security risks: While generally safe, cloud-based EHR systems require continuous efforts to meet digital security requirements.
Pros of On-Site-Hosted EHR/EMR	**Cons of On-Site-Hosted EHR/EMR**
Infrequent expenses: There are no monthly data storage fees; upfront costs include purchasing servers and equipment.	Cost: Initial investment can be high, and ongoing maintenance costs may add up.
Greater speed: On-premise servers can upload and share information faster than remote servers.	Downtime: System updates may require periodic shutdowns, causing inconvenience for staff.
Increased flexibility: User has the ability to choose hardware and software combinations for optimal functionality.	Ongoing maintenance: Health IT staff must actively monitor and maintain the system.
Retain data ownership: Organizations maintain ownership of their medical data.	Data loss: Data loss could occur if the organization ceases operations.
Pros of Remote-Hosted EHR/EMR	**Cons of Remote-Hosted EHR/EMR**
Fast startup: It allows quick implementation without the need for complex hardware and software installations.	Internet reliance: Accessing data requires an internet connection.
Cost savings: It is generally less expensive than physician-hosted EHR software, making it more affordable for small organizations.	Loss of data ownership: Organizations may surrender ownership of their medical data, leading to legal complications.
No maintenance responsibilities: The server owner handles updates and security, saving time and money for healthcare organizations.	No control over maintenance schedule: Updates and maintenance are performed on the vendor's schedule, potentially causing inconvenience.

EHR, electronic health record; EMR, electronic medical record; IT, information technology; SaaS, software as a service.

Source: Adapted from O'Connor, K. (2024, February 23). *The 3 types of EHR systems to choose from.* Eldermark. https://www.eldermark.com/blog/the-3-types-of-ehr-systems-to-choose-from.

practice and is imperative when choosing telehealth and other virtual contact such as secure messaging, including text, email, as well as video. If a vendor fails to offer a BAA, their service may be noncompliant with HIPAA.

    iii. Compliance with HIPAA is also essential. A patient portal that follows HIPAA guidelines enables secure data exchange between the healthcare provider and the patient.

b. Management of patient records can be simplified with EHRs. These tools help digitally arrange patient appointments, track diagnoses and treatments, improve collaboration and productivity, and reduce paperwork and errors.

c. Electronic charting allows healthcare providers to digitally document patient appointments and medical information more efficiently, improving data accuracy and accessibility. EHRs can also exchange information with other healthcare professionals, when necessary, which can result in improved care coordination and reduced administrative burden.

d. Scheduling features streamline the process of booking and managing patient appointments using an EHR. Automatic reminders reduce missed appointments and enhance time management and patient satisfaction. Some allow the patient to self-schedule. The schedule may also integrate with an external calendar, such as Google or iCal.

3. The clinical side: The following may be included or as an add-on:

a. e-Prescribing (eRx) enables the electronic transmission of prescriptions to pharmacies. This increases safety and efficiency by minimizing errors and clarifications required by pharmacists. Other advantages include automating prescription renewal requests and authorizations, accessing more affordable medication options, and reducing prescription drug misuse and abuse.

    i. eRx is required for qualified clinicians participating in the CMS's MIPS program. Different states have varying laws and pharmacy requirements concerning eRx usage.

    ii. Medicare Part D has required eRx for controlled substances since January 1, 2023. The 2008 Ryan Haight Online Pharmacy Consumer Protection Act controls how controlled substances can be prescribed online in the United States, mandating a face-to-face medical assessment by the prescribing provider prior to issuing such prescriptions, with certain exceptions.

    iii. Although numerous EHR systems already include eRx functions, separate eRx options, including the ability to electronically prescribe controlled substances, do exist for those who want eRx as an add-on to their existing system or a stand-alone option. Go to www.surescripts.com to explore an eRx solution that will work well for you and your practice.

    iv. Electronic prescribing of controlled substances (EPCS) and prescription drug monitoring programs (PDMP) are digital systems that keep track of a patient's prescription information so prescribers can review their medication history before prescribing controlled substances. Recent efforts, such as mandating EPCS technology and integrating PDMPs into EHR systems, aim to improve the efficiency of data within PDMPs (Richwine & Everson, 2023).

b. Clinical decision support (CDS) tools are like peripheral guardrails checking for safety in practice. For example, they may provide support for medication management and automatically check for drug–drug interactions and contraindications. They can also be useful in ordering, collecting, reporting, viewing, and interpreting laboratory testing. CDS may be a fundamental function of the EHR, depending on the platform (Rudolf & Dighe, 2019). Today, an EHR that does not contain some type of internal decision support tool is either outdated or very basic in its functionality.

c. Treatment planners allow you to construct detailed notes and treatment plans quickly.

d. Customizable templates allow users to upload their own documents (e.g., consents, demographics, health history, inventories, and questionnaires), which are essential for most. Some systems are limited to the EHR's stock templates like SOAP (**s**ubjective, **o**bjective, **a**ssessment, and **p**lan) notes and common forms.

e. Voice dictation enhances efficiency, reduces administrative burden, and improves documentation quality.

f. Telehealth capabilities may include HIPAA-compliant video and chat features.

g. Patient portals enable patients to become active participants in their care, resulting in better health results. They also improve productivity, decrease paperwork, guarantee data precision, and boost security.

h. Onboarding and patient intake may be integrated and fully customizable to one's practice.

4. The business side: Enhanced business functionalities in EHR systems aid in clinical, administrative, and financial aspects of healthcare practices. EHR systems play a role in not only organizing medical data but also effectively managing different facets of healthcare business operations.

a. Billing, payment processing, and accounting features allow you to securely save credit card details for automatic payments, streamline automated billing, minimize mistakes, and accelerate payment collection without compromising on security. The EHR can assist in coding, submitting, and tracking insurance claims and reimbursements.

b. Collection features handle overdue payments effectively by sending reminders, creating statements, and potentially outsourcing debts to enhance cash flow and organization.

c. Revenue cycle management (RCM) modules follow patient care events from registration to payment completion, simplifying billing, overseeing claims, monitoring denials, and reporting financial results. These tools decrease the time between providing a service and receiving payment, enhance the accuracy of billing, guarantee compliance, and offer financial health analytics.

d. Incorporating marketing tools into EHR systems assists in handling patient and referral source relationships, creating marketing initiatives, and interacting with patients via customized communication.

e. Website services may include add-ons for creating websites that include embedded patient portals, online appointment scheduling, health record access, and educational materials to improve patient involvement and accessibility.

c. Explore and choose an EHR system.
1. Do your research! There are hundreds of different EHR suppliers, each with unique characteristics of their systems. Free publicly available information assistance, such as the software clearinghouse Capterra and Software Advice, can help you narrow down EHR.
2. Investigate the various EHR suppliers available in the marketplace as above.
    a. Search for vendors with a solid reputation, relevant experience, and favorable customer feedback.
    b. Consider their history of performance, the support and training they provide, and their dedication to ensuring data security and compliance with regulatory requirements.
    c. Ask colleagues who are practicing in similar clinical settings and practice sizes about the pros and cons of the system they use. Ask their opinion on value for money, vendor support, functionality, and ease of use.
    d. Read reviews! Both the positive and negative ones will give you material for questions.
3. EHR design: Earlier research found EHR design challenging for clinicians in use. A cross-sectional survey of 282 clinicians from three health systems identified several EHR design and use factors associated with high stress and burnout (Kroth et al., 2019), including:
    a. Information overload
    b. Slow system response times
    c. Excessive data entry
    d. Inability to navigate the system quickly
    e. Note bloat [unnecessarily long cut-and-pasted progress notes]
    f. Interference with the patient–clinician relationship
    g. Fear of missing something, and
    h. Notes geared toward billing. (Kroth et al., 2019, p. 10)
4. Ask the vendors (Box 29.1).
    a. How long has the vendor been in operation? Many EHR vendors are linked to big software developers with a long history in the IT industry. It is best to inquire about the length of time their EHR has been available and the number of updates or versions that have been released since its launch.
    b. Ask about the number of healthcare providers the vendor services, specifically the number of mental health and prescribing providers utilizing their product. The more commonly utilized software is more likely to uphold its existing ONC certification (official recognition by the ONC). Ask if the EHR software meets specific criteria set by the U.S. government. Widely used ONC-certified products are likely to have a bigger support team to help you in case of any issues.
    c. Determining how many psychiatric-mental health professionals utilize their software can offer information about the EHR vendor's commitment to mental health-specific IT unique concerns.
    d. If you are considering an on-site system, ask which computer systems, devices, or hardware are best suited for their EHR platform. Also, ask which PC, Mac, and tablet versions you will need and if they plan to discontinue support or updates for certain systems.
    e. Ensure security of data.
        i. General security considerations
            (a) Could you give us references from customers who have experienced security or backup problems?
            (b) What options are there for addressing security or data loss problems?
            (c) What external certifications or audits does your system hold?
            (d) What measures are taken to guarantee the physical safety of data centers?
            (e) What security protocols can prevent ransomware and cyber threats?
        ii. Data security
            (a) Which security measures safeguard patient information?
            (b) What is the process of encrypting data while it is being transmitted and when it is stored?
            (c) What measures do you take to avoid unauthorized entry?
            (d) Does multifactor authentication receive support?
            (e) What is the frequency of security audits and who carries them out? What are the steps involved in dealing with security breaches?
            (f) How can you guarantee adherence to regulations such as HIPAA?
            (g) What kind of training is given to employees regarding data security? How is the control and monitoring of sensitive data access handled?
            (h) How are security updates and patches controlled and handled?
        iii. Backing up data
            (a) What is the frequency of data backup operations? Where are the backup files stored, and is encryption applied to them?
            (b) How does the data recovery process work when there is a loss?
            (c) Can you share your policy for retaining backups? Do backup and recovery services come with extra charges?
            (d) Does a disaster recovery plan exist, and how frequently is it tested?
            (e) What assurances do you provide for the availability and uptime of data? Is it possible for users to create their own backups of data?
            (f) What is the process for transferring data when transitioning to a new EHR system? What measures does the system take to guarantee accurate and efficient data transfer and entry?
            (g) Explore how functionalities such as auto-complete, error-checking, and data validation contribute to ensuring the accuracy and reliability of the patient records within the system.
    f. The kind of computer you utilize for accessing/managing the EHR relies on the EHR's design and the vendor's offerings. For example, numerous cloud-based EHR systems can work with Windows computers, Mac computers, and/or tablets/smartphones.
        i. Some EHRs are designed specifically for Windows operating systems, while others are tailored for use on tablets or smartphones.
        ii. When choosing an EHR system, make sure to inquire the following from the EHR provider:
            (a) What is the best computer(s), devices, or hardware options for the EHR product?
            (b) What if every iteration of their software is released simultaneously across all platforms

BOX 29.1 QUESTIONS TO ASK ELECTRONIC HEALTH RECORD (EHR) SYSTEM VENDORS

Availability and upkeep of the system
- ☐ Can I see live updates of your website's uptime instead of just seeing static pages?
- ☐ Did the platform ever go offline previously? How long did the outage last, and what caused it? How did you take care of your customers?
- ☐ What types of contingency plans are in place for unforeseen interruptions? In what way will you notify me? What measures will you take to safeguard my information?
- ☐ What is the date of your planned maintenance? What is the frequency and duration?
- ☐ Is there 24/7 guarantee of access to the system and records?

Features and integration of the product
- ☐ Do demos, trials, or freemium options exist?
- ☐ Which system characteristics can be tailored, like templates?
- ☐ Which of my current software tools do you connect with?
- ☐ Will the integration of my current tools be smooth and seamless?
- ☐ Is the system compatible with other systems, such as practice management and hospital systems?

Data management and protection of information
- ☐ If I were to terminate my subscription, would all my data be deleted or restored?
- ☐ Can the data be moved to another product? If so, will it be free of charge?
- ☐ What systems are in place to uphold privacy and guarantee security of patient data?
- ☐ Is it possible to establish access permissions at the individual data element level (such as diagnosis or medication)?
- ☐ Who owns the records?
- ☐ Where are files saved (e.g., at the provider's office; off-site at the vendor's location; on the web through cloud computing)?

Technology requirements
- ☐ What type of hardware is needed to utilize the system?
- ☐ Is it possible for the healthcare provider to remotely access the system from outside the office? If yes, in what way (e.g., browser on regular computer, smartphone, tablet)?
- ☐ In what ways can data be input into the system (e.g., manual entry, voice recognition, structured notes, scanner)?

Assistance and support
- ☐ Is 24/7 support included in the subscription cost, or is it a separate charge?
- ☐ Which customer support method do you primarily use: phone, ticketing, email, or live chat? Are these support methods available 24/7 for free?
- ☐ What kind of resources do you have available for training and putting into practice?
- ☐ Is there continuous technical support available? What do the terms refer to?
- ☐ What is the usual duration for implementation?

Pricing and membership fees
- ☐ What is included in your guarantee?
- ☐ What is the cost of implementing (e.g., software license, installation, training)?
- ☐ What is the expense for maintenance?
- ☐ How much does installation cost?
- ☐ If we determine the platform isn't right for us within 30 days, can we get a refund of the fee?
- ☐ Can the subscription be canceled and a full refund received within the first month?

Conformance and accreditations
- ☐ Can you ensure that your system will meet the federal criteria for "meaningful use"?
- ☐ Have you already submitted or are you planning to submit your product for certification to ensure users are eligible for federal incentives (i.e., ONC-ATCB certified)?

ONC-ATCB, ONC-Authorized Testing and Certification Bodies.

---

and systems, including when version 7.0 is launched on PC, Mac, and Tablet, or when they plan to discontinue support or updates for a particular system?

g. Does the EHR system work on mobile devices and tablets? Due to the increasing reliance on mobile technology, it is important to inquire about the accessibility and functionality of EHRs on smartphones and tablets to enhance convenience and accessibility.

h. The interface of user and ease of use: How simple and easy is it to understand the software?

i. User interface and usability: How user-friendly and intuitive is the software? How computer-savvy are you and your staff?

j. Automation and predictive technology: Ask about the EHR system's built-in automation and predictive technology to assist in overall operations. Automated systems can streamline mental healthcare, from booking appointments to billing and documentation. Predictive technology in EHRs can forecast treatment outcomes, evaluate risks, and anticipate symptom changes for proactive patient care.

k. Interoperability: Certain aspects of the software may be shared with office staff and others, such as scheduling patients, recording information in charts, eRx, integrating lab results, handling billing, coding, and collections. Ensuring seamless sharing of patient data (interoperability) among various staff, providers, and ▶

other systems, as well as secure storage and retrieval of patient records such as diagnosis, treatment plan, progress notes, and generating reports, should be considered according to their role.

l. Segmentation: Ask how the EHR contains or customizes its services to add extra protection for highly sensitive mental health PHI and how it can keep certain data segregated from office staff and others who have access to the patient's information when healthcare policy emphasizes linking healthcare providers via EHR to exchange patient health information for improved decision-making. Methods such as role-based access control (RBAC), data segmentation, and encryption enable the management of shared information, ensuring privacy protections for mental health records.

m. Customization. One size fit none. However, does it have potential with customization? Is it optimized for psychiatric practice? Is the product best for a group practice or solo practice? Some are better for large practices and health systems. EHR vendors can customize workflows, dashboards, and templates to integrate screening tools and outcome measures, for example. Is this built-in or done by the vendor for an extra cost?

n. Integration: Can I integrate my current office management software with the new EHR? Using office management software (OMS) for scheduling and billing is different from using an EHR, which includes patient health information. EHRs can also have OMS functionality. Finding EHRs that will either work with your OMS or migrate your data is possible. Check with the vendor if they have prior experience transferring data from your OMS to their platforms.

o. Workflow: Different EHR systems aid various practices' unique processes, such as patient registration, onboarding, assessment, lab requests, prescriptions, and dispensing, billing, and collections. Asking for specifics about workflow management based on your needs will help you determine how this vendor's system might improve daily tasks.

p. Training: What will I and my staff need to learn to implement the EHR? Different EHR providers offer various training methods for implementing their software, including in-person, online tutorials, webinars, and real-time video sessions. Costs vary, with in-person training usually being more expensive.

q. Support: What support options are available, and what can I expect in terms of availability and response time? Do they offer teaching videos, 24/7 support through phone or chat (including real people vs. chatbots), or designated contact personnel? What are the fees for these services?

   i. Ask about the accessibility and speed of technical support in resolving usability problems. Knowing that you have dedicated support can alleviate worries about handling interface issues.
   ii. Seek support, information, and workarounds from online product-specific community blogs.
   iii. What are the common complaints that users express about the interface? Gaining knowledge of common issues or complaints from current or past users can offer understanding of potential usability problems with the EHR system.

r. Scalability. Can the EHR expand to keep up with your practice's projected growth? With changes such as opening other offices, you will need the transition to be as seamless as possible. A scalable EHR system has a modular design for easy add-on of features, a cloud-based infrastructure for resource adjustments, interoperability with other systems, customization for changing needs, effective data management, and reliable performance with dedicated support and regulatory compliance.

D. Financial considerations

1. Various cloud-based platforms offer monthly or yearly subscriptions. These subscriptions usually charge per user per month. A "user" may only apply to the practitioners, or it could include any staff member that uses the system. Certain larger platforms, particularly those that require downloadable software hosted locally, can be significantly pricier.

2. Determine the overall expenses, including software, hardware, customizing, initial and future training, and ongoing support.

3. What will be the ongoing costs? Licensing cost? Per user or per NPI? What are their subscription models and refund policies if the software does not meet your needs?

4. What are the payment options? Are there any incentives? Discounts? Warrantees? If you are on a monthly plan, what is the commitment?

5. Do they offer a 30- or 90-day free trial? Do they have a-la-carte features at different price points?

6. How do they describe your expected return on investment (ROI)?

E. Analyzing costs and benefits is essential in calculating the ROI of an EHR system.

1. The procedure includes recognizing different costs:
   a. Original buying price
   b. Implementation costs
   c. Training expenses
   d. Continuous maintenance expenses

2. When looking at the advantages, consider the following:
   a. Higher effectiveness
   b. Better billing procedures
   c. Superior patient care
   d. Benefits in meeting regulations.

3. Determine the financial worth of every advantage and add up all expenses to assess the potential ROI within a designated period.

4. To calculate the ROI for an EHR, analyze the costs and potential benefits to make a well-informed decision before making a technology investment.
   a. To find net benefits, use the equation: net benefits = total benefits − total costs. Calculate ROI by dividing the total net benefits by the total costs, multiplying the result by 100, and understanding it as the investment's efficiency.
   b. Considering non-monetary advantages such as having an organized, efficient practice can lead to better patient satisfaction and better care. Safeguarding their information increases trust, potentially leading to more referrals.
   c. Test how changes in your estimates affect the ROI calculation. Then compare the ROI with your investment criteria to decide if buying the EHR system is a good decision. Evaluate the ROI calculation in relation to investment standards to determine the worthiness of making the purchase. This comprehensive financial

assessment guarantees that the decision to invest in an EHR system is well-founded and ensures that costs are in line with the practice's overall value.

DEAL/NO DEAL

A. Can meet functional and data needs either intrinsically or by customization, as above
B. Can facilitate connections with external databases, especially those to be used as mandated by government regulations
C. Provide sufficient level of support for:
    1. Meaningful use (including detailed functions and data), if necessary
    2. Certifications from government-authorized organizations
    3. Government backing for HIPAA and other privacy rules
    4. Implementing security measures by enforcing encryption standards for data protection
D. Assures that the customer has legal ownership of the data
E. Product economically feasible through cost–benefit analysis and predicted ROI
F. Confirmation that the vendor has conducted sufficient testing
G. The volume of their clients, including both typical and psychiatric-mental health-exclusive customers; level of availability to the vendor's clients for feedback and reviews
H. Offers demos, training, free noncommitting trials
I. Can meet deadlines for implementation
J. Help and support available promptly for customization, training, implementation, and troubleshooting
K. Necessary backup either to the cloud, remotely, or in-house of software and data to guarantee system availability and meet response time demands
L. Anticipated downtime something you can live with

CONTRACT NEGOTIATION

Not all EHRs require a long-contracted commitment these days. Some allow you to pay month to month and cancel any time. However, those that require more commitment, especially on-site or remote systems, want your business and are often negotiable. By strategically planning negotiations, you can obtain an EHR system that fits your requirements and provides lasting value and dependability. Prior to engaging in talks with EHR suppliers, make sure you:

A. Have a clear grasp of your unique requirements and outline key features to prioritize.
B. Investigate the vendor's standing and talk to current customers for input.
C. Get quotes from various vendors and leverage competitor prices during negotiations.
D. Place emphasis on the overall cost of owning the product and discuss the importance of including all necessary elements in the proposal.
E. Look for flexibility in contract terms and incorporate clauses allowing for termination in unexpected situations.
F. Ask for demonstrations and trials to evaluate the EHR system before deciding and ask about training and ongoing support options available.
G. Talk about support and maintenance contracts, including service level agreements and updates/upgrades.
H. Get a sense that the vendor is invested in building a lasting partnership and will ensure provisions are made for continuous evaluation.
I. Then go ahead. Complete contracts and agreements with EHR vendor and set up a start time.

PREPARATION OF INFRASTRUCTURE

A. Technical
    1. Evaluate, update, and enhance current hardware and network capacities if needed.
    2. Implement procedures for backing up and restoring data if necessary. Develop protocols for the creation of data backups and disaster recovery processes.

CUSTOMIZING AND INCORPORATING SYSTEMS

A. Tailoring to suit the practice's flow is essential. Expansion and customization utilizing apps can be a remedy to the one-size-fits-none issue, thus meeting the needs of healthcare providers and patients in a rapidly changing landscape (Sheikh et al., 2017).
    1. Customize the EHR system to align with the activities and procedures of the practice.
    2. Templates are provided for typical procedures and documentation.
B. Transfer of data
    1. Organize the transfer of current patient files to the updated system.
    2. Guarantee the preservation of data accuracy and security and maintain confidentiality throughout the migration process.
    3. Collaborate with other systems.
        a. Integrate the EHR with laboratory systems, pharmacy systems, billing software, and more.
        b. Evaluate the ability to work together and exchange data.

LEARNING AND INSTRUCTION

A. Establish a program for comprehensive training.
    1. Create or acquire training materials for various staff positions in the practice.
    2. Plan at least three hands-on training sessions.
    3. Offer assistance for independent learning and problem-solving.
B. Provide continuous assistance and education.
    1. Create a system of support for continuous inquiries and technical problems. Schedule regular refresher courses and system updates.

TRANSITION TO LIVE OPERATIONS AND SUPPORT AFTER IMPLEMENTATION

A. Initial test
    1. Begin by assessing the system in a real-life setting with a limited, supervised team.
    2. Adjust as needed per feedback.
B. Complete execution
    1. Implement the system across the entire practice.
    2. Keep a close watch for any problems or interruptions in the workflow.

C. Assessment and enhancements after implementation
1. Perform routine evaluations to gauge the efficiency of the system and the satisfaction of users.
2. Collect input and modify to enhance utilization of the EHR system.
D. Continuous assistance from suppliers
1. Stay in touch with the EHR vendor for updates, assistance, and problem-solving.
2. Participate in ongoing enhancement procedures as technology and practice requirements change continuously.

ASSESSMENT, EVALUATION, AND ONGOING ENHANCEMENT

A. Evaluation criteria and response
1. Create measurements to assess the influence on practice effectiveness, patient contentment, and medical results.
2. Get feedback from employees and patients on a consistent basis. Make continuous refinements.
   a. a. Make adjustments and improvements according to feedback and performance evaluations.
   b. Stay updated on new EHR features and recommended best practices.
B. Requirements for EHR additions/changes are confirmed during software implementation. This involves changes in functions, interfaces, and data conversion software.
C. Placing orders for hardware such as computers and servers in advance is important.
D. Planning should involve establishing protocols for system failures and disaster recovery and creating timelines for testing, training, conversion, and implementation to ensure a smooth process.
E. Depending on the EHR/EMR, sufficient staffing may be critical to carrying out, testing, and implementation.
F. If participating in the MU program, this will involve evaluating your practice for more data and features. Testing levels consist of unit, integrated, function, and system testing. Vendor/developer testing and customer data testing are both essential. Parallel testing might be necessary during system transitions to guarantee the new system operates as intended.
G. Learning how to use an EHR system can be accomplished through either on-site classes or online training, customized to fit each user's individual work responsibilities.
1. User groups can offer important communication and assistance to EHR users.
2. Continued availability of a demo system is essential for practicing.
H. The process of conversion includes transferring data to the new EHR, creating a strategy to transition to the new system, and guaranteeing data integrity throughout the changeover.
I. A smooth conversion process depends heavily on having effective support from vendors/developers.
J. The vendor should be consulted about continued customization support. It is important to carefully evaluate the vendor's software update process and technical support to guarantee the EHR system operates efficiently.
K. Thorough internet documentation for every EHR feature is imperative, with printed versions for training purposes. Talk to the vendor about customization support, including the time it takes for them to respond to requests. The vendor must thoroughly explain software updates to demonstrate their effect on EHR availability.
L. Technical assistance should be strong, meeting requirements for availability and responsiveness.

LEGAL AND ETHICAL CONSIDERATIONS

A. Maintain compliance. Consistently check and revise procedures to ensure adherence to healthcare laws and regulations. Perform audits regularly and evaluate risks!

RESOURCES

A. For Certified EHR Products & Vendor List, go to americanehr.com/ehr-products.
B. The National Learning Consortium (NLC) is a virtual and evolving body of knowledge and tools designed to support healthcare providers and health IT professionals working toward the implementation, adoption, and meaningful use of certified EHR systems. They have templates to request for proposal (RFP) and other helpful information. Go to https://bphc.hrsa.gov
C. The CMS website has information about EHRs: www.cms.gov/priorities/key-initiatives/e-health/records.
D. MIPS Safety Assurance Factors for EHR Resilience (SAFER) Guides requirements are available from the CMS: www.cms.gov/files/document/cms-safer-guides-infographic-2023.pdf
E. Health Level Seven International (HL7) is a not-for-profit, American National Standards Institute (ANSI)-accredited standards developing organization dedicated to providing a comprehensive framework and related standards for the exchange, integration, sharing, and retrieval of electronic health information that supports clinical practice and the management, delivery, and evaluation of health services.
F. These free software matchmaking companies can connect you with an advisor who specializes in your industry based on your needs. They offer research and online reviews of EHRs and free telephone advice to help narrow the choices.
1. Capterra.com
2. SoftwareAdvice.com
3. ExpertMarket.com
4. EHRinPRACTICE.com

REFERENCES AND BIBLIOGRAPHY

American Psychiatric Association. (n.d.). *EHR: Frequently asked questions.* https://www.psychiatry.org/ehr

Cifuentes, M., Davis, M., Fernald, D., Gunn, R., Dickinson, P., & Cohen, D. J. (2015). Electronic health record challenges, workarounds, and solutions observed in practices integrating behavioral health and primary care. *Journal of the American Board of Family Medicine, 28*(Suppl. 1), S63–S72. https://doi.org/10.3122/jabfm.2015.S1.150133

Garrett, P., & Seidman, J. (2011, January 4). EMR vs. EHR—What is the difference? *HealthITbuzz.* https://www.healthit.gov/buzz-blog/electronic-health-and-medical-records/emr-vs-ehr-difference

Greenberg, S. G. (2019, June 26). *What exactly are the roles of pharmacies in healthcare?.* The Medidex. https://themedidex.com/what-exactly-are-the-roles-of-pharmacies-in-healthcare

Hydrick, M. (n.d.). In J. McCaulley (Ed.), *What is an Electronic Medical Record?* Fast Online Master's. Retrieved April 15, 2024, from https://www.fastonlinemasters.com/faq/what-is-an-electronic-medical-record

Kroth, P. J., Morioka-Douglas, N., Veres, S., Babbott, S., Poplau, S., Qeadan, F., Parshall, C., Corrigan, K., & Linzer, M. (2019). Association of electronic health record design and use factors with clinician stress and burnout. *JAMA Network Open, 2*(8), e199609. https://doi.org/10.1001/jamanetworkopen.2019.9609

Practice Solutions. (n.d.). *Tips for keeping your patient records secure.* https://www.practicesol.com/single-post/tips-for-keeping-your-patient-records-secure

Richwine, C., & Everson, J. (2023, January). *Electronic prescribing of controlled substances and use of prescription drug monitoring programs among office-based physicians, 2019–2021* [ONC Data Brief No. 63].

Office of the National Coordinator for Health Information Technology. https://www.healthit.gov/sites/default/files/2023-01/Electronic%20Prescribing%20of%20Controlled%20Substances%20and%20Use%20of%20PDMP-Data-brief_508.pdf

Ritchie, J., & Welch, B. (2020). Categorization of third-party apps in electronic health record app marketplaces: Systematic search and analysis (Preprint). *JMIR Medical Informatics, 8*(5). https://doi.org/10.2196/16980

Rudolf, J. W., & Dighe, A. S. (2019). Decision support tools within the electronic health record. *Clinics in Laboratory Medicine, 39*(2), 197–213. https://doi.org/10.1016/j.cll.2019.01.001

Sheikh, A., Bates, D. W., Wright, A., & Cresswell, K. (2017). *Key advances in clinical informatics: Transforming health care through health information technology.* Academic Press.

Uzialko, A. (2024, January 23). *Adam Uzialko.* Business News Daily. https://www.businessnewsdaily.com/author/adam-uzialko

TELEHEALTH

INTRODUCTION

Despite our modern perspective, telehealth has existed since before the 1920s when Grandma called her doctor for advice on her sore knees. Telehealth's long history dates back to ancient Egyptians, Greeks, and Romans (Hurst, 2016), when scrolls and hieroglyphs were used to share health information. During the Middle Ages, bonfires were used to exchange bubonic plague information across Europe. The exact date of the use of telemedicine is unknown (Zundel, 1996).

Telehealth's development has advanced in the last few decades, and this increase was especially noticeable throughout the recent pandemic. During the public health emergency (PHE), certain regulatory restrictions that had previously been in place were lifted in order to make the healthcare system more flexible. Licensure barrier relaxation for physicians and nurses increased access to more providers. However, people who were ill or terrified stayed home. They skipped their usual preventive care, and even sick care got sidelined for fear of dying if exposed to the deadly virus. Thankfully, relaxing restrictions to telehealth saved lives and catapulted the field of telehealth into the mainstream.

As telehealth gains acknowledgment as a legitimate cost-saving and convenient alternative to traditional in-person visits, advantages are realized for individuals with various health challenges, limited mobility, and those living far from resources. Those advantages have resulted in vast acceptance from healthcare providers and patients. Telehealth is here to stay. Research now focuses on improving device compatibility and security and enhancing telehealth platforms to improve user experience in accessing electronic health records (EHRs). Telemental health promotes health awareness, mainly through the increased availability of virtual counseling and services during the COVID-19 pandemic. As convenient and user-friendly as it has become, safe and effective integration of telemedicine into healthcare environments requires planning for safe and effective use.

The following information is for information only. Consulting relevant state and federal agencies for additional details and guidance is strongly advised.

DEFINITIONS

A. The federal government, the states, and institutions may define *telehealth* and *telemedicine* differently, but they can broadly be defined as using technology to provide healthcare services when the two parties are not in the same location.

B. While the terms are often used interchangeably, *telehealth* technically encompasses a broader range of services than *telemedicine*, including nonclinical services like training, education, meetings, care coordination, and sharing healthcare information. Telemedicine is more focused on the medical aspects of patient clinical care.

C. The CMS sees telemedicine as a subset of *telehealth*. The CMS defines *telehealth* as "the use of telecommunications and information technology to provide access to health assessment, diagnosis, intervention, consultation, supervision and information across distance" (CMS, n.d.-a, para 1.). It allows the patient and the healthcare provider to communicate with each other from various locations.

D. This communication may be *synchronous*, meaning it occurs in real time between healthcare providers and patients, family members, or colleagues using video conferencing, audio-only telehealth, or secure text messaging to provide care, digital sessions, brief check-ins, or interprofessional consultations. Alternatively, it may be asynchronous.

E. *Asynchronous* forms of telehealth are information exchanges that do not occur in real time, such as encrypted emails, patient data, or lab results. Other forms of asynchronous telehealth may include the following:

1. *Remote patient monitoring (RPM),* such as wearable devices that transmit patient data to the provider, including heart monitors, oximeters, and glucose monitors
2. *Mobile health (mHealth),* such as fitness trackers and mobile reminder apps
3. *Store-and-forward technology,* which involves sending medical information to another practitioner, often a specialist, who then uses it to assess a case or provide a service without interacting in real time

F. The National Institute of Mental Health (NIMH) refers to *telemental* health as using telecommunications or videoconferencing technology to provide mental health services. It is also known as *telepsychiatry* or *telebehavioral* health and is often used interchangeably. In essence, telemedicine, telemental health, telebehavioral, and telepsychiatry are all included in the larger virtual health ecosystem, which includes all aspects of digital and telehealth.

G. *Virtual care, or eHealth,* encompasses various digital technologies, including telehealth services, online appointments, mobile applications, and messaging platforms.

H. *Digital health* refers to technologies such as mobile apps, eRx, wearable devices, and RPM.

I. *Originating site* refers to where the patient is located.

J. *Distant site* means where the provider is located. A *distant provider* is a person who provides telehealth.

K. A HIPAA-covered entity is a health plan, healthcare clearinghouse, or healthcare provider who transmits any health information electronically in connection with a transaction covered by this subchapter (U.S. Department of Health & Human Services, 2021).

L. *Protected Health Information (PHI)* is health information that can identify an individual and is managed by an HIPAA covered entity or business associate (Brown, 2018). In addition to medical details, any other nonmedical information stored in the same specified record collection that can identify—or could potentially be combined with other data to identify—the individual mentioned in the medical information is also considered PHI, according to HIPAA (*HIPAA Journal*, 2023).

M. *Business associate agreement (BAA)* is a written contract specifying each party's responsibilities regarding PHI. HIPAA requires covered entities to work only with business associates who ensure complete protection of PHI. These assurances must be in writing as a contract or other agreement between the covered entity and the business associate (Office for Civil Rights [OCR], 2009).

REGULATORY, COMPLIANCE, AND LEGAL CONSIDERATIONS

A. Telehealth provides healthcare services, coordinates care, collects data, shares information, educates and trains, collects public health information, and accesses EHRs.
B. Modalities include real-time audio alone or audio/video conferencing, mobile technology using apps, RPM, and storing and forward transmitting information.
C. Policy is built around laws, regulations, and guidance, which may be in the form of policy memos issued by the regulatory agency, such as the CMS provider manual. The courts can also develop policies.
D. Telehealth is regulated at the federal and state level.
   1. Federal: Medicare/CMS, HIPAA, Drug Enforcement Administration (DEA), licensure
   2. State: Medicaid, private payers, prescribing, licensure
E. During the PHE, licensure and other regulatory flexibilities were implemented through temporary waivers that dramatically expanded access to healthcare providers. Nurses and physicians could work out of state, and patients could be seen virtually in their homes. Healthcare providers were reimbursed at the same rate for telehealth as in-person visits, and controlled substances could be ordered virtually. Many of the regulations around the technology that had become urgently needed at that time were not enforced but left to the healthcare provider's discretion (OCR, 2020).

FEDERAL

A. Medicare and CMS specifics to telehealth involving reimbursement and coverage include the following:
   1. Before the pandemic, Medicare/CMS policy on telehealth was very restrictive, with limitations on where, what services, who could provide it, and specifics on how.
   2. However, during the unprecedented COVID-19 health crisis and concomitant social distancing and isolation, telehealth was brought out of the shadows to answer the exigent need to provide safe care. Swiftly, numerous executive orders removed barriers through temporary waivers. The PHE ended in May 2023, but most significant waivers remained until December 2024. Out of 70 or more CMS waivers, some have expired, some have been made statutorily permanent, and some sunset in December 2024.
   3. Telehealth has become an essential aspect of healthcare.
B. According to HHS.gov (2023), some changes pertaining to behavioral health were made permanent with the end of the PHE.
   1. Federally qualified health centers (FQHCs) and rural health clinics (RHCs) can serve as distant site providers for behavioral/mental telehealth services.
   2. Medicare patients can receive telehealth services for behavioral/mental healthcare in their homes.
   3. There are no geographic restrictions for the originating site for behavioral/mental telehealth services.
   4. Behavioral/mental telehealth services can be delivered using audio-only communication platforms.
   5. Rural emergency hospitals (REHs) are eligible originating sites for telehealth.
   6. Some services are allowed to be audio-only.
   7. Site limitations were waived.
   8. Others sunset in December 2024:
      a. FQHCs and RHCs can serve as a distant site provider for nonbehavioral/mental telehealth services.
      b. Medicare patients can receive telehealth services in their homes.
      c. There are no geographic restrictions for originating site for nonbehavioral/mental telehealth services.
      d. Some nonbehavioral/mental telehealth services can be delivered using audio-only communication platforms.
      e. An in-person visit within 6 months of an initial behavioral/mental telehealth service, and annually thereafter, is not required.
      f. Telehealh services can be provided by all eligible Medicare providers (U.S. Health Resources and Services Administration [HRSA], n.d., para. 3).
      g. Allowing the provider to use their business address instead of their home address for privacy reasons.
C. There may be another extension. What will be permanent is still up in the air. A federal telehealth-specific bill is unlikely, but telehealth features may be rolled into another bigger bill, such as appropriations. In any case, telehealth will probably be more restrictive than during the pandemic.

STATE

A. Due to the intricate and interconnected state-level regulatory system overseeing healthcare delivery, barriers in one area could obstruct alignment in other areas, hindering the adoption and full utilization of telehealth capabilities. Telehealth is fundamentally a complicated combination of four interconnected areas: the population being served, the service being delivered (including coverage and reimbursement), the healthcare provider delivering the care, and the technology used.
B. States should support the use of telehealth technology to provide covered services within the Medicaid program in a clinically appropriate manner.
   1. States can choose how to cover Medicaid and CHIP services offered through telehealth, allowing for a lot of flexibility. States can choose to decide if they want to use telehealth, which services to include, where it can be used, how it is set up, who can provide services through telehealth, as long as they are qualified under Medicaid regulations, and reimbursement rates. States have complete freedom to choose from a range of Healthcare Common Procedures Coding System (HCPCS) codes and modifiers to distinguish, monitor, and compensate for these services (CMS, n.d.).
C. For specific information, see the CMS "Partner Tools and Toolkits" under the "Resources" section. For information on individual state policies, go to www.cchpca.org to read full policy information by state.

PROFESSIONAL BOARDS STANDARDS AND OVERSIGHT

A. Professional regulation of telehealth has experienced a gradual yet consistent evolution in recent years. Following past uncertainty, numerous states previously silent on the subject are now specifying in legislation or board regulations the conditions under which telehealth can establish a healthcare provider–patient relationship. Frequently, this involves regulations related to licensing, obtaining consent, and prescribing medications (Center for Connected Health Policy [CCHP], n.d.).

B. Regulations require practitioners to adhere to high standards, whether in-person or virtually. Every state has a Nurse Practice Act governing licensing boards that oversee APRNs and other healthcare professionals and uphold high patient care standards.

C. The American Telemedicine Association (ATA) emphasizes the importance of the CMS, Federal Trade Commission (FTC), and DEA in overseeing telehealth and virtual care. The CMS uses evidence to decide which services are covered, while the FTC concentrates on regulating data and safeguarding privacy. The DEA monitors the prescribing of controlled substances, granting temporary waivers because of the pandemic.

D. The U.S. HHS Office of Inspector General (OIG) conducts audits and investigations to combat healthcare fraud in telehealth. Although fraud is present, it is mainly found in telemarketing rather than telehealth.

GENERAL PRINCIPLES

A. HIPAA applies to telehealth regarding the technology used and the usual privacy protections. All PHI exchanges must be encrypted.
B. Privacy risks occur when people cannot control how their health data are collected, used, and shared. Security risks occur when someone gains unauthorized access to a person's health information while it is being collected, transmitted, or stored.
C. These dangers can impact the bond between the patient and the healthcare provider, decreasing adherence and continuity of care.
D. Meet privacy requirements by staying informed about security needs, communicating risks to patients, and implementing safeguards.
E. Confirm identities, utilize unique IDs and passwords, and enable automatic logoff to convey privacy safeguards.
F. Safeguard personal privacy by examining policies, removing files, storing data, and performing security assessments.
G. Health data breaches are expensive and must be examined and disclosed to patients.
H. APRNs must know security features and obtain independent evaluations of their telehealth systems.
I. Discover additional security advice from the Office of the National Coordinator for Health Information Technology (ONC).

BEFORE OFFERING TELEHEALTH

A. Know the laws and regulations regarding telehealth that apply in the originating state.
   1. Every state in the United States has laws that govern the practice of nursing. These laws are defined in the Nursing Practice Act and regulated through licensing boards that oversee APRNs, mandating that they uphold high patient care standards.
   2. Standard of care is a legal phrase that denotes a healthcare provider's responsibility to administer appropriate treatment to a patient based on specific circumstances. This standard of care equally applies to the provision of telehealth services.
B. Licensure: APRNs must be licensed in their own state and be licensed or legally permitted to practice in the state where the patient is located (originating state).
   1. Some states permit out-of-state providers to offer telemedicine services in their state through specific licenses or telehealth exceptions or under certain conditions, such as not establishing an office in that state.
   2. Numerous states have now established interstate compacts to reduce the challenges for healthcare providers in obtaining licenses for telehealth practice in multiple states. These compacts allow them to practice in states without that state's license if they hold a valid license in their home state.
   3. Other states may not have laws explicitly covering telehealth or telemedicine licensing, but they do allow practicing in neighboring states or issuing temporary licenses if certain conditions are met.
   4. According to the HHS, many states are revisiting their licensure process to ensure access. There are various ways a healthcare provider may provide services across state lines:
      a. Obtain a full license in that state.
      b. Check the originating state for temporary practice laws.
      c. See if there is licensure reciprocity in that state.
   5. Join a licensure compact if both the APRN's state and the originating state participate in the multistate licensure compact. The CCHP is currently monitoring six compacts, and Nurse Licensure Compact is included in them.
   6. Apply for a telehealth registration or certificate if available in origination state.
C. The federal government allows the interstate practice of healthcare as permitted under the following:
   1. Specific laws and for particular patient population groups, such as sports teams and the U.S. Department of Veterans Affairs (VA). The Uniform Emergency Volunteer Health Practitioners Act (UEVHPA) is a model law created to facilitate volunteer health professionals' quick mobilization during emergencies and grant reciprocal licensing to responders. Healthcare workers in states that have implemented this Act can sign up in advance or during a crisis to offer volunteer services through various registration systems set up by organizations like the Medical Reserve Corps, disaster relief groups, licensing boards, or national or multistate associations of health professionals.
D. Insurance:
   1. If the APRN plans to practice in multiple states, confirm that the malpractice and liability insurance policy covers all locations and includes telehealth.
   2. Liability insurance may already provide coverage in certain situations, while additional cybersecurity protection may be necessary in others.
   3. Adhering to regulations like HIPAA is essential to protecting patient data and maintaining confidentiality. To ensure privacy, develop secure communication systems and storage solutions that meet HIPAA regulations.
   4. Be aware of state laws and regulations regarding the collection and storage of PHI.
E. Maintaining detailed records of telehealth interactions is essential for clinical, legal, and billing purposes. Documentation should be as thorough as for in-person visits.
F. Consent:
   1. Confirm the patient's identity and location and determine suitability for telehealth.
   2. Reveal any potential conflicts of interest.
   3. The CCHP and the HHS have identified vital legal concepts in telehealth implementation and use.

a. Most states' statutes, administrative codes, and/or Medicaid policies include telehealth-specific informed consent requirements. The requirement for consent may accompany other requirements, such as ensuring the same level of care is delivered via telehealth as expected in person.

b. Before making an appointment with a new patient, the APRN should verify the patient's location and obtain consent to use telehealth services. Then, the APRN should clearly explain the nature, benefits, limitations, and privacy considerations, detailing the characteristics of telemedicine and what to expect.

c. Patients must be assured that the details discussed during the telehealth visit are confidential. They should be provided with specifics about the telehealth services they will receive, such as the technology utilized, possible advantages and disadvantages, privacy concerns, and their rights.

d. Have a conversation with children and teenagers about sharing private information that will not be disclosed to their parents or guardians unless there is a serious potential for danger.

e. Summarize situations in which data can be disclosed to a caregiver, colleague, parent, or any other party.

f. Safeguard patient privacy and security, including actions taken by staff and others. Discuss with the patient the importance of having a secluded and peaceful area for the meeting and utilizing headphones if necessary to maintain confidentiality.

g. Verify if the rest of the household is honoring the patient's privacy requirements.

h. Inform the patient about the data that can and cannot be retrieved by the APRN, such as from the electronic medical record or the state's prescription drug monitoring program (PDMP).

i. If the patient has a background of substance use disorder, inform them that this information will not be documented in their medical record unless further permission is given.

j. Consent may be provided verbally or in written form, depending on the state's regulations.

k. Have clear protocols for emergency management during telehealth sessions, including having local emergency service contacts in the patient's location at hand.

G. Online prescribing:

1. Variations exist among states regarding the utilization of technology in the prescribing process. Most states deem it insufficient to rely solely on an internet/online survey to establish a patient–healthcare provider relationship, as required for prescribing medication in most states.

2. Some but not all states may mandate a physical exam before a prescription is given, and some allow telehealth to be the setting for the examination.

3. Controlled substances:

a. If the APRN is prescribing controlled dangerous substances in more than one state, they will need to have a DEA in each state where services are being provided, including via telehealth (DEA, 2023).

b. As of this writing, the temporary rule authorizes healthcare providers meeting specific criteria to prescribe controlled substances through telehealth.

c. Enacted in 2008, the Ryan Haight Online Pharmacy Consumer Protection Act regulates the Unites States' online prescribing and dispensing of controlled substances. The Act requires at least one in-person medical evaluation before prescribing controlled substances online. The legislation aims to combat the illegal sale and abuse of prescription drugs while supporting legitimate telehealth services.

d. The DEA and HHS have extended PHE telemedicine flexibilities for controlled substance prescribing until December 31, 2024. Until then, practitioners can prescribe controlled substances via telemedicine to patients outside registered facilities. Buprenorphine can be prescribed by qualifying practitioners based on a phone evaluation. APRNs are advised to check their state and federal registers for updates.

e. For as long as the designation of a PHE remains in effect, DEA-registered practitioners may issue prescriptions for all Schedule II to V controlled substances to patients for whom they have not conducted an in-person medical evaluation, provided all of the following conditions are met:

i. The prescription is issued for a legitimate medical purpose by a practitioner acting in the usual course of their professional practice.

ii. Telemedicine communication is conducted using an audiovisual, real-time, two-way interactive communication system.

iii. The practitioner is acting per applicable federal and state laws.

ETHICAL CONSIDERATIONS

A. HIPAA: Healthcare providers and institutions are required by law to protect the privacy of PHI under HIPAA. Healthcare providers and health plans under HIPAA rules must use technology vendors who adhere to the rules and will establish BAA for their video communication products or other remote communication technologies used for telehealth services.

1. Providers have an ethical obligation to discuss privacy and security risks. These discussions can be part of a patient-centered care plan to help ensure confidentiality.

2. Ensure that the quality of care provided via telehealth meets or exceeds the standard of in-person care.

3. Ensure confidentiality.

a. Securing privacy in virtual healthcare services is a new frontier that requires APRNs to be astutely aware and to uphold the same standards of confidentiality as in traditional settings.

b. APRNs must ensure that telehealth technologies comply with privacy laws like the HIPAA of 1996 and maintain the security of store-and-forward systems, which govern how information is stored or transmitted electronically.

c. The APRN must prioritize the privacy of sessions that are conducted remotely. Patients should also be advised that their sessions must take place in a secure location. If others are present during the session, healthcare providers should adhere to in-person protocols for documenting additional attendees' names in the EHR.

d. Practical measures to maintain confidentiality include utilizing background white noise in the designated exam or consultation room and ensuring the healthcare provider and the patient wear earbuds or headphones during the session to prevent others from overhearing the therapeutic interaction.

e. Utilize the telehealth technologies and the EHR system on a password-protected computer dedicated to clinical practice and securely located.

f. Considerations for maintaining confidentiality in EHR systems involve restricting access to authorized personnel, implementing regularly updated individual user passwords, and employing data encryption measures (Basil et al., 2022; HealthIT.gov, n.d.). Additionally, computing devices used to operate the EHR must be safeguarded against unauthorized access by setting up firewalls and using antivirus software (HealthIT.gov, n.d.).

4. Make privacy part of the workflow.
   a. Confirm the identities of everyone present at each telehealth session and communicate how and if any third parties may be involved.
   b. Create unique user identification numbers. Use password-protected platforms. Establish automatic logoffs.
   c. Set up and communicate safeguards to patients.

B. Health Information Technology for Economic and Clinical Health Act (HITECH): Advancements in technology, especially in information technology, are altering individuals' perspectives on time and distance, impacting interactions among people, including and, significantly, patients and their care providers.

1. The HITECH Act motivated healthcare providers to incorporate EHRs and enhance privacy and security measures for healthcare data.
2. This was accomplished by offering financial rewards for adopting EHRs and imposing stricter penalties for not following the HIPAA Privacy and Security Rules.
3. Telehealth uses varying technologies to provide care, adding an extra layer of responsibility to engendering patients' trust in APRNs' competency and ethical conduct.
4. APRNs involved in telehealth are required to:
   a. Ensure the technology is secure and compliant with privacy laws
   b. Acknowledge and deal with technological restrictions
   c. Inform patients of the limitations of telehealth
   d. Document encounters, including assessments, treatment, evaluation, and prescribing medication
   e. Facilitate follow-up care
   f. Offer impartial and precise health information when in the digital realm, such as websites and social media
   g. Endorse quality care standards
   h. Maintain professionalism and adherence to ethical guidelines
   i. Have comprehensive understanding of pertinent technologies
   j. Be skilled in electronic communication with patients in order to provide telehealth services effectively
   k. Maintain a consistent approach to the patient's care
   l. Communicate effectively with other members of the patient's team
   m. Monitor technology advancements and outcomes
   n. Take proactive steps to guarantee safe and efficient telehealth practices for all patients

TECHNOLOGY INFRASTRUCTURE

A. When selecting a telehealth platform, opt for one that is secure, compliant with healthcare regulations, and most importantly user-friendly. It must provide essential functions such as secure video calls, encrypted messaging, and file sharing while remaining user-friendly for healthcare providers and patients.

B. For a messaging platform to be compliant with HIPAA, it must have robust security measures in place, such as data encryption, access controls, and audit controls. Additionally, it must then enter into a BAA with the healthcare provider.

1. Platforms such as iMessage, Facebook/Messenger, FaceTime, WhatsApp, Telegram, and WeChat may have some but not all features and therefore lack HIPAA compliance. Some secure communication platforms for healthcare, such as TigerText and Signal, with appropriate configurations, are available to meet HIPAA requirements in medical settings.
2. HIPAA compliance for two-way, audio-video platforms involves more than just the technology; it also includes implementation and usage within the organization. Commonly used platforms that can adhere to HIPAA regulations and that verify the presence of a BAA for you to enter into include the following:
   a. Zoom For Healthcare: This is a specialized version of the Zoom video conferencing platform designed specifically for the healthcare industry. However, regular Zoom is missing certain security features and there is no BAA included.
   b. Microsoft Teams: This has the capability to be set up in a way that meets HIPAA compliance standards.
   c. Google Meet: This can adhere to HIPAA guidelines when used within Google Workspace (formerly G Suite) designed for healthcare.
3. Types of platforms that are NOT HIPAA-compliant include the following:
   a. Apple Video calls using Apple devices
   b. FaceTime, which is not HIPAA-compliant as they do not offer a BAA

C. Ensure that the APRN, staff, and patients possess the necessary technology, such as computers, smartphones, webcams, and microphones, and the qualified software to conduct telehealth consultations securely and effectively.

D. Selecting a platform from an organization primarily focused on telehealth services is highly recommended. These organizations specialize in telehealth technologies and services, ensuring they are developed with unique healthcare features and meet telemedicine compliance requirements.

E. A reliable, secure, high-speed internet connection is essential for healthcare providers and patients to facilitate high-quality video consultations. The quality of video and audio during consultations is directly affected by the speed and stability of the connection.

F. Access to prompt and efficient technical support is vital to address any technical issues swiftly, ensuring minimal disruption to telehealth services and maintaining stable connectivity throughout consultations.

G. Healthcare providers must stay informed about the latest security standards and regulatory requirements, especially HIPAA compliance, to protect patient data and ensure legal adherence in the delivery of telehealth services.

H. The option to tailor the telehealth platform to suit the needs of the APRN is an added benefit. Personalize the virtual space by looking for features such as branded interfaces, secure audio and video, appointment scheduling, and secure messaging. An interactive platform that offers reminders and educational materials will promote active patient involvement.

I. Secure video may be a feature in the EHR software. Other options for a charge include the following:
   1. Google Meet is HIPAA-compliant under certain conditions, making it suitable for handling electronic PHI through a Google Workspace business plan, as long as it includes HIPAA-compliant features and a Business Associate Addendum. After that, it is crucial to set up the service to align with HIPAA guidelines and ensure employees are trained on properly using Google Meet in accordance with regulations. Search for Google Workspace and Cloud Identity HIPAA Implementation Guide.
J. Cybersecurity is vital. Cyberattacks can result in operational disruptions and compromised EHR security and endanger patient safety. It is essential to consider all aspects of one's health IT network when introducing new technology.
   1. APRNs in small practices frequently do not have internal security personnel and instead depend on outside vendors for cybersecurity assistance. Having knowledge of fundamental cybersecurity concepts enables individuals to ask vendors about relevant information. When incorporating telehealth technology, make sure to adhere to HIPAA regulations and provide extra safeguards for data from medical devices and patient apps. The U.S. Food and Drug Administration (FDA) does not test the cybersecurity of apps and medical devices before they are marketed, so manufacturers must find and reduce risks themselves.
K. The FTC recommends the following:
   1. Update all software, including apps, web browsers, and operating systems, and set updates to happen automatically.
   2. Encrypt devices and media with sensitive information, such as laptops, tablets, smartphones, removable drives, backup tapes, and cloud storage.
   3. Use strong passwords for all devices and do not leave them unattended in public places.
   4. Secure important files by backing them up offline or in the cloud.
   5. Implement multifactor authentication for network access with sensitive information.
   6. Secure your wireless network by changing the default name and password, using WPA2 or WPA3 encryption, and requiring strong passwords.
   7. Train all staff on security measures and create a culture of security.
   8. Have a plan in place for saving data, running the business, and notifying customers in case of a breach. The FTC's Data Breach Response Guide provides steps to take in the event of a breach.
      a. See the "Resources" section for additional guidance.

TRAINING AND SUPPORT

A. Recommendations and reviews are invaluable in choosing the right platform to serve the needs of the APRN and the patients well. Tech support is a must. Ensure that the platform provides 24/7 assistance to address any technical issues swiftly.
B. Several online training workshops cover various aspects of telehealth. They may cover everything from lighting, background, body language, and communication to troubleshooting the technology.
C. Train staff and healthcare providers on how to use telehealth technologies effectively. Include training on troubleshooting common technical issues.
D. Educate patients on accessing and using telehealth services, including scheduling appointments, joining video calls, and managing technical issues.

TELEHEALTH INTEGRATION

A. Many EHRs now offer compliant, integrated video and messaging platforms for telehealth. If not, ensure the telehealth platform integrates well with one's EHR system for seamless patient data management. In either case, consider how compatible the platform will be with current operating systems and devices.
B. Integrate telehealth into existing clinical workflows, streamlining administrative processes such as scheduling, patient intake, documentation, billing, and follow-up care. Patient portals can enhance patient care and autonomy.
C. Consider how a new telehealth solution will impact one's existing health IT network, especially if outside one's current EHR vendor. View networks holistically to ensure that all the "entry" and "exit" points for information coming in and out of the practice are effectively protected (AMA-ASSN, 2017).
D. Understanding cybersecurity basics empowers the APRN to know the most relevant questions when seeking or working with vendors.

PATIENT SELECTION AND CARE COORDINATION

Telebehavioral health has immense potential as a valuable tool, constantly evolving in its application. Hilty et al. (2013), in their landmark study, concluded that "telemental health is effective for diagnosing and evaluating various populations (adult, child, geriatric, ethnic) and for disorders in various environments (emergency, home *health), and appears to be comparable to in-person care*" (p. 444), showing similar results to traditional face-to-face care. In addition, new models of care (i.e., collaborative care, asynchronous, mobile) with equally positive outcomes, telemental health is effective and increases access to care (Hilty et al., 2013).

A. Determining which appointments and patient concerns are suitable for telehealth versus in-person care is crucial. Many patients lack enough medical expertise to know when to visit a behavioral health provider in person or when to opt for telehealth services.
B. Some observations made during telehealth sessions may require an in-person assessment for proper evaluation.
C. Establish protocols for referring patients and handling emergencies during telehealth sessions.
D. Review previous psychiatric records to assess suitability for remote mental health services. Patients with unstable conditions, acute psychosis, active suicidal or homicidal ideations, or domestic violence situations may not be suitable for telehealth.
E. Patients must be comfortable with telemental healthcare and have access to a private space for remote sessions.

F. Collaboration with other members of the healthcare team is necessary.
G. Know the state regulations regarding prescriptions, licensing procedures, and payment for telemedicine treatments in one's own practice state.
H. Extensive preparation is necessary for the effective integration and continued improvement of telehealth services.

PREPARING PATIENTS FOR TELEHEALTH

A. Educate patients on telehealth basics covering types of care offered.
   1. Discuss when telehealth is and is not appropriate or a perfect fit for some individuals.
   2. Options for virtual care include phone, text, email, videoconferencing, and mobile and remote monitoring. Does the patient:
      a. Have access to a computer, smartphone with or tablet with camera?
      b. Have internet with enough broadband to support video as needed?
      c. Have a secure WiFi network?
      d. Need help with setup or getting an email account if needed? Need language help?
   3. Educate patients on similarities/differences from in-person.
   4. Educate patients on the logistics of appointment scheduling, availability, and self-scheduling if available.
   5. Educate patients on the costs and insurance reimbursements and how payments are to be made.
   6. Allow patient control as to switching back to in-person visits.
   7. Discuss the benefits of the convenience of virtual visits.
      a. Convenience: Time and money savings in travel often means less time off work and smoother logistics coordination for things like transportation or childcare. Patients can schedule appointments with less advance notice and at more flexible hours. There is also increased access to services especially for those in remote areas and during emergency care situations. There may be fewer barriers for those hesitant to seek in-person mental healthcare.
   8. Advances in technology: As telemental health services have increased, healthcare providers have become more familiar with evolving videoconferencing technology, with some switching entirely to virtual practices (NIMH, 2023), saving on travel and access to specialists.
   9. Discuss disadvantages or risks with patients.
      a. Access to technology: device and internet connectivity issues. Varying levels of technological quality can affect how services are provided and received. Evolving technology means updating equipment, platforms, and networks for patients. Cameras in users' homes and virtual online platforms pose privacy considerations. Individuals also might be more hesitant to share sensitive personal information with a healthcare provider in a situation where others might hear.
   10. Insurance coverage: The rise in telehealth during the COVID-19 pandemic has led to policy changes to make services accessible to more people. However, it is not known how long such flexibilities will stay in place, and understanding what services are available can be complicated. Coverage and healthcare provider licensure requirements vary from state to state (NIMH, 2023).
   11. Encourage the patient to express their concerns or hesitation about telehealth visits.
   12. Discuss and reassure patient about confidentiality and privacy concerns they may have, as well as potential risks and protections that are in place to mitigate risk.
   13. Discuss the need for a private environment for the patient and the intentional (interpreter, advocate) or accidental presence of other individuals that may be at home.
   14. Patients may need help with technology and assistance with setup.
   15. Since the patient may not be in the same locality as the APRN, it is necessary to discuss an emergency preparedness in the first visit:
      a. Obtain the patient's current location and their full address for telemedicine appointments.
      b. The emergency numbers for the patient's location should be noted as 911 may not always be effective in forwarding calls to a different location.
      c. Obtain emergency contact information for the patient's local healthcare provider and identify a local emergency contact or support person who can assist in times of crisis.
      d. Plans should be established for reconnecting with the patient in case of a disconnected call during an emergency.
      e. Determine the circumstances that would warrant putting the emergency plan into action or requiring a referral to in-person treatment or care.
      f. Appointments should not be missed, especially if there is a possibility of a crisis.
   16. Patients can be given a handout tip sheet on maximizing their telehealth benefits. See "Resources" section for additional resources.
B. Train staff to offer the option of televisits when patients call for appointments. Teach staff how to help patients with technology and to be available to answer questions and to help in maximizing their telehealth visit. Inform patients about technology requirements, assistance with setup, and the potential presence of others.
C. Support patients who do not have internet or phone services.
   1. Patients who lack access to internet service with not enough bandwidth for video may qualify for federal support through the Lifeline program (getinternet.gov).
   2. Many fast food restaurants have free WiFi that reaches the parking lot.
   3. Most public libraries provide access to high-speed internet (and often private rooms; Telehealth.HHS.gov, 2023).

DISPARITIES IN TELEHEALTH

A. Telepsychiatry offers many advantages, particularly in addressing obstacles to mental health services. Telepsychiatry removes geographic obstacles and enhances availability, particularly in areas with scarce resources.
B. By using various communication methods such as online translation services, writing tools, and chat features, telepsychiatry can provide more immediate help, leading to better patient results and making chronic homebound care and hospice care easier to manage.
C. Telepsychiatry is not just a trend, but a promising solution gaining global acceptance due to its cost and efficiency. It

empowers clinicians to reach more patients, fostering patient involvement and self-reliance while delivering high-quality care. Additionally, telepsychiatry helps bring specialized psychiatric services to areas that have limited resources, guaranteeing equal access to mental healthcare regardless of where a person is situated.

D. Nevertheless, it is important to recognize the difficulties that telepsychiatry encounters. Lack of thorough physical examinations can affect the precision of diagnoses and the health of individuals.

E. Technical issues, security concerns, and regulatory complexities pose significant hurdles that need to be overcome.

F. Devoid of the personal connection found in face-to-face sessions, telehealth may actually hinder the therapeutic bond, making it seem less personal.

G. While telepsychiatry shows the potential to decrease disparities in mental health by eliminating obstacles to treatment, ensuring fair and individualized access is still problematic. This is especially true for our most vulnerable populations. Minorities, immigrants, older adults, rural residents, and those encountering barriers due to social determinants of health, including mental illness, require out-of-the-box solutions in addressing issues like limited or absent broadband access and digital illiteracy.

H. A study in the field of telepsychiatry (Connolly et al., 2020) found that, although most patients and healthcare providers welcome telehealth, disparities in health outcomes and healthcare delivery persist across racial and ethnic minorities, individuals with lower incomes and socioeconomic status, older adults, and residents of rural areas (Haimi, 2023).

I. National Telecommunications and Information Administration (NTIA) data indicate that about one in five U.S. households are not connected to the internet at home (Cao & Goldberg, 2022). Those struggling to survive often do not see having technology at home as a priority. Many cannot afford the necessary devices or broadband. Ironically, those who need it most are unable to avail themselves.

J. Therefore, it is imperative for policy makers to prioritize the regulation and support of telepsychiatry programs. This includes enhancing digital infrastructure and providing training in telehealth methods. President Biden's Internet for All initiative was a step in the right direction, aiming to connect every American to affordable, reliable high-speed internet (Cao & Goldberg, 2022). However, funding has halted new applications. By prioritizing these obstacles, telehealth can bridge mental health gaps and improve outcomes for individuals with psychiatric disorders, ultimately advancing mental health equity across diverse populations.

K. Actions APRNs can take to improve accessibility include the following:
  1. Assist patients in finding technology devices and resources where there is free broadband.
    a. Local libraries, which may have private rooms that can be accessed for free or a small fee
    b. Community resources such as nonprofit organizations, religious, schools, or government programs
    c. Donated items from local businesses, Goodwill, or Salvation Army

L. The HHS recommends the following:
  1. Make materials accessible in various formats and languages, including images and simple words for patients with low literacy.
  2. Improve services by measuring patient satisfaction through postvisit surveys.
  3. Use inclusive intake forms that ask about technology access and patient preferences, such as language and pronouns.
  4. Ensure patients have assistive devices for virtual visits and train staff to broaden telehealth access.
  5. Incorporate accessibility options in telehealth programs, like screen readers and closed captioning.
  6. Allocate extra time in virtual appointments for patients needing support.
  7. Utilize technology with equity in mind and involve patients in health equity planning, including sitting on boards or committees and providing input on procedures.
  8. Seek team members with cultural competency and experience in underserved communities and other languages (Telehealth.HHS.gov, n.d.).

REIMBURSEMENT

A. Get to know the billing and reimbursement rules for telehealth services of different insurers, such as Medicare and Medicaid, private insurance, and so forth.

B. Develop clear billing practices for telehealth services and communicate these to patients.
  1. Inform patients that payment options such as PayPal, Zelle, Venmo, CashApp, and other commonly used payment apps, while convenient, are not secure and do not meet HIPAA requirements.
  2. Most EHRs now have integrated payment software specifically focused on ensuring HIPAA compliance. Platform vendors should demonstrate their ability to ensure HIPAA compliance by providing a BAA or HITRUST certificate. To protect data privacy, steer clear of any payment tool that refuses to sign a BAA.
  3. Verify the credit card processing service meets Payment Card Industry Data Security Standards (PCI DSS) standards and can securely manage transactions while protecting PHI. If you choose to use PayPal, make sure to use their services that are compliant with HIPAA regulations and sign a BAA.
  4. Do not use Venmo, Zelle, or Cash App as they are not appropriate for processing HIPAA-compliant payments.

MARKETING

A. Promoting the availability of telehealth to consumers educates them about the option to access care that can be convenient and privately done at home.

B. Use various channels to inform existing and potential patients about your telehealth services, benefits, and how to access them. APRNs can begin by:
  1. Updating website, maintaining an up-to-date clinical practice website with contact information, list of services, and short bios with a photo of the practice's providers
  2. Sending an email, mailing a flyer or letter to patients
  3. Sharing on social media, newspapers, radio
  4. Starting a podcast, YouTube shorts, or reels
  5. Placing brochures or flyers in multiple languages in the waiting room
  6. Giving talks at local community groups and religious organizations
  7. Bringing flyers and business cards to community events, such as health fairs and school or public library events

C. Implement a system for collecting feedback from patients and providers to continuously improve your telehealth services.
D. Online reviews serve as valuable tools for receiving patient feedback and leveraging them for marketing purposes.
E. One effective method to integrate reviews into your practice is by sending patients a link via text or email to review their visit.
F. Another method is to have online reviews directly on the clinical practice website. In today's digital era, potential patients frequently rely on online reviews before choosing services.
G. Additionally, it is important to regularly moderate the reviews to address any areas of concern.
H. Maintain an up-to-date clinical practice website with contact information, list of services, and a short bio with a photo of the mental healthcare providers.
I. Establish partnerships with the local community, such as hospital EDs, primary care providers, faith-based organizations, and schools.
J. Leverage marketing tools such as news outlets, social media platforms, multilingual brochures, and publicizing in community organizations about available telehealth services to address mental health issues.

ADVOCACY FOR TELEHEALTH MOVING FORWARD

A. The ATA is against unnecessary obstacles such as in-person mandates, geographic restrictions, and physical location requirements for telehealth, promoting fair access to virtual healthcare.
B. Telehealth providers may be working from home. Having to reveal their home address as the location of services provided, especially for mental health services, can create security vulnerabilities.
C. Enforcing legal limits on telehealth services ignores medical judgment and technological advancements. Over 95% of Medicare beneficiaries utilize telehealth services from familiar providers. Reports from the OIG indicate low levels of fraud in Medicare telehealth billing.
D. Research suggests telehealth reduces hospital admissions. Audits conducted in Montana and Illinois revealed that Medicaid telehealth reimbursement requirements were followed during the pandemic.

RESOURCES

A. Translating Research into Practice (PDF) from the Health Resources and Services Administration (HRSA)
B. Telehealth Implementation Playbook from the American Medical Association
C. The National Consortium of Telehealth Resource Centers, which provides consultation, resources, and news at no cost to help plan: www.telehealthresourcecenter.org
D. Tip sheet for patients on maximizing telehealth benefits
E. Lifeline program (getinternet.gov): a federal benefit to help individuals and families afford technology useful for telehealth; not currently accepting new applications
F. Telehealth 101: The Learning Series: www.cchpca.org/video-learning-series
G. American Telemedicine Association: offers telemedicine practice guidelines (registration is required) specific to the discipline; also present core standards, assessment, and outcome measurements
H. Center for Connected Health Policy (CCHP): a nonprofit federally designated National Telehealth Policy Resource Center; tracks and offers a policy finder compilation of telehealth-related laws and regulations at the federal level and across all U.S. jurisdictions; one can track telehealth regulations by jurisdiction or by topic
I. Telehealth HHS: almost any guidance on telehealth needed to safely implement telehealth can be found on this government: www.telehealth.HHS.gov/providers
J. Informational Tip Sheets: https://telehealth.hhs.gov/patients
K. State Medicaid & CHIP Telehealth Toolkit Policy Considerations for States Expanding Use of Telehealth: www.Medicaid.gov
L. Partner tools and toolkits (CMS): www.cms.gov/marketplace/in-person-assisters/outreach-education/partner-tools-toolkits

Cybersecurity
A. Top 10 Tips for Cybersecurity: www.healthit.gov
B. Cybersecurity 101: www.ama-assn.org
C. Cybersecurity Basics: www.ftc.gov

Online Course on Telehealth
A. Overview of Law and Ethics. Therapist Development Center: www.therapistdevelopmentcenter.com
B. Online Telehealth 101: The Learning Series: www.cchpca.org/policy-101

REFERENCES AND BIBLIOGRAPHY

American Medical Association. (2017). *Cybersecurity 101: What you need to know*. https://www.ama-assn.org/system/files/2020-06/ama-telehealth-quick-guide-appendix-d3-cybersecurity-101.pdf

American Medical Association. (2019). *1.2.12 ethical practice in telemedicine*. https://code-medical-ethics.ama-assn.org/sites/amacoedb/files/2022-08/1.2.12%20Ethical%20practice%20in%20telemedicine%20--%20background%20reports.pdf

American Nurses Association. (2022). *Psychiatric-mental health nursing: Scope and standards of practice* (3rd ed.).

American Psychiatric Association and American Telemedicine Association. (2022). *Resource document on best practices in synchronous videoconferencing-based telemental health*. https://www.psychiatry.org/getmedia/49f487ae-7b83-416a-8812-b2b25c717f6a/Resource-Document-Telemental-Health-Best-Practices.pdf

Basil, N. N., Ambe, S., Ekhator, C., & Fonkem, E. (2022). Health records database and inherent security concerns: A review of the literature. *Cureus, 14*(10), e30168. https://doi.org/10.7759/cureus.30168

Brown, T. (2018, November 4). *What is covered under HIPAA?* Compliance Home. https://www.compliancehome.com/covered-under-hipaa

Cao, M., & Goldberg, R. (2022, October 5). *Switched off: Why are one in five U.S. households not online?* National Telecommunications and Information Administration, U.S. Department of Commerce. https://www.ntia.gov/blog/2022/switched-why-are-one-five-us-households-not-online

Center for Connected Health Policy. (n.d.). *Professional boards standards*. https://www.cchpca.org/topic/professional-boards-standards/

Center for Connected Health Policy. (2023, September). *Welcome to the policy finder*. https://www.cchpca.org/all-telehealth-policies

Centers for Medicare & Medicaid Services. (n.d.-a). *Healthcare Common Procedure Coding System (HCPCS)*. U.S. Department of Health and Human Services. Updated October 2, 2024. https://www.cms.gov/medicare/coding-billing/healthcare-common-procedure-system

Centers for Medicare & Medicaid Services. (n.d.-b). *Telehealth*. U.S. Department of Health and Human Services. Updated September 10, 2024. Accessed September 11, 2024. https://www.cms.gov/medicare/coverage/telehealth

Chaet, D., Clearfield, R., Sabin, J. E., & Skimming, K. (2017). Ethical practice in telehealth and telemedicine. *Journal of General Internal Medicine, 32*(10), 1136–1140. https://doi.org/10.1007/s11606-017-4082-2

Connolly, S. L., Miller, C. J., Lindsay, J. A., & Bauer, M. S. (2020). A systematic review of providers' attitudes toward telemental health via videoconferencing. *Clinical Psychology: Science and Practice*, *27*(2). https://doi.org/10.1111/cpsp.12311

Drug Enforcement Administration. (2023). *Practitioner's manual: An informational outline of the Controlled Substances Act*. U.S. Department of Justice. https://www.deadiversion.usdoj.gov/GDP/(DEA-DC-071)(EO-DEA226)_Practitioner's_Manual_(final).pdf

Federal Trade Commission. (n.d.). *Cybersecurity for small business*. https://www.ftc.gov/business-guidance/small-businesses/cybersecurity

Garber, K., Chike-Harris, K., Vetter, M. J., Kobeissi, M., Heidesch, T., Arends, R., Teall, A. M., & Rutledge, C. (2023). Telehealth policy and the advanced practice nurse. *The Journal for Nurse Practitioners*, *19*(7), 104655. https://doi.org/10.1016/j.nurpra.2023.104655

Haimi, M. (2023). The tragic paradoxical effect of telemedicine on healthcare disparities—a time for redemption: A narrative review. *BMC Medical Informatics and Decision Making*, *23*(1), 95. https://doi.org/10.1186/s12911-023-02194-4

HealthIT.gov. (n.d.). *Top 10 tips for cybersecurity in health care*. https://www.healthit.gov/sites/default/files/Top_10_Tips_for_Cybersecurity.pdf

Hilty, D. M., Ferrer, D. C., Parish, M. B., Johnston, B., Callahan, E. J., & Yellowlees, P. M. (2013). The effectiveness of telemental health: A 2013 review. *Telemedicine and e-Health*, *19*(6), 444–454. https://doi.org/10.1089/tmj.2013.0075

HIPAA Journal. (2023, February 15). *What is considered PHI under HIPAA? 2023 update*. https://www.hipaajournal.com/considered-phi-hipaa/#:~:text=These%20include%20(but%20are%20not

Health Resources and Services Administration. (n.d.). *Translating research into practice*. https://telehealth.hhs.gov/documents/Translating+Research+into+Practice+Tip+Sheet.pdf

Health Resources and Services Administration. (2023, November 7). *Legal considerations*. https://telehealth.hhs.gov/providers/legal-considerations?utm_campaign=OATannouncements20230321&utm_medium=email&utm_source=govdelivery

Hurst, E. J. (2016). Evolutions in telemedicine: From smoke signals to mobile health solutions. *Journal of Hospital Librarianship*, *16*(2), 174–185. https://doi.org/10.1080/15323269.2016.1150750

Medicaid.gov. (n.d.). *Telehealth*. Centers for Medicare & Medicaid Services. Accessed September 11, 2024. https://www.medicaid.gov/medicaid/benefits/telehealth/index.html

Nagy, L. (2017, April 1). Telehealth: Changing healthcare for humans and animals. Distance Learning. https://www.thefreelibrary.com/Telehealth%3A+Changing+Healthcare+for+Humans+and+Animals.-a0517807614

National Institute of Mental Health. (2023, June). *NIMH» What is telemental health?* https://www.nimh.nih.gov/health/publications/what-is-telemental-health

Office for Civil Rights. (2009, January 7). *Business associates*. U.S. Department of Health and Human Services. https://www.hhs.gov/hipaa/for-professionals/privacy/guidance/business-associates/index.html

Office for Civil Rights. (2020, March 17). *Notification of enforcement discretion for telehealth*. U.S. Department of Health and Human Services. https://www.hhs.gov/hipaa/for-professionals/special-topics/emergency-preparedness/notification-enforcement-discretion-telehealth/index.html

Palmer, C. S., Brown Levey, S. M., Kostiuk, M., Zisner, A. R., Tolle, L. W., Richey, R. M., & Callan, S. (2022). Virtual care for behavioral health conditions. *Primary Care*, *49*(4), 641–657. https://doi.org/10.1016/j.pop.2022.04.008

Philipsen, N. C., & Haynes, D. (2007). The multi-state nursing licensure compact: Making nurses mobile. *The Journal for Nurse Practitioners*, *3*(1), 36–40. https://doi.org/10.1016/j.nurpra.2006.11.004

Rural Health Information Hub. (n.d.). *Marketing considerations for telehealth programs*. https://www.ruralhealthinfo.org/toolkits/telehealth/4/marketing

Russell, D. (Ed.). (2018). *Telemedicine risk management considerations* [White paper]. American Society for Health Care Risk Management. https://www.ashrm.org/sites/default/files/ashrm/TELEMEDICINE-WHITE-PAPER.pdf

Telehealth.HHS.gov. (n.d.). *Health equity in telehealth*. Health Resources and Services Administration. Updated August 20, 2024. Accessed October 8, 2024. https://telehealth.hhs.gov/providers/health-equity-in-telehealth

U.S. Department of Health and Human Services. (n.d.). *Announcing the availability of telehealth*. https://telehealth.hhs.gov/providers/preparing-patients-for-telehealth/announcing-the-availability-of-telehealth

U.S. Health Resources and Services Administration. (n.d.). *Telehealth policy changes after the COVID-19 public health emergency*. Telehealth.HHS.gov. Accessed September 11, 2024. https://telehealth.hhs.gov/providers/telehealth-policy/policy-changes-after-the-covid-19-public-health-emergency

U.S. Department of Health and Human Services. (2021, May 17). *HIPAA for professionals*. https://www.hhs.gov/hipaa/for-professionals/index.html

Zundel, K. M. (1996). Telemedicine: History, applications, and impact on librarianship. *Bulletin of the Medical Library Association*, *84*(1), 71–79. https://www.ncbi.nlm.nih.gov/pmc/articles/PMC226126

30 ADVOCACY, THE LAW, AND MENTAL ILLNESS

Denise Snow

INTRODUCTION

This chapter provides an overview of government-created rights and rules, the concepts of disability, how to obtain and maintain financial benefits for patients, competence versus capacity, and discrimination, as well as policies in place to protect populations. This chapter also by necessity discusses the various systems that patients experience and how the healthcare provider can assist their patients in navigating through these systems.

RIGHTS, RULES, AND REGULATIONS

A. Laws and regulations
 1. A basic understanding of how laws are made is necessary to discuss mental health law.
 2. Laws are the combination of legislation, judicial decisions, and administrative actions, and may be federally, state, or locally enacted.
  a. Administrative agency: An administrative agency is a department of the executive branch that has the authority to implement or administer legislation.
  b. Common law: Common law is the body of law derived from judicial decisions, rather than from statutes or constitutions. It may also be referred to as *case law*. The courts (a branch of government) create laws when a higher court such as the Supreme Court of the United States or a state's highest court makes a decision. That decision is called *stare decisis* and is the law of that jurisdiction.
  c. Institutional policies: These policies govern worksites and identify the institution's goals, operation, and treatment of employees.
  d. Ordinances: Ordinances are laws created by municipalities.
  e. Organizations: These are associations that set standards in a particular area. They may be recognized by the corresponding government body as an accrediting body, such as the not-for-profit organization The Joint Commission (TJC). Although it is not a government agency, they may enforce standards. In the case of TJC, accreditation by an institution is voluntary, but confers Medicare and Medicaid certification on a healthcare facility.
  f. Public health law: Public health law is a statute, ordinance, or code that prescribes sanitary standards and regulation for the purpose of promoting and preserving the community's health. It consists of legislation, regulations, and court decisions enacted by governments at the federal, state, and local levels to protect the public's health.
  g. Regulations: These are the rules or orders that have legal force and are issued by an administrative agency/regulatory body.
  h. Statutes: Statutes are any law passed by a legislative body.
B. Individual right to healthcare under the U.S. Constitution
 1. Nowhere in the U.S. Constitution does it state what "health" is.
 2. The World Health Organization (WHO) describes health as "a state of complete physical, mental, and social well-being and not merely the absence of disease or infirmity" (WHO, 2006, p. 1).
 3. "Health care" allows for the attainment of health, as in the "care, services, or supplies related to the health of an individual." (Yale University, n.d., "Health Care").
 4. There is no right of healthcare explicitly stated in the U.S. Constitution.
  a. Although the Supreme Court has found the right of privacy and bodily integrity, there is no right to access to healthcare, particularly for those who do not have the ability to pay for care.
  b. There may be a right to healthcare but only if the individual can pay for it.
  c. Over the last eight decades, at least two proposals for an amendment to the Constitution have been discussed to give individuals the right to adequate medical care by those who believe that health is a human right.
C. Public health under the U.S. Constitution
 1. While there is no individual right to health and healthcare under the U.S. Constitution, the framers did provide a means for the individual states to protect the public's health through their "police powers."
 2. While there is no exact definition for *police powers*, the term refers to broad governmental regulatory power. As noted in the 1954 U.S. Supreme Court case *Berman v. Parker*, the court stated, "Public safety, public health, morality, peace and quiet, law and order ... are some of the more conspicuous examples of the traditional application of the police power" (*Berman v. Parker*, 1954, p. 348).
 3. The Tenth Amendment states: "the powers not delegated to the United States by the Constitution, nor prohibited by it to the states, are reserved to the states respectively, or to the people" (U.S. Const. amend. X). Therefore, the states' power to regulate public health is broad and only limited by its own state constitution or by a power held exclusively by the federal government.
 4. There has been an increase in federal activity in the last few decades through federal agencies such as environmental standards, food and drug safety, tobacco advertising, and workplace safety, to name but a few.

PAYING FOR CARE: OVERVIEW OF HEALTHCARE COVERAGE

COMMERCIAL INSURANCE

A. Most Americans have commercial/private insurance through employment that covers the employee and their family members.
B. Particularly important is coverage for young adults who may need mental/behavioral healthcare.
C. Before the Affordable Care Act, many health plans and issuers could remove adult children from their parents' coverage due to their age, whether or not they were a student, or where they lived.
D. The Affordable Care Act requires plans and issuers that offer dependent child coverage to make the coverage available until the adult child reaches the age of 26. Many parents and their children who worried about losing health coverage after they graduated from college no longer have to worry.
E. The Affordable Care Act requires plans and issuers that offer dependent child coverage to make the coverage available until the child reaches the age of 26. Both married and unmarried children qualify for this coverage. This rule applies to all plans in the individual market and to all employer plans (Box 30.1).

Financial Issues and Access to Care

A. Commercial insurance issues for healthcare providers
  1. Balance billing
     a. Most patients with commercial insurance are enrolled in a health maintenance organization (HMO).
     b. Depending on the plan, the patient may be able to go out of network (OON) or may be prohibited from using a healthcare provider not in network with the plan.
     c. Patients often are not aware of an additional payment liability from their insurer and this has the potential to create an adversarial event between the healthcare provider and the patient.
     d. For example, a patient comes to the practice and is billed $100. The healthcare provider then bills the patient's HMO as an OON healthcare provider. How does the HMO decide to reimburse the healthcare provider for the services? Will they reimburse $100 (100% of what was billed)?
        i. Unlikely! HMOs reimburse at a rate that should be "reasonable and customary," which is determined by the HMO themselves.
        ii. These rates have been made artificially low by the HMOs themselves or condition the rate on the Medicare rate. Many states maintain databases that show the reasonable and customary rate.
        iii. What are the options to get paid? The practitioner could turn around and *balance-bill* the patient.
     e. *Balance billing* is the term used to describe what a healthcare provider charges over the reimbursement from the insurer.
        i. The problem with balance billing is that it pits the practitioner against the patient and creates an adversarial relationship, diminishing the trust in the patient–healthcare provider relationship. It also puts the practitioner in the unfavorable position of having to send patients to collections for unpaid bills. Alternatively, the practitioner could appeal the reimbursement rate by the HMO by showing the bill is reasonable and customary and their reimbursement is below the standard.
     f. The following are the two common reasons why healthcare providers sue patients:
        i. Kept check: The insurer sends the check to the patient directly but the patient does not give it to the healthcare provider.
        ii. Balance billing: The insurer has paid some of the healthcare provider's charges and tells the patient they are responsible for the rest. These cases often go to collections, and the worst-case scenario is that a judgment is obtained against the patient.
  2. Insurance denials
     a. Private insurance companies often deny treatment plans, diagnostics, and pharmaceuticals.
     b. Individual state departments of insurance set the standards for appealing insurance denials. In most states, any denial from the insurer based on "not medically necessary (medical necessity), experimental or investigational" can be appealed by either the healthcare provider or the patient through the internal appeal process in the insurer's policy plan, or if unsuccessful through the external appeal process. Patients can also appeal denials based on OON.
     c. To appeal the denial based on "not medically necessary," the healthcare provider must show why for this particular patient the proposed treatment plan is correct and that other treatment plans are not appropriate.
     d. To appeal a denial for investigational or experimental, the healthcare provider must show peer-reviewed support for the use and why traditional (frequently less expensive) treatment is not appropriate for this patient.
     e. Healthcare providers can conference with the insurance plan to appeal, and if this does not result in approval then the healthcare provider can submit an appeal to an independent external review board on behalf of the patient that can decide whether the denial was correct.

BOX 30.1 KEY TERMS IN COMMERCIAL INSURANCE

- *Managed care organization (MCO):* An MCO is a healthcare plan that provides a range of health services through a defined network of physicians and hospitals.
- *Health maintenance organization (HMO):* In an HMO, the patient is generally required to choose a primary care provider; referrals go through this healthcare provider. Most require the patient to remain in network.
- *Preferred provider organization (PPO):* A PPO is an insurance plan that lets the patient choose their healthcare provider/hospital.
- *Point-of-service plan (POS):* A POS is an insurance plan that combines the aspects of an HMO and PPO to keep costs lower.
- *Fee for service:* Patients pay out of pocket at the time of service.
- *Self-funded plan:* This is an insurance plan created by entities such as school districts or unions that provide insurance.
- *Copay:* Copay is a set dollar amount the patient must pay when they utilize a service or pharmaceutical.
- *Coinsurance:* This refers to a percentage of the cost of service.
- *Deductible:* This refers to the amount the enrollee of plan must pay each year out of pocket before the insurance the company will pay.

PUBLIC INSURANCE FOR MENTAL HEALTH IN THE UNITED STATES

A. Many patients seeking mental healthcare services will be enrolled in public insurance. Therefore, an overview of public insurance is helpful. Historically, in this country, people with mental health illness ended up in jails or in poor houses. Then in the 1840s, reformers such as Dorothea Dix pushed for more humane treatment of the mentally ill through publicly funded hospitals, which unfortunately resulted in merely warehousing this population.

1. The number of those in state mental hospitals rose until the 1950s when stories appeared about the nightmarish conditions in those hospitals and eventually resulted in social reformers deinstitutionalizing this population and providing community-based treatment.
2. In the 1960s, the U.S. Food and Drug Administration (FDA) approved Thorazine for control of psychosis. This led to the belief inpatient treatment was no longer necessary for medicated patients. The federal Mental Retardation Facilities and Community Health Centers Construction Act of 1963 gave federal money to the states to build community-based treatment centers for individuals with mental illness and developmental disabilities.
3. The unfortunate result of this Act was that many state legislatures used it to justify closing the state mental hospitals. Care centers were never adequately funded and never fully realized.
4. In 1999, the U.S. Supreme Court, in *Olmstead v. L.C.*, held that failing to care for people with mental illness in the least restrictive environment violated the Americans with Disabilities Act, which in turn required states to provide community-based care for those with disabilities.
5. In terms of deinstitutionalization, the number of those with mental illness living in psychiatric hospitals dropped from almost half a million to about 50,0000 by 2000. Treatment availability is limited for the millions of individuals with debilitating mental health illness, furthering instability that results in homelessness and incarceration.
6. Currently, more than 70% of people incarcerated in the United States have at least one diagnosed mental illness or substance use disorder or both, and up to 30% have a serious mental illness (National Judicial Task Force, 2022).

B. In 1965, the Medicare and Medicaid programs were enacted. Medicaid offers healthcare to many qualifying low-income individuals, including adults, children, pregnant women, seniors, and those with disabilities, with around 72.5 million Americans enrolled in the program. States and the federal government share the funding of Medicaid.

1. Federal legislation mandates that states include specific categories of people in Medicaid eligibility. Examples of mandatory groups include low-income families, pregnant women who meet the criteria, children, and individuals who are enrolled in Supplement Security Income (SSI) programs. States can opt for different coverage options and decide to include other groups like individuals getting home- and community-based services and foster care children who do not qualify otherwise (Center for Medicaid and Children's Health Insurance Program [CHIP] Services, n.d.).
    a. The Affordable Care Act allowed the states to extend eligibility to adults with income at or below 133% of the federal poverty level (FPL). Most but not all states chose to expand coverage to adults.
    b. Medicaid is based on income and on an individual's modified adjusted gross income (MAGI), and they must be either citizens or qualified noncitizens.
    c. Additionally, 36 states and the District of Columbia also established a "medically needy program" for individuals with significant health needs whose income is too high to otherwise qualify for Medicaid under other eligibility groups.
    d. Medically needy individuals can still become eligible by "spending down" the amount of income that is above a state's medically needy income standard. Individuals spend down by incurring expenses for medical and remedial care for which they do not have health insurance.
    e. Once an individual's incurred expenses exceed the difference between the individual's income and the state's medically needy income level (the "spenddown" amount), the person can be eligible for Medicaid.
2. The Medicaid program then pays the cost of services that exceeds the expenses the individual had to incur to become eligible. Healthcare providers can check with local legal aid or other advocacy programs to discuss the best way for Medicaid recipients to "spenddown" their overage income in their state. Healthcare providers need to sign up to be a Medicaid healthcare provider in their state. If they do not accept Medicaid as payment, they cannot treat the patient unless the patient agrees to be billed. Medicare is the federally run program for those 65 or older and those who have a permanent disability, such as end-stage renal disease (ESRD) or amyotrophic lateral sclerosis (ALS). Medicare covers approximately 62 million Americans. Doctors need to "opt out" of Medicare if they do not accept Medicare rates for patients. They must let patients know they have opted out of Medicare. They cannot bill for more than 15% over the Medicare rate (a limiting charge).
    a. Mental health providers will often have individuals in their care called "dual eligibles." The category of "dual eligibles" is becoming increasingly important. *Dual eligible* is the term given to individuals with a disability and need the most extensive and expensive care. They are eligible for Medicare when they are found to have a disability; there is a 24-month wait to enroll after being determined by the Social Security Agency that they have a disability. However, many individuals who receive Medicare also need to have Medicaid due to the high copays and the need for medications that Medicare does not cover.

ADVOCACY TIP

Consider suggesting to the patient with Medicare insurance they also enroll in Medicaid so they can save copay and other out-of-pocket costs of care.

DETERMINING DISABILITY

A. Many individuals with mental health illness cannot work and cannot earn income due to their disability. They may be eligible for government benefits to receive monthly income. In most instances, it is the federal government, through the Social Security Administration, that determines if someone has a permanent disability (expected to last or has lasted more than 12 months). This can be a financial lifeline for someone who cannot work.

1. Mental health disorders account for several of the top causes of disability in the United States. According to the 2022 National Survey on Drug Use and Health (Richesson et al., 2023), "among adults aged 18 or older in 2022, 23.1 percent (or 59.3 million people)" suffer from a diagnosable

mental disorder in a given year. Many people suffer from more than one mental disorder at a given time. In particular, depressive illnesses tend to co-occur with substance use and anxiety disorders.

B. There are two programs for individuals with disabilities and they are based on work history.

1. Individuals who have developed a disability but have contributed to Social Security through employment are eligible for benefits under Social Security Disability Insurance, or SSDI. This is commonly known as *SSD*. Once a determination is made that the individual has a permanent disability, they will receive a monthly benefit based on their work history. After 24 months, they will then receive Medicare as their primary insurance benefit.

2. Many of those whose primary disability is mental illness will have sporadic or no work history. For these individuals, monthly disability payments will be from the SSI. It is important to know which type of disability benefit the patient is receiving because the rules and insurance are very different for each. The SSI benefit amount is the same for everyone in the country no matter where they reside—$914/month for 2023. This is the amount calculated to meet the food and shelter needs of individuals with a disability. Importantly, along with the monthly benefit, SSI recipients will receive Medicaid. Therefore, any patient on SSI will also have Medicaid as their insurance.

C. As stated above, disability is determined on a permanent basis. For younger adults, choosing to apply for disability based on their mental status is an extremely difficult decision. The healthcare provider can assist the patient by exploring the potential risk or benefit of applying for disability.

> **ADVOCACY TIP**
>
> Medical documentation is critical to obtaining benefits—fill out forms in a timely manner. Remember that "having a permanent disability" means lasting 12 months or more. If you are not sure if the condition will last that long, be sure and indicate that is unknown until reevaluation.

CAPACITY, COMPETENCY, AND COMMUNICATION

A. *Competence* and *capacity* (short for "decision-making capacity"), terms that are often used interchangeably but are not the same

1. *Competence* is a legal term. Competence is presumed unless a court has determined that an individual is incompetent. A judicial declaration of incompetence may be global, or it may be limited (e.g., to financial matters, personal care, or medical decisions). Every adult is presumed to have capacity to make medical decisions unless there has been a prior court determination that the individual is incompetent, or a court-appointed guardian is authorized to decide about healthcare for the adult. *Decision-making capacity* is a clinical term that is task-specific. A physician may determine that a patient does not have the capacity to make a decision for or against surgery but may have the capacity to decide if they want pain meds.

2. *Capacity* to make medical decisions may be defined in a state's public health statute, but the general concept of capacity is the ability to (a) understand and appreciate the nature of the proposed healthcare, including the benefits of, and alternatives to, the proposed healthcare; and (b) reach an informed decision. The determination of capacity does not mean that the person is free from all mental impairments. If a patient is in a psychiatric unit, special laws may apply and may need court order for medical decisions if the patient is incapacitated.

B. The right to refuse treatment

1. The right to refuse treatment is a liberty interest protected by the due process clauses of the U.S. Constitution. The Patient Self-Determination Act (PSDA) is a federal law, and compliance is mandatory. The purpose of this Act is to ensure that a patient's right to self-determination in healthcare decisions is communicated and protected.

2. Through advance directives such as a medical healthcare proxy, the right to accept or reject medical or surgical treatment is available to adults while competent, so that in the event that such adults become incompetent to make decisions they would more easily continue to control decisions affecting their healthcare.

3. This concept "while competent" when applied to persons with serious mental illness becomes a significant challenge for the healthcare provider. Every adult with decisional capacity has the right to consent to or refuse medical treatment even if that decision will result in the patient's death. But how is this applied to individuals with mental illness that interferes with their judgment, self-interest, self-preservation, and safety?

4. All states have statutes regarding involuntary hospitalization, and most, but not all, have a corresponding law on mandatory outpatient treatment when a person is a danger to themselves or others, or likely to become so. Many statutes explicitly state that the "least restrictive" means should be applied, and court orders are necessary to treat patients against their will.

C. Communication

1. Mental health laws that are meant to be protective can be a barrier to effective treatment plans. For example, the Health Insurance Portability and Accountability Act of 1996 (HIPAA) protects patients' privacy. However, in doing so, it limits what a healthcare provider can learn from the family of the adult patient, such as important history, medical conditions, and past and recent behaviors, which could guide best treatment for the patient.

2. When patients refuse to allow the healthcare provider to communicate with their family, crucial information may be lost, with a cost to the patient and to others.

> **ADVOCACY TIP**
>
> Because capacity can change, consider obtaining a designated healthcare agent/proxy and a power of attorney to document when the patient demonstrates capacity. Both of these documents require a lesser degree of capacity than is needed to make a contract for a sale and they may help avoid guardianship proceeding.

GUARDIANSHIP/CONSERVATORSHIP

A. *Guardianship*, sometimes called *conservatorship*, means obtaining legal authority to make decisions for another person.

B. A guardian is the person appointed by the court to make decisions on behalf of the incapacitated person.

C. A guardianship may be needed over an adult if the adult is incapacitated, meaning the person is unable to take care of self due to mental illness.

D. A guardianship proceeding is held in court and presided over by a judge. The allegedly incapacitated person had the right to be present and to present their objections.

E. The healthcare provider may be called as a witness regarding the person's behavior.

F. If the judge determines the alleged incapacitated person is incompetent, the judge may issue and order for a guardian of the person to make medical decisions or a guardian of the person's property or frequently both.

G. For any order the judge may issue, it must be made in the least restrictive manner.

> **ADVOCACY TIP**
>
> Guardianship proceedings may be avoided if the individual has designated a healthcare agent to make medical decisions and/or a fiduciary agent under a power of attorney to make final decisions while the patient has capacity to do so.

CONCLUSION

Both federal and state laws have been enacted to protect those with mental illness. However, unlike other conditions, there exists a delicate balance of rights and concerns for safety, which may abridge those rights for those with mental illness. As a profession, all providers of mental healthcare have a mandate to advocate for the needs and appropriate treatment for those with mental illness. There is a national shortage of inpatient and outpatient treatment facilities. As a nation, we have increasingly criminalized mental illness. In the United States, people with mental illness are 10 times more likely to be incarcerated than they are to be hospitalized. It is a moral imperative for nurse practitioners to actively advocate for a more humane system of care.

REFERENCES AND BIBLIOGRAPHY

Berman v. Parker, 348 U.S. 26 (1954). https://supreme.justia.com/cases/federal/us/348/26

Centers for Medicare & Medicaid Services. (n.d.). *Eligibility policy*. U.S. Department of Health and Human Services. https://www.medicaid.gov/medicaid/eligibility-policy/index.html

National Judicial Task Force to Examine State Courts' Response to Mental Illness. (2023, January 1). *State courts leading change: Report and recommendations*. State Justice Institute. https://www.ncsc.org/__data/assets/pdf_file/0031/84469/MHTF_State_Courts_Leading_Change.pdf

Olmstead v. L.C., 527 U.S. 581; 119 S.Ct 2176. (1999). https://supreme.justia.com/cases/federal/us/527/581

Richesson, D., Magas, I., Brown, S., & Hoenig, J. M. (2023). *Key substance use and mental health indicators in the United States: Results from the 2022 National Survey on Drug Use and Health*. (HHS Publication No. PEP23-07-01-006, NSDUH Series H-58). Center for Behavioral Health Statistics and Quality, Substance Abuse and Mental Health Services Administration. https://www.samhsa.gov/data/sites/default/files/reports/rpt42731/2022-nsduh-nnr.pdf

Warth, P. (2022, December 5). Unjust punishment: The impact of incarceration on mental health. *New York State Bar Association Journal, 95*, 1. https://nysba.org/unjust-punishment-the-impact-of-incarceration-on-mental-health/

World Health Organization. (2006, October 6). *Constitution of the World Health Organization*. https://apps.who.int/gb/bd/pdf/bd47/en/constitution-en.pdf

Yale University. (n.d.). *HIPAA glossary + terms*. https://hipaa.yale.edu/policies-procedures-forms/hipaa-glossary-terms#:~:text=Health%20Care%20

V SPECIAL CONSIDERATIONS

31 INTERSECTION OF HEALTH COMORBIDITIES AND MENTAL HEALTH

Brenda Marshall, Kathleen T. McCoy, Melanie R. Baker, and Kirsten E. Pancione

INTRODUCTION

Comorbidity refers to the occurrence of two or more illnesses in the same person. The term *psychiatric comorbidity* refers to the occurrence of at least one psychiatric disorder that is coupled with a substance use disorder (SUD). Despite the high prevalence of medical diagnoses in patients with psychiatric lived experiences, recognition and management of comorbidities continues to present challenges for the clinician. Almost 75% of in-hospital patients with psychiatric disorders had one or more medical comorbidity (Goldman et al., 2020). Of importance to the APRN is that comorbidity predicts a poorer clinical outcome in patients with psychiatric disorders. When the clinician adheres only to an unstructured interview rather than a full systems assessment, comorbid illnesses (medical and concurrent psychiatric) may be missed, increasing the patient's risk for a slower recovery and higher negative clinical outcomes. This chapter examines the comorbidities, regardless of which came first—the psychiatric disorder or the medical diagnosis. It also identifies the adverse effects of psychotropic drugs on the different systems. In some cases, there are crossovers, where a disease like COVID-19—primarily a viral respiratory disease—also has neuropsychiatric manifestations. In almost all cases, the morbidity and mortality of patients are increased when coupled with even the most common psychiatric disorders like depression and anxiety. Clinical management and collaboration with the interdisciplinary team improves patient care and supports recovery. Assessment of premedical diagnosis in mental health is imperative in order to determine the best course of treatment to achieve maximum state of mental and physical recovery after diagnosis is confirmed. Any psychiatric comorbidity added to a medical diagnosis will have an impact on the patient's quality of life, as well as an increased caregiver burden and distress.

HEAD AND NECK DISORDERS

A. Tumors and cancer
  1. Head and neck cancer (HNC) treatments often include disfigurement and other life-changing alterations in areas like eating, breathing, and speaking. These added psychosocial stressors can place patients at high risk for psychiatric disorders.
  2. All patients diagnosed with HNC should be routinely screened for psychiatric-mental health disorders.
  3. The prevalence of mental health disorders increases after cancer diagnosis in patients with HNCs (Lee et al., 2019).
  4. A cohort study of approximately 53,000 patients identified a 9% increase in the prevalence of psychiatric disorders post-HNC diagnosis, from 20.6% to 29.9%.
  5. The prevalence of mental health disorders in patients with HNC is higher in females, as well as in those with a history of tobacco use and those with a history of alcohol abuse and dependence.
  6. One of the highest suicide rates in patients with cancer has been found in those diagnosed with HNC.
      a. A person who is diagnosed with tracheal cancer is twice as likely to develop mental health disorders than those who have oral cavity cancer (Lee et al., 2019).
          i. Quality of life issues increase the likelihood of mental health disorders.
          ii. Support for patients with HNC as well as their caregivers is important.
B. Neurologic disorders
  1. Epilepsy
      a. It is not uncommon for persons diagnosed with epilepsy to have their psychiatric disorders undiagnosed and subsequently untreated. Lack of treatment for depression in these patients is assessed at 70% (Goel et al., 2022).
      b. Patients with known seizure disorders are at considerable risk for mental health disorders and require screening for depression, anxiety, and other psychiatric disorders.
      c. Around 50% of patients with epilepsy also have a psychiatric disorder, where either can exacerbate the symptoms of the other (Kanner, 2016).
      d. Depression and anxiety often coexist with epilepsy, especially with those who also have migraine, stroke, traumatic brain injury (TBI), or dementia.
      e. In a person with epilepsy, mental health disorders impact quality of life more than the actual seizures.
      f. Common mental health comorbidities with epilepsy are depression (23%), anxiety disorders (20%), personality change, attention deficit hyperactivity disorder (ADHD), agoraphobia, social phobia, obsessive-compulsive disorder (more rare), psychosis (6%), and cognitive abnormalities (Goel et al., 2022).
  2. Migraine
      a. There is a bidirectional influence between migraine and major depression.
      b. Common comorbidities include depression, panic disorder, anxiety, epilepsy, stroke, and essential tremors.
      c. There is a strong and consistent association with panic disorder.
  3. Stroke
      a. There is a bidirectional relationship between stroke and depression, as each of these conditions impact the other.
      b. Common relevant comorbidities are depression, anxiety, psychosis, or dementia.

c. Poststroke depression can affect about 33% of all stroke survivors and may appear within 5 years of stroke event (Hoyer et al., 2019).
   d. Persons with preexisting affective disorders are at higher risk for stroke.
4. TBI
   a. Post-TBI, the most common psychiatric comorbidities are depression, anxiety, sleep disorders, and panic attacks.
   b. Other comorbidities in cases of TBI include chronic pain, new-onset stroke, posttraumatic seizures or epilepsy, and neuroendocrine dysfunction. Each of these also carries the possibility of a comorbid psychiatric disorder.
5. Parkinson disease
   a. Parkinson disease is the second most common neurodegenerative disease after Alzheimer disease.
   b. Depression is highly correlated with Parkinson disease with about half of the patients followed by anxiety.
   c. Apathy, cognitive disorders, impulse control disorders, psychosis, and anhedonia are also prevalent in Parkinson disease.
   d. Clinical presentation of psychosis is different from what is seen in schizophrenia. It is considered to have indicators for being able to stage and manage Parkinson disease and is often referred to as Parkinson disease psychosis (PDP).
   e. Tripathi et al. (2022) suggest that there be separate diagnosis for the patient with Parkinson who also has apathy, depression, and cognitive dysfunction.
6. Alzheimer disease
   a. Psychiatric and neuropsychiatric comorbidities are common in persons with Alzheimer disease.
   b. Apathy and depression are the most prevalent symptoms, with depression thought to be bidirectional, but anxiety, irritability, agitation, and delusions are also common.

RESPIRATORY DISORDERS

A. Types of respiratory diseases include the following:
   1. Obstructive: bronchial asthma, chronic obstructive pulmonary disease (COPD)
   2. Restrictive: interstitial lung diseases
   3. Infective: pneumonia, tuberculosis (TB), COVID-19
   4. Others: tumors and pleural cavity disorders

B. Lung disease is one of the chronic conditions in medicine that is highly correlated with psychiatric comorbidities. Psychiatric comorbidities in persons with respiratory disorders are seen as possibly modifiable risk factors for premature death.
C. Anxiety and depression in persons with respiratory disease, especially COPD, are both complex and bidirectional.
D. Anxiety, SUD, and depression are the most common psychiatric comorbidities with COPD.
E. Of persons with chronic respiratory diseases, 32% also have a comorbid psychiatric disorder (Sariaslan et al., 2022).
F. Persons with TB and long COVID deal with ongoing stresses that can make them more susceptible to depression and anxiety disorders.
G. Psychiatric comorbidities are associated with increased risk of death in long COVID (Hoertel et al., 2022).

CARDIOVASCULAR DISORDERS

A. Cardiovascular diseases, the leading cause of death around the globe, include any disorder of the heart and blood vessels, including coronary heart disease (CHD), cerebrovascular disease and cerebrovascular accident/stroke (CVD/CVA), rheumatic heart disease, heart arrhythmias, congestive heart failure (CHF), heart valve disease, pericardial disease, cardiomyopathy, and congenital heart disease.
B. CHD, along with mental illnesses, are the leading global causes of morbidity and mortality.
C. Mood disorders, anxiety disorders, posttraumatic stress disorder (PTSD), and stress disorders are commonly seen in patients with co-occurring cardiovascular disease. An increased prevalence of psychiatric disorders in patients with CHD has been identified. The etiology is multifactorial and often bidirectional (De Hert et al., 2018).
D. Developing a psychiatric disorder in a patient with CHD increases the risk of morbidity and mortality. Shen et al. (2022) identified that a sibling who has a diagnosis of a cardiovascular disease is twice as likely to develop a psychiatric disorder in the subsequent year than the sibling who does not have the diagnosis. This underscores the importance of assessing psychiatric symptoms in patients with heart disease.
   1. The risk of depression in patients with CHD is 20%, which increases with severity of CHD.
   2. There is a dose–response correlation between symptoms of depression and cardiac events.
   3. Anxiety (including stress disorders and panic disorder) is common in patients with CHD and is associated with an increase in adverse cardiac events.
   4. PTSD develops in a small number of persons with sudden cardiac events. The symptoms of PTSD appear to diminish over time; however, continuing symptoms of PTSD doubles the risk of another cardiac event or death within 3 years (De Hert et al., 2018).

GASTROINTESTINAL DISORDERS

A. There is a high psychiatric comorbidity in patients diagnosed with functional gastrointestinal disorders (FGIDs).
B. FGIDs arise without a clear pathogenesis but are believed to be due to the gut–brain communication. Of people with FGID, 60% also have comorbid psychiatric illnesses, with depression and anxiety the most common. Symptoms of FGID include the following:
   1. Abdominal pain and bloating
   2. Vomiting
   3. Dysphagia and dyspepsia
   4. Diarrhea and constipation
C. Common gastrointestinal (GI) diseases include the following:
   1. Irritable bowel syndrome (IBS)
   2. Crohn's disease
   3. Celiac disease
   4. Lactose intolerance
   5. Diverticulosis and diverticulitis
   6. Gastroesophageal reflux disease (GERD) and gastroesophageal reflux (GER)
   7. Exocrine pancreatic insufficiency (EPI)
D. The microbiome–gut–brain axis (GBA) is involved in the development of psychiatric comorbidities in GI disorders.

1. There is a bidirectional communication that occurs between the enteric nervous system and the brain.
    a. Influences maintenance of GI homeostasis
    b. Influences motivation and higher levels of cognitive function
2. Disruption between the GBA interactions can result in autism, anxiety, depression, and IBS (Carabotti et al., 2015).

E. The presence of psychiatric symptoms in patients with GI disorders impacts the illness and level of disability, worsening factors like nonadherence to therapy and lifestyle choices, which can result in deleterious outcomes.

F. Common psychiatric symptoms seen in patients with GI disease and FGIDs include the following:
1. It is estimated that persons with GI problems are 7% more likely to have depression and almost 9% more likely to have anxiety (Cantarero-Prieto & Moreno-Mencia, 2022).
2. The prevalence of anxiety and depression is significantly higher in patients with IBS and ulcerative colitis than in the general public without the diagnosis (Shah et al., 2014).

GENITOURINARY DISORDERS

A. Some genitourinary (GU) disorders may be congenital, while others develop later in the life cycle. Some affect all persons, while others affect only those who are assigned male at birth (AMAB) or affect only those assigned female at birth (AFAB).

B. Common GU disorders include the following:
1. AMAB disorders
    a. Benign prostatic hyperplasia (BPH), hydrocele, testicular torsion, and undescended testicle
    b. Prostatitis and erectile dysfunction
    c. Hypospadias (pediatric GU disorder)
    d. Hernia (inguinal and femoral)
    e. Cancers: prostate and testicular
2. AFAB disorders
    a. Vaginal yeast infections
    b. Ovarian cysts, uterine fibroids, and polycystic ovary syndrome (PCOS)
    c. Pelvic inflammatory disease (PID)
    d. Genitourinary syndrome of menopause (GSM)
    e. Cancers: cervical, ovarian, and endometrial
3. Disorders affecting all
    a. Chronic kidney disease (CKD)
    b. Hemolytic uremic syndrome (rare): affects the kidneys and blood clotting functions and can lead to kidney failure; usually a complication of diarrheal infections like *Escherichia coli*.
    c. Cancers: kidney and bladder
    d. Urinary tract infection and interstitial cystitis
    e. Kidney stones
    f. Sexually transmitted infections (STIs; human papillomavirus [HPV], chlamydia, gonorrhea, and HIV)

C. Psychiatric comorbidities in GU disorders include the following:
1. In all cases of GU disorders, imperative to take a thorough sexual and psychiatric history
    a. Adverse childhood experiences (ACEs) and childhood sexual abuse (CSA)
        i. ACEs and CSA can result in long-term GU problems, other physical health problems, as well as poor psychological well-being.
        ii. There is an association between CSA and vulvodynia, dyspareunia, and other dysfunctions and pain in the pelvic floor. The symptoms can take up to 12 years to be identified, but girls with CSA are more likely to have GU problems (Vezuba-Gagon et al., 2020).
2. Cancer diagnosis requiring hormone therapy (AMAB)
    a. AMAB patients with cancer (e.g., prostate, testicular) requiring hormone therapy in addition to the stressors related to fighting cancer may develop depression, anxiety fear, and a sense of guilt.
    b. Depression can impact treatment decisions as well as treatment adherence.
    c. Other GU diagnoses that cause chronic pain (e.g., orchialgia) can increase the incidence of depression and anxiety.
3. Cancer, surgery, and hormone therapy (AFAB)
    a. Cancer survivors often go undiagnosed for their comorbid psychiatric disorders. Of patients with gynecologic cancer, 30% have an increased risk of anxiety and/or depression in the first year postdiagnosis (Ho et al., 2021).
    b. Disfiguring surgeries as well as surgeries that require hormone replacement can result in insomnia and anxiety, but patients often do not seek to receive specialized care. There is a stigma to mental illness even for those who are battling cancer (Ho et al., 2021).
4. Transgender and gender-diverse patients with GU diagnosis
    a. Prejudice and social stigma may marginalize patients who are trans-/diverse-gendered, especially when there are GU problems to be addressed. Knowledge about this population is still limited due to lack of rigorous, longitudinal studies, despite the high prevalence of psychiatric illnesses (James et al., 2020).
    b. Adverse health outcomes include comorbid psychiatric illnesses (anxiety and mood disorders), substance misuse/abuse, nonsuicidal self-injury (NSSI), and suicide attempts.
    c. Increased risk factors for this diverse group include sexual, physical, or emotional abuse, as well as substance use and engagement in sex work.
    d. James et al. (2020) identified the most common psychiatric disorders as depression (>75%), anxiety (>60%), suicidal ideation (>40%), and NSSI (>30%).
5. Other GU diagnosis affecting all genders and comorbid psychiatric syndromes
    a. STI anxiety: The diagnosis of a sexually transmitted disease and the need to alert partners can initiate feelings of depression, shame, anxiety, and isolation. The stigma of an STI can heighten the feeling of shame and prevent the patient from seeking emotional help.
    b. Survivors of GU cancer experience PTSD.
    c. CKD that leads to end-stage renal dysfunction (ESRD) is associated with high levels of comorbid psychiatric disorders (MacRae et al., 2021).
        i. These include depression, anxiety, some neurotic stress-related and somatoform disorders, substance use, mood disorders, schizophrenia, and eating/feeding disorders.
        ii. Schizophrenia or bipolar disorder, depression, and learning disability have the strongest associations with CKD in MacRae et al.'s (2021) study.

iii. Comorbidities impact adherence to treatment, result in poor coping mechanisms, and reduce social support.

MUSCULOSKELETAL DISORDERS

A. Musculoskeletal disorders are injuries or diseases affecting the muscles, tendons, joints, nerves, cartilage, and spinal discs. Rheumatic diseases are included here as they cause severe joint pain.
B. The following are the types of musculoskeletal disorders:
  1. Sprains, strains, tears, tenosynovitis, bursitis, tendonitis
  2. Chronic pain: rheumatic diseases, arthritis, rheumatoid arthritis, psoriatic arthritis, spondylarthritis (a chronic autoimmune disease with articular and systemic features)
  3. Carpal tunnel syndrome
  4. Osteoporosis
  5. Scoliosis
  6. Systemic lupus erythematosus (SLE); musculoskeletal involvement with SLE including arthralgia, arthritis, osteonecrosis, and myopathies, as well as osteoporosis
  7. Dupuytren contracture: musculoskeletal and connective tissue disorder
  8. Tumors/cancer
C. Psychiatric comorbidities in musculoskeletal disorders include the following:
  1. Anxiety and depression are commonly seen in patients who have been diagnosed with sarcoma and other malignant soft tissue and bone cancers.
  2. Chimenti et al. (2021) identified the pathogenetic relationship that may exist between depression and inflammatory arthritis, citing the difficulty in diagnosing for many of the types of arthritis.
     a. Pathogenesis:
        i. Possible role that can be played by the proinflammatory cytokines in autoimmune disease may be responsible for the central nervous system (CNS) symptoms.
        ii. Inflammatory process that affects the hypothalamic–pituitary–adrenal (HPA) axis can have a lowered inhibitory feedback on the patient's corticotropin-releasing hormone (CRH) glucocorticoids.
  3. A bidirectional relationship exists between chronic pain and depression. Pain levels are often related to psychological distress due to the impact that pain has on social activities and social support systems (Ise et al., 2021).
  4. Depressive signs and symptoms reported by persons with inflammatory arthritis include fatigue, asthenia, poor sleep, chronic pain, impaired relationships, shame, guilt, and suicidal ideation.
  5. The impact of these disease entities on quality of life increases the likelihood of depression, anxiety, and suicidal ideation.

INTEGUMENTARY DISORDERS

A. Common diseases of the skin
  1. Acne, hidradenitis suppurativa (HS), psoriasis, rosacea: skin diseases that result in pimples, boils, and/or thickening of the skin
  2. Alopecia areata: hair loss secondary to impaired hair follicles
  3. Atopic dermatitis: itching, redness, crusting, and scaling of skin
  4. Pachyonychia congenita: thickening of the nails and painful foot calluses
  5. Epidermolysis bullosa, pemphigus: disorders resulting in blisters on the skin
  6. Scleroderma: tightening and hardening of the skin that can be harmful to blood and organs in the body
  7. Raynaud phenomenon: a condition where blood vessels do not deliver enough blood to hands and feet
  8. Vitiligo: loss of skin pigment
  9. Allergic reactions and viral symptoms (e.g., sunburn, diaper rash, contact dermatitis, hives, shingles)
  10. Cancer: basal cell carcinoma, squamous cell carcinoma, Merkel cell cancer, and melanoma
B. Associated psychiatric comorbidities with disorders of the skin, where psychiatric disorders are considered the most common comorbid condition in a person with a skin disorder (Shlyankevich et al., 2014)
  1. Background:
     a. Due to the high prevalence of mental health disorders related to dermatologic disorders, there is now a field of study focused on this area called *psychodermatology*.
     b. Skin, as the most visible organ, plays an important role in how a person gauges self-worth. Appearance is tied to both physical and mental well-being.
     c. There is a bidirectional impact between skin health and mental health.
     d. Carniciu et al. (2023) identified the underdiagnosis of secondary psychiatric disorders in people with skin disease. Up to 80% of patients diagnosed with a skin disease will have a secondary psychiatric comorbidity.
  2. Emotional distress accompanied by psychological/psychiatric symptoms:
     a. Depression, anxiety, and suicidal ideation due to ongoing stigmatization
     b. Social anxiety and generalized anxiety, which impact relationships and quality of life
     c. Frequent assessment necessary in children and young adults with skin diseases to identify emotional dysregulation of depression and anxiety due to the stigmatization that can occur
     d. Skin diseases, which can impact a developing identity formation in children and young adults
     e. Coping strategies, which can be impacted in patients experiencing chronic stigmatization due to skin diseases
     f. Self-esteem and body image issues
     g. Substance misuse
     h. Sleep disorders
     i. Impact on sexual health due to the negative influence of the skin disorder

SPECIAL CONSIDERATIONS

SOMATIC CONDITIONS COMMON TO GENETICS/BIRTH THROUGH YOUNG ADULTHOOD

A. Childhood/school age (Pan & Bolte, 2020)
  1. Seizure disorder
  2. Migraine
  3. Immunologic dysregulation
  4. Respiratory and skin disorders (e.g., asthma, allergic rhinitis, atopic eczema)

B. Adolescence/young adulthood (Jameson et al., 2016)
  1. Allergies and hay fever; females have higher rates of somatic conditions.
  2. Severe acne or other skin problems
  3. Headaches and migraines; females have higher rates of somatic conditions.

COMMON RELATED PSYCHIATRIC DISORDERS

A. Seizure disorder
  1. ADHD, depression, anxiety disorders
  2. Conduct disorder
  3. Oppositional defiant disorder
  4. Cognitive impairment

B. Migraine, headaches: bidirectional, stress and migraines, and psychiatric comorbidity as factors for chronic migraines (Radat, 2021)
  1. Major depressive disorder (MDD)
  2. Bipolar disorder
  3. All anxiety disorders

C. Skin problems, similar to general psychiatric disorders for adults
  1. Anxiety
  2. Depression with and without suicidality

D. Immunologic dysregulation with possible genetic disorders
  1. Autism spectrum disorder

E. Specific learning disorders associated with neurodevelopmental disorders (e.g., dyslexia, dyscalculia, speech/language disorders; Khodeir et al., 2020)
  1. ADHD
  2. Conduct disorder
  3. Anxiety
  4. Depression

RESEARCH: YOUTH DEPRESSION WITH SOMATIC DISEASES

A. Leone et al. (2020) conducted a longitudinal study in Sweden with a total of 1,487,964 participants looking across 69 somatic diseases.
  1. Females between 5 and 19 years of age had a first diagnosis of depression and males at 16.7 years.
  2. Age at end of follow-up was between 17 and 31.
  3. Youth depression is related to increased substance misuse, early cardiovascular disease, and premature death.
  4. The results of the study show the following:
      a. Those with youth depression are at higher risk for 66 somatic diseases and early death (Leone et al., 2020).
      b. There is an association between somatic illness and psychiatric illness:
        i. Self-harm (more for girls)
        ii. Sleep disorders
            (a) All-cause mortality, especially by intentional self-harm

INTERVENTIONS

A. All patients require a full and detailed history, including psychiatric history, as well as evaluation for any signs and symptoms of psychiatric disorders.

B. Use of the *Diagnostic and Statistical Manual of Mental Disorders*, Fifth Edition (*DSM-5*; American Psychiatric Association, 2013), Level 1 Cross-Cutting Measure is a facile method to identify general psychiatric symptoms that might be existing in a patient who has come in for a physical concern.

C. Refer to psychiatric specialists (psychiatric nurse practitioner, psychiatrist, social worker) who can work with the team to suggest interventions for the patient and the family/community/caregivers.

D. Everyday interventions for patients and caregivers include the following:
  1. Consider the caregiver's stress: Caregivers working with children and adults with chronic somatic illnesses are also at risk for signs and symptoms of depression, anxiety, and other psychiatric illnesses.
  2. Refer the family to social services for additional support.
  3. Provide activities that are easy to engage in. Suggest the following:
      a. Talk about how they are feeling to somebody (e.g., friend, family, partner, religious leader, someone they trust).
      b. Take care of their daily physical health. Self-care includes eating properly, resting, exercising, and being social.
      c. Find different ways to lower their daily stress level. Identify an online or in-person free program (e.g., yoga, meditation, or taking a leisurely walk).
      d. Find a support group specific to the somatic illness or the level of caregiving.
  4. Reduce the level of stigma attached to the psychiatric signs and symptoms that they might be experiencing. Remind the patient and the caregiver of the importance of seeking professional help.
      a. Therapy can improve quality of life.
      b. Therapy can help develop coping mechanisms.
      c. Professional help can implement pharmacologic interventions to alleviate some of the symptoms.
      d. Professionals can help connect the individual with more support to ease the stress of the physical/somatic disease experience.

REFERENCES AND BIBLIOGRAPHY

American Psychiatric Association. (2013). *Diagnostic and statistical manual of mental disorders* (5th ed.). https://doi.org/10.1176/appi.books.9780890425596

Basu, D., Basu, A., & Ghosh, A. (2018). Assessment of clinical co-morbidities. *Indian Journal of Psychiatry*, 60(Suppl. 4), S457–S465. https://doi.org/10.4103/psychiatry.IndianJPsychiatry_13_18

Cantarero-Prieto, D., & Moreno-Mencia, P. (2022). The effects of gastrointestinal disturbances on the onset of depression and anxiety. *PLoS ONE*, 17(1), e0262712. https://doi.org/10.1371/journal.pone.0262712

Carabotti, M., Scirocco, A., Maselli, M. A., & Severi, C. (2015). The gut-brain axis: Interactions between enteric microbiota, central and enteric nervous systems. *Annals of Gastroenterology*, 28(2), 203–209. PMID: 25830558.

Carniciu, S., Hafi, B., Gkini, M.-A., Tzellos, T., Jafferany, M., & Stamu-O'Brien, C. (2023). Secondary psychiatric disorders and the skin. *Dermatological Reviews*, 4(4), 162–171. https://doi.org/10.1002/der2.211

Chimenti, M. S., Fonti, G. L., Conigliaro, P., Triggianese, P., Bianciardi, E., Coviello, M., Lombardozzi, G., Tarantino, G., Niolu, C., Siracusano, A., & Perricone, R. (2021). The burden of depressive disorders in musculoskeletal diseases: Is there an association between mood and inflammation? *Annals of General Psychiatry*, 20(1), 1. https://doi.org/10.1186/s12991-020-00322-2

De Hert, M., Detraux, J., & Vancampfort, D. (2018). The intriguing relationship between coronary heart disease and mental disorders. *Dialogues in Clinical Neuroscience*, 20(1), 31–40. https://doi.org/10.31887/DCNS.2018.20.1/mdehert

Goel, P., Sing, G., Bansal, V., Sharma, S., Kumar, P., Chaudhry, R., Bansal, N., Chaudhary, A., Sharma, S., & Sander, J. W. (2022). Psychiatric comorbidities among people with epilepsy: A population-based assessment in disadvantaged communities. *Epilepsy & Behavior, 137*(Pt A). https://doi.org/10.1016/j.yebeh.2022.108965

Goldman, M. L., Mangurian, C., Corbeil, T., Wall, M. M., Tang, F., Haselden, M., Essock, S. M., Frimpong, E., Mascayano, F., Radigan, M., Schneider, M., Wang, R., Dixon, L. B., Olfson, M., & Smith, T. E. (2020). Medical comorbid diagnoses among adult psychiatric inpatients. *General Hospital Psychiatry, 66*, 16–23. https://doi.org/10.1016/j.genhosppsych.2020.06.010

Ho, D., Kim, S. Y., Kim, S. I., Kim, S. Y., & Lim, W. J. (2021). Insomnia, anxiety, and depression in patients first diagnosed with female cancer. *Psychiatry Investigation, 18*(8), 755–762. https://doi.org/10.30773/pi.2021.0090

Hoertel, N., Sánchez-Rico, M., Herrera-Morueco, J. J., de la Muela, P., Gulbins, E., Kornhuber, J., Carpinteiro, A., Becker, K. A., Cougoule, C., Limosin, F., on behalf of AP-HP/Université de Paris/INSERM COVID-19 Research Collaboration/AP-HP COVID CDR Initiative/"Entrepôt de Données de Santé" AP-HP Consortium. (2022). Comorbid medical conditions are a key factor to understand the relationship between psychiatric disorders and COVID-19-related mortality: Results from 49,089 COVID-19 inpatients. *Molecular Psychiatry, 27*, 1278–1280. https://doi.org/10.1038/s41380-021-01393-7

Hoyer, C., Schmidt, H., Kranaster, L., & Alonso, A. (2019). Impact of psychiatric comorbidity on the severity, short-term functional outcome, and psychiatric complications after acute stroke. *Neuropsychiatric Diseases and Treatment, 15*, 1823–1831. https://www.tandfonline.com/doi/epdf/10.2147/NDT.S206771?needAccess=true

Ise, M., Nakata, E., Katayama, Y., Hamada, M., Kunisada, T., Fujiwara, T., Nakahara, R., Takihira, S., Sato, K., Akezaki, Y., Senda, M., & Ozaki, T. (2021). Prevalence of psychological distress and its risk factors in patients with primary bone and soft tissue tumors. *Healthcare, 9*(5), 566. https://doi.org/10.3390/healthcare9050566

James, H. A., Chang, A. Y., Imhof, R. L., Sahoo, A., Montenegro, M. M., Imhof, N. R., Gonzalez, C. A., Lteif, A. N., Nippoldt, T. B., & Davidge-Pitts, C. J. (2020). A community-based study of demographics, medical and psychiatric conditions, and gender dysphoria/incongruence treatment in transgender/gender diverse individuals. *Biology of Sex Differences, 11*(1), Article 55. https://doi.org/10.1186/s13293-020-00332-5

Jameson, N. D., Sheppard, B. K., Lateef, T. M., Vande Voort, J. L., He, J.-P., & Merikangas, K. R. (2016). Medical comorbidity of attention-deficit/hyperactivity disorder in US adolescents. *Journal of Child Neurology, 31*(11), 1282–1289. https://doi.org/10.1177/0883073816653782

Kanner, A. (2016). Management of psychiatric and neurological comorbidities in epilepsy. *Nature Reviews Neurology, 12*(2), 106–116. https://doi.org/10.1038/nrneurol.2015.243

Khodeir, M., ElSady, S., & Mohammed, H. (2020). The prevalence of psychiatric comorbid disorders among children with specific learning disorders: A systematic review. *The Egyptian Journal of Otolaryngology, 36*, 1–10. https://doi.org/10.1186/s43163-020-00054-w

Lee, J. H., Ba, D., Liu, G., Leslie, D., Zacharia, B. E., & Goyal, N. (2019). Association of head and neck cancer with mental health disorders in a large insurance claims database. *JAMA Otolaryngology–Head & Neck Surgery, 145*(4), 339–344. https://doi.org/10.1001/jamaoto.2018.4512

Leone, M., Kuja-Halkola, R. Leval, A., D'Onofrio, B. M., Larsson, H., Lichtenstein, P., & Bergen, S. E. (2020). Association of youth depression with subsequent somatic diseases and premature death. *JAMA Psychiatry, 78*(3), 302–310. https://doi.org/10.1001/jamapsychiatry.2020.3786

MacRae, C., Mercer, S., Guthrie, B., & Henderson, D. (2021). Comorbidity in chronic kidney disease: A large cross-sectional study of prevalence in Scottish primary care. *British Journal of General Practice, 71*(704), e243–e249. https://bjgp.org/content/bjgp/71/704/e243.full.pdf

Pan, P., & Bolet, S. (2020). The association between ADHD and physical health: A co-twin control study. *Scientific Reports, 10*(1), 22388. https://doi.org/10.1038/s41598-020-78627-1

Radat, F. (2021). What is the link between migraine and psychiatric disorders? From epidemiology to therapeutics. *Revue Neurologique, 177*(7), 821–826. https://doi.org/10.1016/j.neurol.2021.07.007

Sariaslan, A., Sharpe, M., Larsson, H., Wolf, A., Lichtenstein, P., & Fazel, S. (2022). Psychiatric comorbidity and risk of premature mortality and suicide among those with chronic respiratory diseases, cardiovascular diseases, and diabetes in Sweden: A nationwide matched cohort study of over 1 million patients and their unaffected siblings. *PLoS Medicine, 19*(1). https://doi.org/10.1371/journal.pmed.1003864

Shah, E., Rezaie, A., Riddle, M., & Pimentel, M. (2014). Psychological disorders in gastrointestinal disease: Epiphenomenon, cause or consequence? *Annals of Gastroenterology, 27*(3), 224–230. PMID: 24974805

Shen, Q., Song, H., Aspelund, T., Yu, J., Lu, D., Jakobsdóttir, J., Bergstedt, J., Yi, L., Sullivan, P., Sjölander, A., Ye, W., Fall, K., Fang, F., & Valdimarsdóttir, U. (2022). Cardiovascular disease and subsequent risk of psychiatric disorders: A nationwide sibling-controlled study. *Elife, 11*, e80143. https://doi.org/10.7554/eLife.80143

Shlyankevich, J., Chen, A. J., Kim, G. E., & Kimball, A. B. (2014, December). Hidradenitis suppurativa is a systemic disease with substantial comorbidity burden: A chart-verified case-control analysis. *Journal of the American Academy of Dermatology, 71*(6), 1144–1150. https://doi.org/10.1016/j.jaad.2014.09.012

Tripathi, A., Gupta, P. K., & Bansal, T. (2022). Management of psychiatric disorders in patients with Parkinson's diseases. *Indian Journal of Psychiatry, 64*(Suppl. 2), S330–S343. https://doi.org/10.4103/indianjpsychiatry.indianjpsychiatry_29_22

Vezina-Gagon, P., Bergeron, S., Hébert, M., McDuff, P., Guérin, V., & Daigneault, I. (2020). Childhood sexual abuse, girls' genitourinary diseases and psychiatric comorbidity: A matched-cohort study. *Health Psychology, 40*(2), 104–112. http://dx.doi.org/10.1037/hea0000994

32 SYMPTOM SHARING BETWEEN MEDICAL AND PSYCHIATRIC DISORDERS

Lewis Marshall and Brenda Marshall

INTRODUCTION

Some of the most common symptoms that are classic signs of a psychiatric disorder as well as a metabolic or respiratory disorder are complaints of:

A. Difficulty concentrating
B. Disorientation
C. Confusion
D. Fatigue/exhaustion
E. Mood change
F. Depression—psychomotor retardation
G. Personality changes
H. Changes in sleep habits
I. Social withdrawal
J. Weight gain or loss
K. Visual disturbances
L. A sense of impending doom, or anxiety

When the patient presents with confounding symptoms, where the presenting signs masquerade as an alternative diagnosis, there is a requirement for the practitioner to rely heavily on the clinical assessment as well as symptom exploration. It requires the clinician to become an expert in the art of investigation and deductive analysis. Practitioners must engage in deliberate cognitive debiasing strategies, as too often it is a level of unconscious bias that leads to misdiagnosis. The easy answer is not always the correct one, and it might increase the likelihood that the practitioner could make assumptions reliant on common cognitive preconceptions. The difficulty in making assumptions when faced with these signs is that the practitioner might make a medical diagnosis when the actual problem requires a psychiatric intervention or vice versa. This chapter will examine some of these diagnoses that present confounding symptoms and methods to distinguish them in identifying the differential diagnosis.

As with any diagnostic process, a biopsychosocial approach alongside a complete and thorough intake interview will help avoid a missed or incorrect diagnosis. During the initial assessment, the practitioner will want to determine whether the patient's social and mental functioning prior to onset of symptoms was typical for the patient's life cycle or whether it was atypical. Understanding the family and patient history of both psychiatric and metabolic diseases assists the practitioner in narrowing the likelihood of identifying the wrong, or sometimes concurrent, medical and psychiatric diagnosis.

A practical tool to utilize that can reduce the likelihood of making a cognitive error in the diagnosis of a psychiatric disease rather than a medical one is to take a diagnostic time-out. This is a time to question whether what seems to present as a psychiatric illness might be something else. Utilization of a differential diagnosis checklist and a diagnostic time-out can reduce misdiagnosis that might delay the patient's ability to get potentially lifesaving treatment.

Areas of assessment for disturbances include:

A. Executive function
B. Language
C. Perception
D. Praxis
E. Thought
F. Mood and emotion
G. Behaviors
H. Personality changes

METABOLIC AND AUTOIMMUNE DISEASES

A. The category of metabolic diseases is applied when there is a disruption of the metabolic process, or the process of utilization of energy that the body receives from proteins, carbohydrates, and fats. These disorders affect the body's ability to breakdown and utilize amino acids, lipids, and carbohydrates, and impact the mitochondria, which produce energy for the body.
B. Autoimmune diseases are disorders where the immune system mistakes parts of the body as though they are foreign invaders. Some of the more common autoimmune diseases are lupus, rheumatoid arthritis, celiac disease, type 1 diabetes, and multiple sclerosis (MS).
   1. Specific areas of the body attacked by the immune system can include the blood vessels, the endocrine glands (i.e., thyroid or pancreas), connective tissues, skin, and joints.
   2. Common symptoms of autoimmune disorders that could be mistaken for psychiatric symptoms include fatigue, depression, malaise, and psychomotor retardation.
   3. In cases like MS—one of the most common disabling neurologic diseases that affect young adults and with symptoms that often appear between 20 and 30 years of age—a delay in treatment can have long-lasting consequences.
C. Reduction of these symptoms requires treatment of the specific autoimmune process. If, for example, a person with Hashimoto thyroiditis presents with fatigue, sadness, and psychomotor retardation, treatment with an antidepressant would not alleviate the symptoms; only treating the underactive thyroid would help. The following disorders are the more common metabolic and autoimmune disorders that will be seen in patients as they arrive at the ED, private practice office, and clinic. It does not include all the metabolic diseases; however, when the practitioner sees a change in mood, energy, thought processing, and movement, the age, patient history, patient's family history, and symptom presentation can provide clues to possible differential diagnosis that can be confirmed through testing.

DIAGNOSTIC TESTS FOR METABOLIC DISORDERS
A. Comprehensive metabolic panel (CMP)
B. Lactic acid test

SPECIFIC METABOLIC DISEASES AND THEIR SYMPTOMS

Acromegaly
A. Shares symptoms with depression and memory impairment
B. A rare condition of excess growth hormone (GH) secreting pituitary adenoma in adults; usually presents between the ages of 40 and 50 years; neuropsychological symptoms develop with elevating GH
C. Symptoms:
  1. Patients may begin to experience irritability, agitation, and anxiety prior to the development of physical changes.
  2. Other symptoms include increased size of the hands, feet, and head, with coarsening of facial features, as well as joint pain and headaches.
  3. Due to perceptions of body changes, acromegaly is associated with depression, apathy, mood instability, recent memory impairment, loss of self-esteem, and withdrawal.
D. History and physical examination: pertinent questions to ask if signs and symptoms of acromegaly are present:
  1. Have you noticed any changes in your glove, shoe, or hat size?
  2. Are you noticing any changes in skin, like thickening? Is it harder for people to draw blood for blood tests?
E. Diagnostic tests:
  1. Patients who begin to develop physical changes should have an MRI to look for pituitary adenoma.
  2. Blood tests include elevated serum insulin-like growth factor-1 (IGF-1) and glucose tolerance.
  3. Patients with untreated acromegaly can have neuropsychological symptoms. Short- and long-term memories are most severely impaired. Memory performance decreases as GH and IGF-1 increase. Cognitive testing to evaluate executive function should be performed.
F. Intervention:
  1. Surgery and radiation therapy treat pituitary adenomas.
  2. Medication includes somatostatin analogs and dopamine agonists that reduce GH release and can shrink tumors. GH receptor antagonists block GH from increasing IGF-1.
  3. Actions that improve executive function along with interdisciplinary intervention can improve quality of life.
G. Referral: endocrinologist

Acute Porphyrias
A. Shares symptoms with anxiety, depression, psychosis, and mania/hypomania
B. Genetic metabolic diseases presenting with episodic symptoms brought on by alcohol, medication, infections, menstruation, and fasting
  1. Two adult types: acute intermittent porphyria and porphyria variegate
  2. More common in females, seen after puberty and prior to the age of 60
  3. Prevalence higher in persons with psychiatric disorders
C. Symptoms:
  1. Symptoms can include abdominal pain, nausea, vomiting, constipation, paresthesias, seizures, and coma.
  2. Associated neuropsychological symptoms are episodic and may be confused with depression, bipolar disease, and psychosis.
  3. Behavioral changes, anxiety, depression, hypomania, delirium, or frank psychosis can develop at any point in the disease process, including muteness, catatonia, hypomania, and confusion.
D. History and physical examination: pertinent questions to ask if signs and symptoms of acute porphyrias are present:
  1. Have you experienced episodes of abdominal pain?
  2. Do you know if there are people in your family who have experienced episodes of abdominal pain, mental illness, or premature death?
E. Diagnostic tests:
  1. Blood, urine, and stool testing for porphyrin levels
  2. Genetic tests may be helpful
  3. Neuropsychological testing
F. Intervention:
  1. Treatment depends on the type of porphyria. Medication to reduce porphyrin production can be administered.
  2. Hospitalization may be required for acute episodes.
  3. Early identification and treatment of neuropsychological symptoms is important.
G. Referral: primary care provider and genetic counselor

Anti-N-Methyl-D-Aspartate Receptor Autoimmune Encephalitis
A. Shares symptoms with psychosis or anxiety disorder
B. An inflammation of brain tissues resulting from an immune response
  1. Anti-N-methyl-D-aspartate receptor (NMDAR) affects 1 out of 1.5 million people each year.
  2. It has insidious onset, so neuropsychiatric help might be the patient's first response; however, delay in diagnosis can result in decline in cognitive function, autonomic nervous system (ANS) dysfunction, and involuntary movements.
  3. Neuropsychiatric features are common presenting complaints.
C. Symptoms:
  1. It begins with viral symptoms, then progresses to neuropsychiatric symptoms within 3 months.
  2. Symptoms include rapid pressured speech, tangential language, delusions, insomnia, psychomotor agitation, and seizure-like activity (more common in children).
  3. Differential diagnoses include psychiatric disorder, various encephalitis, brain tumor, drug exposure, or withdrawal symptoms.
D. History and physical examination: pertinent question to ask if signs and symptoms of anti-NMDAR autoimmune encephalitis are present:
  1. Were you recently sick with a virus or viral infection?
E. Diagnostic tests:
  1. Brain MRI and EEG can be normal.
  2. Antibody testing is required in the serum or cerebrospinal fluid.
  3. CT, MRI of the abdomen, and transvaginal ultrasound should be considered due to the high incidence of ovarian teratoma.
F. Intervention:
  1. Early diagnosis is important. Immune suppressive medication, immunoglobulin infusions, and plasmapheresis are first-line treatments.

2. Tumor removal if identified is also first-line.
3. Seizure management can be challenging in these patients.
G. Referral: neurologist

Cushing Syndrome
A. Shares symptoms with depression, mania, and cognitive decline
B. Results from exposure to high levels of cortisol and similar glucocorticoid hormones
   1. Prevalence is about 13 per million each year.
   2. Females are five times more likely to have Cushing syndrome than males.
   3. Symptoms present usually between the ages of 25 and 40 years.
C. Symptoms:
   1. Physical symptoms of Cushing syndrome include weight gain, fatigue, rounding of the face, fat pad at the base of the neck, easy bruising, purple stretch marks on the abdomen primarily, excess facial hair in females, and decreased fertility in males.
   2. Patients with active Cushing syndrome can have impairment in attention, executive function, language, visuospatial processing, intelligence, and memory.
   3. Major depression, mania, anxiety, and cognitive impairment are common.
   4. Patients may have a lower quality of life, and problems with family, social, and work life.
D. History and physical examination: pertinent questions to ask if signs and symptoms of Cushing syndrome are present:
   1. Have you been taking any steroids or corticosteroids recently?
   2. Have you stopped taking steroids or corticosteroids recently?
   3. Have you noticed any changes in your body over the past few years?
E. Diagnostic tests:
   1. There is no specific test for Cushing syndrome. There are two different tests to help diagnose Cushing syndrome: the corticotropin-releasing hormone (CRH) test and the dexamethasone-suppressed corticotropin-releasing hormone (Dex-CRH) test. The Dex-CRH test is a combination of a low-dose dexamethasone suppression test and a CRH stimulation test. The Dex-CRH test differentiates between Cushing syndrome and pseudo-Cushing syndrome.
   2. Testing can be done after treatment to determine severity and any changes in mood and cognitive function.
F. Intervention:
   1. Normalize cortisol levels.
   2. Identify and treat comorbidities, including cardiovascular disease, cognitive and mood disorders, and osteoporosis.
   3. Continued psychiatric treatment may be needed.
G. Referral: endocrinologist

Diabetes Mellitus
A. Shares symptoms with depression and anxiety
B. A group of diseases that affect blood glucose levels
   1. Diabetes Mellitus affects 11.6% of the U.S. population over 18 years of age (38.4 million people).
   2. Diabetes Mellitus affects people of all ages.
   3. Nearly nine million Americans are believed to have undiagnosed diabetes (Centers for Disease Control and Prevention [CDC], 2022).
C. Symptoms:
   1. Symptoms develop slowly as the blood sugar increases.
   2. Early symptoms include increased thirst and urination, blurred vision, and fatigue.
   3. Later symptoms include dry mouth, abdominal pain, shortness of breath, confusion, and loss of consciousness.
   4. Mental health can affect management of diabetes, and diabetes can exacerbate mental health issues. Patients with diabetes are more likely to have depression and exhibit sadness, loss of interest, eating disorders, hopelessness, irritability, and anxiety.
D. History and physical examination: Pertinent questions to ask if signs and symptoms of diabetes mellitus are present:
   1. Have you ever been told you have high blood sugar, or "sugar in your blood"?
   2. Are you thirsty all the time?
   3. Does anyone in your family have high blood sugar or diabetes?
E. Diagnostic tests:
   1. The most common testing includes blood glucose level, ketones, blood pH, and kidney function.
F. Intervention:
   1. Management of blood glucose with diet and medication
   2. Behavioral health management for depression and other mental health symptoms
G. Referral: endocrinologist

Hypothyroidism
A. Shares symptoms with depression, dysphoria, and dementia
B. Characterized by an underactive thyroid with low T4 levels and high thyroid-stimulating hormone (TSH)
   1. Almost 5% of the U.S. population older than 12 years have an underactive thyroid.
   2. It is more common in females than males.
   3. Other conditions that increase the likelihood of hypothyroidism include celiac disease, diabetes, rheumatoid arthritis, Sjögren syndrome, or lupus.
C. Symptoms:
   1. Medical symptoms include fatigue, cold sensitivity, constipation, weight gain, slow heart rate, and irregular menses.
   2. Neuropsychiatric symptoms include cognitive decline, memory loss, dementia, dysphoria, depression, and possibly coma.
D. Diagnostic tests:
   1. Thyroid studies include T3, T4, and TSH.
   2. Elevated TSH and low T4 are common.
   3. Thyroid ultrasound can be helpful.
E. Intervention:
   1. Replacement of thyroid hormone.
F. Referral: endocrinologist

Hyperthyroidism
A. Shares symptoms with mania, depression, and psychosis.
B. Characterized by an overactive thyroid; Graves disease an autoimmune disorder affecting the thyroid and making it hyperactive
   1. Basedow and myxedema psychosis are associated with thyroid disease.

2. Hyperthyroidism can lead to thyrotoxicosis.
3. Hyperthyroidism is prevalent in 1.2% of the U.S. population.
C. Symptoms:
1. Medical symptoms include weight loss, tachycardia, hunger, anxiety, tremors, sweating, sensitivity to heat, sleep disturbance, and thinning brittle hair.
2. Neuropsychiatric symptoms include depression, agitation, acute psychosis, and apathy in older patients.
D. History and physical examination: pertinent questions to ask if signs and symptoms of hyperthyroidism are present:
1. Have you ever been told you have an overactive thyroid?
2. Have you had problems with or been treated for anxiety in the past?
E. Diagnostic tests:
1. Thyroid studies include T3, T4, and TSH.
2. Elevated T4 and low TSH are common.
3. Thyroid ultrasound can be helpful.
F. Intervention:
1. Antithyroid medications such as methimazole and propylthiouracil can be administered.
2. Beta blockers, radioiodine, and thyroidectomy are also used as treatments.
3. Treatment can help reduce neuropsychiatric symptoms.
G. Referral: endocrinologist

HEREDITARY METABOLIC DISEASES (RARE)
A. See Table 32.1 for a summary of symptom sharing across hereditary metabolic diseases and psychiatric conditions.

TABLE 32.1 HEREDITARY METABOLIC DISEASES AND ASSOCIATED PSYCHIATRIC SYMPTOMS

Hereditary Metabolic Disease Diagnosis	Psychiatric Diagnosis	Occurrence	Psychiatric Symptoms	Associated Symptoms
Remethylation disorders	Schizophrenia	Triggering factor (stress)	Delusions, hallucinations	Consciousness disorders, peripheral disease, rapid cognitive decline
Cerebrotendinous xanthomatosis	Schizophrenia	Chronic	Delusions, hallucinations	Dementia, psychiatric disturbances, seizures, progressive neurologic dysfunction
Metachromatic leukodystrophy	Schizophrenia	Chronic late onset	Behavioral disturbances, hallucinations	Loss of motor skills, decreased mental function, memory loss, seizures, loss of bladder and bowel function
GM2 gangliosidosis (Tay–Sachs disease)	Schizophrenia	Chronic late onset	Hallucinations, delusions, depression, cognitive decline	Peripheral symptoms, ataxia
X-linked adrenoleukodystrophy Niemann–Pick type C	Atypical psychosis	Variable	Depression, delusions, behavioral disorders, confusion	Spastic paraplegia, ataxia, abnormal movements, supranuclear gaze palsy
Acute intermittent porphyria	Inebriation, personality disorder, Guillain–Barré disease, bipolar or schizoaffective disorder	Triggering factor (alcohol, smoking, hormonal and dietary changes, fasting, and stress) may be progressive	Behavioral disturbances, impulsivity, depression, mania	Intermittent pain, ataxia, abnormal movements, supranuclear gaze palsy
Wilson disease	Bipolar disorder	Chronic	Depression, behavioral disturbances, impulsivity	Extrapyramidal symptoms, dysarthria, akinesia
Urea cycle disorders	Bipolar disorder		Confusion, behavioral disturbances, hallucinations	Headache, abdominal pain, change in diet
Homocystinuria	Personality disorders	Chronic	Obsessive-compulsive disorder, behavioral disturbances, impulsivity, disinhibition	Ectopia lentis, marfanoid appearance, mental deficiency, thrombosis
Creatinine deficiency syndrome	Personality disorder	Chronic	Behavioral disturbances, aggressiveness	Mental deficiency, language delay, epilepsy, extrapyramidal symptoms

Source: Adapted from Demily, C., & Sedel, F. (2014). Psychiatric manifestations of treatable hereditary metabolic disorders in adults. *Annals of General Psychiatry, 13,* Article 27. https://doi.org/10.1186/s12991-014-0027-x. Retrieved from https://www.ncbi.nlm.nih.gov/pmc/articles/PMC4255667/table/T1/?report=objectonly.

SPECIFIC AUTOIMMUNE DISORDERS

Hashimoto Thyroiditis

A. Shares symptoms with depression, dysphoria, and dementia.
B. Characterized by an underactive thyroid with low T4 levels and high TSH.
    1. The prevalence is 1% to 2% of the U.S. population.
    2. It is more common in females, possibly due to hormonal factors.
C. Symptoms:
    1. Medical symptoms include fatigue, cold sensitivity, constipation, weight gain, slow heart rate, and irregular menses.
    2. Neuropsychiatric symptoms include cognitive decline, memory loss, dementia, dysphoria, depression, and possibly coma.
D. Diagnostic tests:
    1. Thyroid studies include T3, T4, and TSH.
    2. Elevated TSH and low T4 are common.
    3. Thyroid ultrasound can be helpful.
E. Intervention:
    1. Replacement of thyroid hormone
F. Referral: endocrinologist

Type 1 Diabetes

A. Shares symptoms with depression and anxiety
B. A chronic condition characterized by little or no insulin production
    1. Type 1 diabetes accounts for 5% to 10% of all cases of diabetes diagnosed in the United States.
    2. It can occur at any age, but peaks in children 4 to 7 years old and in children 10 to 14 years old.
    3. Persons diagnosed with type 1 diabetes are not overweight; on the contrary, they are usually underweight or of normal weight.
    4. It is not uncommon for the newly diagnosed patient to lose weight before diagnosis.
C. Symptoms:
    1. Medical symptoms include sweating, anxiety, tremor, tachycardia, and confusion, which can be seen with hyper- and hypoglycemic episodes.
    2. Symptoms develop slowly as the blood sugar increases. Early symptoms include increased thirst and urination, blurred vision, and fatigue. Later symptoms include dry mouth, abdominal pain, shortness of breath, confusion, and loss of consciousness.
    3. Hypoglycemia occurs after insulin injection: sweating, shaking, headache, tachycardia, anxiety, tingling, fatigue, and irritability.
    4. It can be bidirectional with glucose changes and anxiety.
    5. Anxiety disorder is higher in the population of patients with type 1 diabetes. Management of the associated anxiety in these patients' response to selective serotonin reuptake inhibitors (SSRIs) and treatment of the anxiety can reduce the patient missing the psychological signs and symptoms of an event of hypoglycemia.
D. Diagnostic tests:
    1. The most common tests include blood glucose level, ketones, blood pH, and kidney function.
E. Intervention:
    1. Management of blood glucose with diet and medication
    2. Behavioral health management for depression and other mental health symptoms
F. Referral: endocrinologist and nutritionist

Atypical Stroke–Stroke Chameleons

A. Shares symptoms with psychosis and delirium
B. Strokes that have symptoms that are not like ischemic strokes and therefore are at risk for misdiagnosis
    1. Patients are likely to present with dizziness, confusion, altered mental status, nausea/vomiting, and an abrupt change in level of consciousness.
    2. The incidence can be as high as 30%.
    3. It is associated with 50% of acute ischemic neurologic events in children with sickle cell disease.
    4. Persons with comorbid psychiatric disease are 20% less likely to get acute thrombolysis treatment for presenting strokes than those without a psychiatric diagnosis.
C. Symptoms:
    1. Medical symptoms include altered mental status, ataxia, dizziness, and visual hallucinations (Charles Bonnet syndrome) such as well-formed animals, grid patterns, and shrubbery. Gerstmann syndrome presents with agraphia, acalculia, finger agnosia, and right-left confusion. Symptoms also include wrist drop, foot drop, and alien limb syndrome.
    2. Psychiatric symptoms include hyperkinetic movement disorders, alien limb, and Anton syndrome, which presents as denial of blindness with confabulation of vision. These patients lack insight.
D. Diagnostic tests:
    1. History, physical exam, neurologic exam including fundoscopy, and psychiatric exam; CT scan or MRI of the brain
    2. Mental status exam, motor exam, language exam with naming
E. Intervention:
    1. Activate the stroke team.
F. Referral: neurologist, autoimmune specialist, and vascular specialist

REFERENCES AND BIBLIOGRAPHY

Centers for Disease Control and Prevention. (n.d.). *Diabetes and mental health*. U.S. Department of Health and Human Services. https://www.cdc.gov/diabetes/living-with/mental-health.html

Centers for Disease Control and Prevention. (2024, May 15). *National Diabetes Statistics Report*. U.S. Department of Health and Human Services. https://www.cdc.gov/diabetes/php/data-research

Demily, C., & Sedel, F. (2014). Psychiatric manifestations of treatable hereditary metabolic disorders in adults. *Annals of General Psychiatry, 13*, 27. https://doi.org/10.1186/s12991-014-0027-x

Leon-Carrion, J., Martin-Rodriguez, J. F., Madrazo-Atutxa, A., Soto-Moreno, A., Venegas-Moreno, E., Torres-Vela, E., Benito-Lopez, P., Gálvez, M. A., Tinahones, F. J., & Leal-Cerro, A. (2010). Evidence of cognitive and neurophysiological impairment in patients with untreated naive acromegaly. *The Journal of Clinical Endocrinology & Metabolism, 95*(9), 4367–4379. https://doi.org/10.1210/jc.2010-0394

Lin, T. Y., Hanna, J., & Ishak, W. W. (2020). Psychiatric symptoms in cushing's syndrome: A systematic review. *Innovations in Clinical Neuroscience, 17*(1–3), 30–35. PMID: 32547845.

Mayo Clinic. (n.d.). *Hypothryroidism (underactive thyroid): Symptoms and causes*. https://www.mayoclinic.org/diseases-conditions/hypothyroidism/symptoms-causes/syc-20350284

National Institute of Diabetes and Digestive and Kidney Diseases. (n.d.). *Cushing's syndrome*. https://www.niddk.nih.gov/health-information/endocrine-diseases/cushings-syndrome#diagnose

Pivonello, R., Simeoli, C., De Martino, M. C., Cozzolino, A., De Leo, M., Iacuaniello, D., Pivonello, C., Negri, M., Pellecchia, M. T., Iasevoli, F., & Colao, A. (2015). Neuropsychiatric disorders in cushing's syndrome. *Frontiers in Neuroscience, 9*, 129. https://doi.org/10.3389/fnins.2015.00129

Roberts, C., McEachern, M., & Mounsey, A. (2020). CSF studies which ultimately led to the possible diagnosis of anti-NMDAR encephalitis. *BMJ Case Reports, 13*(5), e233489. https://doi.org/10.1136/bcr-2019-233489. https://www.ncbi.nlm.nih.gov/pmc/articles/PMC7228146

Samanta, D., & Lui, F. (2023, July 17). *Anti-NMDAR encephalitis*. StatPearls Publishing. https://www.ncbi.nlm.nih.gov/books/NBK551672

Sharma, S. T., Nieman, L. K., & Feelders, R. A. (2015). Comorbidities in cushing's disease. *Pituitary*, 18(2), 188–94. https://doi.org/10.1007/s11102-015-0645-6

Solomon, E., Brănişteanu, D., Dumbravă, A., Solomon, R. G., Kiss, L., Glod, M., & Preda, C. (2019). Executive functioning and quality of life in acromegaly. *Psychology Research and Behavior Management*, 12, 39–44. https://doi.org/10.2147/PRBM.S183950 https://www.niddk.nih.gov/health-information/endocrine-diseases/acromegaly#treat

Xu, L., & Chen, Z. (2021). Anti-NMDA receptor encephalitis misdiagnosed as generalized anxiety disorder: A case report. *Cureus*, 13(12), e20529. https://doi.org/10.7759/cureus.20529

NEUROLOGIC DISORDERS

A. The general category of neurologic disorders encompasses any disorders that affect both the brain and the nerves anywhere within and throughout the body, including the spinal cord. The World Health Organization (WHO) identifies the central and peripheral nervous systems as including the brain and spinal cord, as well as the neuromuscular junction, muscles, and ANS, in addition to the peripheral nerves, nerve roots, and cranial nerves.

B. Changes in the neurologic system can be through genetics; cancers; trauma; invasion of a bacteria, parasite, or virus; or as a result of the response of the immune system.

C. Some of the neurologic disorders that can share symptoms with psychiatric disorders include dementia, delirium, Alzheimer disease, epilepsy, mycobacterial tuberculosis, *Neisseria meningitidis*, HIV, migraine and headache disorders, myasthenia gravis (MG), and Parkinson disease.

D. The field of neuropsychiatry examines these disorders that live at the intersection of neurology and psychiatry.
  1. The resulting effects are often the behavioral symptoms that stem from the onset of physical brain deterioration or dysfunction.
  2. Infusion of psychiatric symptoms, especially during the onset of the neurologic disease process, can confuse the presentation and delay the true diagnosis.

E. As with metabolic diseases, neurologic disorders and psychiatric disorders are not mutually exclusive and can be present simultaneously in the same patient.
  1. Especially with neurologic conditions, brain insult resulting in neurologic symptoms, like seizures in a person with epilepsy, also affects the same parts of the brain regulating mood, perception, and cognition.
  2. Awareness of the disturbances these disorders can produce in affect, cognition, perception, and general behavior makes the treatment of the patient as a whole person imperative.
  3. Some neurologic disorders are also autoimmune disorders. Two examples are MG and MS, which are categorized as chronic, autoimmune, neuromuscular disorders.

F. Presented in this section are disorders that might be seen in the ED, practitioner's office, or clinic. Included in this section is one nonneurologic diagnosis, psychogenic nonepileptic seizures (PNES), as its presentation can be mistaken for a neurologic condition and lead to a misdiagnosis.

SPECIFIC NEUROLOGIC DISORDERS

Delirium/Dementia

A. Shares symptoms with depression, mania, and psychosis

B. Delirium: an acute change in mental status or behavior and can be associated with fever, intoxication, or other conditions; dementia: can be expressed as progressive loss of cognition, memory, and abstract thinking, and personality changes

C. Symptoms:
  1. Symptoms of delirium include confusion, disorientation, agitation, and hallucinations.
  2. Cognitive changes related to dementia include memory loss, word-finding difficulty, visual and spatial problems, and problems with complex tasks.

D. Diagnostic tests:
  1. There are no specific tests to diagnose delirium. Most tests are done to eliminate other causes such as electrolyte imbalance, blood sugar level, and presence of an infectious process.
  2. Conducting a complete history and physical exam is important. Interview significant others. Cognitive and neuropsychological testing of memory, orientation, reasoning, and judgment is also important, as well as of visual perception. CT or MRI of the brain may help rule out some causes such as stroke, bleeding, or mass. Blood tests, which can include thyroid studies, diabetes check, vitamin B_{12}, and inflammatory markers, might be useful.

E. Intervention:
  1. There is no specific treatment for delirium. Treatment of the underlying cause will clear up the delirium.
  2. Some medications are available to slow the progression of dementia, including cholinesterase inhibitors and memantine.

Multiple Sclerosis

A. Shares symptoms with depression, bipolar disorders, pseudobulbar affect, and anxiety

B. A disease of the brain and spinal cord where the immune system attacks the nerve sheath covering, resulting in poor nerve conduction; also an autoimmune disease
  1. Worldwide, over 1.8 million people have MS.
  2. It is most common in young adults and females, although a person can be affected at any age.
  3. The risk of developing MS in the United States is 3.5 per 1,000 (<0.5%).
  4. The risk of developing MS increases when a first-degree relative has the disease.

C. Symptoms:
  1. Symptoms include unilateral numbness or weakness, problems with walking, double vision, dizziness, slurred speech, and cognitive and mood disorders. Memory and attention can also be affected.
  2. Patients have major depression, dysphoria, agitation, anxiety, and suicidal ideations. Symptoms also include disorders of sleep and eating, bipolar disorder, mania, and pseudobulbar affect.

D. Diagnostic tests:
  1. Clinical diagnosis is based on the development of various neurologic symptoms that come and go and are spread over time. A brain MRI is indicated after two or more neurologic attacks lasting 24 hours or more. Spinal tap with evaluation of cerebrospinal fluid may also be indicated.
  2. Depression screening, Folstein Mini-Mental State Examination, and speaking with family members can be helpful.

E. Intervention:
1. Steroids to reduce nerve inflammation; plasmapheresis; medications, which may include agents to reduce relapse rates and slow progression of the disease

F. Referral: neurologist

Myasthenia Gravis

A. Shares symptoms with depression and anxiety

B. An autoimmune disorder with skeletal muscle weakness, especially in muscles controlling the eyes, eyelids, chewing, swallowing, facial expressions, and speaking
1. U.S. prevalence is between 14% and 20% per 100,000.
2. There are approximately 36,000 to 60,000 cases in the United States.

C. Symptoms:
1. Medical symptoms include muscle weakness following physical activity with improvement after resting. Common areas include the eyes and facial muscles involved in chewing and talking. Other symptoms include blurred vision, shortness of breath, and speech problems.
2. Psychiatric symptoms include fatigue, conversion disorder, slower cognitive processing, and slurred speech. Anxiety and depression are common, along with social withdrawal.

D. Diagnostic tests:
1. Clinical diagnosis is based on symptoms. Blood tests for antibodies against nerve synapses are commercially available.
2. Anti-acetylcholine receptor antibody (AChR-Ab) is widely used to diagnose MG.

E. Intervention:
1. There is no known cure for MG.
2. Reduction in symptoms can be achieved with thymectomy, monoclonal antibodies, anticholinesterase agents like mestinon, immunosuppression, plasmapheresis, and intravenous (IV) immunoglobulin for severe cases.

F. Referral: neurologist

Transient Global Amnesia

A. Shares symptoms with anxiety

B. An acute onset of temporary amnesia not associated with seizures; often follows strenuous activity and can be associated with migraines; has also been associated with consumption of polypharmacy and also of benzodiazepines and anticholinergic drugs
1. Incidence is rare, affecting between 23 and 32 people per 100,000 annually.
2. Transient global amnesia (TGA) is more common in individuals over 50 years of age.
3. Differential diagnoses include dissociative fugue, transient ischemic attack (TIA), and transient epileptic amnesia.

C. Symptoms:
1. Symptoms include acute onset of memory loss of several hours. Patients will exhibit repetitive questioning and do not know how they got to where they are or what they were doing right before.

D. Diagnostic tests:
1. Toxicology screens should be done to rule out other causes of amnesia; blood glucose and electrolyte and oxygen levels should be checked.

E. Intervention:
1. Admit to hospital until amnesia resolves. Thiamine may be given since this condition may resemble Wernicke encephalopathy.

F. Referral: neurologist

Epilepsy

A. Shares symptoms with psychosis

B. A disorder of nerve cell activity in the brain, causing chronic seizures
1. Approximately 3.4 million Americans have epilepsy.
2. Approximately 0.6% of American children under the age of 17 years have epilepsy.
3. The highest incidence of epilepsy is in persons over the age of 65 years.

C. Symptoms:
1. Olfactory hallucinations, lip smacking, forgetfulness, and memory loss

D. Diagnostic tests:
1. EEG

E. Intervention:
1. Antiseizure medications
2. Reduction in environmental stimulation
3. Adequate hydration, sleep, and nutrition

F. Referral: neurologist

Psychogenic Nonepileptic Seizures

A. Shares symptoms with epilepsy

B. A conversion disorder in which mental stress is converted into physical symptoms; can be mistaken for epilepsy and treated in urgent care as a seizure disorder, but in fact not caused by abnormal brain electrical activity as epilepsy is
1. Although PNES presents like epilepsy, there is no organic or physical origin for the resulting behavioral and motor response.
2. PNES is not a psychiatric disorder in itself but can be related to anxiety; dissociative disorders; history of sexual, emotional, or physical abuse; excess stress; psychosis; a personality disorder; or a mood disorder.
3. PNES can be activated in times of extreme stress.
4. Many with PNES have experienced trauma, sexual and physical abuse, and neglect.

C. Symptoms:
1. Symptoms include anxiety, panic, fear, depression, psychomotor retardation, ecstasy, and increased sexuality. Patients may have prolonged convulsive seizures and rapid movements of the head, limbs, and torso.
2. Patients may have concurrent psychiatric disorders including depression, posttraumatic stress disorder (PTSD), panic attacks, and personality disorders.

D. Diagnostic tests:
1. Video EEG to monitor movement and brain activity

E. Intervention:
1. Psychotherapy, talk therapy, and cognitive behavioral therapy (CBT)

F. Referral: psychiatric consult

REFERENCES AND BIBLIOGRAPHY

Anathhanam, S., & Hassan, A. (2017). Mimics and chameleons in stroke. *Clinical Medicine, 17*(2), 156–160. https://doi.org/10.7861/clinmedicine.17-2-156

Butler, C., & Zeman, A. Z. J. (2005). Neurological syndromes which can be mistaken for psychiatric conditions. *Journal of Neurological Neurosurgical Psychiatry, 1*(Suppl. 1), i31–i38. https://doi.org/10.1136/jnnp.2004.060459. Accessed from https://jnnp.bmj.com/content/jnnp/76/suppl_1/i31.full.pdf

Cleveland Clinic. (n.d.). *Delirium*. https://my.clevelandclinic.org/health/diseases/15252-delirium

Cleveland Clinic. (n.d.). *Psychogenic nonepileptic seizure (PNES)*. https://my.clevelandclinic.org/health/diseases/24517-psychogenic-nonepileptic-seizure-pnes

Iapoce, C. (2021, December 12). *Atypical stroke linked to half of acute ischemic neurological events in SCD children*. HCP Live. https://www.hcplive.com/view/atypical-stroke-linked-half-acute-ischemic-neurological-events-scd-children

Law, C., Flaherty, C. V., & Bandyopadhyay, S. (2020). A review of psychiatric comorbidity in myasthenia gravis. *Cureus, 12*(7), e9184. https://doi.org/10.7759/cureus.9184

Marshall, B. (2017). *Fast facts for managing patients with a psychiatric disorder: What RNs, NPs, and new psych nurses need to know*. Springer Publishing Company.

Mayo Clinic Staff. (n.d.). *Dementia*. Mayo Clinic. https://www.mayoclinic.org/diseases-conditions/dementia/diagnosis-treatment/drc-20352019

National Institute of Neurological Disorders and Stroke. (n.d.). *Myasthenia gravis*. https://www.ninds.nih.gov/health-information/disorders/myasthenia-gravis

Nehring, S. M., Spurling, B. C., & Kumar, A. (2024, June 22). *Transient global amnesia*. StatPearls Publishing. https://www.ncbi.nlm.nih.gov/books/NBK442001

Rousseff, R. T. (2021). Diagnosis of Myasthenia Gravis. *Journal of Clinical Medicine, 10*(8), 1736. https://doi.org/10.3390/jcm10081736

Wallace, E. J. C., & Liberman, A. L. (2021). Diagnostic challenges in outpatient stroke: Stroke chameleons and atypical stroke syndromes. *Neuropsychiatric Disease and Treatment, 17*, 1469–1480. https://doi.org/10.2147/NDT.S275750. https://www.ncbi.nlm.nih.gov/pmc/articles/PMC8129915

World Health Organization. (2016). *Mental health: Neurological disorders*. https://www.who.int/news-room/questions-and-answers/item/mental-health-neurological-disorders

PHYSICAL TRAUMA

A. The importance of trauma-informed care is examined in Chapter 3, "Trauma-Informed Care"; however, this section will review how trauma to the brain as well as to the body can result in psychiatric symptoms that are secondary to the primary diagnosis of trauma.

B. Trauma, whether from a one-time experience or resulting from repetitive events, presents differently in different individuals.

C. Assault on brain tissues is another type of trauma that can result in psychiatric symptoms, but treatment requires a different intervention to reduce the encephalopathy that is at the origin of the disease process.

SPECIFIC DISORDERS RELATED TO PHYSICAL TRAUMA

Encephalopathies and Traumatic Brain Injury

A. Shares symptoms with PTSD, psychosis, and depression

B. Encephalopathies: a group of conditions that cause brain dysfunction, and include chronic traumatic encephalopathy (CTE; dementia pugilistica) and traumatic brain injury (TBI); CTE and TBI: acute traumas that may be associated with blood loss, significant pain, and distracting injuries

C. Symptoms:
   1. Symptoms include headaches, loss of language, slurred speech, apathy, ataxia, quick to anger, tremors, balance issues, and decreased executive function.
   2. Patients also present with pain, disorientation, confusion, blood loss, and hypoxia.
   3. Cognitive and behavioral changes include memory problems, change in sleep pattern, frustration, and irritability. CTE can also cause problems with impulse control, depression, and confusion.

D. Diagnostic tests:
   1. TBI and CTE require medical and neurologic evaluation. The Acute Concussion Evaluation (ACE) tool and the Sport Concussion Assessment Tool 2 can be used to assess a person with possible TBI/CTE. CT scan and MRI may also be indicated.
   2. Neuropsychological testing to assess brain function, memory, executive function, reaction time, and problem-solving can be helpful.

E. Intervention:
   1. Brain rest and symptom control; prevention from future concussions; medications, which may include pain medication, anticonvulsants, diuretics to reduce pressure in the brain, stimulants, antidepressants, and anti anxiolytics
   2. Rehabilitation, including cognitive rehabilitation

F. Referral: neurologist and trauma specialist

G. Postconcussion syndrome: seen after a mild head injury; usually seen following the head collision, but can emerge a few days later with headaches, lightheadedness, fatigue, and ringing in the ears; may also be accompanied by new onset of tremors
   1. Shares symptoms with substance use withdrawal
   2. Referral to neurologist as well as for neuropsychological testing

Vascular Dementia

A. Shares symptoms with psychosis, depression, and mania/hypomania

B. Caused by interruption of blood and oxygen to the brain, with patients possibly having small, unrecognized strokes or other vascular diseases
   1. Second most common type of dementia
   2. Caused by reduced blood flow to the brain
   3. Rare in persons younger than 65 years of age

C. Symptoms:
   1. Physical symptoms depend on the area of the brain affected. Patients present with problems with speech, gait, and motor function. Epilepsy can be seen in patients with vascular dementia.
   2. There is gradual onset of cognitive decline. Other symptoms include depression, mania, hypomania, and delusions of theft of personal belongings. Patients may also have hallucinations, agitation, apathy, and aggressive behavior.

D. Diagnostic tests:
   1. CT and MRI with changes in the white matter

E. Intervention:
   1. Stroke prevention; control of high blood pressure, diabetes, and arrhythmias

F. Referral: neurologist

REFERENCE AND BIBLIOGRAPHY

National Institute of Neurological Disorders and Stroke. (n.d.). *Traumatic brain injury (TBI)*. https://www.ninds.nih.gov/health-information/disorders/traumatic-brain-injury-tbi

RESPIRATORY DISORDERS

SPECIFIC RESPIRATORY DISORDERS

Carbon Monoxide Poisoning

A. Shares symptoms with substance use disorders (SUD) and psychosis

B. Results from an excess of carbon monoxide (CO) in the blood

1. Patient presents with malaise and shortness of breath as a result of underlying systemic toxicity.
2. The cause is both impaired oxygen delivery and also disrupted oxygen utilization and respiration at the cellular level.
3. Disruption specifically affects organs that require high oxygenation (e.g., heart, brain).
4. Common sources are gas-powered generators, motor vehicles, fire, gas-powered tools, grills and propane stoves, and paint and varnish strippers.
C. Symptoms:
1. Symptoms include agitation, fatigue, dizziness, decreased mental acuity, altered consciousness, seizures, hallucinations, delirium, restlessness, possible echolalia, mutism, ataxia, and bizarre behaviors.
D. Diagnostic tests:
1. Diagnosis is confirmed by measuring the patient's carboxyhemoglobin (COHgb) level.
2. COHgb levels can be tested either in whole blood or by pulse oximeter.
3. It is important to know how much time has elapsed since the patient has left the toxic environment because this will impact the COHgb level.
E. Intervention:
1. Individual hyperbaric oxygen unit (monoplace hyperbaric oxygen unit)
2. Oxygen therapy via mask
F. Referral: primary care provider

Hypoxia/Altitude Sickness
A. Shares symptoms with SUD
B. Occurs when oxygen is insufficient in the body's tissue and homeostasis cannot be maintained
1. There are three syndromes of altitude sickness: acute mountain sickness (AMS), high-altitude cerebral edema (HACE), and high-altitude pulmonary edema (HAPE).
C. Symptoms:
1. Symptoms include depression, disorientation, confusion, anxiety, possible euphoria, short-term memory loss, uncooperative, and cognitive changes.
D. Diagnostic tests:
1. Pulse oximetry to evaluate arterial oxygen saturation (SaO_2), which refers to the amount of oxygen bound to hemoglobin in arterial blood
2. Arterial blood gas (ABG)
3. Imaging
4. Arterial oxygen partial pressure to fractional inspired oxygen ratio ($PaO_2:FiO_2$)
5. Pulmonary function test (PFT)
6. Nocturnal (overnight) trend oximetry
7. 6-minute walk test
8. Hemoglobin
9. EKG
E. Intervention:
1. Treatment depends on the underlying cause and may include inhaled steroids, diuretics, continuous positive airway pressure (CPAP), bilevel positive airway pressure (BiPAP), and mechanical ventilation in acute hypoxia.
F. Referral: pulmonologist

Chronic Obstructive Pulmonary Disease, Chronic Bronchitis, and Emphysema
A. Shares symptoms with anxiety and panic disorders
B. Chronic obstructive pulmonary disease (COPD): the third global leading cause of death; 14 million Americans have emphysema, which is more common in smokers than in nonsmokers
C. Symptoms:
1. Symptoms include panic, anxiety, fear, phobias, and cognitive changes.
D. Diagnostic tests:
1. Chest x-ray
2. CT scan
3. PFT
4. ABG
5. EKG
6. Blood tests and genetic tests
E. Intervention:
1. Inhaled corticosteroids, bronchodilators, antibiotics, anti-inflammatory medications, oxygen therapy, lung volume reduction surgery (LVRS), and smoking cessation programs
F. Referral: pulmonologist

SPECIFIC SLEEP DISORDERS

Sleep Apnea
A. Shares symptoms with depression and anxiety
B. A sleep disorder in which breathing intermittently stops and starts during sleep
1. Sleep apnea is a common condition, with 1 in 16 Americans experiencing some kind of sleep apnea.
2. The prevalence is 15% to 30% in males and 10% to 15% in females.
3. Increasing levels of sleep apnea are believed to be connected to the epidemic of obesity.
C. Symptoms:
1. Symptoms include chronic fatigue, insomnia, hypersomnia, inattention, irritability, moodiness, and headaches
D. Diagnostic tests:
1. Sleep tests
E. Intervention:
1. CPAP machine
F. Referral: pulmonologist

Narcolepsy and Other Sleep Disorders
A. Shares symptoms with anxiety disorder and psychosis
B. A sleep disorder characterized by rapid switch between being awake and sleeping; a lifelong condition without a cure
1. Cataplexy describes sudden loss of muscle tone associated with narcolepsy.
2. There are two types of narcolepsy: one with cataplexy and one without.
C. Symptoms:
1. Symptoms include daytime drowsiness and falling asleep suddenly without warning. Sleeping episodes may last up to a half an hour. Cataplexy is uncontrollable and can be triggered by intense emotions or excitement. Patients may also experience sleep paralysis, hallucinations, and rapid eye movement (REM) sleep behavior disorder.
2. Psychiatric symptoms include anxiety, altered level of consciousness, cataplexy, violent outbursts, and hypnagogic and hypnopompic hallucinations.
D. Diagnostic tests:
1. Tests include nighttime sleep study and multiple sleep latency test (MSLT).

2. The patient's sleep history should be reviewed.
3. Genetic testing for type 1 with cataplexy can be performed, as well as a spinal tap testing for specific proteins in the cerebrospinal fluid.
E. Intervention:
1. Stimulants may be prescribed to improve alertness during the day.
2. Serotonin and norepinephrine reuptake inhibitors (SNRIs) and SSRIs can be used to suppress REM sleep. Some antidepressants can be used for cataplexy.
3. Lifestyle changes may be important, including sticking to a schedule, taking naps, avoiding alcohol, smoking cessation, and exercise.
F. Referral: sleep specialist and neurologist

REFERENCES AND BIBLIOGRAPHY

Marshall, B. (2017). Medical diagnosis and symptom sharing: Respiratory disease. In B. Marshall (Ed.), *Fast facts for managing patients with a psychiatric disorder: What RNs, NPs, and new psych nurses need to know* (pp. 127–136). Springer Publishing Company.

McKee, J., & Brahm, N. (2016). Medical mimics: Differential diagnostic considerations for psychiatric symptoms. *Mental Health Clinician, 6*(6), 289–296. https://doi.org/10.9740/mhc.2016.11.289

VITAMIN DISORDERS

SPECIFIC VITAMIN DEFICIENCIES

Thiamine Deficiency Disorder

A. Shares symptoms with cognitive disorders and psychosis
B. Also known as *Wernicke–Korsakoff syndrome,* which is a neurologic disorder resulting from lack of thiamine (vitamin B_1); Wernicke encephalopathy is the acute phase of the syndrome; thiamine can be depleted due to alcohol abuse, lack of vitamin B1, vomiting, eating disorders, and some chemotherapy
  1. 92% of Americans have some vitamin deficiency.
  2. 50% of Americans have deficiencies in magnesium, vitamin C, and vitamin A.
  3. More than 50% are deficient in vitamin D.
  4. 70% of older Americans are deficient in vitamin D, along with 90% of Americans of color.

C. Symptoms:
1. Physical symptoms include jerky movements of the eyes, double vision, ataxia, disorientation, tachycardia, and postural hypotension.
2. Patients can have confusion, tremors, and amnesia. Delirium may be present in the acute phase. Chronic stages include memory loss and confabulation, and hallucinations may be present.
D. Diagnostic tests:
1. Blood and urinary testing detect other problems. Thiamine blood levels can be checked.
E. Intervention:
1. Replace thiamine and improve hydration and nutrition.
F. Referral: primary care provider

REFERENCES AND BIBLIOGRAPHY

Marshall, B. (2017). Medical diagnosis and symptom sharing: Metabolic disease. In B. Marshall (Ed.), *Fast facts for managing patients with a psychiatric disorder: What RNs, NPs, and new psych nurses need to know* (pp. 117–126). Springer Publishing Company.

McKee, J., & Brahm, N. (2016). Medical mimics: Differential diagnostic considerations for psychiatric symptoms. *Mental Health Clinician, 6*(6), 289–296. https://doi.org/10.9740/mhc.2016.11.289

SUMMARY

Correct diagnosis depends on the clinician's ability to conduct a thorough history and physical, utilize valid/reliable scales, and order appropriate laboratory tests. It requires the healthcare provider to step outside of preconceived, limiting beliefs and question some implicit and explicit biases. Implementing a team-based "diagnostic time-out" as part of patient evaluation, especially for those who present with confounding symptoms, allows for expansion of thought and inclusion of other ideas. The art and science of diagnosing is never a solitary experience. Healthcare providers are responsible for considering all possible causes of the patient's symptoms. To achieve this, clinicians must engage the healthcare team, utilize the resources of the healthcare system, and remain vigilant in the ability to see and respect the patient's uniqueness and desire for recovery.

33 MOVEMENT, NUTRITION, AND MENTAL HEALTH

Katherine J. Roberts

INTRODUCTION

MENTAL WELLNESS AND LIFESTYLE

Determinants of Well-Being and Mental Health Challenges

A. Family history of mental health problems
   1. Mental health challenges are more likely in families where other members have been diagnosed with a disorder.
   2. There is a genetic predisposition to mental health issues.
   3. There is epigenetic inheritance or the transmission of epigenetic markers from one generation to the next, independent of changes to the underlying DNA sequence. Epigenetic modifications can occur due to environmental influences, lifestyle, stress, diet, or exposure to toxins.

B. Life experiences
   1. Trauma
      a. 70% of adults report at least one traumatic event.
      b. More than two-thirds of children report at least one traumatic event by 16 years of age.
   2. Bereavement and loss
      a. Loss of a loved one
      b. Loss of a relationship
   3. Stressful experiences
      a. Chronic stress, whether related to work, school, or home life
      b. Financial stress, such as financial instability and poverty
      c. Pandemic and other world events
   4. Medical conditions
      a. Chronic illness
      b. Traumatic brain injuries, which can affect mood and anxiety disorders

C. Lifestyle
   1. Physical inactivity
   2. Poor diet
   3. Substance use (e.g., substance abuse, withdrawal from substances)

REFERENCES AND BIBLIOGRAPHY

Benjet, C., Bromet, E., Karam, E. G., Kessler, R. C., McLaughlin, K. A., Ruscio, A. M., Shahly, V., Stein, D. J., Petukhova, M., Hill, E., Alonso, J., Atwoli, L., Bunting, B., Bruffaerts, R., Caldas-de-Almeida, J. M., de Girolamo, G., Florescu, S., Gureje, O., Huang, Y., ... Koenen, K. C. (2016). The epidemiology of traumatic event exposure worldwide: Results from the World Mental Health Survey Consortium. *Psychological Medicine, 46*(2), 327–343. https://doi.org/10.1017/S0033291715001981. Epub 2015 Oct 29.

Copeland, W. E., Keeler, G., Angold, A., & Costello, E. J. (2007). Traumatic events and posttraumatic stress in childhood. *Archives Of General Psychiatry, 64*(5), 577–584. https://doi.org/10.1001/archpsyc.64.5.577

PHYSICAL ACTIVITY

A. Research has shown the beneficial effects of physical activity on mental health.
   1. A recent meta-analysis of 97 systematic reviews of 1,039 randomized controlled trials involving 128,119 participants found that physical activity is 1.5 times more effective than medication or cognitive behavioral therapy in reducing mild to moderate symptoms of depression, psychological stress, and anxiety.
   2. A systematic review and meta-analysis of 49 studies found that physical activity is effective in reducing symptoms of anxiety in both clinical and nonclinical populations.
   3. Physical activity has been found to be effective in reducing depression and anxiety.

B. Structured physical activity interventions should be considered a mainstay approach to managing mild to moderate symptoms of depression, anxiety, and psychological distress.
   1. However, physical activity is often not the treatment of choice to manage mental health conditions despite its effectiveness.
   2. Healthcare providers may not be fully aware of the extent that physical activity can benefit mental health or may lack training in prescribing physical activity as a treatment.

C. Promoting physical activity interventions as a treatment for mental health can also improve an individual's physical health, especially since people with mental health conditions are at higher risk of developing physical illness.
   1. Mental illness is associated with 1.4 to 2 times increased risk of obesity, diabetes, and cardiovascular diseases compared with the general population.
   2. People with a diagnosis of physical illness, especially cardiovascular disease, diabetes, and cancer, have a higher risk of developing mental health problems.
   3. When both mental and physical illnesses are present, there is a higher overall rate of morbidity, healthcare utilization, and poorer quality of life.

NEUROPHYSIOLOGIC BENEFITS

A. Physical activity can improve mood in persons with depression.
   1. This is achieved through various neuromolecular mechanisms, including:
      a. Increased expression of neurotrophic factors
      b. Increased availability of serotonin and norepinephrine
      c. Regulation of hypothalamic–pituitary–adrenal axis activity
      d. Reduced systemic inflammation
   2. The neurophysiologic benefits are underscored:
      a. By release of endorphins, which are endogenous substances that serve as natural mood elevators and reduce pain perception
   3. Physical activity has been identified as a pivotal mechanism in stress modulation.
      a. Exercise initially spikes the stress response in the body, but significantly decreases it after.

▶

b. Modulation can be achieved through downregulation of cortisol and facilitation of norepinephrine synthesis, which are hormones integral to the body's stress response system.

BRAIN CHANGES

A. Physical activity promotes the growth of new neurons and increases the size of the hippocampus.
  1. Physical activity benefits the white and gray matter in the brain.

B. Physical activity is correlated with cognitive enhancements.
  1. Improvement in focus
  2. Improvement in memory
  3. Improvement in perception

C. Physical activity induces stimulation of neurochemical processes.
  1. Physical activity contributes to neurogenesis and synaptic plasticity.
  2. Consistent physical activity may ameliorate the onset of neurodegenerative disorders.
     a. Alzheimer disease
     b. Various dementias

PERCEPTION OF SELF

A. Physical activity has been demonstrated to improve self-perception and self-worth.

B. Physical activity can provide a sense of accomplishment.
  1. Self-efficacy, or being able to accomplish a goal, improves self-worth.
  2. Regular engagement in physical activity can increase a person's sense of self-efficacy.

C. Engaging in physical activity increases a person's access to socialization.
  1. Meeting new people is beneficial to those who are feeling lonely or isolated.
     a. Team or group participation mitigates isolation.
     b. Individuals who are part of a team feel a sense of belonging.
  2. Communal integration occurs through group exercise.
     a. Persons who are isolated can achieve a level of integration into their community through participation in group activities.
     b. Persons of shared interest through physical activity can create a sense of community.

SLEEP

A. Sleep problems can contribute to the onset and worsening of mental health challenges.
  1. Lack of sleep or too much sleep is often related to depression and anxiety.
  2. A bidirectional relationship exists with bipolar disorders, schizophrenia, attention deficit hyperactivity disorder (ADHD), and suicidal ideation.

B. The existence of a mental health disorder can increase the difficulty of getting a good night's sleep.
  1. Insomnia, or the inability to fall asleep or stay asleep, is a contributing factor to the worsening of symptoms of mental health challenges.
  2. Hypersomnia, or sleeping too much, can worsen alienation and impact the quality of engagement in activities of daily living.

C. Sleep and physical activity are mutually beneficial.
  1. Engagement in physical activity improves sleep quantity and quality.
  2. Regular physical activity can normalize the circadian rhythm, leading to more consistent sleep patterns.
  3. Sleep can improve physical activity performance and recovery.

D. Moderate to vigorous exercise is also beneficial.
  1. It can increase sleep quality in adults by reducing sleep onset, or the time it takes to fall asleep.
  2. It can decrease the amount of time lying awake in bed during the night.
  3. It can decrease the risk of excessive weight gain, which makes a person less likely to experience symptoms of obstructive sleep apnea.

LIFE STRUCTURES AND DEPENDABILITY

A. Regular exercise schedules provide indispensable structure.
  1. Regular exercise is beneficial to patients contending with mood dysregulation.
  2. Emotional resilience and mood stabilization are additional benefits conferred by physical activity.

B. Engagement in an exercise routine or ritual can provide access to constructive coping mechanisms.
  1. Diverting focus away from maladaptive thought processes
  2. Considered meditation in movement
  3. Release of cortisol during physical activity, which can help in coping with stress
  4. Provides a positive focus during difficult emotional times

C. Regular exercise was recommended as a coping mechanism during the pandemic.
  1. Regular physical activity is associated with a stronger immune system.
  2. Positive exercise changes that were begun during the pandemic improved psychological and physical well-being.
  3. Older adults benefited from engaging in exercise during the pandemic, decreasing their depression and anxiety (Ejiri et al., 2021).

REFERENCES AND BIBLIOGRAPHY

Doherty, A. M., & Gaughran, F. (2014). The interface of physical and mental health. *Social Psychiatry and Psychiatric Epidemiology, 49*(5). https://doi.org/10.1007/s00127-014-0847-7

Ejiri, M., Kawai, H., Kera, T., Ihara, K., Fujiwara, Y., Watanabe, Y., Hirano, H., Kim, H., & Obuchi, S. (2021). Exercise as a coping strategy and its impact on the psychological well-being of Japanese community-dwelling older adults during the COVID-19 pandemic: A longitudinal study. *Psychology of Sport and Exercise, 57*. https://doi.org/10.1016/j.psychsport.2021.102054

Firth, J., Siddiqi, N., Koyanagi, A., Siskind, D., Rosenbaum, S., Galletly, C., Allan, S., Caneo, C., Carney, R., Carvalho, A. F., Chatterton, M. L., Correll, C. U., Curtis, J., Gaughran, F., Heald, A., Hoare, E., Jackson, S. E., Kisely, S., Lovell, K., … Stubbs, B. (2019). The Lancet Psychiatry Commission: A blueprint for protecting physical health in people with mental illness. *The Lancet Psychiatry, 6*(8), 675–712. https://doi.org/10.1016/S2215-0366(19)30132-4

Gujral, S., Aizenstein, H., Reynolds, C. F., Butters, M. A., & Erickson, K. I. (2017). Exercise effects on depression: Possible neural mechanisms. *General Hospital Psychiatry, 49*, 2–10. https://doi.org/10.1016/j.genhosppsych.2017.04.012

Singh, B., Olds, T., Curtis, R., Dumuid, D., Virgara, R., Watson, A., Szeto, K., O'Connor, E., Ferguson, T., Eglitis, E., Miatke, A., Simpson, C. E. M., & Maher, C. (2023). Effectiveness of physical activity interventions for improving depression, anxiety and distress: An overview of systematic reviews. *British Journal of Sports Medicine, 57*(18), 1203–1209. https://doi.org/10.1136/bjsports-2022-106195

Stubbs, B., Koyanagi, A., Hallgren, M., Firth, J., Richards, J., Schuch, F., Rosenbaum, S., Mugisha, J., Veronese, N., Lahti, J., & Vancampfort, D. (2017). Physical activity and anxiety: A perspective from the World Health Survey. *Journal of Affective Disorders, 208*. https://doi.org/10.1016/j.jad.2016.10.028

TYPES OF EXERCISE AND THEIR IMPACT ON MENTAL HEALTH

A. All forms of exercise, including aerobic, strength-based, yoga, Pilates, and tai chi, produce significant mental health benefits.
B. Moderate-intensity and high-intensity exercises have been demonstrated to be more effective than lower intensities in improving mental health.
  1. Low-intensity physical activity may be insufficient in stimulating the neurologic and hormonal changes needed to alleviate depression or anxiety.
  2. High-intensity exercise programs show the most benefits.
C. Different types of physical activity stimulate different physiologic and psychosocial effects.
  1. Exercise is associated with a greater reduction in depression symptoms compared with relaxation or meditation.
  2. Resistance exercise may be the most effective in depression.
  3. Yoga and other mind–body exercises may be the most effective in anxiety.
D. Physical activity can be more effective in reducing mild to moderate symptoms of depression, psychological stress, and anxiety than medication or cognitive behavioral therapy.
E. To improve overall health, the U.S. Department of Health and Human Services recommends 150 minutes or 2.5 hours of moderate aerobic activity a week or 75 minutes of more vigorous activity.

HEALTHCARE PROVIDER RECOMMENDATIONS

A. Healthcare providers, after establishing the safety of any engagement in exercise, can recommend physical activities that improve the individual's mental well-being.
B. Evaluate what barriers might make physical activity difficult for the patient.
  1. Lack of knowledge or skills on how to exercise
  2. Lack of time due to work commitments or caregiving responsibilities
  3. Finances for gym memberships or equipment
  4. Lack of access to parks or recreational areas, unsafe neighborhoods
C. Persons with mental health challenges may have other comorbid diagnoses, which can interfere with their engagement in physical activity.
  1. Consider the age and the medical and physical health limitations of the patient.
  2. Ask the patient what level of engagement is possible.
      a. Assess where the patient is in their behavior change.
      b. Partner with the patient.
      c. Start slowly so that the patient can build self-efficacy and continue with the routine.
  3. Provide a menu of exercises and assess access to venues that are easy for the patient to attend.
      a. Online
      b. In-person
      c. Group
      d. Individual
  4. Although multimodal, moderate- and vigorous-intensity physical activity is the gold standard for improving mental health, recommend this level of activity only when the patient is able to safely engage.
D. Utilize the stages of change model.
  1. Stages of change: precontemplation, contemplation, preparation, action, maintenance, and relapse (Figure 33.1)
      a. Worksheets are available online for free.
      b. The simple Stages of Exercise Change Questionnaire can be used and is readily available on the internet. An example is found on the Exercise Is Medicine website, which is a global health initiative managed by the American College of Sports Medicine (see www.exerciseismedicine.org; American College of Sports Medicine, n.d.).
  2. Precontemplation
      a. Identify patients in precontemplation.
      b. These patients are inactive.
      c. These patients have no thoughts of becoming active.
      d. Move patients out of precontemplation.
          i. Increase the patient's awareness of the impact of physical activity on their mental health.
          ii. Demonstrate curiosity regarding the patient's lack of knowledge about activity and mood.
          iii. Personalize information on the risks and benefits of physical activity.
          iv. Provide a menu of types of things that are considered activity.

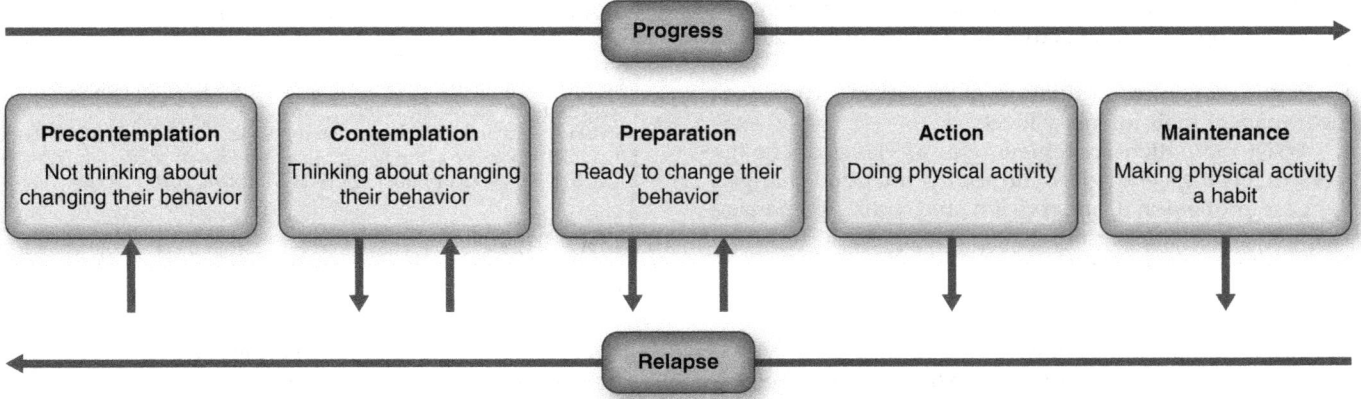

FIGURE 33.1 The stages of change. Progress from precontemplation to maintenance stages is shown. Arrows going down indicate relapse can occur in any stage. The up arrows show that an individual can relapse and go back to any of the three stages: precontemplation, contemplation, and preparation.

3. Contemplation
   a. Individuals in the contemplation stage are inactive but are thinking about becoming active.
   b. Provide motivation and encouragement.
4. Preparation
   a. Individuals in the preparation stage intend to be physically active in the next month.
   b. Develop a concrete action plan.
   c. Set SMART (i.e., specific, measurable, achievable, relevant, and timebound) goals.
   d. Make small changes.
5. Action
   a. Individuals in the action stage are physically active at the recommended levels but have been active for less than 6 months.
   b. This stage has the greatest risk of relapse.
   c. Encourage successful strategies.
   d. Continue to set goals.
6. Maintenance
   a. Individuals in the maintenance stage are physically active at the recommended levels and have been for 6 or more months.
   b. These individuals have created a positive lifestyle habit.
7. Relapse
   a. Individuals in relapse used to be physically active but are no longer.
   b. Successful strategies should be identified.
   c. Barriers should be identified.
   d. Incentives should be provided.

IMPLICATIONS FOR PRACTICE

A. Clinicians can consider physical activity the same way as they would consider pharmaceutical support.
   1. Patients might be more compliant with a "prescription for exercise" when they know the benefits of ongoing engagement.
   2. Clear instructions related to what type of physical activity and how often can help the patient be compliant.
   3. Prescription pads to promote physical activity are available.

B. Clinicians can include family, community, and other environments where the patient routinely spends time.
   1. Increase walking by parking farther from work.
   2. Walk during lunch hour.
   3. Participate or even start a team sport.
   4. Plan family games that include activities of movement.

C. Suggest using a physical activity training plan to maintain compliance.
   1. Provide ongoing evaluation of engagement to assess the impact of their intensity level.
   2. Assist the patient in achieving a safe level of engagement that is high enough to induce the intended changes.

D. Suggest professional supervision and training management, especially in the beginning.
   1. Certified personal trainers
   2. Team sports with a coach
   3. Online supervision

E. Suggest technology and tools.
   1. Utilize technology such as apps to track physical activity.
   2. Use technology such as fitness trackers, pedometers, accelerometers, and heart rate monitors.
   3. Interactive video games that measure and track physical activity are available.

F. Integrate physical activity into psychoeducation and psychotherapy.
   1. Suggest patients keep a training journal.
   2. Have patients evaluate their mood pre- and post-exercise.
   3. Review training and mood assessments during psychoeducation to increase the patient's insight into the relationship between mood and movement.

G. Consider differential acute effects depending on the patient's training history and actual fitness.
   1. Assess if any prior training may have had aspects of trauma.
      a. Gymnasts who were exposed to sexual abuse
      b. High school and college athletes who experienced verbal or physical abuse
      c. Student athletes who were bullied during training periods or in athletic environments
   2. Assess for positive past experiences in engagement in exercise.
      a. Trained subjects experience greater improvements in vigor, positive affect, and less fatigue than non-trained subjects.
      b. Seek encouragement from a teammate, fellow athlete, or coach.
      c. Build positive relationships with others who were engaging in similar physical activities.

H. Be aware of and make use of inexplicit effects.
   1. Social support
   2. Time structure
   3. Therapeutic contact
   4. Positive reinforcement

REFERENCES AND BIBLIOGRAPHY

American College of Sports Medicine. (n.d.). *Exercise is medicine: Healthcare providers' action guide*. Accessed August 31, 2023. https://www.exerciseismedicine.org/assets/page_documents/HCP_Action_Guide.pdf

Cooney, G., Dwan, K., & Mead, G. (2014). Exercise for depression. *JAMA, 311*(23). https://doi.org/10.1001/jama.2014.4930

Piercy, K. L., Troiano, R. P., Ballard, R. M., Carlson, S. A., Fulton, J. E., Galuska, D. A., George, S. M., & Olson, R. D. (2018). The physical activity guidelines for Americans. *JAMA, 320*(19). https://doi.org/10.1001/jama.2018.14854

Prochaska, J. O., & DiClemente, C. C. (1983). Stages and processes of self-change of smoking: Toward an integrative model of change. *Journal of Consulting and Clinical Psychology, 51*(3), 390–395. https://doi.org/10.1037//0022-006x.51.3.390

Reed, G. R., Velicer, W. F., Prochaska, J. O., Rossi, J. S., & Marcus, B. H. (1997). What makes a good staging algorithm: Examples from regular exercise. *American Journal of Health Promotion, 12*(1). https://doi.org/10.4278/0890-1171-12.1.57

Sutton, J. (2020, August 13). *The 6 stages of change: Worksheets for helping your clients*. Positive Psychology. https://positivepsychology.com/stages-of-change-worksheets

Thompson, W. R., Sallis, R., Joy, E., Jaworski, C. A., Stuhr, R. M., & Trilk, J. L. (2020). Exercise is medicine. *American Journal of Lifestyle Medicine, 14*(5), 511–523. https://doi.org/10.1177/1559827620912192

HEALTHY DIET

A. Research supports the association between dietary patterns and mental health outcomes.
   1. A meta-analysis of 21 studies from 10 countries showed an association between dietary patterns and risk of depression.
   2. A systematic review and meta-analysis of observational studies found that healthy dietary patterns were associated with a low risk of depression.

3. A recent longitudinal prospective study involving women enrolled in the Nurses' Health Study II found that eating high amounts of ultraprocessed foods increased the risk of developing depression.

B. People with mental disorders typically excessively consume high-fat and high-sugar foods and have inadequate intake of nutrient-dense foods compared with the general population.
1. The U.S. Department of Agriculture (USDA) Dietary Guidelines state that nutrient-dense foods include vegetables, fruits, whole grains, seafood, eggs, beans, peas, lentils, nuts and seeds, and lean meats and poultry that have little added sugars, saturated fat, and sodium (USDA & U.S. Department of Health and Human Services, 2020).
2. The relationship between poor diet and mental health disorders persists even when controlling for other factors, such as:
   a. Obesity
   b. Lifestyle factors, including physical activity, alcohol, and smoking behavior

C. Excessive consumption of processed foods, including high-fat and high-added-sugar foods, can increase systemic inflammation.
1. Heightened levels of peripheral inflammatory markers are seen in people with severe mental illness.
2. Mental health disorders are associated with increased concentrations of proinflammatory cytokines.
3. Inflammation contributes to both chronic physical and mental illnesses.

D. A healthy diet can promote mental health as well as recovery from mental health challenges.
1. As is the case with promoting physical activity, dietary improvements can be an effective treatment approach for those with mental health disorders and can also benefit the management of comorbidities.
2. Dietary interventions have demonstrated greater improvements in those with moderate to severe depression than social support groups.

DIETS THAT INCREASE RISK OF MENTAL HEALTH DISORDERS

A. Western-style diet or a diet high in processed foods, added sugar, and saturated fat and low in plant foods
1. Ultraprocessed foods
   a. Have many added ingredients such as added sugar, salt, and fat, as well as artificial colors or preservatives
   b. Use ingredients that are not typically used in home cooking
2. Foods containing artificial sweeteners and beverages that are artificially sweetened
   a. Artificial sweeteners elicit purinergic transmission in the brain.
   b. These are involved in the etiopathogenesis of depression.
3. Low amount of whole plant foods, which are high in fiber and polyphenols, leading to loss of gut microbial diversity and function, as well as extinction of important beneficial gut microbes

B. Western-style diet is associated with depression, anxiety, and other mental health issues throughout all stages of life, even in children and adolescents.

C. Western-style diet is associated with lower health-related quality of life.

D. Inflammation has been proposed as the mechanism linking a Western-style diet to mental health.
1. Markers of inflammation are positively correlated with components of a poor diet, and a healthy diet is associated with reduced inflammation.
2. Depression is associated with increased concentrations of proinflammatory cytokines.
3. Inflammatory dietary patterns are high in added sugar, refined grains, red meat, and artificial sweeteners.

DIETS THAT DECREASE RISK OF MENTAL HEALTH DISORDERS

A. A "whole foods" traditional diet that is high in fruits and vegetables has been found to be protective against developing depression, among other mental illnesses.
1. A general positive influence of dietary patterns and mental health is characterized by a higher intake of:
   a. Fruit
   b. Vegetables
   c. Both fruit and vegetable products
2. A high-quality, plant-based diet may be protective against depressive symptoms.
3. Mediterranean-style diet, where there is high consumption of fruits and vegetables, whole grains and legumes, herbs, nuts and seeds, fish and seafood, and limited red meat, can be protective against the development of a mental disorder.
4. Anti-inflammatory dietary patterns reduce the risk of cardiovascular and cerebrovascular diseases.
5. All chronic health conditions are related to chronic inflammation.
   a. Increasing consumption of nutrient-dense foods such as fruits and vegetables is known to reduce systemic inflammation.
   b. Whole food diets have high fiber and have a beneficial effect on the gut microbiota, which is associated with mental health disorders.

NUTRITIONAL SUPPLEMENTATION

A. Some specific nutrients have been shown to have a positive impact on mental health, with omega-3 having the strongest evidentiary support.
1. Omega-3 fatty acids
   a. Omega-3 fatty acids regulate neurotransmission, influence gene expression, and directly affect neurogenesis and neuronal survival.
   b. They act as an antioxidant and have anti-inflammatory properties.
   c. Due to processed foods that have high levels of processed vegetable oils, Western diets are abundant in omega-6 fatty acids and low in omega-3s.
   d. An elevated omega-6 to omega-3 fatty acid ratio has been associated with major depressive disorder.
   e. High levels of omega-3 fatty acids are found in flaxseeds, chia seeds, walnuts, seafood, and fish.
   f. There is a small to modest beneficial effect on depressive symptomology.
2. Folate, along with other B vitamins
   a. These are essential for the methylation cycle, which produces a cofactor crucial for monoamine neurotransmitter synthesis.
   b. The proper function of the methylation cycle reduces homocysteine elevated levels.

i. High levels of homocysteine are linked to cardiovascular disease and depression.
   c. Homocysteine is an amino acid in the blood, and its levels are influenced by genetic factors and diet.
      i. Homocysteine levels can be higher in individuals in which the enzymatic reaction that converts folic acid to the active methyl donor L-5-methyltetrahydrofolate (5-MTHF) does not function properly.
      ii. Folate is found in foods like leafy green vegetables, legumes, nuts, and fortified grains.
      iii. Folate works in tandem with other B vitamins, particularly vitamin B_{12} and vitamin B_6, in the metabolism of homocysteine. Thus, a balanced intake of these vitamins is important in maintaining healthy homocysteine levels.
   d. A homocysteine test may be used to find out if a patient is lacking vitamin B_6, vitamin B_{12}, or folic acid.
3. N-acetylcysteine (nutraceutical form of the amino acid cysteine)
   a. A meta-analysis showed that N-acetylcysteine improved depressive symptoms compared with placebo.
   b. N-acetylcysteine has been shown to increase dopamine release in animal models.

B. Pre/probiotic supplements may serve as potentially useful therapeutic options.
1. There is promising evidence on the potential of probiotics in improving anxiety, depression, and subjective stress in human populations.
2. However, changing the gut microbiota through diet may be more feasible and economically cheaper than probiotic supplementation.

C. Evidence supporting the use of vitamins (such as E, C, or D) and minerals (zinc and magnesium) for any mental disorder is lacking.
1. A study of more than 18,000 people aged 50 or older found that taking 2,000 IU per day of vitamin D for 5 years did not lead to any significant differences in depression scores compared with taking a placebo.

D. Overall, there is limited and inconsistent literature on nutritional supplementation as a treatment for mental disorders.
1. Research is confounded by overall dietary quality.
2. It is difficult to determine the impact of specific nutrients outside of experimental models.

GUT MICROBIOME

A. There is ample evidence that mental disorders are linked to the dysfunction of the gut microbiome, which is the symbiotic bacteria that live within the gastrointestinal system.

B. Bacteria in the gastrointestinal system have the following effects:
1. They influence many aspects of physiology via neural, hormonal, and immunologic pathways.
2. They can disrupt homeostatic regulation and may influence the etiology and pathophysiology of many diseases, including mental disorders.
3. They interact with the central nervous system and emerged as a key player in regulating brain processes and behavior through bidirectional communication, which is referred to as the *microbiota–gut–brain axis*.
4. The concept of "leaky gut," also known as *increased intestinal permeability*, is closely related to the functioning of the gut–brain axis.
   a. Gut permeability markers correlated significantly with interleukin-6, a marker of systemic inflammation.
   b. Gut dysbiosis and the leaky gut may influence several pathways implicated in the biology of major depressive disorders.
   c. Dietary factors, such as fiber-rich foods, probiotics, and prebiotics, can help reverse intestinal leakiness and mucosal damage.

C. Symptoms in the gastrointestinal system have been identified as the most common somatic symptoms associated with mental health disorders.

D. The gut microbiota produces neurotransmitters: gamma-aminobutyric acid, butyric acid, serotonin, dopamine, and short-chain fatty acids.
1. A recent systematic review highlighted the association between gut microbiota composition and major depressive disorder, bipolar disorder, and schizophrenia, providing strong evidence for the relationship between the gut microbiome and mental illness. They found that specific bacterial taxa commonly associated with mental disorders include:
   a. Lower levels of butyrate-producing bacteria that produce short-chain fatty acids
   b. Higher levels of lactic acid-producing bacteria
   c. Higher levels of bacteria associated with glutamate and gamma-aminobutyric acid (GABA) metabolism

E. The gut microbiome should be improved through diet.
1. Diet is a powerful tool in beneficially affecting the gut microbiota.
   a. Eliminate processed foods, added sugars, and artificial sweeteners.
   b. Eat more whole foods, including fruits and vegetables.
   c. Remove foods that may create problems, such as gluten and dairy.
   d. Eat fermented foods such as sauerkraut, kimchi, and pickled foods, which can positively affect the gut microbiome in both the short and long term.
      i. Have been part of the history of the human diet
      ii. Remain part of the dietary practices of most known traditional diets today

HEALTHCARE PROVIDER RECOMMENDATIONS

A. Realize that the evidence linking diet to mental illness has evolved from a focus on specific nutrient deficiencies to an emphasis on overall dietary patterns.
1. The field of nutritional psychiatry has turned its attention to investigating the relationship between dietary patterns and mental health instead of focusing on select nutrients.

B. Existing data consistently support increasing the intake and variety of plant foods and reducing or eliminating ultra-processed foods.
1. Encourage traditional diets based on nutrient-dense whole foods.
2. Consume a plant-based diet that is high in fiber-rich foods, such as fruits, vegetables, whole grains, nuts, and seeds.
3. Choose nutriments that are whole foods, do not come with an ingredients list, or contain minimal additions and mainly other whole food ingredients.
4. Reduce processed foods.
   a. Consider where food is from.

b. Consider how food was made, including what has happened to it before it reaches the table.
5. Reduce high-fat and high added sugar foods.
C. To improve diet, a multifaceted approach involving psychological, environmental, and educational interventions may be needed.
D. Utilize the theory of planned behavior, a social cognitive theory, to improve healthy eating behaviors, increasing consumption of fruits, vegetables, and whole grains.
1. Theory of planned behavior: a theory suggesting that intention is the primary determinant of behavior, which is influenced by attitudes or beliefs about a behavior; subjective norms, which are the beliefs about others' attitudes toward a behavior; and perceived behavioral control, or the perception of to what extent the behavior is under control
2. Enhancing attitude toward healthy eating
   a. Provide education and information about the benefits of healthy eating tailored to the patient's health needs and goals.
   b. Emphasize the positive outcomes of dietary changes, such as improved mental and physical health, improved energy levels, and enhanced overall quality of life.
3. Influencing subjective norms
   a. Encourage social support networks, seeking support from friends, family, or support groups who value healthy eating.
   b. Share success stories of others who have successfully changed their eating habits, which can create a positive and achievable goal.
4. Increasing perceived behavioral control
   a. Build skills such as how to read nutrition labels, healthy cooking techniques, and meal planning.
   b. Help identify potential barriers to changing their eating habits and develop strategies to overcome these barriers.
   c. Build self-efficacy in their belief that they can make and sustain dietary changes through achieving small milestones and celebrating these.
5. Strengthening behavioral intentions
   a. Assist in setting SMART goals.
   b. Develop detailed action plans with the patient, outlining steps to achieve their dietary goals.
6. Facilitating action and maintenance
   a. Monitor progress by scheduling regular check-ins, provide feedback, and make necessary adjustments to the action plan.
   b. Offer ongoing support and encouragement, recognizing that behavior change is a process with ups and downs.
7. Addressing relapse and resilience
   a. Educate about common causes of relapse and strategies to deal with them.
   b. Build resilience by finding ways to cope with setbacks and use them as learning opportunities for future success.
E. Self-regulation strategies have been identified as important in promoting healthy eating behaviors, with the ability to work toward a goal by monitoring and managing thoughts, feelings, and behaviors being critical to changing healthy eating.

IMPLICATIONS FOR PRACTICE
A. Healthcare providers should not only focus on the patient's diet but should also consider the behavioral, psychological, and social factors that influence dietary habits.
B. Ask patients to keep track of their food intake for a week.
1. A food history is essential to understanding whether targeted dietary recommendations could assist in recovery from mental health disorders.
2. Focus on the amount of fruits and vegetables eaten daily. According to the Dietary Guidelines, adults should consume:
   a. 1.5 to 2 cup-equivalents of fruits
      i. About 80% of the U.S. population does not meet the fruit recommendations.
   b. 2 to 3 cup-equivalents of vegetables daily
      i. Almost 90% of the U.S. population does not meet the recommendation for vegetables.
3. Examine how much of the diet is processed and how much is whole nutrient-dense foods.
4. Take into consideration patients' dietary preferences such as paleo, vegan, vegetarian, and any allergies.
5. Develop personalized nutrition plans that consider the patient's lifestyle, cultural preferences, and economic situation.
C. Suggest the patient receive a current blood test to determine whether there are any deficiencies.
1. Individual blood tests are available to test levels of vitamins, minerals, and other nutrients.
D. Encourage behavioral and motivational counseling.
1. Use motivational interviewing techniques to encourage patients to express their thoughts and feelings about diet changes, enhancing their motivation and commitment.
2. Set realistic and achievable dietary goals in collaboration with the patient.
3. Empower the patient to take an active role in their dietary changes, emphasizing the importance of their choices and actions.
4. Be aware of any eating disorders, such as anorexia and bulimia, which can have severe negative impact on mental health.
   a. Individuals with these conditions should seek help from a professional nutritionist and/or mental health provider.
E. Provide education on healthy foods.
1. Provide evidence-based dietary information and education, explaining the importance of nutrition for mental and physical health.
2. Use clear and simple language, avoiding medical jargon.
3. Encourage the use of MyPlate (www.myplate.gov) and Dietary Guidelines for Americans resources (www.dietaryguidelines.gov).
F. Develop skills.
1. Teach practical skills such as:
   a. Reading food labels
   b. Portion control
   c. Meal planning
   d. Healthy cooking techniques
2. Offer cooking demonstrations or workshops.
G. Encourage support system and community engagement.
1. Encourage patients to involve family members or friends in their dietary changes for support.
2. Connect patients with community resources such as nutrition classes, support groups, or community gardens.
H. Conduct regular monitoring and follow-up.
1. Schedule regular follow-ups to monitor progress, provide feedback, and adjust dietary plans as needed.

2. Recognize and celebrate small achievements to boost confidence and motivation.
I. Address barriers to change.
   1. Identify and discuss potential barriers to dietary changes, such as time constraints, limited cooking skills, or budget limitations.
   2. Take into consideration the patient's cultural and socioeconomic background, which can influence food choices and availability.
J. Provide technology and tools (e.g., apps or online platforms for tracking food intake and that provide nutritional information and motivation).
K. Collaborate with other professionals (e.g., nutritionists, dietitians, psychologists, or social workers) for a multidisciplinary approach.

REFERENCES AND BIBLIOGRAPHY

Ajzen, I. (2020). The theory of planned behavior: Frequently asked questions. *Human Behavior and Emerging Technologies, 2*(4). https://doi.org/10.1002/hbe2.195

Appleton, K. M., Voyias, P. D., Sallis, H. M., Dawson, S., Ness, A. R., Churchill, R., & Perry, R. (2021). Omega-3 fatty acids for depression in adults. *Cochrane Database of Systematic Reviews, 11*(11), Article CD004692. https://doi.org/10.1002/14651858.CD004692.pub5

Berding, K., Vlckova, K., Marx, W., Schellekens, H., Stanton, C., Clarke, G., Jacka, F., Dinan, T. G., & Cryan, J. F. (2021). Diet and the microbiota-gut-brain axis: Sowing the seeds of good mental health. *Advances in Nutrition, 12*(4), 1239–1285. https://doi.org/10.1093/advances/nmaa181

Dean, O., Giorlando, F., & Berk, M. (2011). N-acetylcysteine in psychiatry: Current therapeutic evidence and potential mechanisms of action. *Journal of Psychiatry & Neuroscience, 36*(2), 78–86. https://doi.org/10.1503/jpn.100057

Fernandes, B. S., Dean, O. M., Dodd, S., Malhi, G. S., & Berk, M. (2016). N-Acetylcysteine in depressive symptoms and functionality: A systematic review and meta-analysis. *The Journal of Clinical Psychiatry, 77*(4), e457–e466. https://doi.org/10.4088/JCP.15r09984

Firth, J., Stubbs, B., Teasdale, S. B., Ward, P. B., Veronese, N., Shivappa, N., Hebert, J. R., Berk, M., Yung, A. R., & Sarris, J. (2018). Diet as a hot topic in psychiatry: A population-scale study of nutritional intake and inflammatory potential in severe mental illness. *World Psychiatry, 17*(3), 365–367. https://doi.org/10.1002/wps.20571

Guzek, D., Głąbska, D., Groele, B., & Gutkowska, K. (2022). Fruit and vegetable dietary patterns and mental health in women: A systematic review. *Nutrition Reviews, 80*(6), 1357–1370. https://doi.org/10.1093/nutrit/nuab007

Jacka, F. N., O'Neil, A., Opie, R., Itsiopoulos, C., Cotton, S., Mohebbi, M., Castle, D., Dash, S., Mihalopoulos, C., Chatterton, M. L., Brazionis, L., Dean, O. M., Hodge, A. M., & Berk, M. (2017). A randomised controlled trial of dietary improvement for adults with major depression (the "SMILES" trial). *BMC Medicine, 15*, Article 23. https://doi.org/10.1186/s12916-017-0791-y

Lassale, C., Batty, G. D., Baghdadli, A., Jacka, F., Sánchez-Villegas, A., Kivimäki, M., & Akbaraly, T. (2019). Healthy dietary indices and risk of depressive outcomes: A systematic review and meta-analysis of observational studies. *Molecular Psychiatry, 24*(7), 965–986. https://doi.org/10.1038/s41380-018-0237-8

Lee, M. F., Eather, R., & Best, T. (2021). Plant-based dietary quality and depressive symptoms in Australian vegans and vegetarians: A cross-sectional study. *BMJ Nutrition, Prevention & Health, 4*(2), 479. https://doi.org/10.1136/bmjnph-2021-000332

Li, Y., Lv, M. R., Wei, Y. J., Sun, L., Zhang, J. X., Zhang, H. G., & Li, B. (2017). Dietary patterns and depression risk: A meta-analysis. *Psychiatry Research, 253*, 373–382. https://doi.org/10.1016/j.psychres.2017.04.020

McGuinness, A. J., Davis, J. A., Dawson, S. L., Loughman, A., Collier, F., O'Hely, M., Simpson, C. A., Green, J., Marx, W., Hair, C., Guest, G., Mohebbi, M., Berk, M., Stupart, D., Watters, D., & Jacka, F. N. (2022). A systematic review of gut microbiota composition in observational studies of major depressive disorder, bipolar disorder and schizophrenia. *Molecular Psychiatry, 27*(4), 1920–1935. https://doi.org/10.1038/s41380-022-01456-3

Nicolaou, M., Colpo, M., Vermeulen, E., Elstgeest, L. E. M., Cabout, M., Gibson-Smith, D., Knuppel, A., Sini, G., Schoenaker, D. A. J. M., Mishra, G. D., Lok, A., Penninx, B. W. J. H., Bandinelli, S., Brunner, E. J., Zwinderman, A. H., Brouwer, I. A., & Visser, M. (2020). Association of a priori dietary patterns with depressive symptoms: A harmonised meta-analysis of observational studies. *Psychological Medicine, 50*(11), 1872–1883. https://doi.org/10.1017/S0033291719001958

Okereke, O. I., Reynolds, C. F., Mischoulon, D., Chang, G., Vyas, C. M., Cook, N. R., Weinberg, A., Bubes, V., Copeland, T., Friedenberg, G., Lee, I. M., Buring, J. E., & Manson, J. E. (2020). Effect of long-term vitamin D3 supplementation vs. placebo on risk of depression or clinically relevant depressive symptoms and on change in mood scores: A randomized clinical trial. *JAMA, 324*(5), 471–480. https://doi.org/10.1001/jama.2020.10224

O'Neil, A., Quirk, S. E., Housden, S., Brennan, S. L., Williams, L. J., Pasco, J. A., Berk, M., & Jacka, F. N. (2014). Relationship between diet and mental health in children and adolescents: A systematic review. *American Journal of Public Health, 104*(10), e31–e42. https://doi.org/10.2105/AJPH.2014.302110

Samuthpongtorn, C., Nguyen, L. H., Okereke, O. I., Wang, D. D., Song, M., Chan, A. T., & Mehta, R. S. (2023). Consumption of ultraprocessed food and risk of depression. *JAMA Network Open, 6*(9), e2334770. https://doi.org/10.1001/jamanetworkopen.2023.34770

U.S. Department of Agriculture and U.S. Department of Health and Human Services. (2020, December). *Dietary Guidelines for Americans, 2020–2025* (9th ed.). https://www.dietaryguidelines.gov/resources/2020-2025-dietary-guidelines-online-materials

Vajdi, M., & Farhangi, M. A. (2020). A systematic review of the association between dietary patterns and health-related quality of life. *Health and Quality of Life Outcomes, 18*(1), 337. https://doi.org/10.1186/s12955-020-01581-z

34 ETHICAL CONSIDERATIONS FOR THE ADVANCED PRACTICE REGISTERED NURSE

Shaquita Starks, Nia Josiah, and Freida Outlaw

INTRODUCTION

Ethics, a branch of philosophy, can be described as the exploration of the fundamental principles that shape human conduct. *Ethics* is a broad term encompassing the guiding principles that inform one's actions and choices when striving to lead a virtuous life. The origins of ethical study can be traced back to ancient Greek philosophers, namely Socrates, Plato, and Aristotle, all of whom played vital roles in its establishment as a distinct philosophical discipline.

Bioethics, often referred to as *applied ethics*, was designed to address "ought-to questions." As a field, bioethics emerged from interdisciplinary discussions between theologians, philosophers, sociologists, psychologists, scientists, and individuals in the field of law and medicine, and integrated both deontology (adhering to moral rules and professional duties) and utilitarianism (moral righteousness of an action and its ability to maximize happiness for the majority).

Bioethics is commonly conceptualized as an ethical application in the health sciences and is used to address dilemmas or conflicts related to clinical care in healthcare settings. Bioethical dilemmas or conflicts often involve two or more paradoxical options. Such dilemmas are often the most difficult challenges healthcare providers encounter since they often make decisions about competing concerns, such as benefits versus harm, the rights of individuals versus the rights of others, and patient competency, as well as other associated issues. This chapter explores the influence of ethics and bioethics on psychiatric-mental health nursing, tracing the historical foundations and contemporary challenges they face.

REFERENCES AND BIBLIOGRAPHY
Beauchamp, T. L., & Childress, J. F. (2001). *Principles of biomedical ethics*. Oxford University Press.
Chan, S. (2015). A bioethics for all seasons. *Journal of Medical Ethics, 41*(1), 17–21. https://doi.org/10.1136/medethics-2014-102306

HISTORY OF BIOETHICS

A. Certain historical events occurred that facilitated the emergence of bioethics as a discipline, such as the following:
  1. The Nuremberg Trial held physicians associated with the Nazi party accountable for their unethical experiments on humans, leading to the introduction of several essential principles. Of these principles, informed consent was an important concept ensuring that research subjects had the legal capacity to give consent to participate freely and willingly in experiments.
  2. The Tuskegee Syphilis Study in 1932 to 1972, in which African American men were not informed of or offered treatment for syphilis, triggered significant changes in research ethics and the creation of institutional review boards (IRBs) aimed to meet universal ethical standards, adhere to institutional policies, and protect the rights of research participants.
  3. The Declaration of Helsinki, introduced in 1964, stands as a global ethical guideline for unethical human subject research in medicine, crafted by the World Medical Association (WMA), and placed strong emphasis on the principles of beneficence and the reduction of harm to individuals participating in research.
  4. The Belmont Report published in 1979 incorporated the principles of both the Nuremberg and Helsinki reports, leading to the establishment of the Standards for Institutional Review Boards for Clinical Investigations. These standards were mainly focused on the rights of children and adults who are legally determined to be incompetent, thus promoting beneficence and ensuring justice for these specific vulnerable populations. This seminal report laid the groundwork for establishing regulations and formulating ethical guidelines that continue to govern research practices today.

B. Bioethical moral dilemmas healthcare providers encounter are viewed through the lens of the principles of autonomy, beneficence, nonmaleficence, and justice (Table 34.1), while striving to balance the pursuit of scientific progress and medical innovations with the protection of patients' rights, well-being, and broader societal interests.

C. Bioethics serves a vital role in guiding treatment and policy decisions, shaping medical practices, and fostering ethical dialogue to ensure that healthcare and biomedical research align with society's values and respect the dignity of all individuals involved.

REFERENCES AND BIBLIOGRAPHY
Barrett, M. S. (2012). Ethical decision-making: A framework for understanding and resolving mental health dilemmas. In C. M. Ulrich (Ed.), *Nursing ethics in everyday practice*. Nursing Knowledge.
Beauchamp, T. L., & Childress, J. F. (2001). *Principles of biomedical ethics*. Oxford University Press.
Centers for Disease Control and Prevention. (n.d.). *Syphilis study: Effects on research*. U.S. Department of Health and Human Services. https://www.cdc.gov/tuskegee/about/effects-research.html
Czech, H., Druml, C., & Weindling, P. (2018). Medical ethics in the 70 years after the nuremberg code, 1947 to the present. *Wien Klin Wochenschr, 130*(Suppl. 3), 159–253. https://doi.org/10.1007/s00508-018-1343-y
Kumar, N. K. (2013). Informed consent: Past and present. *Perspectives in Clinical Research, 4*(1), 21–25. https://www.ncbi.nlm.nih.gov/pmc/articles/PMC3601698
Nagai, H., Nakazawa, E., & Akabayashi, A. (2022). The creation of the Belmont report and its effect on ethical principles: A historical study. *Monash Bioethics Review, 40*(2), 157–170. https://doi.org/10.1007/s40592-022-00165-5
Shrestha, B., & Dunn, L. (2019). The declaration of Helsinki on medical research involving human subjects: A review of the seventh revision. *Journal of Nepal Health Research Council, 17*(4), 548–552. https://doi.org/10.33314/jnhrc.v17i4.1042

TABLE 34.1 PHILOSOPHICAL PRINCIPLES APPLIED IN BIOETHICS

Autonomy	• The right to self-determination • Providing information to allow patients to make their own decisions
Beneficence	• The promotion of good • Ensuring the patient's best interest and the greater interest of society
Justice	• Equal distribution of benefits • Impartiality to a patient's age, ethnicity, economic status, religion, or sexual orientation
Nonmaleficence	• The avoidance or minimization of harm • Provision of safe, effective, high-quality care

BIOETHICS AND THE HISTORY OF PSYCHIATRY

A. APRNs must understand the historical foundation of the profession of psychiatry to prevent providing unjust treatment, and to deliver sound professional, evidence-based care that demonstrates cultural humility and that respects individuals' fundamental rights, dignity, and freedom.
  1. Theories unsupported by evidence, biased data, collection methods, and accounts of historical unethical treatment shaped the practice of medicine, including psychiatry.
  2. Many beliefs and practices in medicine and nursing in the past were harmful, unsupported by evidence, and void of many ethical principles that violated individuals' autonomy, privacy, and the right to be treated with respect, care, and compassion.
    a. In the late 1800s, Drs. W. M. Bevis, G. Stanley Hall, and Mary O'Malley researched Black people who were enslaved and concluded that depression was a mental illness of elite White people, and that Black people lacked the capacity to experience prolonged sadness and depression. These physicians also suggested that Black people were more prone to developing dementia praecox (schizophrenia); thus, they did not receive equal treatment compared with their White counterparts.
    b. Psychiatric hospitals during the late 1800s would not admit Black people for care. Epidemiology supported their claims, with data showing that free Black people were insane.
    c. The Sixth U.S. Census of 1840 was used to justify slavery by claiming that the rate of "insanity" among Black people in the North, where they were free, was 11 times higher than among those enslaved in the South.
  3. Unethical practices like those previously discussed influenced the treatment of patients with psychiatric disorders, contributed to the ongoing disparities, and possibly influenced how some clinicians continue to view Black people with psychiatric disturbances.
    a. Unsupported claims violated many ethical principles and unfortunately influenced psychiatric education and clinicians' diagnostic reasoning—manifesting as unconscious bias. This implicit bias is harmful, violating the principle of nonmaleficence, but used diagnostic and treatment approaches that justified slavery, which perpetuated punishment rather than promoting the principles of beneficence.
    b. Nontherapeutic treatment continues today as a disproportionate number of Black people compared with White people with mental illnesses or substance use disorders are incarcerated, rather than being provided mental health or substance use treatment.
B. The influence of past beliefs, based on White supremacist, racist notions, is ever-present today and sustains health disparities, including unequal and unethical treatment, especially for individuals with disabilities, older individuals, and racial, ethnic, and gender/sexual minority groups.
C. Persons with mental illnesses are a vulnerable group who may lack the capacity to make sound decisions; therefore, their rights may be easily compromised.
  1. Patients' ability to make decisions needs to be assessed upon initial evaluation.
  2. APRNs must always uphold the highest values and ethical standards to respect people's fundamental human rights and honor and build trust within the patient–healthcare provider relationship to help their patients progress toward optimum recovery.
D. Diagnosis in psychiatry, due to the lack of evidence-based tools at the time, and racial, ethnic, and gender bias, was historically based on the clinician's judgment, which was informed by these factors.
E. The development of the *Diagnostic and Statistical Manual of Mental Disorders* (*DSM*) in 1952 (American Psychiatric Association, 1952) was not the first attempt to formally classify psychopathology in the United States, with some attempts made in the 19th century that were more focused on policy and treatment regulation.
  1. Revisions since the release of the first *DSM* have been informed by research and other venues based on the changing social theories established by social sciences findings.
  2. One such addition was the outline for cultural formulation introduced in the fourth edition of the *DSM* (*DSM-IV*; American Psychiatric Association, 1994), which placed individuals' mental health problems in historical, social, and cultural context. This multicontextual approach, now called the Cultural Formulation Interview (CFI), has been expanded with the *DSM-5-TR* (5th ed., text rev.; American Psychiatric Association, 2022) to improve culturally sensitive assessment, diagnosis, and treatment by focusing clinical attention on the patient's perspective and social context, as well as to curtail ethical misconduct and misjudgment of the patient's culture and tradition, which may decrease misdiagnosis and inappropriate treatment based on biased observations or erroneous beliefs of healthcare providers.
  3. While the changes to the *DSM* are based on scientific strides and humanitarian intent, it is important to measure such claims by the purported objectives to improve diagnosis and treatment following both psychiatry's professed medical identity, and the new dimensions of the discipline and its practice that are enabled by neuroscience, neurotechnology, genetics, the social sciences, and the humanities. As the *DSM* has progressed (now in its fifth edition, the *DSM-5-TR*; American Psychiatric Association, 2022), the involvement of contemporary users—including scholars, researchers, mental health practitioners, patients, and the public—helps ensure a comprehensive approach to diagnosis and optimal patient outcomes as the science evolves.

RESOURCES

A. Discrimination and Racism in the History of Mental Health Care (National Alliance on Mental Illness): www.nami.org/Blogs/NAMI-Blog/July-2020/Discrimination-and-Racism-in-the-History-of-Mental-Health-Care

B. Psychiatry in the Wake: Racism and the Asylumed South (Southern Spaces): https://southernspaces.org/2021/psychiatry-wake-racism-and-asylumed-south

C. "Blacks Are Immune From Mental Illness" (Psychiatric News): https://psychnews.psychiatryonline.org/doi/full/10.1176/appi.pn.2018.5a18

REFERENCES AND BIBLIOGRAPHY

American Psychiatric Association. (1952). *Diagnostic and statistical manual of mental disorders* (1st ed.). Author.

American Psychiatric Association. (1994). *Diagnostic and statistical manual of mental disorders* (4th ed.). Author.

American Psychiatric Association. (2022). *Diagnostic and statistical manual of mental disorders* (5th ed., text rev.). https://doi.org/10.1176/appi.books.9780890425787

Bevis, W. M. (1921). Psychological traits of the southern negro with observations as to some of his psychoses. *The American Journal of Psychiatry, 78*(1), 69–78. https://doi.org/10.1176/ajp.78.1.69

First, M. B., Yousif, L. H., Clarke, D. E., Wang, P. S., Gogtay, N., & Appelbaum, P. S. (2022). *DSM-5-TR*: Overview of what's new and what's changed. *World Psychiatry, 21*(2), 218. https://onlinelibrary.wiley.com/doi/pdf/10.1002/wps.20989

Hall, G. S. (1904). *Adolescence: Its psychology and its relations to physiology, anthropology, sociology, sex, crime, religion, and education* (Vol. 2). Appleton & Company.

Hall, W. J., Chapman, M. V., Lee, K. M., Merino, Y. M., Thomas, T. W., Payne, B. K., Eng, E., Day, S. H., & Coyne-Beasley, T. (2015). Implicit racial/ethnic bias among health care professionals and its influence on health care outcomes: A systematic review. *American Journal of Public Health, 105*(12), e60–e76. https://doi.org/10.2105/AJPH.2015.302903

Kawa, S., & Giordano, J. (2012). A brief historicity of the *Diagnostic and Statistical Manual of Mental Disorders*: Issues and implications for the future of psychiatric canon and practice [Editorial]. *Philosophy, Ethics, and Humanities in Medicine, 7*, Article 2. https://doi.org/10.1186/1747-5341-7-2

Morrison, A. (2021, July 13). 50-year war on drugs imprisoned millions of Black Americans. *The Associated Press*. https://apnews.com/article/war-on-drugs-75e61c224de3a394235df80de7d70b70

O'Malley, M. (1914). Psychosis in the colored race. *The American Journal of Psychiatry, 1*(2), 309–337. https://doi.org/10.1176/ajp.71.2.309

THE ETHICAL FOUNDATIONS OF NURSING PRACTICE

A. U.S. nurses have continued to have the highest ethical rating among the healthcare professions by the general public according to the Gallup poll.

B. Nursing is a professional discipline that requires the provision of personal care informed by scientific, ethical, and aesthetics.

C. Watson's Theory of Human Caring further stressed that nursing is guided by a moral ideal to protect, enhance, and preserve human dignity.

D. The Code of Ethics for Nurses With Interpretive Statements (The Code) outlines the professional expectations for all nurses, based on the ethical principles of autonomy, beneficence, nonmaleficence, and justice. It also stresses the importance of professionalism and maintaining patient confidentiality.

   1. The American Nurses Association's (ANA's) Code of Ethics is essential in articulating professional expectations for nurses as well as informing society about the ethical obligations and duties expected from this group of healthcare providers.

   2. All people come into the profession with formulated virtues, beliefs, values, and ideas based on their own lived experiences, so complying with a professional code of ethics means infusing their ideas with the codes.

   3. The ANA Code of Ethics provides the expectations of a professional caring behavior; however, this code fails to articulate a course of action for nurses when faced with a specific ethical dilemma.

   4. Without a framework to guide the decision-making process, nurses' personal virtues and beliefs may influence their decisions. The nature of this difficult process explains how two ethically sound nurses can disagree about a clinical course of action since in ethical decision-making there are often, as we have noted, at least two compelling equally right or wrong choices, rather than a clear, objective and formulated right or wrong choice.

E. Ethical decision-making is especially challenging in psychiatry, which is the foundation of theory and practice of psychiatric-mental health nursing. Therefore, APRNs face unique ethical moral dilemmas related to not only their personal beliefs and values, but also to historical beliefs held by others, including physicians, other healthcare providers, theologians, and scientists, that mental illness lacks a biological basis and is a fictitious illness characterized by a moral failing based on individual character deficits.

   1. These beliefs in moral failure were rooted in pseudoscience, racism, and mistreatment of racial, ethnic, and gender/sexual minority groups, and women embraced by the society at large.

   2. Psychiatric-mental health practice is the only healthcare delivery specialty that, as previously noted, has been largely subjective and continues to be influenced by society in areas of diagnostic decision-making, where healthcare providers are asked to make decisions about patient rights, such as individual competence, decision-making, and culpability.

F. Ethical issues in mental health have also occurred in women with serious mental illness (SMI) during the perinatal period. Often, clinicians discontinue psychotherapeutic medications during pregnancy that may increase the risk of poor outcomes for the infant and the mother, or fail to incorporate the mother with SMI in the decision-making process. Box 34.1 depicts an ethical dilemma regarding a woman with SMI and questionable pregnancy.

RESOURCES

A. The Nursing Code of Ethics: Its Value, Its History: https://ojin.nursingworld.org/MainMenuCategories/ANAMarketplace/ANAPeriodicals/OJIN/TableofContents/Vol-20-2015/No2-May-2015/The-Nursing-Code-of-Ethics-Its-Value-Its-History.html

B. Ethics and Human Rights (ANA): www.nursingworld.org/practice-policy/nursing-excellence/ethics

REFERENCES AND BIBLIOGRAPHY

American Nurses Association. (2015). *Code of ethics for nurses with interpretive statements*. American Nurses Association. https://www.nursingworld.org/practice-policy/nursing-excellence/ethics/code-of-ethics-for-nurses

Barrett, M. S. (2012). Ethical decision-making: A framework for understanding and resolving mental health dilemmas. In C. M. Ulrich (Ed.), *Nursing ethics in everyday practice*. Nursing Knowledge.

Brenan, M. (2023, January 10). *Nurses retain top ethics rating in U.S., but below 2020 high*. Gallup. https://news.gallup.com/poll/467804/nurses-retain-top-ethics-rating-below-2020-high.aspx

BOX 34.1 CASE STUDY: WOMAN WITH BIPOLAR DISORDER AND UNCONFIRMED PREGNANCY

M.J. is a 27-year-old, African American woman with bipolar II disorder, first diagnosed in college, who is brought to the psychiatric ED by her mother. She is highly religious, practicing the Pentecostal faith, and does not believe in abortion. Her mother is hoping that she will be admitted to the hospital "before she goes wild." She reports that M.J. cannot keep a job! Over the past 6 weeks, she reports that M.J. has been up around the clock, does not appear tired, constantly moves, rearranges furniture, and cleans the house. She moves items in and outside of the house daily to clean and sanitize them. She has told her boyfriend that she wants to "have a lot of sex even though she is upset with him." M.J. told the APRN: "There is nothing wrong with me. The government is watching my every move!" She says that she has not been able to sleep "because of the neighbors." She says that they talk loudly at night and that she and the baby will "fix that" because babies "wake everyone up at night too!" Her mom seems confused by this comment, saying that M.J. and her boyfriend have no children and that M.J. is not pregnant to her knowledge. Her mother states: "I don't know why she is talking about a baby! I know she is bipolar, but this is pretty crazy; she does not have a baby!" M.J. states that her thoughts are like the "Hartsfield airport!" and that she has "no problem keeping up" with the different "planes coming and going." The patient says that she stopped taking all of her medications about 3 months ago. "I cannot take the lithium, I just do not like it. I don't want it." She has no illicit drug or alcohol use history and no history of suicidal ideation or attempts, or homicidal ideation or attempts.

On the mental status exam, M.J. is a neatly dressed, overweight woman who appears older than her stated age. She is cooperative with the clinical interview and asks that her mom step out of the room when she is talking with the APRN. Her speech is rapid and loud, with a euphoric affect. Her thought form is tangential. She denies auditory or visual hallucinations and reports no thoughts or past attempts of self-harm. M.J. tells the APRN: "I got Bipolar II, I ain't got no Bipolar I—I ain't that messed up. Never have been! Nope! I am so good right now." She does not want to be admitted to the hospital, despite her mom's request, but says she will go to see her psychiatrist the next day. When you ask her if she is pregnant, she tells you, "I might be, I might not be. If I am, I am not getting an abortion!"

Haddad, L. M., & Geiger, R. A. (2023, August 14). *Nursing ethical considerations*. StatPearls Publishing. https://www.ncbi.nlm.nih.gov/books/NBK526054

Ozan, D. Y., Okumus. H., Lash, A. A. (2015). Implementation of Watson's theory of human caring: A case study. *International Journal of Caring Sciences*, 8(1), 25. https://www.internationaljournalofcaringsciences.org/docs/4-Lash%20-%20Original.pdf

Pajnkihar, M., McKenna, H. P., Štiglic, G., & Vrbnjak, D. (2017). Fit for practice: Analysis and evaluation of Watson's theory of human caring. *Nursing Science Quarterly*, 30(3), 243–252. https://doi.org/10.1177/0894318417708409

ETHICAL DECISION-MAKING FOR PATIENTS WITH MENTAL ILLNESS AND UNCONFIRMED PREGNANCY

A. Ethical considerations and treatment plan development: The scenario in Box 34.1 presents both clinical and ethical issues that the APRN must consider when developing a treatment plan for M.J., a 27-year-old patient diagnosed with bipolar II disorder with psychotic features. The complexities of her condition and the ethical principles of autonomy, beneficence, nonmaleficence, and justice must guide the APRN's approach. Although her mother provides essential information, she is not M.J.'s legal conservator, so M.J.'s autonomy remains a critical factor in decision-making. The following section will explain how the APRN can develop a comprehensive treatment plan in light of these ethical principles and clinical details.

B. Here are a select number of decisions the APRN must make, keeping in mind ethical principles:
  1. Does the patient need to be hospitalized?
  2. Does she want/need to have a pregnancy test?
  3. Does she give consent to have lithium levels drawn?

C. The APRN needs to start their ethical decision-making by first centering on the patient and providing the same choices and information as they would to a person without a mental health disorder. This includes the following:
  1. Including the patient in the treatment plan to maintain their autonomy
  2. Assessing the patient's decision-making capacity
  3. Eliciting the patient's beliefs about their current condition and ways to manage the disorder

D. In the dilemma presented in Box 34.1, the APRN faces many ethical dilemmas, including the following:
  1. The APRN must uphold the autonomy of the patient, whose decision-making capacity upon examination appears to be impaired.
  2. If the patient is pregnant, the APRN is obligated to protect the fetus. A decision must also be made regarding the risks and benefits of using psychotropic medications, the potential effect on the developing fetus, and the potential adverse fetal outcomes if psychiatric treatment is withheld.
  3. The APRN must also consider that this patient may have taken lithium, which is teratogenic.

E. To apply the principle of autonomy, the patient needs to be given every opportunity to make their own decision. However, APRNs are often obligated to determine the patient's decision-making capacity. Ultimately, treatment and nontreatment both carry risks, and this can be a challenging decision for an APRN if the patient has active symptoms impacting cognition and judgment.

F. Steps the APRN can take include first noting that all adult patients are presumed to have decision-making capacity despite their psychological state until further assessment proves otherwise.

G. A person's capacity to make decisions depends on their ability to do the following:
  1. Understand the information being presented (comprehension)
  2. Understand the relevance of the information presented in context (appreciation)
  3. Manipulate information rationally, weighing risks and benefits (reasoning)
  4. Clearly and consistently communicate decisions (choice)

H. To promote autonomy, the APRN could start by correcting any factual errors by supplementing the patient's knowledge and explaining their clinical judgment. They could also disclose recommendations about all available treatment options based on the patient's condition, while respecting and helping the patient identify their values and beliefs.

I. The APRN desiring to apply the principle of nonmaleficence, seeking to "do no harm" to the patient in the scenario, needs to be concerned that the patient might have taken lithium. Because her pregnancy status has not been confirmed, the APRN will order a pregnancy test due to the teratogenicity of lithium. However, the APRN would need to teach this information to the patient and assess the patient's level of understanding of the situation and whether it aligns with the patient's beliefs and values.

RESOURCES

A. Our National Network of Perinatal Psychiatry Access Programs (UMass Chan): www.umassmed.edu/lifeline4moms/Access-Programs
B. Maternal Mental Health (World Health Organization): www.who.int/teams/mental-health-and-substance-use/promotion-prevention/maternal-mental-health
C. Caring for Pregnant Women: A Psychiatrist's Guide (American Psychiatric Association): www.psychiatry.org/news-room/apa-blogs/caring-for-pregnant-women-a-psychiatrists-guide

REFERENCES AND BIBLIOGRAPHY

Jeste, D. V., Eglit, G. M. L., Palmer, B. W., Martinis, J. G., Blanck, P., Saks, E. R. (2018). Supported decision making in serious mental illness. *Psychiatry, 81*(1), 28–40. https://doi.org/10.1080/00332747.2017.1324697

McCullough, L. B., Chervenak, F. A., & Coverdale, J. H. (2016). Managing care of an intrapartum patient with agitation and psychosis: Ethical and legal implications. *AMA Journal of Ethics, 8*(3), 209–214. https://doi.org/ 10.1001/journalofethics.2016.18.3.ecas2-1603

Varkey, B. (2021). Principles of clinical ethics and their application to practice. *Medical Principles and Practice, 30*(1), 17–28. https://doi.org/10.1159/000509119

DECISION-MAKING FOR PATIENTS WITH SEVERE MENTAL ILLNESS

A. Because the patient described in Box 34.1 has a severe mental illness and the pregnancy test was positive, the decision has to be made about the possible impact of lithium on the fetus. The APRN applying the principle of autonomy seeks to allow the patient to make her own decision and could therefore pursue interventions to employ (a) assisted, (b) supported, or (c) surrogate decision-making.

  1. Assisted decision-making: The APRN identifies impairments that they need to address to restore the patient's decision-making capacity using respectful persuasion in alignment with clinical recommendations to achieve favorable outcomes. In this case, the mania the patient is experiencing needs to be managed before she can engage in the decision-making process. Restoration of the patient's decision-making capacity could be accomplished with the use of psychotropics or other evidence-based treatments.
  2. Supported decision-making: This involves the patient enlisting family members, friends, and other trusted individuals or entities (e.g., National Alliance on Mental Illness [NAMI] or community health workers and therapists) to promote autonomy and augment the patient's decision-making capacity. This type of decision-making provides a less restrictive alternative to guardianship. These enlisted individuals generally know and understand the wishes of the patient and can make decisions based on the patient's desires.
  3. Surrogate decision-making: If assisted or supported decision-making fails to be effective, the APRN needs to then consult with the applicable state laws to identify and prioritize potential surrogate decision-makers who can identify the patient's values and beliefs and make decisions accordingly. If the patient's wishes are not known, the surrogate decision-maker needs to make decisions based on the patient's best interest, which is a beneficence-based standard. Ethical decision-making for pregnant patients with mental illness is a complex process. APRNs must balance the patient's autonomy with the need to protect the fetus. They must also consider the patient's decision-making capacity and seek interventions to promote autonomy whenever possible.

RESOURCE

A. Shared Decision Making: Empowering People Living With Mental Illness (National Alliance on Mental Illness): www.nami.org/nami-news/shared-decision-making-empowering-people-living-with-mental-illness

CONCLUSION: ETHICAL IMPERATIVE TODAY

A. APRNs need to exercise the principle of autonomy to ensure patients have the necessary information to make informed decisions about their care despite their mental health status or level of judgment and/or insight about their condition.
B. Patients must be educated and encouraged to actively participate in their care even if it means sometimes being supported by others.
C. APRNs hold a great responsibility for the safety of their patients, themselves, and others. Psychiatric-mental health nurse practitioners (PMHNPs) are responsible for being honest, truthful, and transparent with their patients and being open to communication about treatment options, risks and benefits of mental health interventions, and potential adverse outcomes. Any urge to provide false information or to use coercive methods when delivering care to patients must be avoided.
D. All patients deserve the right to receive the best care that encompasses the principles of justice and fairness regardless of race, ethnicity, gender, age, and sexual orientation. Therefore, APRNs must advocate for and provide equitable care and ensure that their patients have access to evidence-based mental healthcare. APRNs must understand that a mental health disorder does not exclude individuals from being treated with respect and dignity.
E. Bioethical principles must be practiced to ensure patients' rights are protected and respected, and ensure that APRNs embody professionalism, are legally protected, and act with integrity in the best interest of their patients. By understanding the codes and standards outlined by the ANA and being aware of how history has influenced the field, APRNs can ensure that their practice is ethically sound.

35 CAREGIVER AND END-OF-LIFE ISSUES

Denise Snow

INTRODUCTION

The term *carer*, or *informal carer*, is widely used in health-related policy and research and refers to unpaid caring, usually by family members or close friends, for someone who is ill, is frail, or has a disability. However, most of these millions of unpaid carers will not recognize themselves as such and will describe themselves simply as "family" or "friend" and may thus be best termed *family caregiver*.

THE CAREGIVER'S BURDEN

A. Increasingly, families are performing medical care tasks in the home that in the past would have been performed by licensed professionals (AARP & National Alliance for Caregiving, 2020).
B. Dr. Lynn Hallarman, a palliative care doctor, described her own experience with caregiving: "The intensity of caregiving maps directly to the deteriorating daily function of the care recipient.... One week, a caregiver can be assisting with the basics of daily living for a recipient with moderate functional impairments, and the next week can be in charge of managing the totality of a person's bodily needs" (Hallarman, 2021, pp. 791–792).
C. Hospitalization may result when the needs of the loved ones become more than the caregiver can provide, despite the stated desires of the individual at end of life.
D. Patients' needs change day-to-day, often occurring with a fall and other common hospitalizations such as pneumonia or urinary tract infection.
E. Family members of individuals with chronic illness may not recognize a decline in their loved one as they provide daily care and may be surprised to learn from the healthcare provider the extent of decline. The healthcare provider can clarify the prognosis and the likely course of the illness/stage of dying.
F. The aging U.S. population has tremendous impact on healthcare dynamics, particularly for those with long-term care needs.
  1. Most aging individuals rely on family and friends for assistance—whether out of a sense of love, loyalty, or obligation, or because there is simply no one else to help.
  2. As more individuals are living into their 90s, children who would be caregivers for their parents may be well into their 70s.
  3. Commonly, one older adult spouse has the sole responsibility of caring for their partner with a disability.
G. Clinicians have a professional responsibility to support caregivers as they become key in long-term care.
  1. More than one in five Americans (21.3%) are caregivers, having provided care to an adult or child with special needs at some time in the past 12 months (AARP & National Alliance for Caregiving, 2020). This reflects 53 million adults serving as caregivers in the United States, an increase from the estimated 43.5 million caregivers in 2015.
  2. Many caregivers take on this role without adequate and affordable services and support in place.
  3. Caregivers may be providing assistance with activities of daily living (ADLs) and instrumental activities of daily living (IADLs), in addition to managing complex medical conditions of those who receive long-term care.
  4. Fewer than one-third of caregivers report receiving paid help. Family caregivers must navigate complicated systems and coordinate care across various services.
  5. Many caregivers have no alternative to being the sole provider of care. Eligibility for long-term care services in the current healthcare system is convoluted, complex, costly, and can be frustrating. Even in cases of eligibility for long-term care services through programs such as Medicaid, fewer individuals pursue this type of work. Homecare agencies report that in many rural areas there are no aides available. Hourly pay is often twice the national minimum wage, and transportation to the recipient's home may be a barrier.
H. While many caregivers feel their role has given them a sense of purpose or meaning, they are also often exhausted. Providing around-the-clock care is physically demanding. Caregivers may suffer from loss of sleep, with no respite from their task, and for many this can be isolating. Providing full-time care to another restricts the caregiver's ability to meet their own health needs. The stress of caregiving may exacerbate health issues, especially for aging caregivers. Compounding physical and emotional strain, family caregivers may experience financial strain through diminished employment related to caregiving and paying for services on behalf of the care recipient, which can have long-term implications on the caregiver's financial security. According to an AARP survey:
  1. 1 in 5 caregivers report high financial strain as a result of caregiving.
  2. 4 in 10 have experienced at least one financial impact as a result of their caregiving.
  3. 3 in 10 have stopped saving.
  4. 1 in 4 have taken on more debt.
  5. 1 in 4 have used up their personal short-term savings.
  6. 2 in 10 have left bills unpaid or paid them late.
  7. 1 in 10 have been unable to afford basic expenses like food (AARP & National Alliance for Caregiving, 2020, p. 7).

COMMUNITY-BASED CARE

A. Many if not most individuals experiencing declining health through chronic and acute health conditions have a definite preference for remaining in their homes rather than prolonged hospitalization, rehabilitation, and skilled nursing facilities.
B. The shift in healthcare to community-based settings rather than institutional care settings puts additional pressure on families to fill the gaps in long-term and end-of-life care.
C. From a policy perspective, at first glance, it appears that use of family caregivers reduces costs for community-based

care. However, family caregivers who cannot care for themselves may become unavailable to care for others; likewise, caregivers have their own financial, health, and wellness needs. As caregivers' health and finances erode, the cost of community-based care may very well become greater rather than reduced.

D. Many family caregivers rely on health professionals for information and support needs related to caring for the recipient, such as how to keep the recipient safe at home and navigating systems for services and completing the necessary forms and paperwork. Very few caregivers report having conversations with health professionals about what they need to care for their recipient or to support their own well-being.

E. It is critical to identify the psychological and physical stress involved in giving care, especially when the need for care is 24 hours 7 days a week. However, as professionals, it is equally critical to avoid assumptions about those who give "informal" care. Most caregivers do not describe the care they give as *informal* as this term may be perceived by some as being less important than "paid" care. Also often overlooked is the sense of self-worth by those providing care. Caring, especially in the end-of-life scenario, is often accompanied by a mix of stress and self-satisfaction in providing care and comfort to a loved one. Equally important considerations include cultural variations, age or gender of the carer precare relationship, and the presence of other sources of support in the family and community. Practitioners involved with end-of-life treatment plans are well-versed in including the family in any plan of care.

ADVOCATING FOR THE CAREGIVERS

A. End-of-life care recipients may require more care than the family or friend caregiver can provide. If a patient has been placed on home hospice, Medicare will provide resources such as intermittent visits from a nurse and a personal care aide for several hours per week. Often, this is insufficient to meet the needs of the end-of-life patient and the family has few choices to supplement the care.

   1. A personal care aide may be privately hired by contacting a homecare agency; the patient or the caregiver will then be responsible for paying for the aide services out of pocket on an hourly basis.

   2. Patients and caregivers may apply for Medicaid long-term care under the "Medically Needy" category. Note that most states have enacted this category of Medicaid. If approved, Medicaid will assess the individual's homecare needs and provide a personal care aide to meet those needs. However, Medicaid is needs-based and has both an income level and a resource level of eligibility. State by state guidelines on eligibility can be found on the Medicaid.gov website.

B. Providing care to individuals with serious illness requires the ability to have difficult but critical discussions with families regarding end of life and the eventuality of "letting go." These discussions may be facilitated by skilled social workers, case managers, and/or faith-based leaders. Having these discussions with professionals may relieve family members of the burden of this role.

   1. There are several ways the healthcare provider can initiate these discussions, but remaining open and available to the family is key.

BOX 35.1 RESOURCES FOR FAMILY CAREGIVERS

Family Caregiver Alliance: *National Center on Caregiving*
(415) 434-3388 | (800) 445-8106
Website: www.caregiver.org
Email: info@caregiver.org
CareNav: https://fca.cacrc.org/login

Services by state: www.caregiver.org/connecting-caregivers/services-by-state

Aging Life Care Association (formerly National Association of Professional Geriatric Care Managers)
This professional group offers a listing of care managers nationwide.
www.aginglifecare.org

Compassion and Choices
www.compassionandchoices.org

National Hospice and Palliative Care Organization
www.nhpco.org

Hospice Foundation of America
www.hospicefoundation.org

Five Wishes: *Aging with Dignity*
Five Wishes is a document that helps you express how you want to be treated in the event you become seriously ill and unable to speak for yourself.
www.agingwithdignity.org

National POLST
Objective information provided about this advanced care planning tool. Offers a current POLST (portable medical order) program map by state and a downloadable POLST form.
www.polst.org

---

   2. Sensitivity to the stress of the family caregiver will enable the healthcare professional to provide information and support to the family regarding treatment options, do not resuscitate (DNR) orders, advance directives such as a living will, and physician orders for life sustaining treatment (POLST), which allow the individual to state whether or not they want to be resuscitated, and whether or not they would want a feeding tube, ventilator, and other treatments (Box 35.1).

   3. It is critical that the decisions reflect the individual's personal values and beliefs. Having these difficult and painful conversations allows the family time to process feelings of doubt, guilt, or blame that may surface within the family dynamic.

REFERENCES AND BIBLIOGRAPHY

AARP & National Alliance for Caregiving. (2020, May). *2020 report: Caregiving in the U.S.* https://www.aarp.org/content/dam/aarp/ppi/2020/05/full-report-caregiving-in-the-united-states.doi.10.26419-2Fppi.00103.001.pdf

Greenwood, N., McKevitt, C., & Milne, A. (2018). Time to rebalance and reconsider: Are we pathologising informal, family carers? *Journal of the Royal Society of Medicine, 111*(7), 253–254 https://doi.org/1177/0141076818779204

Hallarman, L. (2021). The great escape—a physician confronts family caregiving during the COVID-19 pandemic. *JAMA Neurology, 78*(7), 791–792. https://doi.org/10.1001/jamaneurol.2021.1170

U.S. Census Bureau. (2022, June 30). *Nation continues to age as it becomes more diverse* [Press release]. https://www.census.gov/newsroom/press-releases/2022/population-estimates-characteristics.html

APPENDIX: CODING REFERENCE FOR PSYCHIATRIC CONDITIONS

Complete codes will need to be assessed by use of the *International Classification of Diseases*, 11th Revision (*ICD-11*; World Health Organization, 2019), coding tool, and for the *Diagnostic and Statistical Manual of Mental Disorders*, Fifth Edition, Text Revision (*DSM-5-TR*; American Psychiatric Association, 2022), please refer to the *DSM-5-TR* manual for coding related to acuity. Codes listed in the following table are reflective of the least acute diagnosis.

The *ICD-11* was officially launched by the World Health Organization in 2019; however, the United States has not yet adopted it for clinical or billing use.

The *ICD-11* is accessible worldwide, yet the implementation process in the United States is expected to be gradual, necessitating updates to systems, training, and regulatory changes. At this printing, the *ICD-10-CM* (10th Revision, Clinical Modification) is the prevailing standard in the United States for health records and insurance claims.

Disorder, Condition, or Problem	ICD-11 Code(s)	DSM-5-TR Diagnostic Code(s)
Alcohol Use Disorder	6C40.Z	F10.10, F10.20
Anorexia Nervosa	6B80.Z	F50.01, F50.02
Antisocial Personality Disorder	6D10.0–6D11	F60.2
Anxiety Disorders	6B00–6B0Z	F41.1
Avoidant Personality Disorder	6D10.0–6D10.Z	F60.6
Avoidant/Restrictive Food Intake Disorder	6B83	F50.8
Binge Eating Disorder	6B82	F50.8
Bipolar Disorder I	6A60Z	F06.33, F06.34, F31
Bipolar Disorder II	6A61.Z	F31.81
Borderline Personality Disorder	6D10.Z	F60.3
Brief Psychotic Disorder	6A23.Z	F23
Bulimia Nervosa	6B81.Z	F50.2
Cannabis Use Disorder	6C41.Z	F10.10, F12.10
Circadian Rhythm Sleep–Wake Disorders	7A60–7A6Z	G47.20–G47.24, G47.26
Conversion Disorder (Functional Neurological Symptom Disorder)	6B60.Z	F44.4–F44.7
Cyclothymic Disorders	6A62	F34.0
Delirium	6D70.0–6D70.Z	F05.9 unspecified
Delusional Disorder	6A24.Z	F22
Dependent Personality Disorder	6D10	F60.7
Dissociative Identity Disorder	6B64	F44.81
Eating Disorder, Other Specified	6B8Y	F50.8
Eating Disorder, Unspecified	6B8Z	F50.9
Factitious Disorder	6D5.Z	F68.10
Generalized Anxiety Disorder	6B00	F41.1
Hallucinogen Use Disorder	6C49	F16.10, F16.20
Histrionic Personality Disorder	6D10.Z	F60.4

(continued)

Disorder, Condition, or Problem	ICD-11 Code(s)	DSM-5-TR Diagnostic Code(s)
Illness Anxiety Disorder	6B23.Z	F45.21
Insomnia	7A00, 7A01, 7A0Z	G47.00
Major Depressive Disorder	6A70–6A7Y	F32.0–F32.5, F32.9
Mild Neurocognitive Disorders	6D71	G31.84
Narcissistic Personality Disorder	6D10.Z	F60.81
Narcolepsy	7A20.0–7A20.Z	G47.411, G47.419, G47.429
Obsessive-Compulsive Disorder	6B20, 6B2Y, 6B2Z	F42
Opioid Use Disorder	6C43.Z	F11.10, F11.20
Panic Disorder	6B01	F41.0
Parasomnias	7B0Y, 7B0Z	
Persistent Depressive Disorder (Dysthymia)	6A72	F34.1
Personality Disorder, Unspecified	6D10.Z	F60.9
Phobias	6B0Z, 6B03	F40.218, F40.228, F40.230–233, F40.248, F40.298
Pica	6B84	F50.8, F98.3
Posttraumatic Stress Disorder	6B40, 6B41	F43.10
Premenstrual Dysphoric Disorder	GA34.41	N94.3
Psychotic Disorder Due to Another Medical Condition	6G4G.6	F06.0, F06.2
Restless Legs Syndrome	7A80	G25.81
Rumination Disorder	6B85	F98.21
Schizoaffective Disorder	6A21.Z	F25.0, F25.1
Schizoid Personality Disorder	6D10.Z	F60.1
Schizophrenia	6A20.Z	F20.9
Schizophreniform Disorder		F20.81
Selective Mutism	6B06	F94.0
Separation Anxiety Disorder	6B05	F93.0
Sleep Disordered Breathing/Obstructive Sleep Apnea	7A41	G47.33
Social Anxiety Disorder	6B04	F40.10
Somatic Symptom Disorder	6C20.Z	F45.1
Somatic Symptoms, Other Specified/Unspecified	6C20.Z	F45.8
Stimulant Use Disorder	6C46.Z	F15.10, F15.20
Substance-Induced Bipolar and Related Disorder		F19.180, F19.280, F19.980
Substance-Induced Psychotic Disorders	6C4G.6, 6C4F.6, 6C4E.6	
Substance-Induced Psychotic Disorders, Alcohol (Alcohol-Induced Psychotic Disorder, Unspecified)	6C40.6Z	F10.159, F10.259, F10.959
Substance-Induced Psychotic Disorders, Amphetamine (Stimulant-Induced Psychotic Disorder Including Amphetamines, Methamphetamine, or Methcathinone, Unspecified)	6C46.6Z	F15.159, F15.259, F15.959

(continued)

Disorder, Condition, or Problem	ICD-11 Code(s)	DSM-5-TR Diagnostic Code(s)
Substance-Induced Psychotic Disorders, Cannabis (Cannabis-Induced Psychotic Disorder)	6C41.6	F12.159, F12.259, F12.959
Substance-Induced Psychotic Disorders, Cocaine (Cocaine-Induced Psychotic Disorder, Unspecified)	6C45.6Z	F14.159, F14.259, F14.959
Substance-Induced Psychotic Disorders, Inhalant (Volatile Inhalant-Induced Psychotic Disorder)	6C4B.6	F18.159, F18.259, F18.959
Substance-Induced Psychotic Disorders, Other (Psychotic Disorder Induced by Unknown or Unspecified Psychoactive Substance)	6C4G.6	F19.159, F19.259, F19.959
Substance-Induced Psychotic Disorders, Other Hallucinogen (Hallucinogen-Induced Psychotic Disorder)	6C49.5	F16.159, F16.259, F16.959
Substance-Induced Psychotic Disorders, Phencyclidine (Dissociative Drug-Induced Psychotic Disorder Including Ketamine or PCP)	6C4D.5	F16.159, F16.259, F16.959
Substance-Induced Psychotic Disorders, Sedative, Hypnotic, or Anxiolytic (Sedative-, Hypnotic- or Anxiolytic-Induced Psychotic Disorder)	6C44.6	F13.159, F13.259, F16.959
Tobacco Use Disorder	6C4A.1Z	F17.200, F17.203, Z72.0

REFERENCES

American Psychiatric Association. (2022). *Diagnostic and statistical manual of mental disorders* (5th ed.; text rev.). https://doi.org/10.1176/appi.books.9780890425787

National Center for Health Statistics. (2015). *International statistical classification of diseases* (10th rev.; clinical modification). Centers for Disease Control and Prevention; World Health Organization. https://www.cdc.gov/nchs/icd/icd-10-cm/index.html

World Health Organization. (n.d.). *ICD-11 coding tool*. https://icd.who.int/ct/icd11_mms/en/release

World Health Organization. (2019). *International statistical classification of diseases* (11th rev.). https://icd.who.int

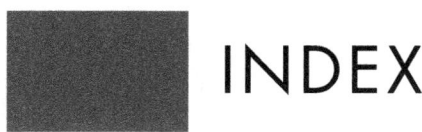

INDEX

abnormal illness behavior concept, 253
acceptance and commitment therapy (ACT), 422
accountable care organizations (ACOs), 7
acetylcholinesterase (AChE) inhibitors, 77
acromegaly, 478
actigraphy, 215
active listening, 12
acute porphyrias, 478
acute psychiatric care setting
  challenges and tools, 413–414
  clinical decision-making process, 413–414
  clinicians education and training, 407
  collaborative care and referrals, 414–415
  cultural diversity, 404
  healthcare professionals attitudes, 406
  individual and group therapy, 403
  inpatient, 414–415
  lack of knowledge, 405
  legislative reform and advocacy, 407–408
  mental illness, 411–412
  mood disorders, 404
  myths and biases, 404
  negative attitudes, 406
  outpatient, 415
  patient and family engagement, 412–413
  persons with mental illness, 407
  psychiatric emergencies, 404–405
  psychoeducation, 403
  research, 408–409
  risk and protective factors, 409–411
  shame, 405
  stigma, 405, 407
  therapeutic interventions, 406–407
  violence risk, 405
adjustment disorders, 44, 57–58, 249
Administration on Aging (AoA), 348
administrative agency, 464
adolescents. *See also* children and adolescents
  development, 326–327
  generalized anxiety disorder, 119
  illness anxiety disorder, 121
  mental health problems, 327–329
  obsessive-compulsive disorder, 124
  panic disorder, 126
  stages, 328
aducanumab, late life psychosis, 77
Adult ADHD Self-Report Scale, 45
adult psychiatric assessment
  active listening, 35
  chief complaint, 35
  developmental history, 38–39
  educational history, 40
  family history, 40
  general medical history, 37–38
  history of present illness, 35–36
  history of psychiatric illness, 36–37
  history of substance use, 37
  informed consent, 35
  mental status examination, 41
  observation, 35
  occupational history, 40
  patient identification, 35
  psychosocial history, 39
  questionnaires/rating scales, 42
  rapport building, 34, 35
  risk assessment, 42
  sociocultural history, 39–40
advanced practice registered nurses (APRNs)
  barriers to, 7
  ethical decision-making, 498–499
  ethical foundations, 497
  private psychiatric APRN practice
    behavioral health, 434
    benefits, 429
    business evaluation, 442–443
    business plan/outcomes, 439–442
    competitive analysis, 434–435
    diagnosis, 437–439
    economic assessment, 434
    executive function skills, 431
    experience assessment, 431–432
    family circumstances, 432
    federal regulatory laws, 432–433
    goals and plans, 441
    ideal patient, 434
    implementation, 442
    interprofessional collaboration, 432
    leadership skills assessment, 431
    location considerations, 433–434
    market analysis, 433
    marketing and advertising, 441–442
    moral compass, 431
    motivation and goals assessment, 430–431
    needs assessment, 433–435
    office, 435–437
    patient benefits, 429–430
    payment models, 435
    personal financial style, 431
    plan development, 430–433
    professional limitations, 432
    risk management, 442
    self-assessment, 430
adverse childhood experiences (ACEs), 19, 21
Adverse Childhood Experiences Questionnaire, 45
advocacy, telehealth, 462
Affordable Care Act, 465
aging and older adult populations
  APRN challenges and tools, 346–348
  assessment, 344–345
  community care settings, 342, 343
  data analysis, 345
  diagnostic uncertainties, 346
  end-of-life care decisions, 347
  family-centered care, 345–346
  healthcare system navigation, 347
  partnerships and referrals, 348
  protective factors, 344
  reassessment, 345
  resource limitations, 346–347
  resources, 348–349
  risk factors, 343–344
  unconscious biases and myths, 342–343
alcohol behavioral couples therapy (ABCT), 268
alcohol use disorder (AUD), 265–269
  definition, 265
  diagnosis and screenings, 266
  older adults, 268
  pregnancy, 268–269
  prevalence, 266
  psychosocial interventions, 267–268
  treatment, 266–268
  young individuals, 268
Alcohol Use Disorders Identification Test (AUDIT), 44
Alcoholics Anonymous (AA), 267
allostatic load, 190
alopecia areata, 474
alternative payment models (APMs), 433
altitude sickness, 485
Altman Self-Rating Mania Scale (ASRM), 90
Alzheimer disease, 472
Alzheimer's Association, 349
ambivalence, 263
amenorrhea, 145
American Academy of Child and Adolescent Psychiatry, 26
American Association of Retired Persons (AARP), 348
American healthcare model, 315
American Nurses Credentialing Center (ANCC), 3
American Psychiatric Nurses Association (APNA), 4
anorexia nervosa (AN)
  comorbidities, 150
  definitions, 138
  diagnostic criteria, 146
  differential diagnoses, 144
  incidence, 139
  pathogenesis, 139
Antecedent-Behavior-Consequence (ABC) chart, 363
antidepressants
  anxiety disorders, 82
  dissociative disorders, 116
  eating disorders, 152

anti-N-methyl-D-aspartate receptor (NMDAR) autoimmune encephalitis, 478–479
anti-N-methyl-D-aspartate receptor (NMDAR) encephalitis, 191
antipsychotics
　for brief psychotic disorder, 285–287
　for dissociative disorders, 116
antisocial personality disorder, 197–198
anxiety disorders (ADs), 144
　autonomic symptoms, 114
　brain and mind symptoms, 114
　chest and abdominal symptoms, 114
　classification, 113
　clinical features, 82
　definition, 81, 113
　dissociative disorders, 115–117
　environmental and psychological risk factors, 82
　environmental factors, 114
　etiology, 81, 114
　family history, 114
　generalized anxiety disorder (GAD), 117–119
　generalized/nonspecific symptoms, 114
　geriatrics, 81–82
　illness anxiety disorder (IAD), 119–121
　incidence, 113
　medication-induced, 121–122
　neurobiology, 114
　obsessive-compulsive disorder (OCD), 122–124
　panic disorder, 124–126
　pediatrics, 53–56
　phobias, 126–128
　physical complaints, 113
　physical examination, 115
　posttraumatic stress disorder, 128–131
　predisposing/risk factors, 113
　prevalence, 81, 114
　psychological complaints, 113
　psychometric tools, 115
　racial discrimination, 114
　screening tools, 44
　selective mutism, 131–132
　separation anxiety disorder, 132–134
　social anxiety disorder, 134–136
　substance use, 114
　treatment, 82
anxiolytics
　for generalized anxiety disorder, 118
　for posttraumatic stress disorder, 129
applied behavioral analysis (ABA), 104–105
APRNs. *See* advanced practice registered nurses
Ask Suicide-Screening Questions (ASQ), 65, 68, 169
assigned female at birth (AFAB), 473
assigned male at birth (AMAB), 473
assisted decision-making, 499
atopic dermatitis, 474
attention deficit hyperactivity disorder (ADHD), 351, 359–360

adults assessments, 91–92
pediatric assessments, 91
pediatrics, 60
screening questions, 60
atypical stroke–stroke chameleons, 481
Autism Diagnostic Observation Schedule, Second Edition (ADOS-2), 356
autism spectrum disorder (ASD), 104, 359, 365–366
　pediatrics, 60–61
　screening questions, 61
Autism Spectrum Quotient (AQ), 355
autocratic leadership, 431
autoimmune diseases, 481
automatic thoughts, 95
avoidant personality disorder, 199–200
avoidant/restrictive food intake disorder (ARFID), 71
　comorbidities, 150
　definition, 137–138
　diagnostic criteria, 148
　differential diagnoses, 144
　incidence and prevalence, 139

balance billing, 465
Beck Depression Inventory (BDI), 44
Beck Depression Inventory 2 (BDI-2), 90
behavior modification, eating disorders, 152
behavior theory, 131
behavior therapy, somatization disorder, 83
behavioral and emotional disorders, 45
behavioral and psychological symptoms in dementia (BPSD), 77
Behavioral Risk Factor Surveillance System (BRFSS), 19
benzodiazepines, 79, 281
　for anxiety disorders, 82
　for generalized anxiety disorder, 118
beta-blockers, 116
binge eating, 71
binge eating disorders (BEDs)
　comorbidities, 150
　definitions, 138
　diagnostic criteria, 147–148
　differential diagnoses, 144
　incidence, 139
　pathogenesis, 140
binge/intoxication stage, drug addiction, 176
bioethics, 495
　history, 495
　philosophical principles, 496
biopsychosocial (BPS) model, 49, 239, 262
bipolar disorder
　consultation and referral, 160–161
　definition, 157
　diagnostic tests and screening, 158
　differential diagnosis, 158
　follow-up, 160
　incidence, 157
　partners/family, 161
　pathogenesis, 157

　patient teaching, 158
　pediatrics, 53, 161
　physical examination, 158
　predisposing factors, 157
　pregnancy, 161
　signs and symptoms, 157
　subjective data, 158
　treatment, 158–160
　types, 157
bizarre delusions, 289
blast-related TBI, 398–399
body dysmorphic disorder (BDD), 250, 257
body language, 6
body mass index (BMI), 38
bone densitometry, feeding and eating disorders, 143
borderline personality disorder (BPD), 25, 96, 144, 246
　complaints, 201
　consultation and referrals, 202
　definition, 200
　diagnostic tests and screening, 201
　differential diagnosis, 201
　follow-up, 202
　medication management, 202
　pathogenesis, 200
　pediatrics, 202
　physical examination, 201
　predisposing factors, 200–201
　prevalence and incidence, 200
　signs and symptoms, 201
　treatment, 201–202
Borderline Personality Screener (BPS), 45
Brain Research Through Advancing Innovative Neurotechnologies (BRAIN), 420
Brief Addiction Monitor (BAM), 44
Brief Psychiatric Rating Scale (BPRS), 85, 293
brief psychotic disorder
　antipsychotics, 285–287
　consultation and referrals, 285
　definition, 283
　diagnostic tests and screening, 284
　differential diagnosis, 284
　follow-up, 285
　geriatrics/older adults, 288, 290
　partners/family, 288
　pathogenesis, 284
　patient teaching, 285
　pediatrics, 288
　physical examination, 284
　predisposing factors, 284
　pregnancy, 288
　prevalence, 284
　signs and symptoms, 284
　subjective data, 284
　treatment, 284–285
Brief Screener for Alcohol, Tobacco, and Other Drugs (BSTAD), 89
brief strategic family therapy (BSFT), alcohol use disorder, 267
Brown Attention-Deficit Disorder Scales (BADDS), 92

bulimia nervosa (BN)
  comorbidities, 150
  definitions, 138
  diagnostic criteria, 146–147
  differential diagnoses, 144
  incidence, 139
  pathogenesis, 140
  risk factors, 147
  severity, 147
bullying, 314
buprenorphine, 179–180, 272–274, 276–277
business associate agreement (BAA), 454–455
buspirone, 118, 129

CAGE Questionnaire, 44
Calgary Depression Scale for Schizophrenia (CDSS), 293
Camouflaging Autistic Traits Questionnaire (CAT-Q), 355
cannabis use disorder (CUD), 269–270
capacity, medical decision, 467
carbon monoxide (CO) poisoning, 484–485
cardiovascular disease, 472
caregiver
  advocating, 501
  burden, 500
  community-based care, 500–501
carer, 500
Car, Relax, Alone, Forget, Friends, Trouble (CRAFFT) assessment scale, 44, 70, 89
case formulation, 42–43
cataplexy, 485
catatonia, 283, 365
Center for Youth Wellness Adverse Childhood Experiences Questionnaires (ACE-Qs), 332
Centers for Medicare & Medicaid Services (CMS), 433
cerebral palsy (CP), 350
challenging behaviors, 361
change talk, 264, 337
chief complaint, in assesment, 35
child study team (CST), 329
childhood/juvenile arthritis, 350
childhood sexual abuse (CSA), 473
children and adolescents
  advanced practice registered nurse, 335
  adverse childhood experiences, 331–332
  collaboration, 330–331
  confidentiality, 329–330
  development, 326–327
  evidence-based practice, 336
  HEADSS assessment, 332–333
  healthcare decision-making capacity, 329
  mental health problems, 327–329
  mental healthcare and primary care providers partnership, 335–336
  motivational interviewing, 336–340
  preventive care, 326
  trauma, 331–333
  trauma-informed care to practice, 335
  treatment adherence, 333–334
  unconscious biases and myths, 331
Children's Health Insurance Program (CHIP), 433, 441
cholestasis, pregnancy, 178
chronic homelessness, 369–370
chronic obstructive pulmonary disease (COPD), 485
chronic sleep disorders, 216
chronic traumatic encephalopathy (CTE), 484
cigarette smoking, 38
circadian rhythm sleep–wake disorder, 225–226
clarification, 14
classical conditioning, 104
clichés, nontherapeutic communication, 15
clinical decision support (CDS) tools, 448
Clinical Global Impression for Schizoaffective Disorder Scale (CGI-SCA), 293
Clinical Global Impression-Severity Scale (CGI-S), 408–409
Clinical Laboratory Improvement Amendments of 1988 (CLIA), 440
Clinical Opioid Withdrawal Scale (COWS), 271, 272
closed-ended questioning, 14
cloud-based systems, 445
coalition, 105
cognitive behavioral groups, 107
cognitive behavioral skills therapy (CBST), community care, 422
cognitive behavioral therapy (CBT)
  components, 95
  constructs, 94
  overview, 94
  somatization disorder, 83
  substance use disorders, 264–265
  training and certification, 95
cognitive behavioral therapy for eating disorders (CBT-ED), 152
cognitive disorders, screening tools, 45
cognitive distortions, 95, 265
cognitive restructuring, 95
coinsurance, 465
collaborative care model, 435
collective trauma, 23
Columbia-Suicide Severity Rating Scale (C-SSRS), 44
commercial/private insurance, 465
common law, 464
communication disorders (CD), 351
communication process, 9–10
  cultural considerations, 15–16
  nontherapeutic, 14–15
Communities of Healing program, 155
community care, 500–501
  CHANGE tool and action, 419
  community assessment, 418–419
  definition, 417
  healthcare cost, 423
  individual providers and agencies, 421–422
  inpatient vs. outpatient care, 417–418
  mental healthcare, 420
  protective factors, 421
  research and assistance organizations, 420–421
  risk factors, 421
  treatment disparity, 418
community health workers (CHWs), 386
Community Mental Health Act (CMHA), 417
community outreach center (COC), 387
community outreach programs, 386–387
comorbidities and mental health, 471
  cardiovascular disease, 472
  gastrointestinal disorders, 472–473
  genitourinary disorders, 473–474
  head and neck disorders, 471–472
  integumentary disorders, 474
  interventions, 475
  learning disorders, 475
  migraine and headaches, 475
  musculoskeletal disorders, 474
  respiratory diseases, 472
  seizure disorder, 475
  somatic conditions, 474–475
competence, 10, 467
complementary and alternative medicine (CAM)
  alcohol use disorder, 268
  dissociative disorders, 116
  generalized anxiety disorder, 118
  posttraumatic stress disorder, 130
  tobacco use disorder, 280
complex posttraumatic stress disorder (CPTSD), 24, 25
comprehensive resource model (CRM), 103
compulsions, 122
conditioned response (CR), 104
conditioned stimulus (CS), 104
conduct disorder (CD)
  assessment questions, 63
  maladaptive and antisocial behaviors, 63
  pediatrics, 62–63
  screening tools for, 63
Conners' Adult ADHD Rating Scales (CAARS™), 91–92
conservatorship, 467
contingency management, alcohol use disorder, 268
conversion disorder, 59, 239–244
coordinated entry system (CES), 386
copay, 465
coronary heart disease (CHD), 472
corrosive disadvantage, 16
Council for Affordable Quality Healthcare (CAQH), 441
countertransference, 100
COVID-19 pandemic, homelessness, 373–375
credibility, 11

Cross-Cutting Symptom Checklists, 44
cultural competence, 305, 395–396
cultural competence model (CCM), 305
cultural competency
    homeless and indigent populations, 381–382
    veterans and survivors of war, 392–395
cultural considerations
    clinical practice, 305–306
    cultural competence, 305
    cultural humility, 305
    psychiatric medications, 306
    treatment plans, 306
Cultural Formulation Interview (CFI), 87, 496
    informant version, 87
    supplementary modules, 87
Cultural Formulation Interview-With Patient, 86–87
cultural humility, 305
culture, 10, 15
Cushing syndrome, 479
cybernetics, 106
cyclothymia, 161–162

Danger Assessment Tools (DATools), 44
delirium, 482
    clinical presentation, 77–78
    etiology, 77
    history, 77
    incidence, 77
    in older adults, 77–78
    prevalence, 77
    treatment, 78
delusional disorder, 257, 288–290
    consultation and referrals, 285
    definition, 288–289
    diagnostic tests and screening, 289
    differential diagnosis, 289
    follow-up, 290
    incidence, 289
    partners/family, 290
    pathogenesis, 289
    patient teaching, 290
    pediatrics, 290
    predisposing factors, 289
    pregnancy, 290
    signs and symptoms, 289
    subjective data, 289
    treatment, 290
delusions, 282–283, 364
democratic leadership, 431
depression
    children, 90–91
    geriatrics, 89–90
    major depressive disorder, 162–168
    perinatal, 182–189
    persistent depressive disorder, 168–170
    postpartum, 189–194
depressive disorders, 257
dermatologic issues, 38
development disorders, 45
Developmental Behavior Checklist (DBC-A), 363

developmental history, 38–39, 51
diabetes mellitus, 479
diagnosis formulation, 42
Diagnostic and Statistical Manual of Mental Disorders, Fifth Edition (*DSM-5*), 85–86
diagnostic overshadowing, 361
dialectical behavioral therapy (DBT), 96–97, 152
disengage family, 105
disorganized thinking and speech, 283
dissociative disorders, 242
    consultation and referral, 117
    definition, 115
    diagnostic tests and screening, 116
    dissociative identity disorder, 115
    follow-up, 116–117
    geriatrics/older adults, 117
    pathogenesis, 115
    patient teaching, 116
    pediatrics and adolescents, 117
    physical examination, 116
    predisposing factors, 115–116
    prevalence, 115
    subjective reports, 116
    transgender individuals, 117
    treatment, 116
    veterans and minority, 117
dissociative identity disorder, 115
distress tolerance, 96
documentation burden, APRNs, 347
Down syndrome, 360
Drug Abuse Screening Test (DAST), 89, 272
drug addiction, 175–176
dual eligibles, 466
Dupuytren contracture, 474

eating disorders (EDs), 45
    complaints and characteristics, 140–141
    definitions, 138
    incidence and prevalence, 139
    pediatrics, 70–71
    predisposing factors, 140
    therapies, 152
Edinburgh Postnatal Depression Scale (EPDS), 90, 184, 185
educational history, 40
egosyntonic/egodystonic beliefs, 364
Eldercare Locator, 349
electroconvulsive therapy (ECT), 81
electronic data interchange (EDI), 440
electronic health record (EHR)
    assessment and evaluation, 453
    cloud-based systems, 445
    confidentiality, 445
    contract negotiation, 452
    customizing and incorporating systems, 452
    design, 449
    vs. electronic medical record, 446
    essential functionality and features, 447–448
    financial considerations, 451

    learning and instruction, 452
    legal and ethical considerations, 453
    live operations and support, 452–453
    on-premise, 445
    planning stage, 445–452
    pros and cons, 447
    questions to ask, 450
    remotely hosted, 445
    resources, 453
    scalability, 451
electronic medical record (EMR), 445
    vs. electronic health record (EHR), 446
    pros and cons, 447
    types, 445
electronic prescribing of controlled substances (EPCS), 448
emergency shelters, 384
emotion regulation, 96
emotional and psychological stress, APRNs, 348
emotionally focused family therapy (EFT), 106
empathy, 16
empathy fatigue, 16
employer identification number (EIN), private psychiatric APRN practice, 440
encephalopathies, 484
endocrine disease, 38
endocrine disorders, 145
enmeshed family, 105
environmental management, 6–7
epilepsy, 350, 360, 471, 483
e-Prescribing (eRx), 448
Erikson's psychosocial developmental stages and behavioral indicators, 326, 327
erotomanic delusion, 289
ethical and legal challenges, APRNs, 347
ethical decision-making
    mental illness and unconfirmed pregnancy, 498
    severe mental illness, 499
ethics, 495
ethos, 9
excessive questioning, nontherapeutic communication, 15
exercises
    healthcare provider recommendations, 489–490
    high-intensity, 489
    moderate-intensity, 489
    types, 489
exploration, 14
eye contact, cultural considerations, 15
eye movement desensitization and reprocessing (EMDR) therapy, 102

factitious disorder (FD), 58, 244–248
    complaints, 245
    consultation and referrals, 247
    definition, 244–245
    diagnostic tests and screening, 246
    differential diagnoses, 246

follow-up, 247
geriatrics/older adults, 247
partners/family, 247
pathogenesis, 245
patient teaching, 247
pediatrics, 247
physical examination, 245–246
predisposing factors, 245
pregnancy, 247
prevalence, 245
signs and symptoms, 245
subjective data, 245
treatments, 246–247
factitious disorder imposed on another (FDIA), 244
faith-based organizations, 349
Families Empowered and Supporting Treatment of Eating Disorders (F.E.A.S.T.), 155
families/significant others
  acute psychiatric care setting, 412–413
  alcohol use disorder, 267
  assessments, 45
  caregiver, 500, 501
  generalized anxiety disorder (GAD), 119
  history, 40, 52
  illness anxiety disorder (IAD), 121
  obsessive-compulsive disorder (OCD), 124
  panic disorder, 126
  phobias, 128
  posttraumatic stress disorder, 130–131
  selective mutism, 132
  social anxiety disorder, 136
family behavioral therapy (FBT), 267
family-centered care, aging, 345–346
family systems theory, 105
family therapy approaches, 105–106, 152
fear disorders, 82
federal housing policies, 372
federal regulatory laws, 432–433
feeding and eating disorders (FEDs)
  comorbidities, 145, 150
  complaints and characteristics, 140–141
  consultation and referrals, 154
  definitions, 137–138
  diagnostic criteria, 146–150
  diagnostic tests and screening, 142–143
  differential diagnosis, 144–146
  follow-up, 153–154
  general treatments and interventions, 151–153
  geriatrics, 155
  incidence and prevalence, 138–139
  LGBTQ+ population, 155
  pathogenesis, 139–140
  patient teaching, 152–153
  pediatrics, 154
  physical examination, 141–142
  predisposing factors, 140
  pregnancy and infertility, 154
  prevalence, 137
  subjective data, 141
  treatment plan, 150–151

fetal alcoholic syndrome, 268
firearm-related violence, 22–23
folate, 491–492
forensic assertive community team/ treatment (FACT), 422
Freedom of Access to Clinic Entrances Act (FACE Act), 323
Friendship Line at Institute on Aging, 349
full opioid agonists, 272
functional gastrointestinal disorders (FGIDs), 472–473
functional neurologic symptom disorder (FND), 59, 257
  complaints, 240
  consultation and referrals, 243
  definition, 239
  diagnostic tests and screening, 240–241
  differential diagnoses, 241–242
  follow-up, 243
  geriatrics/older adults, 243
  incidence, 239–240
  partners/family, 243
  pathogenesis, 240
  patient teaching, 242–243
  pediatrics, 243
  physical examination, 240
  predisposing factors, 240
  pregnancy, 243
  signs and symptoms, 240
  subjective data, 240
  treatment, 242

GAIN Short Screener (GSS), 45
gastrointestinal disorders, 472–473
gender-affirming care, 310
gender-affirming hormone therapy (GAHT), 319
gender dysphoria (GD), 64
General Anxiety Disorder-7 (GAD-7), 44, 87
General Health Questionnaire, 12-Item, (GHQ-12), 408
generalized anxiety disorder (GAD), 117–119, 249, 257
  common complaints, 118
  consultation and referral, 119
  definition, 117
  diagnostic tests and screening, 118
  differential diagnosis, 118
  families, 119
  follow-up, 119
  geriatrics/older adults, 119
  incidence, 118
  minority/underrepresented individuals, 119
  pathogenesis, 118
  patient teaching, 119
  pediatrics, 54
  pediatrics and adolescents, 119
  physical examination, 118
  predisposing/risk factors, 118
  signs and symptoms, 117–118
  subjective reports, 118
  transgender individuals, 119

treatment, 118
veterans, 119
generational trauma, 23
Geriatric Depression Scale (GDS), 45, 90
geriatric psychiatric assessment
  anxiety disorders, 81–82
  conduct assessment, 75
  diagnosis-directed questions, 75–76
  differential evaluation, 75–76
  external time-limited computer algorithms, 75
  late life psychosis, 76–77
  medical diagnostic interviews, 75
  mild cognitive impairment (MCI), 79–80
  mood disorders, 80–81
  sleep disorders, 78–79
  somatization disorder, 83
  structured interview, 76
geriatrics
  avoidant personality disorder, 200
  brief psychotic disorder, 288
  circadian rhythm sleep-wake disorder, 226
  cyclothymia, 162
  delusional disorder, 290
  factitious disorder (FD), 247
  feeding and eating disorders, 155
  functional neurologic symptom disorder, 243
  generalized anxiety disorder, 119
  histrionic personality disorder, 205
  illness anxiety disorder (IAD), 121, 251
  insomnia, 229
  major depressive disorder, 168
  narcissistic personality disorder, 207
  narcolepsy, 231
  obsessive-compulsive disorder (OCD), 124
  obsessive-compulsive personality disorder, 208
  obstructive sleep apnea, 237
  opioid use disorder (OUD), 276–277
  panic disorder, 126
  paranoid personality disorder, 211
  parasomnias, 233
  persistent depressive disorder, 170
  phobias, 128
  posttraumatic stress disorder (PTSD), 130
  psychological factors affecting other medical conditions, 255
  restless legs syndrome, 235
  schizoaffective disorder, 294
  schizoid personality disorder, 214
  schizophrenia, 298
  schizophreniform disorder, 299
  sleep disorder, 224
  social anxiety disorder, 136
  somatic symptom disorder, 259
  substance/medication-induced psychotic disorder, 301
gestational diabetes, feeding and eating disorders, 154
gifted children, 351
global homelessness, 373

glymphatic system (GS), 215
grandiose delusion, 289
Grit Scale measures, 430
grossly disorganized or abnormal motor behavior, 283
group therapy, 106–107
guardianship, 467
gut microbiome, 492

hallucinations, 282
hallucinogen use disorder (HUD), 269–270
hallucinogens, 269, 270
Hamilton Anxiety Rating Scale (HAM-A), 44
Hamilton Depression Rating Scale (HAMD), 90
Hamilton Rating Scale for Depression (HAM-D), 45
Hashimoto thyroiditis, 481
head and neck disorders, 471–472
head, eyes, ears, nose, throat (HEENT), 38
health advocacy, homelessness, 377–378
Health Information Technology for Economic and Clinical Health Act (HITECH), 458
Health Insurance Portability and Accountability Act (HIPAA), 43, 321, 432, 457–458
health maintenance organization (HMO), 465
health-risk behaviors, trauma, 20
healthcare coverage, commercial/private insurance, 465
Healthcare for the Homeless, 384
healthcare literacy, homeless, 382
healthcare provider, 16
healthy diet
  gut microbiome, 492
  healthcare provider recommendations, 492–493
  mental health disorders, 491
  nutritional supplementation, 491–492
  processed foods, 491
hearing loss, military, 394
hereditary metabolic diseases, 480
historical trauma, 23
histrionic personality disorder, 204–205
homeless and indigent populations
  APRN challenges, 389–390
  assessment and outreach interventions, 384–388
  barriers to care, 380–381
  community care, 423
  community health APRNs, 386
  community outreach programs, 386–387
  COVID-19 pandemic, 373–375
  crisis intervention, 390
  cultural competency, 381–382
  data collection, 382–384
  definition, 369–370
  demographic characteristics, 371
  gender and ethnicity, 370
  global, 373
  health advocacy, 377–378
  health hazard, 378–379
  housing instability, 372
  incidence, 370
  interprofessional collaboration, 390
  intimate partner violence (IPV), 376
  life cycle of service, 394
  mental and physical illness, 375
  mental health, 376
  mental illness, 371
  mobile clinics, 388
  myths, 380
  pathways, 371–376
  prevalence, 370
  racial inequities, 372–373
  reduced life expectancy, 379
  risk factors and protective factors, 384
  safety assessments, 385–386
  social determinants of health (SDH), 375–376
  socioeconomic programs, 384
  street medicine, 387–388
  substance use disorder, 376
  systemic racism, 382
  telehealth, 390–391
  therapeutic rapport, 385
  trauma-informed care, 385
  treatment plan modalities, 388–389
homeostasis, 106
Homestead Act, 372
homocysteine, 492
Hospital Elder Life Program (HELP), 78
Hospital Readmissions Reduction Program (HRRP), 433
housing assistance programs, 384
Housing Fast program, 423
"Housing First" approach, 400
housing instability, 372
human-caused disasters, 22–23
hyperthyroidism, 479–480
hypochondriasis, 248
hypothyroidism, 479
hypoxia, 485

identity, 308
illness anxiety disorder (IAD), 58–59, 240, 254, 257
  complaints, 248
  consultation and referral, 121, 250
  definition, 119–120, 248
  diagnostic tests and screening, 120, 249
  differential diagnoses, 120, 249–250
  families/significant others, 121
  follow-up, 121
  geriatrics/older adults, 121, 251
  incidence, 120, 248
  minority/underrepresented individuals, 121
  partners/family, 251
  pathogenesis, 120, 248
  patient education, 120–121, 250
  pediatrics, 250–251
  pediatrics and adolescents, 121
  physical examination, 120, 249
  predisposing/risk factors, 120, 248
  pregnancy, 251
  prevalence, 120
  signs and symptoms, 248
  subjective data, 249
  transgender individuals, 121
  treatment, 120, 250
  veterans, 121
Illness Attitude Scales (IAS), 249
implicit bias, cultural considerations, 15–16
In Transition program, service members, 400
incoherent speech, 365
Individual Education Program/Plan (IEP), 328
informal carer, 500
informed consent, 35
inpatient psychiatric units, 403
insomnia, 227–229
  complaints, 227
  consultation and referrals, 229
  definition, 227
  diagnostic tests and screening, 228
  differential diagnoses, 228
  follow-up, 228–229
  geriatrics, 229
  partners/family, 229
  pathogenesis, 227
  patient teaching, 228
  pediatrics, 229
  pharmacologic treatment, 79
  physical examination, 228
  predisposing factors, 227
  pregnancy, 229
  signs and symptoms, 227
  subjective data, 227–228
  treatment, 228
institutional policies, 464
insurance denials, 465
integumentary disorders, 474
intellectual disability (ID), 351, 359
  assessor challenges, 364
  autistic spectrum disorder, 365
  behavior assessment, 365
  biological investigations, 362
  biopsychosocial approaches, 367
  challenging behaviors, 361
  classification system, 360
  definition, 359–360
  delusions, 364
  diagnosis, 363
  diagnostic overshadowing, 361
  egosyntonic/egodystonic beliefs, 364
  hallucination assessment, 364–365
  history, 362
  informant history, 362
  interview, 362
  medication treatments, 363
  mental health, 359
  multidisciplinary approach, 367
  negative psychotic symptoms, 365
  nurse practitioner and tools, 366–367
  observations, 362

prevalence, 360–361
psychiatric assessment, 361–365
psychological interventions, 363
psychotic illnesses, 364
rating instruments, 362–363
research, 367
risk factors, 361
schizophrenia, 365
thought assessment, 365
intensive outpatient programs (IOP), 422
International Society of Psychiatric-Mental Health Nurses (ISPN), 4
International Trauma Questionnaire (ITQ), 45
interpersonal challenges, APRNs, 348
interpersonal therapy (IPT), 97–98, 152
interprofessional collaboration, 432
intimate partner violence (IPV), 21, 376
isotonitazene, 281

Joint Commission, The, 9, 404, 408, 464
judgment, 41

Katz Index of Independence in Activities of Daily Living (Katz ADL Index), 45
kidney function test, feeding and eating disorders, 143

la belle indifference, 59, 240
laissez-faire leadership, 431
late life psychosis
  definition, 76
  etiology, 76
  incidence, 76
  prevalence, 76
  treatments, 77
leadership skills assessment, 431
leaky gut, 492
Leininger's sunrise model, 305
LGBTQ+ individuals
  American healthcare model, 315
  assessment needs, 315–317
  bullying, 314
  clinical referrals, 324
  community-level risk factors, 314–315
  community resources, 324–325
  disclosures, 321
  disinformation and bias, 309–311
  economic constraints to access, 323
  families, 319–320
  family-level factors, 314
  feeding and eating disorders, 155
  gender-affirming care, 317–319
  health disparities, 312–313
  historical perspective, 308–309
  identity, 308
  inclusive terminology, 317
  individual-level factors, 314
  institutional and state regulations, 320–321
  minority stress model, 313
  research, 311–312

  resilience factors, 314
  risk and resilience factors, 315
  social connectedness, 315
  surgical intervention, 319
  trans youth families, 321–322
  universal risk factors, 313–314
Liebowitz Social Anxiety Scale (LSAS), 87
lifestyle modifications, anxiety disorders, 82
limited liability corporation (LLC), 437
lisdexamfetamine, 152
liver function tests, feeding and eating disorders, 143
logos, 9
Long-Term Care Ombudsman Program, 349
lung disease, 472

Maintaining Internal Systems and Strengthening Integrated Outside Networks (MISSION) Act, 392
major depressive disorder (MDD), 144, 250
  consultation and referrals, 167–168
  definition, 162
  diagnostic tests and screening, 163–164
  differential diagnosis, 164
  follow-up, 167
  geriatrics, 168
  incidence, 162
  partners/family, 168
  pathogenesis, 162–163
  patient teaching, 167
  pediatrics, 53, 168
  physical examination, 163
  predisposing factors, 163
  pregnancy, 168
  signs and symptoms, 163
  subjective data, 163
  treatment, 164–167
malingering, 246
managed care organization (MCO), 465
mania/hypomania, 53, 91
Marital Status Inventory (MSI), 45
Massachusetts Child Psychiatry Access Program (MCPAP) for Moms, 185, 187
Meals on Wheels America, 349
measurement-based care (MBC), 408
Medicaid program, 466
medical history, 37–38
medical respite programs (MRP), 384
medically assisted opioid withdrawal, 272–273
Medicare Access and CHIP Reauthorization Act (MACRA), 433
medication history, 38
medication-induced anxiety disorder
  consultation and referral, 122
  definition, 121
  differential diagnosis, 122
  follow-up, 119
  incidence, 121
  patient teaching, 119

  physical examination, 122
  predisposing/risk factors, 121–122
  subjective reports, 122
melatonin receptor agonist, 79
memantine, 77
mental health and illness. *See also* intellectual disability
  child and adolescent patients, 49–50, 327–329
  commercial/private insurance, 465
  community care, 420
  decision-making capacity, 467
  disability determination, 466–467
  homelessness, 371, 375
  intellectual disability (*see* intellectual disability)
  laws and regulations, 464
  public insurance, 465–466
  veterans, 396–399
Mental Health First Aid (MHFA), 423
Mental Health Gap Action Program (mh-GAP), 423
mental health law, 464
mental health respite programs (MHRP), 384
mental retardation, 359
mental status exam (MSE), 41, 44, 72, 83
mental wellness and lifestyle, 487
metabolic disease
  acromegaly, 478
  acute porphyrias, 478
  anti-N-methyl-D-aspartate receptor autoimmune encephalitis, 478–479
  Cushing syndrome, 479
  diabetes mellitus, 479
  diagnostic tests, 478
  hereditary metabolic diseases, 480
  hyperthyroidism, 479–480
  hypothyroidism, 479
methadone, 179–180, 272–275, 276, 277
Michigan Alcohol Screening Test (MAST), 44
migraine, 471
mild cognitive impairment (MCI), 79–80
military
  active component, 393
  cultural competence, 395–396
  culture, 392–395
  ethos strengths and vulnerabilities, 393
  exposures, 394
  family, 394–395
  language, 393
  norms, 393
  organization, 393
  ranks, 393–394
  reserve component, 393
  as social group, 393
  values and symbols, 393
  and veteran healthcare, 395
military occupational specialty (MOS), 394
military sexual trauma (MST), 21–22
  screening and assessment, 397
  stigma-related barriers, 397

military sexual trauma (MST) (cont.)
  traditional logistical barriers, 397
  treatment and resources, 397–398
  veterans, 397–398
mindful-based therapy, somatization disorder, 83
mindfulness, 96
Mini-Mental State Examination (MMSE), 44
Mini Psychiatric Assessment Schedule for Adult with Developmental Disability (PAS -ADD), 363
minority/underrepresented individuals
  generalized anxiety disorder (GAD), 119
  illness anxiety disorder (IAD), 121
  obsessive-compulsive disorder (OCD), 124
  panic disorder, 126
  phobias, 128
  posttraumatic stress disorder (PTSD), 130
  selective mutism, 132
  social anxiety disorder, 136
miracle question, 14
mobile clinics, 388
mobile health (mHealth), 454
Montreal Cognitive Assessment (MoCA), 83
mood and affect, mental status exam, 41
Mood Disorder Questionnaire (MDQ), 45
mood disorders
  bipolar disorder, 157–161
  cyclothymic disorder, 161–162
  definition, 80
  differential diagnosis, 81
  etiology, 80
  geriatrics, 89
  incidence, 81
  pediatrics, 53
  prevalence, 80–81
  screening tools, 44–45
  treatment guidelines, 81
motivational interviewing (MI), 28, 98–99
  children and adolescents, 336–340
  elements, 338
  opioid use disorder, 178
  principles, 338–339
  substance use disorders, 263–264
motor disorders (MD), 351
movement disorders, screening tools, 45
Multidimensional Assessment of Interoceptive Awareness-Version 2 (MAIA-2), 355
multidimensional family therapy (MDFT), 267
multiple sclerosis, 482–483
multiple sleep latency testing (MSLT), 215
Munchausen syndrome, 245
muscular dystrophy, pediatrics, 350
musculoskeletal disorders, 474
myasthenia gravis, 483

N-acetylcysteine, 492
naloxone, 179, 272, 274–275, 276
narcissistic personality disorder
  complaints, 205–206
  consultation and referrals, 207
  definition, 205
  diagnostic tests and screening, 206
  differential diagnosis, 206
  follow-up, 207
  pathogenesis, 205
  physical examination, 206
  predisposing factors, 205
  prevalence and incidence, 205
  signs and symptoms, 206
  subjective data, 206
  treatment, 206–207
narcolepsy, 485
narrative exposure therapy (NET), 103
National Association for Males with Eating Disorders (N.A.M.E.D.), 155
National Association of Anorexia Nervosa and Associated Disorders (ANAD), 155
National Council on Aging (NCOA), 348
National Elder Law Foundation (NELF), 349
National Institute of Mental Health (NIMH), 420–421
National Institute on Aging, 349
National Licensure Compact for APRNs (NLC-APRN), 7
National Patient Safety Goal (NPSG), 408
National Plan and Provider Enumeration System (NPPES), 440
national provider identification (NPI), 440
negative transference, 100
neurodevelopmental disorders, childhood, 350–351
neurodiversity, 353
neurologic disorders, 471–472
  delirium/dementia, 482
  epilepsy, 483
  multiple sclerosis, 482–483
  myasthenia gravis, 483
  psychogenic nonepileptic seizures, 483
  transient global amnesia, 483
neurologic history, 38
neurotransmitters, 190
nicotine, 279
nicotine inhaler, 280
nicotine replacement therapy (NRT), 279–280
nicotine transdermal system, 280
nonbenzodiazepine, 79, 221, 226, 228
nonnicotine-containing products, 280
non-rapid eye movement (NREM) sleep, 216
nonsuicidal self-injurious behaviors (NSSIs), 65
nontherapeutic communication, 14–15
nonverbal behavior visual cues, 10
No Surprises Act, 433
Nuremberg Trial, 495
nurse psychotherapist, 93

nutritional deficiencies, 145, 154
nutritional supplementation, 491–492

obsessions, 122
obsessive-compulsive disorder (OCD), 257
  consultation and referral, 122
  definition, 122
  diagnostic tests and screening, 123
  differential diagnosis, 123
  families/significant others, 124
  follow-up, 124
  geriatrics/older adults, 124
  minority/underrepresented individuals, 124
  pathophysiology, 122
  patient teaching, 124
  pediatrics, 56–57
  pediatrics and adolescents, 124
  physical examination, 123
  prevalence, 123
  subjective reports, 123
  transgender individuals, 124
  veterans, 124
obsessive-compulsive personality disorder, 207–208
obstructive sleep apnea (OSA), 38, 235–237
  complaints, 236
  consultation and referrals, 237
  definition, 235
  diagnostic tests and screening, 236
  differential diagnoses, 236
  follow-up, 237
  incidence, 235–236
  pathogenesis, 236
  patient teaching, 237
  pediatrics, 237
  physical examination, 236
  predisposing factors, 236
  prevalence, 235
  signs and symptoms, 236
  subjective data, 236
  treatment, 236–237
occupational history, 40
olanzapine, 116, 152, 159, 202, 286–287
older adults. *See* geriatrics
omega-3 fatty acids, 491
open-ended questioning, 14
operant conditioning, 104
Opioid Risk Tool (ORT), 272
Opioid Risk Tool-Opioid Use Disorder (ORT-OUD), 89
opioid use disorder (OUD), 271–277
  airway management, 272
  body systems, 177
  consultation and referrals, 181
  definition, 175, 271
  diagnostic tests and screening, 177–178, 271–272
  differential diagnosis, 178
  emergency naloxone, 179, 272
  follow-up care, 181
  geriatrics, 276–277

hospitalized patients, 276, 277
incidence, 175, 271
medically assisted opioid withdrawal, 272–273
medication-assisted treatment (MAT), 273–275
neonatal intensive care unit (NICU), 275
pathogenesis, 175–176
patient teaching, 179–180
pediatrics, 276
pharmacologic treatment, 272
physical examination, 177
pregnancy, 276
psychosocial rehabilitation, 275
signs and symptoms, 177, 271
subjective data, 177
treatment, 178–180
oppositional defiant disorder (ODD)
  pediatrics, 61–62
  screening questions, 62
  symptoms, 61
other specified feeding and eating disorder (OSFED)
  definition, 138
  diagnostic criteria, 149

pachyonychia congenita, 474
panic disorder (PD), 249–250, 257
  consultation and referral, 126
  definition, 124–125
  diagnostic tests and screening, 125
  differential diagnosis, 125
  families/significant others, 126
  follow-up, 126
  geriatrics/older adults, 126
  minority/underrepresented individuals, 126
  pathogenesis, 125
  patient teaching, 126
  pediatrics, 55
  pediatrics and adolescents, 126
  physical examination, 125
  predisposing factors, 125
  subjective reports, 125
  transgender individuals, 126
  veterans, 126
paranoid personality disorder, 210–211
paraphrasing, therapeutic communication, 14
parasomnias, 231–233
Parental Stress Index (PSI), 45
parentification, 106
Parkinson disease, 472
partners/family, 437
  brief psychotic disorder, 288
  circadian rhythm sleep-wake disorder, 226
  delusional disorder, 290
  factitious disorder (FD), 247
  functional neurologic symptom disorder, 243
  illness anxiety disorder, 251
  insomnia, 229
  major depressive disorder, 168

narcolepsy, 231
obstructive sleep apnea, 237
parasomnias, 233
psychological factors affecting other medical conditions, 255
restless legs syndrome (RLS), 235
schizoaffective disorder, 294
schizophrenia, 298
schizophreniform disorder, 299
sleep disorder, 224
somatic symptom disorder, 259
substance/medication-induced psychotic disorder, 301
pathos, 9
patient-centered care, eating disorders, 151–152
patient-centered medical home (PCMH), 7, 423
Patient Health Questionnaire-2 (PHQ-2), 53, 90
Patient Health Questionnaire-9 (PHQ-9), 45, 53, 89–91, 293, 408
Patient Health Questionnaire 15-Item Subscale (PHQ-15), 256
Patient Navigator Program, 7
Patient Protection and Affordable Care Act (PPACA), 7
Patient-Reported Outcomes Measurement Information System (PROMIS)-Anxiety—Short Form, 87
Patient Safety and Quality Improvement Act of 2005 (PSQUIA), 433
Patient Self-Determination Act (PSDA), 467
pediatric psychiatric assessment
  assessment process, 47–48
  biopsychosocial model, 49
  current and past medications, 52
  developmental history, 51
  family psychiatric history, 52
  formulation phase, 74
  history of presenting illness, 50–51
  history taking, 49
  information-gathering phase, 50–52
  mental status exam (MSE), 72, 73
  physical health assessment, 72–74
  preparation, 50
  protective factors, 49
  psychiatric history, 52
  review of systems, 53–74
  social history, 51–52
  therapeutic rapport, 50
pediatrics
  antisocial personality disorder, 198
  bipolar disorder, 161
  borderline personality disorder, 202
  brief psychotic disorder, 288
  cannabis use disorder, 270
  circadian rhythm sleep-wake disorder, 226
  cyclothymia, 162
  delusional disorder, 290
  factitious disorder (FD), 247
  feeding and eating disorders, 154

functional neurologic symptom disorder, 243
generalized anxiety disorder (GAD), 119
hallucinogen use disorder (HUD), 270
histrionic personality disorder, 205
illness anxiety disorder, 121, 250–251
insomnia, 229
major depressive disorder, 168
narcolepsy, 231
obsessive-compulsive disorder (OCD), 124
obstructive sleep apnea, 237
opioid use disorder, 276
panic disorder, 126
parasomnias, 233
persistent depressive disorder, 170
phobias, 128
posttraumatic stress disorder, 130
psychological factors affecting other medical conditions, 254
restless legs syndrome, 234
schizoaffective disorder, 294
schizophrenia, 298
schizophreniform disorder, 299
selective mutism, 132
sleep disorder, 223
somatic symptom disorder, 259
substance/medication-induced psychotic disorder, 301
tobacco use disorder, 281
peer support model, 27–28
Penn State Worry Questionnaire (PSWQ), 87–88
perceptual disturbances, 41
perinatal depression, 182–189
  complaints, 183, 184
  consultation and referrals, 187
  definition, 182
  diagnostic tests and screening, 184–185
  differential diagnosis, 185
  follow-up, 187
  incidence, 182–183
  pathogenesis, 183
  patient teaching, 187
  physical examination, 184
  predisposing factors, 183
  risk factors, 183
  signs and symptoms, 183–184
  subjective data, 184
  treatment, 186–188
perinatal mental health
  mood disorders, 182–189
  opioid use disorder, 175–181
permanent housing programs, 384
persecutory delusion, 289
persistent depressive disorder (PDD)
  consultation and referrals, 170
  definition, 168
  diagnostic tests and screening, 169
  differential diagnosis, 169
  follow-up, 169
  geriatrics, 170
  incidence, 168

persistent depressive disorder (PDD) (cont.)
  partners/family, 170
  pathogenesis, 168
  patient teaching, 169
  pediatrics, 170
  physical examination, 163
  predisposing factors, 168
  signs and symptoms, 168–169
  subjective data, 169
  treatment, 169, 170
persistent postconcussive syndrome, 398
Personal Information Protection and Electronic Documents Act (PIPEDA), 49
personality disorders, 45, 196
  antisocial personality disorder, 197–198
  avoidant personality disorder, 199–200
  borderline personality disorder, 200–202
  dependent personality disorder, 202–204
  diagnostic criteria, 197
  histrionic personality disorder, 204–205
  narcissistic personality disorder, 205–207
  obsessive-compulsive personality disorder, 207–208
  other specific personality disorders, 209–210
  paranoid personality disorder, 210–211
  schizoid personality disorder, 212–214
  unspecified, 212
Personality Inventory for DSM-5 (PID-5), 45
person-centered psychotherapy, 107–108
phencyclidine-type substances, 281
phenethylamines, 281
phobias, 126–128
  consultation and referral, 128
  definition, 126
  diagnostic tests and screening, 127
  differential diagnosis, 127
  etiology, 126
  families/significant others, 128
  follow-up, 128
  geriatrics/older adults, 128
  minority/underrepresented individuals, 128
  patient teaching, 127–128
  pediatrics and adolescents, 128
  physical examination, 127
  predisposing factors, 127
  subjective reports, 127
  transgender individuals, 128
  veterans, 128
physical activity
  brain changes, 488
  life structures and dependability, 488
  neurophysiologic benefits, 487–488
  self-perception, 488
  sleep problems, 488
  structured, 487
physical and mental disabilities, pediatrics, 360
  APRN challenges, 357

assessment, 354–356
cerebral palsy (CP), 350
childhood/juvenile arthritis, 350
definition, 350
epilepsy, 350
etiology, 350
neurodevelopmental disorders, 350–351
parents, collaboration with, 351–353
prevalence, 350, 351
problem-solving approach, 353
profile based approach, 353–354
spina bifida, 350
spinal cord injury, 350
strength-based approach, 356–357
physical health, pediatrics, 72–74
physical illness, homelessness, 375
physical touch, cultural considerations, 15
physical trauma, 484
pica, 137
  comorbidities, 150
  diagnostic criteria, 149
  differential diagnoses, 144
  prevalence, 138
point-of-service plan (POS), 465
police powers, 464
polysomnography (PSG), 215, 236
positive transference, 100
postconcussion syndrome, 484
postpartum depression (PPD)
  anxiety, 192
  complaints, 190–191
  consultation and referrals, 194
  definition, 190
  diagnostic tests and screening, 191
  differential diagnosis, 191
  follow-up, 194
  pathogenesis, 190
  patient teaching, 193–194
  physical examination, 191
  vs. postpartum psychosis, 192
  predisposing factors, 190
  prevalence and incidence, 190
  signs and symptoms, 191, 192
  subjective data, 191
  treatment, 192–193
poststroke depression, 472
posttraumatic stress disorder (PTSD), 128–131, 472
  comorbid with major depressive disorder, 22
  consultation and referral, 130
  definition, 128
  diagnostic criteria, 18
  diagnostic tests and screening, 129
  differential diagnosis, 129
  families/significant others, 130–131
  follow-up, 130
  geriatrics/older adult patients, 130
  incidence, 128–129
  minority/underrepresented individuals, 130
  pathogenesis, 129
  patient teaching, 130
  pediatrics and adolescents, 130

physical examination, 129
physical signs, 129
predisposing factors, 129
prevalence, 21
psychological symptoms, 129
subjective reports, 129
treatment plan, 129–130
veterans, 22, 130, 398
Posttraumatic Stress Disorder Checklist (PCL-5), 45
poverty, community care, 423
prebiotic/probiotic supplements, 492
preferred provider organization (PPO), 465
pregnancy
  alcohol use disorder, 268–269
  bipolar disorder, 161
  brief psychotic disorder, 288
  cannabis use disorder, 270
  circadian rhythm sleep-wake disorder, 226
  cyclothymia, 162
  delusional disorder, 290
  feeding and eating disorders, 154
  functional neurologic symptom disorder, 243
  illness anxiety disorder, 251
  insomnia, 229
  major depressive disorder, 168
  narcolepsy, 231
  obstructive sleep apnea, 237
  opioid use disorder, 276
  psychological factors affecting other medical conditions, 254
  restless legs syndrome, 234–235
  schizoaffective disorder, 294
  schizophrenia, 298
  schizophreniform disorder, 299
  sleep disorder, 223–224
  somatic symptom disorder, 259
  substance/medication-induced psychotic disorder, 301
  tobacco use disorder, 281
Pregnancy and Lactation Labeling Rule (PLLR), 186
premenstrual dysphoric disorder (PMDD)
  consultation and referrals, 173
  definition, 171
  diagnostic tests and screening, 172
  differential diagnosis, 172
  follow-up, 173
  incidence, 168
  pathogenesis, 171
  patient teaching, 172
  physical examination, 171–172
  predisposing factors, 171
  signs and symptoms, 171
  subjective data, 171
  treatment, 172
preoccupation/anticipation stage, drug addiction, 176
prescription drug monitoring programs (PDMP), 448
professional limited liability company (PLLC), 437

INDEX

projective questioning, 14
Protected Health Information (PHI), 454
Protection and Advocacy for Individuals with Mental Illness (PAIMI) Program, 407–408
pseudocyesis, 252
psychiatric assessment
   adult (*see* adult psychiatric assessment)
   case formulation, 42–43
   clinical interview, 43–44
   components, 33
   consultation, 34
   diagnosis formulation, 42
   diagnosis-specific scales, 87–92
   goals, 33
   initial symptom assessment scales, 85–87
   inpatient settings, 34
   objectives, 33
   outpatient settings, 34
   privacy and confidentiality, 43
   purpose, 33
   resources, 43–45
   technology and telehealth, 42–43
psychiatric comorbidity, 471
psychiatric conditions, coding reference, 503–505
psychiatric-mental health clinical nurse specialist (PMHCNS), 4
Psychiatric-Mental Health Nurse-Board Certified (PMH-BC™), 4
psychiatric-mental health nurse practitioners (PMHNPs), 4, 242, 335
   education and training, 93
   scope and standards of practice, 94
psychiatric-mental health nursing
   certification, 4–5
   development of, 3
   history, 3–4
   scope and standards, 5
   tools, 6–7
psychiatric-mental health registered nurses (PMHRNs), 94
psychoanalysis, 99–100
psychodynamic theory, 107, 131
psychodynamic therapy, 100–101
psychoeducation, 95
   groups, 107
   sleep disorder, 220
   somatization disorder, 83
psychogenic nonepileptic seizures (PNES), 483
psychological factors affecting other medical conditions (PF-AMC), 253–255
   consultation and referrals, 254
   definition, 252
   differential diagnosis, 253–254
   geriatrics/older adults, 255
   incidence, 253
   partners/family, 255
   pathogenesis, 253
   patient teaching, 254
   pediatrics, 254
   predisposing factors, 253
   pregnancy, 254
   prevalence, 253
   subjective data, 253
   treatments, 254
psychometric tools, 293
psychomotor agitation, 405
psychopharmacology, 6, 129
psychosis, pediatrics, 57
psychosocial history, 39
psychotherapy, 6
   applied behavioral analysis, 104–105
   cognitive behavioral therapy (CBT), 94–95
   dialectical behavioral therapy (DBT), 96–97
   for dissociative disorders, 116
   documentation, 108–109
   family therapy approaches, 105–106
   functional neurologic symptom disorder, 243
   group therapy, 106–107
   interpersonal therapy, 97–98
   motivational interviewing (MI), 98–99
   older adults, 108
   pediatrics, 108
   person-centered psychotherapy, 107–108
   for posttraumatic stress disorder, 130
   psychoanalysis, 99–100
   psychodynamic therapy, 100–101
   somatic symptom disorder (SSD), 258
psychotic disorder
   another medical condition, 291–292
   brief psychotic disorder, 283–288
   delusional disorder, 288–290
   schizophreniform disorder, 298–299
   substance/medication-induced psychotic disorder, 299–301
psychotropic drugs, 6
public health law, 464
Purnell model for cultural competence, 305

Quality of Life Scale (QOLS), 45

racially driven microaggressions, 23
rapid eye movement (REM) sleep, 216
Rapid Mood Screener (RMS), 90, 293
rapport building, pediatric assessment, 50
Raynaud phenomenon, 474
refeeding syndrome, 150
reflections, 14, 264
Reframing Aging Initiative, 342
remote patient monitoring (RPM), 454
respiratory disorders, 472, 484–486
Response to Intervention (RTI) approach, 356
restating, 14
restless legs syndrome (RLS), 233–235
   complaints, 234
   consultation and referrals, 234
   definition, 233
   diagnostic tests and screening, 234
   differential diagnoses, 234
   follow-up, 234
   geriatrics, 235
   incidence, 233
   partners/family, 235
   pathogenesis, 233
   patient teaching, 234
   pediatrics, 234
   physical examination, 234
   predisposing factors, 233–234
   pregnancy, 234–235
   signs and symptoms, 234
   subjective data, 234
   treatment plan, 234
Revised Child Anxiety and Depression Scale (RCADS), 88
Ritvo Autism Asperger Diagnostic Scale (RAADS), 45
Ritvo Autism Asperger Diagnostic Scale-Revised (RAADS-R), 355
rumination disorder, 137
   comorbidities, 150
   diagnostic criteria, 148–149
   differential diagnoses, 144
   prevalence, 138–139

Satisfaction With Life Scale (SWLS), 45
schizoaffective disorder, 292–294
   consultation and referrals, 294
   definition, 292
   diagnostic tests and screening, 284
   differential diagnosis, 293
   follow-up care, 294
   geriatrics/older adult, 294
   partners/family, 294
   pathogenesis, 292–293
   pediatrics, 294
   predisposing factors, 293
   pregnancy, 294
   prevalence, 292
   psychoeducation, 294
   signs and symptoms, 293
   subjective data, 293
   treatment, 293–294
schizoid personality disorder, 212–214
schizophrenia, 144, 295–298, 365
   consultation and referrals, 297
   definition, 295
   diagnostic tests and screening, 296
   differential diagnosis, 296
   follow-up, 297
   geriatrics/older adult, 298
   incidence, 295
   partners/family, 298
   pathogenesis, 295
   patient teaching, 297
   pediatrics, 298
   physical examination, 296
   predisposing factors, 295
   pregnancy, 298
   signs and symptoms, 295
   subjective data, 295–296
   treatment modalities, 296–297
schizophreniform disorder, 298–299

S-corp, 437
Screen for Child Anxiety Related Emotional Disorders (SCARED), 88
Screening to Brief Intervention (S2BI), 89
selective mutism
　consultation and referral, 132
　definition, 131
　diagnostic tests and screening, 132
　differential diagnosis, 132
　families/significant others, 132
　minority/underrepresented individuals, 132
　pathogenesis, 131
　pediatrics, 55–56
　pediatrics and adolescents, 132
　physical examination, 131–132
　predisposing factors, 131
　prevalence, 131
　psychoeducation, 132
　subjective reports, 131
　treatment, 132
selective serotonin reuptake inhibitors (SSRIs), 81
　for illness anxiety disorder (IAD), 120
　for posttraumatic stress disorder, 129
self-awareness, 6
self-funded plan, 465
self-harming behaviors, 423
self-help groups, 107
self-neglect, 343
semaglutide, 152
senior centers, 349
Senior Companions Program, 349
sensory processing disorder (SPD), 351
separation anxiety disorder, 132–134
　consultation and referral, 134
　definition, 132
　diagnostic tests and screening, 133
　differential diagnosis, 133
　etiology, 133
　follow-up, 134
　incidence, 132–133
　pathogenesis, 133
　pediatrics, 54–55
　physical examination, 133
　predisposing factors, 133
　psychoeducation, 134
　subjective reports, 133
　treatment, 134
serious mental illness (SMI), 497
serotonin and norepinephrine reuptake inhibitors (SNRIs)
　for illness anxiety disorder (IAD), 120
　for posttraumatic stress disorder, 129
Severity Measure for Depression, 90
sexual and reproductive history, 38
shared decision-making (SDM), 7
sheltered homelessness, 369
Short Health Anxiety Inventory (SHAI), 88
short-term sleep disorder, 216
silence, therapeutic communication, 12
skills development groups, 107
sleep apnea, 485

sleep diary/log, 218
sleep disorder
　clinical presentation, 216–217
　complaints, 215, 217
　consultation and referrals, 223
　definition, 78, 215
　diagnostic classification, 216
　diagnostic tests and screening, 215–216, 218
　differential diagnoses, 79, 218–219
　etiology, 78
　follow-up, 223
　geriatrics, 224
　incidence, 78, 217
　insomnia, 227–229
　narcolepsy, 230–231
　obstructive sleep apnea, 235–237
　parasomnias, 231–233
　partners/family, 224
　pathogenesis, 217
　patient teaching, 220, 223
　pediatrics, 223
　physical examination, 218
　predisposing factors, 215, 217
　pregnancy, 223–224
　prevalence, 78
　relaxation techniques, 220
　restless legs syndrome (RLS), 233–235
　signs and symptoms, 217
　sleep cycles, 216
　sleep patterns, 217
　sleep stages, 216
　specialized treatment plans, 220
　stimulus control therapy, 220
　subjective data, 218
　treatment plan, 79, 219–223
sleep hygiene, 219–220
sleep problems, 488
SMART goals. See Specific, Measurable, Achievable, Realistic, and Timebound goals
social affirmation, 318
social anxiety disorder (SAD)
　consultation and referral, 135–136
　definition, 134
　diagnostic tests and screening, 135
　differential diagnosis, 135
　families/significant others, 136
　follow-up, 135
　geriatrics/older adults, 136
　incidence, 134
　minority/underrepresented individuals, 136
　pathogenesis, 134
　pediatrics, 55
　physical examination, 135
　predisposing factors, 134
　psychoeducation, 135
　subjective reports, 135
　treatment, 135
　veterans, 136
　youth, 136
social determinants of health (SDH), homelessness, 375–376

social history, pediatrics, 51–52
social interaction, 9
Social Security Disability Insurance (SSDI), 467
sociocultural history, 39–40
Socratic dialogue, 95
sole proprietorship, 437
somatic delusions, 289
Somatic Experiencing® (SE) therapy, 103
somatic symptom and related disorders (SSRDs)
　biopsychosocial (BPS) model, 239
　factitious disorder (FD), 244–248
　functional neurologic symptom disorder, 239–244
　illness anxiety disorder, 248–251
　other specified/unspecified, 252
　somatic symptom disorder, 255–259
somatic symptom disorder (SSD), 240, 246, 249
　consultation and referrals, 258
　definition, 255
　diagnosis and screenings, 256
　differential diagnosis, 257
　geriatrics/older adults, 259
　incidence, 255–256
　partners/family, 259
　pathogenesis, 256
　patient teaching, 258
　pediatrics, 58–59, 259
　physical examination, 256
　predisposing factors, 256
　pregnancy, 259
　psychotherapy, 258
　signs and symptoms, 256
　subjective data, 256
　treatment, 257
Somatic Symptom Scale-8 (SSS-8), 59, 256
somatization disorder, geriatrics, 83
specific learning disorder (SLD), 351
Specific, Measurable, Achievable, Realistic, and Timebound (SMART) goals, 439
specific phobia, pediatrics, 56
Spence Children's Anxiety Scale, 88
spina bifida, 350
spinal cord injury, pediatrics, 350
stereotype threat, 16
stimulant use disorder, 278–279
strategic family therapy, 106
street medicine, 387–388
Strengths, Weaknesses, Opportunities, and Threats (SWOT) analysis, 437, 438
stroke, 471–472
Structured Clinical Interview for *DSM-5* (SCID-5), 87
Structured Clinical Interview for *DSM-5* Alternative Model for Personality Disorders (SCID-5-AMPD), 44
Structured Clinical Interview for *DSM-5* Disorders—Clinician Version (SCID-5-CV), 43

Structured Clinical Interview for *DSM-5* Personality Disorders (SCID-5-PD), 44
Substance Abuse and Mental Health Services Administration (SAMHSA), 18, 181
substance-induced bipolar and related disorders, 173–174
substance use disorders (SUDs), 144
  alcohol use disorder, 265–269
  biopsychosocial model, 262
  cannabis use disorder, 269–270
  change talk vs. sustain talk, 264
  cognitive behavioral therapy, 264–265
  community care, 423
  definition, 261
  designer drugs, 281
  disasters, 261–262
  geriatrics, 88–89
  harm reduction approaches, 262
  homelessness, 376
  incidence, 261
  motivational interviewing (MI), 263–264
  nonpharmaceutical treatment, 262–265
  opioid use disorder, 271–277
  pediatrics, 69–70
  prevalence, 261
  screening tools, 44
  stimulant use disorder, 278–279
  tobacco use disorder (TUD), 279–281
Substance Use Risk Profile-Pregnancy Scale (SURP-P), 178
suicidal behavior
  acute psychiatric care setting, 410–411
  Ask Suicide-Screening Questions (ASQ), 65, 68, 169
  community care, 423
  disposition planning, 67, 69
  narcissistic personality disorder, 207
  risk assessment interview, 65–67
  risk factors, 65
  screening for, 65
  veterans, 396–397
  warning signs, 65
suicidality, 44
summarization, 14
support groups, 107
supported decision-making, 499
Supporting Partnerships for Anti-Racist Communities (SPARC) Initiative, 373
surrogate decision-making, 499
sustain talk, 264
SWOT analysis. See Strengths, Weaknesses, Opportunities, and Threats analysis
synthetic cathinones, 281
synthetic/semisynthetic opioid, 272
systemic lupus erythematosus (SLE), 474
systemic racism, 372, 382

tax identification number (TIN), private psychiatric APRN practice, 440
team-based integrative behavioral healthcare (IBH), 435

telehealth, 42–43
  advocacy, 462
  asynchronous forms, 454
  consent, 456–457
  definitions, 454–455
  disparities, 460–461
  electronic health record integration, 459
  ethical considerations, 457–458
  federal and state level, 455
  homeless and indigent populations, 390–391
  insurance, 456
  licensure, 456
  marketing, 461–462
  online prescribing, 457
  patient preparation, 460
  patient selection and care coordination, 459–460
  professional boards standards, 455–456
  reimbursement, 461
  technology infrastructure, 458–459
  training and support, 459
telemedicine, 454
temporary housing models (THM), 384
therapeutic agent, healthcare provider as, 16
therapeutic communication
  channels, 11–12
  decoding, 10
  developmental level, 11
  disease process, 10–11
  encoding, 9
  environmental factors, 11
  factors affecting, 10–12
  feedback, 10
  healthcare provider factors, 11
  mediums, 11
  message, 10
  nonverbal behavior visual cues, 10
  outcomes, 9
  patient-centered factors, 10
  receiver, 10
  sender, 9
  social interaction, 9
  techniques, 12–14
  verbal and nonverbal cues, 12
thiamine deficiency disorder, 486
thought broadcasting, 289
thought disorders
  classification, 282–283
  delusions, 282–283
  negative symptoms, 283
  positive, 282
thought process and content, 41
3,4-methylenedioxy methamphetamine (MDMA), 129
thyroid function test, feeding disorders, 143
Tobacco, Alcohol, Prescription Medications, and Other Substances (TAPS) Tool, 88–89
tobacco use disorder (TUD), 279–281
  definition, 279
  diagnosis and screenings, 279

pediatrics, 281
pregnancy, 281
prevalence, 279
signs and symptoms, 279
smokers of color, 281
treatment, 279–280
topiramate, eating disorders, 152
transcultural nursing model, 305
transdisciplinary practice, 7
transformational leadership, 431
transgender individuals
  generalized anxiety disorder, 119
  illness anxiety disorder (IAD), 121
  obsessive-compulsive disorder (OCD), 124
  panic disorder, 126
transgender obsessive-compulsive disorder (TOCD), 124
transient global amnesia (TGA), 483
transient sleep disorder, 216
transinstitutionalization, 6
transitional housing (TH), 384
trauma-informed care
  adverse childhood experiences, 19, 21
  collaboration and mutuality, 28
  cultural, historical, and gender issues, 28
  effects, 18–19
  elements, 24–26
  empowerment, voice, and choice, 28
  epidemiology and etiology, 20–23
  experiences, 18
  health outcomes, 19
  health-risk behaviors, 20
  homeless and indigent populations, 385
  human-caused disasters, 22–23
  intimate partner violence, 21
  military-related trauma, 21–22
  natural disasters, 22
  neurobiological changes, 20
  neuroendocrine changes, 20
  organizational policies and procedures, 28–29
  peer support, 27–28
  practical recommendations, 28–29
  prevalence, 24
  principles, 27–28
  recognition, 25–26
  responding, 26
  safety, 27
  screening tools, 26
  structural changes, 20
  traumatic event, 18
  trustworthiness and transparency, 27
trauma-informed cognitive behavioral therapy (TI-CBT), 103–104
trauma-informed therapies
  Adverse Childhood Experiences (ACEs) Scale, 101
  EMDR treatment, 102
  Somatic Experiencing® (SE) therapy, 103
  trauma-informed cognitive behavioral therapy, 103–104

trauma screening tools, 45
traumatic brain injury (TBI), 472, 484
   blast-related, 398–399
   direct and indirect traumatic forces, 398
   incidence, 398
   persistent postconcussive syndrome, 398
   repetitive mild, 399
   screening and assessment, 399
   secondary injuries, 398
   severity, 398
   treatment and resources, 399
   veterans, 398–399
traumatic event, 18
Tuskegee Syphilis Study, 495
12-Item General Health Questionnaire (GHQ-12), 408
type 1 diabetes, 481

unconditioned stimulus (US), 104
unsheltered homelessness, 369
unspecified feeding and eating disorder (UFED)
   definitions, 138
   diagnostic criteria, 149
U.S. Preventive Services Task Force (USPSTF), 26

Vanderbilt ADHD Diagnostic Parent Rating Scale (VADPRS), 91, 355–356
Vanderbilt ADHD Diagnostic Teacher Rating Scale (VADTRS), 91
vascular dementia, 484
vascular depression hypothesis, 80
Veterans Affairs (VA) services for seniors, 349
veterans and survivors of war. *See also* military
   definition, 392
   dissociative disorders, 117
   generalized anxiety disorder, 119
   healthcare, 395
   illness anxiety disorder (IAD), 121
   mental health disorders, 396–399
   military cultural competencies, 392–395
   military organization, 393
   obsessive-compulsive disorder, 124
   panic disorder, 126
   posttraumatic stress disorder, 130
   referral sources, 400
   social anxiety disorder, 136
violence risk assessment tools, 44
virtual care, 454
vitamin disorders, 486

weekly individual therapy, 96
Wernicke–Korsakoff syndrome, 486
Whiteley Index (WI-7), 249
withdrawal/negative affect stage, drug addiction, 176
worry/distress disorders, 82

xylazine, 281

Young Mania Rating Scale (YMRS), 293

Zung Self-Rating Anxiety Scale, 44, 192
Zung Self-Rating Depression Scale, 45, 184